PATHOLOGY OF INCIPIENT NEOPLASIA

Pathology of
Incipient Neoplasia
Third Edition

Edited by
DONALD EARL HENSON, M.D.
Program Director
Cancer Biomarkers Research Group
Division of Cancer Prevention
National Cancer Institute
Bethesda, Maryland

Adjunct Associate Professor of Pathology
Department of Pathology
Uniformed Services University of the Health Sciences
Bethesda, Maryland

JORGE ALBORES-SAAVEDRA, M.D.
Professor of Pathology
Director, Division of Anatomic Pathology
Phillip O'Bryan Montgomery, Jr., M.D. Professorship
in Surgical Pathology
Department of Pathology
University of Texas Southwestern Medical Center
Parkland Health & Hospital System
Zale Lipshy University Hospital
Dallas, Texas

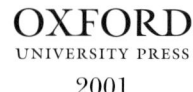
OXFORD
UNIVERSITY PRESS
2001

OXFORD
UNIVERSITY PRESS

Oxford   New York
Athens   Auckland   Bangkok   Bogotá   Buenos Aires   Calcutta
Cape Town   Chennai   Dar es Salaam   Delhi   Florence   Hong Kong   Istanbul
Karachi   Kuala Lumpur   Madrid   Melbourne   Mexico City   Mumbai
Nairobi   Paris   São Paulo   Shanghai   Singapore   Taipei   Tokyo   Toronto   Warsaw
and associated companies in
Berlin   Ibadan

Published by Oxford University Press, Inc.
198 Madison Avenue, New York, New York 10016

Oxford is a registered trademark of Oxford University Press

Library of Congress Cataloging-in-Publication Data
Pathology of incipient neoplasia /
edited by Donald Earl Henson, Jorge Albores-Saavedra.—3rd ed.
p. ; cm.   Includes bibliographical references and index.
ISBN 0-19-512338-7
1. Precancerous conditions.
I. Henson, Donald Earl. II. Albores-Saavedra, Jorge.
[DNLM: 1. Neoplasms—pathology.
2. Precancerous Conditions—pathology
QZ 200   P2965 2000]   RC262.P38 2000   616.99'207—dc21   99-052562

The science of medicine is a rapidly changing field. As new research and clinical experience broaden our knowledge, changes in treatment and drug therapy do occur. The authors and the publisher of this work have checked with sources believed to be reliable in their efforts to provide information that is accurate and complete, and in accordance with the standards accepted at the time of publication. However, in light of the possibility of human error or changes in the practice of medicine, neither the author, nor the publisher, nor any other party who has been involved in the preparation or publication of this work warrants that the information contained herein is in every respect accurate or complete. Readers are encouraged to confirm the information contained herein with other reliable sources, and are strongly advised to check the product information sheet provided by the pharmaceutical company for each drug they plan to administer.

1 3 5 7 9 8 6 4 2

Printed in Hong Kong
on acid-free paper

PREFACE

The fact that many malignant tumors have a morphologically recognizable precursor lesion has implications for the early diagnosis and control of cancer. Because these lesions do not cause symptoms, their presence is often unsuspected clinically. Early diagnosis, therefore, provides the best opportunity for cure, and thus efforts to find these lesions by screening, by careful examination of individuals known to be at high risk, and by sophisticated diagnostic techniques are justified. Already, the number of early lesions seen by pathologists has increased. Unfortunately, a lack of experience with these lesions and a lack of uniform histologic criteria for precursors in many organs can make diagnostic interpretation difficult. Even after a diagnosis has been made, uncertainties may remain because, in many cases, therapeutic strategics are empirical and even controversial.

It is evident that physicians need a better understanding of the early phases of neoplasia to provide optimal treatment and patient care. Thus far, experimental models for the study of early cancer have not provided sufficient data that pathologists can use to solve the diagnostic problems caused by these lesions.

As long as the etiology of most human malignant neoplasms remains unknown and effective prevention interventions are unavailable, the most practical method of reducing morbidity and mortality is the detection of early lesions. It is therefore reasonable to assume that in the future more early cancers will be found and treated.

In the third edition of this book, we have attempted to bring together all of the information available on the clinicopathologic features of early lesions in most human organs and tissues. Because this field is broad and controversial, such a task cannot be accomplished by one individual. Therefore, we have asked highly qualified pathologists to summarize their knowledge. Their chapters reflect their own interests, experiences, and concerns, and provide information specific to each site. We want to acknowledge their contributions and thank them for their time and creative efforts. This book is essentially their collective work. It is our hope that pathologists, oncologists, and all physicians interested in the diagnosis, natural history, and treatment of the early stages of cancer will find the third edition as useful and stimulating as previous editions.

Bethesda, Maryland   D.E.H.
Dallas, Texas   J.A.-S.
January 2000

CONTENTS

Contributors

JORGE ALBORES-SAAVEDRA, M.D.
Division of Anatomic Pathology
Department of Pathology
University of Texas Southwestern Medical
    Center
Parkland Health and Hospital System/
    Zale Lipshy University Hospital
Dallas, TX

MAHUL B. AMIN, M.D.
Director of Surgical Pathology
Emory University Hospital
Atlanta, GA

DONALD A. ANTONIOLI, M.D.
Harvard Medical School
Beth Israel Deaconess Medical Center
Children's Hospital
Boston, MA

ALBERTO G. AYALA, M.D.
Department of Pathology
University of Texas M.D. Anderson Cancer
    Center
Houston, TX

MICHAEL W. BEATY, M.D.
Hematopathology Section, Laboratory of
    Pathology
National Cancer Institute
Bethesda, MD

J. BRUCE BECKWITH, M.D., HonFRCPath(UK)
Pathology & Human Anatomy
Loma Linda University
Loma Linda, CA

DEBRA A. BELL, M.D.
Department of Pathology
Massachusetts General Hospital
Boston, MA

KEVIN E. BOVE, M.D.
Department of Pathology
University of Cincinnati College of Medicine
Children's Hospital Research Foundation
Cincinnati, OH

DENNIS K. BURNS, M.D.
Department of Pathology
University of Texas Southwestern Medical
    Center
Dallas, TX

CAROLYN C. COMPTON, M.D., PH.D.
Department of Pathology
Harvard Medical School
Massachusetts General Hospital
Boston, MA

PELAYO CORREA, M.D.
Department of Pathology
Louisiana State University Medical Center
Staff Charity Hospital
New Orleans, LA

BOGDAN CZERNIAK, M.D., PH.D.
Department of Pathology
The University of Texas MD Anderson
    Cancer Center
Houston, TX

ENRIQUE DE ALAVA, M.D., PH.D.
Associate Professor of Pathology
Universidad de Navarra
Pamplona, SPAIN

RUBY DELGADO, M.D.
Department of Pathology
Memorial Sloan-Kettering Cancer Center
New York, NY

JOHN N. EBLE, M.D.
Department of Pathology
Richard L. Roudebush V.A. Medical Center
Indianapolis, IN

MICHAEL GILCREASE, M.D.
Department of Pathology
University of Texas Southwestern Medical
    Center
Parkland Health and Hospital System/
    Zale Zipshy University Hospital
Dallas, TX

DONALD EARL HENSON, M.D.
Cancer Biomarkers Research Group
Division of Cancer Prevention
National Cancer Institute
Bethesda, MD

R. NICK HOGAN, M.D., PH.D.
Department of Ophthalmology and
    Pathology
University of Texas Southwestern Medical
    Center
Dallas, TX

RALPH H. HRUBAN, M.D.
Departments of Pathology and Oncology
The Johns Hopkins University School of
    Medicine
Baltimore, MD

CARRIE Y. INWARDS, M.D.
Division of Anatomic Pathology
Mayo Clinic and Mayo Foundation
Mayo Medical School
Rochester, MN

KAMAL G. ISHAK, M.D., PH.D.
Department of Hepatic & Gastrointestinal
    Pathology
Armed Forces Institute of Pathology
Washington, DC

ELAINE S. JAFFE, M.D.
Hematopathology Section
Laboratory of Pathology
National Cancer Institute
Bethesda, MD

ROBERT J. KURMAN, MD
Departments of Pathology and Gynecology
    & Obstetrics
Division of Gynecologic Pathology
The Johns Hopkins University School of
    Medicine
Baltimore, MD

CHARLES R. LASSMAN, M.D., PH.D.
Department of Pathology
University of California at Los Angeles
Los Angeles, CA

KLAUS J. LEWIN, M.D.
Department of Pathology
University of California at Los Angeles
Los Angeles, CA

RUTH A. LININGER, M.D., M.P.H.
Department of Pathology and Laboratory
    Medicine
University of North Carolina School of
    Medicine
Chapel Hill, NC

MARIO A. LUNA, M.D.
Department of Anatomic Pathology
The University of Texas MD Anderson
    Cancer Center
Houston, TX

KEYLA PINEDA-DABOIN, M.D.
Department of Pathology
The University of Texas MD Anderson
    Cancer Center
Houston, TX

VICTOR G. PRIETO, M.D., PH.D.
Head, Dermatopathology
Department of Pathology and Medicine
University of Texas MD Anderson Cancer
    Center
Houston, TX

LUIS REQUENA, M.D., PH.D.
Department of Dermatology
Universidad Autonoma
Fundacion Jimenez Diaz
Madrid, Spain

ROBERT R. RICKERT, M.D.
Department of Pathology
St. Barnabas Medical Center
University of Medicine and Dentistry
    New Jersey
Livingston, NJ

JAE Y. RO, M.D.
Division of Pathology
University of Texas System Cancer Center
M.D. Anderson Hospital and Tumor
    Institute
Houston, TX

BRIGITTE M. RONNETT, M.D.
Departments of Pathology and Obstetrics/
    Gynecology
The Johns Hopkins University School of
    Medicine
Baltimore, MD

ELISABETH J. RUSHING, M.D.
Department of Pathology
The University of Texas Southwestern
    Medical Center
Dallas, TX

ROBERT E. SCULLY, M.D.
Department of Pathology
Massachusetts General Hospital
Boston, MA

CHRISTOPHER RICHARD SHEA, M.D.
Associate Professor of Pathology and
    Medicine
Director of Dermatopathology
Duke University Medical Center
Durham, NC

MARK E. SHERMAN, M.D.
Departments of Pathology and Gynecology
    & Obstetrics
The Johns Hopkins University School of
    Medicine
Baltimore, MD

EIICHI TAHARA, M.D., PH.D., FRCPATH
Department of Pathology
Hiroshima University School of Medicine
Hiroshima, JAPAN

FATTANEH A. TAVASSOLI, M.D.
Department of Gynecologic and Breast
    Pathology
Armed Forces Institute of Pathology
Washington, DC

WILLIAM D. TRAVIS, M.D.
Department of Pulmonary and Mediastinal
    Pathology
Armed Forces Institute of Pathology
Washington, DC

THOMAS M. ULBRIGHT, M.D.
Director of Anatomic Pathology
Department of Pathology
Indiana University
Indianapolis, IN

K. KRISHNAN UNNI, M.D.
Mayo Medical School
Division of Anatomic Pathology
Mayo Clinic and Mayo Foundation
Rochester, MN

ROBB E. WILENTZ, M.D.
Department of Pathology
The Johns Hopkins University School of
    Medicine
Baltimore, MD

PATHOLOGY OF INCIPIENT NEOPLASIA

1

INTRODUCTION

Donald Earl Henson and Jorge Albores-Saavedra

For many anatomic sites, the diagnosis of cancer is being made earlier as smaller lesions are now found more often (Cady et al., 1996). This has been the result of both public awareness and the systematic application of early detection programs. Squamous-cell carcinoma *in situ* of the uterine cervix is now more common than its invasive counterpart (Sherman and Kurman, 1998), and a new disease, carcinoma *in situ* of the breast, has emerged as a result of screening. The routine use of prostate-specific antigen (PSA) testing in men has resulted in the increased detection of early prostate cancer and prostate intraepithelial neoplasia (Bostwick, 1996; Bostwick and Aquilina, 1996; Mettlin et al., 1993). Genetic testing has also contributed to the detection of incipient neoplastic lesions in a variety of organs. If these trends continue and new screening tests are developed, we may be able to eliminate the invasive forms of most malignant epithelial tumors without even knowing their cause. In fact, because of prophylactic polypectomy and perhaps changes in the diet, a reduction in the incidence of colonic adenocarcinomas has recently been reported in the U.S.

Although there is reasonable expectation that molecular biology will eventually provide the tools to separate early neoplastic from non-neoplastic lesions, the fact remains that use of the light microscope still provides the basis for diagnosis. In some organs, such as the gallbladder, pancreas, and lung, precursor lesions of invasive carcinoma have been well characterized, however, we

do not yet have practical cost-effective clinical tools for detection. Recognition of precursor lesions in these organs is often due to an incidental surgical or autopsy finding.

"Incipient neoplasia" refers to those lesions that have been associated with early neoplastic development. In general, they include hyperplasia, atypical hyperplasia, metaplasia, various forms of dysplasia, carcinoma *in situ*, and even microinvasive carcinoma. These lesions occur not only along epithelial surfaces, such as in the breast, skin, or urinary bladder, but also as complications of other lesions, such as polyps, cysts, benign tumors, and even chronic inflammatory conditions (Riddell, 1976). Other types of lesions are also found in this group, such as biliary papillomatosis which histologically shows complex papillary structures that are often difficult to separate from papillary carcinoma. Concepts of incipient neoplasia occurring in mesenchymal and lymphoid tissues have not been defined, but progress has been made with some of the precursors found in these anatomic sites.

The term "incipient" does not imply that cancer is always the final outcome. Rather, the term refers to well-defined histologic changes that have an increased probability or risk for cancer. This risk varies in different age-groups, in different races, with different lesions, and with other factors. In other words, most of the lesions described in this book are the histological risk factors for cancer.

Incipient neoplasia is the borderline that

separates normal-appearing tissue from invasive cancer. It should serve, therefore, as an integrating focus for the study of cancer, including its mechanisms of development, mechanisms of progression, and biological manifestations, such as dedifferentiation and genetic instability. The study of invasive cancer has often focused on the end result, the outcome, which is nearly always predictable, whereas the behavior of an incipient lesion is often difficult to predict. Years may be required for incipient lesions to progress to invasive cancer (Brockie et al., 1998; Lininger et al., 1998).

In humans, our knowledge of the pathology of malignant tumors is largely based on the invasive forms of cancer. Less is known about the early or preclinical stages of tumor development. Most of our information about early cancer is limited to those sites in which the preclinical stages can be detected through direct investigation, such as endoscopy or cytology. Continued progress in radiology may enable us to image very small lesions or even to detect "field changes" in deep-seated organs.

A number of changes occur in the incipient lesions as they progress to malignant behavior. Although these changes have been recognized at the cellular level of analysis, they are also found at the more complex molecular genetic level. For example, K-*ras* mutations, which are found in more than 80% of invasive carcinomas of the pancreas, have also been detected in hyperplastic, atypical hyperplastic, and even in normal pancreatic ducts (Moskaluk et al., 1997; Sugio et al., 1997). But with our present knowledge, it is still uncertain at which stage the neoplastic change is reached, or at what point it is no longer reversible (Bajardi, 1984), even at the molecular genetic level.

Morphologically, incipient epithelial lesions often follow a sequence from hyperplasia to dysplasia to *in situ* carcinoma. Most likely, this sequence reflects continued genetic instability, that is, an increased rate of unrepaired DNA damage with the formation of abnormal genomic variants (Boone et al., 1997; Minna et al., 1997). However, there is morphologic evidence that not all lesions follow the full sequence, and that some may even reverse direction. For example, in the stomach, endocrine cell hyperplasia, which can occur in the mucosa of the gastric body

in patients with pernicious anemia, is reversible if the trophic stimulus that results from G cell hyperplasia in the antrum is removed (Kern et al., 1990). Furthermore, with some malignant tumors, the sequence may not start with hyperplasia but instead follow the routes from adenoma to invasive carcinoma or, alternatively, from dysplasia to invasive carcinoma. Regardless of the sequence, the same uncertainties continue to confront pathologists as they histologically interpret these lesions even for the most common ones such as those in the breast and uterine cervix (Rosai, 1991; Schnitt and Connolly, 1997). As our histologic criteria become better defined and our diagnostic ability increases, the separation of incidental reactive lesions from those that are truly preneoplastic or even neoplastic will become less problematic.

Furthermore, the time required to complete the sequence from hyperplasia to invasive cancer varies. In some patients, lesions seem to require years to progress, whereas in others only a short time is needed. In fact, for some lesions the full sequence may not even be evident morphologically. For others, the evidence supporting the full sequence is weak. We all have seen invasive cancers that arise directly from normal-appearing epithelium. In addition, early carcinoma can be superimposed on atypical epithelial proliferations. Superimposition is seen, for example, with actinic keratosis of the skin or with the atypical lesions of mucous membranes. Since these variations in sequential morphology must be the result of various sequential genetic changes, the same issues that currently confront pathologists will also confront molecular biologists as they seek to unravel the neoplastic process.

Questions have arisen regarding the nature of these incipient lesions—questions that do not always apply to the corresponding invasive cancers. These questions refer to the morphologic and genetic determinants of progression, regression, dormancy, invasivness, and so forth, all of which have bearing on treatment and prognosis. All pathologists have seen atypical hyperplastic lesions in the breast, but with our current knowledge, we cannot predict with certainty the future growth potential or invasive capacity of such lesions (Fitzgibbons et al., 1998). In some sites, especially in the uterine cervix, the chances of regression or progression seem to correlate with specific types of papilloma virus.

In some sites, such as soft tissue, the brain, and lymphoid system, the histologic precursors of malignant tumors are virtually unknown. In other sites, embryonal rests may serve as a precursor. Wilms' tumor, for example, seems to arise from hamartomatous remnants in the kidney (Bove and McAdams, 1976). In fact, the kidney is one the few organs in which embryonal rests have been documented to give rise to malignant tumors.

Incipient neoplasia also includes the concept of minimal cancer. Originally introduced for small breast cancers less than 0.5 cm, this concept expresses uncertainty about the behavior and treatment of small or microinvasive cancers as well as in situ lesions. In the liver, cancers less than 3 cm are considered small. In the lung, certain small carcinoid neoplasms have been designated as tumorlets. In the kidney, clear-cell tumors less than 3 cm were originally considered benign. The term "minimal" as applied to small carcinomas is vague and even misleading because it can refer either to size or behavior or both. Basal cell carcinomas of the skin can grow to a large size and never metastasize. Mucinous cystic tumors of the pancreas that show dyplastic or even in situ changes follow a benign clinical course (Wilentz et al., 1999). In this respect, these cancers are also minimal from a biologic point of view.

In practice, many diagnostic terms have been applied to incipient lesions. Of necessity, they all convey a mixture of diagnostic and prognostic meanings. These terms include "atypical hyperplasia," "mild, moderate, or severe dysplasia," "high-grade intraepithelial lesion," "minimal deviation melanoma," "epithelial atypias," "borderline tumors," "grade one-half carcinomas," "intraepithelial neoplasia," and "minimal cancer." Most of these terms express our inability to relate the morphologic changes observed to their subsequent biologic behavior. They all, however, reflect some concern on the part of pathologists about the potential for future growth and invasion. Clearly, the biological potential of incipient lesions has an effect on our terminology. The term "dysplasia," for example, as used in cases of inflammatory bowel disease, has been redefined as an unequivocal neoplas-

tic alteration equivalent to carcinoma in situ (Riddell et al., 1983). The new definition is based on knowledge about the potential outcome of the in situ lesions, and not on pure morphology.

For practical reasons, the incipient stages of neoplastic development are classified morphologically. Other classifications are possible which may incorporate changes in DNA sequences, oncogene amplification, production of growth-stimulating factors, extent of aneuploidy, extent of heterogeneity, and extent of accumulated genetic damage (Thiberville et al., 1995). To be useful, these other definitions must be associated with outcome. Mutations have been found in potential precursor lesions. For example, p53 gene mutations have been found in cases of atypical alveolar hyperplasia of the lung (Slebos et al., 1998) and in the non-neoplastic mucosa of the stomach showing intestinal metaplasia (Ochiai et al., 1996). However, the relation between the mutations found in the precursor lesions and in the corresponding invasive cancers remains to be determined.

Above all, it is important that we determine whether the sequence is a continuous or discontinuous process, since this will influence our concepts of progression. At the morphologic level, many of these lesions form a continuum, which is why it is often difficult for pathologists to separate benign from malignant lesions or to predict the biological potential. For therapeutic reasons, it is also important to know whether the ultimate biologic potential is predetermined in the incipient lesion or whether it unfolds over time by chance or random processes. If the incipient lesion is cancer from its inception, then such information should be considered in any therapeutic strategy.

Pathologists have long recognized that incipient lesions are often multifocal, which, from a practical perspective, is important for the design of treatment and follow-up strategies. For example, medullary carcinoma in situ of the thyroid (C cell hyperplasia) in patients with the MEN II syndrome is usually bilateral, and therefore a total thyroidectomy is the treatment of choice (Perry et al., 1996). In dealing with incipient lesions, pathologists should think in terms of field changes as well as limited or focal changes. They should bear in mind that precursor lesions are often found in the vicinity of malignant tumors, especially those of epithelial origin. For example, one recent contribution to our understanding of the origin of germ cell tumors was achieved by a careful study of testes removed from patients with invasive germ cell tumors. Intratubular germ cell neoplasia, which is found in a high proportion of testes with invasive cancer, is now considered to be a true precursor lesion.

In some anatomic sites, metaplasia may presage cancer, because it seems to make tissue more susceptible to malignant transformation. Intestinal metaplasia of the stomach, for example, often precedes invasive carcinoma. Although metaplasia is often considered a response to injury, its position in the sequence is uncertain. Nonetheless, metaplasia, at least in some sites, is considered a precancerous lesion—for example, in Barrett's esophagus. It may even influence the histologic type of invasive cancer that eventually develops. In the gallbladder, intestinal metaplasia is thought to give rise to intestinal-type carcinomas, and in the uterine cervix and the lung, squamous metaplasia gives rise to squamous cell carcinomas.

Even though the terms "dysplasia" and "carcinoma *in situ*" describe changes occurring in epithelium, analogous changes that precede neoplasia probably occur in nonepithelial sites, such as in lymph nodes or in soft tissues. Although little is known about these changes, it seems reasonable to assume that every cancer has its own precancer. Presumably, incipient lesions in nonepithelial sites also follow a similar sequence from hyperplasia to invasive cancer. Nonetheless, known precursor lesions can assume a variety of morphologic changes. In soft tissue, for instance, chronic lymphedema may lead to the proliferation of small lymphatic channels, which may eventually progress to a lymphangiosarcoma. Neurofibromatosis, a condition that may give rise to malignant schwannomas, is discussed in detail in the chapter on soft tissue tumors (Chap. 25). Chondrosarcomas have been known to arise in benign cartilaginous tumors. Lymphoid hyperplasia, such as that seen in Hashimoto's thyroiditis and in the stomach in association with chromic gastritis, appears to be a precursor of lymphomas in these organs. For some cancers, the precursor is a benign tumor. For other cancers the precursor is a benign condition such as immunodeficiency or its complication. Many adenocarcinomas of the colon or of the ampulla of Vater originate from villous adenomas.

In addition to morphology, there are other differences between precancerous lesions and the corresponding invasive tumors. Precancerous lesions are often multiple and may occupy wide areas of the surface mucosa, especially in hollow organs such as the urinary bladder or gallbladder (Albores-Saavedra et al., 2000). In most sites, they are more common than the corresponding invasive cancers. In Gardner's syndrome, for instance, the colon contains hundreds of polyps, but only one, or at most several, evolves into invasive cancer, although given time, all may progress to malignancy. Even colonic polyps, the precursors of invasive cancer, are far more common than invasive carcinomas of the colon. Autopsy studies have shown that 8% of adults harbor polyps more than 0.5 cm in diameter, and 4% have polyps more than 1 cm in diameter (Arminski and McLean, 1964). In the skin, pigmented nevi are more common than malignant melanomas, and actinic keratoses are more prevalent than squamous cell carcinomas. For these reasons, incipient lesions may represent a separate disease category that is distinct from invasive forms of cancer.

From a clinical perspective, early lesions can have consequences beyond the everyday work of pathologists. These lesions involve treatment regimens that include extent of surgery, follow-up strategies, and cost of care. Although we will not discuss here all the issues related to these lesions, knowledge of their biology and extent clearly relates to the question of whether the cancer can be treated by local means alone, such as limited resection, or by extensive, mutilating surgery. The use of new prognostic markers, such as aneuploidy, increased production of growth factors, expression of tumor-associated antigens, and activation of protooncogenes, may hold promise for guiding appropriate treatment, even for incipient lesions. However, the prognostic value of these new markers must first be confirmed, and their practical benefit must be established against a background of conventional morphology on which medical decisions have traditionally been made.

The purpose of this book is to describe these incipient lesions and to provide morphologic criteria for their diagnosis and progression as well as clues useful in the differential diagnosis. Because microscopic identification is subjective, problems of diagnoses will remain until histologic markers are found that can accurately predict progression. In the meantime, pathologists, as consultants in patient management, must still provide some estimate about the natural history of these lesions and their propensity for invasion, based on traditional staining and histologic criteria.

REFERENCES

Albores-Saavedra J, Henson DE, Klimstra D. Tumors of the Gallbladder, Extrahepatic Bile Ducts and Ampulla of Vater. Tumor Atlas, Series 3. Armed Forces Institute of Pathology, Washington DC. 2000.

Arminski, TC, McLean DW. (1964) Incidence and distribution of adenomatous polyps of the colon and rectum based on 1000 autopsy examinations. Dis Colon Rectum 7:249–261.

Bajardi F. (1984) Histogenesis of spontaneous regression of cervical intraepithelial neoplasias. Cancer 54:616–619.

Boone CW, Bacus JW, Bacus JV, Steele VE, Kelloff GJ. (1997) Properties of intraepithelial neoplasia relevant to the development of cancer chemopreventive agents. J Cell Biochem Suppl 28–29; 1–20.

Bostwick DG. (1996) Prospective origins of prostate carcinoma. Prostate intraepithelial neoplasia and atypical adenomatous hyperplasia. Cancer 78:330–336.

Bostwick DG, Aquilina JW. (1996) Prostate intraepithelial neoplasia (PIN) and other prostatic lesions as risk factors and surrogate endpoints for cancer chemoprevention trials. J Cell Biochem Suppl 25: 156–164.

Bove KE, McAdams J. (1976) The nephroblastomatosis complex and its relation to Wilms' tumor, a clinicopathologic treatise. In: Perspectives in Pediatric Pathology, Vol. 3 (Rosenberg HS, Bolande RP, eds.) pp. 185–223. Chicago, Yearbook Medical Publishers.

Brockie E, Anand A, Albores-Saavedra J. (1998) Progression of atypical ductal hyperplasia/carcinoma in situ of the pancreas to invasive adenocarcinoma. Ann Diagn Pathol 2:286–292.

Cady B, Stone MD, Schuler JG, Thakur R, Wanner MA, Lavin PT. (1996) The new era in breast cancer. Invasion, size, and nodal involvement dramatically decreasing as a result of mammographic screening. Arch Surg 131:301–308.

Fitzgibbons PL, Henson DE, Hutter RVP. (1998) Benign breast changes and the risk for subsequent breast cancer. Arch Pathol Lab Med 122:1053–1055.

Kern SE, Yardley JH, Lazenby AJ, Boitnott JK, Yang VW, Bayless TM, Sitzmann JV. (1990) Reversal by antrec-tomy of endocrine cell hyperplasia in the gastric body in pernicious anemia: a morphometric study. Mod Pathol 3:561–566.

Lininger RA, Fujii H, Man Y, Gabrielson E, Tavassoli FA. (1998) Comparison of loss of heterozygosity in primary and recurrent ductal carcinoma in situ of the breast. Mod Pathol 11:1151–1159.

Mettlin C, Jones G, Averette H, Gusberg SB, Murphy GP. (1993) Defining and updating the American Cancer Society for the cancer-related checkup: prostate and endometrial cancers. CA Cancer J Clin 43:42–46.

Minna JD, Sekido Y, Fong KM, Gazdar AF. (1997) Molecular biology of lung cancer. In: Cancer: Principles and Practice of Oncology, 5th ed., (DeVita VT Jr, Hellman S, Rosenberg SA, eds.) Lippincott-Raven, Philadelphia

Moskaluk CA, Hruban RH, Kern SE. (1997) p16 and K-ras gene mutations in the intraductal precursors of human pancreatic adenocarcinoma. Cancer Res 57:2140–2143.

Ochiai A, Yamauchi Y, Hirohashi S. (1996) p53 mutations in the non-neoplastic mucosa of the human stomach showing intestinal metaplasia. Int J Cancer 69:28–33.

Perry A, Molberg K, Albores-Saavedra J. (1996) Physiologic versus neoplastic C-cell hyperplasia of the thyroid. Cancer 77:750–756.

Riddell RH. (1976) The precarcinomatous phase of ulcerative colitis. Curr Topic Pathol 63:179–219.

Riddell RH, Goldman H, Ransohoff DF, Appelman HD, Fenoglio CM, Haggitt RC, Ahren C, Correa P, Hamilton SR, Morson BC, et al. (1983) Dysplasia in inflammatory bowel disease: standardized classification with provisional clinical applications. Hum Pathol 14;931–968.

Rosai J. (1991) Borderline epithelial lesions of the breast. Am J Surg Pathol 15:209–221.

Schnitt SJ, Connolly JL. (1997) Classification of ductal carcinoma in situ: striving for clinical relevance in the era of breast conserving therapy. Hum Pathol 28:877–880.

Sherman ME, Kurman RJ. (1998) Intraepithelial carcinoma of the cervix: reflections on half a century of progress. Cancer 83:2243–2246.

Slebos RJ, Baas IO, Clement MJ, Offerhaus GJ, Askin FB, Hruban RH, Westra HW. (1998) p53 alterations in atypical alveolar hyperplasia of the human lung. Hum Pathol 29:801–808.

Sugio K, Molberg K, Albores-Saavedra J, et al. (1997) K-ras mutations and allelic loss at 5q and 18q in the development of human pancreatic cancer. Int J Pancreatol 21:205–217.

Thiberville L, Payne P, Vielkinds J, LeRiche J, Horsman D, Nouvet G, Palcic G, Lam S. (1995) Evidence of cumulative gene losses with progression of premalignant epithelial lesions to carcinoma of the bronchus. Cancer Res 55:5133–5139.

Wilentz RE, Albores-Saavedra J, Talamini MA, Yeo CJ, Hruban RH. (1999) Pathologic examination accurately predicts prognosis in mucinous cystic neoplasms of the pancreas. Am J Surg Pathol 23:1328–1339.

2

SKIN: EPIDERMAL AND ADNEXAL EPITHELIUM

Luis Requena

In the skin, incipient malignant neoplasms other than melanoma *in situ* represent forms of carcinoma *in situ*. Classically, they have been considered "precursors" (Brownstein, 1979), "premalignant lesions" (Pinkus and Mehregan, 1980), or "precanceroses" (Sober and Burstein, 1995), but they actually are malignant neoplasms confined to the epidermis, consisting either of epidermal keratinocytes or adnexal epithelial cells. Each of those lesions may extend from the epidermis into the dermis, and from there may metastasize, a phenomenon that qualifies them as malignant. But they are malignant from the very beginning and their potential to kill by destruction locally or by metastases widely results from their capability to involve deeper structures of the skin, and not from any tendency to "malignant degeneration" or "malignant transformation".

Usually, the term "carcinoma *in situ* of the skin" refers to a variant of squamous cell carcinoma confined to the epidermis and the epithelium of the adnexa, which is characterized histopathologically by atypical keratinocytes that display crowded, pleomorphic nuclei, many of them in mitosis, and abnormal cornification in the form of dyskeratotic cells. This type of squamous cell carcinoma *in situ*, also known as *Bowen's disease*, is not the only variant of cutaneous carcinoma *in situ*. Other forms of incipient malignant epithelial neoplasms involve the epidermis and/or the epithelium of the adnexa. Furthermore, most of those malignant neoplasms are primarily of the skin, but there

are rare instances in which epidermotropically metastatic carcinomas may mimic primary cutaneous carcinoma *in situ*. The different variants of incipient malignant neoplasms of the skin, other than melanoma *in situ*, are described in this chapter and listed in Table 2–1. They have been classified according to their presumed type of differentiation.

INCIPIENT MALIGNANT NEOPLASMS WITH SQUAMOUS DIFFERENTIATION

SOLAR KERATOSIS

Solar keratosis, also known as *actinic keratosis* or *senile keratosis*, is the most common expression of squamous cell carcinoma *in situ* of the skin. It appears on sun-exposed sites, especially of persons who have a fair complexion and who have been exposed for long periods to the ultraviolet radiation of the sun (Pinkus and Mehregan, 1980).

Clinically, solar keratoses are ill-defined, erythematous, scaly papules. The sites affected most are the dorsa of hands, forearms, the face, and bald zones of the scalp in men. In most patients the lesions are numerous. When the keratotic component of them is removed, a hyperemic base with bleeding points becomes apparent. The keratotic part may become so thick that the lesion assumes the appearance of a cutaneous horn. This type of solar keratosis is encountered especially on the dorsa of forearms and

Table 2–1. Incipient Malignant Neoplasms of the Skin Other Than Melanoma *in Situ* and Simulators of Them

Incipient malignant neoplasms with squamous cell differentiation

Skin
  Solar keratosis
  Bowen's disease
  Arsenical keratosis
  Radiation keratosis
  PUVA keratosis

Mucous membranes and mucocutaneous junctions
  Solar cheilitis
  Erythroplasia of Queyrat
  Bowenoid papulosis

Incipient malignant neoplasms with follicular differentiation
  Superficial basal cell carcinoma

Incipient malignant neoplasms with sebaceous differentiation
  Intraepidermal sebaceous carcinoma

Incipient malignant neoplasms with eccrine and apocrine differentiation
  Malignant hidroacanthoma simplex
    (intraepidermal porocarcinoma)
  Extramammary Paget's disease

Epidermotropically metastatic carcinomas that may mimic carcinoma *in situ* of the skin
  Mammary Paget's disease
  Other forms of epidermotropically metastatic
    carcinoma

dermis, where nuclei are large and pleomorphic, as well as crowded (Fig. 2–1). Sometimes, this altered basal layer is separated from the rest of the epidermis by a cleft (Pinkus and Mehregan, 1980). At this time, the solar keratosis is not yet evident clinically, because the epidermis is stratified in an orderly arrangement, and the granular and cornified layers are mostly normal. In time, the process comes to affect the other layers of the epidermis, by disordered maturation, loss of the granular layer at least focally, and parakeratosis above atypical epidermal keratinocytes. When parakeratosis is present, the solar keratosis becomes apparent clinically as a rough-surface keratosis. The epidermis is slightly thickened by buds composed of cells whose nuclei are crowded and larger and more pleomorphic than those of normal keratinocytes. In rare instances, the rete pattern is attenuated, the epidermis being thinner than normal, and composed of only three or four layers of large atypical keratinocytes covered by parakeratosis, so-called *atrophic solar keratoses* (Maize et al., 1998). At the opposite end of the spectrum is *hypertrophic solar keratosis*, in which the surface epithelium is mostly composed of prominent, compact parakeratosis (Fig. 2–2), although there is also irregular downward extension of broad rete of the epidermis (Billano and Little, 1982; Rabkin and Weems, 1987). A thick solar keratosis should be not confused with changes of lichen simplex chronicus superimposed in a solar keratosis due to long-term rubbing or scratching.

hands (Billano and Little, 1982; Rabkin and Weems, 1987).

Histopathologically, the earliest findings in solar keratosis are abnormalities confined to keratinocytes in the basal layer of the epi-

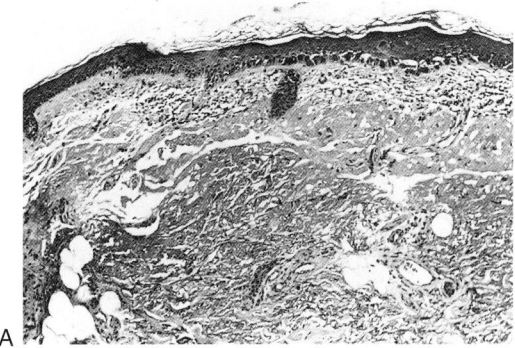
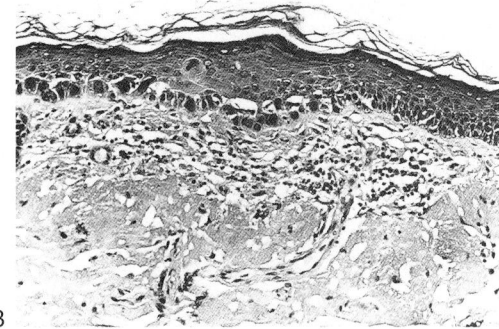

A   B

Figure 2–1. Subclinical solar keratosis. *A:* Low-power view shows atypical keratinocytes in the basal layer of the epidermis and intense solar elastosis in the dermis. *B:* Higher magnification demonstrates atypical keratinocytes with large and hyperchromatic nuclei in the basal layer of the epidermis. Note the normal appearance of the upper layers of the epidermis, including the cornified cells, which appeared basophilic, orthokeratotic, and with a basket-weave arrangement.

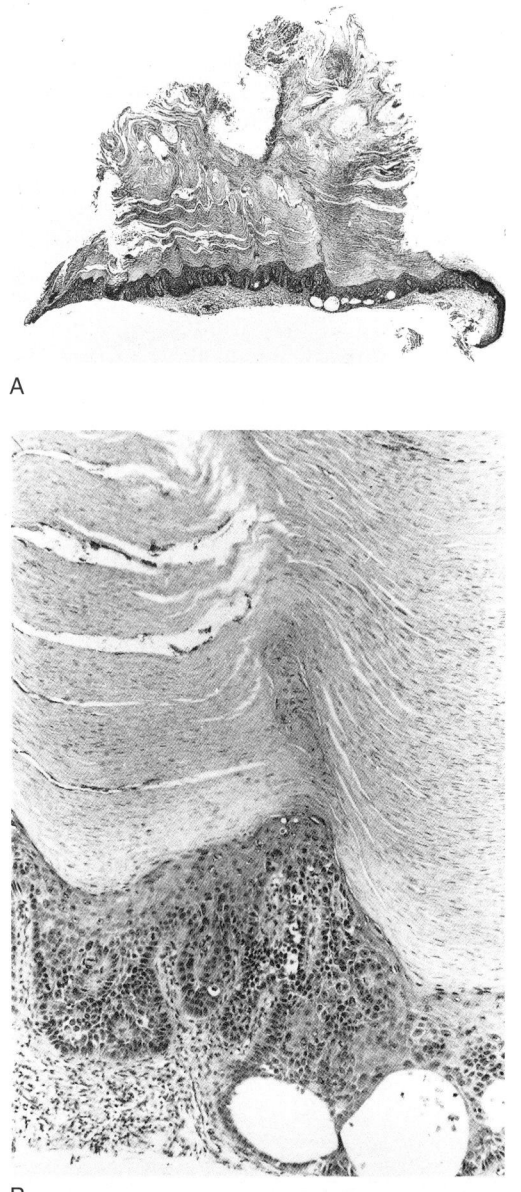

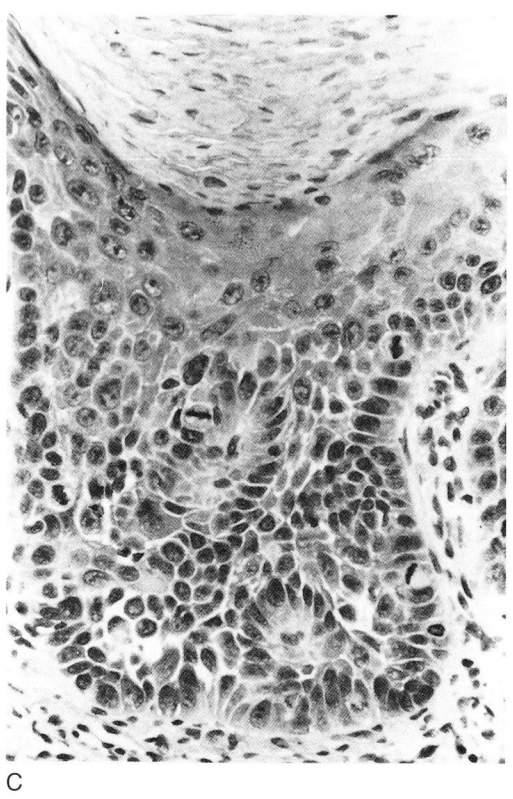

Figure 2–2. Hypertrophic solar keratosis. *A:* Scanning power view shows a hyperkeratotic lesion. *B:* The hyperkeratosis is composed of parakeratotic cornified cells. Note the absence of granular layer. *C:* The epidermis at the base of the lesion has atypical keratinocytes and several mitotic figures.

In the latter situation, vertical collagen bundles and dilated blood vessels are seen in dermal papillae (Billano and Little, 1982).

A highly characteristic histopathologic feature of solar keratosis is the presence of a sharp line of separation between the atypical keratinocytes of the involved epidermis and the intraepidermal portion of the adnexal epithelium; the intraepidermal segment of the eccrine ducts (acrosyringia) and the intraepidermal part of the infundibula (acrotrichia) are spared by the process.

Thus, a sharp line of separation is evident between normal keratinocytes of acrosyringia and acrotrichia and atypical epidermal cells of solar keratosis. Usually, this line is not entirely vertical but oblique, because normal epithelium of the intraepidermal portion of the adnexa extends laterally like an umbrella covering atypical cells of the epidermis, which spare adnexal epithelium (Pinkus, 1958). The contrast is still more evident in the cornified layer, where the spared intraepidermal portion of adnexal epithe-

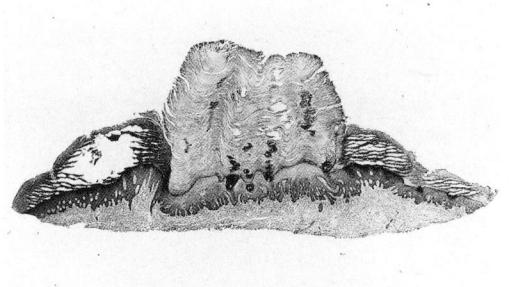

A

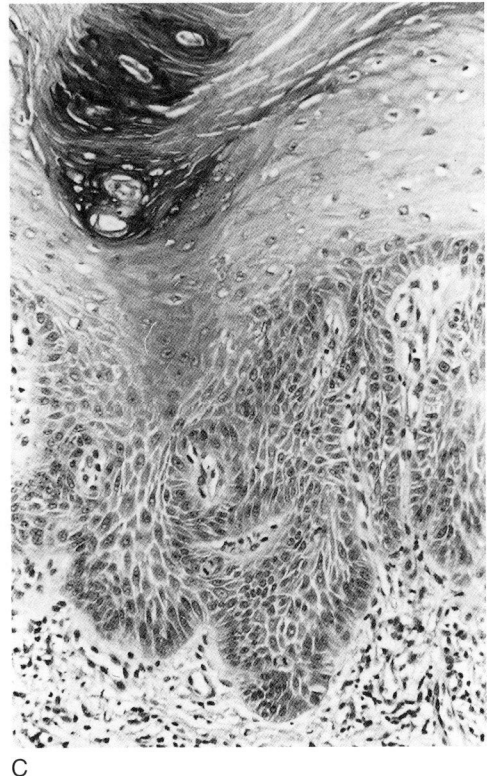

C

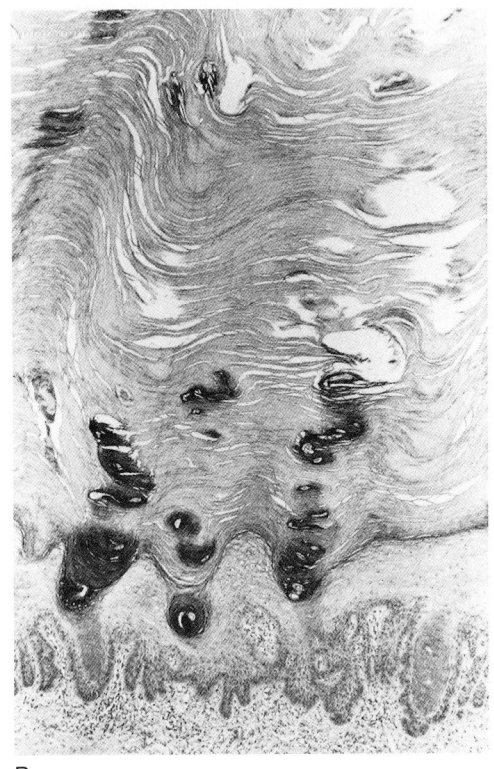

B

Figure 2–3. Hypertrophic solar keratosis. *A:* Scanning power view shows a hyperkeratotic lesion. *B:* Columns of orthokeratotic basophilic corneocytes of the acrosyringia within the eosinophilic parakeratotic layer. *C:* The basal layer of the epidermis has atypical keratinocytes with hyperchromatic and crowded nuclei.

lium shows a well-formed granular layer and at that level the cornified layer is composed of basket-weave orthokeratotic basophilic corneocytes, whereas the horny layer covering atypical cells of the epidermis exhibits compact eosinophilic parakeratosis. When the cornified layer is thicker, as in a thick solar keratosis, alternating blue columns of orthokeratotic corneocytes of the acrosyringia and acrotrichia are evident within the eosinophilic parakeratotic layer (Fig. 2–3). However, in long-term solar keratoses, atypical keratinocytes may also involve the in-

fundibular portion of follicles (Goldberg et al., 1994; Pinkus, 1958).

Several variants of solar keratosis have been reported. The hypertrophic and atrophic types have been described above. In *acantholytic solar keratosis* there is exaggeration of suprabasal clefts that are often seen in lesions of solar keratosis (Fig. 2–4), as well as acantholysis of atypical keratinocytes and dyskeratotic cells that are seen within the clefts (Carapeto and Garcia Perez, 1974; Lever and Marks, 1989). Usually, atypical keratinocytes are also evident in upper lay-

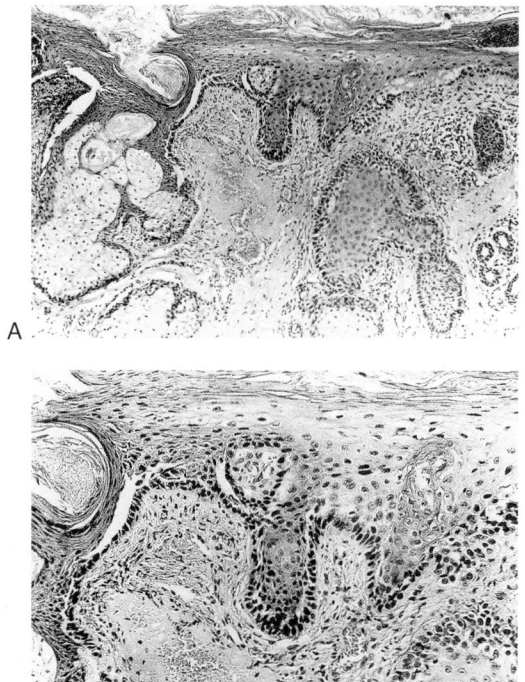

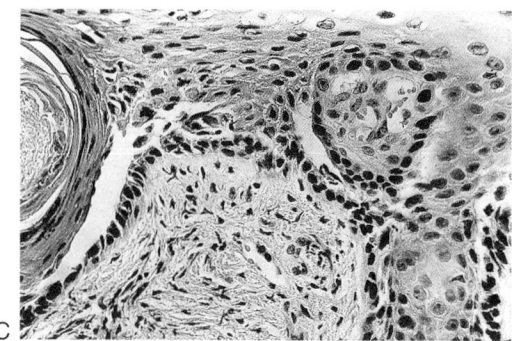

Figure 2–4. Acantholytic solar keratosis. *A:* A cleft separates the basal layer from the upper layers of the epidermis. *B:* Higher magnification demonstrates suprabasal clefting as well as the parakeratotic cornified layer and the absence of granular layer. *C:* Atypical keratinocytes, with hyperchromatic nuclei, are more evident in the basal layer of the epidermis.

ers of the epidermis, and buds of large and pleomorphic cells extend from the lower part of the epidermis into the dermis. Acantholytic solar keratosis should be not confused with *epidermolytic solar keratosis*, which is epidermolytic hyperkeratosis in a solar keratosis (Ackerman and Reed, 1973). In rare instances, solar keratosis may appear as a pigmented lesion because of the abundant melanin within it and numerous melanophages in the papillary dermis (Dinehart and Sanchez, 1988; James et al., 1978). Some authors consider lichen planus-like keratosis to be a variant of solar keratosis (Maize et al., 1998), but in our view this lesion is better interpreted as a solar lentigo or an incipient seborrheic keratosis that has attracted to it a lichenoid infiltrate and prominent necrosis of single keratinocytes in the form of Civatte bodies (Shapiro and Ackerman, 1966). However, sometimes authentic solar keratoses show a lichenoid infiltrate composed mostly of lymphocytes and plasma cells along atypical cells of dermoepidermal junction (Tan and Marks, 1982). Some authors have used the term "bowenoid solar keratosis" to refer to those solar keratoses in which the keratinocytic atypia involve the full thickness of the epi-

dermis (James et al., 1978). Atypia seems to be more prominent in solar keratoses in patients who are immunosuppressed (Price et al., 1988).

The dermal changes of solar keratosis include elastosis in the upper dermis, which consists of basophilic degeneration of collagen bundles of the papillary dermis that appear as thick blue fibers, although usually a thin band of the upper papillary dermis is spared, and an infiltrate of inflammatory cells of variable intensity composed mostly of lymphocytes and plasma cells and arranged in a lichenoid or perivascular pattern (Pinkus and Mehregan, 1980).

Lesions of solar keratosis show an immunohistochemical profile of cytokeratins and involucrin similar to that of normal epidermis (Ichikawa et al., 1995). Nuclear morphometric studies, however, have demonstrated that neoplastic cells of solar keratosis show kariometric features commonly found in cells of carcinomas (Bozzo et al., 1998), are aneuploid (Biesterfeld et al., 1995), and express mutant p53 protein (Sim et al., 1992a; Taguchi et al., 1994); bcl-2 protein expression has been reported by some authors (Nakagawa, et al., 1994) and denied by others (Mills, 1997).

Some authors have calculated that at least 10%–20% of solar keratoses, if left untreated, gradually "transform" into squamous cell carcinomas (Pinkus and Mehregan, 1980), although controversy exits in the literature about the boundary that separates solar keratosis and squamous cell carcinoma (Jones, 1984). The most frequent histopathologic criteria proposed to separate solar keratosis from squamous-cell carcinoma are the protrusion of atypical cells into the dermis and the detachment of neoplastic aggregations of keratinocytes from the lower layers of the epidermis (Jones, 1984). However, serial sections occasionally demonstrate that these apparently detached nests of atypical keratinocytes are surrounded by basement membrane and connected to buds of abnormal keratinocytes. The distinction between an intraepidermal solar keratosis and a squamous cell carcinoma involving the dermis is important for prognosis, but, in our opinion, solar keratosis, conceptually, is already a squamous cell carcinoma, albeit in its embryonic stage of development.

The main histopathologic differential diagnosis for solar keratosis is Bowen's disease. Usually, the distinction between these two variants of squamous cell carcinoma *in situ* of the skin may be established with confidence. In Bowen's disease the basal layer of the epidermis is spared by the neoplastic process and consists of a sharply defined line composed of a single layer of small basaloid cells cells compressed by overlying, larger atypical cells that nearly involve all suprabasal layers. Other differential features that favor Bowen's disease are the involvement of the intraepidermal segment of adnexal epithelium and the basaloid appearance of the neoplastic cells with crowded and hyperchromatic nuclei, and the premature cornification in the form of dyskeratotic cells.

BOWEN'S DISEASE

Bowen's disease, like solar keratosis, is another variant of squamous cell carcinoma *in situ* of the skin. It may appear both on sun-exposed and unexposed areas of the skin. Classically, lesions on unexposed areas have been thought to be related to ingestion of inorganic arsenic (Yeh, 1973), but they may be also seen in patients with no history of arsenic intake. Several studies support an etiologic role of different types of human papillomavirus (HPV) in the histogenesis of Bowen's disease, especially in some anatomic locations. Recent investigations using different DNA hybridization techniques have identified HPV-2 (Pfister and Haneke, 1984), HPV-16 (de Villiers et al., 1986; Ikenberg et al., 1983; Kawashima et al., 1990; Kettler et al., 1990; Mcgrae et al., 1993; Moy et al., 1989; Ostrow et al., 1987; Sau et al. 1994., Stone et al., 1987), HPV-20 (Shamanin et al., 1994), HPV-33 (Deguchi et al., 1998; Kawashima et al., 1990), HPV-34 (Kawashima et al., 1986), and genital-mucosal human papillomaviruses types HPV-31, -54, -58, -61, 62, and -73 (Mitsuishi et al., 1997) in lesions of Bowen's disease involving genital skin, hands, and periungual areas. Some HPV types have been also detected in lesions of Bowen's disease involving nongenital and nonvolar areas of the skin (Collina et al., 1995). Some authors, however, have failed to demonstrate DNA of HPVs in extragenital lesions of Bowen's disease (Lu et al., 1996).

Clinically Bowen's disease consists of a slowly growing erythematous, well-demarcated patch, with irregular borders and a scaling, crusted surface. A first glance, a patch of Bowen's disease may resemble lesions of superficial basal cell carcinoma, but it differs from them by the absence of a fine pearly border. The lesion may be solitary or multiple, and the lower extremities, face, and upper trunk are the sites most frequently involved (Cox, 1994), although lesions have described elsewere, including on the nail bed (Baran and Gormley, 1987; Coskey et al., 1972; Mikhail, 1974; Sau et al., 1994), lip (Biediger et al., 1995), nipple (Venkataseshan et al., 1994), palm (Jacyk, 1980; Wagers et al., 1973), sole (Grekin and Swanson, 1984), and eyelid (McCallum et al., 1975). Multiple pigmented lesions originally reported as Bowen's disease of the anogenital region are probably better interpreted as examples of bowenoid papulosis (see below). Lesions of Bowen's disease involving the mucosa of the glans penis are traditionally referred to as erythroplasia of Queyrat (see below). Usually a patch of Bowen's disease remains as carcinoma *in situ* for years, but the presence of ulceration with indurated borders indicates that the lesion has extended further into the dermis. Although some investigators have proposed a relationship between Bowen's disease and internal cancer (Epstein, 1960; Graham and Helwig, 1959; Miki et al., 1982; Petreka et al., 1961), recent well-controlled studies have failed to demonstrate such a relationship (Arbesman and Ransohoff, 1987; Chuang and Reizner, 1988; Reymann et al., 1988).

Several histopathologic variants of Bowen's disease have been described, including both architectural and cytologic types, and more than one pattern may be found in different zones of the same lesion (Strayer and Santa Cruz, 1980). Histopathologic features in common to all these variants include nearly full-thickness epidermal atypia, crowded nuclei, increased nuclear/cytoplasmic ratio of neoplastic keratinocytes, and parakeratosis (Fig. 2–5). In contrast to solar keratosis, early lesions of Bowen's disease appear to spare the basal layer of the epidermis, but the basal cells often have columnar nuclei arranged in a palisade ("eye-lines sign"). The intraepidermal portion of adnexal epithelium (acrotrichia and acrosyringia) is usually involved by Bowen's disease, and sometimes neoplastic cells extend down along the adnexal epithelium (Argenyi et al., 1990; Hunter, 1977). The involvement of infundibula and the distal segment of eccrine

ducts is an important cause of treatment failure in Bowen's disease when superficial methods of destruction, such as freezing or the application of 5-fluorouracil ointment, are used. These measurements only destroy the epidermis, which is replaced by neoplastic epithelium of underlying or adjacent involved adnexa.

Architectural variants of Bowen's disease include psoriasiform, atrophic, verrucous-hyperkeratotic, irregular, and nesting types, or a combination of two or more of these in the same lesion (Strayer and Santa Cruz, 1980). The psoriasiform type shows uniform acanthosis, with elongated and thickened rete ridges composed of atypical keratinocytes and covered by parakeratosis (Fig. 2–6). Atrophic Bowen's disease is an unusual type that consists of pronounced thinning of the epidermis, which appears to be composed of only three or four layers of atypical keratinocytes covered by parakeratosis. In the verrucous-hyperkeratotic type there are prominent papillomatous projections of neoplastic epidermis and marked hyperkeratosis (Fig. 2–7). In rare instances, lesions of Bowen's disease show a nesting pattern (pagetoid Bowen's disease), which is characterized by sharply delimited clusters of

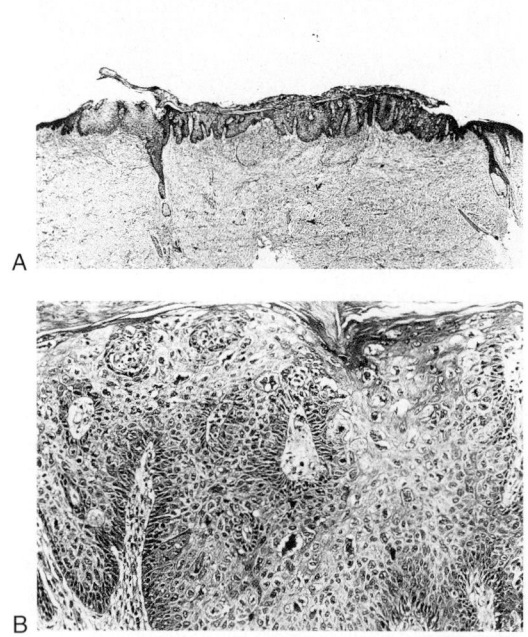

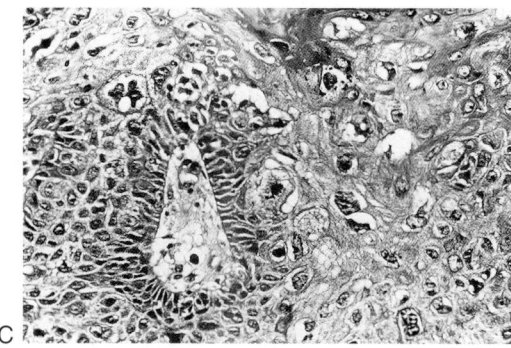

Figure 2–5. Bowen's disease. *A:* Low-power view demonstrates an acanthotic and hyperkeratotic lesion. *B:* Higher magnification shows atypical keratinocytes at all levels of the epidermis. *C:* Still higher magnification shows the pleomorphic and hyperchromatic nuclei of the neoplastic keratinocytes.

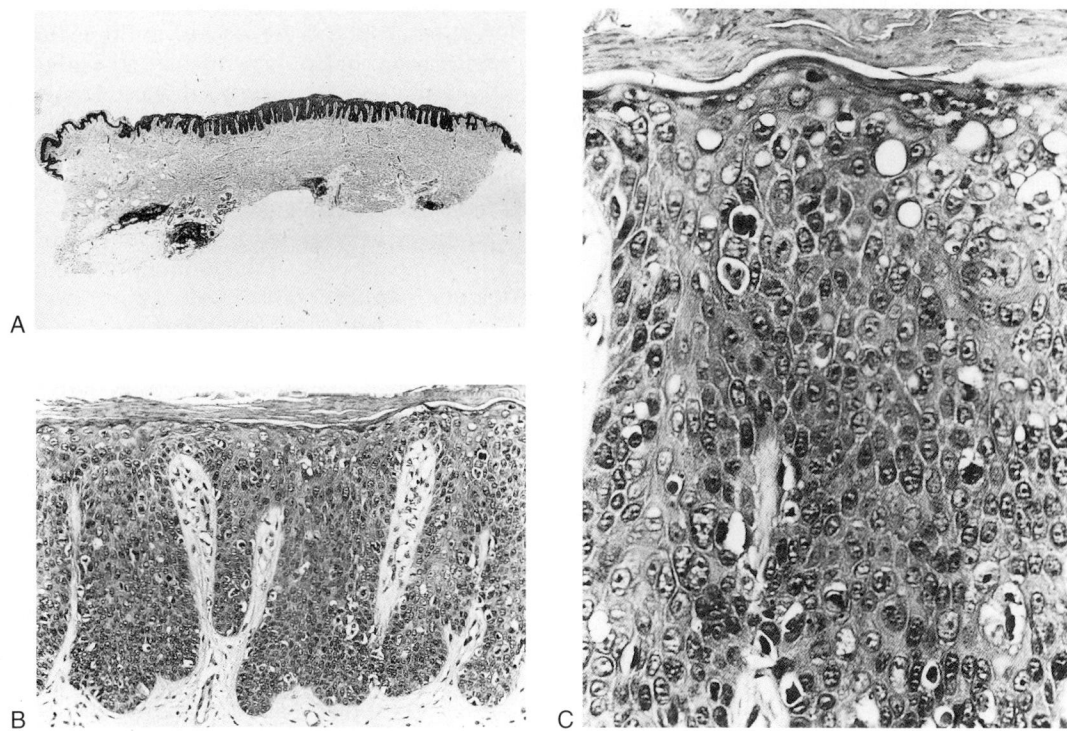

Figure 2–6. Psoriasiform Bowen's disease. *A:* Scanning magnification shows a psoriasiform epidermis. *B:* This psoriasiform epidermis displays full-thickness atypia. *C:* Higher magnification shows atypical and pleomorphic keratinocytes covered by parakeratosis.

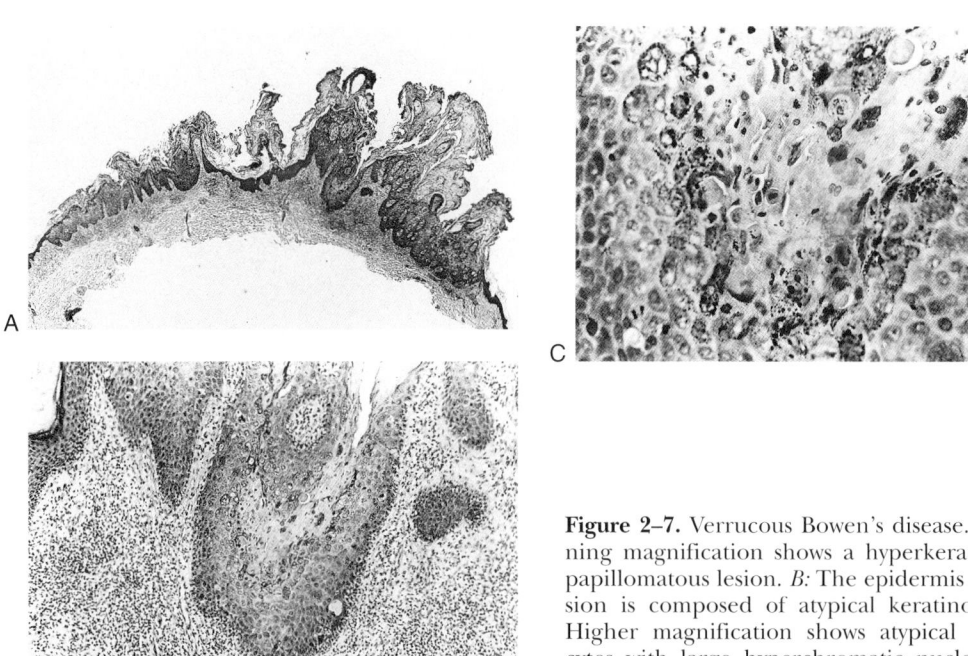

Figure 2–7. Verrucous Bowen's disease. *A:* Scanning magnification shows a hyperkeratotic and papillomatous lesion. *B:* The epidermis of the lesion is composed of atypical keratinocytes. *C:* Higher magnification shows atypical keratinocytes with large hyperchromatic nuclei, coarse keratohyalin granules, and dyskeratotic cells.

neoplastic cells within an otherwise normal epidermis (Fig. 2–8; Raiten et al., 1976). Often, neoplastic cells within the nests show a clear-cell appearance (clear-cell Bowen's disease). Probably some examples of Bowen's disease with nesting pattern were included in the dated concept of intraepidermal epithelioma of Borst-Jadassohn, which is now considered to be a histopathologic pattern characterized by sharply defined nests of morphologically different keratinocytes within the epidermis that may be seen, in addition to Bowen's disease, in a series of different lesions, including seborrheic keratosis, hidroacanthoma simplex, solar keratosis, and epidermal nevi (Steffen and Ackerman, 1985).

From a cytologic point of view, atypical vacuolated keratinocytes, dyskeratoses with large eosinophilic cytoplasm, "monster cells" with large and hyperchromatic nuclei, randomly distributed atypical suprabasal mitotic figures, and neoplastic multinucleated giant cells are characteristic of Bowen's disease. These cytologic features were described in the two cases of the seminal description by Bowen (1912). This cytologic variant, traditionally referred to as classic Bowen's disease, is the most frequently described and illustrated type in textbooks of dermatology and

dermatopathology. In our experience, however, basaloid Bowen's disease, another cytologic variant of Bowen's disease, is at least as frequent as classic Bowen's disease. Basaloid Bowen's disease was described by Achille Civatte many years ago (Civatte, 1936), but it has received little attention in the literature. It consists of plaque-like, irregular acanthotic epidermis, with obliterated rete ridges, which appears composed of small, monomorphous basaloid keratinocytes, with large, hyperchromatic, and crowded nuclei surrounded by scant cytoplasm (Fig. 2–9). In sections stained by hematoxylin and eosin, the epidermis has a dark blue rather than light eosinophilic cast because of the deeply stained and closely crowded nuclei of neoplastic cells. Basaloid Bowen's disease usually shows relatively monomorphous nuclei and dyskeratotic cells. Neoplastic multinucleated giant cells are absent, and the diagnosis may not be thought of at first glance. In these cases, the crowded nuclei of neoplastic epidermis contrasts with the adjacent normal, more eosinophilic epidermis. In the pigmented variant of Bowen's disease, melanin is present in individual neoplastic cells and melanophages are situated in the underlying papillary dermis (Ragi et al., 1988). Some authors have described dendritic arborizations

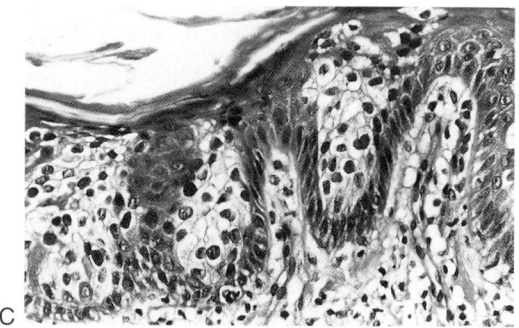

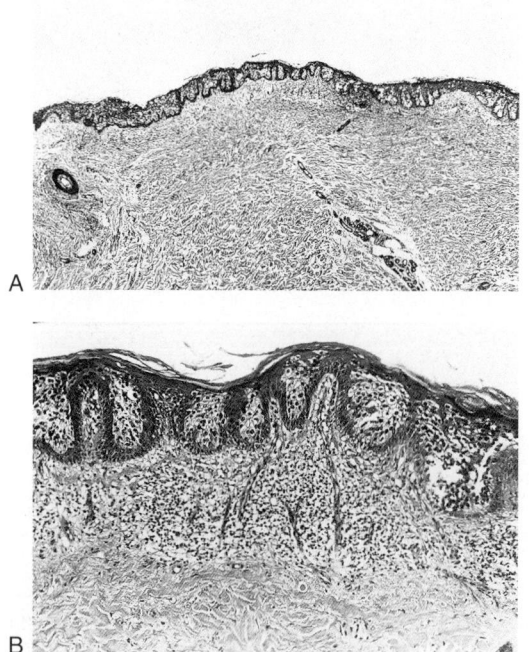

Figure 2–8. Pagetoid Bowen's disease. *A:* Scanning power. *B:* Multiple nests of clear cells are seen within the epidermis. Note the spared basal layer of the epidermis. *C:* Many of these clear cells show large, hyperchromatic, and pleomorphic nuclei.

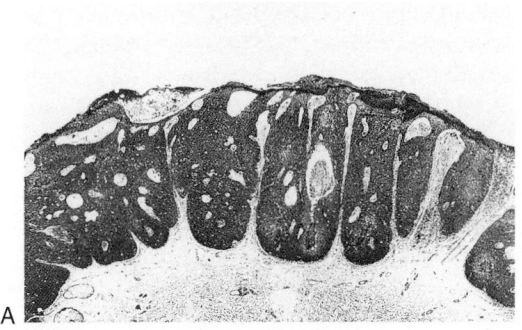

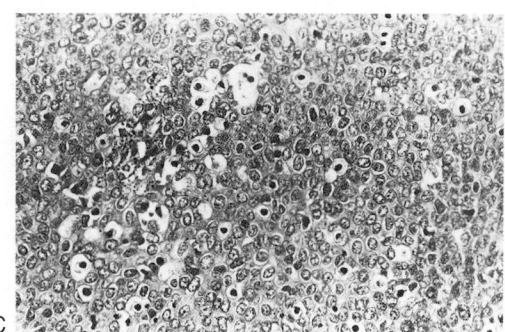

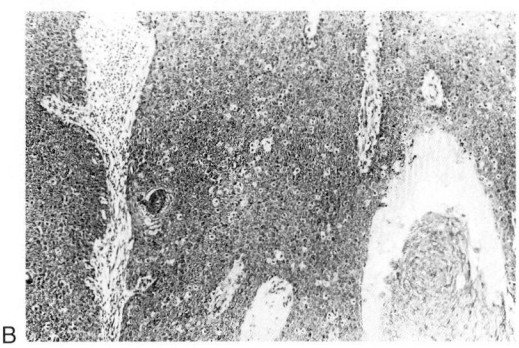

Figure 2–9. Basaloid Bowen's disease. *A:* Low-power view shows an irregular acanthotic epidermis. *B:* This epidermis is composed of basaloid cells. *C:* Higher magnification shows atypical keratinocytes with large, hyperchromatic, and crowded nuclei. Note the presence of several mitotic figures as well as many individual necrotic keratinocytes.

of melanocytes among neoplastic cells (Strayer and Santa Cruz, 1980). Finally, mucinous and sebaceous metaplasia have been also described in lesions of Bowen's disease, which, according to Fulling et al. (1981), "suggest a spectrum of patterns of differentiation available to keratinocytes in squamous carcinoma." In our opinion, however, it is unlikely that true sebaceous differentiation can occur in a squamous cell carcinoma.

The dermis of lesions of Bowen's disease usually shows prominent vascularity and an infiltrate of inflammatory cells of variable intensity, composed mainly of lymphocytes. The presence of solar elastosis depends of the location of the lesion and the intensity of sun damage. Small deposits of amyloid (Strayer and Santa Cruz, 1980) and areas of regression (Murata et al., 1996) have been also described.

It has been stated that Bowen's disesase may extend into the dermis in 3%–5% (Goldes and Kao, 1989; Kao and Graham, 1986) or 8% (Kao, 1986) of untreated cases, and the metastatic potential for these lesions has been stated to be as high as 13% (Kao, 1986). Some authors have described sebaceous (Jacobs et al., 1986) and sweat gland (Saida et al., 1989) differentiation in lesions

of Bowen's disease extending to the dermis, but in our opinion, those lesions are better interpreted as undifferentiated sebaceous carcinoma *in situ* that eventually became invasive carcinoma, and as undifferentiated eccrine (or apocrine) ductal carcinoma *in situ* that become invasive.

In the differential diagnosis between Bowen's disease and solar keratosis, the basal layer of Bowen's disease is composed of columnar cells arranged in a palisade, whereas that is not the case in solar keratosis. Another differential feature is the presence of buds of atypical keratinocytes that extend down the upper portion of eccrine dermal ducts and infundibula in solar keratosis (Pinkus, 1958), whereas in Bowen's disease atypical keratinocytes are seen within the epithelium of infundibula (Hunter, 1977) and upper eccrine ducts (Argenyi et al., 1990; Peralta et al., 1983). Bowenoid papulosis of the genitalia (see below) may be indistinguishable histopathologically from Bowen's disease, although atypia is usually more focal in lesions of bowenoid papulosis and often there are cytologic signs suggestive of HPV infection, such as basophilic inclusions in the cytoplasm of neoplastic cells or koilocytes. In pagetoid Bowen's disease, both the keratinocytes themselves and the pattern of their arrangement resemble changes of extramammary Paget's disease. Unlike extramammary Paget's disease, however, pagetoid Bowen's disease is marked by signs of altered cornification, such as dyskeratotic cells and parakeratosis. Furthermore, in pagetoid Bowen's disease there is no mucin within the cytoplasm of neoplastic cells and no formation of tubules, in contrast to authentic extramammary Paget's disease (Raiten et al., 1976). Immunohistochemistry is also helpful in this distinction, because Paget cells of extramammary Paget's disease stain for carcinoembryonic antigen (CEA), the results of which are negative in Bowen's disease (Guldhammer and Nrgaard, 1986). Neoplastic cells of extramammary Paget's disease and those of Bowen's disease also show a different immunohistochemical profile for cytokeratins (Shah et al., 1987), although the keratin distribution in lesions of Bowen's disease is variable from lesion to lesion (Ichikawa et al., 1995). Neoplastic cells of Bowen's disease show a diffuse pattern of immunostaining for nuclear proliferating antigens (Baum et al., 1994; Geary and Cooper, 1992; Szekeres and de Giacomoni, 1994), and, as in solar keratosis, they are aneuploid (Biesterfeld et al., 1995) and express mutant p53 protein (Hughes and Robinson, 1995; Sim et al., 1992b; Szekeres and de Giacomoni, 1994), and bcl-2 protein (Nakagawa et al., 1994). Overexpression of p53 seems to be higher in cases of Bowen's disease induced by chronic exposure to arsenic (Kuo et al., 1997).

ARSENICAL KERATOSIS

Patients with a history of chronic arsenic intake may develop keratotic lesions on the palms and soles that are indistinguishable histopathologically from those of Bowen's disease, although usually these lesions show less atypia and more prominent hyperkeratosis and papillomatosis (Yeh, 1973). Often, these patients also have multiple lesions of other forms of cutaneous carcinoma, mainly located on the trunk, including basal cell carcinoma and squamous cell carcinoma (Wong et al., 1998). They are also at higher risk for visceral carcinoma (Miki et al., 1982), with bronchial and genitourinary carcinomas being the most frequent internal

malignancies (Fierz, 1965; Sommers and McManus, 1953).

RADIATION KERATOSIS

In the times past, radiologists, radiotherapists, dentists, and other individuals exposed professionally to small amounts of X-ray irradiation over long periods of time developed keratotic lesions on the dorsum of the hands. These lesions, known as *radiation keratoses*, are surrounded by atrophic skin that displays telangiectasia and hyperpigmented and hypopigmented areas.

Histopathologically, radiation keratoses show variable epidermal thickness, with hyperkeratosis and disordered maturation of keratinocytes. Usually atypical and hyperchromatic keratinocytes and scattered dyskeratotic cells are seen at different levels of the epidermis, although radiation keratosis may be identical to solar keratosis in terms of epithelial changes. In the dermis, however, there are changes similar to those of chronic radiodermatitis—namely, homogenization of the collagen bundles, telangiectatic vessels, some of them with thickened eosinophilic walls, and atypical stellate fibroblasts with large and hyperchromatic nuclei (Jacobi and Burgoon, 1985). Folliculosebaceous structures are absent or reduced in number, but the arrector pili muscles remain intact. When radiation keratosis progresses to squamous cell carcinoma, the neoplasm is often composed of spindle cells (Kao, 1990).

PUVA KERATOSIS

This is a specific type of keratosis that appears in patients receiving long-term treatment with psoralens and ultraviolet-A radiation (PUVA) for psoriasis, mycosis fungoides, and other dermatologic disorders. These patients develop raised keratotic papules with a broad base, located mainly on the trunk and thighs. Histopathologically, PUVA keratoses consist of circumscribed areas of acanthosis and papillomatosis, hyperkeratosis with focal parakeratosis, necrotic keratinocytes disposed as solitary units in the spinous layer, and slight atypia of keratinocytes (van Praag et al., 1993). In two rare instances, hypopigmented PUVA keratoses have been described (Morison et al., 1991). PUVA keratoses may be associated with an increased risk for nonmelanoma skin cancer (McKenna et al., 1996; van Praag et al., 1993).

Solar Cheilitis

Solar keratosis involving the mucocutaneous junction of the lower lip is known as *solar cheilitis*. The lesion presents itself as a diffuse scaling of the entire lower lip or as focal areas of hyperkeratosis (Picascia and Robinson, 1987). Sometimes, solar cheilitis appears as a white patch of leukoplakia on the vermillon border of the lower lip (Gibson and Perry, 1985). Histopathologically, lesions of solar cheilitis show acanthosis with disordered maturation of epidermal cells, hyperkeratosis, and parakeratosis (Cataldo and Doku, 1981; Nicolau and Balus, 1964; Schmitt and Folsom, 1968). Sometimes, buds of epidermal keratinocytes like those of cutaneous solar keratosis are seen in solar cheilitis (Picascia and Robinson, 1987). Cytological atypia varies from case to case, but usually abnormal mitoses and bizarre keratinocytes with pleomorphic nuclei are absent, making diagnosis of carcinoma difficult (Koten et al., 1967). The dermis shows solar elastosis and an infiltrate of inflammatory cells with many plasma cells (Koten et al., 1967; Nicolau and Balus, 1964).

Erythroplasia of Queyrat

Bowen's disease involving the mucosa of the glans penis is called *erythroplasia of Queyrat*. The process appears most commonly in uncircumcised elderly males and clinically consists of a well-circumscribed erythematous plaque with a bright red shiny surface. Occasionally, the inner surface of the prepuce also is involved. Induration or ulceration indicates that the process has extended into the dermis. Histopathologically, the findings are identical to those of cutaneous Bowen's disease (Mikhail, 1980; Sonnex et al., 1982). It has been postulated that when erythroplasia of Queyrat becomes invasive it has a greater metastatic potential than that of a squamous cell carcinoma that begins as Bowen's disease (Graham and Helwig, 1973; Mikhail, 1980). Red plaques involving the oral mucosa with histopathologic features of squamous cell carcinoma *in situ* have been designated *erythroplakia of the oral cavity* (Shafer and Waldron, 1975).

Bowenoid Papulosis

Bowenoid papulosis was first described by Lloyd in 1970 as "multicentric pigmented Bowen's disease of the groin" (Lloyd, 1970), but was recognized as a distinctive entity and termed *bowenoid papulosis* a few years later (Kopf and Bart, 1977; Wade et al., 1978, 1979). The lesions consist of papules or plaques like condylomata acuminata that involve genital skin. Most patients are young, sexually active individuals and have multiple lesions (Patterson et al., 1986; Schwartz and Janniger, 1991). In females, lesions on the vulva are often pigmented. The cause of this process is certainly viral, because DNA sequences of HPV-16 have been identified in most cases (Grosshans and Grossmann, 1985; Ikenberg et al., 1983; Lookingbill et al., 1987; Obalek et al., 1986), although examples of bowenoid papulosis due to HPV-18, -31, -32, -34, -35, -39, -42, -48, -51–54, or mixed infections have also been reported (Abdennader et al., 1989; Cobb, 1990; Favre et al., 1990; Obalek et al., 1986; Penneys et al., 1984; Rüdlinger et al., 1989). All these HPV types are commonly detected in genital malignant neoplasms (Matsukura and Sugase, 1995), and these patients seem to have a specific suppression of natural cell-mediated cytotoxicity against HPV-infected cells (Malejczyk et al., 1989). Bowenoid papulosis has also been described in patients with acquired immunodeficiency syndrome (AIDS) (Rüdlinger and Buchmann, 1989) and hairy cell leukemia (Lebbe et al., 1993).

Histopathologically, bowenoid papulosis is characterized by nearly full-thickness atypia of epidermal keratinocytes, disordered maturation of keratinocytes, and crowded hyperchromatic nuclei of keratinocytes. There may be atypical mitotic figures, individual necrotic cells, and dyskeratotic cells scattered at all levels of the epidermis (Fig. 2–10). All of these features are identical to those of Bowen's disease and the histopathologic differential diagnosis between these two disorders may sometimes be impossible without consideration of clinical aspects. Some authors, however, have proposed that

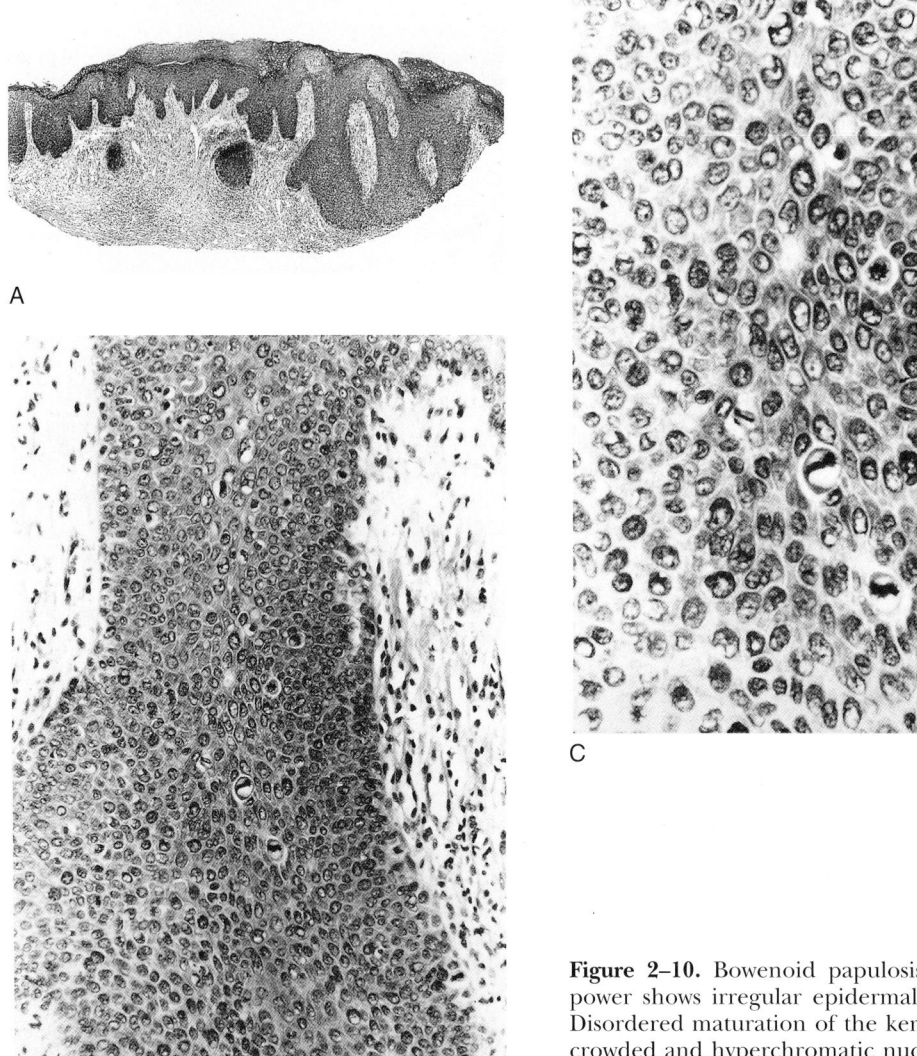

Figure 2–10. Bowenoid papulosis. *A:* Scanning power shows irregular epidermal acanthosis. *B:* Disordered maturation of the keratinocytes with crowded and hyperchromatic nuclei. *C:* Atypical keratinocytes and several mitotic figures.

histologic features in favor of a diagnosis of bowenoid papulosis over that of Bowen's disease are a general architecture of the lesion like that of condyloma acuminatum, atypia restricted to foci rather than the full thickness of the epidermis, numerous metaphase mitoses, and sparing of the intraepidermal segments of adnexal epithelium (Patterson et al., 1986). Furthermore, some investigators have reported significant differences in cytomorphometric studies between lesions of Bowen's disease and bowenoid papulosis (Olemans et al., 1994).

The evolution of the lesions is variable and cases of spontaneous regression have been occasionally described, especially in young women (Friedrich, 1972; Skinner et al., 1973). Some examples of bowenoid papulosis have progressed to squamous cell carcinoma that involves the dermis (Obalek et al., 1986; Rüdlinger and Buchmann, 1989). Overexpression of p53 tumor suppressor protein has been noted in neoplastic cells of bowenoid papulosis. Some of these cells also contained HPV-DNA (Ranki et al., 1995), but in other studies, p53 overexpression and HPV-DNA were detected in separate keratinocytes (Lassus and Ranki, 1996). No mutations of the tumor-suppressor gene *p53* have been identified, which suggests that *p53* mutations are not important in the carcinogenesis of bowenoid papulosis (Castren et al., 1998). In any event, bowenoid papulosis should be considered a peculiar variant of squamous cell carcinoma *in situ* of the skin, a conclusion that is supported by histomorphologic studies and DNA ploidy analysis (Böcking et al., 1989). Close follow-up of patients is therefore essential.

INCIPENT MALIGNANT NEOPLASMS WITH FOLLICULAR DIFFERENTIATION

SUPERFICIAL BASAL CELL CARCINOMA

We consider basal cell carcinoma to be the malignant counterpart of *trichoblastoma*, a malignant neoplasm of follicular germinative cells. Although most examples of basal cell carcinoma are nodular in type and are nearly always undifferentiated, three types of basal cell carcinoma show indubitable signs of follicular differentiation; superficial basal cell carcinoma, fibroepithelial basal cell carcinoma, and infundibulocystic basal cell carcinoma (Ackerman et al., 1993). Clinically,

superficial basal cell carcinoma appears as an erythematous plaque that spreads slowly and has a slightly raised, thread-like papular margin. The surface shows scaly, crusted, and eroded areas, and foci of pigmentation are also often seen. These features cause the lesion to resemble Paget's disease of the nipple, and for that reason superficial basal cell carcinoma is also named *pagetoid basal cell carcinoma*. The denomination of multicentric basal cell carcinoma for this variant is inaccurate, because three-dimensional reconstructive studies have shown that all of the apparently separated aggregations of neoplastic cells are actually interconnected (Lang et al., 1987). This clinicopathological variant is found mainly on the trunk of adult or elderly persons and sometimes multiple lesions are present in the same patient.

Histopathologically, superficial basal cell carcinoma is composed of follicular germinative cells clustered in aggregations of variable sizes and shapes attached to the undersurface of the epidermis. It is usually confined to a thickened papillary dermis (Fig. 2–11). In the aggregations, the nuclei of neoplastic cells are aligned in a palisade at the periphery and clefts form between the aggregations and adjacent altered stroma.

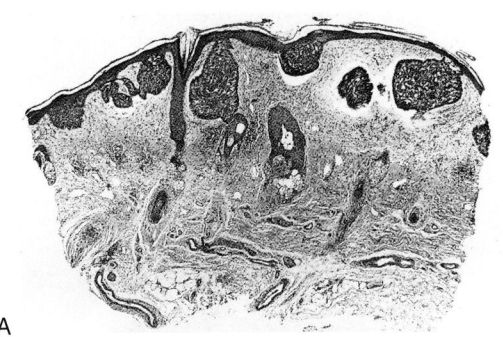

A

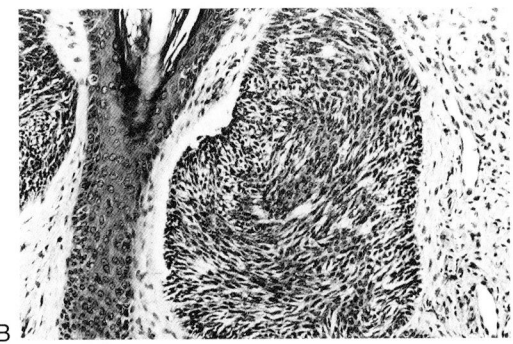

B

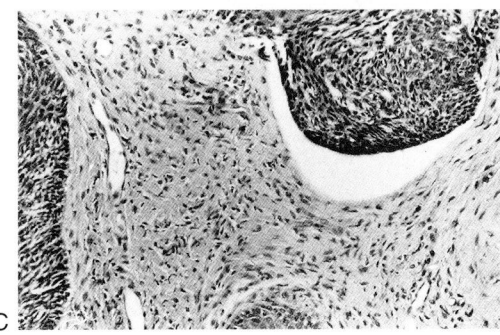

C

Figure 2–11. Superficial basal cell carcinoma. *A:* Low-power view shows aggregations of basaloid neoplastic cells attached to the undersurface of the epidermis. *B:* Higher magnification of an aggregation of basaloid neoplastic cells with a palisade at the periphery. *C:* Clefting between the aggregation of neoplastic cells and adjacent altered stroma.

Individual necrotic cells and mitotic figures are often seen within the aggregations of neoplastic cells. In rare instances, acantholysis has been reported to have been found within aggregations of a superficial basal cell carcinoma (Mehregan, 1979). This, however, is unlikely. The stroma consists of delicated fibrillary bundles of collagen, abundant mucin, and dilated venules. Features of what seems to be regression are sometimes seen in sections of specimens of superficial basal cell carcinoma. They consist of areas of lymphocytic inflammatory infiltrate, intermingled with melanophages and Civatte bodies that result from necrotic neoplastic cells, and vertically oriented capillaries in a thickened fibrotic papillary dermis (Curson and Weedon, 1979). Some of the neoplastic aggregations have crescentic or bulbous shapes resembling follicular germs in an embryo, but there is no accompanying follicular papilla. In rare instances, however, neoplastic aggregations of a superficial basal cell carcinoma show a more advanced degree of follicular differentiation, and they appear surrounded by whorls of fibrocytes and fibrillary collagen such as those of perifollicular sheaths or associated with a rudimentary follicular bulbs and papilla (Sanchez Yus et al., 1989).

From an immunohistochemical perspective, basal cell carcinomas express a pattern of cytokeratins similar to that of keratinocytes of the basal layer of the epidermis (Kariniemi et al., 1984b; Markey et al., 1992). They also show immunostaining for cytokeratins found only in follicular epithelium, supporting a follicular differentiation for this neoplasm (Kariniemi et al., 1984b; Shimizu et al., 1989). Neoplastic cells also express a diffuse staining pattern of the apoptosis-suppressing oncogene protein bcl-2, which is not found in squamous cell carcinomas and is expressed only in the peripheral layer of trichoblastomas (Cerroni and Kerl, 1994; Crowson et al., 1996; Mills, 1997; Morales-Ducret et al., 1995; Nakagawa et al., 1994; Smoller et al., 1994; Verhaegh et al., 1995). Basal cell carcinomas also express immunoreactivity for the murine monoclonal antibody VM-1, which stains the keratinocytes of the basal layer of the normal human epidermis (Oseroff et al., 1983), and for Ber EP4, another monoclonal antibody that recognizes an epithelial gly-copolypeptide antigen and is negative in squamous cell carcinoma (Tellechea et al., 1993). In contrast, neoplastic cells of basal cell carcinoma do not express involucrin and CD44, which are usually found in the neoplastic cells of squamous cell carcinoma (Hale et al., 1995; Prieto et al., 1995; Said et al., 1984). A peripheral ring of immunostaining with peanut agglutinin is seen around neoplastic aggregations of basal cell carcinoma (Vigneswaran et al., 1987), but not around trichoblastoma aggregations (Haneke, 1995). CD34 antibody stains the fibrocytes of the stroma in trichoblastoma, but not those of basal cell carcinoma (Kirchmann et al., 1994). In our opinion, all these immunohistochemical investigations are not necessary for the practical purpose of diagnosis of basal cell carcinoma, as it can be distinguished from squamous cell carcinoma and from trichoblastoma with hematoxylin-eosin staining alone. Squamous cell carcinoma is composed of cells with more eosinophilic cytoplasm that show evidence of abnormal keratinization in the form of "horn pearls" and atypical dyskeratotic. Trichoblastoma is a benign neoplasm of germinative follicular cells that has the silhouette of a benign neoplasm in which the stroma composed of abundant fibrocytes and connective tissue resembles perifollicular sheath. In our view, the main histopathologic differential diagnosis of superficial basal cell carcinoma is the induction of primitive follicles often seen on the undersurface of the epidermis above dermatofibromas, and a large variety of inflammatory, hyperplastic, and neoplastic skin conditions that involve the upper part of the dermis. These basaloid proliferations with follicular differentiation closely simulate superficial basal cell carcinoma, and immunohistochemical investigations have demonstrated that they show unusual patterns of cytokeratin expression, including cytokeratins K6 and K16, proteins often associated with epidermal proliferative disorders but not present in normal epidermis (Stoler et al., 1989). Furthermore, basaloid proliferations overlying dermatofibromas and neoplastic aggregations of basal cell carcinoma show similar patterns of expression for β-2-microglobulin (Rosen et al., 1993) and metallothionein (Rosen et al., 1997). However, differential diagnosis between the basaloid proliferations in the epidermis overlying dermatofibroma and an authentic superficial basal cell carcinoma may be established on the basis of the nature of the dermal proliferation; its altered stroma is responsible for the inductive changes seen in the epidermis (Requena et al., 1996b). In our opinion, the case described as "intraepidermal pilar epithelioma" (Ito et al., 1988) is better interpreted as an example of seborrheic keratosis that has a nested pattern, rather than as an intraepidermal basal cell carcinoma with follicular differentiation.

Superficial basal cell carcinoma can be thought of as a basal cell carcinoma *in situ* that remains confined to the papillary dermis for a long time before it extends deeper and into reticular dermis. This variant may be adequately treated by superficial electrocoagulation and curettage with a low rate of persistent neoplasm.

INCIPIENT MALIGNANT NEOPLASMS WITH SEBACEOUS DIFFERENTIATION

Intraepidermal Sebaceous Carcinoma

In rare instances, neoplastic aggregations of an extraocular sebaceous carcinoma are confined within the epidermis and/or adnexal epithelium; the neoplasm may then be considered to be a sebaceous carcinoma *in situ* (Jacobs et al., 1986; Oka and Katsumata, 1990; Steffen and Ackerman, 1994d; Wick et al., 1985). In those cases, the neoplasm is composed of circumscribed aggregations of immature nonvacuolated sebocytes that are intermingled with mature, vacuolated, foamy sebocytes and sebaceous ductal structures that sport a corrugated eosinophilic luminal cuticle. Within the intraepidermal nests there is disordered arrangement of neoplastic cells, many individual necrotic cells or massive necrosis, numerous atypical mitotic figures, and pleomorphic and crowded nuclei. In general, more differentiated sebocytes tend to be situated in the center of the aggregations of neoplastic cells.

Immunohistochemically, neoplastic cells of sebaceous carcinoma express positivity for epithelial membrane antigen and human milk fat lobule antigen, but they do not express immunostaining for carcinoembryonic antigen, S-100 protein, or gross cystic disease fluid protein-15 (Ansai et al., 1993).

Histopathologic differential diagnosis of intraepidermal sebaceous carcinoma includes the rare examples of seborrheic keratosis with sebaceous differentiation, and superficial variants of sebaceous adenoma and sebaceoma, which are benign neoplasms with sebaceous differentiation that exhibit all the cytologic and architectural attributes of the benign neoplasms that they are (Steffen and Ackerman, 1994b,c,e). Another lesion that should be considered is the so-called *superficial epithelioma with sebaceous differentiation* (Friedman et al., 1987; Kato and Ueno, 1992; Rothko et al., 1980; Toyoda et al., 1998; Vaughan and Sau, 1990), a benign neoplasm with sebaceous differentiation that has been designated by others as reticulated acanthoma with sebaceous differentiation (Steffen and Ackerman, 1994a). This neoplasm is characterized histopatologically by an exoendophytic epithelial proliferation with a papillated surface and reticulated configuration. It is composed of strands and lobules of basophilic keratinocytes that contain nests of mature and immature sebocytes and ductal sebaceous structures within aggregations of basaloid cells or at the bases of distorted rete ridges. Intraepidermal sebaceous carcinoma should also be differentiated from the pagetoid "spread" seen in many specimens of ocular sebaceous carcinoma, the pagetoid sebocytes being scattered in a pagetoid pattern within the epidermis of the eyelid and conjuntival epithelium (Rao et al., 1982; Wolfe et al., 1984). These cases should be not interpreted as examples of ocular sebaceous carcinoma *in situ* that extend to the dermis but as epidermotropic pagetoid spread within the epidermis of eyelid and conjunctival epithelium from a sebaceous carcinoma present in sebaceous lobules of the dermis. The intraepidermal pagetoid "spread" from a sebaceous carcinoma has been not described in extraocular cases. Ocular sebaceous carcinoma probably does not arise from cells of the conjunctival epithelium or from epidermis of the eyelids but from sebaceous glands within the dermis or the meibomian glands of the tarsal plate; to the best of our knowledge, no examples of ocular sebaceous carcinoma *in situ* have been recorded.

Sebaceous carcinoma involving the dermis is a highly malignant neoplasm, capable of metastasizing widely and causing death in cases of both ocular and extraocular location (Jenson, 1990; King et al., 1979; Wick et al., 1985). If an intraepidermal sebaceous carcinoma is completely excised and stromal infiltration has not occurred, the patient will be cured.

INCIPIENT MALIGNANT NEOPLASMS WITH ECCRINE AND APOCRINE DIFFERENTIATION

Malignant Hidroacanthoma Simplex (Intraepidermal Porocarcinoma)

Poromas are benign neoplasms composed of poroid and cuticular cells that resemble those that make up the uppermost part of the eccrine and apocrine ducts. On the basis of their architectural pattern, four histopathologic variants are recognized; hidroacanthoma simplex or intraepidermal poroma, when well-circumscribed nests of poroid and cuticular cells are confined within the epidermis; dermal duct tumor, when discrete neoplastic aggregations are within the dermis; classic poroma, when neoplastic strands and lobules of poroid and cuticular cells are connected with the epidermis and from there extend into the dermis; and poroid hidradenoma, which is a wholly intradermal neoplasm with both solid and cystic components (Abenoza and Ackerman, 1990). The four poroid neoplasms are closely related to one another; when step sections are cut throughout a particular specimen, it becomes evident that a sharp demarcation among the different variants is often not possible. Examples of poromas combining the four histopathologic subtypes in the same neoplasm are well documented in the literature (Kakinuma et al., 1994). Since the original description by Pinkus and Rogin in 1956 (Pinkus and Rogin, et al., 1956), poroma has invariably been considered to be a neoplasm with eccrine differentiation. But more recently, examples of poroid neoplasms showing features of follicular and/or sebaceous differentiation

have been interpreted as poromas with apocrine differentiation on the basis of the common embryologic origin of the three elements of the folliculosebaceous-apocrine unit (Harvell et al., 1996; Requena et al., 1998a).

Malignant hidroacanthoma simplex is a porocarcinoma whose neoplastic aggregations are confined within the thickness of the epidermis or the epithelium of preexisting adnexa, a porocarcinoma *in situ*. Only a few examples of this rare neoplasm have been reported in the literature (Bardach, 1978; Ishikawa, 1971; Kitamura et al., 1983; Mehregan et al., 1983; Miyashita and Suzuki, 1993; Moreno et al., 1984; Pique et al., 1995; Ruffieux and Ramelet, 1985; Smith and Coburn, 1956; Takano et al., Zina et al., 1982). It is also likely that most porocarcinomas begin as a malignant hidroacanthoma simplex or prorocarcinoma *in situ*, before involving the dermis. The clinical appearance of the reported lesions of malignant hidroacanthoma simplex has been variable, with some of them being nodular, whereas others were keratotic plaques. The lesions were situated on the lower half of the body, mainly the legs. The duration of the lesions before excision ranged from 1 to 30 years (Moreno et al., 1984; Ruffieux and Ramelet, 1985). In some cases, the neoplasm was ulcerated. The two most frequent clinical diagnoses made were Bowen's disease or seborrheic keratosis.

Histopathologically, malignant hidroacanthoma simplex has the silhouette of a malignant neoplasm, as it is asymmetric, and poorly circumscribed, and intraepidermal neoplastic aggregations vary considerably in sizes and shapes. Because massive necrosis is a frequent finding in both poromas and porocarcinomas, that feature alone is not helpful in distinguishing between these two neoplasms. At higher magnification, neoplastic aggregations of malignant hidroacanthoma simplex can be seen to consists of two types of cells, poroid and cuticular, but sometimes the neoplasm is so undifferentiated that the two types of cells are usually no longer recognizable as such. Nuclei are crowded, hyperchromatic, and often pleomorphic. Some neoplastic cells are necrotic, and some may exhibit atypical mitoses. Although most aggregations are solid, tubular structures appear in others within zones of cuticular cells (Fig. 2–12).

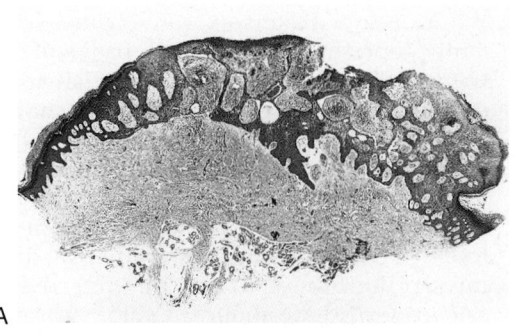

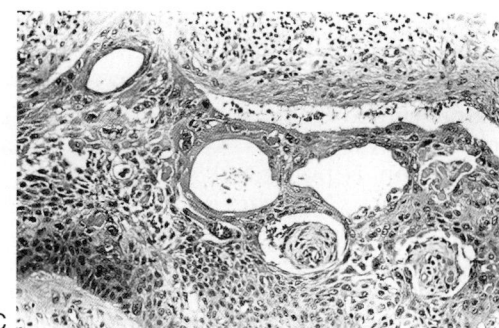

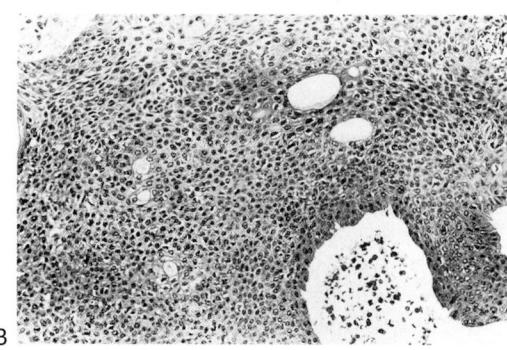

Figure 2–12. Intraepidermal porocarcinoma. *A:* Scanning view showing irregular acanthotic epidermis. *B:* Poroid cells with crowded nuclei and two small ductal structures surrounded by cuticular cells. *C:* Ductal structures surrounded by atypical cuticular cells.

It should be recalled that the presence of intraepidermal nests of porocarcinoma is not unequivocal evidence of a primary, rather than a metastatic, nature of porocarcinoma, because there are several published examples of epidermotropically metastatic porocarcinomas (see below).

Enzyme histochemical investigations of porocarcinoma have shown positivity for amylophosphorylase and succinic dehydrogenase (Claudy et al., 1983; Puttick et al., 1986). Ductal structures within the areas of cuticular cells express immunohistochemical reactivity for carcinoembryonic antigen and epithelial membrane antigen (Moreno et al., 1984; Pique et al., 1995; Puttick et al., 1986; Requena et al., 1990; Swanson et al., 1987). Other immunohistochemical attributes of neoplastic cells of porocarcinoma include expression of cytokeratins, antibody Leu-M1, and blood isoantigens A, B, and H (blood group I; Swanson et al., 1987). Holden and co-workers reported loss of membrane β-2-microglobulin from cell membranes of the neoplastic cells of porocarcinoma (Holden et al., 1984). Porocarcinomas have a significantly high proportion of neoplastic cells that express proliferating cell nuclear antigen (Tateyama et al., 1995).

Some cases of malignant hidroacanthoma simplex have been claimed to have originated in a preexisting benign intraepidermal poroma (Bardach, 1978; Ishikawa, 1971; Puttick et al., 1986; Ruffieux and Ramelet, 1985; Shaw et al., 1982; Zina et al., 1982). Clinical signs that have been proposed as suggestive of development of malignant transformation within a preexisting hidroacanthoma simplex include ulceration, bleeding, pain, sudden growth within few months, and, sometimes, a multinodular pattern within a single lesion. However, most cases of malignant hidroacanthoma simplex originate *de novo.* Malignant hidroacanthoma simplex is a porocorcarcinoma *in situ,* and complete excision of the neoplasm is curative. When porocarcinoma involves the dermis, metastases often appear in the form of satellite epidermotropic ones in regional lymph nodes or as widespread metastatic disease. Some patients have died as a consequence of metastases from porocarcinoma (Snow and Reizner, 1992).

EXTRAMAMMARY PAGET'S DISEASE

In our view, extramammary Paget's disease is a primary carcinoma with apocrine differentiation that begins within the epidermis. From here it extends first into epithelial structures of the adnexa and, uncommonly, and only after many years, into the dermis, from which it may metastasize. We consider extramammary Paget's disease to be an apocrine adenocarcinoma *in situ* of the skin. This conclusion is predicated on the cytologic characteristics of Paget cells, such as the presence, episodically, of signs of "decapitation" secretion, abundant intracytoplasmic mucin that sometimes results in the formation of signet-ring cells, and the occasional finding of lipofuscin. Furthermore, some intraepidermal tubules in examples of extramammary Paget's disease exhibit signs of decapitation secretion. This constellation of findings favors an apocrine nature of the neoplastic cells of extramammary Paget's disease (Requena et al., 1998b).

Extramammary Paget's disease presents as a solitary reddish patch. The surface may be scaly and is sometimes covered by small crusts and erosions. Pruritus is the most prominent symptom. Pigmented and depigmented lesions have also been described (Kakinuma et al., 1994). Extramammary Paget's disease occurs more frequently in women than in men, and the vulva is the most common site (Fenn et al., 1971; Fetherston and Friedrich, 1972; Gunn and Gallagher, 1980; Jones et al., 1979; Koss et al., 1968; Lee et al., 1977; Taki et al., 1971; Woodruff, 1955), followed by the scrotum (Crocker, 1889; Hamm et al., 1986; Koh and Nazarina, 1995), perianal area (Helwig and Graham, 1963; Merot et al., 1985), and axilla (Jones et al., 1979; Mazoujian et al., 1984). Less often, lesions of extramammary Paget's disease have been described on the groin (Hamm et al., 1986), buttock (Jones et al., 1979), pubis (Jones et al., 1979), knee (de Blois et al., 1984), penis (Crocker, 1889; Mitsudo et al., 1981), chest (Kao et al., 1986; Saida and Iwata, 1987), back (Inada et al., 1985), external ear canal (Fligiel and Kaneko, 1975), tongue (Changus et al., 1971), oral mucosa (Theaker, 1988), umbilicus (Remond et al., 1993), and abdomen (Onishi and Ohara, 1996). Rare presentations are extramammary Paget's disease in a supernumerary nipple (Martin et al., 1994) and concurrent involvement of both axilla and the genital region (Imakado et al., 1991; Kawatsu and Miki, 1971). The lesions reputed to be extramammary Paget's disease on the eyelid (Knauer and Whorton, 1963;

Whorton and Patterson, 1955) almost certainly represent examples of pagetoid intraepithelial sebaceous carcinoma that arose in underlying sebaceous glands (Rao et al., 1982).

Histopathologically, lesions of extramammary Paget's disease show atypical large epithelial cells scattered as solitary units at all levels of the epidermis and epithelial structures of the adnexa. These cells, referred to as *Paget's cells*, have abundant pale cytoplasm and large round pleomorphic nuclei, sometimes with prominent nucleoli (Fig. 2–13). Paget's cells show a bluish cast in their cytoplasm, reflecting the presence of abundant mucin, and sometimes these cells have an eccentric nucleus and the appearance of a signet ring (Ordoñez et al., 1987; Roth et al., 1977). In early lesions, atypical epithelial cells proliferate in the lower layers of the epidermis as single units, but later the entire thickness of the epidermis may be involved with the formation of intraepidermal nests and small glandular structures lined by epithelial neoplastic cells showing decapitation secretion in their luminal border (Fig. 2–14). Authentic tubular structures should not be confused with pseudotubules resulting from necrosis in the center of aggregations. In time, Paget's cells are also found in the epithelial structures of adnexa, the eccrine ducts and folliculosebaceous units (Fig. 2–15). Extramammary Paget's disease tends to remain as an apocrine adenocarcinoma *in situ* for long periods of time, but in rare instances and after many years, Paget's cells may descend into the dermis or the lamina propria of the mucosa (Evans and Neven, 1991; Hawley et al., 1991; Jones et al., 1979) and may metastasize from there.

In contrast with most cases of mammary Paget's disease, neoplastic cells of extramammary Paget's disease contain abundant mucin, and therefore show positive staining with mucicarmin, alcian blue at pH 2.5, colloidal iron, and periodic acid-Schiff (PAS) (Fig. 2–16; Glasgow et al., 1987; Helm et al., 1992; Ordoñez et al., 1987; Sitakalin and Ackerman, 1985). Histoenzymatic studies have not contributed to elucidation of the histogenesis of Paget's cells in extramammary Paget's disease, because the presence of both eccrine and apocrine enzymes has been demonstrated (Kanitakis, 1985). Through immunohistochemical techniques,

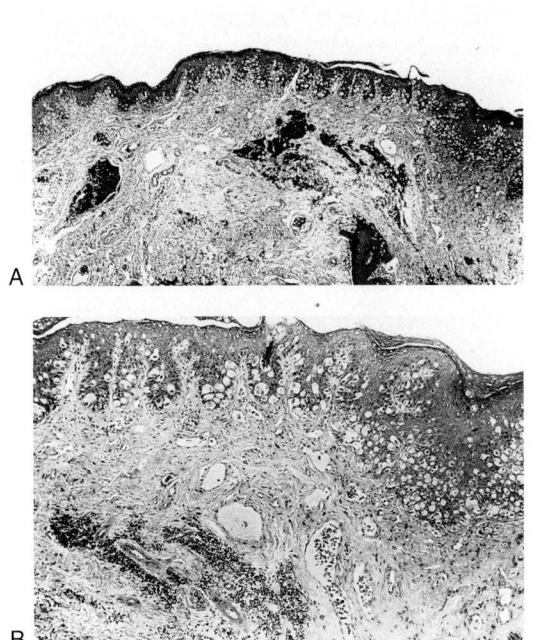

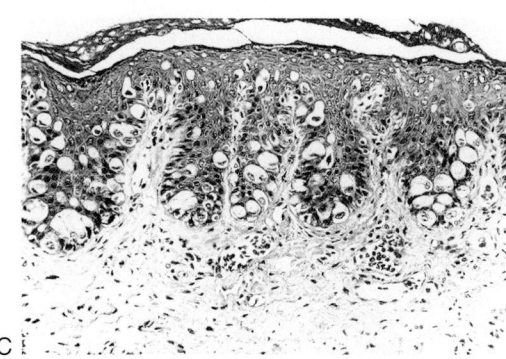

Figure 2–13. Extramammary Paget's disease. *A:* Low-power view showing clear cells scattered as solitary units at all levels of the epidermis. *B:* Higher magnification demonstrates that neoplastic cells have abundant pale cytoplasm. *C:* Still higher magnification shows that Paget's cells have abundant pale cytoplasm and large pleomorphic nuclei.

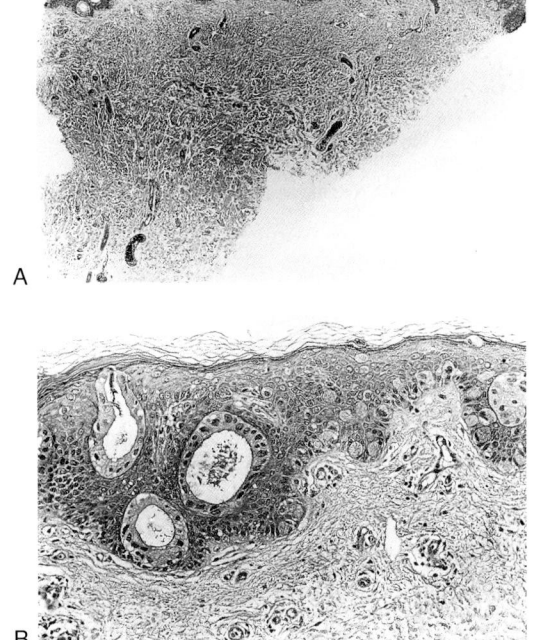

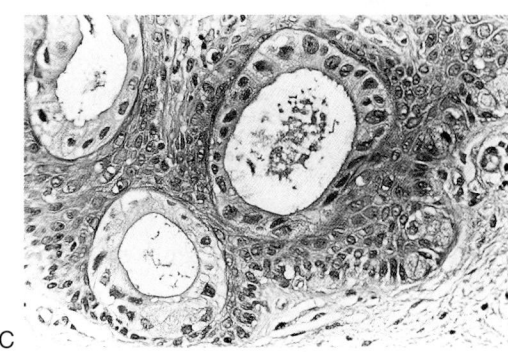

Figure 2–14. Extramammary Paget's disease. *A:* Scanning power shows clear cells scattered at all levels of the epidermis. *B:* Glandular structures within the epidermis. *C:* Epithelial cells lining the glandular structures have a columnar shape with large nuclei and abundant cytoplasm with a bluish cast because of the presence of mucin.

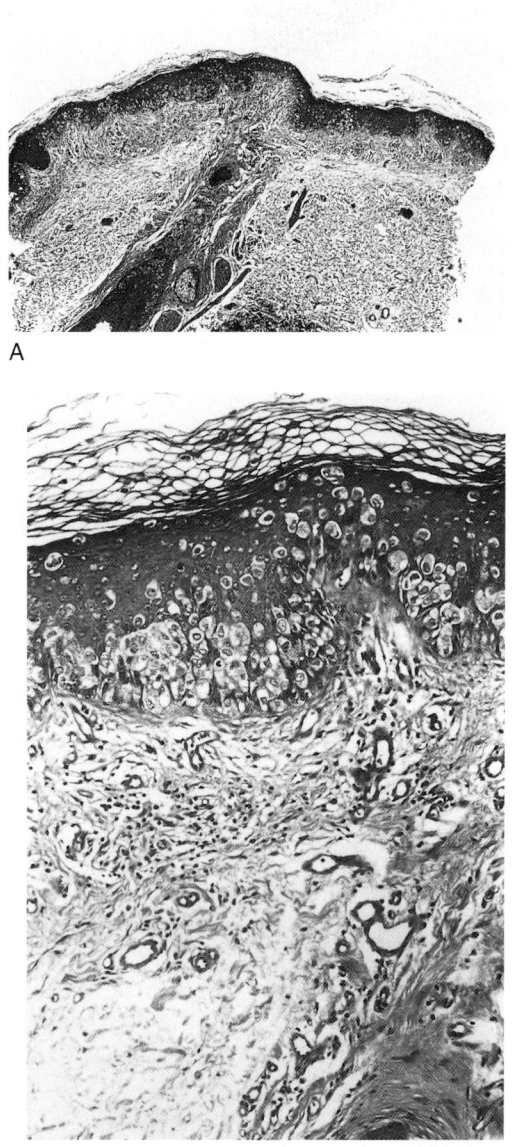

A

B

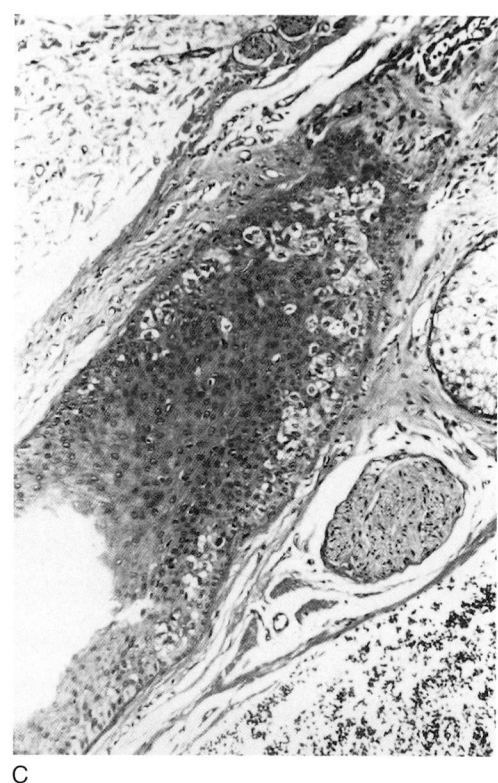

C

Figure 2–15. Extramammary Paget's disease. *A:* Low-power view shows pale cells scattered at all levels of the epidermis. *B:* Paget's cells within the epidermis show abundant pale cytoplasm. *C:* Paget's cells also involved the epithelium of the outer sheath of the hair follicle.

Paget's cells of extramammary Paget's disease express reactivity for CEA (Fig. 2–17; Battles et al., 1997; Guarner et al., 1989; Helm et al., 1992; Kariniemi et al., 1984a; Mazoujian et al., 1984; Nadji et al., 1982; Vanstapel et al., 1984; Yamamura et al., 1993), epithelial membrane antigen (Anthony et al., 1986; Guarner et al., 1989; Russell Jones et al., 1989; Yamamura et al., 1993), gross cystic disease fluid protein-15 (de Blois et al., 1984; Kohler and Smoller, 1996; Mazoujian et al., 1984; Merot et al.,

1985), low-molecular-weight cytokeratins (Fig. 2–18; Alguacil-Garcia and O'Connor, 1989; Battles et al., 1997; Guarner et al., 1989; Helm et al., 1992; Kariniemi et al., 1995; Miller et al., 1992; Moll and Moll, 1985; Nagle et al., 1985; Tazawa et al., 1988), tumor marker antibodies Ca 15-3 and Ka-93, but not antibody Ca 19-9 (Tsuji, 1995), ovarian carcinoma antigen MLV-2 (Mariani-Constantini et al., 1985), estrogen receptors (Lloveras et al., 1991), and lectins (Ookusa et al., 1985; Tamaki et al., 1985). Paget cells

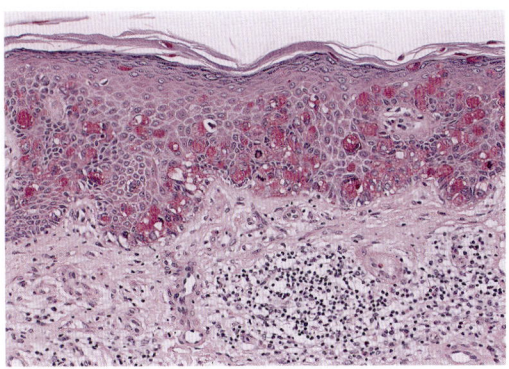

Figure 2–16. Extramammary Paget's disease. Paget's cells were PAS positive.

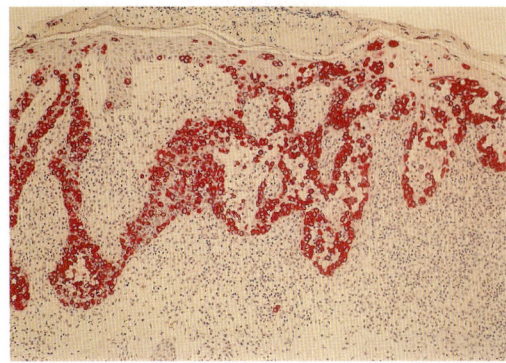

Figure 2–18. Extramammary Paget's disease. Paget's cells expressed immunohistochemical reactivity for low molecular weight (CAM 5.2) cytokeratins.

of extramammary Paget's disease do not express CD44 and S-100 protein (Battles et al., 1997; Glasgow et al., 1987; Guarner et al., 1989; Miller et al., 1992; Tsuji, 1995). All these immunohistochemical investigations, however, have failed to clarify the histogenesis of Paget cells in extramammary Paget's disease. Although the nature of extramammary Paget's disease remains controversial, there are four major theories about it. (*1*) It is an apocrine adenocarcinoma that arises in glandular structures of the dermis and extends from there to the epidermis (Boehm and Morris, 1971; Crocker, 1989; Koss et al., 1968; Lee et al., 1977; Mitsudo et al., 1981; Ordoñez et al., 1987). (*2*) It is a metastasis to the skin from a distant carcinoma (Weiner, 1937). (*3*) It is a primary carcinoma

of a nearby epithelium (rectum, cervix, bladder, or prostate) and extends by continuity to the skin (Defegu et al., 1986; McKee and Hertogs, 1980; Ojeda et al., 1987; Saruk et al., 1984; Sasaki et al., 1990; Takeshita et al., 1978; Tuck and Williams, 1985; Turner, 1980; Yoell and Price, 1960). (*4*) It is an adenocarcinoma that begins in the epidermis (Evans and Neven, 1991; Fetherson and Friedrich, 1972; Helwig and Graham, 1963; Jones et al., 1979; Mazoujian et al., 1984; Merot et al., 1985; Murrel and McMullan, 1962; Nadji et al., 1982; Taki and Janovski, 1961; Urabe et al., 1990; Woodruff, 1955; Yamamoto et al., 1993). We concur with the latter opinion—namely, that it is a primary apocrine carcinoma that begins in the epidermis (Requena et al., 1998b).

The differential diagnosis of extramammary Paget's disease includes a series of disparate processes characterized histopathologically by large cells with pale cytoplasm scattered within the epidermis and the epithelium of the adnexa. Clear cell papulosis of the skin is a rare benign disorder, described only in Oriental children, that is clinically characterized by keratotic papules on the chest and abdomen, and histopathologically consists of clear monomorphous cells scattered within the epidermis. Immunohistochemically, neoplastic cells of clear cell papulosis express the same immunohistochemical profile as that for Paget cells of extramammary Paget's disease, but they do not contain mucin, neither nests of pale cells nor tubular structures are formed, and clear cells

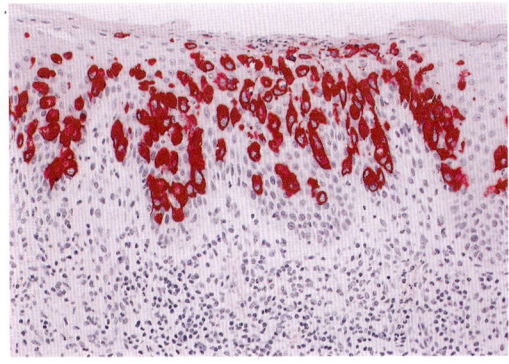

Figure 2–17. Extramammary Paget's disease. Paget's cells expressed immunoreactivity for CEA.

are monomorphous without evidence of cytologic atypia. Clear cell papulosis seems to be a benign counterpart of extramammary Paget's disease (Kuo et al., 1987, 1995; Lee and Chao, 1998). Paget cells have also been described within the epidermis of a cutaneous hamartoma (Pierard-Franchimont et al., 1991). Mammary Paget's disease is also characterized histopathologically by large round cells with pale-staining cytoplasm scattered at all levels of the epidermis and epithelial structures of the adnexa of the mammary areola. However, mammary Paget's disese does not originate in the epidermis, but is an intraductal carcinoma of the breast that extends by continuity through lactiferous ducts into the epidermis of the areola. In short, mammary Paget's disease is a specific type of epidermotropically metastatic carcinoma (see below). In contrast with extramammary Paget's disease, Paget cells of mammary Paget's disease do not contain mucin, signet-ring cells and tubular structures are rare or absent, and, if the biopsy specimen is generous enough, an intraductal carcinoma is often seen within the underlying lactiferous ducts.

In rare instances, adenocarcinomas of the rectum, urethra, cervix, and bladder may extend, in continuity, into adjacent epidermis of genital and perianal skin, and they may mimic extramammary Paget's disease both clinically and histopathologically. In the literature, these cases have been reported as extramammary Paget's disease associated with corresponding visceral carcinoma, but in our opinion, they are not examples of true extramammary Paget's disease but rather represent epidermotropic metastatic carcinomas with a poor prognosis (see below). The histopathologic differential diagnosis between these cases of epidermotropically metastatic adenocarcinoma and authentic extramammary Paget's disease is difficult and may be impossible. Therefore, an extensive search for an underlying adenocarcinoma in adjacent viscera should be performed before a diagnosis of extramammary Paget's disease of genital or perianal skin is established. In any event, these cases of epidermotropically metastatic adenocarcinoma usually show intraepidermal tubular structures whose histopathologic character reflects the nature of the primary adenocarcinoma. Some authors have proposed that

gross cystic disease fluid protein-15 immunohistochemical reactivity enables distinction between true extramammary Paget's disease and an epidermotropically metastatic carcinoma, as positivity for this antibody indicates authentic extramammary Paget's disease (Kohler and Smoller, 1996). In the same sense, other authors have postulated that negativity for PAS, alcian blue, and CEA, and positivity for cytokeratin 20 indicate extension by continuity of neoplastic cells from an adjacent organ rather than authentic extramammary Paget's disease (Battles et al., 1997). There are also cases described as extramammary Paget's disease of the scrotum or umbilicus associated with prostatic adenocarcinoma (we interpret them to be epidermotropically metastatic carcinomas from the prostate) in which the intraepidermal neoplastic cells expressed immunoreactivity for prostate-specific antigen (PSA) in some examples (Allan et al., 1998; Perez et al., 1989) but not in others (Remond et al., 1993). Pagetoid melanoma *in situ* is characterized histopathologically by proliferation of neoplastic melanocytes that have large, round nuclei and abundant pale-staining cytoplasm containing dusty melanin. These pagetoid melanocytes are arranged in a pagetoid pattern within the epidermis, simulating extramammary Paget's disease. Pagetoid melanoma *in situ* may be distinguished form extramammary Paget's disease; because the proliferation of atypical melanocytes begins at the dermoepidermal junction, they do not contain mucin and never form acini. Immunohistochemistry is helpful in extreme cases, as neoplastic melanocytes of pagetoid melanoma *in situ* usually express S-100 protein and HMB-45 markers, which are negative in extramammary Paget's disease (Glasgow et al., 1987; Guldhammer and Nrgaard, 1986; Reed et al., 1990; Shah et al., 1987). Pagetoid Bowen's disease may also mimic extramammary Paget's disease, but neoplastic cells of this histopathologic variant of squamous cell carcinoma *in situ* of the skin always show some sign of cornification, such as dyskeratoses or parakeratosis, they do not contain mucin, and there is no tendency toward formation of tubules (Raiten et al., 1976). Pagetoid reticulosis, also known as *Woringer-Kolopp disease,* is a morphological expression of mycosis fungoides characterized clinically by a solitary lesion and histopathologically by prominent epidermotropism of neoplastic lymphocytes. The differential diagnosis with extramammary Paget's disease is straightforward: neoplastic cells within the epidermis in pagetoid reticulosis are not epithelial cells with pale large cytoplasm, but atypical lymphocytes with hyperchromatic nuclei and scant cytoplasm (Burns et al., 1995). Histiocitosis X may also simulate extramammary Paget's disesase in terms of both architectural pattern and cytologic features, but cells of histiocytosis X are neoplastic Langerhans cells, with reniform nuclei and amphophilic cytoplasm (Wells, 1979).

Extramammary Paget's disease usually follows a benign clinical course and often remains localized for many years as an indo-lent erythematous plaque that extends horizontally within the epidermis and the epithelial structures of the adnexa. In rare instances, the plaque becomes thickened, indicating involvement of the dermis, and from there may metastasize to regional lymph nodes (Hart and Millman, 1977). Usually, the lesion extends beyond the clinically involved area, and for that reason, extramammary Paget's disease often persists at a local site after what had seemed to be complete surgical excision (Anthony et al., 1986). Alternative therapies include Mohs' micrographic surgery (Mohs and Blanchard et al., 1979) and local radiotherapy (Burrows et al., 1995). Apparent spontaneous regression has been reported after partial surgical excision (Archer et al., 1987).

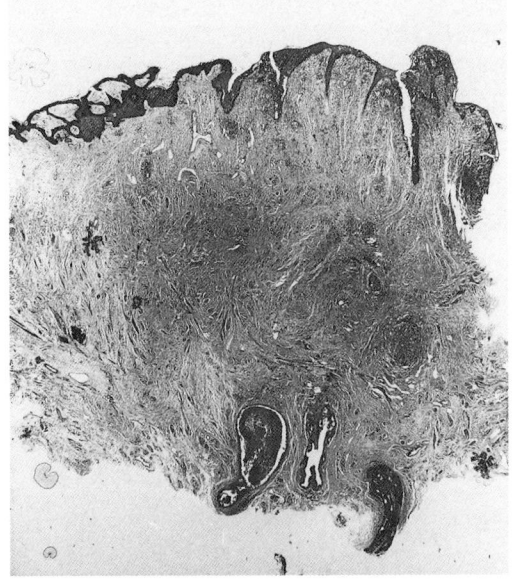

A

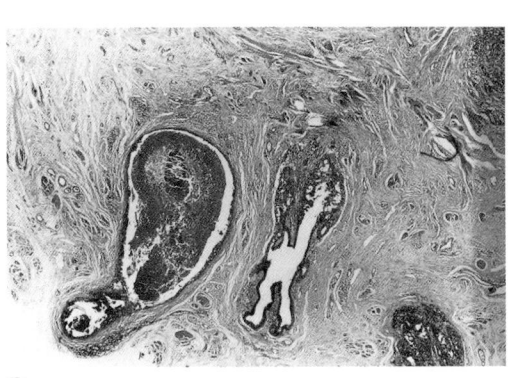

C

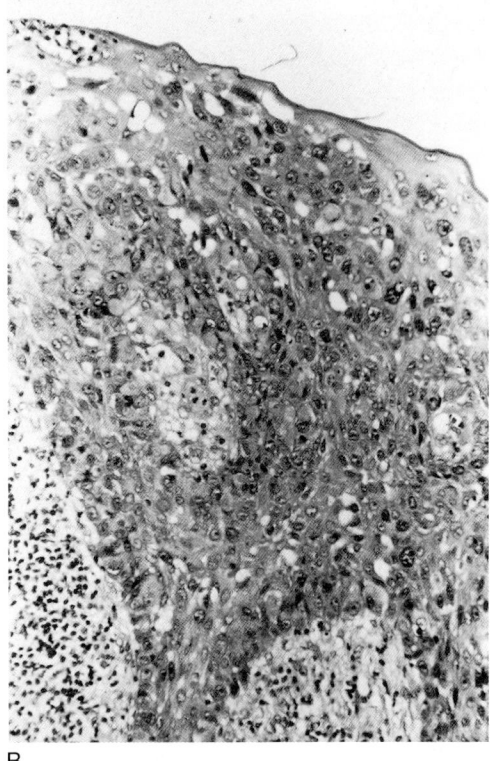

B

Figure 2–19. Mammary Paget's disease. *A:* Low-power view. *B:* Atypical cells scattered as solitary units at all levels of the epidermis. *C:* Intraductal mammary carcinoma within the underlying lactiferous ducts.

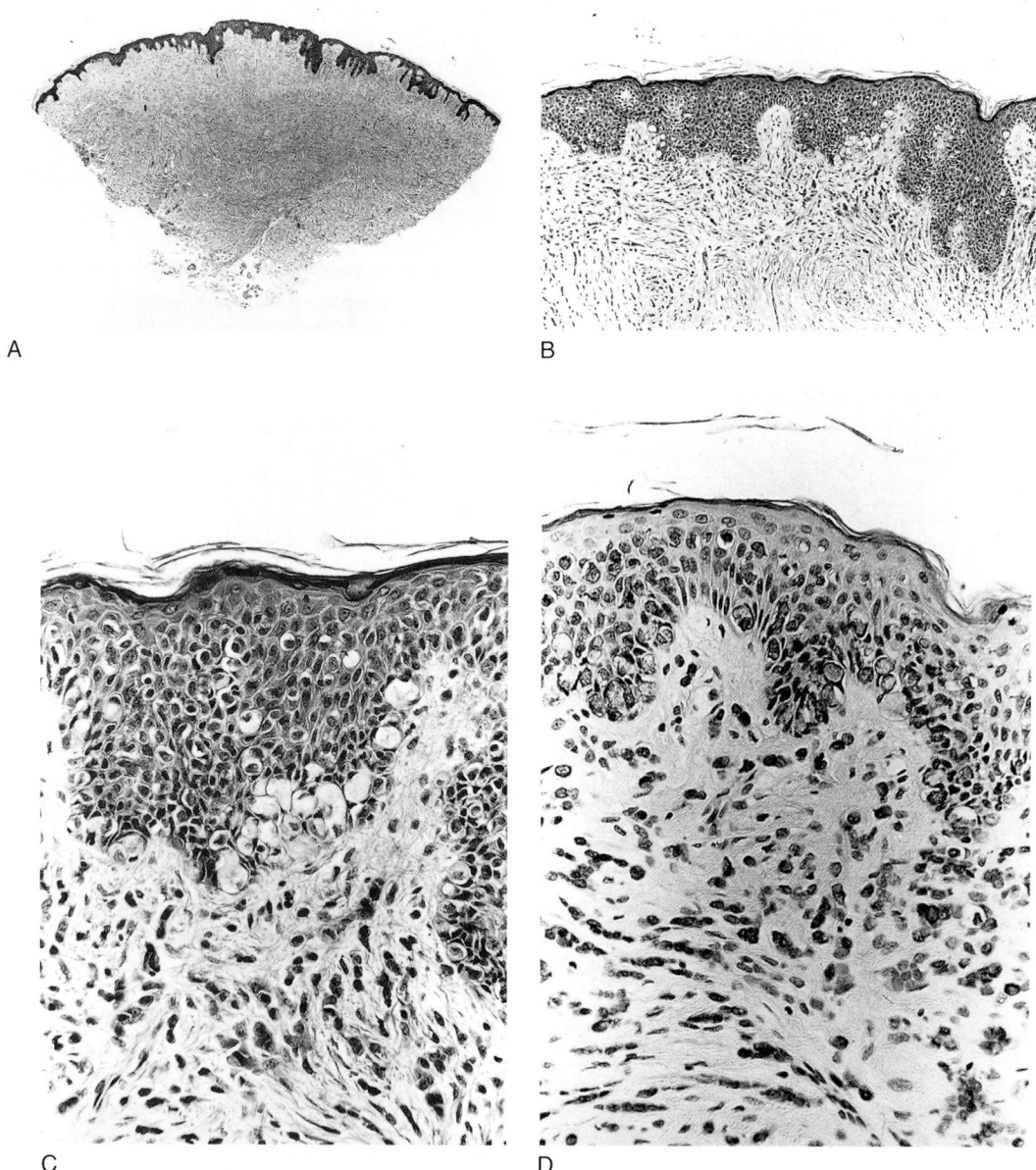

Figure 2–20. Epidermotropically metastatic carcinoma. Primary neoplasm was mammary carcinoma and multiple cutaneous metastases appeared on the chest wall. *A:* Scanning power. *B:* Neoplastic cells with abundant pale cytoplasm are seen at the lower layers of the epidermis. Note cords of neoplastic cells involving the dermis. *C:* Higher magnification demonstrates the pagetoid appearance of the intraepidermal neoplastic cells. *D:* Cytokeratins of low molecular weight (CAM 5.2) express immunoreactivity both in intraepidemal pagetoid cells and in neoplastic cells of the dermis. (*Continued*)

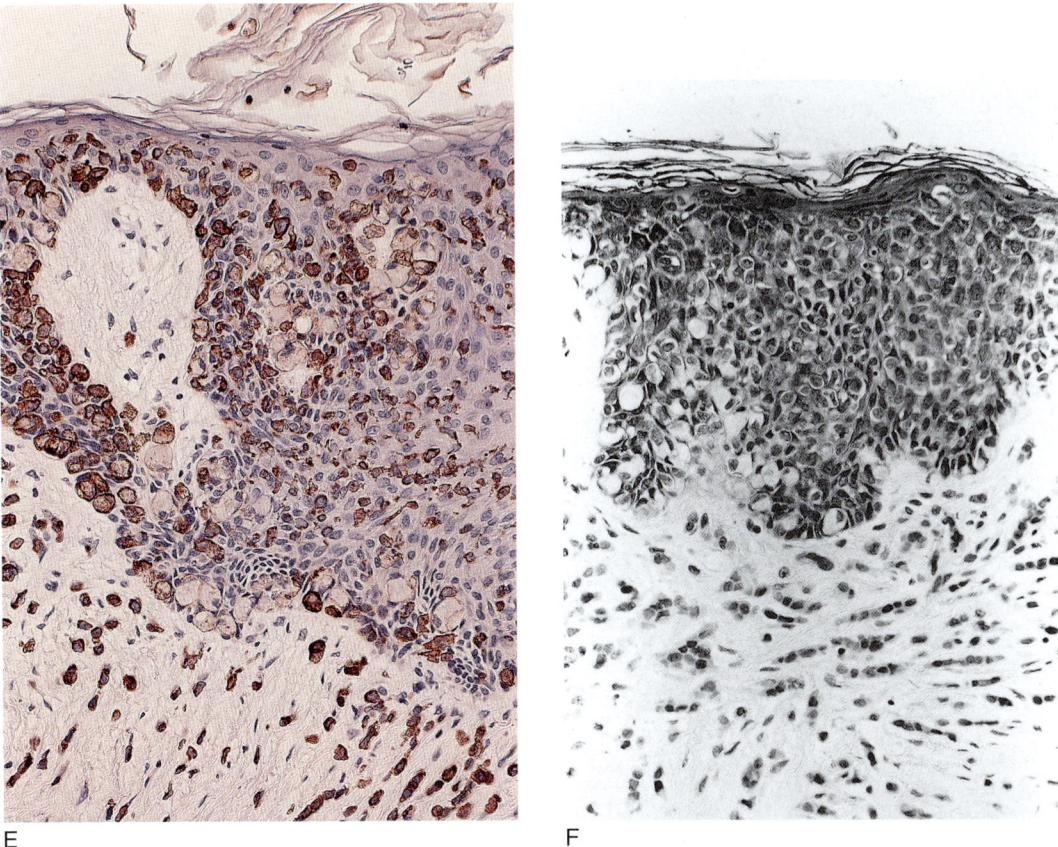

E   F

Figure 2–20. (*Continued*) *E:* Carcinoembryonic antigen is also immunohistochemically demonstrated both in the intraepidermal neoplastic pagetoid cells and in neoplastic cells of the dermis. *F:* Cytokeratins of high molecular weight (EAB-902 cytokeratins) are negative in pagetoid intraepidermal neoplastic cells. Note positive immunostaining in keratinocytes of the upper layers of the epidermis.

EPIDERMOTROPIC METASTATIC CARCINOMAS THAT MAY MIMIC CARCINOMA *IN SITU* OF THE SKIN

MAMMARY PAGET'S DISEASE

Mammary Paget's disease is a peculiar form of epidermotropically metastatic carcinoma in which neoplastic cells of an intraductal breast carcinoma ascend lactiferous ducts to reach the epidermis of the nipple and areola. In fact, mammary and extramammary Paget's disease are completely different processes; extramammary Paget's disease is an apocrine carcinoma *in situ*, in which neoplastic cells proliferate first within the epidermis and then descend infundibula and eccrine ducts, whereas in mammary Paget's disease, neoplastic cells of an intraductal carcinoma ascend the lactiferous ducts to reach the epidermis. Clinically, mammary Paget's disease appears as a reddish patch covered by scale crusts involving the areola. Often, on palpation, a nodule is discovered in the underlying breast parenchyma. As in extramammary Paget's disease, histopathologic study of an areola affected by mammary Paget's disease shows large epithelial cells with atypical nuclei and abundant pale cytoplasm disposed both as solitary units or in collections at all levels of the epidermis. However, differential diagnosis between mammary and extramammary Paget's disease may be established. Signet-ring cells containing cytoplasmic mucin and tubular structures are hardly observed in mammary Paget's disease, and often an intraductal carcinoma may be

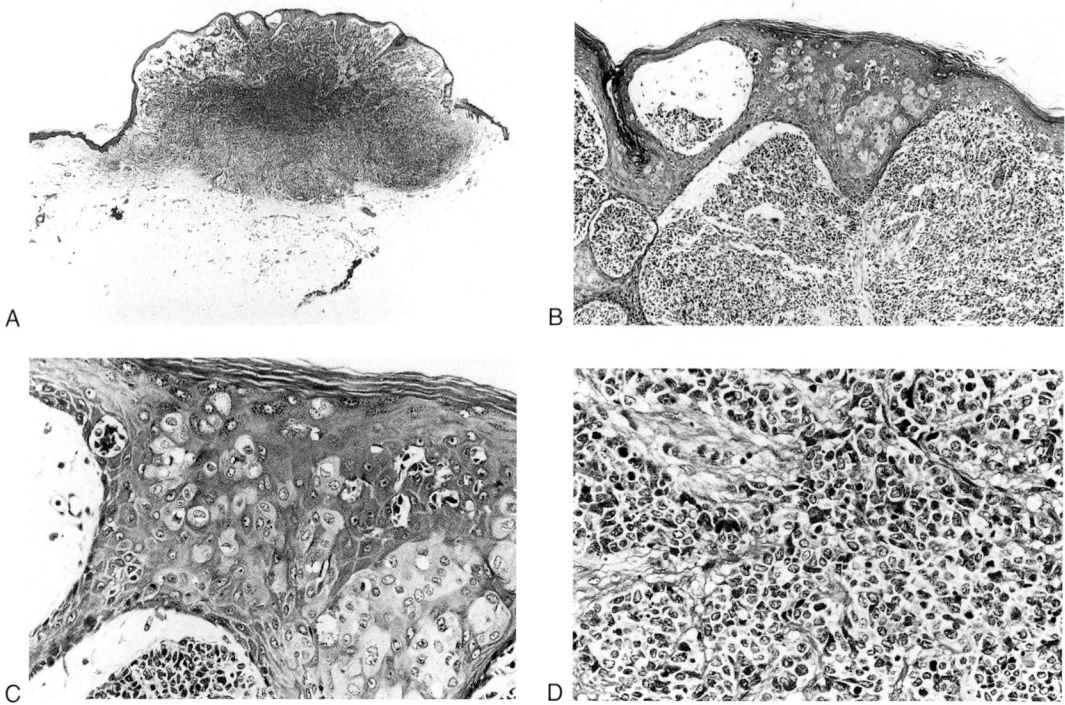

Figure 2–21. Merkel cell carcinoma with epidermal involvement. *A:* Scanning power of the neoplasm. *B:* Nests of neoplastic cells within the epidermis. *C:* Higher maginification demonstrates discrete nests of neoplastic cells with small hyperchromatic nuclei within the epidermis. *D:* Characteristic neoplastic cells of Merkel cell carcinoma in the dermis.

discovered within the underlying lactiferous ducts of the same biopsy specimen (Fig. 2–19). Biologically, these two processes are completely different; neoplastic cells of extramammary Paget's disease tend to remain *in situ* for a long time or even the lifetime of the patient, whereas neoplastic cells of mammary Paget's disease may infiltrate the breast stroma and give rise to metastasis.

OTHER FORMS OF EPIDERMOTROPICALLY METASTATIC CARCINOMA

As stated previously, a particular variant of epidermotropically metastatic carcinoma occurs when a primary carcinoma in an organ continuous with the skin, e.g., the rectum, cervix, urethra, bladder, or prostate, extends into the epidermis of the perianal or genital skin. These cases are often described as extramammary Paget's disease involving the genital or perianal skin associated with the corresponding underlying carcinoma (De-

fegu et al., 1986; McKee and Hertogs, 1980; Ojeda et al., 1987; Saruk et al., 1984; Sasaki et al., 1990; Takeshita et al., 1978; Tuck and Williams, 1985; Turner, 1980; Yoell and Price, 1960). In our view, however, these are not examples of authentic extramammary Paget's disease but are carcinomas of neighboring viscera that "metastasize" by continuity to the epidermis of the genital or perianal skin. In contrast with true extramammary Paget's disease, these epidermotropically metastasizing carcinomas have a poor prognosis, and widespread metastatic disease often appears shortly after.

But epidermotropically metastatic carcinomas are not exclusive of mammary Paget's disease or the genital and perianal skin involved from carcinomas of rectum, cervix, bladder, prostate, or urethra. There also are examples of epidermotropically metastatic carcinomas in extramammary and extragenital areas of the skin that originated in cutaneous squamous cell carcinomas (Weldner and Foucar, 1985), porocarcinomas

(Landa and Winkelmann, 1991; Pinkus and Mehregan, 1963), colon carcinomas (Aguilar et al., 1991), breast carcinomas (Fig. 2–20; Aguilar et al., 1991; Manteaux et al., 1992; Requena et al., 1996a), and laryngeal carcinoma (Aguilar et al., 1991). Furthermore, epidermotropism may be seen in the epidermis overlying primary neuroendocrine Merkel cell carcinomas of the skin (Fig. 2–21; Gillham et al., 1991; LeBoit et al., 1992; Rocamora et al., 1987), and sebaceous carcinoma of the eyelid (Rao et al., 1982; Wolfe et al., 1984). The distinction between extramammary Paget's disease and epidermotropically metastatic carcinoma can be established without difficulty. Epidermotropically metastatic carcinomas, in addition to having pagetoid cells in pagetoid pattern within the epidemis, also show the stereotypical findings of cutaneous metastases involving the dermis—namely, solid aggregations of neoplastic cells, tubular structures of metastatic adenocarcinoma, strands of neoplastic cells between collagen bundles of the dermis, or neoplastic cells within blood or lymphatic vessels of the dermis.

REFERENCES

Abdennader S, Lessana-Leibowitch M, Pelisse M. (1989) An atypical case of penile carcinoma in situ associated with human papillomavirus DNA type 18. *J Am Acad Dermatol* 20:887–889.

Abenoza P, Ackerman AB. (1990) Poromas. In: *Neoplasms with Eccrine Differentiation*, pp. 113–185. Lea & Febiger, Philadelphia.

Ackerman AB, de Viragh PA, Chongchitnant N. (1993) Basal-cell carcinoma with follicular differentiation. In: *Neoplasms with Follicular Differentiation*, pp. 605–658. Lea & Febiger, Philadelphia.

Ackerman AB, Reed RJ. (1973) Epidermolytic variant of solar keratosis. *Arch Dermatol* 107:104–106.

Aguilar A, Schoendorff C, Lopez MJ, Ambrojo P, Requena L, Sanchez Yus E. (1991) Epidermotropic metastases from internal carcinomas. *Am J Dermatopathol* 13:452–458.

Alguacil-Garcia A, O'Connor R. (1989) Mucin-negative biopsy of extra-mammary Paget's disease. A diagnostic problem. *Histopathology* 15: 429–431.

Allan SJR, McLaren K, Aldridge RD. (1998) Paget's disease of the scrotum: a case exhibiting positive prostate-specific antigen staining and associated prostatic adenocarcinoma. *Br J Dermatol* 138:689–691.

Ansai S, Hashimoto H, Aoki T, et al. (1993) A histochemical and immunohistochemical study of extraocular sebaceous carcinoma. *Histopathology* 22:127–133.

Anthony PP, Freeman K, Warin AP. (1986) Extramammary Paget's disease. *Clin Exp Dermatol* 11:387–395.

Arbessman H, Ransohoff DF. (1987) Is Bowen's disease a predictor for the development of internal malignancy? A methodological critique of the literature. *JAMA* 257:516–518.

Archer CB, Louback JB, MacDonald DM. (1987) Spontaneous regression of perianal extramammary Paget's disease after partial surgical excision. *Arch Dermatol* 123:379–382.

Argenyi ZB, Hughes AM, Balogh K, Vo T-L. (1990) Cancerization of eccrine sweat ducts in Bowen's disease as studied by light microscopy, DNA spectrophotometry and immunohistochemistry. *Am J Dermatopathol* 12:433–440.

Baran RL, Gormley DE. (1987) Polydactylous Bowen's disease of the nail. *J Am Acad Dermatol* 17:201–204.

Bardach H. (1978) Hidroacanthoma simplex with in situ porocarcinoma: a case suggesting malignant transformation. *J Cutan Pathol* 5:236–248.

Battles OE, Page DL, Johnson JE. (1997) Cytokeratins, CEA, and mucin histochemistry in the diagnosis and characterization of extramammary Paget's disease. *Am J Clin Pathol* 108:6–12.

Baum HP, Meurer I, Unteregger G. (1994) Expression of proliferation-associated proteins (proliferating cell nuclear antigen and Ki-67 antigen) in Bowen's disease. *Br J Dermatol* 131:231–236.

Biediger TL, Grabski WJ, McCollough ML. (1995) Bilateral pigmented Bowen's disease of the lower lip. *Int J Dermatol* 34:116–118.

Biesterfeld S, Pennings K, Grussendorf-Conen EI, Böcking A. (1995) Aneuploidy in actinic keratosis and Bowen's disease—increased risk for invasive squamous cell carcinoma? *Br J Dermatol* 133:557–560.

Billano RA, Little WP. (1982) Hypertrophic actinic keratosis. *J Am Acad Dermatol* 7:484–489.

Böcking A, Chatelain R, Salterberg A, et al. (1989) Bowenoid papulosis. Classification as a low-grade in situ carcinoma of the epidermis on the basis of histomorphologic and DNA ploidy studies. *Anal Quant Cytol Histol* 11:419–425.

Boehm F, Morris JM. (1971) Paget's disease and apocrine gland carcinoma of the vulva. *Obstet Gynecol* 38:185–192.

Bowen JT. (1912) Precancerous dermatoses: a study of two cases of chronic atypical epithelial proliferations. *J Cutan Dis* 30:241–255.

Bozzo PD, Vaught LC, Alberts DS, Thompson D, Bartels PH. (1998) Nuclear morphometry in solar keratosis. *Anal Quant Cytol Histol* 20:21–28.

Brownstein MH. (1979) The precursors of cutaneous squamous cell carcinoma (review) *Int J Dermatol* 18:1–16.

Burns MK, Chan LS, Cooper KD. (1995) Woringer-Kolopp disease (localized pagetoid reticulosis) or unilesional mycosis fungoides? An analysis of eight cases with benign disease. *Arch Dermatol* 131:325–329.

Burrows NP, Jones DH, Hudson PM, Pye RJ. (1995) Treatment of extramammary Paget's disease by radiotherapy. *Br J Dermatol* 132:970–972.

Carapeto FJ, Garcia Perez A. (1974) Acantholytic keratosis. *Dermatologica* 148:233–239.

Castren K, Vahakangas K, Heikkinen E, Ranki A. (1998) Absence of p53 mutations in benign and pre-malignant male genital lesions with over-expressed p53 protein. *Int J Cancer* 31:674–678.

Cataldo E, Doku HC. (1981) Solar cheilitis. *J Dermatol Surg Oncol* 7:989–995.

Cerroni L, Kerl H. (1994) Aberrant *bcl*-2 protein expression provides a possible mechanism of neoplastic cell growth in cutaneous basal cell carcinoma. *J Cutan Pathol* 21:398–403.

Changus GW, Yonan TN, Bartolome JS. (1971) Extramammary Paget's disease of the tongue. *Lanryngoscope* 81:1621–1625.

Chuang T-Y, Reizner GT. (1988) Bowen's disease and internal malignancy. A matched case–control study. *J Am Acad Dermatol* 19:47–51.

Civatte A. (1936) Dermatoses précancereuses. In: *Nouvelle Pratique Dermatologique*, Vol. VI. (Darier J, Sabouraud R, Gougerot H, Milian H, Pautrier G, Ravaut P, Sézary A, Simon C, eds.) pp. 636–663. Masson et Cie, Paris.

Claudy AL, Garcier F, Kanitakis J. (1983) Eccrine porocarcinoma: ultrastructural and immunologic study. *J Dermatol* 1983;11:282–286.

Cobb MW. (1990) Human papillomavirus infection. *J Am Acad Dermatol* 22:547–566.

Collina G, Rossi E, Bettelli S, Cook MG, Cesinaro AM, Trentini GP. (1995) Detection of human papillomavirus in extragenital Bowen's disease using in situ hybridization and polymerase chain reaction. *Am J Dermatopathol* 17:236–241.

Coskey RJ, Mehregan A, Fosnaugh R. (1972) Bowen's disease of the nail bed. *Arch Dermatol* 106:79–80.

Cox NH. (1994) Body site distribution of Bowen's disease. *Br J Dermatol* 130:714–716.

Crocker HR. (1889) Paget's disease affecting the scrotum and penis. *Trans Pathol Soc Lond* 40:187–191.

Crowson AN, Magro CM, Kadin ME, Stranc M. (1996) Differential expression of the *bcl*-2 oncogene in human basal cell carcinoma. *Hum Pathol* 7:355–359.

Curson C, Weedon D. (1979) Spontaneous regression in basal cell carcinomas. *J Cutan Pathol* 6:432–437.

De Blois GG, Patterson JW, Hunter SB. (1984) Extramammary Paget's disease arising in knee region in association with sweat gland carcinoma. *Arch Pathol Lab Med* 108:713–716.

Degefu S, O'Quinn AB, Dhurandhar HN. (1986) Paget's disease of the vulva and urogenital malignancies: a case report and review of the literature. *Gynecol Oncol* 25:347–354.

Deguchi M, Tomioka Y, Mizugaki M, Tagami H. (1998) Detection of human papillomavirus type 33 DNA in extragenital Bowen's disease with polymerase chain reaction. *Dermatology* 196:292–294.

de Villiers E-M, Schneider A, Gross G, zur Hausen H. (1986) Analysis of benign and malignant urogenital tumors for human papillomavirus infection by labelling cellular DNA. *Med Microbiol Immunol (Berl)* 174:281–286.

Dinehart SM, Sanchez RL. (1988) Spreading pigmented actinic keratosis. An electron microscopic study. *Arch Dermatol* 124:680–683.

Epstein E. (1960) Association of Bowen's disease with visceral cancer. *Arch Dermatol* 80:349–351.

Evans AT, Neven P. (1991) Invasive adenocarcinoma arising in extramammary Paget's disease of the vulva. *Histopathology* 18:355–360.

Favre M, Kremsdorf D, Jablonska S, et al. (1990) Two human papillomavirus types (HPV 54 and 55) characterized from genital tumors illustrate the plurality of genital HPVs. *Int J Cancer* 45:40–46.

Fenn ME, Morley GW, Abell MR. (1971) Paget's disease of the vulva. *Obstet Gynecol* 38:660–670.

Fetherston WC, Friedrich EG. (1972) The origin and significance of vulvar Paget's disease. *Obstet Gynecol* 39:735–744.

Fierz U. (1965) Katamnestische Untersuchungen über die Nebenwirkungen der Therapie mit anorganischem Arsen bei Hautkrankheiten. *Dermatologica* 131:41–58.

Fligiel Z, Kaneko M. (1975) Extramammary Paget's disease of the external ear canal in association with ceruminous carcinoma. *Cancer* 36:1072–1076.

Friedman KJ, Boudreau S, Farmer ER. (1987) Superficial epithelioma with sebaceous differentiation. *J Cutan Pathol* 14:193–197.

Friedrich EG Jr. (1972) Reversible vulvar atypia. *Obstet Gynecol* 39:173–181.

Fulling KH, Strayer DS, Santa Cruz DJ. (1981) Adnexal metaplasia in carcinoma *in situ* of the skin. *J Cutan Pathol* 8:79–88.

Geary WA, Cooper PH. (1992) Proliferating cell nuclear antigen (PCNA) in common epidermal lesions. *J Cutan Pathol* 19:458–468.

Gibson LE, Perry HO. (1985) Skin lesions from sun exposure: a treatment guide. *Geriatrics* 40:87–92.

Gillham SL, Morrison RG, Hurt MA. (1991) Epidermotropic neuroendocrine carcinoma. Immunohistochemical differentiation from simulators, including malignant melanoma. *J Cutan Pathol* 18:120–127.

Glasgow BJ, Wen DR, Al-Jitawi S, Cochran AJ. (1987) Antibody to S-100 protein aids the separation of pagetoid melanoma from mammary and extramammary Paget's disease. *J Cutan Pathol* 14:223–226.

Goldberg LH, Joseph AK, Tschen JA. (1994) Proliferative actinic keratosis. *Int J Dermatol* 33:341–345.

Goldes JA, Kao GF. (1989) Premalignant lesions of the skin. In: *Principles of Dermatologic Surgery* (Roenigk RK, Roegnigk HH, eds.) pp. 563–590. Marcel Dekker, New York.

Graham JH, Helwig EB. (1959) Bowen's disease and its relationship to systemic cancer. *Arch Dermatol* 80:133–159.

Graham JH, Helwig EB. (1973) Erythroplasia of Queyrat. A clinicopathologic and histochemical study. *Cancer* 32:1396–1414.

Grekin RC, Swanson NA. (1984) Verrucous Bowen's disease of the plantar foot. *J Dermatol Surg Oncol* 10:734–736.

Grosshans E, Grossmann L. (1985) Bowenoid papulosis. *Arch Dermatol* 121:858–863.

Guarner J, Cohen C, DeRose PB. (1989) Histogenesis of extramammary and mammary Paget cells. An immunohistochemical study. *Am J Dermatopathol* 11:313–318.

Guldhammer B, Nrgaard T. (1986) The differential diagnosis of intraepidermal malignant lesions using immunohistochemistry. *Am J Dermatopathol* 8:295–301.

Gunn RA, Gallagher HS. (1980) Vulvar Paget's disease: a topographic study. *Cancer* 46:590–594.

Hale LP, Patel DD, Clark RE, Haynes BF. (1995) Distribution of CD44 variant isomorfs in human skin: differential expression in components of benign and malignant epithelia. *J Cutan Pathol* 22:536–545.

Hamm H, Vroom TM, Czarnetzki BM. (1986) Extramammary Paget's cells: further evidence of sweat gland derivation. *J Am Acad Dermatol* 15:1275–1281.

Haneke E. (1995) Differentiation of basal cell carcinoma from trichoepithelioma by lectin histochemistry. *Br J Dermatol* 132:1024–1025.

Hart WR, Millman JB. (1977) Progression of intraepithelial Paget's disease of the vulva to invasive carcinoma. *Cancer* 40:2333–2337.

Harvell JD, Kerschmann RL, LeBoit PE. (1996) Eccrine or apocrine poroma? Six poromas with divergent adnexal differentiation. *Am J Dermatopathol* 18:1–9.

Hawley IC, Husain F, Pryse-Davies J. (1991) Extramammary Paget's disease of the vulva with dermal invasion and vulval intra-epithelial neoplasia. *Histopathology* 18:374–376.

Helm KF, Goellner JR, Peters MS. (1992) Immunohistochemical stains in extramammary Paget's disease. *Am J Dermatopathol* 14:402–407.

Helwig EB, Graham JH. (1963) Anogenital (extramammary) Paget's disease: a clinicopathological study. *Cancer* 16:387–403.

Holden CA, Shaw M, McKee PH, et al. (1984) Loss of membrane beta-2-microglobulin in eccrine porocarcinoma. *Arch Dermatol* 120:732–735.

Hughes JH, Robinson RA. (1995) p53 expression in Bowen's disease and microinvasive squamous cell carcinoma of the skin. *Mod Pathol* 8:526–529.

Hunter GA. (1977) Follicular Bowen's disease. *Br J Dermatol* 97 (Suppl 15):20.

Ichikawa E, Watanabe S, Otsuka F. (1995) Immunohistochemical localization of keratins and involucrin in solar keratosis and Bowen's disease. *Am J Dermatopathol* 17:151–157.

Ikenberg H, Gissmann L, Gross G, Grussendorf-Conen E-I, zur Hausen H. (1983) Human papillomavirus type-16-related DNA in genital Bowen's disease and in bowenoid papulosis. *Int J Cancer* 32:563–565.

Imakado S, Abe M, Okuno T, et al. (1991) Two cases of genital Paget's disease with bilateral axillary involvement: mutability of axillary lesions. *Arch Dermatol* 127:1243.

Inada LS, Kohno T, Sakai I, et al. (1985) A case of extramammary Paget's disease on the back. *Jpn J Clin Dermatol* 39:685–691.

Ishikawa K. (1971) Malignant hidroacanthoma simplex. *Arch Dermatol* 104:529–532.

Ito M, Tazawa T, Shimizu N, Saito A, Sato Y, Nonaka N. (1988) Intraepidermal pilar epithelioma: a new dermatopathologic interpretation of a skin tumor. *J Am Acad Dermatol* 18:123–132.

Jacobs DM, Sandles LG, LeBoit PE. (1986) Sebaceous carcinoma arising from Bowen's disease of the vulva. *Arch Dermatol* 122:1191–1193.

Jacoby RA, Burgoon CF Jr. (1985) Atypical fibroblasts as a clue to radiation injury. *Am J Dermatopathol* 7:53–56.

Jacyk WK. (1980) Bowen's disease of the palm. Report of a case in an African. *Dermatologica* 161:285–287.

James MP, Wells GC, Whimster IW. (1978) Spreading pigmented actinic keratoses. *Br J Dermatol* 98:373–379.

Jensen ML. (1990) Extraocular sebaceous carcinoma of the skin with visceral metastases: case report. *J Cutan Pathol* 17:117–121.

Jones RE Jr. (1984) What is the boundary that separates a thick solar keratosis and a thin squamous cell carcinoma? *Am J Dermatopathol* 6:301–306.

Jones RE Jr, Austin C, Ackerman AB. (1979) Extramammary Paget's disease: a critical reexamination. *Am J Dermatopathol* 1:101–132.

Kakinuma H, Iwasawa U, Kurakata N, Suzuki H. (1994) A case of extramammary Paget's disease with depigmented macules as the sole manifestation. *Br J Dermatol* 130:102–105.

Kakinuma H, Miyamoto R, Iwasawa U, Baba S, Suzuki H. (1994) Three subtypes of poroid neoplasia in a single lesion: eccrine poroma, hidroacanthoma simplex, and dermal duct tumor. Histologic, histochemical, and ultrastructural findings. *Am J Dermatopathol* 16:66–72.

Kanitakis J. (1985) La maladie de Paget extramammaire. *Ann Dermatol Venereol* 112:75–87.

Kao GF. (1986) Carcinoma arising in Bowen's disease. *Arch Dermatol* 122:1124–1126.

Kao GF. (1990) Precancerous lesions and carcinoma in situ. In: *Pathology of the Skin* (Farmer ER, Hood AF, eds.) pp. 550–567. Appleton & Lange, Norwalk.

Kao GF, Graham JH. (1986) Premalignant cutaneous disorders of the head and neck. In: *Otolaryngology*, Vol. 5 (England, GM, ed.) pp. 1–20. Harper & Row, Philadelphia.

Kao GF, Graham JH, Helwig EB. (1986) Paget's disease of the ectopic breast with an underlying intraductal carcinoma: report of a case. *J Cutan Pathol* 13:59–66.

Kariniemi AL, Forsman L, Wahlstrom T, et al. (1984a) Expression of differentiation antigens in mammary and extramammary Paget's disease. *Br J Dermatol* 110:203–210.

Kariniemi AL, Holthofer H, Vartio T, Virtanen I. (1984b) Cellular differentiation of basal cell carcinoma studied with fluorescent lectins and cytokeratin antibodies. *J Cutan Pathol* 11:541–548.

Kariniemi AL, Ramaekers F, Lehto VP, et al. (1995) Paget cells express cytokeratins of glandular epithelia. *Br J Dermatol* 112:179–183.

Kato N, Ueno H. (1992) Superficial epithelioma with sebaceous differentiation. *J Dermatol* 19:190–194.

Kawashima M, Favre M, Obalek S, Jablonska S, Orth G. (1990) Premalignant lesions and cancers of the skin in the general population: evaluation of the role of human papillomaviruses. *J Invest Dermatol* 95:537–542.

Kawashima M, Jablonska S, Favre M, Obalek S, Croissant O, Orth G. (1986) Characterization of a new type of human papillomavirus found in a lesion of Bowen's disease of the skin. *J Virol* 57:688–692.

Kawatsu T, Miki Y. (1971) Triple extramammary Paget's disease. *Arch Dermatol* 104:316–319.

Kettler AH, Rutledge M, Tschen JA, Buffone G. (1990) Detection of human papillomavirus in nongenital Bowen's disease by in situ DNA hybridization. *Arch Dermatol* 126:777–781.

King DT, Hirose FM, Gurevitch AW. (1979) Sebaceous carcinoma of the skin with visceral metastases. *Arch Dermatol* 115:862–863.

Kirchmann TTT, Prieto VG, Smoller BR. (1994) CD34 staining pattern distinguishes basal cell carcinoma from trichoepithelioma. *Arch Dermatol* 130:589–592.

Kitamura K, Kinehara M, Tamura N, et al. (1983) Hidroacanthoma simplex with invasive growth. *Cutis* 32:83–88.

Knauer WJ Jr, Whorton CM. (1963) Extramammary Paget's disease originating in Moll's glands of the lids. *Trans Am Acad Ophthalmol Otolaryngol* 67:829–833.

Koh KBH, Nazarina AR. (1995) Paget's disease of the scrotum: report of a case with underlying carcinoma of the prostate. *Br J Dermatol* 133:306–307.

Kohler S, Smoller BR. (1996) Gross cystic disease fluid protein-15 reactivity in extramammary Paget's disease with and without associated internal malignancy. *Am J Dermatopathol* 18:118–123.

Kopf AW, Bart RS. (1977) Tumor conference No. 11: multicentric bowenoid papules of the penis: a new entity? *J Dermatol Surg Oncol* 3:265–269.

Koss LG, Ladinsky S, Brockunier A. (1968) Paget's disease of the vulva: report of 10 cases. *Obstet Gynecol* 31:513–525.

Koten JW, Verhagen ARHB, Frank GL. (1967) Histopathology of actinic cheilitis. *Dermatologica* 135:465–471.

Kuo TT, Chan HL, Hsueh S. (1987) Clear cell papulosis of the skin. *Am J Surg Pathol* 11:827–834.

Kuo TT, Hu S, Lo SK, Chan H. (1997) p53 expression and proliferative activity in Bowen's disease with or without chronic arsenic exposure. *Hum Pathol* 28:786–790.

Kuo TT, Huang CL, Chan HL, et al. (1995) Clear cell papulosis: report of three cases of a newly recognized disease. *J Am Acad Dermatol* 33:230–233.

Landa NG, Winkelmann RK. (1991) Epidermotropically eccrine porocarcinoma. *J Am Acad Dermatol* 24:27–31.

Lang PG Jr, McKelvey AC, Nicholson JH. (1987) Three-dimensional reconstruction of superficial multicentric basal cell carcinoma using serial sections and a computer. *Am J Dermatopathol* 9:198–203.

Lassus J, Ranki A. (1996) Simultaneously detected aberrant p53 tumor suppressor protein and HPV-DNA localize mostly in separate keratinocytes in anogenital and common warts. *Exp Dermatol* 5:72–78.

Lebbe C, Rybojad M, Ochonisky S, et al. (1993) Extensive human papillomavirus-related disease (bowenoid papulosis, Bowen's disease, and squamous cell carcinoma) in a patient with hairy cell leukemia: clinical and immunologic evaluation after an interferon alfa trial. *J Am Acad Dermatol* 29:644–646.

LeBoit PE, Crutcher WA, Shapiro PE. (1992) Pagetoid intraepidermal spread in Merkel cell (primary neuroendocrine) carcinoma of the skin. *Am J Surg Pathol* 16:584–592.

Lee JYY, Chao SC. (1998) Clear cell papulosis of the skin. *Br J Dermatol* 138:678–683.

Lee SC, Roth LM, Ehrlich C, Hall JA. (1977) Extramammary Paget's disease of the vulva: a clinicopathologic study of 13 cases. *Cancer* 39:2540–2549.

Lever L, Marks R. (1989) The significance of the Darier-like solar keratosis and acantholytic changes in preneoplastic lesions of the epidermis. *Br J Dermatol* 120:383–389.

Lloveras B, Googe PB, Goldberg DE, Bhan AK. (1991) Estrogen receptors in skin appendage tumors and extramammary Paget's disease. *Mod Pathol* 4:487–490.

Lloyd KM. (1970) Multicentric pigmented Bowen's disease of the groin. *Arch Dermatol* 101:48–51.

Lookingbill DP, Kreider JW, Howett MK, et al. (1987) Human papillomavirus type 16 in bowenoid papulosis, intraoral papillomas, and squamous cell carcinoma of the tongue. *Arch Dermatol* 123:363–368.

Lu S, Syrjanen K, Havu VK, Syrjanen S. (1996) Failure to demonstrate human papillomavirus (HPV) involvement in Bowen's disease of the skin. *Arch Dermatol Res* 289:40–45.

Maize JC, Burgdorf WH, Hurt MA, LeBoit PE, Metcalf JS, Smith P. (1998) Actinic keratosis. In: *Cutaneous Pathology*, pp. 461–464. Churchill-Livingstone, Philadelphia.

Malejczyk J, Majewski S, Jablonska S, et al. (1989) Abrogated NK-cell lysis of human papillomavirus (HPV)-16 bearing keratinocytes in patients with precancerous and cancerous HPV-induced anogenital lesions. *Int J Cancer* 43:209–214.

Manteaux A, Cohen PR, Rapini RP. (1992) Zosteriform and epidermotropic metastasis. Report of two cases. *J Dermatol Surg Oncol* 18:97–100.

Mariani-Constantini R, Andreola S, Rilke F. (1985) Tumour-associated antigens in mammary and extramammary Paget's disease. *Virchows Arch A* 405:333–340.

Markey AC, Lane EB, MacDonald DM, Leigh IM. (1992) Keratin expression in basal cell carcinomas. *Br J Dermatol* 126:154–160.

Martin VG, Pellettiere EV, Gress D, Miller AW. (1994) Paget's disease in an adolescent arising in a supernumerary nipple. *J Cutan Pathol* 21:283–286.

Matsukura T, Sugase M. (1995) Identification of genital human papillomaviruses in cervical biopsy specimens: segregation of specific virus types in specific clinicopathologic lesions. *Int J Cancer* 61:13–22.

Mazoujian G, Pinkus GS, Haagensen DE. (1984) Extramammary Paget's disease—evidence for an apocrine origin: an immunoperoxidase study of gross cystic disease fluid protein-15, carcinoembryonic antigen and keratin proteins. *Am J Surg Pathol* 8:43–50.

McCallum DI, Kinmont PDC, Williams DW, et al. (1975) Intra-epidermal carcinoma of the eyelid margin. *Br J Dermatol* 93:239–252.

Mcgrae JD Jr, Greer CE, Manos MM. (1993) Multiple Bowen's disease of the fingers associated with human papilloma virus type 16. *Int J Dermatol* 32:104–107.

McKee PH, Hertogs KT. (1980) Endocervical adenocarcinoma and vulval Paget's disease: a significant association. *Br J Dermatol* 103:443–448.

McKenna KE, Patterson CC, Handley J, et al. (1996) Cutaneous neoplasia following PUVA therapy for psoriasis. *Br J Dermatol* 134:639–642.

Mehregan AH. (1979) Acantholysis in basal cell epithelioma. *J Cutan Pathol* 6:280–283.

Mehregan AH, Hashimoto K, Rahbari H. (1983) Eccrine adenocarcinoma. A clinicopathologic study of 35 cases. *Arch Dermatol* 119:104–114.

Merot Y, Mazoujian G, Pinkus G, et al. (1985) Extramammary Paget's disease of the perianal regions: evidence of apocrine derivation. *Arch Dermatol* 121:750–752.

Mikhail GR. (1974) Bowen disease and squamous cell carcinoma of the nail bed. *Arch Dermatol* 110:267–270.

Mikhail GR. (1980) Cancers, precancers, and pseudocancers on the male genitalia. A review of clinical appearances, histopathology, and management. *J Dermatol Surg Oncol* 6:1027–1035.

Miki Y, Kawatsu T, Matsuda K, et al. (1982) Cutaneous and pulmonary cancers associated with Bowen's disease. *J Am Acad Dermatol* 6:26–31.

Miller LR, McCunniff AJ, Randall ME. (1992) An immunohistochemical study of perianal Paget's disease. Possible origins and clinical implications. *Cancer* 69:2166–2171.

Mills AE. (1997) Solar keratosis can be distinguished from superficial basal cell carcinoma by expression of bcl-2. *Am J Dermatopathol* 19:443–445.

Mitsudo S, Nakanishi I, Koss LG. (1981) Paget's disease of the penis and adjacent skin: its association with fatal sweat gland carcinoma. *Arch Pathol Lab Med* 105:518–520.

Mitsuishi T, Sata T, Matsukura T, Iwasaki T, Kawashima M. (1997) The presence of mucosal human papillomavirus in Bowen's disease of the hands. *Cancer* 79:1911–1917.

Miyashita M, Suzuki H. (1993) *In situ* porocarcinoma: a case with malignant expression in clear tumor cells. *Int J Dermatol* 32:749–750.

Mohs FE, Blanchard L. (1979) Microscopically controlled surgery for extramammary Paget's disease. *Arch Dermatol* 115:706–708.

Moll I, Moll R. (1985) Cells of extramammary Paget's disease express cytokeratins different from those of epidermal cells. *J Invest Dermatol* 84:3–8.

Morales-Ducret CRJ, van de Rijn M, LeBrun DP, Smoller BR. (1995) *bcl-2* expression in primary malignancies of the skin. *Arch Dermatol* 131:909–912.

Moreno A, Salvatella N, Guix M, et al. (1984) Malignant hidroacanthoma simplex. A light-microscopic, ultrastructural, and immunohistochemical study of 2 cases. *Dermatologica* 169:161–166.

Morison WL, Kerker BJ, Tunnessen WW, Farmer ER. (1991) Disseminated hypopigmented keratoses. *Arch Dermatol* 127:848–850.

Moy RL, Eliezri YD, Nuovo GJ, Zitelli JA, Bennett RG, Silverstein S. (1989) Human papillomavirus type 16 DNA in periungual squamous cell carcinomas. *JAMA* 261:2669–2673.

Murata Y, Kumano K, Sashikata T. (1996) Partial spontaneous regression of Bowen's disease. *Arch Dermatol* 132:429–432.

Murrel TW, McMullan FH. (1962) Extramammary Paget's disease. *Arch Dermatol* 85:600–613.

Nadji M, Morales AR, Girtanner TE, et al. (1982) Paget's disease of the skin: a unifying concept of histogenesis. *Cancer* 50:2203–2206.

Nagle RB, Lucas DO, McDaniel KM, et al. (1985) New evidence linking mammary and extramammary Paget's cells to a common cell phenotype. *Am J Clin Pathol* 83:431–438.

Nakagawa K, Yamamura K, Maeda S, Ichihashi M. (1994) Bcl-2 expression in epidermal keratinocytic diseases. *Cancer* 74:1720–1724.

Nicolau SG, Balus L. (1964) Chronic actinic cheilitis and cancer of the lower lip. *Br J Dermatol* 76:278–289.

Obalek S, Jablonska S, Beaudenon S, et al. (1986) Bowenoid papulosis of the male and female genitalia: risk of cervical neoplasia. *J Am Acad Dermatol* 14:433–444.

Ojeda VJ, Heenan PJ, Watson SH. (1987) Paget's disease of the groin associated with adenocarcinoma of the urinary bladder. *J Cutan Pathol* 14:227–231.

Oka K, Katsumata M. (1990) Intraepidermal sebaceous carcinoma: case report. *Dermatologica* 180:181–185.

Olemans C, Pierard-Franchimont C, Delvenner P, Pierard GE. (1994) Comparative karyometry in Bowen's disease and bowenoid papulosis. Derivation of nuclear atypia index. *Anal Quant Cytol Histol* 16:284–286.

Onishi Y, Ohara K. (1996) Ectopic extramammary Paget's disease affecting the upper abdomen. *Br J Dermatol* 134:958–961.

Ookusa Y, Takata K, Nagashima M, et al. (1985) Lectin-binding patterns in extramammary Paget's disease by horseradish peroxidase (HRP)-labeling method-specific staining with *Dolichos biflorus* agglutinin (DBA). *Arch Dermatol Res* 277:65–70.

Ordoñez NG, Awalt H, Mackay B. (1987) Mammary and extramammary Paget's disease. An immunocytochemical and ultrastructural study. *Cancer* 59:1173–1183.

Oseroff AR, Roth R, Lipman S, Morhenn VB. (1983) Use of a murine monoclonal antibody which binds to malignant keratinocytes to detect tumor cells in microscopically controlled surgery. *J Am Acad Dermatol* 8:616–619.

Ostrow RS, Manias D, Mitchell AJ, Stawowy L, Faras AJ. (1987) Epidermodysplasia verruciformis: a case associated with primary lymphatic dysplasia, depressed cell-mediated immunity, and Bowen's disease containing human papillomavirus 16 DNA. *Arch Dermatol* 123:1511–1516.

Patterson JW, Kao GF, Graham JH, et al. (1986) Bowenoid papulosis: a clinicopathologic study with ultrastructural observations. *Cancer* 57:823–836.

Penneys NS, Mogollon RJ, Nadji M, Gould E. (1984) Papillomavirus common antigens. *Arch Dermatol* 120:859–861.

Peralta OC, Barr RJ, Romansky SG. (1983) Mixed carcinoma *in situ*: an immunohistochemical study. *J Cutan Pathol* 10:350–358.

Perez MA, LaRossa DD, Tomaszewski JE. (1989) Paget's disease primarily involving the scrotum. *Cancer* 63:970–975.

Peterka ES, Lynch FW, Goltz RW. (1961) An association between Bowen's disease and internal cancer. *Arch Dermatol* 84:623–629.

Pfister H, Haneke E. (1984) Demonstration of human papilloma virus type 2 DNA in Bowen's disease. *Arch Dermatol Res* 276:123–125.

Picascia DD, Robinson JK. (1987) Actinic cheilitis: a review of the etiology, differential diagnosis, and treatment. *J Am Acad Dermatol* 17:255–264.

Pierard-Franchimont C, Laso Dosal F, Arrese Estrada J, Pierard GE. (1991) Cutaneous hamartoma with pagetoid cells. *Am J Dermatopathol* 13:158–161.

Pique E, Olivares M, Espinel ML, et al. (1995) Malignant hidroacanthoma simplex. A case report and literature review. *Dermatology* 190:72–76.

Pinkus H. (1958) Keratosis senilis. *Am J Clin Pathol* 29:193–207.

Pinkus H, Mehregan AH. (1963) Epidermotropic eccrine carcinoma. *Arch Dermatol* 88:587–606.

Pinkus H, Mehregan AH. (1980) Premalignant skin lesions. *Clin Plast Surg* 7:289–300.

Pinkus H, Rogin JR. (1956) Eccrine poroma: tumors exhibiting features of the epidermal sweat duct unit. *Arch Dermatol* 74:511–521.

Price ML, Tidman MJ, Fagg NLK, et al. (1988) Distinctive epidermal atypia in immunosuppression-associated cutaneous malignancy. *Histopathology* 13:89–94.

Prieto VG, Reed JA, McNutt S, et al. (1995) Differential expression of CD44 in malignant cutaneous epithelial neoplasms. *Am J Dermatopathol* 17:447–451.

Puttick L, Ince P, Comaish JS. (1986) Three cases of eccrine porocarcinoma. *Br J Dermatol* 115:111–116.

Rabkin MS, Weems WS. (1987) Hyperplastic acral keratoses—association with invasive squamous cell carcinoma. *J Dermatol Surg Oncol* 13:1223–1228.

Ragi G, Turner MS, Klein LE, Stoll HL Jr. (1988) Pigmented Bowen's disease and review of 420 Bowen's disease lesions. *J Dermatol Surg Oncol* 14:765–769.

Raiten K, Paniago-Pereira C, Ackerman AB. (1976) Pagetoid Bowen's disease vs. extramammary Paget's disease. *J Dermatol Surg Oncol* 2:24–25.

Ranki A, Lassus J, Niemi KM. (1995) Relation of p53 tumor suppressor protein expression to human papillomavirus (HPV) DNA and to cellular atypia in male genital warts and in premalignant lesions. *Acta Dermatol Venereol (Stockh)* 75:180–186.

Rao NA, Hidayat A, McLean IW, Zimmerman LE. (1982) Sebaceous carcinomas of the ocular adnexa: a clinicopathologic study of 104 cases with five-year follow-up data. *Hum Pathol* 13:113–122.

Reed W, Oppedal BR, Eeg Larsen T. (1990) Immunohistology is valuable in distinguishing between Paget's disease, Bowen's disease and superficial spreading malignant melanoma. *Histopathology* 16:583–588.

Remond B, Aractingi S, Blanc F, et al. (1993) Umbilical Paget's disease and prostatic carcinoma. *Br J Dermatol* 128:448–450.

Requena L, Kiryu H, Ackerman AB. (1998a) Apocrine poroma. In: *Neoplasms with Apocrine Differentiation*, pp. 545–561. Lippincott-Raven, Philadelphia.

Requena L, Kiryu H, Ackerman AB. (1998b) Extramammary Paget's disease. In: *Neoplasms with Apocrine Differentiation*, pp. 961–1020. Lippincott-Raven, Philadelphia.

Requena L, Sanchez M, Aguilar A, et al. (1990) Periungual porocarcinoma. *Dermatologica* 180:177–180.

Requena L, Sanchez Yus E, Nuñez C, White CR Jr, Sangueza OP. (1996a) Epidermotropically metastatic breast carcinomas. Rare histopathologic variants mimicking melanoma and Paget's disease. *Am J Dermatopathol* 18:385–395.

Requena L, Sanchez Yus E, Simon P, del Rio E. (1996b) Induction of cutaneous hyperplasias by altered stroma. *Am J Dermatopathol* 18:248–268.

Reymann F, Ravnborg L, Schou G, et al. (1988) Bowen's disease and internal malignant diseases. A study of 581 patients. *Arch Dermatol* 124:677–679.

Rocamora A, Badia N, Vives R, Carrillo R, Ulloa J, Ledo A. (1987) Epidermotropic primary neuroendocrine (Merkel cell) carcinoma of the skin with Pautrier-like microabscesses. *J Am Acad Dermatol* 16:1163–1168.

Rosen K, Haerslev T, Huo-Jensen K, Jacobsen GK. (1997) Metallothionein expression in basaloid proliferations overlying dermatofibromas and in basal cell carcinomas. *Br J Dermatol* 136:30–34.

Rosen K, Hou-Jensen K, Wederlin O. (1993) Altered expression of beta-2-microglobulin in basaloid pro-

liferations overlying dermatofibromas. *Acta Dermatol Venereol (Stockh)* 73:419–421.

Roth LM, Lee SC, Erlich CE. (1977) Paget's disease of the vulva. A histogenetic study of five cases including ultrastructural observations and review of the literature. *Am J Surg Pathol* 1:193–206.

Rothko K, Farmer ER, Zeligman I. (1980) Superficial epithelioma with sebaceous differentiation. *Arch Dermatol* 116:329–331.

Rüdlinger R, Buchmann P. (1989) HPV 16-positive bowenoid papulosis and squamous-cell carcinoma of the anus in an HIV-positive man. *Dis Colon Rectum* 32:1042–1045.

Rüdlinger R, Grob R, Yu YX, Schnyder UW. (1989) Human papillomavirus-35-positive bowenoid papulosis of the anogenital area and concurrent human papillomavirus-35-positive verruca with bowenoid papulosis of the periungual area. *Arch Dermatol* 125:655–659.

Ruffieux C, Ramelet A. (1985) Porocarcinome eccrine: présentation de 4 cas. *Dermatologica* 170:202–206.

Russell Jones R, Spaull J, Gusterson B. (1989) The histogenesis of mammary and extramammary Paget's disease. *Histopathology* 14:409–416.

Said JW, Sassoon AF, Shintaku IP, Banks-Schlegel S. (1984) Involucrin in squamous and basal cell carcinomas of the skin: an immunohistochemical study. *J Invest Dermatol* 82:449–452.

Saida T, Iwata M. (1987) Ectopic extramammary Paget's affecting the lower anterior aspect of the chest. *J Am Acad Dermatol* 17:910–913.

Saida T, Okabe Y, Uhara H. (1989) Bowen's disease with invasive carcinoma showing sweat gland differentiation. *J Cutan Pathol* 16:222–226.

Sanchez Yus E, Simon P, Requena L, Ambrojo P. (1989) Basal cell carcinoma with follicular differentiation. *Am J Dermatopathol* 11:505–507.

Saruk M, Olsen TG, Lucky PA. (1984) Metastatic epidermotropic squamous cell carcinoma of the vagina. *J Am Acad Dermatol* 11:353–356.

Sasaki M, Terada J, Nakanuma Y, et al. (1990) Anorectal mucinous adenocarcinoma associated with latent perianal Paget's disease. *Am J Gastroenterol* 85:199–202.

Sau P, McMarlin SL, Sperling LC, Katz R. (1994) Bowen's disease of the nail bed and periungual area: a clinicopathological analysis of seven cases. *Arch Dermatol* 130:204–209.

Schmitt CK, Folsom TC. (1968) Histologic evaluation of degenerative changes of the lower lip. *J Oral Surg* 26:51–56.

Schwartz RA, Janniger CK. (1991) Bowenoid papulosis. *J Am Acad Dermatol* 24:261–264.

Shafer WG, Waldrom CA. (1975) Erythroplakia of the oral cavity. *Cancer* 36:1021–1028.

Shah KD, Tabibzadeh SS, Gerber MA. (1987) Immunohistochemical distinction of Paget's disease from Bowen's disease and superficial spreading melanoma with the use of monoclonal cytokeratin antibodies. *Am J Clin Pathol* 88:689–695.

Shamanin V, Glover M, Rausch C, Proby C, Leigh IM, zur Hausen H, et al. (1994) Specific types of human papillomavirus found in benign proliferations and carcinomas of the skin in immunosuppressed patients. *Cancer Res* 54:4610–4613.

Shapiro L, Ackerman AB. (1966) Solitary lichen planus-like keratosis. *Dermatologica* 132:386–392.

Shaw M, McKee PH, Lowe D, Black MM. (1982) Malignant eccrine seroma: a study of twenty-seven cases. *Br J Dermatol* 107:675–680.

Shimizu N, Ito M, Tazawa T, Sato Y. (1989) Immunohistochemical study of keratin expression in certain cutaneous epithelial neoplasms. Basal cell carcinoma, pilomatricoma, and seborrheic keratosis. *Am J Dermatopathol* 11:534–540.

Sim CS, Slater S, McKee PH. (1992a) Mutant p53 expression in solar keratosis: an immunohistochemical study. *J Cutan Pathol* 19:302–308.

Sim CS, Slater S, McKee PH. (1992b) Mutant p53 is expressed in Bowen's disease. *Am J Dermatopathol* 14:195–199.

Sitakalin C, Ackerman AB. (1985) Mammary and extramammary Paget's disease. *Am J Dermatopathol* 7:335–340.

Skinner MS, Sternberg WH, Ichinose H, et al. (1973) Spontaneous regression of bowenoid atypia of the vulva. *Obstet Gynecol* 42:40–46.

Smith JLS, Coburn JG. (1956) Hidroacanthoma simplex: an assessment of a selected group of intraepidermal basal cell epitheliomata and of their malignant homologues. *Br J Dermatol* 68:400–418.

Smoller BR, van de Rijn M, Lebrun D, Warnke RA. (1994) bcl-2 expression reliably distinguishes trichoepitheliomas from basal cell carcinomas. *Br J Dermatol* 131:28–31.

Snow SN, Reizner GT. (1992) Eccrine porocarcinoma of the face. *J Am Acad Dermatol* 27:306–311.

Sober AJ, Burstein JM. (1995) Precursors to skin cancer. *Cancer* 75:645–650.

Sommers SC, McManus RG. (1953) Multiple arsenical cancers of skin and internal organs. *Cancer* 6:347–359.

Sonnex TS, Ralfs IG, Plaza de Lanza M, Dawber RPR. (1982) Treatment of erythroplasia of Queyrat with liquid nitrogen cryosurgery. *Br J Dermatol* 106:581–584.

Steffen C, Ackerman AB. (1985) Intraepidermal epithelioma of Borst-Jadassohn. *Am J Dermatopathol* 7:5–24.

Steffen C, Ackerman AB. (1994a) Reticulated acanthoma with sebaceous differentiation. In: *Neoplasms with Sebaceous Differentiation*, pp. 449–467. Lea & Febiger, Philadelphia.

Steffen C, Ackerman AB. (1994b) Sebaceoma. In : *Neoplasms with Sebaceous Differentiation*, pp. 385–431. Lea & Febiger, Philadelphia.

Steffen C, Ackerman AB. (1994c) Sebeceous adenoma. In: *Neoplasms with Sebaceous Differentiation*, pp. 349–382. Lea & Febiger, Philadelphia.

Steffen C, Ackerman AB. (1994d) Sebaceous carcinoma. In: *Neoplasms with Sebaceous Differentiation*, pp. 487–574. Lea & Febiger, Philadelphia.

Steffen C, Ackerman AB. (1994e) Seborrheic keratosis with sebaceous differentiation. In: *Neoplasms with Sebaceous Differentiation*, pp. 433–446. Lea & Febiger, Philadelphia.

Stoler A, Duvic M, Fuchs E. (1989) Unusual patterns of keratin expression in the overlying epidermis of patients with dermatofibromas: biochemical alterations in the epidermis as a consequence of dermal tumors. *J Invest Dermatol* 93:728–738.

Stone MS, Noonan CA, Tschen J, Bruce S. (1987) Bowen's disease of the feet: presence of human papillomavirus 16 DNA in tumor tissue. *Arch Dermatol* 123:1517–1520.

Strayer DS, Santa Cruz DJ. (1980) Carcinoma *in situ* of the skin: a review of histopathology. *J Cutan Pathol* 7:244–259.

Swanson PE, Cherwitz DL, Neumann MP, et al. (1987) Eccrine sweat gland carcinoma. *J Cutan Pathol* 14:15–22.

Szekeres G, de Giacomoni P. (1994) Ki-67 and p53 expression in cutaneous Bowen's disease: an immunohistochemical study of fixed-embedded tissue sections. *Acta Dermatol Venereol (Stockh)* 74:95–97.

Taguchi M, Watanabe S, Yashima K, Murakami Y, Sekiya T, Ikeda S. (1994) Aberrations of the tumor suppresor p53 gene and p53 protein in solar keratosis in human skin. *J Invest Dermatol* 103:500–503.

Takano Y, Nisimura M, Urabe A, et al. (1989) Malignant hidroacanthoma simplex. *J Dermatol* 16:405–408.

Takeshita K, Izumoi S, Ebuchi M, et al. (1978) A case of rectal carcinoma concomitant with pagetoid lesion in the perianal region. *Gastroenterol Jpn* 13:85–95.

Taki I, Janovski NA. (1961) Paget's disease of the vulva: presentation and histochemical study of four cases. *Obstet Gynecol* 18:385–402.

Tamaki K, Hino H, Ohara K, Furue M. (1985) Lectin-binding sites in Paget's disease. *Br J Dermatol* 113:17–24.

Tan CY, Marks R. (1982) Lichenoid solar keratosis—prevalence and immunologic findings. *J Invest Dermatol* 79:365–367.

Tateyama H, Eimoto T, Tada T, et al. (1995) P53 protein and proliferating cell nuclear antigen in eccrine poroma and porocarcinoma. An immunohistochemical study. *Am J Dermatopathol* 17:457–464.

Tazawa T, Ito M, Fujiwara H, et al. (1988) Immunologic characteristics of keratins in extramammary Paget's disease. *Arch Dermatol* 124:1063–1068.

Tellechea O, Reis JP, Domingues JC, Poiares Baptista A. (1993) Monoclonal antibody Ber EP4 distinguishes basal-cell carcinoma from squamous-cell carcinoma of the skin. *Am J Dermatopathol* 15:452–455.

Theaker JM. (1988) Extramammary Paget's disease of the oral mucosa with in situ carcinoma of the minor salivary gland ducts. *Am J Surg Pathol* 12:890–895.

Toyoda M, Shoji T, Morohashi M, Bhawan J. (1998) Benign sebaceous neoplasm with prominent epidermal component. *Am J Dermatopathol* 20:194–198.

Tsuji T. (1995) Mammary and extramammary Paget's disease: expression of Ca 15-3, Ka-93, Ca 19-9 and CD44 in Paget cells and adjacent normal skin. *Br J Dermatol* 132:7–14.

Tuck SM, Williams A. (1985) Paget's disease of the vulva complicated by bladder carcinoma: case report. *Br J Obstet Gynecol* 92:416–418.

Turner AG. (1980) Pagetoid lesions associated with carcinoma of the bladder. *J Urol* 123:124–126.

Urabe A, Matsukuma A, Shimizu N, et al. (1990) Extramammary Paget's disease: comparative histologic studies of intraductal carcinoma of the breast and apocrine adenocarcinoma. *J Cutan Pathol* 17:257–265.

van Praag MCG, Bavinck JNB, Bergman W, et al. (1993) PUVA keratosis. A clinical and histopathologic entity associated with an increased risk for nonmelanoma skin cancer. *J Am Acad Dermatol* 28:412–417.

Vanstapel MJ, Gatter KC, de Wolf-Peeters C, et al. (1984) Immunohistochemical study of mammary and extramammary Paget's disease. *Histopathology* 8:1013–1023.

Vaughan TK, Sau P. (1990) Superficial epithelioma with sebaceous differentiation. *J Am Acad Dermatol* 23:760–762.

Venkataseshan VS, Budd DC, Kin DU, Hutter RVP. (1994) Intraepidermal squamous carcinoma (Bowen's disease) of the nipple. *Hum Pathol* 25:1371–1374.

Verhaegh MEJM, Sanders CJG, Arends JW, Neumann HAM. (1995) Expression of the apoptosis-suppressing protein Bcl-2 in non-melanoma skin cancer. *Br J Dermatol* 132:740–744.

Vigneswaran N, Haneke E, Peters KP. (1987) Peanut agglutinin immunohistochemistry of basal cell carcinoma. *J Cutan Pathol* 14:147–153.

Wade TR, Kopf AW, Ackerman AB. (1978) Bowenoid papulosis of the penis. *Cancer* 42:1890–1903.

Wade TR, Kopf AW, Ackerman AB. (1979) Bowenoid papulosis of the genitalia. *Arch Dermatol* 115:306–308.

Wagers LT, Shapiro L, Kroll JJ. (1973) Bowen disease of the hand. *Arch Dermatol* 107:745–746.

Weiner HA. (1937) Paget's disease of the skin and its relation to carcinoma of the apocrine sweat glands. *Am J Cancer* 31:373–403.

Weldner N, Foucar E. (1985) Epidermotropic metastatic squamous cell carcinoma. Report of two cases showing histologic continuity between epidermis and metastasis. *Arch Dermatol* 121:1041–1043.

Wells GC. (1979) The pathology of adult type Letterer-Siwe disease. *Clin Exp Dermatol* 4:407–412.

Whorton CM, Patterson JB. (1955) Carcinoma of the Moll's glands with extramammary Paget's disease of the eyelid. *Cancer* 8:1009–1015.

Wick MR, Goellner JR, Wolfe JT, et al. (1985) Adnexal carcinomas of the skin. II. Extraocular sebaceous carcinoma. *Cancer* 56:1163–1172.

Wolfe JT III, Campbell RJ, Yeatts RP, et al. (1984) Sebaceous carcinoma of the eyelid. Errors in clinical and pathologic diagnosis. *Am J Surg Pathol* 8:597–606.

Wong SS, Tan KC, Goh CL. (1998) Cutaneous manifestations of chronic arsenicism: review of seventeen cases. *J Am Acad Dermatol* 38:179–185.

Woodruff JD. (1955) Paget's disease of the vulva: review, report of two cases. *Obstet Gynecol* 5:175–185.

Yamamoto O, Haratake J, Hisaoka M, Asahi M, Bhanan J. (1993) A unique case of apocrine carcinoma on the male pubic skin: histopathologic and ultrastructural observations. *J Cutan Pathol* 20:378–383.

Yamamura T, Honda T, Matsui Y, et al. (1993) Ultrastructural study of extramammary Paget's disease—histologically showing transition from bowenoid pattern to Paget's disease pattern. *Br J Dermatol* 128:189–193.

Yeh S. (1973) Skin cancer in chronic arsenicism. *Hum Pathol* 4:469–485.

Yoell JH, Price WG. (1960) Paget's disease of the perineal skin with associated adenocarcinoma. *Arch Dermatol* 82:986–991.

Zina AM, Bundino S, Pippione M. (1982) Pigmented hidroacanthoma simplex with porocarcinoma: light and electron microscopic study of a case. *J Cutan Pathol* 9:104–112.

3

SKIN: MELANOMA

Victor G. Prieto and Christopher R. Shea

Melanoma is the skin cancer with highest mortality. Since there is no cure for advanced disease, it is crucial to detect melanoma in early stages, when it is either *in situ* (confined to the epidermis) or superficially invasive (Breslow thickness <1 mm). For such lesions, around 95% are cured by complete surgical removal (NIH 1992). Exposure to ultraviolet radiation (UVR) is a major risk factor for melanoma (de Gruijl, 1999). Other factors are fair skin, history of sunburn, blue or green eyes, and red hair. Also considered to be risk factors are the number of typical acquired, congenital, or atypical (dysplastic) nevi, and of ephelides, and lentigines. Immunosuppression, and personal and family history of melanoma are associated with increased risk of melanoma. The incidence of reported melanoma cases has risen strikingly over the past several decades. Although part of this increment may be due to increased awareness or changes in diagnostic criteria, there also seems to be a real increase (Dennis, 1999).

Compared with visceral tumors, whose presence often goes undetected until they cause symptoms, skin lesions are easily observed by patient, family, and doctor. For that very reason, lesions that are grossly suspicious for early changes of melanoma are likely to undergo biopsy. Moreover, the small size (<1 cm) of most such lesions permits a relatively easy complete surgical removal.

Thus, with the exception of melanoma arising in large congenital nevi, the initial biopsy usually alters irrevocably the natural history of atypical melanocytic lesions. Therefore, to deduce the pathogenetic sequence we must rely on inferences from statistical associations of melanoma with certain nonmalignant (or premalignant) melanocytic lesions; from known common etiologic factors, especially UVR; and from spatial proximity of fully evolved (malignant) and evolving (dysplastic) atypia within particular lesions. This chapter briefly reviews these developments, with emphasis on the histopathologic recognition of melanoma, its simulants, and precursors.

MELANOCYTIC LESIONS OTHER THAN NEVI AND MELANOMA

Melanocytic lesions range from functional hyperactivity of epidermal melanocytes (ephelis), through benign proliferation of single epidermal melanocytes (lentigo), to benign proliferation of structurally altered, nested melanocytes (nevi) of the epidermis, dermis, or both, and atypical proliferations of solitary or nested melanocytes.

A freckle, or *ephelis*, is a localized macule of epidermal hyperpigmentation due to increased melanin biosynthesis by melanocytes that are normal in number and morphology. Ephelides occur predominantly on sun-ex-

41

posed skin of fair-skinned people having poor ability to tan, particularly in red-haired people. These individuals' skin and hair contain pheomelanin, an ineffective sunscreen whose photoreactions may generate mutagenic free radicals. Ephelides darken in response to sun exposure in summer and fade in winter, presumably reflecting aberrant regulation of melanogenesis in response to UVR. Ephelides are an independent risk factor for melanoma, probably because of the common pathogenesis of chronic UVR exposure in a genetically susceptible host; ephelides themselves probably do not evolve into melanoma.

A *lentigo* is a persistent, circumscribed macule of epidermal hyperpigmentation. Histopathologically, a *lentigo simplex* exhibits hyperpigmentation and acanthosis of the epidermal keratinocytes. Most studies report an increased number of basilar melanocytes in lentigines, but the increase may be too subtle for detection by routine histology, thus requiring specialized techniques (e.g., DOPA histochemistry or immunohistochemistry). Some authors use the term *nevoid lentigo* for lesions having a definite expansion in melanocyte number by routine light microscopy, but lacking nests as seen in nevi proper. *Solar lentigo* is a somewhat different lesion having club-shaped rete ridges and prominent dermal solar elastosis and showing histologic overlap with pigmented actinic keratosis. Lentigines are not generally considered precursors of melanoma. The controversial term *lentiginous* may refer to arrangement of melanocytes as solitary units (rather than nests) at the epidermal basal layer (rather than suprabasal); alternatively, it may indicate elongation of rete ridges and epidermal hyperpigmentation. Because of this ambiguity, we prefer to avoid the term lentiginous whenever possible.

MELANOCYTIC NEVI

The term *nevus*, related to the Latin *nativus* ("of birth"), should strictly refer to congenital lesions; however, about 99% of melanocytic nevi as presently defined are acquired, not congenital, in origin. Moreover, "nevus" may denote a malformation or hamartoma, as in nevus sebaceus, connective tissue nevus, etc. Following the most common use, in this chapter "nevus" refers to congenital or acquired, benign neoplasms of melanocytes or their close relatives (so-called nevomelanocytes or nevus cells) that have a tendency to form nests. Melanocytic nevi are the most common human neoplasms; an average white adult has 10 or more, depending on age. According to the most commonly held concept, nevi may originate at the dermal–epidermal junction and progressively descend into the dermis over time (*Abtropfung*) (Unna, 1893). This idea is supported by the age-dependent stratification of nevus types. Thus, in youth, most nevi are located at the dermal–epidermal junction; subsequently compound nevi (with both junctional and intradermal components) predominate, and intradermal nevi are most common in later adult life. Many nevi disappear in old age, perhaps being replaced by fibrous tissue, fat, or mucin. A rival theory proposes that nevi may originate from dermal cells that subsequently populate the epidermis (*Hochsteigerung*) (Cramer, 1991). It has been suggested that melanocytes may be derived from pluripotential cells in the nerve-sheath precursor stage of the melanocytic differentiation pathway.[5] By this concept, "mature" melanocytes are those with pigment (end stage of differentiation) while the "immature" melanocytes are those dermal spindle cells resembling Schwann cells. Finally, some authors have proposed that nevi may originate from either the epidermis or the dermis (Masson, 1951). The morphologic changes described above are also expressed at the molecular level (see Immunohistochemistry below).

The earliest stages of nevus development have rarely been studied. The term *nevus incipiens* is proposed for lesions combining theques of junctional nevus cells with features of lentigo simplex, suggesting a common histogenetic pathway (Mehregan, 1986). In our experience, incipient nevi provided from a pigmented lesions clinic may have striking architectural disorder, including prominent intraepidermal single-cell growth and suprabasal (pagetoid) spread. It is not known whether these "atypical" features are unique to patients with a dysplastic nevus/melanoma diathesis, as opposed to being a developmental phenotype common to all nevi at their incipient stage.

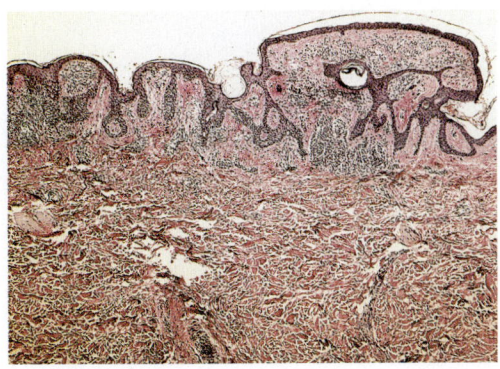

Figure 3–1. Melanoma arising in nevus. The right-hand side shows an exophytic growth, without significant inflammatory infiltrate (Fig. 3–2A). In contrast, the left-hand side shows a much flatter epidermis with a dense lymphocytic infiltrate (Fig. 3–2B).

MELANOMA ARISING IN NEVUS

The number of nevi is an independent risk factor for melanoma (Holly et al., 1987). However, because nevi are so prevalent whereas melanomas are much less common, simple arithmetic proves that the vast majority of nevi are not premalignant. However, some nevi do eventuate into melanoma, as shown histologically by coexistence of nevus and melanoma in surgical specimens (Rhodes et al., 1983). Precursor nevi are identified in contiguity with melanoma in 5%–35% of all cases, and associated melanocytic dysplasia is observed in up to about 40% (Ackerman et al., 1994; Elder et al., 1993; Maize and Ackerman, 1987; Figs. 3–1 and 3–2). In addition, it is possible that a precursor nevus may have been completely overrun and obliterated by the subsequent melanoma in some additional cases. However, it seems that many melanomas originate from epidermal melanocytes so the nevus is not an obligatory stage in the pathogenesis of melanoma.

Particular types of nevus are especially likely to give rise to melanoma. The atypical/dysplastic/Clark nevus is discussed below. Large (>20 cm) congenital nevi have a 10% or more lifetime risk of developing melanoma (DeDavid et al., 1997). Notably, melanoma may arise from the intradermal component of congenital nevi (Rhodes et al., 1981; Tajima et al., 1994), whereas *de novo* melanoma usually originates from the epidermis and only later invades the dermis. Because of this potential for occult transformation, some authors propose that even small congenital nevi should be completely

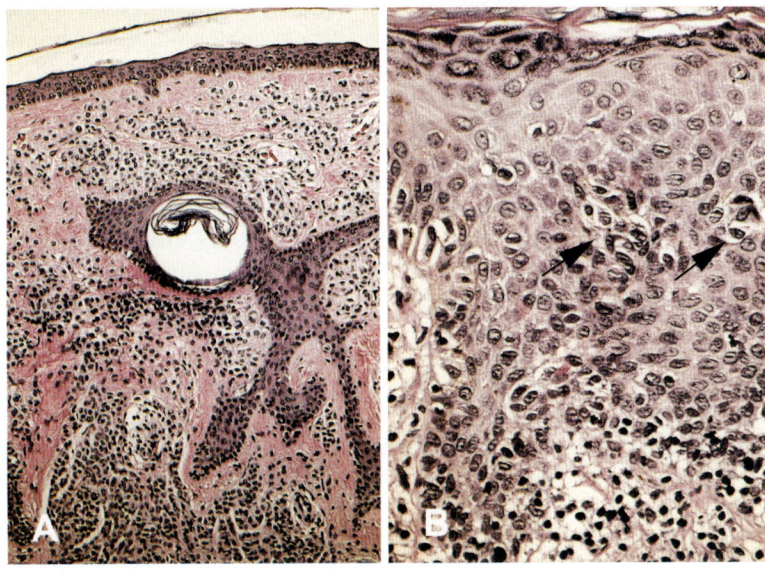

Figure 3–2. Melanoma arising in nevus. *A*: Nevus: dermal nests of melanocytes with uniform nuclei. The overlying epidermis has hyperplasia (elongation of rete ridges and horn pseudocyst). *B*: Melanoma: the flat area has a proliferation of large melanocytes arranged in single cells along the epidermis (pagetoid upward migration; arrows). Note the dense lymphocytic infiltrate.

excised to prevent malignancy. However, un-like large congenital lesions, medium-sized congenital nevi only rarely develop mela-noma (Sahin et al., 1998). Ironically, small to medium-sized nevi, at low risk for malig-nant transformation, are relatively easy to re-move *in toto*, whereas the more risky, large congenital nevi pose a formidable surgical problem. Histologically, congenital lesions show melanocytes arranged as nests or sin-gle cells deep in the dermis, around skin ad-nexae. The finding of infiltration of the arrector pili muscle by nevus cells is a very specific finding indicating a congenital ori-gin. It is important not to overinterpret the presence of single-cell growth and focal cy-tologic atypia in the superficial portion of congenital nevi and consider it as melanoma arising in a nevus (Hurwitz and Buckel, 1997).

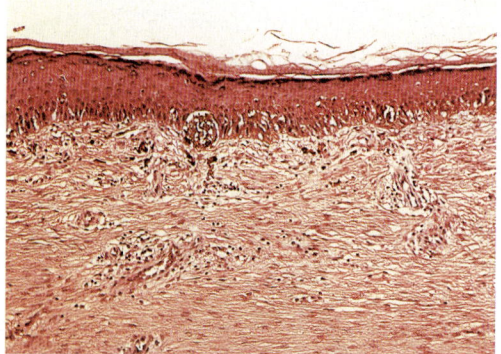

Figure 3–3. Recurrent news: irregular, confluent proliferation of large melanocytes as nests and single cells, with focal pagetoid upward migra-tion. Note the scar (horizontal bundles of colla-gen and a lymphocytic infiltrate) in the under-lying dermis.

NEVI SIMULATING MELANOMA

Recurrent nevi regrow following partial surgi-cal removal because of recolonization of the epidermis by melanocytes from follicles, ec-crine ducts, adjacent epidermis, or dermis (Park et al., 1987). Histologically, they may simulate melanoma, showing strikingly con-fluent growth of junctional melanocytes, focal suprabasal (pagetoid) spread of melan-ocytes, and dermal fibrosis reminiscent of re-gression (Kornberg and Ackerman, 1975; Fig. 3–3). Pathologic recognition is facili-tated by noting a banal nevus remnant deep to the zone of fibrosis, and confinement of the disorderly architecture to the area di-rectly overlying the dermal scar. In prob-lematic cases, immunohistochemistry can be helpful (MP Hoang et al., unpublished re-sults) (analysis of "maturation" with HMB45 and anti-Ki-67, see below).

Suprabasal (pagetoid) melanocytosis simulat-ing melanoma has also been described in nevi following UVR exposure (Tronnier et al., 1995). The presence of suprabasal dyskeratinocytes (sunburn cells) and the lack of high-grade atypia are helpful clues. Nevi of *acral skin* (e.g., palms, soles) (Boyd and Rapini, 1994; Celemente et al., 1995; Fallowfield et al., 1994) and genital (*vulvar*) nevi may contain confluent, basal, single melanocytes, in an architectural pattern sim-ulating melanoma. Moreover, suprabasal

(pagetoid) melanocytosis is common in acral nevi and does not necessarily indicate malignancy. Diagnosis of acral/mucosal mel-anoma requires significant cytologic atypia, asymmetry, inflammatory infiltrates, and dermal mitotic figures. Clinical–pathologic correlation is also important; a high index of suspicion for melanoma is appropriate for acral lesions of recent onset in older patients, or those >1 cm in diameter. Conservative, complete excision should be considered for atypical acral pigmented lesions.

Desmoplastic nevus is a lesion that mimics dermatofibroma, because of the prominent fibrosis of the stroma. Also, desmoplastic ne-vus may resemble desmoplastic melanoma, as they both have dermal atypical cells (Figs. 3–4 and 3–5). However, desmoplastic nevi are infrequently located on the head or neck (a common site for desmoplastic mela-noma), they lack mitotic figures, have sig-nificantly fewer Ki-67-reactive cells, and exhibit a gradient in HMB-45 expression, di-minishing toward the deep area of the le-sions (see Immunohistochemistry; Harris et al., 1990).

Spitz (spindled and epithelioid cell) nevus is a perennial concern (Binder et al., 1998). Spitz first introduced this lesion under the name "melanoma of childhood," and one of her initial cases was actually a malignant melanoma that metastasized fatally (Spitz, 1948). However, Spitz nevi can usually be dis-tinguished from melanoma by their symme-try, sharp circumscription, scant pagetoid

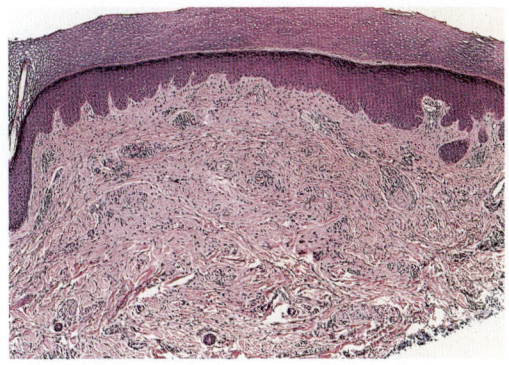

Figure 3–4. Characteristic morphology of desmoplastic nevus. At low power, the presence of hyperkeratosis, acanthosis, and dermal fibrosis resembles a dermatofibroma. Note the symmetry of the lesion.

spread, Kamino bodies (Kamino et al., 1979) cohesiveness of nests with peripheral clefts, minimal melanin pigment, vertical orientation of junctional nests ("raining down" or "bunches of bananas" appearance), cytologic maturation, "breaking up" of nests to disperse as single cells among deeper collagen bundles, and edema and telangiectasia of the dermis (Figs. 3–6 and 3–7). Lesions lacking the above features, or exhibiting necrosis, intralesional transformation (biphasic pattern), or deep mitotic figures raise the possibility of Spitzoid melanoma (Figs. 3–8 and 3–9; Handfield-Jones and Smith, 1996; Walsh et al., 1998) an area in which consensus is only partial (Barnhill et al., 1999). Complete excision of all atypical Spitzoid lesions seems prudent. We recommend conservative but complete primary excision of even routine-appearing Spitz nevi if clinically feasible, because key features including circumscription and symmetry cannot be reliably evaluated in lesions extending to the margins.

The term *ancient nevus* has been proposed for unusual, biphasic, intradermal pigmented lesions exhibiting asymmetry at scanning magnification (Kerl et al., 1998), because these contain both common nevus cells and cells with large, pleomorphic nuclei, scattered deep mitotic figures, and "degenerative" sclerosis and hemorrhage. At least one of the original cases reportedly developed metastasis (communication at the Annual Meeting of the American Society of Dermatopathology). Additional long-term follow-up of additional cases will be required before this concept is validated.

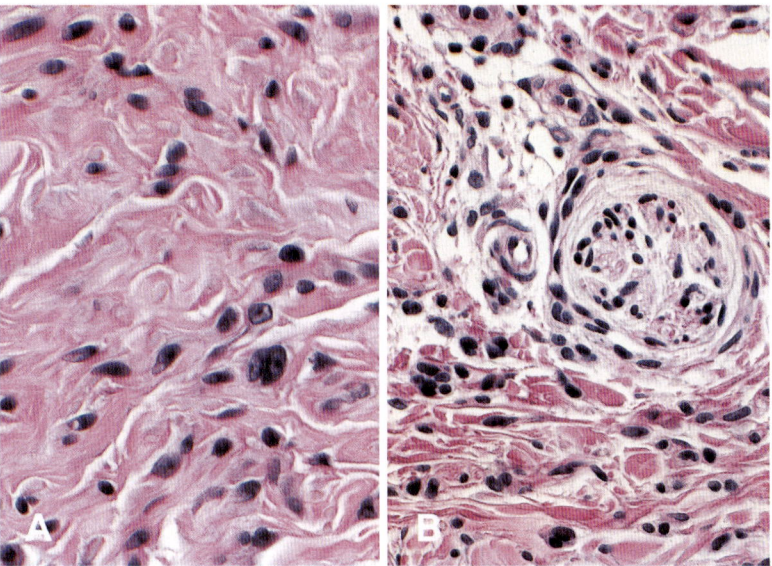

Figure 3–5. Desmoplastic nevus. *A:* In the dermal component, some of the cells display large, hyperchromatic nuclei with prominent nucleoli. Mitotic figures are not identified. Intervening collagen is thick, keloidal type, such as in dermatofibroma. *B:* Perineural arrangement is common in desmoplastic nevi.

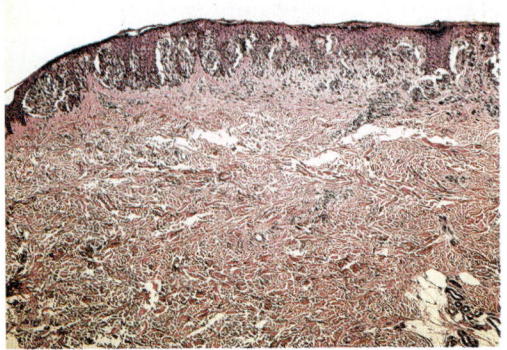

Figure 3–6. Epithelioid and spindle cell (Spitz) nevus. Note the circumscription and symmetry of the lesion. Junctional nests are evenly distributed and arranged perpendicular to the epidermal surface. Most nests are separated from the surrounding epidermis by vertical clefts.

Proliferative nodules in congenital nevi may be biopsied because of clinically evident growth and nodularity, raising the concern of possible melanoma. Proliferative nodules generally occur in the first year of life within large congenital nevi, and the diagnosis should be made with great caution in older patients. Histologically, they contain a discrete nodule with expansile architecture, mitotic figures, and some cytologic atypia. Distinction from melanoma arising in congenital nevus rests on a gradual transition to the typical nevus areas at the periphery, and lack of extensive necrosis, atypical mitotic

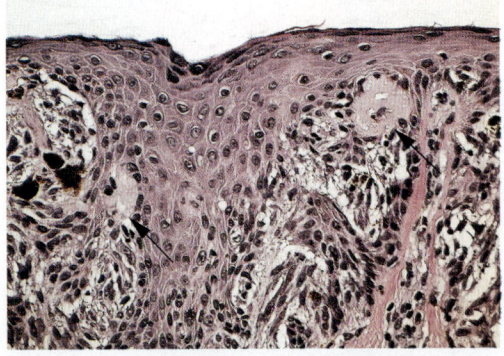

Figure 3–7. Spitz nevus. Junctional nests are similar in size, predominantly along the rete ridges. There are numerous eosinophilic bodies (Kamino bodies). Pagetoid upward migration is not evident.

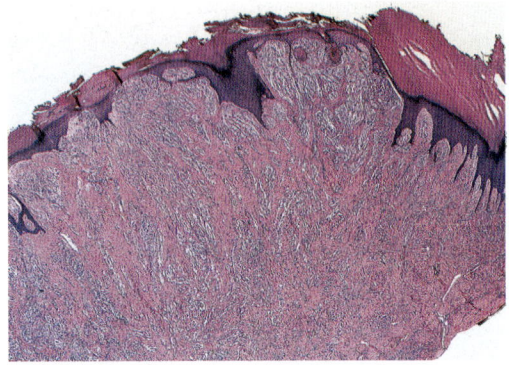

Figure 3–8. Spitzoid melanoma. Exo- and endophytic lesion with epidermal hyperplasia. The lesion extends to both peripheral and deep margins so symmetry and circumscription cannot be fully evaluated.

figures, or associated inflammatory infiltrate. All proliferative nodules require close clinical follow-up, because of the possibility of childhood melanoma, a rare but important tumor (Ceballos et al., 1995; Ruiz-Maldonado and Orozco-Covarrubias, 1997; Scalzo et al., 1997), usually arising from a congenital nevus. Metastases may rarely occur even from relatively thin primary childhood melanomas (Scalzo et al., 1997).

MELANOMAS SIMULATING NEVI

The term *nevoid melanoma* has been used for melanomas deceptively composed of relatively small tumor cells, which at first glance seem to be nevus cells but which exhibit nuclear atypia and deep mitotic figures. Lesions exhibiting strong HMB-45 labeling in the deep dermal component, especially when combined with evidence of cell proliferation (e.g., Ki-67 or PCNA expression; see below), may be nevoid melanomas rather than nevi (McNutt et al., 1995). Some melanomas exhibit a *paradoxical maturation* pattern mimicking benign nevi. We recently studied these tumors, using histologic, cytomorphometric, and immunohistochemical techniques (Ruhoy et al., 2000). Compared with conventional melanoma and common compound nevi, this group of melanomas with paradoxical maturation had features intermediate to both. With increasing depth, paradoxically maturing melanomas had

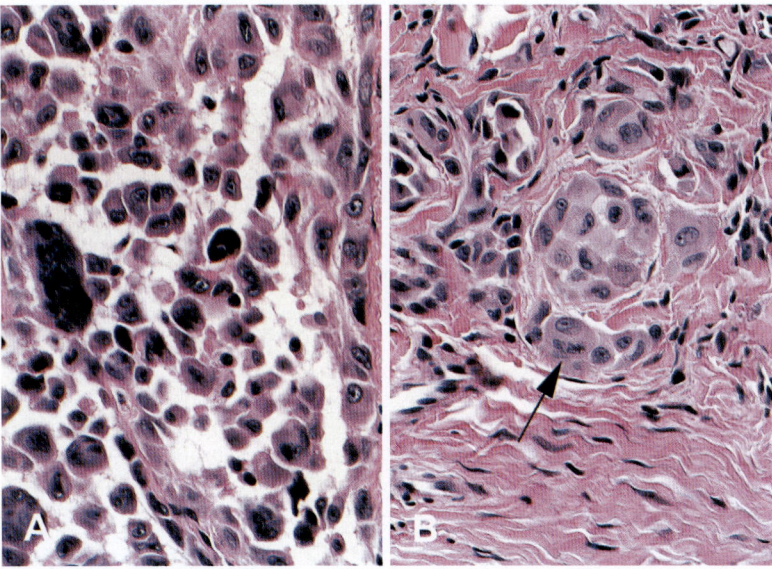

Figure 3–9. Spitzoid melanoma. *A*: Upper dermis. Poorly cohesive cells with pleomorphic, hyperchromatic nuclei and central, prominent nucleoli (Spitzoid morphology). Multinucleated forms are present. *B*: Lower dermis. Cells are still very large with evident nucleoli. Mitotic figures can be identified in these deep regions (arrow).

smaller nuclear and cellular areas and decreased expression of Ki-67, gp100 (with HMB-45), and tyrosinase. Still, in contrast to compound nevi, mitotic figures and melanin pigment can be detected in the deep portions of this type of melanoma.

Certain metastatic melanomas closely resemble nevi. This is particularly true of epidermotropic metastases (Abernethy et al., 1994; Heenan and Clay, 1991), including epidermotropic metastatic melanoma with paradoxical maturation (Ruhoy et al., 2000) and dermal metastases simulating blue nevi (Busam, 1999).

ATYPICAL, DYSPLASTIC, OR CLARK NEVUS

These terms are synonymous; the National Institutes of Health (NIH) Consensus Conference recommended dropping "dysplastic nevus," and proposed instead using "nevus with architectural disorder and cytologic atypia." (National Institutes of Health, 1992). By any name, much controversy has attended this concept, but in essence it is simple: a nevus that resembles melanoma, clinically and histologically. Points of clinical similarity include large size (generally >5

mm), poor circumscription, border irregularity, a play of colors, and asymmetry. The first challenge posed by atypical nevi is to discriminate them clinically from melanoma so that unnecessary excisions are avoided. Rapidly evolving techniques, such as dermoscopy (magnifying lens applied directly to the skin surface) (Andreassi et al., 1999), telespectrophotometry (analysis of color variation) (Bono et al., 1999), ultrasonic imaging and macroscopic spectral imaging (Solivetti et al., 1998; Yang et al., 1999) may help clinicians make this distinction.

Atypical nevi occur at a prevalence of 2%–9% in unselected white populations in most series. One outlying study reported that 53% of white adults had such lesions, but the inclusion criteria for diagnosis were broad; even small lesions were included, and there was no requirement for cytologic atypia (Piepkorn et al., 1989). Overinclusive diagnosis is to be avoided, lest the concept be diluted to the point that it loses all meaning. This would be unfortunate, for nevi with clinical and histologic atypia represent a strong, independent risk factor for development of melanoma (Tucker et al., 1997). This is true whether atypical nevi occur sporadically or in the context of a melanoma-prone familial predisposition (so-called dysplastic nevus syndrome) (Clark et al., 1978). Moreover, this association shows a dose–response relationship, with melanoma risk rising proportionately with the number of atypical nevi present. Apart from this role as a risk factor, atypical nevi may act as a precursor lesion to melanoma; molecular studies have detected similar genetic changes in both atypical nevi and melanoma, as discussed below.

The histopathologic features of atypical nevi comprise abnormalities in architecture, host response, and cytology (Figs. 3–10 to 3–12). There is general consensus on architectural criteria (Hastrup et al., 1994), including bridging of rete ridges, lateral extension of the junctional component ("shoulder"), and location of nests along sides of rete ridges. Cytologic features are the major source of controversy. Some authors insist that cytologic atypia is a *sine qua non* (Barnhill et al., 1990), while others consider atypia less important (Rivers et al., 1990). In our view, cytologic atypia is a highly variable feature in lesions clinically considered to be atypical nevi and showing host–response and architectural features of this diagnosis. Moreover, both the degree of cytologic atypia and the extent of architectural disorder vary widely and tend to be positively correlated with each other. Thus the architecture-versus-cytology controversy may reflect a false dichotomy. In a series of 166 consecutive atypical nevi, we found that about 85% of lesions fell into mild–moderate categories with regard to both cytologic

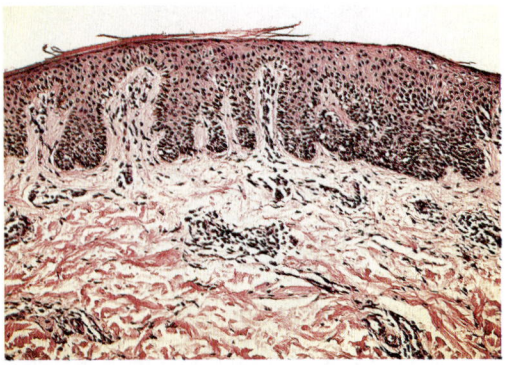

Figure 3–11. Atypical/Clark nevus. Fusion of rete ridges. Note the host response (dermal fibrosis, lymphocytic infiltrate, melanophages, and increased number of capillaries).

atypia and architectural disorder; the remaining minority had a higher degree of atypical features suggesting (but falling short of diagnostic criteria for) melanoma (Shea et al., 1999).

Atypical nevi may occur because of abnormalities in DNA repair in response to UVR, as shown *in vitro* (Moriwaki et al., 1997). Patients with dysplastic nevus syndrome have chromosomal instability, which is documented in normal skin, atypical nevi, and blood lymphocytes. Atypical nevi contain increased amounts of pheomelanin compared with common nevi, which might increase their susceptibility to UVR damage (Salopek et al., 1991). Shifts among these melanin types may reflect changes in pig-

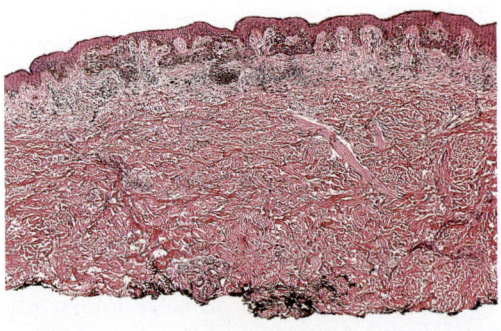

Figure 3–10. Atypical/Clark nevus. Relatively small lesion. Irregularly sized and shaped junctional nests. Note the inflammatory infiltrate and the fusion of rete ridges ("bridging").

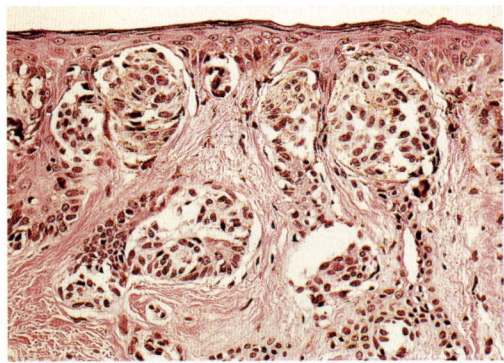

Figure 3–12. Atypical/Clark nevus. This particular lesion has marked cytologic atypia. A diagnosis of nevus is favored because of the nested pattern of growth and lack of pagetoid upward migration.

ment regulatory genes, such as that for the melanocortin-1 receptor (Suzuki et al., 1999).

EARLY/INCIPIENT MELANOMA

Early melanoma has been arbitrarily defined as those lesions with Breslow thickness <1 mm, measured from the top of the granular layer (or base of the ulcer in ulcerated lesions) to the deepest tumor cell. Some such lesions also are in so-called radial growth phase (RGP), considered to have little if any potential for metastasis. By definition, all melanoma *in situ* (MIS) (Clark level I) and some superficially invasive lesions (Clark level II involving but not filling or expanding the papillary dermis) are in RGP. Beyond this point, some authors think that melanoma enters a tumorigenic phase (vertical growth phase, or VGP) (Elder et al., 1984).

Melanoma in situ is defined as melanoma confined to the epidermis, without involvement of the dermis. It has an excellent prognosis, since it can almost always be cured by simple excision. Since MIS has a very low rate of metastasis, and to reduce the psychological charge that a diagnosis of melanoma conveys to the patient, some authors have proposed the use of other terms, such as *atypical melanocytic proliferation.* An expert panel from the U.K. examined interobserver agreement in the diagnosis of 95 melanocytic neoplasms, including many "borderline" lesions (Cook et al., 1996), and attempted to develop common definitions. There was a good overall agreement regarding benignity versus malignancy, but subclassifications as to degree of atypia or depth of invasion were more problematic. Specifically, the distinction between severe junctional atypia and MIS could not be made reliably. The authors therefore recommended combining these two diagnoses into one category of melanocytic intraepidermal neoplasia, in analogy to the practice used for severe cervical dysplasia/carcinoma *in situ*. However, in our experience, the term MIS has the virtue of seeming to convey an appropriate sense of urgency, but not of dire outcome, to most clinicians.

Melanoma *in situ* may exhibit several morphologic patterns. Lentigo-maligna-type MIS occurs in sun-exposed areas, mostly in elderly individuals. It is characterized by den-

dritic, large or small, round melanocytes with hyperchromatic nuclei, either as single cells or in nests, involving predominantly the basal layer of the epidermis and extending into skin adnexae. The epidermis itself is usually atrophic (flat) and there is actinic elastosis in the dermis. Both superficial spreading (predominantly nested growth with significant pagetoid upward migration) and acral-lentiginous (dendritic cells with less extensive pagetoid upward migration) patterns can be seen in MIS.

It is important to examine the dermis beneath lesions of MIS to determine the possible presence of regression (defined as fibrosis, a lymphocytic infiltrate, and melanophages). Such lesions may correspond to previously invasive melanomas in which the dermal component regressed to a point where no melanoma cells are identified in the dermis.

Since most MIS, lentigo maligna type, occur in sun-exposed skin, it sometimes becomes difficult to distinguish between a background phenomenon of actinic damage with atypical melanocytes and frank MIS. In specimens with solar elastosis (morphologic indication of actinic damage), the presence of a confluent growth of melanocytes (either with large nuclei and prominent nucleoli or with small, hyperchromatic nuclei) along the dermal–epidermal junction also involving the skin adnexae is indicative of MIS (Ackerman, 1985). Also, since many specimens from elderly individuals are taken from the face (e.g., to rule out basal cell carcinoma, actinic keratosis, etc.), one should keep in mind that the specimen may also contain MIS, lentigo maligna type. Therefore, in such situations, it is essential to examine the epidermis adjacent to the main lesion for the presence of concurrent MIS.

In the *early melanomas* (<1 mm in Breslow thickness), the overall survival after complete excision is >90% at 5 years. There has been considerable research to identify those features that correlate with a higher risk of metastasis in these early lesions. Apart from preliminary data from some molecular studies (see below), the main histologic features correlating with worse prognosis in thin melanomas are higher Breslow thickness, presence of ulceration, presence of vertical growth phase, presence of regression, and presence of satellitosis (nests of melanoma cells separate from the main lesion). Therefore, these data should probably be included in pathology reports.

CONCEPT OF MELANOMA PROGRESSION

As in other fields of oncology, there may be a progression of molecular and cellular events that accompany the transformation from benign (melanocytes) and malignant cells (melanoma cells). A similar process has been documented in squamous lesions of the genitalia (progression of epithelial dysplasia to carcinoma *in situ,* and to invasive carcinoma) and in the large intestine (adenomatous polyp, adenocarcinoma *in situ,* and invasive adenocarcinoma) (Fearon and Vogelstein, 1990). Although some authors adamantly refuse the idea of melanoma progression (Ackerman, 1994), it has been proposed that melanocytes in the epidermis proliferate, forming nevi (either common or atypical), some of which may transform into melanoma *in situ*, proliferate, and invade the dermis. It has been proposed that a qualitative change from nontumorigenic to tumorigenic type of growth then occurs in the dermis. This change would be present at some point before the tumor cells fill and expand the papillary dermis (features defining Clark level III). When the melanoma

cells form nests in the dermis that are larger than any given intraepidermal nest or mitotic figures are detected in the dermis, those thin melanomas are classified as *vertical growth phase* (VGP). Although this is a somewhat arbitrary distinction, it is true that most of the early melanomas that subsequently develop metastasis fulfill the criteria for VGP.

Note, however, that the risk of progression of any given nevus to frank melanoma is very low. Even clinically atypical (dysplastic) nevi are generally stable, as assessed by serial photography; conversely, a persistent change in a pigmented lesion's size, shape, or color is a high-risk marker for melanoma. The major exception is the expected life-cycle pattern of common nevi, believed to undergo a change from junctional to compound to intradermal location. Moreover, nevi are not an obligatory step in development of melanoma, most of which apparently arise from epidermal melanocytes.

Despite the existence of a spectrum of melanocytic atypia, ranging from banal nevi to outright melanoma, we believe that the experienced pathologist can confidently render a diagnosis of nevus versus melanoma in most cases encountered in routine practice (Tables 3–1 and 3–2). We make this assertion despite a widely cited study (Farmer et al., 1996), wherein eight experts reviewed 37 cases of melanoma or of nevus

Table 3–1. Histologic Features Distinguishing Nevus from Melanoma: Intraepidermal Component

Histologic feature	Nevus	Melanoma
Architecture[a]		
Symmetry	Present	Usually absent
Circumscription (both ends)	Present	Usually absent
Cohesiveness of nests (>50% of lesion)	Present[b]	Usually absent
Pagetoid spread (extensive or at periphery)	Absent[c]	Mostly present
Single cell growth	Mostly absent	Usually present
Confluent growth (>50% of lesion)	Absent	Present
Cytology[a]		
Hyperchromasia of nuclei	Absent	Present
Enlarged nuclei[d]	Absent	Present
Visible, macronucleolus	Absent[e]	Present
Large cytoplasm	Absent[e]	Present

[a]For any of these features, atypical nevi (AN) can have the characteristics of nevus or of melanoma (see text).

[b]Spitz nevus has cohesive nests that pull en masse from the surrounding epidermis.

[c]Spitz nevus can have migration of nests with transepidermal elimination.

[d]Larger than twice the size of basal keratinocyte nuclei.

[e]Present in Spitz nevus.

Table 3–2. Histologic Features Distinguishing Nevus from Melanoma: Dermal Component

Histologic feature	Nevus	Melanoma
Architecture[a]		
Symmetry	Present	Usually absent
Melanin	Only superficial[b]	Throughout
Confluent growth	Only superficial	Also at base
Ulceration	Absent[c]	May be present
Cytology[a]		
Maturation	Present	Absent[d]
Prominent nucleolus	Absent[e]	Usually present
Mitotic figures (deep)	Absent	Usually present
Atypical mitotic figures	Absent	May be present
Other dermal features		
Lymphoid infiltrate	Halo and AN	Usually present
Fibrosis	AN	Mostly present
Melanophages	Halo, AN, BN	Mostly present
Number of AgNOR[f]	Low	High

[a]For any of these features, atypical/Clark nevi (AN) can have the characteristics of nevus or of melanoma (see text).

[b]Blue nevus (BN) has abundant pigment throughout the lesion.

[c]Except for cases with a previous trauma.

[d]There is a subset of melanomas with paradoxical maturation (see text). Nevoid melanoma may also show maturation.

[e]Present in Spitz nevus.

[f]Silver-stained nucleolar organizing regions.

sharing features with melanoma, and were asked to classify them as malignant, indeterminate, or benign. Only moderate concordance was observed, and complete agreement was obtained in only 30% of cases. The discordance may in part be the result of case selection at the high end of the spectrum (where concordance regarding malignancy versus benignity is most problematic). Moreover, lack of definition among participants about whether dysplastic/atypical lesions should be considered benign, indeterminate, or malignant may have exaggerated the reported discordance, through semantic differences.

MOLECULAR PATHOGENESIS OF MELANOCYTIC DYSPLASIA AND MELANOMA

Several genetic changes are associated with the proposed melanoma progression. An early hint as to the molecular pathogenesis of melanoma was the detection of anomalies in chromosome 1 (1p36) in patients with the dysplastic nevus syndrome/familial melanoma. Such families also exhibit abnormalities in at least a second gene, in chromosome 9, that encodes an inhibitor of a kinase involved in the cell cycle, named $p16^{INK4a}$ (Liggett and Sidransky, 1998) or cyclin-dependent kinase inhibitor-2 (CDKN2A). Loss of p16 expression correlates with melanoma progression (Reed et al., 1995). Loss of heterozygosity for p16 appears to be an early event in the proposed progression sequence, having also been reported in atypical nevi; this finding supports a common pathogenesis with melanoma. In families carrying mutations in the gene for p16, the presence of clinically atypical nevi was correlated with an earlier onset of melanoma (Hashemi et al., 1999). The addition of activating mutations in N-*ras* to melanoma cells already containing mutations in p16 may induce the VGP phenotype. Such N-*ras* mutations are common in melanomas from sun-exposed skin but are rare in mucosal melanomas (Jiveskog et al., 1998).

A number of genes show relatively consistent mutations in thick melanomas, correlating with a decreased survival. Among them are c-myc (nuclear protein required for transition from G_1 to S phase), p53 (gatekeeper protein preventing cell proliferation after DNA damage), bcl-2 (anti-apoptotic factor), transforming growth factor-β (TGF-β, protein involved in angiogenesis and wound healing), CD40 (receptor that induces escape from apoptosis), and the cyclin-dependent kinase inhibitors p27 and p21 (KIP1 and Waf-1/SDI-1, respectively) (Bales et al., 1999). Enzymes that degrade collagen have been proposed to facilitate permeation of the dermis and access to blood vessels. Among those, collagenases-1 and -3 are expressed in invasive and metastatic but not in *in situ* melanomas (Airola et al., 1999). Similarly, some integrins (molecules involved in cell-to-cell recognition), such as the beta3 subunit of the vitronectin receptor, are first detected in VGP melanomas (Hsu et al., 1998), as is interleukin-8 (IL-8) (Singh et al., 1999). Since tumors must recruit new vessels in order to grow, it seems obvious that there should be secretion of angiogenic factors at some point. Some studies have shown increased vascularity in VGP versus radial growth phase melanomas (Erhard et al., 1997). Two candidate proteins are vascular endothelial growth factor (VEGF) and basic fibroblast growth factor (b-FGF), which have mitogenic effects on endothelial cells. By immunohistochemistry or *in situ* hybridization, b-FGF is expressed in invasive but not *in situ* melanomas (Reed et al., 1994). Related to angiogenesis, there is a correlation between the number of mast cells (which contain high quantities of angiogenic factors) and invasiveness in melanomas.

Because of the need for sufficient tissue, most genetic changes have been described in advanced lesions, either deeply invasive primary lesions or metastatic lesions, or in cell lines. Generally, only small quantities of tissue are available for analysis in common nevi, atypical nevi, and early malignant melanoma. Breakthrough techniques such as laser microdissection enable removal and analysis of minute quantities of tissue potentially allowing molecular analysis of the earliest stages of incipient melanoma. Briefly, paraffin sections are lightly stained with eosin (which does not significantly damage the cellular DNA and RNA) and then covered with a transparent film. Then, by exposing the tissue to the laser beam under microscopic observation, a discrete portion of the film is attached to the selected area (as few as three cells), which can be separated. Then, appropriate techniques such as comparative genomic hybridization can be applied to analyze different molecular changes. This approach has been used to detect chromosomal differences between RGP and VGP melanoma (Bastian et al., 1998; Wiltshire et al., 1995). These studies have demonstrated losses of chromosomes 9 and 10 early in melanoma progression and gains of chromosome 7 later. Using similar techniques, we found an alteration in Chr 20q13, in an area where a gene involved in chromosome function (aurora2, STK15, or STK6) is located. This modification is present in superficial melanomas and in dysplastic nevi, but not in common nevi, and may therefore be important in early malignant transformation (V. G. Prieto and C. R. Shea, unpublished results).

IMMUNOHISTOCHEMISTRY

The advent of immunohistochemical markers of cell proliferation has profoundly influenced the study of all tumor pathology, including dermatopathology. The use of antibodies against antigens typically expressed in melanocytic cells, such as S-100 protein,

Table 3–3. Immunohistochemical Features Distinguishing Nevus from Melanoma

Expression of	Nevus	Melanoma
gp100 (with HMB45)	Superficial region[a]	Throughout
Tyrosinase	Superficial region[a]	Throughout
Peripherin	Superficial region[a]	Throughout
Ki-67 (nuclear, proliferation marker)	Rare at base	Throughout

Analysis of expression of these markers helps to determine the presence of "maturation" in the dermal component of melanocytic lesions.

[a]Throughout in blue nevi.

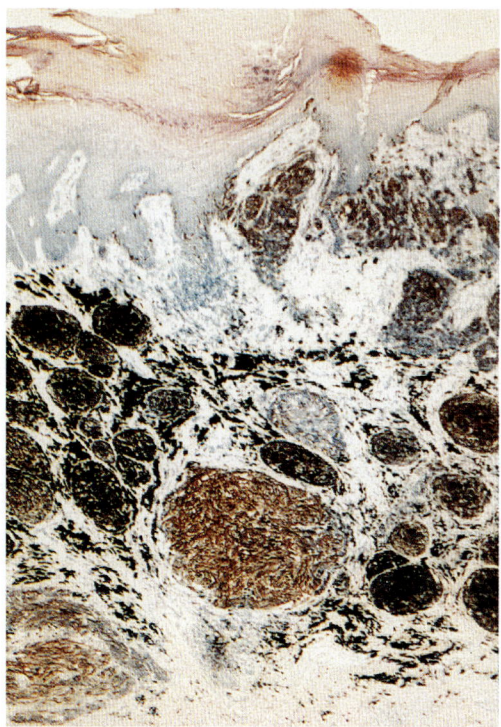

Figure 3–13. Acral lentiginous melanoma. Notice the strong expression of gp100 (brown color) through-out the lesion, including deep dermal nests (lack of immunophenotypic maturation). The use of Giemsa as counterstain enables distinction between the reaction product (diaminobenzidine, brown) and melanin (green). (HMB45[anti-gp100]; Diaminobenzidine; Giemsa as counterstain).

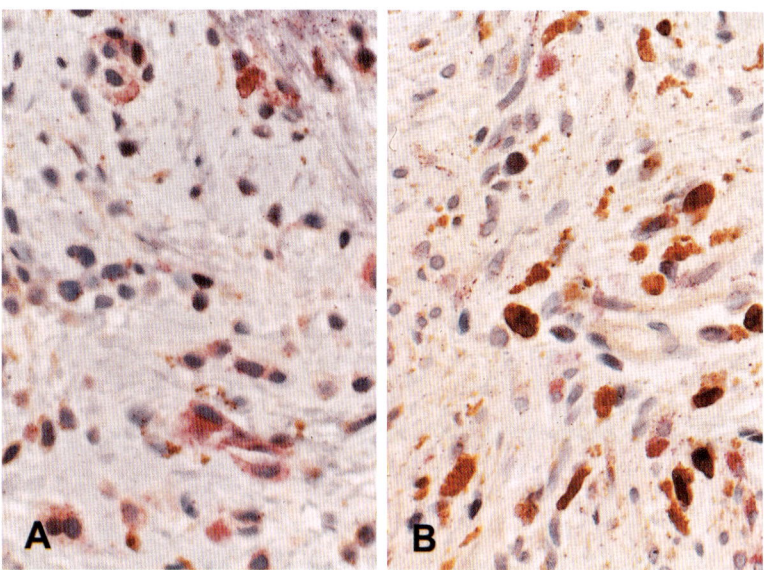

Figure 3–14. Comparison of expression of proliferation marker (Ki-67) and gp100 (with HMB45) in the deep dermal regions of nevus (*A*) and melanoma (*B*). In contrast to nevus, many cells in melanoma maintain expression of the proliferation marker throughout the lesion (Double immunoperoxidase technique: HMB45, fast red, and anti-Ki67, diaminobenzidine, brown).

gp100 (detected with HMB45), or MART-1 (melanoma antigen recognized by T (cells), allows confirmation of melanocytic lineage in a given neoplasm. For example, in small biopsies, immunohistochemical analysis may be helpful in distinguishing pigmented basal cell carcinoma from small cell melanoma (Prieto et al., 1996). Also, when examining sentinel node specimens, use of immunohistochemistry may help in the detection of small clusters of or even single melanoma cells within the lymph node (White and Loggie, 1999).

A controversial field is the use of immunohistochemistry for the differential diagnosis of melanoma and nevus. Although some authors reject this approach, we strongly feel that, in selected cases and along with clinical and histologic criteria, immunohistochemical data are helpful in the diagnosis of melanocytic lesions (Table 3–3). An example is the assessment of maturation in the dermal components. Superficial, round, type-A nevus cells share many immunohistochemical markers with neurons whereas the deep, spindle, type-C nevus cells resemble Schwann cells (Prieto et al., 1997; Reed et al., 1999). This morphology is reflected in the decreased expression of gp100 by those melanocytes located at the base of the nevus and not in melanomas (Bacchi et al., 1996; Fig. 3–13). Also, the almost universal lack of mitotic figures in the deep regions of nevi correlates with the very sparse expression of proliferation markers (Ki-67) by the more deeply located melanocytes in nevi; the validity of this observation has been corroborated by a clinicopathologic study (Rudolph et al., 1997). Of 384 melanocytic lesions, common, dysplastic, and Spitz nevi exhibited reactivity in <6% of cells, generally disposed at the dermal–epidermal junction or in the more superficial dermal compartment. In contrast, melanomas did not show this orderly pattern but instead had a random pattern of immunoreactivity and a mean growth fraction of 16.4%, with increased concentration at the deep tumor borders (Fig. 3–14). Using the Ki-S5 expression pattern as a guide, these authors reclassified 112 lesions that had posed diagnostic problems on routine histology; on subsequent clinical review, systemic progression was demonstrated in 70.7% of the cases finally classified as melanoma and in none of those finally classified as benign lesions. This highly significant result indicates the potential clinical usefulness of this approach.

REFERENCES

Abernethy JL, Soyer HP, Kerl H, Jorizzo JL, White WL. (1994) Epidermotropic metastatic malignant melanoma simulating melanoma in situ. A report of 10 examples from two patients. *Am J Surg Pathol* 18:1140–1149.

Ackerman AB. (1985) Malignant melanoma in situ: the flat, curable stage of malignant melanoma. *Pathology* 17:298–300.

Ackerman AB, Cerroni L, Kerl H. (1994) Melanoma in association with a nevus. *Pitfalls in Histopathologic Diagnosis of Malignant Melanoma*. Lea & Febiger, Philadelphia, pp. 142–143.

Airola K, Karonen T, Vaalamo M, et al. (1999) Expression of collagenases-1 and -3 and their inhibitors TIMP-1 and -3 correlates with the level of invasion in malignant melanomas. *Br J Cancer* 80:733–743.

Andreassi L, Perotti R, Rubegni P, et al. (1999) Digital dermoscopy analysis for the differentiation of atypical nevi and early melanoma - A new quantitative semiology. *Arch Dermatol* 135:1459–1465.

Bacchi CE, Bonetti F, Pea M, Martignoni G, Gown AM. (1996) HMB-45: a review. *Appl Immunohistochem* 4:73–85.

Bales ES, Dietrich C, Bandyopadhyay D, et al. (1999) High levels of expression of p27(KIP1) and cyclin E in invasive primary malignant melanomas. *J Invest Dermatol* 113:1039–1046.

Barnhill RL, Argenyi ZB, From L, et al. (1999) Atypical Spitz nevi/tumors: lack of consensus for diagnosis, discrimination from melanoma, and prediction of outcome. *Hum Pathol* 30:513–520.

Barnhill RL, Roush GC, Duray PH. (1990) Correlation of histologic features and cytoplasmic features with nuclear atypia in atypical (dysplastic) nevi. *Hum Pathol* 21:50–58.

Bastian BC, LeBoit PE, Hamm H, Brocker EB, Pinkel D. (1998) Chromosomal gains and losses in primary cutaneous melanomas detected by comparative genomic hybridization. *Cancer Res* 58:2170–2175.

Binder SW, Ansong C, Paul E, Cochran AJ. (1998) The histology and differential diagnosis of Spitz nevus. *Semin Diagn Pathol* 10:36–46.

Bono A, Tomatis S, Bartoli C, et al. (1999) The ABCD system of melanoma detection: a spectrophotometric analysis of the asymmetry, border, color, and dimension. *Cancer* 85:72–77.

Boyd AS, Rapini RP. (1994) Acral melanocytic neoplasms: a histologic analysis of 158 lesions. *J Am Acad Dermatol* 31:740–745.

Busam KJ. (1999) Metastatic melanoma to the skin simulating blue nevus. *Am J Surg Pathol* 23:276–282.

Ceballos PI, Ruiz-Maldonado R, Mihm MC Jr. (1995) Melanoma in children. *N Engl J Med* 332:656–662.

Clark WH, Jr, Reimer RR, Greene M, Ainsworth AM, Mastrangelo MJ. (1978) Origin of familial malignant melanomas from heritable melanocytic lesions. 'The B-K mole syndrome'. *Arch Dermatol* 114:732–738.

Clemente C, Zurrida S, Bartoli C, Bono A, Collini P, Rilke F. (1995) Acral-lentiginous naevus of plantar skin. *Histopathology* 27:549–555.

Cook MG, Clarke TJ, Humphreys S, et al. (1996) The evaluation of diagnostic and prognostic criteria and the terminology of thin cutaneous malignant melanoma by the CRC Melanoma Pathology Panel. *Histopathology* 28:497–512.

Cramer SF. (1991) The origin of epidermal melanocytes. Implications for the histogenesis of nevi and melanomas. *Arch Pathol Lab Med* 115:115–119.

DeDavid M, Orlow SJ, Provost N, et al. (1997) A study of large congenital melanocytic nevi and associated malignant melanomas: review of cases in the New York University Registry and the world literature. *J Am Acad Dermatol* 36:409–416.

de Gruijl FR. (1999) Skin cancer and solar UV radiation. *Eur J Cancer* 35:2003–2009.

Dennis LK. (1999) Analysis of the melanoma epidemic, both apparent and real - Data from the 1973 through 1994 surveillance, epidemiology, and end results program registry. *Arch Dermatol* 135:275–280.

Elder DE, Clark WH, Jr., Elenitsas R, Guerry Dt, Halpern AC. (1993) The early and intermediate precursor lesions of tumor progression in the melanocytic system: common acquired nevi and atypical (dysplastic) nevi. *Semin Diagn Pathol* 10:18–35.

Elder DE, Guerry Dt, Epstein MN, et al. (1984) Invasive malignant melanomas lacking competence for metastasis. *Am J Dermatopathol* 6 Suppl:55–61.

Erhard H, Rietveld FJ, van Altena MC, Brocker EB, Ruiter DJ, de Waal RM. (1997) Transition of horizontal to vertical growth phase melanoma is accompanied by induction of vascular endothelial growth factor expression and angiogenesis. *Melanoma Res* 7:S19–26.

Fallowfield ME, Collina G, Cook MG. (1994) Melanocytic lesions of the palm and sole. *Histopathology* 24:463–467.

Farmer ER, Gonin R, Hanna MP. (1996) Discordance in the histopathologic diagnosis of melanoma and melanocytic nevi between expert pathologists. *Hum Pathol* 27:528–531.

Fearon ER, Vogelstein B. (1990) A genetic model for colorectal tumorigenesis. *Cell* 61:750–767.

Fujita M, Norris DA, Yagi H, et al. (1999) Overexpression of mutant ras in human melanoma increases invasiveness, proliferation and anchorage-independent growth in vitro and induces tumour formation and cachexia in vivo. *Melanoma Res* 9:279–291.

Goldstein AM, Goldin LR, Dracopoli NC, Clark WH, Jr., Tucker MA. (1996) Two-locus linkage analysis of cutaneous malignant melanoma/dysplastic nevi. *Am J Hum Genet* 58:1050–1056.

Handfield-Jones SE, Smith NP. (1996) Malignant melanoma in childhood. *Br J Dermatol* 134:607–616.

Harris GR, Shea CR, Horenstein MG, Reed JA, Burchette JL, Prieto VG. (1999) Desmoplastic (sclerotic) nevus: an underrecognized entity that resembles dermatofibroma and desmoplastic melanoma. *Am J Surg Pathol* 23:786–794.

Hashemi J, Linder S, Platz A, Hansson J. (1999) Melanoma development in relation to nonfunctional p16/INK4A protein and dysplastic naevus syndrome in Swedish melanoma kindreds. *Melanoma Res* 9:21–30.

Hastrup N, Clemmensen OJ, Spaun E, K. S. (1994) Dysplastic naevus; histological criteria and their inter-observer reproducibility. *Histopathology* 24:503–509.

Heenan PJ, Clay CD. (1991) Epidermotropic metastatic melanoma simulating multiple primary melanomas. *Am J Dermatopathol* 13:396–402.

Holly EA, Kelly JW, Shpall SN, Chiu SH. (1987) Number of melanocytic nevi as a major risk factor for malignant melanoma. *J Am Acad Dermatol* 17:459–468.

Hsu MY, Shih DT, Meier FE, et al. (1998) Adenoviral gene transfer of beta3 integrin subunit induces conversion from radial to vertical growth phase in primary human melanoma. *Am J Pathol* 153:1435–1442.

Hurwitz RM, Buckel LJ. (1997) Superficial congenital compound melanocytic nevus. Another pitfall in the diagnosis of malignant melanoma. *Dermatol Surg* 23:897–900.

Jiveskog S, Ragnarsson-Olding B, Platz A, Ringborg U. (1998) N-ras mutations are common in melanomas from sun-exposed skin of humans but rare in mucosal membranes or unexposed skin. *J Invest Dermatol* 111:757–761.

Kamino H, Flotte TJ, Misheloff E, Greco MA, Ackerman AB. (1979) Eosinophilic globules in Spitz's nevi. New findings and a diagnostic sign. *Am J Dermatopathol* 1:319–324.

Kerl H, Soyer HP, Cerroni L, Wolf IH, Ackerman AB. (1998) Ancient melanocytic nevus. *Semin Diagn Pathol* 15:210–215.

Kornberg R, Ackerman AB. (1975) Pseudomelanoma: recurrent melanocytic nevus following partial surgical removal. *Arch Dermatol* 111:1588–1590.

Liggett WHJ, Sidransky D. (1998) Role of the p16 tumor suppressor gene in cancer. *J Clin Oncol* 16:1197–1206.

Maize JC, Ackerman AB. (1987) Malignant melanoma. Pigmented Lesions of the Skin. Clinicopathologic Correlations. p. 165. Lea & Febiger, Philadelphia.

Masson P. (1951) My conception of cellular nevi. *Cancer* 4:9–38.

McNutt NS, Urmacher C, Hakimian J, Hoss DM, Lugo J. (1995) Nevoid malignant melanoma: morphologic patterns and immunohistochemical reactivity. *J Cutan Pathol* 22:502–517.

Mehregan AH. (1986) Melanocytic tumors and malformations. Pinkus' Guide to Dermatopathology, 4th Ed. pp. 396–397. Appleton-Century-Crofts, Norwalk, CT.

Moriwaki SI, Tarone RE, Tucker MA, Goldstein AM, Kraemer KH. (1997) Hypermutability of UV-treated plasmids in dysplastic nevus/familial melanoma cell lines. *Cancer Res* 57:4637–4641.

National Institutes of Health. (1992) NIH Consensus Conference. Diagnosis and treatment of early melanoma. *JAMA* 268:1314–1319.

Park HK, Leonard DD, Arrington JH, Lund HZ. (1987) Recurrent melanocytic nevi. Clinical and histologic review of 175 cases. *J Am Acad Dermatol* 17:285–292.

Piepkorn M, Meyer LJ, Goldgar D, et al. (1989) The dysplastic melanocytic nevus: a prevalent lesion that correlates poorly with clinical phenotype. *J Am Acad Dermatol.* 20:407–415.

Prieto VG, Lugo J, McNutt NS. (1996) Intermediate- and low-molecular-weight keratin detection with the monoclonal antibody MNF116. An immunohistochemical study on 232 paraffin-embedded cutaneous lesions. *J Cutan Pathol* 23:234–241.

Prieto VG, McNutt NS, Lugo J, Reed JA. (1997) The intermediate filament peripherin is expressed in cutaneous melanocytic lesions. *J Cutan Pathol* 24:145–150.

Reed JA, Finnerty B, Albino AP. (1999) Divergent cellular differentiation pathways during the invasive stage of cutaneous malignant melanoma progression. *Am J Pathol* 155:549–555.

Reed JA, Loganzo F, Shea CR, et al. (1995) Loss of expression of the p16/cyclin-dependent kinase inhibitor 2 tumor suppressor gene in melanocytic lesions correlates with invasive stage of tumor progression. *Cancer Res* 55:2713–2718.

Reed JA, McNutt NS, Albino AP. (1994) Differential expression of basic fibroblast growth factor (bFGF) in melanocytic lesions demonstrated by in situ hybridization: implications for tumor progression. *Am J Pathol* 144:329–336.

Rhodes AR, Harrist TJ, Day CL, Mihm MC, Jr., Fitzpatrick TB, Sober AJ. (1983) Dysplastic melanocytic nevi in histologic association with 234 primary cutaneous melanomas. *J Am Acad Dermatol* 9:563–574.

Rhodes AR, Wood WC, Sober AJ, Mihm MC, Jr. (1981) Nonepidermal origin of malignant melanoma associated with a giant congenital nevocellular nevus. *Plast Reconstr Surg* 67:782–790.

Rivers JK, Cockerell CJ, McBride A. (1990) Quantification of histologic features of dysplastic nevi. *Am J Dermatopathol* 12:42–50.

Rudolph P, Schubert C, Schubert B, Parwaresch R. (1997) Proliferation marker Ki-S5 as a diagnostic tool in melanocytic lesions. *J Am Acad Dermatol* 37:169–178.

Ruhoy SM, Prieto VG, Eliason SL, Grichnik JM, Burchette JL, Shea CR. (2000) Malignant melanoma with paradoxical maturation. *Am J Surg Pathol* 24:in press.

Ruiz-Maldonado R, Orozco-Covarrubias M. (1997) Malignant melanoma in children. A review. *Arch Dermatol* 133:363–371.

Sahin S, Levin L, Kopf AW, et al. (1998) Risk of melanoma in medium-sized congenital melanocytic nevi: a follow-up study. *J Am Acad Dermatol* 39:428–433.

Salopek TG, Yamada K, Ito S, Jimbow K. (1991) Dysplastic melanocytic nevi contain high levels of pheomelanin: quantitative comparison of pheomelanin/eumelanin levels between normal skin, common nevi, and dysplastic nevi. *Pigment Cell Res* 4:172–179.

Scalzo DA, Hida CA, Toth G, Sober AJ, Mihm MC, Jr. (1997) Childhood melanoma: a clinicopathological study of 22 cases. *Melanoma Res* 7:63–68.

Shea CR, Vollmer RT, Prieto VG. (1999) Grading architectural disorder and cytologic atypia in melanocytic nevi. *Hum Pathol* 30:500–505.

Singh RK, Varney ML, Bucana CD, Johansson SL. (1999) Expression of interleukin-8 in primary and metastatic malignant melanoma of the skin. *Melanoma Res* 9:383–387.

Solivetti FM, Thorel MF, Di Luca Sidozzi A, Bucher S, Donati P, Panichelli V. (1998) Role of high-definition and high frequency ultrasonography in determining tumor thickness in cutaneous malignant melanoma. *Radiolog Med* 96:558–561.

Spitz S. (1948) Melanomas of childhoood. *Am J Pathol* 24:591–609.

Suzuki I, Im S, Tada A, et al. (1999) Participation of the melanocortin-1 receptor in the UV control of pigmentation. *J Invest Dermatol Symp Proc* 4:29–34.

Tajima Y, Nakahima T, Sugano I, Nagao K, Kondo Y. (1994) Malignant melanoma within an intradermal nevus. *Am J Dermatopathol* 16:301–306.

Tronnier M, Smolle J, Wolff HH. (1995) Ultraviolet irradiation induces acute changes in melanocytic nevi. *J Invest Dermatol* 104:475–478.

Tucker MA, Halpern A, Holly EA, et al. (1997) Clinically recognized dysplastic nevi. A central risk factor for cutaneous melanoma. *JAMA* 277:1439–1444.

Unna PG. (1893) Naevi und Naevocarcinome. *Berlin Klin Wochenschr* 30:14–16.

Walsh N, Crotty K, Palmer A, McCarthy S. (1998) Spitz nevus versus spitzoid malignant melanoma: an evaluation of the current distinguishing histopathologic criteria. *Hum Pathol* 29:1105–1112.

White WL, Loggie BW. (1999) Sentinel lymphadenectomy in the management of primary cutaneous malignant melanoma. *Dermatol Clin* 17:645–655.

Wiltshire RN, Duray P, Bittner ML, et al. (1995) Direct visualization of the clonal progression of primary cutaneous melanoma: application of tissue microdissection and comparative genomic hybridization. *Cancer Res* 55:3954–3957.

Yang P, Farkas DL, Kirkwood JM, Abernethy JL, Edington HD, Becker D. (1999) Macroscopic spectral imaging and gene expression analysis of the early stages of melanoma. *Mol Med* 5:785–794.

4

UPPER AERODIGESTIVE TRACT

Mario A. Luna and Keyla Pineda-Daboin

Head and neck cancer is estimated to account for 30,300 new cases and 8,000 deaths in 1998 in the U.S. (Landis et al., 1997). Head and neck cancer represents 12% of all cancers seen at the community level and constitutes one-third of malignant neoplasms seen in cancer centers. The advent of endoscopy has allowed the "at-risk" mucosa of the upper aerodigestive tract (UADT) to be visualized, thus permitting identification and biopsy of a greater number of precancerous lesions and microcancers. Despite their anatomic contiguity, cancers and precancerous lesions of the UADT are a disparate and morphologically diverse group. Although the risk factors for these lesions, as a group, have been studied fairly extensively, the biology of the lesions, their interactions with the host, and other remaining mysteries of carcinogenesis need to be solved.

This chapter addresses the morphology of potentially malignant lesions of the UADT, their malignant transformation, and some advanced methods with which to identify those cases that are at high risk of becoming malignant. Also discussed are incipient carcinomas, special lesions of the UADT that have a strong tendency to transform into more aggressive malignancy, and the occurrence of second malignant tumors in patients with primary head and neck carcinomas.

SQUAMOUS CELL CARCINOMAS OF THE UPPER AERODIGESTIVE TRACT

Squamous cell carcinoma of the UADT represents a heterogeneous group of cancers (Table 4–1) with different biologic behaviors. The largest proportion of tumors arises in the larynx (20.9%), followed by the oral cavity, including the lips (17.6%), and the oropharynx (12.3%). The largest percentage of cases (27.0%) appears in the 60- to 69-year age-group, and men with the disease outnumber women by approximately 1.5:1. The disease is still most prevalent in white patients, but the incidence in African Americans and Hispanics increased 10% from 1985–1989 to 1990–1994. Most patients with squamous cell carcinoma of the UADT, regardless of ethnicity, are heavy smokers and drinkers (64%) (Hoffman et al., 1998).

Local control of cancer has improved; the drop in the death rate from local and regional recurrence of treated cancer has been accompanied by more failures from either distant metastasis or the development of second primary cancers (Landis et al., 1997). Notably, patients with squamous cell carcinoma of the UADT have a high probably of developing multiple carcinomas in various mucosa, a tendency now recognized as causing therapeutic failures (Schwartz et al., 1994).

MULTIPLE PRIMARY MALIGNANT TUMORS

The mucosa of the UADT can be regarded as a "field of growth" vulnerable to the traditional carcinogens (e.g., tobacco, alcohol) that can induce malignant transformation. The potential exists, therefore, for multiple areas of malignancy and premalignancy to develop simultaneously or metachronously in the same patient. The mucosa at risk in-

Table 4–1. Variants of Squamous Cell
Carcinoma of the Upper Aerodigestive Tract

Conventional squamous cell carcinoma with varying
   levels of differentiation

Verrucous squamous cell carcinoma and hybrid
   verrucous squamous cell carcinoma

Sarcomatoid (metaplastic) squamous cell carcinoma

Basaloid squamous cell carcinoma

Adenosquamous carcinoma

Adenoid squamous cell carcinoma and acantholytic/
   squamous cell carcinoma

Papillary squamous cell carcinoma

Lymphoepithelial (nasopharyngeal-type) carcinoma

cludes that lining the oral cavity, oropharynx, hypopharynx, larynx, bronchial tree, and esophagus, whereas the mucosa of the paranasal sinuses, nose, and nasopharynx do not seem to be affected by the same carcinogens.

Of patients who have head and neck cancers, 10%–20% either have or will develop additional primary cancers during their life (Schwartz et al., 1994). Most arise in other head and neck sites, in the lungs, or in the esophagus. Recognizing this phenomenon is important because the discovery of a second primary tumor could alter the initial therapeutic approach to the index tumor, represent a more aggressive, life-threatening neoplasm, or compromise previously successful treatment.

Multiple carcinomas are classified according to their temporal appearance as either synchronous or metachronous. However, these terms are used inconsistently. Some authors define *synchronous carcinomas* as neoplasms that are diagnosed at the same time or within 6 months of identification of the primary lesion and *metachronous neoplasms* as those that develop more than 6 months after the index tumor. Others use the term "synchronous carcinoma" for neoplasms that are identified only during the initial evaluation of the index tumor.

Prospective endoscopic studies of head and neck cancer patients indicate that additional simultaneous primary tumors will be found during workup of the index tumor in almost 20% of cases (Schwartz et al., 1994). Gluckman and colleagues observed that the average interval between the diagnosis of the first and second metachronous carcinoma

(i.e., those appearing 6 months or more after the index tumor) was 26 months, with a range of 8 months to 6 years (Gluckman et al., 1980).

The incidence of second primary tumors seems to depend on the anatomic site of the first one. Schwartz and colleagues found that the incidence of a second primary tumor ranged from 10% for squamous cell carcinoma of the mobile portion of the tongue to 46% for carcinoma of the base of the tongue (Schwartz et al., 1994). Derrick and others concluded that patients with supraglottic carcinoma are at higher risk for the development of a secondary primary tumor than patients with glottic carcinoma (Derrick et al., 1980). McGuirt et al. (1982) found that subsequent primary tumors were nearly evenly distributed among the head and neck, esophagus, and lungs. Patients with lung or esophageal cancer have a much lower cure, i.e., considerably fewer patients with cancer at these sites will survive long enough to remain at risk for the development of a second primary cancer in a head-and-neck site.

Despite variation in the incidence of second primary cancers, clinicians should be aware that a patient with one head and neck epidermoid carcinoma is at high risk for the development of a second primary tumor nearby. Moreover, the second primary tumor will most likely be the cause of death. In McGuirt's series, only 7 of 52 patients survived a second cancer to develop a third; only 3 patients had a fourth primary tumor develop (McGuirt et al., 1982). Thus, new symptoms should not always be attributed to the original tumor.

We studied causes of death for patients with head and neck cancer for two separate decades by comparing the autopsy reports from 1955 to 1965 with those from 1973 to 1983 (Goepfert, 1984). Between these two periods, the proportion of deaths caused by distant metastasis increased from 17% to 32.3%. Death from uncontrolled tumors above the clavicle dropped from 30% to 15.3%, and fatal treatment complications dropped from 24.7% to 10.5%. On the other hand, the proportion of deaths caused by unrelated nonmalignant disease increased from 14.7% to 27.7%, and deaths caused by second malignant tumors remained at 14.2% (Goepfert, 1984).

POTENTIALLY MALIGNANT LESIONS OF THE UPPER AERODIGESTIVE TRACT

DEFINITION

Precancerosis describes a pathological condition of the UADT mucosa from which a malignant tumor develops more often than from other benign epithelial lesions. According to one definition, a precancerous lesion of the squamous epithelium is characterized by cellular atypia and loss of normal maturation and stratification, short of carcinoma *in situ* (Shanmugaratnam et al., 1991). Others believe that any benign hyperplastic aberration with surface keratosis is precancerous, and still others consider exclusively carcinoma *in situ* (CIS) to be precancerous.

The concept of precancer assumes that the development of invasive cancer is preceded by a slow process during which the normal epithelium passes through various stages of hyperplasia, sometimes followed after several years by malignant change limited to the surface epithelium. Implicit in the term is the concept that irreversible molecular events have already taken place that lead to invasive cancer. Since this is impossible to determine, the term "potentially malignant" is preferable to precancerous or premalignant (Johnson et al., 1993).

The natural history of neoplastic development in experimental models, and presumably in humans as well, can be separated into three stages: initiation, promotion, and progression (Pitot, 1982). The last stage can be divided into two substages, the first including epithelial abnormalities that potentially can progress into an invasive neoplasm, dysplasia, or CIS, and the second characterized by the presence of an invasive carcinoma. Because the natural history of neoplastic development occurs subclinically, arriving at an accurate diagnosis early in the process may be impossible even with direct microscopic endoscopy. Invasive carcinoma, however, can be distinguished by clinical means and subsequently confirmed by histopathologic examination. Precise identification of epithelial abnormalities of the mucosa requires that surgeons and histopathologists work together to evaluate the microscopic features of a biopsy specimen (Ferlito, 1995).

In any event, cancer arises from a cell that has been altered in such a way as to undergo fundamental genetic changes that endow the cell with aggressive behavior as manifested in its clinical and biological features. Advancements in molecular pathology have contributed to the understanding of the underlying processes but have rendered some classic clinical terms inappropriate for describing histologic features. For example, clinicians use the term "leukoplakia" to indicate any white plaque or patch, but this term is not suitable for histological diagnosis. Also not suitable are the terms "erythroplakia," for reddish patches of raised epithelium; "erythroleukoplakia," for mixed forms of white and red mucosal changes; or "pachydermia" for large areas involved by leukoplakia. These conditions are common to all mucous membranes that contain epithelium that is normally of the nonkeratinized, stratified squamous type. Despite the considerable effort expended to define the supposed differences between keratosis, hyperkeratosis, leukoplakia, and pachydermia, these terms seem to describe mere variants of a single type of reactive keratotic change that the histologic term "keratosis" would most appropriately denote (Fig. 4–1).

Nevertheless, some so-called precancerous lesions will regress or stop in the progression toward cancer; others that are indistinguishable in their macroscopic and microscopic features will become malignant because of various noxious exogenic and endogenic influences (Decosse, 1983). The fundamental questions with regard to potentially malignant lesions are when and under what conditions do benign hyperplastic aberrations of the UADT epithelium become malignant.

CLASSIFICATION AND HISTOLOGY

Although neither the clinical nor the histologic classifications are entirely satisfactory, changes in the squamous epithelium of the UADT can be grouped under the following headings:

- Keratosis-hyperplasia
- Dysplasia: low grade (mild)
- Dysplasia: moderate grade (moderate)

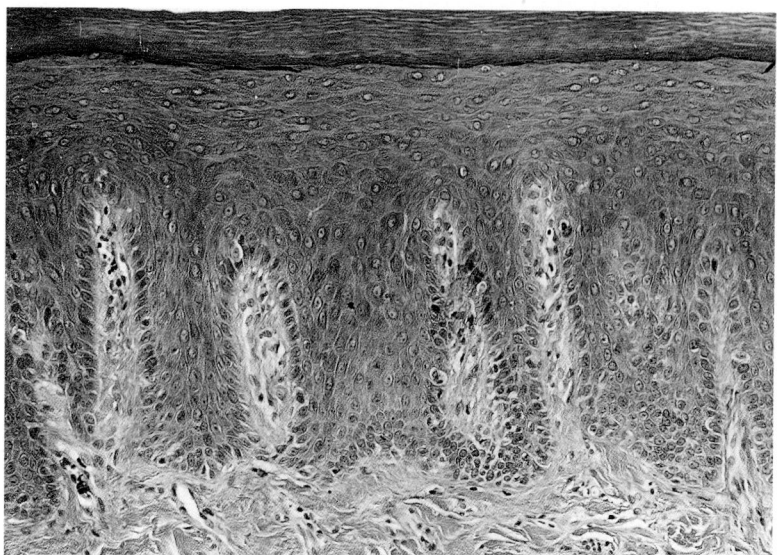

Figure 4–1. Keratosis. Orderly maturation and no evidence of abnormalities associated with dysplasia are present. Hyperkeratosis is visible in the superficial layer.

- Dysplasia: high grade (severe)
- Carcinoma *in situ* (CIS)

These headings represent an attempt to assign risk to various histologic abnormalities thought to be typical of the progression from normal epithelium to cancer. However, the biological behavior of epithelial hyperplasia differs according to its location in the UADT. For example, more than 20 classifications have been proposed for epithelial hyperplasia of the larynx (Kambic and Gale, 1995). Most cancer centers use a classification system similar to that proposed by the World Health Organization (WHO) in 1991 (Shanmurgaratama et al., 1991).

In the oral cavity, the histologic classification of potentially malignant lesions is less complicated, but the clinical classifications are still not universally accepted. Most cancer centers use the WHO classification of dysplasia for histologic diagnosis (Shanmurgaratama et al., 1991) and use the WHO definitions of clinical leukoplakia (Axell et al., 1984, 1996; WHO, 1978) for clinical diagnosis.

The traditional term "dysplasia" seems to have been replaced by "intraepithelial neoplasia," because the epithelial changes are considered to be the morphologic manifestation of a neoplastic process. In this chapter, the terms "squamous intraepithelial neoplasm" (SIN) and "dysplasia" are used interchangeably.

HISTOLOGIC APPEARANCE OF POTENTIALLY MALIGNANT LESIONS

Three grades of dysplasia, or SIN, are recognized on the basis of the extent of nuclear abnormalities and the proportion of epithelial thickness showing loss of normal stratification. Dysplasia coexists with invasive carcinoma; the potential for developing invasive carcinoma increases with the grade of dysplasia (Table 4–2). Following are descriptions of typical histologic features of mild, moderate, and severe dysplasia and those of CIS.

Mild Dysplasia (SIN I)

Squamous intraepithelial neoplasm grade I is characterized by slight nuclear abnormalities that are most marked in the basal third of the epithelial layer and are minimal in the upper layers, where the cells show maturation and stratification. A few normal mitoses may be seen in the parabasal layers but no abnormal mitoses are found. Keratosis and chronic inflammation are usually present. These lesions should be distinguished from squamous cell hyperplasia (Fig. 4–2).

Moderate Dysplasia (SIN II)

In moderate dysplasia, nuclear abnormalities are more marked than in mild dysplasia and the nucleoli tend to be prominent; these changes are most marked in the lower two-thirds of the epithelium. Moderate nuclear

Table 4–2. Morphological Features of Epithelial Dysplasia

Organizational Features	Cytologic Features
Drop-shaped rete processes	Increased number of mitotic figures
Cellular pleomorphism	Mitoses in upper layers of the epithelium
Loss of polarity of the basal cells	Increased nuclear-cytoplasmic ratio
Several layers of basaloid cells	Anisonucleosis
Cell crowding	Abnormal mitoses
Reduced intercellular cohesion	Nuclear hyperchromatism
Keratinization of single cells or cell groups	Enlarged nucleoli
Irregular epithelial stratification	

abnormalities may persist up to the surface, but cell maturation and stratification are evident in the upper layers. Normal mitoses are present in the parabasal and intermediate layers but no abnormal mitoses are present. These lesions may be associated with keratosis (Fig. 4–3).

Severe Dysplasia (SIN III)

Severely dysplastic epithelia show marked nuclear abnormalities and loss of maturation involving more than two-thirds of the epithelial layer, with some stratification of the most superficial layers. Nuclear pleomorphism is common, and some of the cells may contain bizarre nuclei. Nucleoli can be prominent in some areas but in others the entire nucleus is hyperchromatic. Mitoses are found high up in the epithelium, and atypical mitoses may be present. The cells are generally not as crowded as in classic CIS and are usually more differentiated, with intercellular bridges connecting the atypical cells. Evidence of some maturation and strat-

ification of the cells in the most superficial layers distinguishes these lesions from CIS (Fig. 4–4). The SIN grade III lesions are frequently associated with keratosis. Severe dysplasia carries the same high risk for the development of invasive carcinoma as CIS and is therefore grouped with CIS for clinical purposes.

Carcinoma *In Situ*

In CIS the full thickness of the squamous epithelium shows the cellular features of carcinoma without stromal invasion. Carcinoma *in situ* is usually of the large cell keratinizing type; the epithelial cells have markedly abnormal hyperchromatic nuclei and variable cytoplasmic keratinization that closely resembles severe dysplasia (Fig. 4–5). Some cells may have scanty cytoplasm and show minimial or no evidence of squamous differentiation (Fig. 4–6). Mitoses occur high up in the epithelium; atypical mitoses may be present. These lesions can extend into the

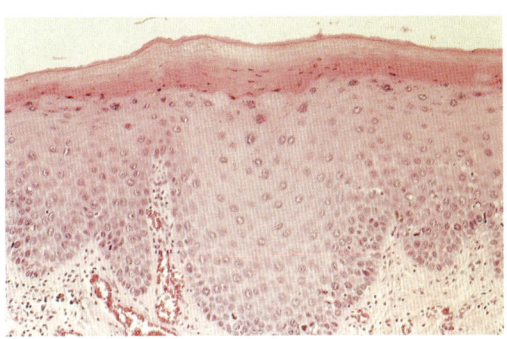

Figure 4–2. Mild dysplasia, or SIN 1. Enlarged hyperchromasia nuclei can be seen crowding in the lower third of the epithelium.

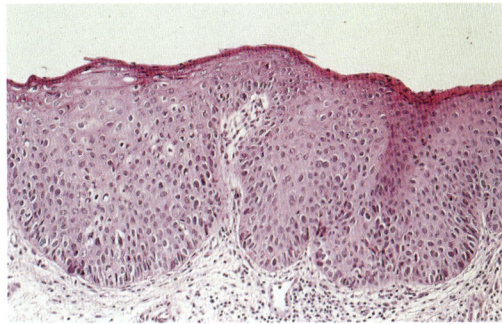

Figure 4–3. Moderate epithelial dysplasia, or SIN 2. Nuclear hyperchromia, pleomorphism, and cellular crowding involve about half of the epithelial thickness.

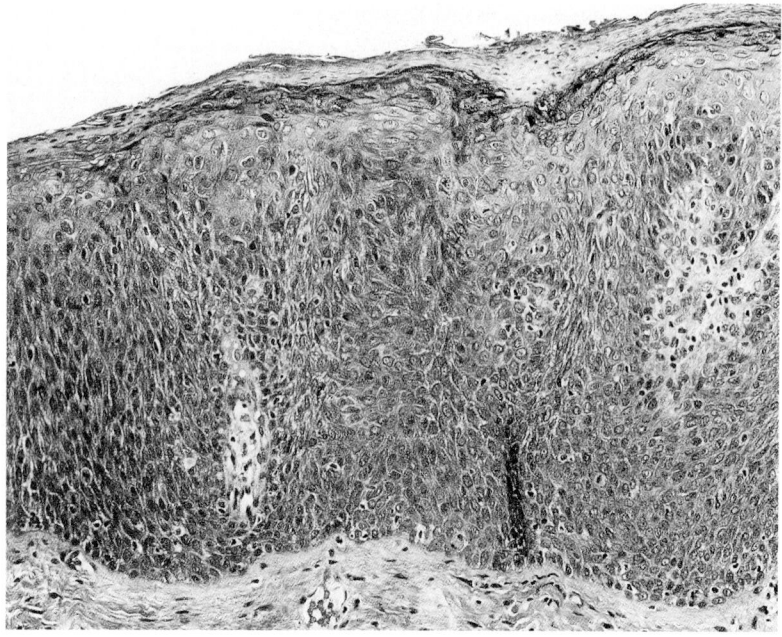

Figure 4–4. Severe epithelial dysplasia, or SIN 3, showing marked loss of cellular organization and polarity, and enlarged and hyperchromic nuclei involving more than two-thirds of the epithelial thickness. Flattened and matured cells are present at the epithelial surface.

ducts of adjacent seromucinous glands, but the basement membrane is intact.

OTHER POTENTIALLY MALIGNANT LESIONS

Clinical Oral Leukoplakia

Of all leukoplakias of the UADT, 80% are found in the oral cavity; most of the remaining 20% are found on the vocal cords and are more aptly termed "laryngeal keratosis" (Bouquot and Whitaker, 1994; Kam-

bic and Gale, 1986). In 1996 an international working group redefined *oral leukoplakia* as "a predominantly white lesion of the oral mucosa that cannot be characterized as any other definable lesion; some oral leukoplakias will transform into cancer" (Axell et al., 1996). This group also recommended that a distinction be made between a provisional (clinical) and a definitive diagnosis of leukoplakia. A *definitive* diagnosis of oral leukoplakia comes after its identification and elimination of suspected etiologic factors, and is for lesions lasting more than 2–4

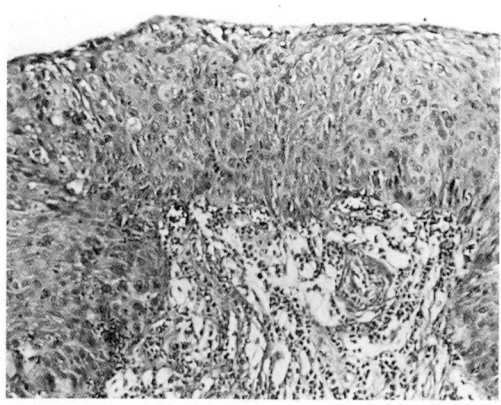

Figure 4–5. Carcinoma *in situ.* Dysplastic changes extend throughout the entire thickness of the epithelium.

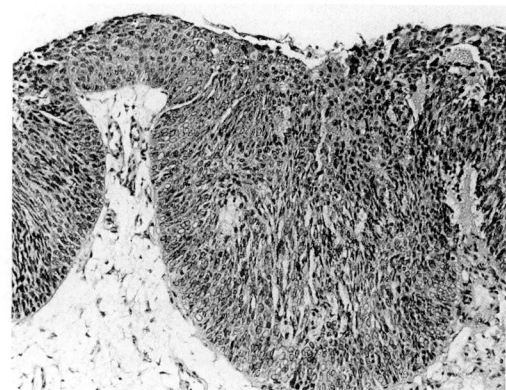

Figure 4–6. Carcinoma *in situ* composed of poorly differentiated cells with no keratinization.

weeks. A biopsy with histopathologic examination is required to rule out any other definable lesion and to assess the extent of dysplasia. If carcinoma (*in situ* or invasive) is found in a biopsy specimen of an oral leukoplakia, then the *provisional* diagnosis of leukoplakia should be replaced by the definitive histopathologic diagnosis.

Schepman et al. (1996) tested the revised definition of oral leukoplakia and the distinction between the provisional and definitive diagnoses and found both to be suitable for epidemiologic studies. The 0.6% prevalence of provisional leukoplakia was reduced to 0.2% after definitive diagnoses by histologic examination.

Proliferative Verrucous Leukoplakia

In 1985, Hansen and associates (1985) described a unique form of oral leukoplakia that was called "proliferative verrucous leukoplakia" (PVL) (Fig. 4–7). Clinically, PVL

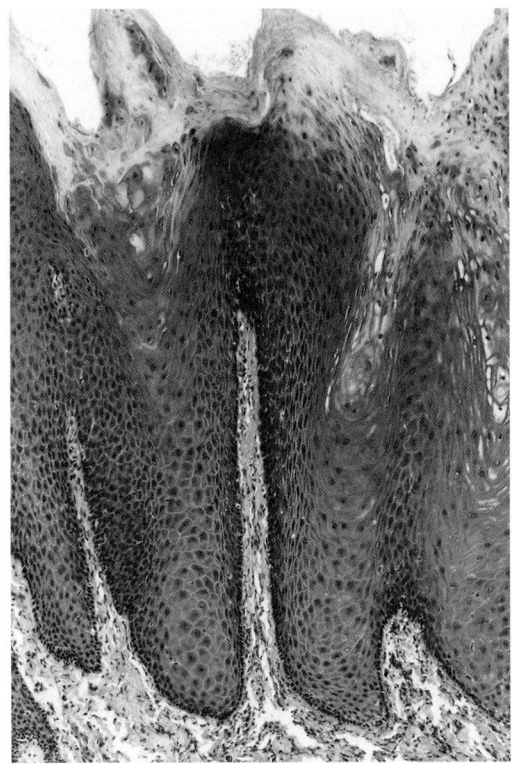

Figure 4–7. Proliferative verrucous leukoplakia. The epithelium is considerably thickened with surface keratinization, papillomatosis, and basal cell proliferation with hyperchromic nuclei and dropping of rete ridges.

presented as a progressive, expanding exophytic/verrucal white lesion. Of the 30 patients studied, 83% of the men and 50% of the women smoked, but the women manifested the disorder four times as much as men.

The microscopic appearance of PVL varies depending on the stage of the lesions. Early PVL appears as a benign hyperkeratosis that is indistinguishable from other simple, benign keratotic lesions. Over time, the condition progresses to a papillary, exophytic proliferation that resembles localized lesions of verrucous leukoplakia or "verrucous hyperplasia." In later stages, this papillary proliferation grows downward to produce well-differentiated squamous epithelium with broad, blunt rete ridges. This epithelium then invades the underlying lamina propria. At this stage, PVL is indistinguishable from verrucous carcinoma. In the final stages, the invading epithelium becomes less differentiated, transforming into an unequivocal squamous cell carcinoma. Because of the variable clinical and histopathologic appearance of PVL, careful correlation of clinical and histological findings is required for its diagnosis.

Lesions from Smokeless Tobacco

Tobacco chewing is the practice of placing a portion of leaf, plug, cake, or threads of tobacco between the cheek and gingiva after it has been chewed. Snuff dipping, on the other hand, involves placing a pinch of powdered or cut tobacco between the cheek or lip and the gingiva or beneath the tongue.

The histologic changes associated with the use of smokeless tobacco vary with the type and geographic origin of the product, but snuff-related lesions have some common features. The epithelium is nearly always thickened because of a vacuolated surface layer that occasionally contains remnants of cell nuclei (Fig. 4–8). This change is associated more often with the use of Scandinavian wet snuff rather than with the dry, weakly alkaline snuff used in the U.S. (Axell, 1993; Bouquot and Schroeder, 1993; Thomas and Kearsley, 1937). The koilocytosis and chevron pattern of keratinization present in many snuff-related lesions are regarded as distinctive findings associated with tobacco use. Occasionally present are subepithelial changes such as a plasma cell inflammatory

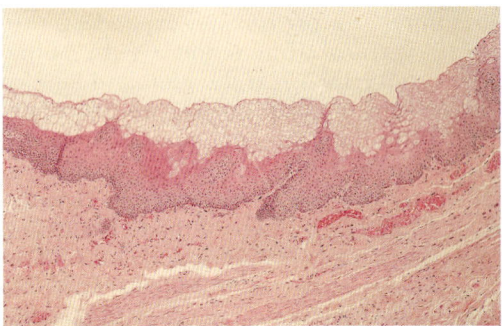

Figure 4–8. Smokeless tobacco lesion. Hyperkeratosis and prominent intracellular edema are present but no dysplasia.

reaction or hyalinization parallel to the surface of the epithelium.

Oral Lichen Planus

Lichen planus afflicts 14% of Americans under the age of 75 years (Batsakis et al., 1994), although only 1 in 100 seeks medical attention for the disorder. Oral lichen planus is less common, with an estimated prevalence of about 1% or 2%. It can occur with or without skin involvement (Batsakis et al., 1994). Oral lesions are characteristically bilaterally symmetrical and are more constant, over time, than those of the skin. Palatal or sublingual involvement is rare, but oral candidiasis is frequent (Batsakis et al., 1994).

Common features of oral lichen planus (Fig. 4–9) include hyperparakeratosis and hyperorthokeratosis, with a dense, band-like lymphoid cell infiltration near the epithelial basement membrane and superficial stroma. Basal epithelial cells often show liquefactive degenerative obliteration or effacement of the epithelial–stromal junction and a sawtooth configuration of the rete ridges. A narrow eosinophilic band adjacent to the basement epithelial membrane is often noted, as is fibrinogen. Eosinophilic ovoid (colloid or civette) bodies and necrotic keratinocytes are occasionally seen at the basal cell level or within the inflammatory infiltrate. Epithelial maturation and cytomorphology are normal (Krutchkoff and Eisenberg, 1985).

DIFFERENTIAL DIAGNOSIS OF POTENTIALLY MALIGNANT LESIONS

Inflammatory and other nonmalignant lesions may be associated with hyperplasia and dysplasia of the overlying squamous epithelium the so-called pseudoepitheliomatous hyperplasia (Fig. 4–10). Because changes such as these are typical of tuberculosis and granular cell tumor, careful examination of the lamina propria is essential in any biopsy sample showing atypical epithelial changes. Particular care should be taken with laryn-

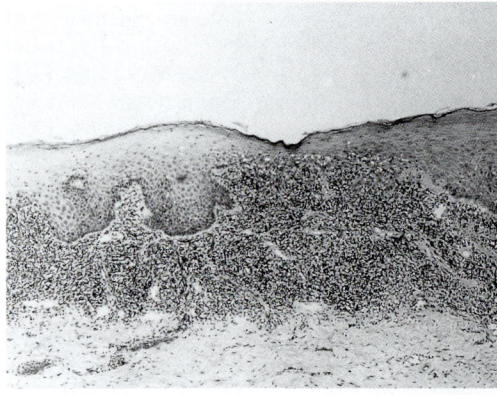

Figure 4–9. Lichen planus. Hyperorthokeratosis and band-like inflammatory infiltrate are present but no dysplasia.

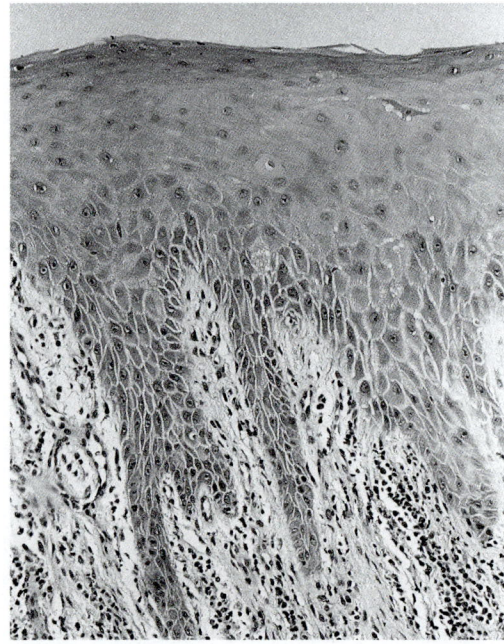

Figure 4–10. Pseudoepitheliomatous hyperplasia. Thin, elongated, branched and pointed rete ridges are visible.

geal samples, since the amount of material available is often small and the histologic features of tuberculosis may be nonspecific. Information about the patient's clinical history, particularly with regard to previous lesions of the larynx and their treatment, is important for two reasons. First, the site of a previous biopsy may show dysplasia that mimics a precancerous lesion. Second, previous irradiation is one of the most common causes of dysplastic change in the UADT mucosa. This change, which can be severe, is unrelated to malignant transformation.

The presence of carcinomatous tissue below the surface of the covering epithelium does not always indicate invasive carcinoma. The CIS often develops all the way to the columnar cells of the ducts of the seromucinous glands in the larynx. The columnar cells may degenerate or disappear near the lesion, a condition that could be misinterpreted as a focus of invasive squamous cell carcinoma.

MALIGNANT TRANSFORMATION OF SQUAMOUS INTRAEPITHELIAL NEOPLASMS (SIN) AND OTHER LESIONS

Most investigators accept the fact that epithelial dysplasia of the UADT can progress to squamous cell carcinoma in some patients. However, meaningful comparisons of studies that chart this progression over time require that two obstacles be overcome: differences in therapeutic approaches to dysplasia and the lack of specific, reproducible criteria for grading dysplasia (Lippman et al., 1993; Lumerman et al., 1995; Pindborg et al., 1985).

EPITHELIAL DYSPLASIA OF THE ORAL CAVITY

Studies have been published on the biologic behavior of epithelial displasia of the oral cavity (OED) (Table 4–3). Mincer and others (1972) studied 56 patients who had either moderate or severe dysplasia or CIS. Of the 45 patients for whom follow-up information was available, 20 had surgical excision of the dysplasias, and 7 of them (35%) had recurrence. Ten patients in the follow-up group (22%) had no treatment and showed no clinical changes in up to 8 years. Lesions in five other patients (11%) either disappeared or shrank without treatment other than the biopsy; lesions in five others (11%) grew or became more severe in up to 8 years of follow-up; and the remaining five patients developed squamous cell carcinoma in up to 7 years. Dysplastic leukoplakias showed malignant transformation in an average of 8.1 years.

In a series of 61 Danish patients with premalignant oral lesions (Vedtofte et al., 1987), 47 patients with epithelial dysplasia were treated by excision and followed for an average of 3.9 years (range 1 to 5 years). Invasive squamous cell carcinoma developed in 3 patients during this period. In another study, 7 (16%) of 44 patients with OED developed invasive squamous cell carcinoma within a mean follow-up period of 33.6 months (Lumerman et al., 1995). Interestingly, 2 (3.7%) of the 54 biopsy specimens were from clinically and histologically verrucous hyperplasia with mild dysplasia.

Table 4–3. Published Cases of Oral Epithelial Dysplasia that Transformed to Invasive Squamous Cell Carcinoma

Reference	Cases n	Transformed Invasive Squamous Cell Carcinoma n (%)	Transformation Time (years)
Mincer et al. (1972)	45	5 (11.0)	Up to 8
Banoczy and Csiba (1976)	68	9 (13.2)	1–20
			Mean 6.3
Pindborg et al. (1977)	61	4 (6.6)	Up to 7
Silverman et al. (1984)	22	8 (36.6)	Mean 8.1
Lumerman et al. (1995)	44	7 (16.0)	Up to 6.5
Total	240	33 (13.8)	

Modified from Lumerman et al. 1995.

In summary, evidence from the five studies of OED (Table 4–3) shows that 33 (13.8%) of 240 patients developed invasive squamous cell carcinoma within a follow-up period of up to 20 years.

DYSPLASIA OF THE LARYNX

Moderate epithelial dysplasia of the laryngeal mucosa has a significant risk of malignant transformation. Hojslet et al. (1989) found that risk to be the same (40%) as that of the combined group of severe dysplasia/CIS lesions. Hellquist et al. (1982) and Riera Velasco et al. (1987) corroborated this level of risk, although their transformation rates were lower (20%) (Table 4–4). Hojslet et al. (1989), Bosatra et al. (1997), and Blackwell et al. (1995) cautioned that even mild epithelial dysplasia bears a 4% risk of malignant transformation.

CARCINOMA IN SITU OF THE UPPER AERODIGESTIVE TRACT

Carcinoma *in situ* without adjacent invasive squamous cell carcinoma represented 13.1% of all UADT carcinomas diagnosed from 1935 through 1984 in residents of Rochester, Minnesota (Bouquot et al., 1988). The most common site was the vermillion border of the lip, followed by the oral cavity, pharynx, larynx, and nasal/paranasal region. The average age of patients with CIS was 60 years, and men were affected almost eight times more often than women. Almost all afflicted individuals smoked and a high proportion abused alcohol as well. Published values for progression of CIS to invasive carcinoma range from 3.5% to 25% for laryngeal CIS and from 11.1% to 50.0% for oral cavity CIS (Bouquot et al., 1988).

Carcinoma *In Situ* of the Larynx

This condition has been followed more extensively than CIS of other UADT sites, in part because three-fourths of the 468 patients with UADT CIS followed after diagnosis have had laryngeal involvement (Bouquot and Gnepp, 1991). Up to 20% of laryngeal CIS lesions become invasive (Table 4–3), with untreated cases transforming at the highest rates (33.3% to 90.0%) (Bouquot and Gnepp, 1991).

Because of differences in the criteria for diagnosing laryngeal dysplasia and CIS, some authors have recommended a classification system similar to the SIN system described earlier. In this system, laryngeal intraepithelial neoplasia grade I (LIN I) denotes mild epithelial dysplasia; LIN II, moderate dysplasia; and LIN III, severe dysplasia or CIS. Use of this system should improve comparability among diagnostic protocols (Bouquot and Gnepp, 1991).

OTHER POTENTIALLY MALIGNANT LESIONS

Clinical Oral Leukoplakia

The presence of oral leukoplakia increases the risk of developing oral carcinoma (Axell et al., 1996). However, specifics are lacking as to the time, course of progression, and the influence of a variety of cofactors. In a prospective study of 257 patients with oral

Table 4–4. Malignant Transformation of Laryngeal Intraepithelial Lesions

Reference	Type and Degree of Dysplasia	Patients n	Patients with Subsequent Carcinoma n (%)	Follow-up Period
Kambic and Gale (1995)	Simple	2757	7 (0.3)	15 years
	Atypical	105	10 (9.5)	15 years
Crissman and Zarbo (1991)	Keratosis without atypia	362	5 (1.4)	
	Keratosis with atypia	230	31 (13.5)	
	CIS/severe dysplasia	367	46 (12.5)	
Riera Velasco et al. (1987)	Keratosis	46	1 (2.2)	123 months
	Moderate	31	6 (19.3)	37 months
	Severe	5	1 (20.0)	110 months
	CIS	5	1 (20.0)	14 months

CIS, carcinoma *in situ*.

leukoplakia who were followed for an average of 8.1 years, 37 (15.7%) of the 235 patients without microscopic epithelial dysplasia developed oral carcinomas, and 8 (36.4%) of the 22 patients with leukoplakia and microscopic epithelial dysplasia developed oral carcinomas (Silverman et al., 1996).

Proliferative Verrucous Leukoplakia

Silverman and Gorsky (1997) studied 54 patients with PVL, 17 of whom were included in a report by Hansen et al. (1985). The patients were followed prospectively for an average of 11.6 years after the initial biopsy. The demographics of the 54 patients were slightly different from those of the original 17 patients; women still outnumbered men 4 to 1, and the mean age at diagnosis was 62 years. Seventy percent of the 54 patients developed a squamous cell carcinoma at a previous site of PVL (mean time of occurrence, 7.7 years), and 21 patients died of their carcinomas. Interestingly, only 17 of the 54 patients used tobacco in any form. This high rate of malignant transformation would likely be even higher if the follow-up period were extended. The 50% mortality rate by the time of the 1997 report (Silverman and Gorsky, 1997) also would likely be higher if the observation period was extended.

Lesions from Smokeless Tobacco

One factor associated with the high incidence of oral cancer in India is the widespread use of smokeless tobacco. Oral cancer rates in India have been cited as being predictive of future trends in the U.S. if the use of smokeless tobacco continues to increase (Bouquot and Whitaker, 1994).

Although a correlation has been established between the use of snuff and clinical changes in the oral mucosa, the presence or extent of dysplasia is difficult to predict. In a study of 323 patients who had dipped snuff for an average of 9.5 years (Kaugers et al., 1989) only 17 developed premalignant or malignant lesions. Almost all of the epithelial dysplasias were either focally mild or mild, and only one was severe; only 1 of the 323 subjects developed squamous cell carcinoma. In another study, Kaugers et al. (1991) estimated that the mean duration of exposure to smokeless tobacco at the time of diagnosis of dysplasia or carcinoma was 48.6 years.

Wray and McGuirt (1993) reviewed 128 patients with oral cavity carcinoma who also used smokeless tobacco but not other tobacco products or alcohol. Most of the subjects were white women whose average age was 78 years; 78% had used smokeless tobacco for 40 years or more, and 26% had a second oral cavity tumor appear at a new site more than 2 years after having been treated for the index carcinoma. Eighty percent of the carcinomas were located where the quid was held between the cheek and gum; others were located on the tonsil, retromolar trigone, floor of the mouth, and lip. Clinical leukoplakia, erythroplakia, or both were associated with carcinoma in 40% of the cases. Moreover, 39% of the patients were known to have had leukoplakia either before or after treatment of their cancer. Most of the carcinomas were moderately to well differentiated.

Nearly all studies involving Scandinavian subjects report that mucosal lesions can be reversed when the subjects stop using smokeless tobacco. However, the demographic characteristics of Scandinavian users of smokeless tobacco were distinctly different from those described by Kaugers et al. (1989, 1991) and Wray and McGuirt (1993), and also from the typical, much younger smokeless-tobacco user of today in the U.S. Nevertheless, these studies do demonstrate the adverse effects of long-term use of smokeless tobacco.

Oral Lichen Planus

Whether oral lichen planus can undergo malignant change has been debated for almost 80 years. Estimates of the frequency of this change have ranged from 0% to 12.5% depending on the subject population and the criteria used to define lichen planus (Batsakis et al., 1994). In a critical review of 220 cases of reported malignant transformation, Krutchkoff et al. (1978) found only 15 that satisfied the criteria. Discrepancies were also noted with regard to epithelial dysplasia in oral lichen planus and the rate at which carcinoma developed.

Clearly, the criteria for diagnosing lichen planus have not been uniformly applied, nor have the diagnostic results always been accurate. Nevertheless, follow-up studies (mean period 5.33 years) of 1955 patients with oral lichen planus have shown a rather consistent overall cancer frequency of 2.8% (Batsakis et al., 1994). The small but clinically important premalignant potential of oral lichen planus was validated by Barnard et al. (1993). In a study of 241 patients with histologically confirmed oral lichen planus, 9 (3.7%) were found to have developed well-differentiated invasive carcinoma or CIS near areas of lichen planus.

AUXILIARY AND ADVANCED DIAGNOSTIC METHODS

The use of light microscopy for assessing dysplasia can give both false-positive results (overestimation of malignant potential) and false-negative results (underestimation of malignant potential). Bosatra and colleagues (1997) have estimated that 3% of patients with oral lesions and 4% of patients with laryngeal lesions classified as mild dysplasia by light-microscopic histology may develop carcinoma later. Recent efforts to develop other methods for assessing dysplasia have led to new applications of cytological and histological techniques as well as chemical or functional analyses. Some of these techniques are described below.

PROLIFERATION MARKERS

Markers of cell proliferation including the number of argyrophilic nucleolar organizer regions (Ag-NOR) and the presence of proliferating cell nuclear antigen (PCNA) and the Ki-67 (Mib-1) antigen have been used to study keratosis, SIN, and CIS of the UADT (Coltera et al., 1992; Cör et al., 1997; Hirsch et al., 1992; Shin et al., 1993; Zidar et al., 1996). The Ag-NOR technique alone cannot distinguish an individual dysplastic lesion or CIS of the UADT (Ashworth and Helliwell, 1988; Cör et al., 1997; Hirsh et al., 1992), and Ki-67 seems to identify SIN more precisely than does PCNA (Cör et al., 1997; Coltera et al., 1992; Zidar et al., 1996). In general, the presence and extent of these markers correspond to the histologic grade of mucosal SIN, and thus the extent of proliferative activity can be used to assess the risk of progression to overt carcinoma (Cör et al., 1997; Jones et al., 1994; Zidar et al., 1996).

DNA HISTOGRAMS

Crissman and Fu (1986) used DNA analysis to study six patients with extensive intraepithelial alterations of the laryngeal mucosa. DNA histograms were generated from Feulgen-stained tissue sections by means of spectrophotometric microscopy. Aneuploid DNA indicative of neoplastic transformation was found in all six cases. Crissman and Zarbo (1991) later used image analysis to assess the DNA content of 56 laryngeal glottic biopsy specimens with a spectrum of SIN (Crissman and Farbo, 1991). Aneuploidy was observed in all specimens graded SIN II and SIN III, and all had prominent keratinization. These authors concluded that atypical DNA distribution can reveal malignant transformation earlier than morphologic criteria.

Cytophotometric analysis of nuclear DNA has also been applied to oral dysplasia (Abdel-Salam et al., 1987, 1990). When Saku and Sato (1983) investigated the predictive value of DNA histograms in oral precancerous lesions, they found that those lesions that developed into carcinomas showed a particular DNA pattern regardless of their degree of dysplasia. By analyzing cytologic smears, Doseva and co-workers (1984) found that samples from leukoplakia and lichen planus that later transformed to invasive carcinoma showed hypodiploid and hypertetraploid DNA distribution patterns.

IMMUNOHISTOCHEMISTRY

The value of immunohistochemistry comes from the ability to apply a wide variety of techniques (e.g., immunofluorescence, immunoperoxidase, and avidin-biotin complex techniques) to paraffin-embedded sections of fixed tissue in order to visualize constituents of the cells and tissues. In studies of premalignant and malignant lesions, epithelial surface antigens such as blood groups and differentiation products such as desmosomes are reduced or lost as the cells progress from dysplasia.

Both the nucleus and cytoplasmic structure develop changes during malignant transformation. Cytokeratins in non-neoplastic squamous laryngeal epithelium typically are expressed as intermediate and high molecular weight, but not as low-molecular-weight species. Moreover, cells in the basal layer of stratified squamous cell epithelium contain keratins of molecular mass up to 58 kD, whereas the higher-molecular-weight keratins are found in more superficial layers. Accordingly, the superficial layers are strongly positive for AE1, AE3, and K8.12 monoclonal antibodies, the suprabasal cells are weakly positive, and the basal layer is usually negative. Reactivity in the lower layers for K8.63, which recognizes the highest-molecular-weight keratin, is positive only in hyperkeratosis. On the other hand, CAM5.2, a monoclonal antibody directed against low molecular weight cytokeratins (i.e., the 8-, 18-, and 19-polypeptide units), is always negative in non-neoplastic squamous cells. Thus CAM5.2-positive staining can be a good marker for malignant transformation in stratified epithelium (Cardesa et al., 1997; Mallofre et al., 1993).

Genetic Alterations

Tumor Suppressor Genes

P53 overexpression and mutation. Of the known tumor suppressor genes (TSG), *p53* has been the most intensively investigated in tumors of various organs including the UADT. Theoretically, a mutant of *p53* that is ineffective in suppressing tumor development may accumulate in premalignant and malignant tissues. Unfortunately, mutant *p53* cannot as yet be selectively labeled by immunohistochemistry, and thus other states may be associated with elevations in normal or wild-type *p53*. On the other hand, abnormalities in *p53* have been reported in cancer and adjacent dysplasia, and *p53* may prove to be a useful marker of potential malignancy.

The functional inactivation of *p53* through mutation or allelic loss plays an important part in the development of various human neoplasms (Marshall, 1991). An intranuclear mutant *p53* has been shown to abolish the tumor suppressor activity of the protein and to have a dominant effect on cell proliferation (Harris, 1990). Others have suggested that *p53* mutations are an early event in the development of squamous cell carcinomas of the head and neck (El-Naggar et al., 1995b).

In one study, accumulated *p53* protein was detected by immunohistochemistry in 89%

of oral leukoplaktic lesions excised from 40 patients (of whom 30 were smokers) but was not found in normal oral mucosa from 7 nonsmoking control subjects (Lippman et al., 1995). In samples positive for p53, the amounts of p53 were highest in the basal cell layers, lower in the parabasal layers, and absent in superficial layers, findings that correlated inversely with cellular differentiation and directly with cellular proliferation. The extent of positive staining in these lesions also correlated with increasing histological severity. Interestingly, an inverse relation was observed between high levels of p53 protein and response to retinoid acid treatment. Oral cavity exposure to carcinogens, especially tobacco, may disrupt p53 function in some oral epithelial cells and promotes regional clonal outgrowth (Lippman et al., 1995).

An immunohistochemical analysis of 89 cases of established squamous cell carcinoma of the larynx (Cardesa et al., 1997) showed no correlation with prognosis or with clinicopathological features. However, p53 accumulation was identified in 32% of low-grade dysplasia samples and in 50% of CIS samples, which suggests that p53 accumulation may reflect early changes in the development of squamous cell carcinoma. Specifically, clusters of p53-positive cells were seen in metaplastic squamous epithelium, just above the basal layer. These cells were morphologically indistinguishable from the surrounding p53-negative cells by hematoxylin-eosin staining. In contrast, in high-grade dysplasia and CIS, p53 staining was present throughout the entire thickness of the epithelium and was accompanied by alterations in the size and shape of the nuclei. Staining was also more intense in high-grade lesions than in low-grade ones (Nadal et al., 1995). Other authors have reported similar changes in p53 in early laryngeal lesions (Dolcetti et al., 1992; Gale et al., 1993).

Rowley and co-workers recently observed p53 protein overexpressed in seven of nine oral dysplastic lesions and found *p53* mutations in exons 5 and 6 in four of these lesions as well. However, the overexpression and the mutations were not always coexistent, suggesting that gene mutation may be only one mechanism responsible for stabilization of the p53 protein (Rowley et al., 1998). Studies that include immunohistochemical tests of p53 expression, *p53* gene mutations, and other factors in large numbers of premalignant oral lesions are required to resolve these discrepancies and clarify the underlying mechanisms (Landers et al., 1997).

Inactivation of the *p16* tumor suppressor gene. Potentially malignant head and neck lesions have also been studied for alterations in the *p16* tumor suppressor gene (Gallo et al., 1997; Liggett et al., 1996; Papadimitrakopoulou et al., 1997; van der Riet et al., 1994). Allelic loss at the site of *p16* has been found as frequently in potentially malignant head and neck lesions as in invasive head and neck cancers. Inactivation of *p16* is thought to be one of the earliest specific genetic events in the head and neck cancer pathway, occurring before *p53* inactivation (van der Riet et al., 1994). Detection of *p16* inactivation may be important in identifying premalignant lesions at high risk for malignant transformation. Further evidence pointing to the importance of the *p16* gene has been provided by *in vitro* studies in which p16 DNA introduced into head and neck cancer cell lines led to marked inhibition of cell growth (Liggett et al., 1996).

In a recent study (Papadimitrakopoulou et al., 1997), loss of p16 expression was found in 28 biopsies obtained from 17 patients with premalignant oral lesions (of a total 74 biopsies from 36 patients). A correlation was found between loss of heterozygosity (LOH) at 9p21 and loss of p16 expression by immunohistochemistry, supporting the concept that precancerous laryngeal lesions lacking p16 protein but overexpressing p53 were prone to progress to invasive cancer (Gallo et al., 1997). These results suggest that inactivation of the *p16* tumor suppressor gene is an early step toward malignant transformation in head and neck tissues.

Cytogenetics

Head and neck squamous cell carcinoma arises from a clonal population of cells that accumulate many genetic alterations over a multistep process (Carey et al., 1993). Traditional and newer cytogenetic techniques such as fluorescence *in situ* hybridization (FISH) and comparative genomic hybridization have been used to detect chromosomal abnormalities in potentially malignant oral lesions (Barrera et al., 1998).

Lee et al. (1993) examined formalin-fixed, paraffin-embedded tissue sections of oral leukoplakia lesions from 13 patients using specific probes for chromosomes 7 and 17. With this technique, normal somatic cells should produce two signals, although many normal cells in tissue sections may exhibit only one. Cells with more than two signals were seen in all lesions examined (range 0.5%–38.2%). In lesions from 12 of the 13 patients, more than 1% of the cells had more than two chromosome signals; in contrast, none of the normal control areas (lymphocytes in the same sections) or control samples (oral mucosa samples from normal volunteers) had more than 1% cells exhibiting two signals. These data indicate that most oral lesions contain abnormal chromosomal alterations that may presage the development of oral cancer (Lee et al., 1993).

Loss of Heterozygosity

Frequently found in multiple chromosomal loci in head and neck squamous cell cancer, loss of heterozygosity (LOH) may indicate the presence of tumor suppressor genes at these loci. Loss of heterozygosity has been studied in potentially malignant lesions of the oral cavity by several groups (El Naggar et al., 1995a; Mao et al., 1996b; Roz et al., 1996). In one study, LOH was found at two loci (9q21 and 3p14) in 51% of the patients studied, suggesting that losses of genetic material at these sites are frequent early events in head and neck cancer. In a series of 37 patients with potentially malignant lesions of the oral cavity, 7 of 19 patients who had LOH in their lesions developed squamous cell carcinoma, whereas only 1 of 18 patients without LOH developed carcinoma (Mao et al., 1996b).

Field Defect in the Upper Aerodigestive Tract

Patients with head and neck squamous cell cancer often present with metachronous or even synchronous neoplasms of the UADT that sometimes have a common clonal origin (Worsham et al., 1995a). Allelic losses also have been demonstrated in preinvasive and in invasive head and neck carcinomas (El-Naggar et al., 1995a). These findings support the existence of a "field defect" in the UADT. The concept that epithelial cells at several sites can transform independently has been recognized for some time at other tumor sites, such as the bladder, and may also apply to the UADT, particularly to the oral cavity (Sidransky et al., 1992; Waridel et al., 1997). Detection of genetic alterations in preinvasive tumors, i.e., early in tumor progression, may have potential clinical applications.

Cyclin D1 and Cyclin-Dependent Kinase Inhibitors

Cyclin-dependent kinase inhibitors have gained interest because of their putative potential for tumor suppression (Chen et al., 1995). The *p21* gene, which encodes one of these kinase inhibitors, is usually overexpressed in squamous cell carcinoma of the UADT. In normal epithelium, p21 is expressed in a few intermediate cells but not in basal or superficial layers; in SIN, p21 expression is present throughout the entire mucosal thickness (Cardesa et al., 1997; Fernandez et al., 1996). Amplification and subsequent overexpression of cyclin D1 appear in late-stage tumors and are therefore unlikely to affect the malignant transformation (Jares et al., 1994).

Reactivation of Telomerase

Activation of telomerase, associated with elongation of telomeres and cell immortalization (Soria et al., 1998), has been detected frequently in head and neck tumors, but not in most normal tissues. Telomerase activity has been found in more than half of oral leukoplakia lesions. Mutirangura and others (1996) also found an association between telomerase activity and the degree of dysplasia in oral leukoplakia lesions. In another series, all of the dysplastic and hyperplastic lesions adjacent to primary head and neck squamous cell carcinomas were telomerase positive, but none of the normal tissues were positive. This finding suggests that telomerase may be activated early in the tumorigenesis process (Mao et al., 1996a). Deactivation of telomerase may be a useful clinical marker for cancer risk assessment, particularly for the oral cavity. Antitelomerase drugs may even be a future treatment option (Mao et al., 1996a).

Other Biological Markers and Molecular Techniques

Other biological markers that have attracted study in the progression of potentially malignant lesions of the UADT include various markers of cell angiogenesis, cell–cell adhesion (such as E-cadherin), and enzymes such as the metalloproteinases, metalloproteinase inhibitors, and collagenases (Rowley et al., 1998). The roll of retinoic acid receptors is also being studied in the progression and treatment of potentially malignant lesions of the UADT (Lotan et al., 1995). Microsatellite instability (MI) has been observed in 23%–35% of potentially malignant lesions of the oral cavity (Mao et al., 1996a,b). However, the meaning of this finding is unclear for potentially malignant lesions of the head and neck.

MALIGNANT LESIONS OF THE UPPER AERODIGESTIVE TRACT

MICROINVASIVE SQUAMOUS CELL CARCINOMA

Distinct from potentially malignant lesions or from CIS is the superficially invasive or *microinvasive squamous cell carcinoma* (MIC), in which the integrity of the basement membrane is violated and a few scattered foci of neoplastic cells have invaded the underlying stroma. Given the presence of vascular spaces high in the lamina propria, even limited numbers of invading cells have access to blood vessels, the lymphatic system, and nerves, which could result in metastatic disease.

The depth of invasion at which a cancer is considered to be microinvasive is controversial and depends on the invasion site (Table 4–5). Kleinsasser and Glanz (1982) considered the defining depth of invasion for the vocal cords to be about 3 mm. For the oral cavity, Platz et al. (1982) specified that superficial invasion means less than 5 mm. Lederer and Managetta (1982) distinguished between carcinoma with pushing invasive borders (5 mm) and those with thin irregular infiltrative borders (3 mm). For the tongue and the floor of the mouth, limits for MIC have been named as 2 mm (Spiro et al., 1986), 1.5 (Mohit-Tabatabai et al., 1986),

Table 4.5. Requisite Invasion Depths for Microinvasive Squamous Cell Carcinoma in Head and Neck Sites

Reference	Patients n	Primary Site	Defining Thickness (mm)	Thickness Related to
McGavran et al. (1974)	15	Vocal cord	<3	Recurrence, survival
Kleinsasser and Glanz et al. (1982)	?	Vocal cord	<3	Recurrence, LN status
Lederer and Managetta (1982)	11	Oral cavity	<3	Recurrence, survival
Platz et al. (1982)	318	Oral cavity	<5	Survival
Spiro et al. (1986)	105	Tongue, FOM	<3	LN status, survival
Moore et al. (1986)	45	UADT	<3	Survival
Mohit-Tabatabai et al. (1986)	57	FOM	<1.5	LN status
Brown et al. (1989)	25	Tongue, FOM	<3	LN status and survival
Close et al. (1989)	65	Oral cavity, oropharynx	<5	No correlation
Rasgon et al. (1989)	22	Oral cavity, oropharynx	<5	LN status
Fakih et al. (1989)	51	Tongue	<4	LN status, not survival
Borges et al. (1989)	57	Oral cavity	<5	LN status
	20	Stages I, II	<5	No correlation
Morton et al. (1994)	26	Tongue <3 cm in diameter	<3	No correlation with LN status or survival
Fukano et al. (1996)	34	Tongue	<3	LN status

FOM, floor of mouth; LN, lymph node; UADT, upper aerodigestive tract.

and 3 mm (Brown et al., 1989). A more recent limit for MIC of the tongue is 5 mm (Fukano et al., 1996). Whatever the exact number, tumor thickness seems to correlate with survival, cervical lymph node metastasis, and perineural invasion.

The MIC thickness, i.e., the total depth of the tumor, can be difficult to measure. For example, tumors that are ulcerated should be measured from the floor of the ulcer to the deepest extent of growth; exophytic neoplasms should be measured from the height of the surface of the adjacent normal mucosa to the deepest-reaching front of invasion (Brown et al., 1989; Fukano et al., 1996; Moore et al., 1986). Brown and others noted four general problems in measurement: poor sampling of the lesion; apparent variations in thickness due to changes in the angle of sectioning; tangential cuts; and finally, errors in sectioning the tumor (Brown et al., 1989). Histologically, the earliest stages of infiltration can be recognized easily in most but not all cases; for some, the pathologist must judge whether the carcinoma is invasive or not.

In general, the diagnosis of MIC is based on the presence of one or more nests of malignant cells penetrating through the basement membrane of the mucosa (Fig. 4–11). This focal disruption of the basement membrane means that the margin of the invading nests is ragged, flanked by an intact basement membrane on either side. A desmoplastic response is often present in the adjacent stroma, as well as an inflammatory infiltrate composed of lymphocytes and plasma cells surrounding the tips of the invasive epithelium. The two main patterns of invasion both involve nests of epithelial cells, one with pushing borders (Fig. 4–12) and the other with thin irregular infiltrative borders (Fig. 4–13.) The overlying mucosa can show CIS, SIN of various degrees, or occasionally, normal tissue. Vascular or lymphatic invasion is not observed in the vocal cords, probably because Reinke's space is relatively free of vessels. In the oral cavity and oropharynx, occasional vascular invasion and metastasis to cervical lymph nodes can be present especially for MIC of the tongue and the floor of the mouth (Table 4–5).

With regard to prognosis, MIC of the vocal cords recurred locally in 6 of 15 patients in one study (McGavran et al., 1974) but in no patients in another study (Kleinsasser and Glanz, 1982). In other regions of the UADT, the few patients who had recurrent

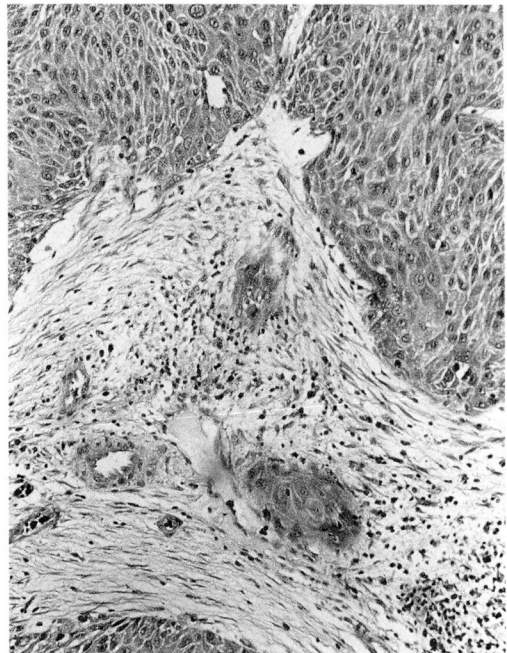

Figure 4–11. Microinvasive carcinoma. Nests of malignant cells are present in the stroma. A desmoplastic reaction can be seen.

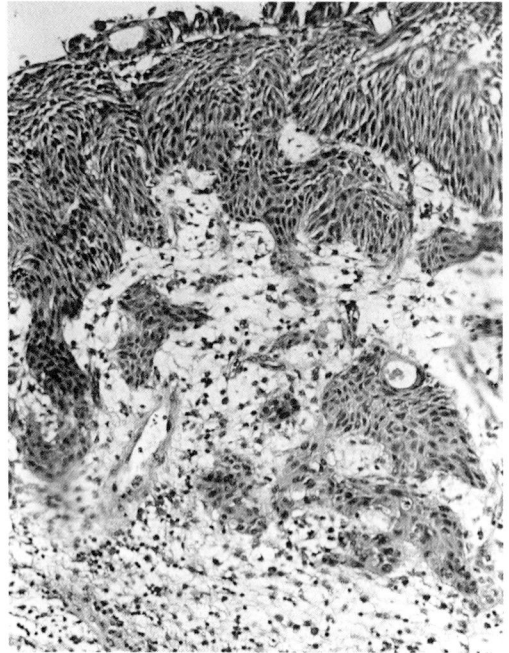

Figure 4–12. Microinvasive carcinoma with limited infiltration of the stroma by large nests of neoplastic cells. The epithelium may show morphologic features of severe dysplasia or carcinoma *in situ.*

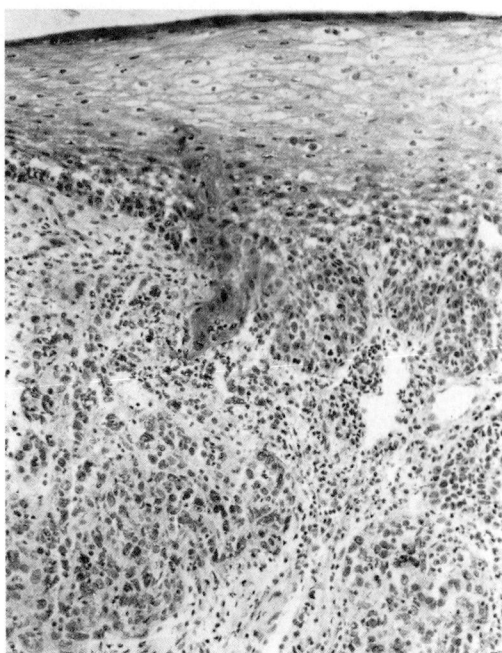

Figure 4–13. Microinvasive carcinoma showing stromal invasion by poorly differentiated cells with irregular infiltrative borders. Normal epithelium overlies the carcinoma.

MIC were treated successfully (Brown et al., 1989; Spiro et al., 1986). Few patients with MIC of the tongue or the floor of mouth have died of their carcinoma; Brown and associates reported one patient who died of local recurrence of MIC carcinoma (Brown et al., 1989). Spiro and co-workers reported one patient with a 1-mm-thick carcinoma who developed cervical lymph node metastasis and died within 14 months with uncontrolled neck disease, despite having had a radical neck dissection and postoperative radiotherapy (Spiro et al., 1986). No cervical metastases have been reported from MIC of the vocal cords (Kleinsasser and Glantz, 1982; McGavran et al., 1974).

MICROCARCINOMA

The concept of microcarcinoma evolved from that of MIC, and includes the surface diameter and histological grade of the neoplasm. However, a single definition of microcarcinoma has not been established, but rather, depends on the site of the lesion. In the vocal cords, a microcarcinoma is defined

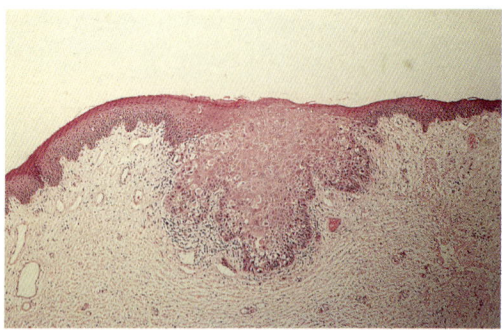

Figure 4–14. Microcarcinoma of the upper aerodigestive tract. The diameter of the carcinoma is small, the cells are well differentiated, and the invasion is superficial.

as a carcinoma of no more than 10 × 10 mm surface area and no more than 3 mm deep (Kleinsasser and Glanz, 1982; Fig. 4–14). In the oral mucosa, the superficial extension of a microcarcinoma is limited to 2 cm in diameter; its depth of invasion should not exceed 3 mm for carcinomas with thin, infiltrating borders and 5 mm for those with blunt, pushing borders, and it should be moderately or well differentiated histologically (Lederer and Managetta, 1982). Microcarcinoma has a substantially better prognosis than the more advanced T1 carcinoma. In one study, none of 11 patients with microcarcinoma had died or had signs of recurrence or metastasis 18–40 months after excision; however, of the 8 patients with advanced T1 carcinomas, 3 died and 1 had metastatic disease in the same period (Lederer and Managetta, 1982). In another study of MIC in the vocal cords, none of the lesions that fulfilled the criteria for microcarcinoma recurred or metastasized (Kleinsasser and Glanz, 1982).

PAPILLOMAS OF THE UPPER AERODIGESTIVE TRACT

SCHNEIDERIAN (SINONASAL TRACT) PAPILLOMAS

A *papilloma* is a benign exophytic neoplastic proliferation arising from an epithelial surface. In sinonasal papillomas, the tissue of origin is the respiratory (Schneiderian) mucosa of the nasal cavity and the adjacent

paranasal sinus cavities (Michaels and Young, 1995). Statistically, papillomas account for 10% of all sinonasal tract neoplasms, benign and malignant, in the Otolaryngologic Tumor Registry of the Armed Forces Institute of Pathology. The median age of subjects with sinonasal papilloma was 35 years (range, 11–85 years); tumor occurrence in subjects younger than 21 years of age was rare. The male-to-female ratio was 5:1 (Hyams, 1971).

Microscopically, the most common sinonasal papilloma is the so-called inverted papilloma, which is restricted to those tumors that arise from the lateral nasal cavity wall or paranasal sinus. Scanning or low-power microscopic examination reveals surface epithelial proliferation pushing or inverting into the underlying submucosal myxomatous stroma (Fig. 4–15). The neoplastic element is a proliferating, uniform, nonkeratinizing stratified epidermoid or squamous epithelial cell (Michaels and Young, 1995). Keratin production is rare; prominent kerating, particularly on the tumor surface, is suggestive of a more aggressive squamous cell neoplastic process, such as a verrucous carcinoma or a well-differentiated squamous cell carcinoma.

The fungiform or exophytic type constitutes 20%–40% of sinonasal tract papillomas and arises almost exclusively in the nasal septum, except for rare cases that originate along the posterior turbinate surface. The architecture consists of a narrow pedicle of attachment and an exophytic, tree-like benign epidermoid (squamous) neoplastic proliferation (Fig. 4–16).

The least common histologic type is the cylindrical cell papilloma, which constitutes 10%–20% of sinonasal papillomas. This particular neoplastic proliferation is formed by uniform, benign tall columnar cells with eosinophilic granular cytoplasms arranged in a pseudostratified pattern (Fig. 4–17). These cylindrical cell papillomas occur only on the lateral nasal wall or paranasal sinuses. Their architecture, like that of the inverted papilloma, involves tumor inversion into a myxomatous fibrous stroma.

Malignant Transformation
Schneiderian papillomas, especially those arising in the lateral wall of the nasal cavity, have been associated with carcinoma. However, association does not imply evolution;

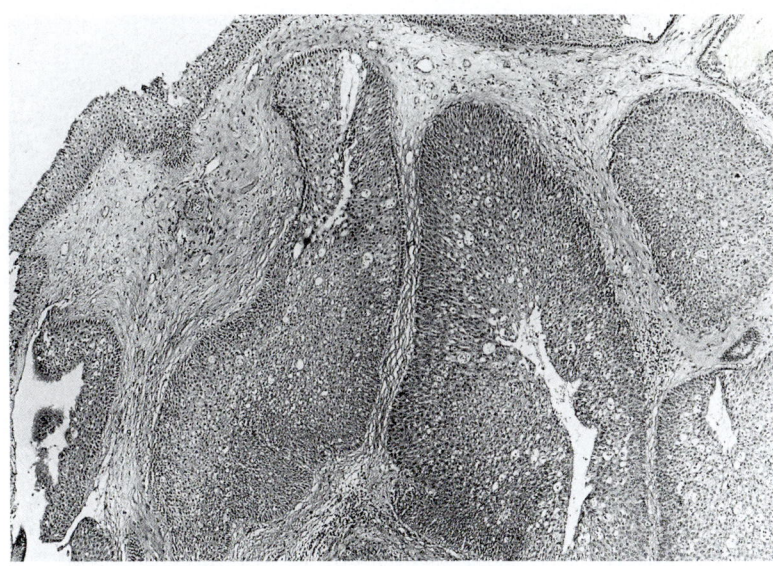

Figure 4–15. Inverted papilloma with typical histologic characteristics. The inverted epithelium extends into underlying stroma. Microscopic mucous cysts are scattered throughout epithelium.

although the reported frequencies may be alarming, the number of examples is small. In the most definitive study, carcinoma was associated with inverted papillomas in 19 cases (13%) (Hyams, 1971); a similar frequency was found for cylindrical cell papilloma (Ward et al., 1990).

Schneiderian papilloma and carcinoma can coexist in 3 ways: *(1)* the carcinoma and papilloma can occupy the same anatomical region, with no evidence that the papilloma has given rise to cancer; *(2)* the Schneiderian papilloma can have within it a focus of *in situ* or invasive carcinoma (synchronous carcinoma); or *(3)* the carcinoma can develop at the site of a previously excised nonrecurrent papilloma (metachronous carcinoma).

Most of the neoplasms associated with Schneiderian papilloma are epidermoid carcinomas, including nonkeratinizing squamous cell carcinomas, although verrucous, mucoepidermoid, spindle-cell, undifferentiated clear-cell carcinomas and adenocarcinomas have been found as well (Benninger et al., 1990; Snyder and Perzin, 1972) (Fig. 4–18).

No histologic change has been found in a Schneiderian papilloma that heralds the advent of carcinoma. However, two potentially useful markers are available for this purpose: one is the loss of ABO blood group antigens and the other is the presence of human

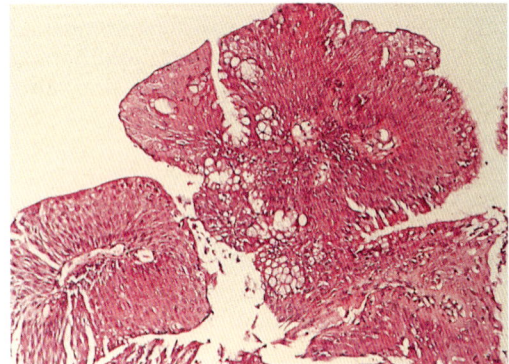

Figure 4–16. A typical fungiform papilloma exophytic growth pattern.

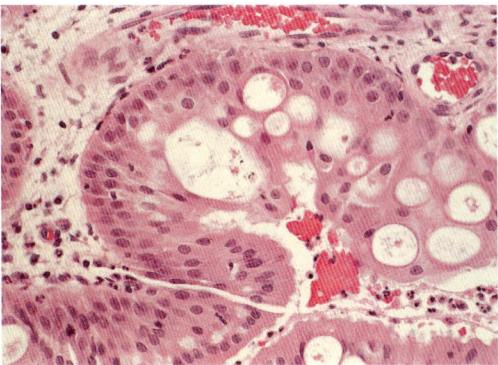

Figure 4–17. Cylindrical cell papilloma. The neoplastic cells are tall, columnar, and uniform with eosinophilic cytoplasm. Focal stratification is present.

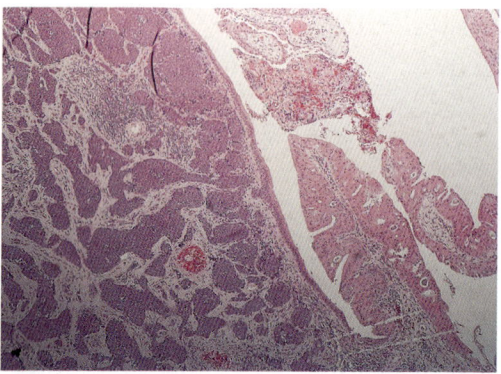

Figure 4–18. Typical cylindrical cell papilloma continuous with an undifferentiated carcinoma.

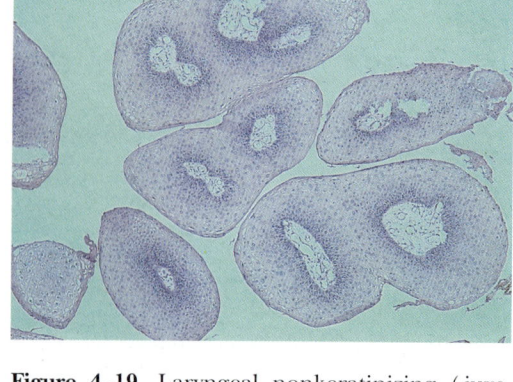

Figure 4–19. Laryngeal nonkeratinizing (juvenile) papilloma. Lack of keratinization and basal cell hyperplasia are visible.

papillomavirus (HPV)-16 or HPV-18 DNA (Beck et al., 1995; Brandwein et al., 1989; Feinmesser et al., 1985). More recently, strongly positive p53 immunoreactivity has been equated with a six-fold increase in the risk of developing carcinoma (Mirza et al., 1998). Schneiderian papillomas that are not associated with HPV infection or p53 reactivity seem to manifest a less aggressive biologic course than those that are (Mirza et al., 1998).

LARYNGEAL PAPILLOMAS

Nonkeratinizing (Juvenile) Papillomas

The lesions attributed to papillomavirus infection of mucosal cells have a characteristic gross and histologic appearance. In the larynx, these lesions occur mainly on the true vocal cords, the false vocal cords, and in the anterior commissure. Lesions may extend upward onto the epiglottis, pharyngeal walls, and soft palate, and also subglottically into the trachea and bronchi (see below). Involvement of the esophagus below the cricopharyngeus muscle is rare.

Histologically, papillomas contain all of the typical epithelial cell layers, but in an exaggerated squamous growth pattern. The sessile or papillary configuration is produced through a combination of cell proliferation and an increase in submucosal capillaries, which are arrayed in fibrovascular cores (Fig. 4–19). Secondary and tertiary branching of the epithelial-covered stalks

also contribute to the papillomatous appearance.

Atypical Papillomas

In the typical laryngeal papilloma, histologic evidence of proliferative cellular activity is confined to the deepest part of the epithelium and is rarely accompanied by a mitotic figure or cellular pleomorphism (Quick et al., 1979).

Invasive Papillomas

A small percentage of patients with laryngeal, tracheal, or bronchial papillomatosis have lesions that extend beyond the mucosa into the adjacent soft tissue, pulmonary, or thyroid parenchyma, or even the skin. This locally aggressive behavior is not accompanied by the traditional cytologic criterion of malignant transformation or metastasis. The extramucosal extensions are usually continuous with surface or intraluminal papilloma (Fig. 4–20). Nearly all invasive papillomas of the larynx have undergone radiotherapy (Fechner et al., 1974; Fechner and Fitz-Hugh, 1980).

Malignancy and Papillomas

One factor that undeniably promotes malignant change in laryngeal papillomas is X-irradiation, particularly of juvenile papillomas. This finding supports the theory of initiation and promotion in the genesis of carcinomas and also acknowledges the relation between radiation and invasive papillomas of the larynx. In 101 cases of juvenile laryngeal papilloma studied at the Mayo

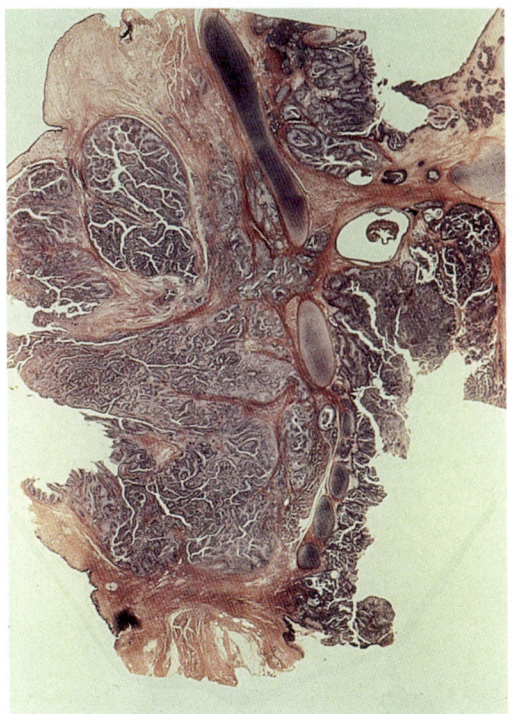

Figure 4–20. Whole-organ section of an invasive laryngeal papilloma. The lesion has extended outside the larynx.

Clinic, 6 of 43 (14%) patients treated with radiotherapy as children developed squamous cell carcinoma of the larynx before 30 years of age (Majoros et al., 1963). A more recent review (Rodriguez-Jurado et al., 1996) revealed only 17 cases of laryngeal papillomatosis coexisting with lung carcinoma in patients who neither smoked nor were exposed to radiation (Rodriguez et al., 1996). Of the six of these patients who had virology studies, five were found to be positive for HPV-11 (Rodriguez et al., 1996).

Keratinizing (Adult) Papillomas

Two types of benign laryngeal papilloma exist in adults. One is a nonkeratinizing lesion, the light-microscopic appearance and biologic behavior of which resemble those of childhood or juvenile-onset papillomas (Fig. 4–19). These nonkeratinized papillomas occasionally show signs of viral genesis characteristic of true papillomas. The other type is a keratinizing or cornifying lesion, which is almost always present as a solitary laryngeal lesion (Fig. 4–21) (Capper et al., 1982; Kleinsasser et al., 1973). Keratinizing papillomas are found almost exclusively in adults. The extent of surface keratinization varies. Their malignant potential is unclear.

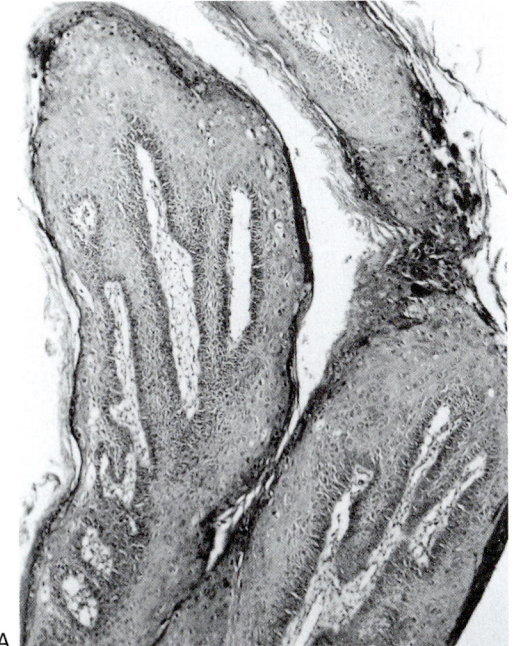

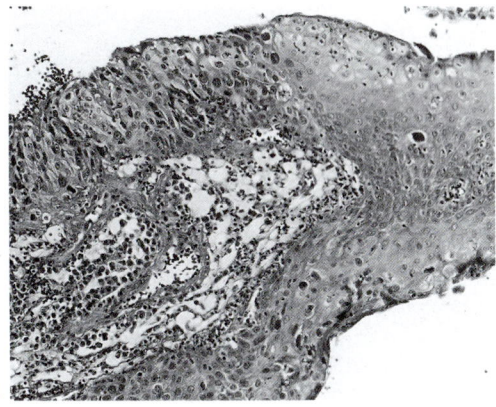

Figure 4–21. Keratinizing laryngeal papilloma. *A:* Keratinization or cornification of the superficial layers is present. *B:* Marked nuclear irregularity, cellular atypia, and CIS are visible.

PAPILLARY SQUAMOUS
CELL CARCINOMA

Papillary squamous cell carcinoma is the least understood of all types of squamous cell carcinoma that occur in the UADT (Table 4–1), largely because of its low incidence (Crissman et al., 1988). In fact, with the exception of three reports (Crissman et al., 1988; Suarez et al., 1999; Thompson et al., 1994) papillary squamous cell carcinoma is not recognized as a distinct entity in the contemporary literature. In summarizing the histopathologic criteria for papillary squamous cell neoplasms of the UADT, Crissman and others (1988) found abnormal cellular DNA but not HPV infection. The tumors were most often found in the oropharynx, the hypopharynx, the larynx, and the sinonasal tract. They originated from a background of hyperplastic, nonkeratinizing, papillomatous mucosa that in 34% of cases showed progressive dysplasia. This type of carcinoma predominated in men by a ratio of 2:1. The average age at diagnosis was 66 years, with a range of 24 to 89 years.

Pathologically, papillary carcinomas are papillary in gross appearance, friable, soft, and pink to gray. Tumor size can range from 0.2 to 4.0 cm. Hematoxylin and eosin staining reveals exophytic proliferation and multiple papillary projections from a central fibrovascular core that is covered with a malignant epithelium (Fig. 4–22). This surface epithelium resembles intraepithelial neoplasia or high-grade dysplasia. The epithelial cells are basaloid and immature with nu-

merous mitoses (Fig. 4–23). Keratinization is rarely observed in individual cells, and surface keratosis is not seen in any papillary carcinomas. All papillary carcinomas have fibrovascular cores with varying degrees of vascular prominence.

The HPV has been found in 29% of papillary carcinomas by *in situ* hybridization and in 43% by polymerase chain reaction (PCR) (Suarez et al., 1999); 70% stained for the p53 protein. Nuclear staining varied considerably among both individual tumors and categories of lesions (Suarez et al., 1999). Of the 25 patients who could be evaluated, 11 (44%) died of these carcinomas after single or multiple recurrences. In terms of site, sinonasal papillary squamous cell carcinomas were the most lethal (Suarez et al., 1999).

VERRUCOUS CARCINOMA

The term "verrucous carcinoma" was first applied in 1948 to describe a highly differentiated type of squamous carcinoma of the oral cavity with a unique biologic behavior and characteristic gross and histologic changes (Ackerman, 1948). Verrucous carcinoma appears primarily in the sixth through eighth decades of life and is rare in patients less than 35 years of age (Bouquot, 1998; Kraus and Perez-Mesa, 1966; Orvidas et al., 1998). The lesions appear most often in the mucous membranes of the head and neck, especially the oral cavity and larynx. In a review of 105 cases, lesions were distrib-

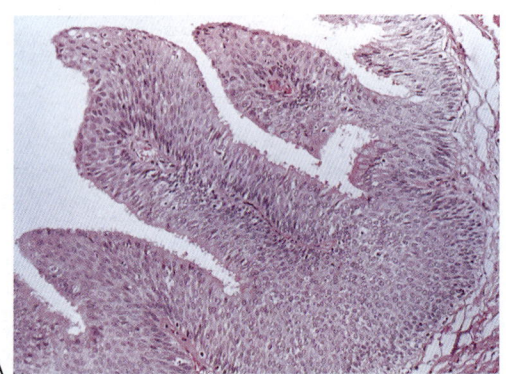
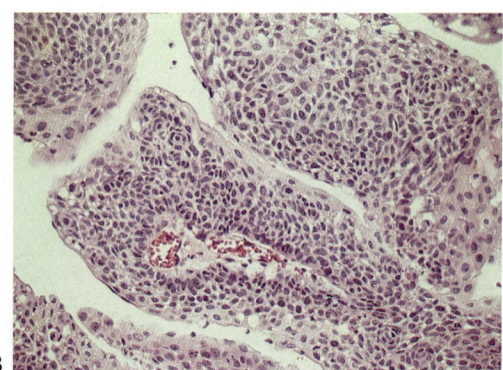

A   B

Figure 4–22. Papillary squamous cell carcinoma. *A:* Fibrovascular cores lined with atypical epithelial cells (H&E, × 20). *B:* Mucosa with full-thickness replacement by cells with marked nuclear irregularity and atypia.

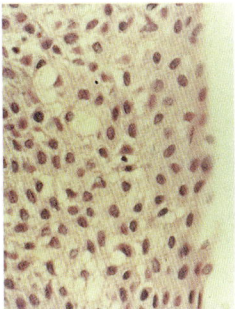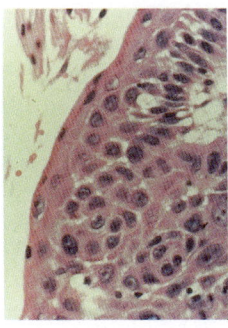

Figure 4–23. Laryngeal papillary squamous cell carcinoma (*right*) and nonkeratinizing laryngeal papilloma (*left*). Marked nuclear irregularity and cellular atypia are visible in the carcinoma.

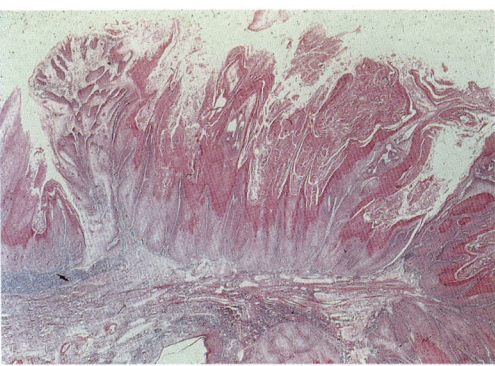

Figure 4–24. Verrucous carcinoma with marked thickened epithelium with pushing or blunt deep margin of invasion and prominent surface keratinization.

uted as follows: oral cavity, 73%; larynx, 11%; glans penis, 8%; nasal fossa, 4%; vulva, 1%; vagina, 1%; scrotum, 1%; and perineum, 1% percent (Kraus and Perez-Mesa, 1966). The diagnostic criteria for verrucous squamous cell carcinoma are listed in Table 4–6.

Microscopically, verrucous carcinoma is broadly based and locally invasive, with a warty, densely keratinized surface (Fig. 4–24). The deep margin is sharply circumscribed, pushing rather than infiltrating, and is composed of bulbous, well-oriented, rete ridges, often with central degeneration (Fig. 4–25). An inflammatory infiltrate is typically but not always present in the adjacent

stroma; this infiltrate consists predominantly of lymphocytes and plasma cells. Histologically, verrucous carcinoma is composed of very well–differentiated squamous epithelial cells that lack the usual cytologic criteria for malignant transformation. The individual cells have uniform vesicular nuclei and abundant cytoplasm. Atypia, pleomorphism, and hyperchromatism are not apparent, but epithelial pearls and small cysts are often seen. If any atypia is present, the lesion should be classified as a well-differentiated papillary squamous cell carcinoma. Vascular and perineural invasion are absent; invasion of these structures is sufficient grounds to question the diagnosis; and additional sections should be submitted to exclude a well-differentiated squamous cell carcinoma or hybrid verrucous carcinoma, in which areas of a less differentiated carcinoma exist within the verrucous carcinoma (Fig. 4–26).

The presence of HPV-18 in verrucous car-

Table 4–6. Diagnostic Criteria for Verrucous Squamous Cell Carcinoma

Male

Elderly

Use of tobacco products

Poor oral hygiene

Lesion in buccal mucosa, gingiva, or glottis

Fungating or exophytic densely keratinized warty surface

Histological criteria

Advancing, pushing, and well-circumscribed deep margin composed of bulbous rete ridges

Deeply projecting cleft-like spaces with cystic degeneration of the central portion of the bulbous projection

High degree of cellular differentiation

Absence of cytologic features of malignancy

Prominent stromal chronic inflammatory reaction

Absence of vascular or perineural invasion

Nonmetastatic behavior

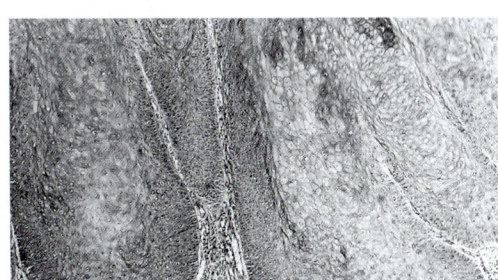

Figure 4–25. Verrucous carcinoma. Cellular atypia and submucosa inflammatory response are minimal.

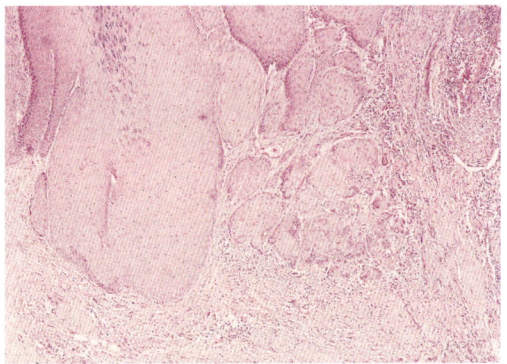

Figure 4–26. Hybrid verrucous carcinoma. A focus of conventional squamous carcinoma is present within otherwise typical verrucous carcinoma.

cinoma of the oral cavity has been detected by PCR in 40% of cases in one series (Noble-Topham et al., 1993). The etiologic and prognostic significance of this finding is as yet unknown. Accumulation of *p53* protein was observed in 50% and overexpression of cyclin D1 in 60% of verrucous carcinomas of the oral cavity in another study (Gimenez-Conti et al., 1996). However, no change in staining for the retinoblastoma (Rb) protein was found, suggesting that Rb may be functionally inactivated by overexpression of cyclin D1 or HPV infection (Gimenez-Conti et al., 1996).

DIFFERENTIAL DIAGNOSIS

The differential diagnosis of verrucous carcinoma includes squamous papilloma, conventional well-differentiated squamous carcinoma, condyloma accuminatum, verruca vulgaris, and pseudoepitheliomatous hyperplasia. The lack of extensive surface keratinization or bulbous rete ridges in squamous papilloma can be used to distinguish it from verrucous carcinoma. The presence of small columns and foci of cells with anaplastic cytologic features, as well as infiltrative margins, signifies squamous cell carcinoma of the conventional type, regardless of how "warty" the surface may be. Verrucous carcinoma can be distinguished from condyloma accuminatum by the absence of a central connective-tissue support in the papillary processes of a verrucous carcinoma; condyloma accuminatum is also associated with vacuolated epithelial cells and branched rete ridges.

Pseudoepitheliomatous hyperplasia does not have the "cauliflower" appearance of verrucous carcinoma and the rete ridges are elongated, branched, thin, and pointed instead of being bulbous.

Finally, verrucous carcinoma can be distinguished from verrucous hyperplasia by the depth of the verrucous process (Shear and Pindborg, 1980). The surface projections are identical in both type of lesions, but verrucous hyperplasia does not extend into the underlying connective tissue as deeply as verrucous carcinoma, and the hyperplastic epithelium remains largely on top of the normal epithelium.

Fechner and Mills (1982) described seven patients who had exophytic keratotic lesions of the larynx that were morphologically indistiguishable from verruca vulgaris of the skin. Verrucous carcinoma has a dense keratotic layer and lacks both the prominent granular cell layer and the large keratohyaline granules characteristic of verruca vulgaris (Fig. 4–27). Moreover, in verrucous carcinoma the rete ridges are bulbous and extend deeply into the stroma; in verruca vulgaris, the rete ridges are thin, pointed,

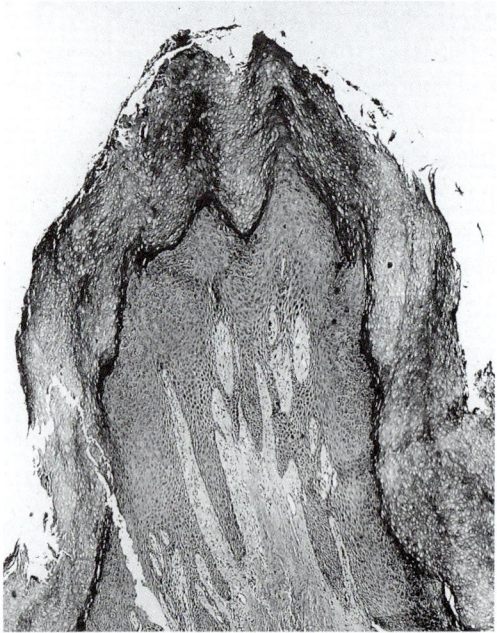

Figure 4–27. Laryngeal verruca vulgaris, with prominent granular cell layer, large keratohyaline granules, and thin, pointy rete ridges separated by abundant stromal tissue.

and often separated by large amounts of stromal connective tissue. Also, verrucous carcinoma is broad based, whereas the papillomatous projections in verruca vulgaris usually radiate out from central hub-like spokes on a wheel (Fechner and Mills, 1982).

ANAPLASTIC TRANSFORMATION

Radiation therapy for verrucous carcinoma has been linked to anaplastic transformation of the tumor. Two review articles published in the 1970s (Biller et al., 1971; Demian et al., 1976) reported a 30% incidence of anaplastic transformation after irradiation. However, these reviews covered only the series in which anaplastic transformation had been reported. A more extensive review that included all patients with verrucous carcinoma who had been treated with radiotherapy found the incidence of anaplastic transformation to be 10.7% (Schwade et al., 1976). A later, more thorough review of published cases of anaplastic transformation revealed that only four cases had been properly documented. Moreover, six other cases were found in which a verrucous carcinoma was transformed to a less well-differentiated form of squamous carcinoma either spontaneously or after surgery (McDonald et al., 1982). The concept that radiation therapy has been blamed for a transformation process that could occur without it was supported indirectly by results from another series in which 12 patients treated with radiation showed no evidence of anaplastic transformation (Medina et al., 1984).

The mechanism of anaplastic transformation, whether occurring spontaneously or in response to radiation, has not been explained satisfactorily. One theory holds that the anaplastic carcinoma occurs *de novo* (Proffitt et al., 1970); another possibility is that a small area of less well–differentiated squamous carcinoma may be missed or hidden within the biopsy or surgical specimens. Verrucous carcinomas are often large, extensive lesions; not one case of postradiation anaplastic transformation reported by Perez and associates (1966) measured less than 4 cm. Small areas of less well–differentiated carcinoma may well be missed in sectioning the excised tissue. Foci of less well–differentiated squamous carcinoma, within

otherwise classic verrucous carcinoma, have been identified in 3 of 7 patients with laryngeal verrucous carcinoma, in 20 of 104 patients with verrucous carcinoma of the oral cavity, and in 6 of 53 patients with verrucous carcinoma of the larynx (Batsakis et al., 1982; Medina et al., 1984; Orvidas et al., 1998). Hybrid carcinomas such as these are of considerable interest in the phenomenon of anaplastic transformation.

In summary, although irradiated verrucous carcinomas have unquestionably became transformed into more aggressive carcinomas, this transformation also has been documented in verrucous carcinoma that has been either surgically treated or untreated.

REFERENCES

Abdel-Salam M, Mayall BH, Chew K, Siverman S, Greenspan JS. (1990) Which oral lesions will become malignant? An image cytometric study. *Oral Surg Oral Med Oral Pathol* 69:345–350.

Abdel-Salam M, Mayall BH, Hansen LS, Chen K, Greenspan JS. (1987) Nuclear DNA analysis of oral hyperplasia and dysplasia using image cytometry. *J Oral Pathol* 16:431–435.

Ackerman LV. (1948) Verrucous carcinoma of the oral cavity. *Surgery* 23:670–678.

Ashworth MT, Helliwell TR. (1988) Nucleolar organizer regions in benign, dysplastic and malignant laryngeal squamous epithelium [Abstract] *J Pathol* 154: 64–65(A).

Axell T. (1993) Oral mucosal changes related to smokeless tobacco usage: research findings in Scandinavia. *Oral Oncol Eur J Cancer* 29B:299–302.

Axell T, Holmstrup P, Kramer IRH, Pindborg JJ, Shear M. (1984) International seminar on oral leukoplakia and associated lesions related to tobacco habits. *Community Dent Oral Epidemiol* 12:145–154.

Axell T, Pindborg JJ, Smith CJ, van der Wael I. (1996) International Collaborative Group on Oral White Lesions. Oral white lesions with special reference to pre-cancerous and tobacco-related lesions: conclusions of an international symposium held in Uppsala, Sweden, May 18–21 1994. *J Oral Pathol Med* 25:49–54.

Banoczy J, Csiba A. (1976) Occurrence of epithelial dysplasia in oral leukoplakia: analysis and follow up of 120 cases. *Oral Surg Oral Med Oral Pathol* 42:766–774.

Barnard NA, Scully C, Eveson JW, Cunningam S, Porter SR. (1993) Oral cancer development in patients with oral lichen planus. *J Oral Pathol Med* 22:421–424.

Barrera JE, Ai H, Pan Z, Meyers AD, Varella-Garcia M. (1998) Malignancy detection by molecular cytogenetics in clinically normal mucosa adjacent to head and neck tumors. *Arch Otolaryngol Head Neck Surg* 124:847–851.

Batsakis JG, Cleary KR, Cho K-J. (1994) Lichen planus and lichenoid lesions of the oral cavity. *Ann Otol Rhinol Laryngol* 103:495–497.

Batsakis JG, Hybels R, Crissman JD, Rice DH. (1982) The pathology of head and neck tumors: verrucous carcinoma, part 15. *Head Neck Surg* 5:29–38.

Beck JC, McClatchey KD, Lesperance MM, Esclamado RM, Carey TE, Bradford ER. (1995) Presence of human papillomavirus predicts recurrence of inverted papilloma. *Otolaryngol Head Neck Surg* 113:49–55.

Benninger MS, Roberts YK, Sebek BA, Levine HL, Tucker HM, Lavertu P. (1990) Inverted papillomas and associated squamous cell carcinomas. *Otolaryngol Head Neck Surg* 103:457–461,

Biller HF, Ogura JH, Bauer WC. (1971) Verrucous cancer of the larynx. *Laryngoscope* 81:1323–1329.

Blackwell KE, Fu Y-S, Calcaterra TC. (1995) Laryngeal dysplasia. A clinicopathologic study. *Cancer* 75:457–463.

Borges AM, Shrikhande SS, Ganesh B. (1989) Surgical pathology of squamous carcinoma of the oral cavity: its impact on management. *Semin Surg Oncol* 5:310–317.

Bosatra A, Bussani R, Silvestri F. (1997) From epithelial dysplasia to squamous carcinoma in the head and neck region: an epidemiological assessment. *Acta Otolaryngol (Stockh) Suppl* 527:47–48.

Bouquot JE. (1998) Oral verrucous carcinoma. Incidence in two U.S. populations. *Oral Surg Oral Med Oral Pathol Oral Radiol Endod* 86:318–324.

Bouquot JE, Gnepp DR. (1991) Laryngeal precancer—a review of the literature, commentary and comparison with oral leukoplakia. *Head Neck* 13:488–497.

Bouquot JE, Kurland LT, Weiland LH. (1988) Carcinoma in situ of the upper aerodigestive tract. Incidence, time trends, and follow-up in Rochester, Minnesota, 1935–1984. *Cancer* 61:1691–1698.

Bouquot JS, Schroeder K. (1993) Oral leukoplakia and smokeless tobacco keratosis are two separate and distinctive precancers. *Oral Surg Oral Med Oral Pathol* 76:588–589.

Bouquot JE, Whitaker SB. (1994) Oral leukoplakia—rationale for diagnosis and diagnosis and prognosis of its clinical subtypes or "phases." *Quintessence Int* 25:133–140.

Brandwein M, Steinberg B, Thung S, Biller H, Dilorenzo T, Galli R. (1989) Human papillomavirus 6/11 and 16/18 in Schneiderian inverted papillomas. In situ hybridization with human papillomavirus RNA probes. *Cancer* 63:1708–1713.

Brown B, Barnes L, Mazariegos J. (1989) Prognostic factors in mobile tongue and floor of the mouth carcinoma. *Cancer* 64:1195–1202.

Capper JWR, Bailey CM, Michaels L. (1982) Squamous papillomas of the larynx in adults: a review of 63 cases. *Clin Otolaryngol* 7:138–139.

Cardesa A, Nadal A, Jares P, Mallofré C, Fernández P, Campo E, Transerra J. (1997) Hyperplastic lesions of the larynx. Experience of the Barcelona group. *Acta Otolaryngol (Stockh) Suppl* 527:43–46.

Carey TE, Van Dyke DL, Worsham MJ. (1993) Nonrandom chromosomes aberrations and clonal populations in head and neck cancer. *Anticancer Res* 13:2561–2568.

Chen YQ, Cipriano SC, Arenkiel JM, Miller IR. (1995) Tumor suppression by p21 WAF1. *Cancer Res* 55:4536–4539.

Close LG, Brown PM, Vuitch MF, Reisch J, Schaefer SD. (1989) Microvascular invasion and survival in cancer of the oral cavity and oropharynx. *Arch Otolaryngol Head Neck Surg* 115:1304–1309.

Coltrera MD, Zarbo RJ, Sakr WA, Gown AM. (1992) Markers for dysplasia of upper aerodigestive tract. *Am J Pathol* 141:817–825.

Cör A, Gale N, Kambic V. (1997) Quantitative pathology of laryngeal epithelial hyperplastic lesions. *Acta Otolaryngol (Stochk) Suppl* 527:57–61.

Crissman JD, Fu YS. (1986) Intraepithelial neoplasia of the larynx: a clinicopathologic study of six cases with DNA analysis. *Arch Otolaryngol Head Neck Surg* 112:522–528.

Crissman JD, Kessis T, Shah KV. (1988) Squamous papillary neoplasia of the adult upper aerodigestive tract. *Hum Pathol* 19:1387–1396.

Crissman JD, Zarbo RJ. (1991) Quantitation of DNA ploidy in squamous intraepithelial neoplasia of the larynx. *Arch Otolaryngol Head Neck Surg* 117:182–188.

Decosse JJ. (1983) Precancer an overview. *Cancer Surv* 2:347–357.

Demian SDE, Bushkin FL, Echevarria RA. (1976) Perineural invasion and anaplastic transformation of verrucous carcinoma. *Cancer* 32:395–401.

Derrick J, Wagenfeld MB, Harwood AR. (1980) Second primary respiratory tract malignancies in glottic carcinoma. *Cancer* 46:1833–1840.

Dolcetti R, Doglioni C, Maestro R. (1992) p53 overexpression is an early event in the development of human squamous-cell carcinoma of the larynx: genetic and prognostic implications. *Int J Cancer* 52:178–182.

Doseva Đ, Christov K, Kristeva A. (1984) DNA content in reactive hyperplasia, precancerosis, and carcinomas of the oral cavity. A cytophotometric study. *Acta Histochem* 75:113–119.

El-Naggar AK, Hurr K, Batsakis JG, Luna MA, Goepfert H, Huff V. (1995a) Sequential loss of heterozygosity at microsatellite motifs in preinvasive and invasive head and neck squamous carcinoma. *Cancer Res* 55:2656–2659.

El-Naggar AK, Lai S, Luna MA, Zhou XD, Weber RS, Goepfert H, Batsakis JG. (1995b) Sequential p53 mutation analysis of pre-invasive and invasive head and neck squamous carcinoma. *Int J Cancer* 64:196–201.

Fakih AR, Rao RS, Borges AM, Patel AR. (1989) Elective versus therapeutic neck dissection in early carcinoma of the tongue. *Am J Surg* 158:309–313.

Fechner RE, Goepfert H, Alford BR. (1974) Invasive laryngeal papillomatosis. *Arch Otolaryngol* 99:147–151.

Fechner RE, Mills SE. (1982) Verrucous vulgaris of the larynx. *Am J Surg Pathol* 6:357–362.

Fechner RE, Ritz-Hugh GS. (1980) Invasive tracheal papillomatosis. *Am J Surg Pathol* 4:79–86.

Feinmesser R, Gay I, Wiesel JM, Ben-Bassat H. (1985) Malignant transformation in inverted papilloma. *Ann Otol Rhinol Laryngol* 94:39–43.

Ferlito A. (1995) The natural history of early vocal cord cancer. *Acta Otolaryngol (Stockh)* 155:345–347.

Fernandez PL, Jares P, Nadal A. (1996) p21 (WAFI) expression in laryngeal carcinomas: correlation with histological and clinical parameters. *Mod Pathol* 9:101A.

Fukano H, Matsuura H, Hasegawa Y, Nakamura S. (1996) Depth of invasion as a predictive factor for cervical lymph node metastasis in tongue carcinoma. *Head Neck* 19:205–210.

Gale N, Poljak M, Kambic V, Ferluga D. (1993) Abnormal *p53* expression in benign and malignant laryngeal hyperplastic lesions. *Pathol Res Pract* 189:701–705.

Gallo O, Santucci M, Franchi A. (1997) Cumulative prognostic value of p16/CDKN2 and p53 oncoprotein expression in premalignant laryngeal lesions. *J Natl Cancer Inst* 89:1161–1163.

Gimenez-Conti IB, Collet AM, Lanfranchi H, Itoiz ME, Luna MA, Xu HJ, Benedict WF, Conti CJ. (1996) p53, Rb, and cyclin D1 expression in human oral verrucous carcinomas. *Cancer* 78:17–23.

Gluckman JL, Crissman JD, Donegan JO. (1980) Multicentric squamous-cell carcinoma of the upper aerodigestive tract. *Head Neck Surg* 3:90–96.

Goepfert H. (1984) Are we making any progress? *Arch Otolaryngol* 110:562–563.

Hansen LS, Olson JA, Silverman S Jr. (1985) Proliferative verrucous leukoplakia: a long-term study of 30 patients. *Oral Surg Oral Med Oral Pathol* 60:285–298.

Harris AL. (1990) Mutant p53—the commonest genetic abnormality in human cancer? *J Pathol* 162:5–6.

Hellquist H, Lundgren J, Olofsson J. (1982) Hyperplasia, keratosis, dysplasia, and carcinoma in situ of the vocal cords—a follow-up study. *Clin Otolaryngol* 7:11–27.

Hirsch SM, DuCant J, Caldarelli DD, Hutchinson JC, Coon JS. (1992) Nucleolar organizer regions in squamous cell carcinoma of the head and neck. *Laryngoscope* 102:39–44.

Hoffman HT, Karnell LH, Funk GF, Robinson RA, Mench HR. (1998) The national cancer data base report on cancer of the head and neck. *Arch Otolaryngol Head Neck Surg* 124:951–962.

Hojslet PE, Nielsen VM, Palvio D. (1989) Premalignant lesions of the larynx. *Acta Otolaryngol (Stockh)* 107:150–155.

Hyams VJ. (1971) Papillomas of the nasal cavity and paranasal sinuses. A clinicopathological study of 315 cases. *Ann Otol Rhinol Laryngol* 80:192–206.

Jares P, Fernandez PL, Campo E, Nadal A, Bosch F, Aiza G, Nayach I, Trasetrata J, Cardesa A. (1994) PRAD-1/cyclin D1 gene amplification correlates with messenger RNA overexpression and tumor progression in human laryngeal carcinomas. *Cancer Res* 54:4813–4817.

Johnson NW, Ranasinghe AW, Warnakulasuriya KAAS. (1993) Potentially malignant lesions and conditions of the mouth and oropharynx: natural history–cellular and molecular markers of risk. *Eur J Cancer Prev* (Suppl 2) 2:31–51.

Jones K, Lodge-Rigal D, Reddick R. (1992) Prognostic factors in the recurrence of stage I and II squamous cell cancer of the oral cavity. *Arch Otolaryngol Head Neck Surg* 118:483–485.

Jones AS, Roland NJ, Caslin W, Cooke TG, Cooke ID, Forster G. (1994) A comparison of cellular proliferation markers in squamous cell carcinoma of the head and neck. *J Laryngol Otol* 108:859–864.

Kambic V, Gale N. (1986) Significance of keratosis and dyskeratosis for classifying hyperplastic aberrations of laryngeal mucosa. *Am J Otolaryngol* 7:323–333.

Kambic V, Gale N. (1995) *Epithelial Hyperplastic Lesions of the Larynx.* Elsevier, Amsterdam.

Kaugars GE, Brandt RB, Chan W, Carcaise-Edinbora P. (1991) Evaluation of risk factors in smokeless tobacco-associated oral lesions. *Oral Surg Oral Med Oral Pathol* 72:326–331.

Kaugars GE, Mehailescu WL, Gunsolley JC. (1989) Smokeless tobacco use and oral epithelial dysplasia. *Cancer* 64:1527–1530.

Kleinsasser D, Oliviera E, Cruz G. (1973) Juvenile and adult kehlkopfpapillome. *HNO* 21:97–106.

Kleinsasser O, Glanz H. (1982) Microcarcinoma and microinvasive carcinoma of the vocal cords. *Clin Oncol* 1:479–487.

Kraus FT, Perez Mesa C. (1966) Verrucous carcinoma: clinical and pathologic study of 105 cases involving oral cavity, larynx and genitalia. *Cancer* 19:26–38.

Krutchkoff DJ, Cutter L, Laskowski S. (1978) Oral lichen planus: the evidence regarding potential malignant transformation. *J Oral Pathol* 7:1–7.

Krutchkoff DJ, Eisenberg E. (1985) Lichenoid dysplasia: a distinct histopathologic entity. *Oral Surg Oral Med Oral Pathol* 60:308–315.

Landers JE, Cassel SL, George DL. (1997) Translational enhancement of mdm2 oncogene expresion in human tumor containing a stabilized wild-type p53 protein. *Cancer Res* 57:3562–3568.

Landis SH, Murray T, Bolden S, Wingo PA. (1997) Cancer statistics 1998. *CA Cancer J Clin* 48:6–29.

Lederer B, Managetta B. (1982) Morphological aspects of minimal invasive carcinoma (microcarcinoma) of the oral mucosa. *Clin Oncol* 1:475–478.

Lee JS, Kim SY, Hong WK, Lippman SM, Ro JY, Gay ML, Hittelman WN. (1993) Detection of chromosome polysomy in oral leukoplakia, a premalignant lesion. *J Natl Cancer Inst* 85:1951–1954.

Liggett WH, Sewell DA, Rocco J, Ahrendt SA, Koch WM, Didransky D. (1996) p16 and p16B are potent growth suppressors of head and neck squamous carcinoma cells in vivo. *Cancer Res* 56:4119–4123.

Lippman SM, Batsakis JG, Toth BB. (1993) Comparison of low-dose isotretinoin with beta carotene to prevent oral carcinogenesis. *N Engl J Med* 328:15–20.

Lippman SM, Shin DM, Lee JJ. (1995) p53 and retinoid chemoprevention of oral carcinogenesis. *Cancer Res* 55:16–19.

Lotan, R, Xu XC, Lee JS. (1995) Expression of retinoic acid receptor in premalignant oral lesions and its up-regulation by isotretinoin. *N Engl J Med* 332:1405–1410.

Lumerman H, Freedman P, Kerpel S. (1995) Oral epithelial dysplasia and the development of invasive squamous carcinoma. *Oral Surg Oral Med Oral Pathol* 79:321–329.

Majoros M, Devine KD, Parkhill EM. (1963) Malignant transformation of benign laryngeal papillomas in children after radiation therapy. *Surg Clin North Am* 43:1049–1061.

Mallofré C, Cardesa A, Campo E. (1993) Expression of cytokeratins in squamous cell carcinomas of the larynx: immunohistochemical analysis and correlation with prognostic factors. *Pathol Res Pract* 189:275–282.

Mao L, El-Naggar AK, Fan Y-H, Lee JS, Lippman SM, Kayser S, Lotan R, Hong WK. (1996a) Telomerase activity in head and neck squamous cell carcinoma and adjacent tissues. *Cancer Res* 56:5600–5604.

Mao L, Lee JS, Fan YH. (1996b) Frequent microsatellite alterations at chromosomes 9p21 and 3p14 in oral premalignant lesions and their value in cancer risk assessment. *Nat Med* 2:682–685.

Marshall CJ. (1991) Tumor suppressor genes. *Cell* 64:313–326.

McDonald JS, Crissman JD, Gluckman JL. (1982) Verrucous carcinoma of the oral cavity. *Head Neck Surg* 5:22–28.

McGavran MH, Stutsman AC, Ogura JH. (1974) Superficially invasive epidermoid carcinoma of the true vocal cord. *Can J Otol* 34:526–527.

McGuirt WF, Matthews B, Koufman JA. (1982) Multiple simultaneous tumors in patients with head and neck cancer: a prospective, sequential panendoscopic study. *Cancer* 50:1195–1199.

Medina JE, Dichtel W, Luna MA. (1984) Verrucous-squamous carcinomas of the oral cavity. A clinico-pathologic study of 104 cases. *Arch Otolaryngol* 110: 437–440.

Michaels L, Young M. (1995) Histogenesis of papillomas of the nose and paranasal sinuses. *Arch Pathol Lab Med* 119:821–826.

Mincer HH, Coleman SA, Hopkins KP. (1972) Observation on the clinical characteristics of oral lesions showing histologic epithelial dysplasia. *Oral Surg Oral Med Oral Pathol* 33:389–399.

Mirza N, Montonel K, Sato Y, Kroger H, Kennedy DW. (1998) Identification of p53 and human papilloma virus in Schneiderian papilloma. *Laryngoscope* 108:487–501.

Mohit-Tabatabai MA, Sobel MJ, Rush BF. (1986) Relation of thickness of floor of mouth stage I and II cancers to regional metastasis. *Am J Surg* 152: 351–353.

Moore C, Kuhns JG, Greenberg R.A. (1986) Thickness as prognostic aid in upper aerodigestive tract cancer. *Arch Surg* 121:1410–1414.

Morton RP, Ferguson CM, Lambie NK, Whitlock RML. (1994) Tumor thickness in early tongue cancer. *Arch Otolaryngol Head Neck Surg* 120:717–720.

Mutirangura A, Supiyaphun P, Trirekapan S, Sriuranpong V, Sakuntabhai A, Yenrudi S, Voravud N. (1996) Telomerase activity in oral leukoplakia and head and neck squamous cell carcinoma. *Cancer Res* 56:3530–3533.

Nadal A, Campo E, Pinto J, Mallofre C, Valacin A, Arias C, Traserra J, Cardesa A. (1995) p53 expression in normal, dysplastic and neoplastic laryngeal epithelium. Absence of a correlation with prognostic factors. *J Pathol* 175:181–188.

Noble-Topham SE, Fliss DM, Hartwick RWJ, McLachlin CM, Freeman JL, Noyck AM, Andrulis IL. (1993) Detection and typing of human papillomavirus in verrucous carcinoma of the oral cavity using the polymerase chain reaction. *Arch Otolaryngol Head Neck Surg* 119:1299–1304.

Orvidas LJ, Olsen KD, Lewis JE, Suman VJ. (1998) Verrucous carcinoma of the larynx: a review of 53 patients. *Head Neck Surg* 21:197–263.

Papadimitrakopoulou V, Izzo J, Lippman SM, Lee JS, Fan YH, Clayman G, Ro JY, Hittelman WN, Lotan R, Hong WK, Mao L. (1997) Frequent inactivation of p16INK4a in oral premalignant lesions. *Oncogene* 14:1799–1803.

Perez CA, Kraus FT, Evans JC, Powers WE. (1966) Anaplastic transformation in verrucous carcinoma of the oral cavity after radiation therapy. *Radiology* 86:108–115.

Pindborg JJ, Daftary DK, Mehta FS. (1977) A follow-up study of sixty-one oral dysplastic precancerous lesions in Indian-villagers. *Oral Surg Oral Med Oral Pathol* 43:383–390.

Pindborg JJ, Reibel J, Holmstrup P. (1985) Subjectivity in evaluating oral epithelial dysplasia, carcinoma in situ and initial carcinoma. *J Oral Pathol* 14:698–708.

Pitot NC. (1982) The natural history of neoplastic development: the relation of experimental models to human cancer. *Cancer* 49:1206–1211.

Platz H, Fries R, Hudec M, Min Tjoa A, Wagner RR. (1982) Prognostic relevance of minimal invasion in carcinomas of the oral cavity: a retrospective DOSAK study. *Clin Oncol* 1:467–473.

Proffitt SD, Spooner TR, Kosek JC. (1970) Origin of undifferentiated neoplasm from verrucous carcinoma of oral cavity following irradiation. *Cancer* 26:389–393.

Quick CA, Foucar E, Dehner LP. (1979) Frequency and significance of epithelial atypia in laryngeal papillomatosis. *Laryngoscope* 89:550–560.

Rasgon B, Cruz R, Hilsinger R. (1989) Relation of lymph-node metastasis to histopathologic appearance in oral cavity and oropharyngeal carcinoma: a case series and literature review. *Laryngoscope* 99: 1103–1110.

Riera Velasco JR, Suárez Nieto C, Pedrero de Bustos C, Alvarez Marcos C. (1987) Premalignant lesions of the larynx: pathological prognostic factors. *J Otolaryngol* 16:367–370.

Rodriguez-Jurado R, Sanz CR, Luna MA. (1996) Papilomatosis respiratoria recurrente y carcinoma broncogénico multicéntrico asociado a HPV 11/6 presentación de un caso y revisión de la literatura. *Patologia (Mex)* 39:11–18.

Rowley H. (1998) The molecular genetics of head and neck cancer. *J Laryngol Otol* 112:607–612.

Rowley H, Sherrington P, Helliwell TR, Kinsella A, Jones AS. (1998) p53 expression and p53 gene mutation in oral cancer and dysplasia. *Otolaryngol Head Neck Surg* 118:115–123.

Roz L, Wu CL, Porter S, Scully C, Speight P, Read A, Sloan P, Thakker N. (1996) Allelic imbalance on chromosome 3p in oral dysplastic lesions: an early event in oral carcinogenesis. *Cancer Res* 56:1228–1231.

Saku T, Sato E. (1983) Prediction of malignant change in oral precancerous lesions by DNA cytofluorometry. *J Oral Pathol* 12:90–102.

Schepman KP, van der Meij EH, Smeele LE, van der Waal I. (1996) Prevalence study of oral white lesions with special reference to a new definition of oral leucoplakia. *Oral Oncol Eur J Cancer* 32B:416–419.

Schwade JG, Wara WM, Dedo HH, Phillips TL. (1976) Radiotherapy for verrucous carcinoma. *Radiology* 120:677–679.

Schwartz LH, Ozsahin M, Zhang GN, Touboul E, De Vataire F, Andolenko JP, Saint-Guily JL, Laugier A, Schlienger M. (1994) Synchronous and metachronous head and neck carcinomas. *Cancer* 74:1933–1938.

Shanmugaratnam K, in collaboration with Sabin LH, et al. (1991) *Histological Typing of Tumors of the Upper Respiratory Tract and Ear*, 2nd ed., pp. 26–28. Springer-Verlag, Berlin.

Shear M, Pindborg JJ. (1980) Verrucous hyperplasia of the oral mucosa. *Cancer* 46:1855–1862.

Shin DM, Voravud N, Ro JY, Lee JS, Hong WK, Hittelman WN. (1993) Sequential increases in proliferating cell nuclear antigen expression in head and neck tumorigenesis: a potential biomarker. *J Natl Cancer Inst* 85:971–978.

Sidransky D, Preisinger AC, Frost P, Oyasu T, Vogelstein B. (1992) Clonal origin of bladder cancer. *N Engl J Med* 326:737–740.

Silverman S Jr, Gorsky M. (1997) Proliferative verrucous leukoplakia. A follow-up of 54 cases. *Oral Surg Oral Med Oral Pathol Oral Radiol Endod* 84:154–157.

Silverman S, Gorsky M, Kaugars GE. (1996) Leukoplakia, dysplasia, and malignant transformation. *Oral Surg Oral Med Oral Pathol* 82:177.

Silverman S, Gorsky M, Lozada F. (1984) Oral leukoplakia and malignant transformation: a follow-up study of 257 patients. *Cancer* 53:563–568.

Snyder RN, Perzin KH. (1972) Papillomatosis of nasal cavity and paranasal sinuses (inverted papilloma, squamous papilloma): a clinicopathologic study. *Cancer* 30:688–690.

Soria JC, Vielh P, El-Naggar AK. (1998) Telomerase activity in cancer: a magic bullet or a mirage? *Adv Anat Pathol* 5:86–94.

Spiro R, Huvos A, Wong G. (1986) Predictive value of tumor thickness in squamous carcinoma confined to the tongue and floor of the mouth. *Am J Surg* 152:345–350.

Suarez P, Adler-Storhz K, Luna MA, El-Naggar AK, Abdul-Karim FW, Batsakis JG. (2000) Papillary squamous cell carcinoma of the upper aerodigestive tract: a clinicopathologic and molecular study. *Head Neck Surg* (In Press).

Thomas S, Kearsley J. (1937) Betel quid and oral cancer: a review. *Eur J Cancer Oral Oncol B* 29B:251–255.

Thompson LDR, Wenig BM, Heffner DK, Gnepp DR. (1994) Exophytic and papillary squamous cell carcinomas of the larynx: a clinicopathologic series of 105 cases. [abstract]. *Mod Pathol* 10:117A.

van der Riet P, Nawroz H, Hruban RH, Corio R, Tokino K, Koch WM, Sidransky D. (1994) Frequent loss of chromosome 9p21-22 early in head and neck carcer progression. *Cancer Res* 54:1156–1158.

Vedtofte P, Holmstrup P, Horting-Hanson E, Pindborg JJ. (1987) Surgical treatment of premalignant lesions of the oral mucosa. *Int J Oral Maxillofac Surg* 16:656–664.

Ward BE, Fechner RE, Mills SE. (1990) Carcinoma arising in oncocytic Schneiderian papilloma. *Am J Surg Pathol* 14:364–369.

Waridel F, Estreicher A, Bron L, Flaman JM, Fontolliet C, Monnier P, Frebourg T, Iggo R. (1997) Field cancerization and polyclonal *p53* mutation in the upper aerodigestive tract. *Oncogene* 14:163–169.

World Health Organization (WHO) Collaborating Center for Oral Precancerous Lesions. (1978) Definition of leukoplakia and related lesions: an aid to studies on oral precancer. *Oral Surg Oral Med Oral Pathol* 46:518–539.

Worsham MJ, Wolman SR, Carey TE, Zarbo RJ, Benninger MS, Van Dyke DI. (1995) Common clonal origin of synchronous primary head and neck squamous cell carcinomas. *Hum Pathol* 26:251–261.

Wray A, McGuint WF. (1993) Smokeless tobacco usage associated with oral carcinoma. Incidence, treatment, outcome. *Arch Otolaryngol Head Neck Surg* 119:929–933.

Zidar N, Gale N, Cör A, Kambie V. (1996) Expression of Ki-67 antigen and proliferative cell nuclear antigen in benign and malignant epithelial lesions of the larynx. *J Laryngol Otol* 110:440–445.

5

SALIVARY GLAND

Ruby Delgado and Jorge Albores-Saavedra

Salivary gland neoplasms are unique for the variety of tumor types and subtypes they encompass and the cytoarchitectural and biological complexity that characterizes them. Theories of histogenesis have been advanced, which follow in chronological order. *1* The stem cell or reserve cell gives rise to all tumor types; however, this putative cell has not been identified. *2* In the semipluripotential bicellular reserve cell hypothesis one class of tumors arises from the intercalated duct cells and another set from basal cells associated with the excretory duct. This theory has proven to be conceptually attractive given its correlation with tumors displaying low-grade and high-grade behaviors, respectively. However, its validity has been questioned in favor of *3* the multicellular theory, whereby each cell type is capable of undergoing neoplastic transformation. Besides the unresolved histogenesis, insights into several intriguing observations, such as the more common occurrence of tumors in the parotid gland, the inverse correlation between incidence of malignancy and salivary gland size, and the greater frequency of salivary gland malignancies in children, have not been set forth.

The diversity of salivary gland neoplasms, the frequency with which they show overlapping features, their proclivity toward undergoing metaplasia, and the occurrence of hybrid tumors, indicate that these neoplasms may have an inherently plastic genome. This is further suggested by the potential of some tumor types to transform or progress into higher-grade neoplasms. This transformation may occur along the line(s) of differentiation of the native tumor (e.g., salivary duct carcinoma and/or myoepithelial carcinoma arising from a pleomorphic adenoma), result from transdifferentiation (e.g., adenoid cystic carcinoma arising in a pleomorphic adenoma), or are preceded by metaplasia (e.g., squamous cell carcinoma arising in Warthin's tumor). Because there are varying pathways of transformation, a single benign precursor lesion may give rise to different malignant tumor types (Table 5–1). Conversely, a malignant tumor type may have more than one benign precursor (Table 5–2). Malignant transformation may occur *de novo*, particularly in the setting of a long-standing tumor, or it may accompany or follow tumor recurrence. Malignancy may be manifested mainly by an invasive growth, with minimal accompanying cytological atypia, or by overt cytological malignancy. Tumor progression may ensue through progressive acquisition of a higher cytological grade or by abrupt dedifferentiation.

MALIGNANT TRANSFORMATION OF PLEOMORPHIC ADENOMA

Pleomorphic adenoma (benign mixed tumor), the most common type of salivary gland neoplasm involving both major and

Table 5–1. Benign Precursors of Malignant Neoplasms

Benign Precursor	Malignant Neoplasms
Pleomorphic adenoma	Salivary duct carcinoma
	Malignant myoepithelioma
	(myoepithelial carcinoma)
	Mucoepidermoid carcinoma
	Adenoid cystic carcinoma
	Polymorphous low-grade adenocarcinoma
	Epithelial-myoepithelial carcinoma
	Carcinosarcoma
Basal cell adenoma	Basal cell adenocarcinoma
(mainly membranous subtype)	Salivary duct carcinoma
	? Adenoid cystic carcinoma
Benign myoepithelioma	Malignant myoepithelioma
	(myoepithelial carcinoma)
Oncocytoma	Malignant oncocytoma
	(oncocytic carcinoma)
Warthin's tumor	Oncocytic adenocarcinoma
	Squamous cell carcinoma
	Mucoepidermoid carcinoma
Sebaceous lymphadenoma	Sebaceous lymphadenocarcinoma
Benign lymphoepithelial lesion	Malignant lymphoepithelial lesion
	(lymphoepithelial carcinoma)
Parotid duct cyst	Mucoepidermoid carcinoma
Mucus retention cyst of	
minor salivary glands	

minor salivary glands, is also the best recognized precursor lesion of salivary gland malignancies (Table 5–3). Malignant transformation may occur *de novo*, in the setting of a long-standing pleomorphic adenoma, but is more frequently associated with recurrent pleomorphic adenomas. It is uncertain whether recurrence allows for the acquisition of malignant phenotype, or if recurring tumors harbor an inherent biologic propensity to both recur and undergo malignant transformation (Auclair and Ellis, 1996). On rare occasion a pleomorphic adenoma may undergo submicroscopic malignant transformation and display metastatic behavior, so-called metastasizing pleomorphic adenoma.

RECURRENT PLEOMORPHIC ADENOMA

Pleomorphic adenomas have the propensity to recur once or multiple times. Tumor recurrence is often the result of inadequate excision and/or tumor rupture and spillage during removal (Phillips and Olsen, 1995)

Table 5–2. Precursors of Malignant Neoplasms

Malignant Neoplasm	Precursors
Malignant myoepithelioma	Pleomorphic adenoma
(myoepithelial carcinoma)	Benign myoepithelioma
High-grade	Pleomorphic adenoma
salivary duct carcinoma	Basal cell adenoma
	Low-grade salivary duct carcinoma
Malignant salivary gland	Carcinoma ex pleomorphic adenoma
tumors with osteoclast-like	Carcinoma with osteosarcoma ex pleomorphic adenoma
Giant cells	High-grade salivary duct carcinoma
	High-grade myoepithelial carcinoma
	High-grade mucoepidermoid carcinoma

Table 5–3. Pleomorphic Adenoma–Related Lesions

Pleomorphic adenoma

Recurrent pleomorphic adenoma

? Atypical/dysplastic Pleomorphic adenoma

Carcinoma ex pleomorphic adenoma
    In situ, intracapsular, noninvasive
    Minimally invasive (<8 mm beyond capsule)
    Invasive (>8 mm beyond capsule)

Carcinosarcoma ex pleomorphic adenoma

Metastasizing pleomorphic adenoma

and usually occurs in the distribution of the primary procedure. Less likely, multicentricity and metachronous tumor development may account for surgical failure (Buchman et al., 1994). The incidence of recurrence increases with the size of the primary tumor, which may be related to the difficulty in its removal. Like their primary counterparts, recurrent pleomorphic adenomas are slow growing tumors. The interval between primary excision and detection of recurrence is 6–10 years (Phillips and Olsen, 1995; Laskawi et al., 1998). The interval appears to be longer when pleomorphic adenoma recurs as a solitary lesion than when it recurs as multiple nodules, the latter being the most common pattern of recurrence (Fig. 5–1; Laskawi et al., 1998). There is a correlation between the patient's age at the time of appearance of the primary pleomorphic adenoma and its tendency to recur. Recurrence is more likely in those patients who de-

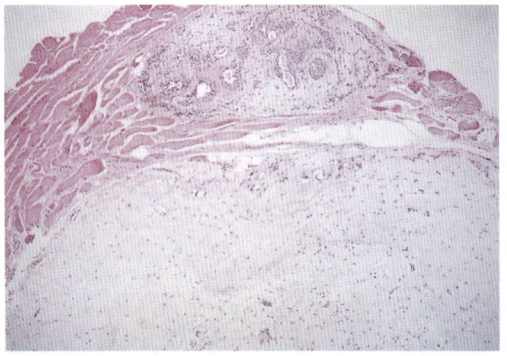

Figure 5–1. Recurrent pleomorphic adenoma. Two well-demarcated nodules are seen within skeletal muscle. The larger nodule is predominantly myxoid while the smaller contains ductal structures.

velop their primary tumor at an earlier age (McGregor et al., 1988). Patients with multiple recurrences are also significantly younger than those with only one. This has been attributed to a greater 'growth potency' of tumor cells in younger patients (Laskawi et al., 1998).

Regardless of their greater frequency, pleomorphic adenomas tend to recur more than other benign tumors of salivary gland (Laskawi et al., 1998). This may be due to their tendency toward capsular ingrowth or bosselation with protuberant outgrowths or pseudopod projections that extend beyond the main tumor. These may be left behind, particularly when enucleation or marginal excision is attempted, thus explaining the often multinodular nature of the recurrence. Alternatively, rupture of a myxoid pleomorphic adenoma may seed the operation site. The occurrence of pseudopodia outside the pseudocapsule remains a more significant risk factor for local recurrence (Henriksson et al., 1998; Natvig and Soberg, 1994). Because of the apparent capsule around pleomorphic adenomas, historically enucleation of the tumor has been the initial treatment of choice (Jackson et al., 1993). However, pleomorphic adenoma has at best a pseudocapsule of compressed glandular parenchyma (Clairmont et al., 1977) which might be closely approached or violated during surgery, particularly in large tumors. In small tumors, the condensation of peripheral fibrous tissue is still minimal (Clairmont et al., 1977); which may also contribute to inadequate excision. For these reasons, an unacceptable number of recurrences have followed enucleation. This practice was abandoned in favor of surgical procedures through which the tumor is excised with normal surrounding tissue, the aim being that the first excision be decisive (Jackson et al., 1993). Superficial or total parotidectomy with preservation of facial nerve is indicated for tumors arising in the superficial or deep lobes of the parotid gland, respectively. Pleomorphic adenomas arising from the deep lobe of the parotid seem to recur with less frequency. This is less likely a variation in innate biological behavior than the result of their anatomical location (Fliss et al., 1992). The space occupied by deep lobe tumors is more firmly enclosed and stimulates more reaction in the surrounding tissues. Consequently, deep lobe tumors have thicker pseudocapsules and less capsular penetration by tumor. In addition, deep lobe tumors are discovered later than those in the superficial lobes as they take longer to manifest clinically, hence there is more time for the capsule to mature. Aggressive treatment of the recurrent tumor is also advocated since the incidence of malignant transformation increases in recurrent tumors (Jackson et al., 1993). Proliferation activity has been reported to be markedly higher in the epithelial component of recurrent adenomas then that of nonrecurrent tumors. (Bankamp and Blerhoff, 1999). Treatment of recurrent pleomorphic adenoma should be aggressive removal of all tumor nodules and surrounding gland and scar tissue as soon as recurrence is detected. Recurrences are associated with malignant transformation and the unlikely possibility of metastasizing behavior. Complete surgical resection of primary tumor precludes transformation of residual tumor. Local recurrence after complete excision of pleomorphic adenomas is unusual; approximately one-half of such cases turn out to have been malignant (Qureshi et al., 1994).

Carcinoma ex Pleomorphic Adenoma

Malignant transformation of pleomorphic adenoma, variably referred to as carcinoma ex pleomorphic adenoma, carcinoma arising in pleomorphic adenoma, or malignant mixed tumor, occurs in approximately 6.2% of pleomorphic adenomas (Gnepp, 1993). It occurs either *de novo* after long periods of latency in a long-standing pleomorphic or in association with recurrent pleomorphic adenomas (Gnepp, 1993; LiVolsi and Perzin, 1977; Table 5–4). The risk of malignant

Table 5–4. Factors Associated with Increased Risk of Malignant Transformation of Pleomorphic Adenoma

Long-standing pleomorphic adenoma

Recurrent pleomorphic adenoma

Large tumor size (>5 cm)

Occurrence in submandibular gland

Older patient age

Prominent stromal hyalinization with calcification

change is increased in recurrent disease (Jackson et al., 1993). In one series, up to two-thirds of the patients whose mixed tumor transformed to carcinoma had recurrence (Auclair and Ellis, 1996). Consequently, the usual age at diagnosis is older than that for pleomorphic adenomas. Most pleomorphic adenomas are detected between the fourth and sixth decades, and carcinomas ex pleomorphic adenomas between the sixth and eighth decades. Factors associated with an increased incidence of malignant transformation are tumor size greater than 2 cm, tumors located in the deep lobe of the parotid, and when arising in recurrent tumors, in solitary mass as opposed to multiple recurrent nodules; all of these factors imply longer evolution (Phillips and Olsen, 1995). The incidence of malignant change may actually be greater since the malignant component may obliterate the underlying adenoma (Spiro et al., 1977). In the absence of such histological evidence, a history of sudden increase in size of a mass that has been present for some time is suggestive of an origin in a benign adenoma (McCluggage et al., 1998). A characteristic history for carcinoma ex pleomorphic adenoma is recent, rapid growth or development of facial nerve paralysis accompanying a long-standing salivary gland mass (Wenig et al., 1992).

The site of occurrence of carcinoma ex pleomorphic adenoma follows the distribution of pleomorphic adenomas—mainly the parotid gland among major salivary glands and palate among minor salivary glands (Gnepp, 1993). However, a slightly greater-than-expected proportion of submandibular, sublingual, and nonpalatal minor salivary gland tumors has been reported. The characteristic presentation of a mass with recent, rapid growth is seen in only a minority of patients. Most present with a painless mass. Facial nerve palsy and skin fixation are variable. More than half of the patients have fixation of their tumors to adjacent tissue. In general, the average size of carcinoma ex pleomorphic adenoma is more than twice as large as its benign counterpart. While most pleomorphic adenomas are less than 5 cm, half of carcinomas ex pleomorphic adenomas are greater than 5 cm. Grossly, carcinoma ex pleomorphic adenoma is poorly circumscribed and may be extensively infiltrative. Clinical findings at initial diagnosis that indicate a greater likelihood of malignant transformation are occurrence in the submandibular gland, older patient age, and large tumor size (Auclair and Ellis, 1996; Table 5–4).

Malignant transformation of any or both of the components of pleomorphic adenoma, epithelial and myoepithelial, may occur. Although the myoepithelial component predominates in most pleomorphic adenomas, most malignancies are along the epithelial line of differentiation—more specifically, salivary duct carcinomas. In addition, all major histologic salivary gland tumor types have been reported (Table 5–1) singly or in combination (Gnepp, 1993). Polymorphous low-grade adenocarcinoma, primarily a tumor of minor salivary glands, occurs in the major salivary glands in the form of a carcinoma ex pleomorphic adenoma.

The diagnosis of carcinoma ex pleomorphic adenoma requires the presence of unequivocal malignancy (Allen et al., 1994; Auclair and Ellis, 1996). Morphologic features of malignancy include invasiveness, necrosis, atypical mitoses, cellular anaplasia and pleomorphism, and architectural atypia, such as back-to-back glands and overgrowth of sheets of cells (Gnepp, 1993). Necrosis and increased mitotic activity are worrisome features but not indicative *per se* of malignancy (Gnepp, 1993). Similarly, hypercellularity has not been predictive of malignancy (Auclair and Ellis, 1996). True invasion into parenchyma or supporting stroma must be distinguished from capsular violation, that is, tumor cell penetration into or perforation through fibrous pseudocapsule (Auclair and Ellis, 1996). Capsular violation, however, is associated with recurrence, which indirectly increases the risk of malignancy. Necrosis may be related to history of manipulation, such as fine-needle aspiration biopsy. Central necrosis of a lesion with a narrow peripheral rim of viable tissue is suggestive of an ischemic or infarctive cause, particularly when accompanied by abrupt initiation of severe pain (Allen et al., 1994). Mitotic activity and some degree of atypia is not unexpected in areas adjacent to necrosis, whether spontaneous or induced. The increased mitotic activity may be the result of cytokines produced in response to necrotic tissue.

The proportion of carcinoma may vary from focal and confined within the pleomorphic adenoma to widely invasive. Presumably, it may obliterate the underlying pleomorphic adenoma. Thus, sampling may account for the variation in incidence of carcinoma ex pleomorphic adenomas among different series.

Carcinomas ex pleomorphic adenomas may be classified according to tumor type and grade, and degree of invasion, the latter considered to be of greater prognostic significance. Tumors with malignant foci confined within the underlying pleomorphic adenoma are variably termed *in situ*, intracapsular, intralesional, or noninvasive (Brandwein et al., 1996; LiVolsi and Perzin, 1977). In invasive tumors the extent of invasion beyond the pleomorphic adenoma capsule seems to determine biological behavior (Tortoledo et al., 1984). Tumors extending greater than 8 mm beyond the capsule behave aggressively, whereas those less than 8 mm have an excellent prognosis. Invasion is measured in a perpendicular plane from the outer limit of the fibrous capsule or from the residual benign component (most often the chondroid matrix) nearest the capsule to the most distant infiltrative edge of the carcinoma. Microscopic invasion may be present as discontinuous satellite tumor nodules (Brandwein et al., 1996). Thus, invasive carcinomas ex pleomorphic adenomas may be subclassified as minimally invasive when less than 8 mm and invasive (widely invasive) if greater than 8 mm. Among the former, when invasion exceeds 6 mm the tumor is more likely to recur and to metastasize to lymph nodes. Noninvasive and minimally invasive carcinomas ex pleomorphic adenomas are viewed as low-grade carcinomas, and invasive ones as high-grade carcinomas, *regardless of histologic tumor grade* (Brandwein et al., 1996). The former may be treated with complete excision and the latter with wide-local excision, lymph node dissection, and adjuvant radiotherapy. The scope of this treatment underscores the importance of adequate and extensive sampling when malignancy is encountered in a pleomorphic adenoma. Only the carcinomatous component is expected in the metastasis (Gnepp, 1993). A rare case in which the lymph node metastases contained both benign and malignant elements has been reported (Mini, 1993).

Salivary duct carcinoma, the most common tumor type arising in pleomorphic adenomas, is evidenced by atypia (plump eosinophilic cells with increased nuclear cytoplasmic ratio and prominent nucleoli) and mitotic activity of the ductal luminal cells (Gnepp, 1993; Brandwein et al., 1996). In its most incipient form, these cells are contained by the myoepithelial cells rimming the ductal structures from which they arise. It is this lesion that best qualifies for carcinoma *in situ* ex pleomorphic adenoma (Fig. 5–2). Salivary duct carcinoma ex pleomorphic adenoma usually arises within a background of fibrosed hyalinized stroma. Architectural changes characterizing the underlying pleomorphic adenoma, from which carcinoma originates, include diffuse hyalinization, minimal chondromyxoid matrix, and a zoning effect of central, small, cellular strands progressing to peripheral, angular, duct-like structures in the subcapsular region that are variably sized and dilated (Brandwein et al., 1996). Therefore, features that should arouse suspicion of malignant change in pleomorphic adenoma are cytologic and nuclear atypia, increased mitotic figures among the epithelial elements, and

excessive hyalinization and calcification of the stroma with isolation of epithelial elements (Clark et al., 1993; Brandwein, 1996; Table 5–4). Hyperchromatic, cytologically atypical cells embedded in a hyaline stromal matrix have been purported to be the earliest microscopic evidence of malignant transformation (Spiro et al., 1977). Whether they are called carcinoma *in situ* ex pleomorphic adenoma or atypical or dysplastic pleomorphic adenomas, tumors exhibiting these features warrant extra assurance that all of the tumor is removed and that the patient be carefully followed (Auclair and Ellis, 1996).

The pathogenetic mechanisms by which malignancy occurs are unknown, but at least two neoplasia-related genes have been implicated—c-*erb*B-2 protooncogene, which encodes a transmembrane putative growth factor receptor, and the *p53* tumor suppressor gene, which encodes a nuclear phosphoprotein thought to regulate proliferation of normal cells (Kamio, 1996). C-erbB-2 accumulation or overexpression is preferentially associated with high-grade carcinomatous components, mostly salivary duct carcinoma (Fig. 5–3), arising from a pleomorphic adenoma; low-grade histologic subtypes are neg-

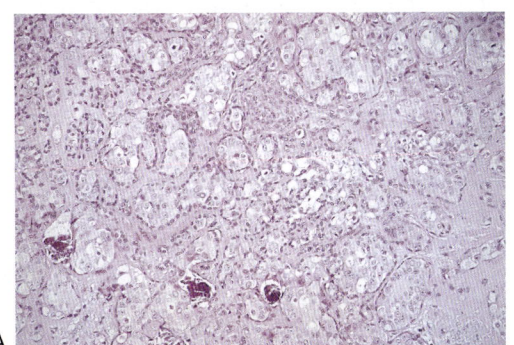

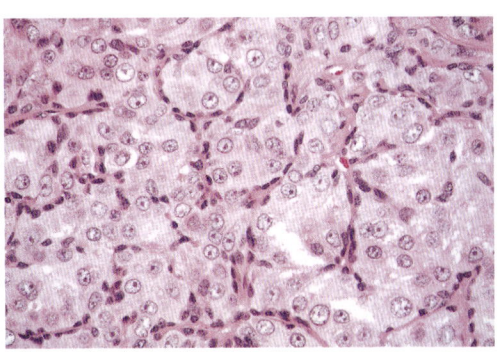

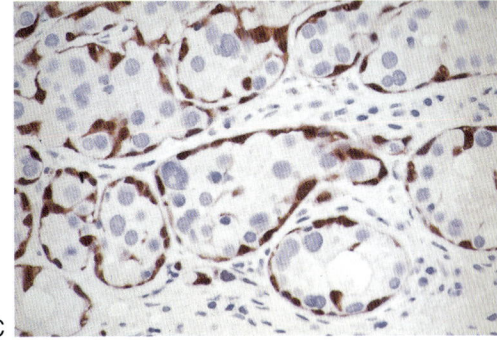

Figure 5–2 *A:* High-grade salivary ductal carcinoma *in situ* arising in pleomorphic adenoma. The neoplastic cells are confined to multiple ductal structures embedded in a hyalinized stroma. Microcalcifications are seen. *B:* Higher magnification of salivary ductal carcinoma *in situ* in pleomorphic adenoma. Plump eosinophilic malignant cells having large vesicular nuclei and prominent nucleoli are surrounded by myoepithelial cells. *C:* Salivary ductal carcinoma *in situ* in pleomorphic adenoma. The S-100 protein highlights the native myoepithelial cells.

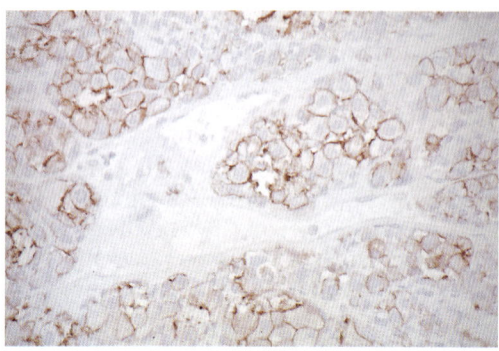

Figure 5–3. C-erb-2 overexpression in high-grade salivary duct carcinoma arising in pleomorphic adenoma. The neoplastic cells show the characteristic membrane reactivity.

ative. This suggests both a specific relation between c-*erb*B-2 gene amplification and a putative pathway of malignant transformation of pleomorphic adenoma, and the existence of more than one pathway in the process of malignant transformation of pleomorphic adenomas. Furthermore, this finding may have prognostic value in carcinoma ex pleomorphic adenoma (Costa Rosa et al., 1996; Müller et al., 1994; Sugano et al., 1992). Oncoprotein p53 expression appears more commonly as a late event, being present in the carcinoma but not in the antecedent pleomorphic adenoma (Righi et al., 1994; Li et al., 1997). Mutation of the *p53* tumor suppressor gene, however, may occur as an early event in the malignant transformation in some pleomorphic adenomas, as it is detected at an early precancerous stage (Deguchi et al., 1993; Righi et al., 1994; Yamamoto et al., 1998). Coexpression of c-erbB-2 and p53 correlates with high cell proliferative activity and may play an important part in the late stage of tumor progression (Kamio, 1996).

CARCINOSARCOMA EX PLEOMORPHIC ADENOMA

Carcinosarcoma ex pleomorphic adenoma, or true malignant mixed tumors, are biphasic tumors in which both epithelial and mesenchymal components fulfill histological criteria of malignancy. True malignant mixed tumors may arise from preexisting or coexisting pleomorphic adenomas or via an intermediate carcinoma ex pleomorphic adenoma (Blockage and Feddersen, 1995; Garner et al., 1989; Gnepp, 1993). Most involve the parotid gland, followed by the submandibular gland and palate (Latkovitch, 1998). In most reported cases there is prior history of a recurrent pleomorphic adenoma or histologic evidence of pleomorphic adenoma (Alvarez-Cañas and Rodilla, 1996; Latkovitch and Johnson, 1998).

Consistent with the putative origin of true malignant mixed tumors from a benign pleomorphic adenoma is the finding that the sarcomatous element is most often a chondrosarcoma and the epithelial element is most often a high-grade salivary duct carcinoma (Hellquist and Michaels, 1986; Stephen et al., 1986). Chondrosarcoma is followed by osteosarcoma, fibrosarcoma, malignant fibrous histiocytoma, and rhabdomyosarcoma (Gandour-Edwards et al., 1994; Latkovitch and Johnson, 1998). Areas of dedifferentiated chondrosarcoma have also been described (Stephen et al., 1986). The carcinomatous component may also be undifferentiated carcinoma or squamous carcinoma. The sarcomatous element usually predominates (Gnepp, 1993; Stephen et al., 1986). As in carcinoma ex pleomorphic adenoma, prominent stromal hyalinization, often associated with diffuse calcification, is commonly seen (Stephen et al., 1986). When these tumors metastasize, both components almost always metastasize together. True malignant mixed tumor is an aggressive, often rapidly lethal neoplasm. Collision tumors or metastatic disease should always be excluded when making the diagnosis of true malignant mixed tumor (Latkovitch and Johnson, 1998). Salivary gland carcinosarcomas de novo occur rarely and their composition departs from that of true malignant mixed tumors (Latkovitch and Johnson, 1998).

METASTASIZING PLEOMORPHIC ADENOMA

Metastasizing pleomorphic adenoma refers to the phenomenon in which a histologically benign pleomorphic adenoma inexplicably metastasizes without having undergone prior histologically detectable malignant transformation; that is, the metastases are also histologically benign. Although pleomorphic adenoma is the most common salivary gland neoplasm, only approximately 50 cases of metastasizing pleomorphic adenomas have been reported, thus they are rare tumors. Reviews on this entity have failed to identify specific features in the primary pleomorphic adenomas that may be predictive of metastasis (Wenig et al., 1992). However, most patients have had at least one but often two or more local recurrences prior to onset of metastasis (Wenig et al., 1992). This has raised the possibility that intravascular or intralymphatic spread associated with surgical manipulation may account for or contribute to this phenomenon (Klijanienko et al., 1997; Goodisson et al., 1999) and has led others to believe that recurrences reflect an inherent aggressive biological behavior (Qureshi et al., 1994).

The primary tumor follows the distribution for pleomorphic adenomas, the most common sites being the parotid gland and palate. Most metastases are detected between 6 and 52 years after excision of the primary tumor (Wenig et al., 1992). Metastases can occur simultaneously with an episode of recurrence or may follow it (Wenig et al., 1992). The most common sites of metastasis are bone, lung, and regional lymph nodes (Wenig et al., 1992; Klijanienko et al., 1997), as for other major salivary malignancies (Batsakis, 1982; Schreibstein et al., 1995). The histologic appearance of the metastatic foci are nearly identical with the primary or recurrent neoplasm with only slight variation in the proportions of epithelial-to-myxochondroid components, cellularity, cellular pleomorphism, and mitotic activity (Wenig et al., 1992). Like the primary lesions, most metastatic lesions are slow-growing and amenable to local resection. A minority of patients has succumbed to disseminated disease; perhaps this is the reason for why the adjective "benign" was removed from metastasizing pleomorphic adenoma, the name previously given this entity (Klijanienko et al., 1997; Wenig et al., 1992). Death in these patients usually occurred between 2 and 8 years after presentation. Recurrences are treated with resection. Radiotherapy has been given but its value is questioned.

The mechanisms underlying such unlikely behavior remain unknown. Human pleomorphic adenomas have been successfully transplanted to nude mice with definite but slow increases in graft size and no change in histologic pattern (Barfoed et al., 1986). Tumorigenicity in the nude mouse model is used by some laboratories as the final criterion for transformation/malignancy. Of interest in this regard is the instance of a pleomorphic adenoma of the parotid gland following an unusually rapid and aggressive course in a heart transplant immunosuppressed patient (Sampson et al., 1998). Two years after excision of the parotid tumor, the patient presented (without prior local recurrence) with widely metastatic pleomorphic adenoma, which resulted in rapid mortality within 6 months. Also worth mentioning is the observation that cytogenetics performed on a metastasizing pleomorphic adenoma revealed the presence of unbalanced translocations, in contrast to the balanced translocations that characterize conventional pleomorphic adenomas. Thus, it seems that a combination of host factors, tumor properties, and surgical manipulation may be at play. Given its rarity, interpretation of a lesion as metastasizing pleomorphic adenoma requires extensive sampling of all resected material for evidence of malignancy (Wenig et al., 1992).

SALIVARY DUCT CARCINOMA

The term *salivary duct carcinoma* has been restricted to tumors composed predominantly or exclusively of ductal cells with formation of distended salivary duct structures and comprises two variants: high-grade salivary duct carcinoma and low-grade salivary duct carcinoma (Table 5–5). High-grade salivary duct carcinoma usually occurs *de novo*; however, it can also result from (1) malignant transformation of a preexisting pleomorphic adenoma or basal cell adenoma—carcinoma ex adenoma—and (2) the biological progression of a low-grade salivary duct carcinoma (Table 5–6). In turn, high-grade salivary duct carcinoma can undergo tumor progression to a sarcomatoid carcinoma. Low-grade salivary duct carcinoma is a recently described entity with no known precursors.

Table 5–5. Distinguishing Histopathologic Features of Low-Grade and High-Grade Salivary Duct Carcinoma

	Low-Grade SDC	High-Grade SDC
Predominant growth	Intraductal	Invasive
Intraductal growth pattern	Pseudocribriform with slit-like spaces, solid, and cystically dilated; focal architectural atypia	Cribriform with geometric spaces
Comedo necrosis	Absent	Frequent
Calcification	Present (psammoma bodies)	Only associated with comedo necrosis
Cell arrangement	Loose to overlapping	Rigid
Cell shape	Predominantly ovoid	Predominantly polygonal
Cytoplasmic borders	Indistinct	Well defined
Cytoplasm	Dense pale to bright eosinophilic	Powdery eosinophilic
Nuclei	Oval, low-grade	Round to oval, moderate to high-grade
Chromatin	Normochromatic	Vesicular
Nucleoli	Identifiable	Prominent
Mitotic figures	Negligible	Present
Cellular composition	Heterogenous; ductal, apocrine, vacuolated	Monomorphous: ductal
Myoepithelial component	Peripheral: rim	Peripheral: scattered
Immunohistochemistry	S-100 + HMW-CK-903 +	S-100 − HMW-CK-903 ±

SDC, salivary duct carcinoma.

HIGH-GRADE SALIVARY DUCT CARCINOMA; PREINVASIVE AND PREMALIGNANT LESIONS

High-grade salivary duct carcinoma (so designated because of its resemblance to mammary duct carcinoma) *de novo* is the most common clinicopathologic form and is believed to originate from the excretory or interlobular ducts of the major salivary glands (Afzelius et al., 1987; Batsakis and Luna,

Table 5–6. Salivary Duct Carcinoma

High-grade salivary duct carcinoma
Intraductal
Predominantly intraductal or minimally invasive
Predominantly invasive or invasive
With sarcomatoid transformation

High-grade salivary duct carcinoma ex pleomorphic adenoma in situ
Noninvasive, intracapsular
Minimally invasive (<8 mm)
Invasive (>8 mm)

Low-grade salivary duct carcinoma
Without high-grade component
With high-grade component

1989; Brandwein et al., 1990; Colmenero et al., 1993; Delgado et al., 1993; Garland et al., 1984; Grenko et al., 1995; Hui et al., 1986; Kleinsasser et al., 1968; Lewis et al., 1996; Luna et al., 1987; Yoshihara, 1994). The preinvasive, *in situ*, or intraductal phase characteristically displays a cribriform growth pattern associated with comedonecrosis (Fig. 5–4A). Micropapillary or solid patterns may coexist. *In situ* spread may occur both along the major ducts, with transition from normal duct to intraductal tumor noted (Fig. 5–4B), or within the salivary gland lobules (cancerization of the lobules). High-grade salivary duct neoplasia is distinguished by large, polygonal cells with granular to powdery eosinophilic cytoplasm, well-defined cell borders, intermediate to high-grade nuclei with prominent nuclear membranes, and macronucleoli. Apical snouts are frequently seen. Multinucleation and anaplasia may be present. Mitotic activity ranges from moderate to high. The neoplastic ducts are surrounded by hyalinized stroma and may be rimmed by slit-like vascular channels. In addition to showing immunoreactivity with the conventional markers of adenocarcinoma

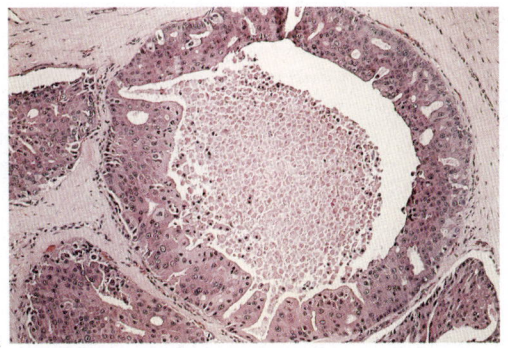 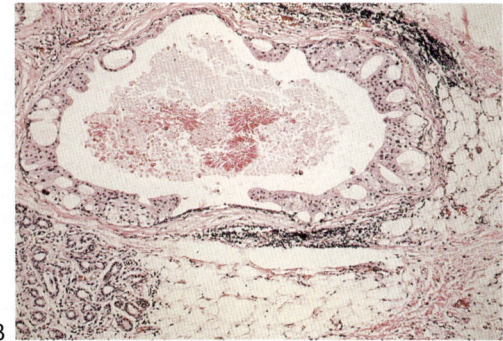

Figure 5–4. *A:* High-grade salivary duct carcinoma. Typical appearance of intraductal phase displaying a cribriform growth pattern and comedonecrosis. Note the characteristic granular to powdery eosinophilic cytoplasm. *B:* High-grade salivary duct carcinoma. Transition from normal to neoplastic epithelium is seen in intraductal carcinoma involving excretory duct.

(carcinoembryonic antigen, Leu-M1 and epithelial membrane antigen), the tumor cells are positive for BRST-1, GCDFP-15 (gross cystic disease fluid protein), and B72.3 antibodies. Notably, they do not express estrogen (ER) or progesterone receptors (PR) (Delgado et al., 1993; Lewis et al., 1996) but show diffuse reactivity for androgen receptor (Kapadia and Barnes, 1998). Ductal neoplastic cells are also negative for S-100 protein antibody (Delgado et al., 1993; Lewis et al., 1996). Ultrastructurally, the intraductal component is characterized by closely apposed polygonal to columnar cells with interdigitating lateral cell membranes, luminal microvilli, and distinct intercellular lumen formation. One tumor from our series was conspicuous for prominent basal membrane invaginations associated with vertically aligned mitochondria, features that distinguish striated ducts (Delgado et al., 1993). Scattered and attenuated myoepithelial cells may be identified by immunohistochemistry and electron microscopy, in keeping with an intraductal proliferation.

The characteristic appearance of intraductal carcinoma, with its reiterated striking resemblance to mammary duct carcinoma, is the distinguishing feature that enables ready recognition of a tumor as salivary duct carcinoma. Although most high-grade salivary duct carcinomas are predominantly invasive on presentation, the invasive component, and even the metastases (Fig. 5–5), may recapitulate the appearance of an intraductal carcinoma. While this provides a diagnostic advantage, it becomes necessary

to perform immunohistochemical stains (in particular, smooth muscle actin and calponin) in an attempt to confirm the presence of myoepithelial cells, albeit rare and attenuated, prior to entertaining the possibility of a predominantly or purely intraductal salivary duct carcinoma in the primary site. In this regard, it is important to distinguish intraductal basal staining from periductal linear staining; the former would correspond to myoepithelial cells, whereas the latter appears to represent a tight cuff of myofibroblasts associated with infiltrating glands (Prasad et al., 1999). The invasive component of high-grade salivary duct carcinoma may vary from well-formed ductal structures with mimicry of intraductal carcinoma as previously mentioned, to sheets or cords of cells with only focal lumen formation embedded in a desmoplastic stroma.

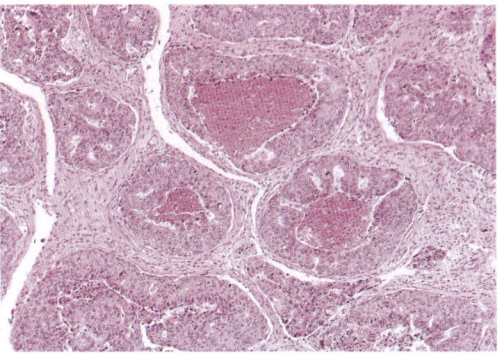

Figure 5–5. High-grade salivary duct carcinoma. Lymph node metastases are mimicking an intraductal carcinoma.

Varying degrees of dysplastic changes may be identified in the major ducts surrounding a high-grade salivary duct carcinoma (Brandwein et al., 1990; Delgado et al., 1993), a finding consistent with the expected evolution of intraductal dysplasia, intraductal carcinoma (*in situ*) to invasive ductal carcinoma. Nevertheless, compared with its breast counterpart, the prototypic duct carcinoma, high-grade salivary duct carcinoma, demonstrates a propensity for a short intraductal growth phase and early stromal invasion. Although explanation for such behavior may be forthcoming, several observations, extrapolated mostly from studies related to breast carcinoma, are worth mentioning here. Salivary duct carcinoma shows a preponderance of the comedocarcinoma pattern, which is reflective of a high proliferative capacity. In the breast this intraductal subtype has been proposed to be more closely related to invasive ductal carcinoma prognostically than to intraductal carcinoma. Periductal neovascularization, which is presumably a result of tumor-induced angiogenesis and has been underscored as a prerequisite for microinvasion, was a focal conspicuous finding in several tumors in our series (Delgado et al., 1993). There have been reports of high-grade salivary duct carcinoma showing distinct membrane positivity for c-erbB-2. Overexpression of c-erbB-2 oncoprotein in breast is associated with poor prognosis (Félix et al., 1996; Hellquist et al., 1994). More recently, enhanced expression of CD44v6 has been noted in salivary duct carcinoma (Kapadia and Barnes, 1998). CD44 is a family of cell adhesion glycoproteins that is involved in two of the three steps of the invasive cascade: adhesion to the extracellular matrix and motility (Herrera-Gayol and Jothy, 1999). CD44 splice variants, especially those containing the v6 domain, are assumed to play a critical role in the malignant progression of many human tumors. Thus, overexpression of CD44v6 may be linked to salivary duct carcinogenesis (Kapadia and Barnes, 1998). In contrast, p53 is infrequently overexpressed in salivary duct carcinoma (Hellquist et al., 1994).

High-grade salivary duct carcinoma arises more frequently in the parotid, but it may also involve submandibular and minor salivary glands (Epivatinos et al., 1995; Kumar et al., 1993; Lewis et al., 1996). One tumor arose from the extraglandular portion of Stensen's duct (Delgado et al., 1993). It has a male preponderance and occurs most often in patients over the age of 50 years. Most tumors behave in a high-grade fashion, with local recurrence, early regional and distant metastases, leading to death within 3 years. A minority have followed a less aggressive course on the basis of minimal or absent invasion after total parotidectomy; subtotal parotid resection led to recurrence (Anderson et al., 1992; Delgado et al., 1993). These tumors were either purely intraductal or predominantly intraductal as confirmed by myoepithelial markers. Despite multiple efforts, no clinically useful prognostic factors have been found for most high-grade salivary duct carcinomas (Barnes et al., 1994; Colmenero et al., 1993; Lewis et al., 1996), except possibly for the proliferative activity as evaluated by Ki-67 (Hellquist et al., 1994; Martinez-Barba et al., 1997). A combination of radical resection with ipsilateral lymph node dissection and postoperative radiotherapy is the recommended therapy.

High-Grade Salivary Duct Carcinoma ex Adenoma

High-grade salivary duct carcinoma is the most common histologic tumor type to arise from a pleomorphic adenoma (Delgado et al., 1993; Grenko et al., 1995; Lewis et al., 1996; Grenko et al., 1996; Tortoledo et al., 1984), and the second most common to arise from a basal cell adenoma (Nagao et al., 1997).

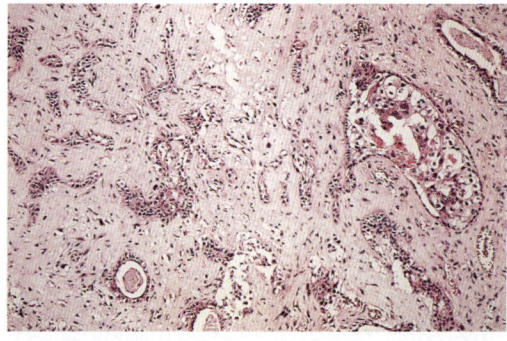

Figure 5–6. High-grade salivary ductal carcinoma arising in pleomorphic adenoma. Low-power view of a pleomorphic adenoma shows a single ductal structure distended by malignant cells of a high-grade salivary duct carcinoma.

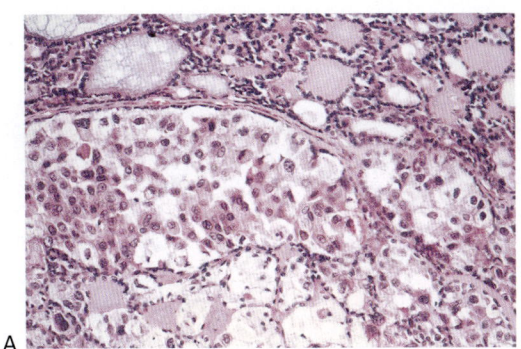 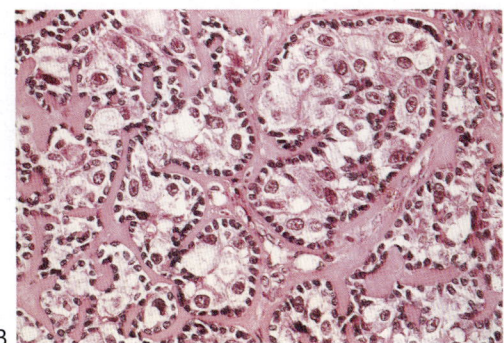

A   B

Figure 5–7. *A:* High-grade salivary ductal carcinoma (center) arising in basal cell adenoma. *B:* Another field of tumor shown in A. The neoplastic cells contain large nuclei with prominent nucleoli. A continuous layer of myoepithelial cells is seen at the periphery of the ducts.

Whereas high-grade salivary duct carcinoma *de novo* seems to arise from the excretory or interlobular ducts, carcinoma ex adenoma appears to originate from the ductal structures that make up each type of adenoma—pleomorphic or basal cell. Salivary duct carcinoma ex adenoma may exhibit the characteristic cribriform architecture, however, in the early stages the carcinomatous component conforms to the underlying architecture of the maternal adenoma. This morphological variant, *salivary ductal carcinoma*, is contained by the myoepithelial layer of the pleomorphic adenoma (Fig. 5–6) or the myoepithelial/basal cell layer of the basal cell adenoma (Fig. 5–7; also discussed in the corresponding sections Pleomorphic Adenoma and Basal Cell Adenoma). Interestingly, we have seen a case in which high-grade salivary duct carcinoma arose both within a pleomorphic adenoma as well as from major ducts surrounding it (Delgado et al., 1993).

HIGH-GRADE TRANSFORMATION OF LOW-GRADE SALIVARY DUCT CARCINOMA

High-grade salivary duct carcinoma arising from a low-grade salivary duct carcinoma (Table 5–5), a recently described entity, is less well recognized (Delgado et al., 1996). Low-grade salivary duct carcinoma is mainly an intraductal proliferative lesion showing a bland to low-grade cytoarchitecture. It is characterized by the proliferation of salivary duct structures exhibiting three main patterns of growth which may coexist in varying

proportions: *(1)* Cystically dilated ducts lined by delicate micropapillae, tufts, or plaque-like intraluminal projections, composed of cuboidal to small columnar cells exhibiting conspicuous intracytoplasmic vacuolization (Fig. 5–8); *(2)* ducts filled and distended by a solid or pseudocribriform (fenestrated) cellular proliferation consisting of ovoid to cuboidal cells with dense pale to bright eosinophilic cytoplasm, indistinct cell borders, and oval nuclei with finely dispersed chromatin and pinpoint nucleoli (Fig. 5–9A); or *(3)* ducts exhibiting architectural atypia. Whereas high-grade salivary duct carcinoma resembles intermediate or high-grade intraductal carcinoma of the breast, low-grade salivary duct carcinoma spans an appearance reminiscent of florid to atypical ductal hyperplasia to low-grade intraductal carcinoma. Low-grade salivary duct carcinomas characteristically coexpress S-100 pro-

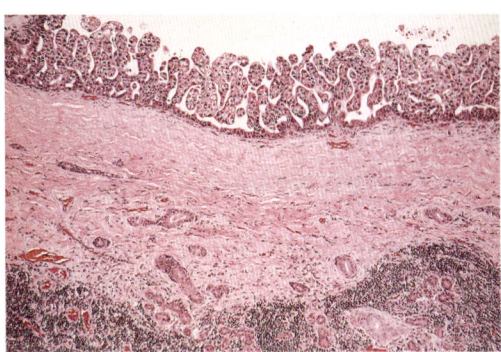

Figure 5–8. Low-grade salivary duct carcinoma. A micropapillary pattern composed of cuboidal cells exhibiting cytoplasmic vacuolization.

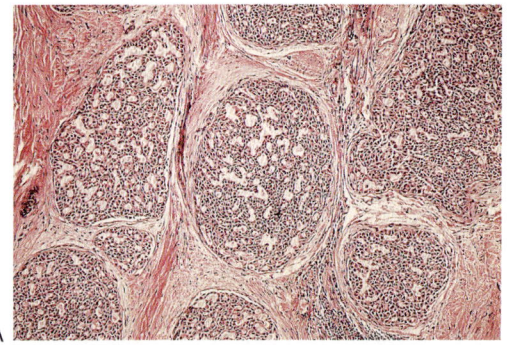

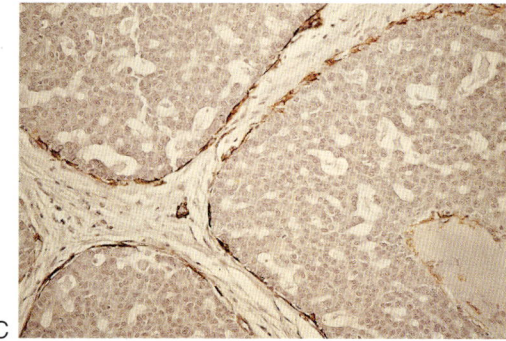

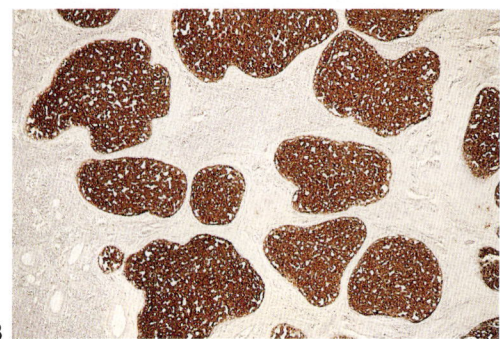

Figure 5–9. *A:* Low-grade salivary duct carcinoma showing the characteristic pseudocribriform (fenestrated) pattern, reminiscent of florid ductal hyperplasia of the breast. *B:* Low-grade salivary duct carcinoma. Strong and diffuse reactivity for S-100 protein is shown. *C:* Low-grade salivary duct carcinoma. The distended ducts filled with tumor cells are silhouetted by a continuous layer of myoepithelial cells that show immunoreactivity for smooth muscle actin.

tein and high-molecular-weight cytokeratin (CK903 or 34BE12) and appear to show differentiation toward an intercalated duct cell phenotype (Fig. 5–9B). A peripheral rim of myoepithelial cells is identified (by immunohistochemistry and ultrastructure) in the involved ducts, in a pattern indicative of a myoepithelial layer of preexisting ducts involved in intraductal neoplastic proliferation (Fig. 5–9C). An alternative possibility is that low-grade salivary duct carcinoma consists of a highly organized bicellular ductal/myoepithelial growth. Low-grade salivary duct carcinoma is histologically, ultrastructurally, and immunophenotypically distinct and appears to represent the low-grade end of the spectrum of salivary duct neoplasia. However, it has demonstrated the capacity to evolve to a high-grade salivary duct carcinoma. In one case progression was evidenced by the acquisition of a higher cytologic grade accompanied by focal microinvasion (Fig. 5–10) (Delgado et al., 1996).

Thus far, low-grade salivary duct carcinoma has occurred in the parotid glands of adult patients, with no gender predilection. Total parotidectomy appears to have been curative.

SARCOMATOID TRANSFORMATION OF HIGH-GRADE SALIVARY DUCT CARCINOMA

Transformation into a sarcomatoid or anaplastic carcinoma is regarded as a morphological manifestation of tumor progression and provides further evidence of salivary duct carcinoma's propensity for biological aggressiveness. The natural history of sali-

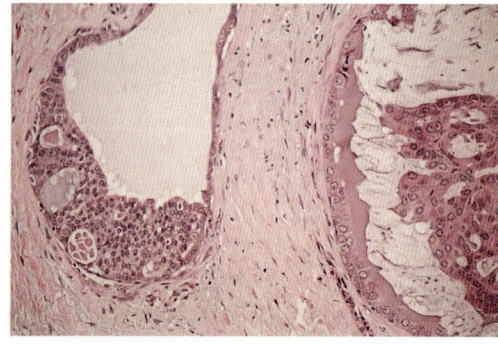

Figure 5–10. Tumor progression in low-grade salivary duct carcinoma. Focus showing a higher cytological grade (*right*) as compared to low-grade salivary duct carcinoma (*left*) (Table 5–5).

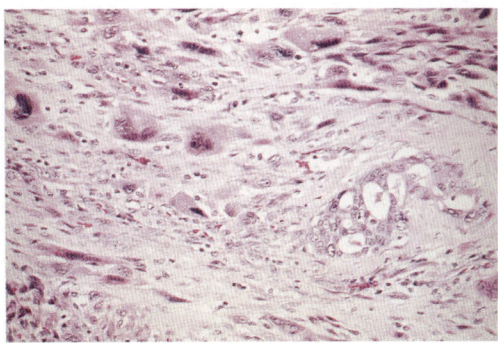

Figure 5–11. High-grade salivary duct carcinoma with sarcomatoid features. The epithelial island shows cribriform features and the sarcomatoid component consists of spindle cells with large pleomorphic nuclei.

vary duct carcinoma should be kept in mind, especially when confronted with presumptive primary salivary gland sarcomas or carcinosarcomas. Extensive sampling of such cases may result in identification of foci diagnostic of salivary duct carcinoma (Fig. 5–11). We saw one case of sarcomatoid salivary duct carcinoma in which both components, high-grade and low-grade salivary duct carcinoma, were identified.

CARCINOMA EX BASAL CELL ADENOMA

Compared to carcinoma ex pleomorphic adenoma, carcinomas arising in basal cell adenomas are rare (Chen, 1985; Luna et al., 1989; Nagao et al., 1997). They occur in the distribution of basal cell adenoma, primarily in the parotid gland, and less commonly in the submandibular gland (Luna et al., 1989). Carcinomas ex basal cell adenoma are diagnosed around a decade later than their benign counterparts and are usually twice their size (Luna et al., 1989; Nagao et al., 1997). These findings support their evolution from a pre-existing, and often long-standing, precursor neoplasm (Luna et al., 1989).

The dual composition of basal cell adenomas may not be readily apparent at light microscopy, hence their alternate designation of monomorphic adenomas. However, immunohistochemical and ultrastructural studies have demonstrated that basal cell adenomas are composed of luminal (ductal) and basal/myoepithelial cells (Ogawa et al., 1990). The degree of differentiation, proportion, and arrangement of these different types of tumor cells are responsible for the variety of histologic patterns that characterize basal cell adenoma. In contrast to carcinomas arising in pleomorphic adenomas, which more commonly show ductal (luminal) differentiation, malignant transformation of a basal cell adenoma usually proceeds along the basal cell line of differentiation and becomes manifest as a malignant basaloid tumor, the *basal cell adenocarcinoma* (Nagao et al., 1997). Malignant transformation along luminal lines occurs rarely and in the form of a non-basaloid tumor, mainly as a morphological variant of *salivary duct carcinoma* (Nagao et al., 1997). As will be discussed below malignant basaloid tumors arising in basal cell adenomas are by definition characterized by an invasive outgrowth beyond the adenoma (Luna et al., 1989; Nagao et al., 1997). Nonbasaloid, salivary duct carcinomas may be confined to basal cell adenoma (Nagao et al., 1997).

Of the four subtypes of basal cell adenoma, tubular, trabecular, solid, and membranous, it is the latter which has the highest risk of undergoing malignant change (Luna et al., 1989; Batsakis & Luna, 1991; Nagao et al., 1998a; Muller & Barnes, 1996). Other notable features distinguish membranous basal cell adenomas: the influence of myoepithelium is believed to be less in these tumors, they lack encapsulation, are often multifocal, recur frequently, and can be part of a salivary gland-cutaneous tumor diathesis (Batsakis et al., 1991). They have also been reported to arise from intranodal salivary tissues (Luna et al., 1987b). It becomes apparent that membranous basal cell adenoma shows a distinct biological behavior that sets it apart from other basal cell adenoma subtypes.

Basal cell adenocarcinoma, whether arising *de novo* or via evolution from a pre-existing basal cell adenoma, is essentially the malignant counterpart of basal cell adenoma (Luna et al., 1989; Batsakis and Luna, 1991; Ellis et al., 1990). As defined by the WHO it is "an epithelial neoplasm that has cytological characteristics of basal cell adenoma but morphological growth pattern indicative of malignancy" (Seifert et al., 1991). The distinctive diagnostic feature that separates it from basal cell adenoma is namely, invasive growth (McCluggage, et al., 1995; Ellis and Wiscovitch., 1990; Nagao et al., 1997). Basal cell adenocarcinoma may show only minimal deviation of cytoarchitecture from that of basal cell adenoma, or may be overtly malignant (Batsakis and Luna, 1991).

Like their benign counterpart, basal cell adenocarcinomas may exhibit four architectural patterns, trabecular, tubular, solid, and membranous (Nagao et al., 1998a). However, the solid pattern or subtype is the predominant in basal cell adenocarcinoma, being comprised of solid basaloid cell nests of varying sizes (Nagao et al., 1998a; Muller and Barnes, 1996; Ellis and Wiscovitch, 1990; Atula et al., 1993). Basal cell adenocarcinomas are also composed by a dual population (peripheral small cells with hyperchromatic nuclei and larger, central cells with pale vesicular nuclei, occasionally prominent nucleoli, and more cytoplasm, both cell types with indistinct cell borders) (Nagao et al., 1998a; Ellis and Wiscovitch, 1990; McCluggage et al., 1995; Muller and Barnes, 1996), but the palisade-like arrangement of tumor cells at the periphery is less conspicuous than in basal cell adenoma (Nagao et al., 1998a; Ellis and Wiscovitch, 1990; Muller and Barnes,1996). In contrast to the circumscribed, expanding and pushing growth pattern that is typical of benign adenomas, basal cell adenocarcinomas demonstrate invasion by strands and islands of tumor cells that extend from the main tumor mass into the normal acinar lobules or into adjacent periglandular soft tissues and dermis (Ellis and Wiscovitch, 1990). However, because membranous basal cell adenoma is typically unencapsulated (except for those arising in lymph nodes), multifocal and has an infiltrative appearance, this feature alone cannot be relied on to support a diagnosis of malignancy (Batsakis and Luna, 1991; Muller and Barnes, 1996). Therefore, other features must be sought. These include, necrosis, either comedo type or spotty, increased mitotic activity (> 4 mitotic figures /10 HPFs are indicative of malignancy), loss of polarity, cellular and nuclear pleomorphism, and perineural and intravascular invasion (Nagao et al., 1998a; McCluggage et al., 1995; Batsakis and Luna, 1991).

Recently, immunohistochemistry has been reported useful in distinguishing a basal cell adenoma from its malignant counterpart.. A Ki-67 labeling index of > 5%, nuclear expression of p53 in > 10% of tumor cells, expression of epidermal growth factor in also > 10% of tumor cells, and loss of bcl-2 expression, all support the diagnosis of basal cell adenocarcinoma (Nagao et al., 1998a). Basal cell adenomas have been characterized by positivity, predominantly in basal cells, for bcl-2, a protein associated with stem cells committed to differentiation and morphogenesis. Loss of bcl-2 immunoreactivity and alterations in p53 seem to accompany malignant transformation to basal cell adenocarcinoma (Nagao et al., 1998a).

Like basal cell adenocarcinoma arising *de novo*, carcinoma ex basal cell adenoma is a low grade malignancy with a high recurrence rate, requiring wide local excison with adequate margins, but with infrequent regional or distant metastases (Luna et al., 1989; Batsakis and Luna, 1991; Ellis and Wiscovitch, 1990; Nagao, 1998a; Muller and Barnes, 1996). Lymph node metastases are uncommon such that cervical dissection is usually not warranted. Although the majority of basal cell adenocarcinomas are of the solid type it has been suggested that recognizing this solid variant may have prognostic significance (Muller and Barnes, 1996). It has shown a disproportionate propensity for perineural and intravascular growth and has given rise to regional or systemic metastases (Ellis and Wiscovitch, 1990).

The salivary gland-cutaneous tumor diathesis or syndrome refers to the coexistence of salivary gland tumors (mainly, basal cell adenomas or basal cell adenocarcinomas occuring in parotid gland) and skin adnexal tumors (usually cylindromas, but also trichoepitheliomas and eccrine spiradenoma) (Ferrandiz et al., 1985; Herbst and Utz, 1984; Headington et al., 1977; Batsakis and Brannon, 1981; Batskis and Luna, 1991). Involvement of parotid gland may be bilateral and multifocal. The basal cell adenoma is almost always of the membranous type, and is associated with the syndrome in 25%–38% of the cases (Muller and Barnes, 1996). Incidentally, because of the histologic resemblance of membranous basal cell adenoma to counterpart tumors arising from skin adnexa, particularly to the eccrine cylindroma, this adenoma subtype has also been refered to as *dermal analogue adenoma* (Batsakis and Brannon, 1981). The basal cell adenocarcinoma is usually of the solid type, either de novo (Batsakis and Luna) or ex basal cell adenoma (Luna et al., 1989). Approximately 10% of basal cell adenocarcinomas are associated with the syndrome, that is, the frequency of coexisting skin lesions is one-third to one-half that observed in membranous basal cell adenoma (Muller and Barnes, 1996; Ellisand Wiscovitch, 1990; Batsakis and Luna, 1991). The association between certain basal cell adenomas and skin adnexal tumors can be explained by their histogenetic relationship (Batsakis and Brannon, 1981). Both the skin adnexae and salivary glands arise from germinal epithelium of ectodermal origin that pushes or invades an investing mesenchyme. Lobular development, tubulo-acinar formation and cytodifferentiation follow during later stages of embryonic life and early postnatal period. One of the significant modifiers of salivary gland and skin adnexae morphogenesis is the epithelial-mesenchyme interaction, which is mediated by an epithelial derived basal lamina. In fact the localization and accumulation of the mucopolysaccharide-containing lamina is likely integral to the final branching morphogenesis and architecture. The analogous salivary gland and skin adnexal tumors, membranous basal cell adenoma and eccrine cylindroma, share an exaggerated basal lamina. Perhaps the target of this syndrome is a pluripotential cell, a basic component of both, salivary intercalated and eccrine glandular ducts (Schmidt et al., 1991).

Basal cell adenoma has also been proposed as a possible benign counterpart or precursor for *adenoid cystic carcinoma*, another basaloid malignant tumor (McCluggage et al., 1995; Bernacchi et al., 1974; Atula et al., 1993; Muller and Barnes, 1996). Some authors prefer to view basal cell adenoma-adenoid cystic carcinoma as hybrid tumors (Muller and Barnes, 1996; Ellisand Wiscovitch, 1990). Thus, histogenetic correlations among basaloid tumors are still controversial (Nagao et al., 1997).

Salivary duct carcinoma arising in basal cell adenomas resembles salivary duct carcinoma ex pleomorphic adenoma, albeit its less frequent occurence. It may exhibit the classic histomorphology of cribriform ducts with comedonecrosis (Nagao et al., 1997). Alternatively, it may arise in the morphological pattern of salivary ductal carcinoma. This is characterized by the appearance, ususaly multifocal, of atypical and mitotically active large, plump eosinophilic cells with large vesicular nuclei and prominent nucleoli (Nagao et al., 1997). Initially, these cells replace the tubules, trabeculae, and nests and are contained within them by a peripheral rim of basal/myoepithelial cells, representing the in situ phase (Fig. 5–7). At a later stage, they become invasive into a hyalinized stroma, where they are unaccompanied by basal/myoepithelial cells (Nagao et al., 1997). As in salivary ductal carcinoma ex pleomorphic adenoma, these carcinoma cells can be highlighted by c-erbB-2 and BRST-1 immunostains (Nagao et al., 1997). In addition, in carcinoma ex basal cell adenoma, non-neoplastic cells express bcl-2, whereas neoplastic cells are negative (Nagao et al., 1998). As gathered from the few cases reported and from our experience, salivary duct carcinoma can arise in membranous and nonmembranous basal cell adenomas. Unlike basal cell adenocarcinoma ex adenoma, which is by definitiion invasive, salivary duct carcinoma may be confined within the adenomas. That is they may be non-invasive (intracapsular) or invasive (Nagao et al., 1998). Presumably, these tumors may be subclassified into minimally invasive and widely invasive according to Tortoledo's criteria for carcinomas ex pleomorphic adenoma, and expect a similar prognosis. However, we caution against applying these criteria to carcinomas arising in membranous basal cell adenoma, given the typical lack of encapsulation, multifocality, and inherently distinct biological behavior of this precursor.

MALIGNANT MYOEPITHELIOMA (MYOEPITHELIAL CARCINOMA)

Myoepithelial cells play an active role in the histogenesis of many salivary gland neoplasms and exert a major influence on their behavior (Batsakis and El-Naggar, 1999). Strategically located between luminal epithelium and basement membrane, they are capable of inducing epithelial differentiation and morphogenesis on one side, and of synthesizing and maintaining basement membrane, an invasive restrictive matrix, on the other. That is, myoepithelial cells may exert paracrine effects on glandular epithelium and also regulate the progression of ductal carcinoma *in situ* to invasive carcinoma. As a result, salivary gland carcinomas in which there is histopathologic (light, ultrastructural, and immunohistochemical) evidence of active participation of myoepithelial cells behave in a low-grade fashion, as compared to carcinomas without myoepithelial participation (Table 5–7). Moreover, the myoepithelial cell is believed to be a natural tumor suppressor. The myoepithelial cell resists malignant transformation and even in a transformed state it resists further progression and usually displays low-grade biologic behavior. Thus, it is not surprising that although myoepithelial cells are an important and even predominant element in many salivary gland tumor histologic types, pure myoepithelial tumors are rare, representing less than 1% of all salivary gland tumors (Seifert 1991). Furthermore, the inherent myoepithelial properties are likely to contribute to most myoepithelial neoplasms being benign or of a low-grade nature (Sternlicht and Barsky, 1997). Malignant myoepitheliomas (myoepithelial carcinoma) comprise only about 10% of myoepitheliomas.

It is not uncommon for malignant myoepitheliomas (myoepithelial carcinoma) to arise from an underlying (myoepithelial-rich) benign tumor, which may be either a pleomorphic adenoma or a benign myoepithelioma. Given its frequency, pleomorphic adenoma is the major precursor for malignant myoepithelioma (myoepithelial carcinoma). However, it must be acknowledged that distinction between a pleomorphic adenoma with myoepithelial predominance and

Table 5–7. Myoepithelial Participation in Salivary Gland Carcinomas

---

Carcinomas with integral myoepithelial participation
Adenoid cystic (tubular, cribriform)
Epithelial-myoepithelial carcinoma

Carcinomas without significant myoepithelial participation
Adenoid cystic (solid)
High-grade mucoepidermoid carcinoma
High-grade salivary duct carcinoma

Modified from Batsakis and El-Naggar, 1999.

a benign myoepithelioma is somewhat imprecise. In fact, some consider myoepithelioma to represent the end of the morphological spectrum of a pleomorphic adenoma (Simpson et al., 1995). Others have proposed that distinction of myoepithelioma from pleomorphic adenoma be based on the proportion of myoepithelial and ductal cells (Dardick et al., 1989). When the latter component is less than 10% the tumor is a myoepithelioma. Biologically, pleomorphic adenomas appear to have a significantly higher rate of recurrences and malignant change (Alos et al., 1996). There is a tendency for malignant myoepithelioma (myoepithelial carcinoma) to involve the parotid gland when arising from a pleomorphic adenoma (Alos et al., 1996; DiPalma et al., 1991; DiPalma and Guzzo, 1993; McCluggage et al., 1998; Singh et al., 1988; Suzuki et al., 1998; Tortoledo et al., 1984), and to involve minor salivary glands when arising from a benign myoepithelioma (Alos et al., 1996; Bombi et al., 1996). Malignant myoepithelioma (myoepithelial carcinoma) appears to be a low-grade malignancy when arising in a pleomorphic adenoma, and is more aggressive with a higher metastatic potential when arising *de novo* (DiPalma and Guzzo, 1993).

Malignant transformation may become manifest in two forms. The terms "malignant myoepithelioma" and "myoepithelial carcinoma," although used interchangeably, may be useful to describe these two forms. *Malignant myoepithelioma* may be virtually indistinguishable from its benign counterpart but displays an invasive growth (DiPalma and Guzzo, 1993). This may be seen as discontinuous tumor nests in surrounding glandular parenchyma or periglandular soft tissues, in unencapsulated myoepitheliomas (Fig. 5–12), or as extracapsular extension in encapsulated ones (Nagao et al., 1998C). Perineural or vascular invasion may also indicate its malignant nature. Malignant myoepitheliomas arising from a benign myoepithelioma or pleomorphic adenoma may recur several times before the diagnosis of malignancy is rendered (Bombi et al., 1996; DiPalma and Guzzo, 1993). Proliferative activity may be useful in the differential diagnosis between benign myoepithelioma and malignant myoepithelioma. A Ki-67 labeling index greater than 10% or more than 7

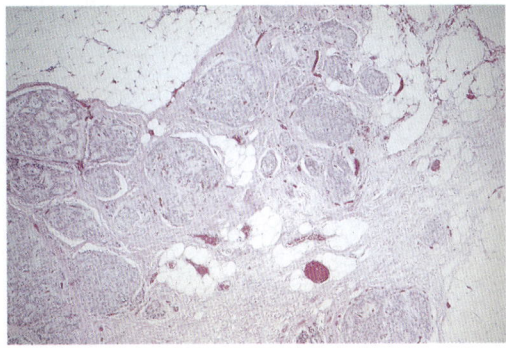

Figure 5–12. Malignant myoepithelioma. Multiple nodules of bland-appearing myoepithelial cells extend into fibroadipose tisssue adjacent to the parotid gland.

mitotic figures/10 high-power fields are reported to be diagnostic of malignant myoepithelioma (Nagao et al., 1998C). This form of myoepithelial malignancy behaves in a low-grade fashion.

In contrast, other malignant myoepithelial neoplasms demonstrate cellular and nuclear pleomorphism, increased mitotic activity, and necrosis, in addition to an invasive growth pattern; the term *myoepithelial carcinoma* seems best suited for these high-grade, overtly malignant tumors (Fig. 5–13; Nagao et al., 1998C). Myoepithelial carcinomas may be highly anaplastic, the myoepithelial nature of which may remain unrecognized if not thought of and confirmed by immunohistochemical markers or ultrastructure. When arising from pleomorphic adenomas, myoepithelial carcinomas

may be combined with other carcinomatous component. Failure to recognize its myoepithelial nature will result in an erroneous diagnosis of sarcoma or carcinosarcoma.

Of the several phenotypes that myoepithelial cells may adopt, spindled and epithelioid cells have emerged as common predominant components in malignant myoepitheliomas (myoepithelial carcinomas) (Alos et al., 1996). Malignant myoepitheliomas (myoepithelial carcinomas) with a predominance of plasmacytoid variants are extremely rare (Suzuki et al., 1998). Cell type does not appear to influence prognosis (Nagao et al., 1998C). The clear cell variant of malignant myoepithelioma, which characteristically exhibits foci of squamous metaplasia and hyaline deposits of basement membrane–like extracellular matrix material and collagenous spherules, must be distinguished from an epithelial–myoepithelial carcinoma with a predominant myoepithelial component (Michal et al., 1996).

In essence, myoepithelial neoplasms are composed of modified myoepithelial cells in various stages of differentiation (Alos et al., 1996; Nagao et al., 1998C). Unlike the native myoepithelial cell, neoplastic myoepithelial cells may show only partial immunophenotypic expression and ultrastructural evidence of myoepithelial differentiation. Recognition of myoepithelial neoplasms should take into account such modifications, particularly in malignant ones, because dedifferentiation adds difficulty to the identification of myoepithelial cells (Alos et al., 1996). There is as yet no

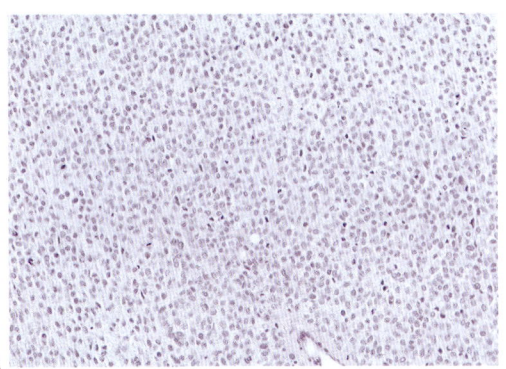
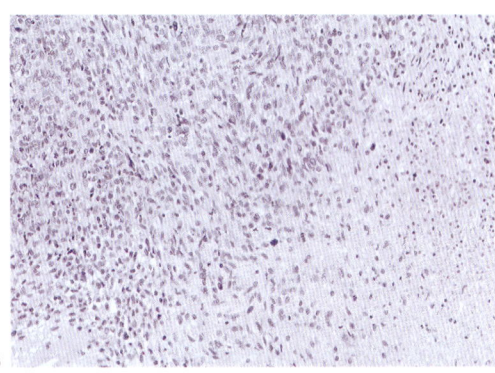

A B

Figure 5–13 *A:* Myoepithelial carcinoma. The tumor is densely cellular and shows predominantly round cells with numerous mitotic figures. *B:* In this field the tumor is composed of spindle-shaped cells and shows necrosis.

consensus regarding the acceptable minimum criteria for recognition of benign or malignant myoepithelial neoplasms (Nagao et al., 1998C; Simpson et al., 1995). In particular, the existence of a plasmacytoid subtype of myoepithelioma, lacking immunohistochemical and ultrastructural evidence of myogenous differentiation, has been questioned (Bombi et al., 1996; Franquemont and Mills, 1993). Ultrastructurally, myofilaments with or without focal densities, which are specific of normal myoepithelial cells, are not a usual finding in neoplastic myoepithelial cells; however, intermediate intracytoplasmic filaments, basal lamina, small desmosomes, and tight junctions are (Alos et al., 1996). The apparent absence of myofilaments should not exclude a diagnosis of myoepithelioma (Dardick, 1996). Among the myoepithelial markers, cytokeratin 14, S-100, vimentin, and calponin (de Araujo et al., 1994; Nagao et al., 1998C; Savera et al., 1997) are the most sensitive for determining neoplastic myoepithelial differentiation. It appears that malignant myoepitheliomas with highly developed myoepithelial characteristics, immunoreactive to most myoepithelial markers, have a low malignant potential (Nagao et al., 1998C). Conversely, the loss of the myoepithelial phenotype, such as may occur in a myoepithelial carcinoma, yields a more aggressive carcinoma with enhanced invasive and metastatic capability (Batsakis and El-Naggar, 1999).

ONCOCYTIC NEOPLASIA AND ASSOCIATED LESIONS

Primary salivary oncocytic lesions comprise a morphologic and biological spectrum of lesions that range from metaplasia and hyperplasia to benign and malignant neoplasia (Table 5–8). Morphological criteria for each one of these lesions have been established, with the caveat that their true biological nature still remains uncertain.

As evidenced by ultrastructural studies, the oncocytic phenotype (transformed large polygonal cells with intensely eosinophilic granular cytoplasm) is given by a striking cytoplasmic accumulation of mitochondria. The proportion of cytoplasmic volume oc-

Table 5–8. Salivary Oncocytic Lesions

Oncocytic neoplasia
  Age-related oncocytic metaplasia/oncocytosis
  Multinodular oncocytic hyperplasia
  Multinodular oncocytic hyperplasia (clear cell)
    oncocytoma
  Oncocytoma
  Malignant oncocytoma (oncocytic carcinoma)
Diffuse oncocytosis
Oncocytic salivary gland tumor

cupied by mitochondria in oncocytes has been estimated to be 60% (Hartwick and Batsakis, 1990). The mitochondria are remarkable for their abnormalities in size, shape, and cristae structure (Davy et al., 1994). A clear cell variant of the oncocyte has been recognized. The clear cell phenotype is given by the intracytoplasmic accumulation of monoparticulate glycogen with margination of the mitochondria (Davy et al., 1994). The degree of extraction of the glycogen during fixation and processing accounts for the variation in the extent of the clear cell component. In salivary oncocytic lesions there may be a predominance of either the typical oncocyte (mitochondria-rich) or the clear cell oncocyte (glycogen-rich) or an admixture of both. A transitional or intermediate form of oncocyte having many mitochondria and a limited accumulation of glycogen is not uncommon. Therefore, in addition to the unexplained excessive number of mitochondria, oncocytic lesions display another histologic facet—namely, excess glycogen production, for which there is currently no explanation (Davy et al., 1994).

The cause of the aberrant mitochondrial biogenesis and its relation to tumorigenesis are still obscure. Oncocytes were originally thought to represent a degenerative or senescent process, especially because oncocytes can be observed in otherwise normal glands from aging patients (Thompson et al., 1996). Oncocytes were considered to represent an age-related, "convergent" or "common final pathway" of differentiation of normal cells due to functional exhaustion of mitochondrial enzymes and subsequent compensatory mitochondrial hyperplasia (Chang and Harawi, 1992). This hypothesis, however, raises the quandary of a senescent cell as the candidate precursor of oncocytic neoplasia (Brandwein and Huvos, 1991). A more accepted view is that the compensatory increase in mitochondrial content is the result of a defect in the energy production machinery of the cell. To put this into context, the following review of mitochondrial biology is pertinent (Tallini, 1998):

Mitochondrial DNA (mtDNA) comprises less than 1% of the total DNA in eukaryotic cells but is a distinct species with its own genetic code and a circular molecular structure similar to that of a plasmid. The entire sequence of mtDNA has been characterized and encodes for 13 proteins (all essential components for the mitochondrial oxidative phosphorylation process), 2 ribosomal RNA and 22 transfer RNA. Both ribosomal and transfer RNAs are specific for mitochondrial protein synthesis, which is at least in part independent of that occurring in the cytoplasm of eukaryotic cells. This is in keeping with the hypothesis that mitochondria are the result of the endosymbiotic evolution of bacteria specialized in oxidative phosphorylation within eukaryotic cells. During phylogenesis, however, control of the respiratory function has been progressively taken over by the nuclear genes which in humans encode for 90% of the mitochondrial respiratory chain proteins and for the enzymes necessary for mtDNA replication and transcription. Unlike nuclear DNA, mtDNA molecules are not protected by histones and other proteins and lack a DNA repair system (Chang et al., 1992). In contrast, they are exposed to the damaging effect of oxygen free radicals, a natural by-product of mitochondrial oxidative phosphorylation. As a result, mt DNA has a high mutation rate, estimated at approximately 10 times that for nuclear DNA.

Therefore, alterations of mtDNA, in the form of deletions or point mutations, may underlie the deficit in energy production and result in the abnormal accumulation of mitochondria. In this sense, oncocytes would represent the manifestation of a primary mitochondrial disease or "mitochondriopathy." The existence and the relevance of specific mtDNA alterations in oncocytes require further investigation. Another interesting possibility is that the abnormal accumulation of mitochondria is driven by alteration(s) of the nuclear genes that normally control the replication of mitochondria (Tallini, 1998).

As demonstrated by ultrastructure and im-munohistochemistry, oncocytic lesions in the salivary glands appear to be composed of ductal and/or acinar cells, with minimal, if any, participation of myoepithelial cells (Thompson et al., 1996). Besides electron microscopy, histochemical (PTAH) and, as of recently, immunohistochemical (antimitochondrial antibodies) stains (Shintaku and Honda, 1997) have proven useful to confirm an oncocytic nature.

The most common and perhaps the earliest of the salivary oncocytic lesions, *oncocytic metaplasia*, transformation of the underlying salivary gland ductal and acinar epithelium, appears with increasing age. Salivary oncocytic foci, also referred to as *oncocytosis*, are rare before age 50 and almost universal by age 70. This age-related oncocytic metaplasia *per se* is an incidental finding of no clinical significance. However, it is of interest to note that most oncocytic lesions of the salivary gland are predominantly observed in older adults around the sixth to eighth decades of life, in keeping with the natural history of oncocytic metaplasia. Thus it seems that the emergence of oncocytosis signals the onset of a predisposition toward the development of oncocytic proliferations. Conceivably, in some cases oncocytosis (with the exception of the diffuse form of oncocytosis described below) may represent the emergence of neoplasia itself.

Diffuse oncocytosis (Palmer et al., 1990; Seifert, 1991; Dardick, 1996) designates a condition in which oncocytic metaplasia diffusely involves acinar and ductal cells over a considerable portion of the gland. The underlying lobar architecture of the gland is retained, and interlobular ducts are identifiable among the extensively involved acini. There is uniform enlargement of the gland within the thin capsule and within the septae (Vigliani and Genetta, 1982). Characteristically, there is a lack of discrete nodular formation. This criterion is of relevance since diffuse oncocytosis is regarded as a rare non-neoplastic, intracellular metabolic disorder with mitochondriopathy (Seifert, 1991). Hence, it is excluded from the list of lesions associated with salivary oncocytic neoplasia (Table 5–8). The process is most commonly unilateral and involves the parotid gland.

Multifocal nodular oncocytic hyperplasia (multifocal oncocytic adenomatous hyperplasia) (Brandwein and Huvos, 1991; Dardick, 1996; Palmer et al., 1990; Seifert 1991; Sørensen et al., 1986) consists of multiple circumscribed and usually unencapsulated, nodules of oncocytes scattered throughout the gland (Fig. 5–14). Uninvolved salivary gland parenchyma is usually present between the oncocytic foci. The oncocytic nodules may contain inclusions of salivary gland parenchyma. The nodules are the result of multifocal oncocytic proliferations originating from the ductal system. Oncocytic buds may be seen originating from the ductal epithelium unrelated to the nodules (Palmer et al., 1990; Seifert and Sobin, 1991). Normal acini may be included at the periphery of large nodules and their presence may be a useful feature in distinguishing between this lesion and oncocytoma (Palmer et al., 1990).

This lesion is characteristically associated with clear cell change (Brandwein and Huvos, 1991; Dardick, 1996; Palmer et al., 1990; Sørensen et al., 1986; Fig. 5–15). The nodules consisting mainly of clear cells often with small groups of cells forming discrete satellite foci. It is assumed that oncocytoma can arise by confluent or expansive growth and later formation of a capsule (Seifert and Sobin, 1991). There is an increasing gradation in the mean ages of presentation of multinodular oncocytic hyperplasia alone and multinodular oncocytic hyperplasia with oncocytoma, which lends support to the suggestion that some cases of oncocytomas may arise by a process of progressive enlargement

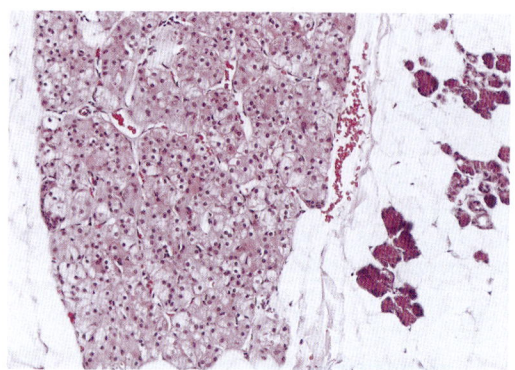

Figure 5–15. Higher magnification of oncocytic nodule containing clear cells.

of one of the nodules of oncocytic cells (Palmer et al., 1990). This process may be unilateral or bilateral and usually involves the parotid gland. Familial (and bilateral) occurrence has been reported (Sørensen et al., 1986), with an earlier age of presentation.

Oncocytoma is a discrete nodule that usually has a thin fibrous capsule, but this may be incomplete or absent. The tumor cells are disposed in cords, sheets, or acini or in organoid growth pattern. They may have little internal fibrous stroma, thin fibrovascular septa, or a sinusoidal capillary-like network. Tumor cells are polygonal to angular or rectangular in shape, and may have a mosaic or a layered and crowded appearance. Lightly and darkly stained cells are noted and intermixed. Oncocytes have pyknotic nuclei or vesicular nuclei with prominent nucleoli. Mild degrees of cellular and nuclear atypia are acceptable in oncocytomas. Focal goblet cell, squamous, or sebaceous differentiation may be identified. Some tumors show central, infarctive-type necrosis with cystic degeneration. Cystic degeneration in oncocytomas (Thompson et al., 1996) may be a consequence of a previous fine-needle aspiration. In addition, tumor cells that contain numerous mitochondria probably have a high oxygen tension requirement that the vascular supply may not be able to support, and hence show a tendency toward cystic degeneration. Cystic oncocytomas should be distinguished from cysts with simple lining of columnar oncocytes that are best classified as cystadenomas. There may be small glandular lumens or

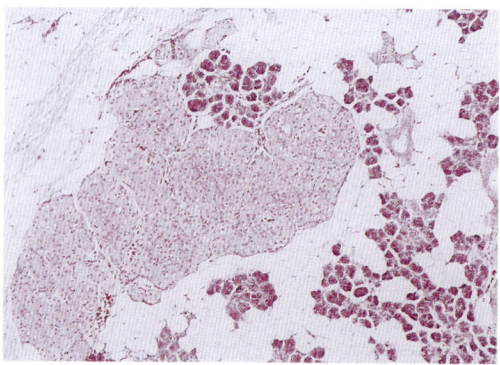

Figure 5–14. Multifocal nodular oncocytic hyperplasia. A well-defined unencapsulated nodule of clear oncocytic cells is surrounded by normal parotid gland.

scattered duct-like structures, but oncocytomas lack the intralobular ducts of normal gland, which distinguishes them from multinodular oncocytic hyperplasia. Oncocytomas arising in otherwise normal glands show typical light and dark oncocytes, whereas oncocytomas found in association with multinodular oncocytic hyperplasia contain predominantly clear cells similar to those present in the nodules (Palmer et al., 1990). Conversely, clear cell oncocytomas usually arise in a background of multinodular oncocytic hyperplasia or clear cell oncocytosis, variably sized aggregates of clear cell oncocytes irregularly scattered throughout or within the salivary gland parenchyma (Ellis, 1988). Transition from oncocytic ductal cells to clear cells may also be evidenced.

Despite the common occurrence of age-related oncocytic metaplasia, oncocytomas are rare, representing less than 1% of the salivary gland tumors (Brandwein and Huvos, 1991). It is important to clarify that although Warthin's tumor, the second most common benign salivary gland tumor, is composed of oncocytes, it is not regarded in the spectrum of oncocytic neoplasia. Its distinctive morphology (papillocystic, rather than solid, lined by columnar cells and accompanied by lymphoid stroma) and its seemingly different histogenesis and pathogenesis have warranted the designation of Warthin's tumor its own category. Nevertheless, hybrid lesions with components of oncocytoma and Warthin's tumor may occur. Most oncocytomas occur in the parotid gland, a minority in the submandibular gland, and less often they may be found in the cervical lymph nodes or in relation to minor salivary glands. As for other salivary oncocytic lesions, most occur in patients between the sixth and eighth decades. Interestingly, patients with a history of radiation exposure had a younger age at presentation (Brandwein and Huvos, 1991). Bilaterality may occur especially in association with clear cell oncocytomas (Brandwein and Huvos, 1991).

Malignant oncocytomas may occur *de novo* or may arise from a benign oncocytoma (Ardekian et al., 1999). Malignancy may manifest itself in two biological forms (Dardick, 1996). One form mainly deviates from oncocytoma by demonstrating an infiltrative, rather than expansive, growth into surrounding salivary gland parenchyma, around nerves and vessels, as well as into soft tissues, bone, and muscle. The term *locally aggressive oncocytoma* or *atypical oncocytoma* has been applied to designate tumors with these features. The second form is an overtly cytologically *malignant oncocytoma (oncocytic carcinoma)* with cellular and nuclear pleomorphism, frequent and abnormal mitoses, and perineural, intravascular, and intralymphatic invasion. Necrosis of both apoptotic and confluent types has been reported as a prominent feature in malignant oncocytomas (Félix et al., 1993). These tumors may give rise to regional lymph node metastasis and distant metastasis, may recur, and rarely have been fatal. Most malignant oncocytomas involve the parotid gland, with rare examples of malignant submandibular oncocytic tumors reported. A significantly higher occurrence of lymph node metastasis was found among patients with tumors located in the submandibular gland than among those having tumors in the parotid (Ardekian et al., 1999). Malignant oncocytomas are rare tumors, comprising approximately 5% of the oncocytomas.

Diagnosis of primary oncocytic tumors requires the exclusion other benign and malignant salivary gland tumors showing prominent oncocytic change. The most common among the former is pleomorphic adenoma. Distinction lies in the overall thicker capsule and the presence of significant internal fibrous or chondromyxoid stroma in pleomorphic adenoma (Ferreiro and Stylopoulos, 1995; Palmer et al., 1990). Occasionally, a rim of pleomorphic adenoma may be present (Ferreiro and Stylopoulos, 1995). A later age of presentation has been reported for pleomorphic adenomas with oncocytic change than that of most pleomorphic adenomas (Palmer et al., 1990). Oncocytic mucoepidermoid carcinoma is the most common tumor mimicking a primary oncocytic carcinoma (Jahan-Parwar et al., 1999; Ferreiro and Stylopoulos, 1995). Most of the oncocytic mucoepidermoid carcinomas have been low grade (Jahan-Parwar, et al., 1999). The heterogenous cellular composition (goblet mucous, squamous, intermediate, clear, columnar (Jahan-Parwar, et al., 1999) aids in the differential diagnosis (Ferreiro and Stylopoulos, 1995). However, it must be kept in mind that oncocytomas may show goblet cells and squamous foci (Dardick, 1996). Clear cell oncocytic elements have not been found in association with mucoepidermoid carcinomas (Jahan-Parwar, et al., 1999). Oncocytic differentiation has been also reported in trabecular cell adenoma, polymorphous low-grade adenocarcinoma, acinic cell carcinoma, and myoepithelioma (Jahan-Parwar, et al., 1999; Skalova et al., 1999). Adequate sampling of salivary oncocytic lesions is warranted to rule out other tumor types, especially since most primary oncocytic tumors are benign (Ferreiro and Stylopoulos, 1995). It is believed that most reported oncocytic carcinomas represent other entities (Ferreiro and Stylopoulos, 1995).

From a review of the literature several general observations may be drawn regarding salivary oncocytic lesions. Most primary oncocytic lesions occur in older adults, involve the parotid—primarily the superficial lobe, except for multinodular oncocytic hyperplasia that may encompass the deep lobe—and most are benign. In addition, they may be segregated according to their predominant oncocyte phenotype, typical (mitochondria-rich) or clear cell (glycogen-rich). The *clear cell oncocyte* is associated with clear cell oncocytosis and multinodular oncocytic hyperplasia, the likely precursors of the clear cell oncocytoma. Clear cell oncocytoma is regarded as a benign lesion. The rare recurrences have been attributed to incomplete resection or to multifocality. It is considered to be perhaps the only benign clear cell tumor arising in the salivary glands. This indolent behavior may have two obvious explanations. Since most clear cell oncocytomas arise in a background of multifocal nodular hyperplasia, it is possible that some of the so-called oncocytomas are in actuality hyperplastic nodules. (The impossibility of distinguishing between dominant hyperplastic nodules and neoplasia is a well-known peculiarity of oncocytic lesions in general.) Another is that malignant clear cell oncocytomas have been misinterpreted as other salivary clear cell malignancies. The *typical oncocyte* is associated with age-related oncocytic metaplasia/oncocytosis, benign oncocytoma, malignant oncocytoma (oncocytic carcinoma), and oncocytic change in other tumor types. This again may stem from fail-

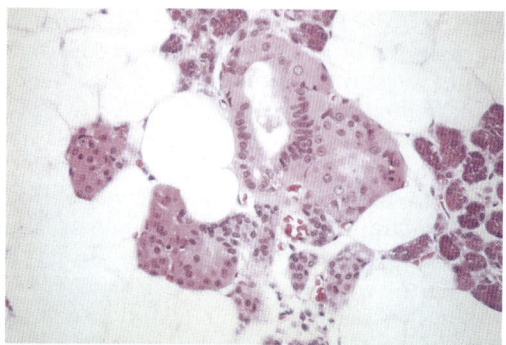

Figure 5–16. Early oncocytic metaplasia and budding. The oncocytic cells appear to arise from a ductal structure and extend into the acini.

ure to recognize a clear cell variant in the latter two settings. However, if these associations are confirmed, then it would seem that there are at least two pathways in salivary oncocytic tumorigenesis.

Recognition of oncocytosis is of importance when accompanying a salivary gland tumor. Theoretically it might aid in distinguishing a primary salivary oncocytic neoplasm from other primary or metastatic tumors. On the other hand, it may be misconstrued for invasive foci, leading to an erroneous diagnosis of malignancy (clear cell oncocytosis is typically misinterpreted as acinic cell carcinoma) or, in the setting of malignancy, lead to overinterpreting the extent of local invasion. Searching for early oncocytic budding from ductal epithelium may help in the identification of oncocytosis (Fig. 5–16).

MALIGNANT TRANSFORMATION OF WARTHIN'S TUMOR

Warthin's tumor, the second most common benign salivary gland neoplasm, is known for its frequent multifocality, bilateral occurrence, and coexistence with other tumors. Perhaps a surgical pathologist's most common encounter with incipient neoplasia of salivary glands is the incidental microscopic Warthin's tumor noted in parotidectomy specimens performed for other reasons. Additional small Warthin's tumors appear to be quite common, even in parotid glands resected for this tumor (Dardick, 1996; Lam et al., 1994).

Carcinomas arising in a Warthin's tumor are extremely rare, their incidence having been estimated to be 0.3% of all Warthin's tumors (Gunduz et al., 1999). The diagnosis of malignant Warthin's tumor implies the exclusion of two more common events: *(1)* the coexistence of another definable malignant salivary gland tumor, this being the most common form of malignancy associated with Warthin's tumor (Batsakis, 1987; Dardick, 1996; Ellis et al., 1991); and *(2)* a metastasis to the lymphoid component (Ellis et al., 1991; Therkildsen et al., 1992). A recent history of rapid enlargement in a long-standing mass (Gunduz et al., 1999) and the histological relationship of the malignant component to the benign epithelium, with transitional changes between them (Bengoechea et al., 1989), support a malignant Warthin tumor. Oncocytic adenocarcinoma is the most common histologic type of malignant Warthin tumor, followed by squamous cell carcinoma and mucoepidermoid carcinoma.

It has been suggested from observations that certain disturbances in epithelial growth such as metaplasia, hyperplastic arrangements, and dysplasia, precede the development of carcinoma in Warthin tumor (Nagao et al., 1998b). Malignant transformation into a squamous cell carcinoma is believed to be preceded by squamous metaplasia, a well-known feature in Warthin's tumors (Damjanov et al., 1983; Gunduz et al., 1999; Therkildsen et al., 1992). A gradual transition from cylindrical cells rich in mitochondria to flattened squamous cells with fewer cytoplasmic organelles has been demonstrated ultrastructurally. Similarly, metaplasia to squamous or goblet cells occurring in the epithelial components of Warthin's tumor are linked to the histogenesis of mucoepidermoid carcinoma (Nagao et al., 1998b). Because secondary metaplastic changes are not uncommon and may follow ischemia or infarction (Gunduz et al., 1999), a diagnosis of malignancy requires the evidence of stromal invasion or metastases (Ellis et al., 1991; Nagao et al., 1998b). In particular, necrotizing squamous/mucinous metaplasia may simulate a low-grade mucoepidermoid carcinoma (Taxy, 1992). In addition to epithelial malignant transformation, malignant lymphomas arising from a lymphoid component of Warthin's tumors have been reported (Ellis et al., 1991).

SEBACEOUS LYMPHADENOCARCINOMA ASSOCIATED WITH SEBACEOUS LYMPHADENOMA

Despite the fact that sebaceous differentiation is a common finding in major salivary glands, primary salivary gland sebaceous tumors are rare (Gnepp, 1983; Gnepp and Brannon, 1984). The few cases described under the term sebaceous lymphadenocarcinoma have consisted of typical sebaceous lymphadenoma with carcinoma either admixed with the benign component or adjacent to it. The malignant phase may be sebaceous carcinoma, solid variant of adenoid cystic carcinoma, epithelial–myoepithelial carcinoma, or adenocarcinoma not otherwise specified (NOS). These tumors most likely originate from the ductal elements commonly found in sebaceous lymphadenomas. They have occurred in the parotid gland and periparotid lymph node of patients in the seventh decade. Both at least a 20 year history and a 1-month history of an asymptomatic mass were elicited. As in Warthin's tumor, sebaceous lymphadenoma is believed to arise from ectopic salivary gland inclusions in lymph nodes (Fig. 5–17).

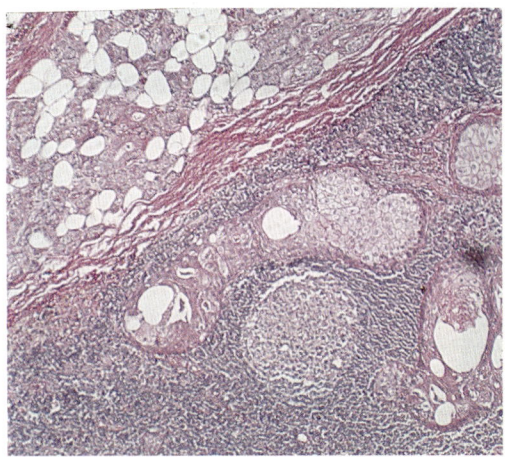

Figure 5–17. Sebaceous lymphadenoma of parotid gland. Both the sebaceous cells and the lymphoid component are clearly shown.

LYMPHOEPITHELIAL
CARCINOMA

Salivary lymphoepithelial carcinoma is a rare tumor that is unique among the salivary gland neoplasms for its specific association with the Epstein-Barr virus (EBV) (Abdulla, 1996; Chan et al., 1994), a human herpes virus. It is histologically indistinguishable from nasopharyngeal undifferentiated carcinoma, being composed of syncytial epithelial islands of large cells with indistinct cell borders, vesicular nuclei, and prominent nucleoli, admixed with a prominent lymphoid stroma. The major salivary glands appear to be the exclusive sites of origin, with the parotid gland leading the submandibular gland by a 7:1 ratio (Cleary and Batsakis, 1990). Unlike nasopharyngeal undifferentiated carcinoma, in which EBV can be consistently demonstrated in the tumor, irrespective of the ethnic origin of the patient, the association of lymphoepithelial carcinoma of salivary gland with EBV is largely restricted to the Eskimo (Innu) population of Greenland, Northern Canada and Alaska, and to the southern Chinese population, including Taiwanese (Chan et al., 1994; Cleary and Batsakis, 1990; Gaffey and Weiss, 1992; Hamilton-Dutoit et al., 1991; Kuo and Hsueh, 1997; Saw et al., 1986; Tsai et al., 1996). The fact that Eskimos have an exceptionally high incidence of lymphoepithelial carcinomas of the salivary gland strengthens the causal role of EBV in the development of this tumor. Given the ubiquitous nature of EBV and the high rate of infection worldwide—with salivary gland ductal epithelium known to be a reservoir for EBV replication (Chan et al., 1994; Raab-Traub et al., 1991)—it is likely that genetic predisposition or environmental or nutritional factors underlie this geographic association (Christiansen et al., 1995). There have been only isolated case reports of primary lymphoepithelial carcinomas in patients of non-Eskimo extraction in which EBV has also been detected (Abdulla, 1996; Kotsianti et al., 1996).

The pathogenetic link between EBV and lymphoepithelial carcinoma was initially suggested by the high titers of antibodies against EBV-related antigens found in the sera of patients harboring these tumors (Cleary and Batsakis, 1990). It has been confirmed by the detection of EBV nuclear antigen (EBNA); EBV DNA; EBV mRNA; EBV-encoded RNAs (EBERs), nontranslated small RNAs present in cells that are latently infected by EBV; and latent membrane protein (LMP) viral oncoprotein, the EBV transforming gene product, in the tumors (Chan et al., 1994; Clift et al., 1987; Huang et al., 1988; Leung et al., 1995; Saemundsen et al., 1982). With *in situ* hybridization, EBV genomes and EBER transcripts have been detected in the neoplastic epithelial cells and not in the lymphoid stroma or in residual benign salivary epithelium (Christiansen et al., 1995; Hamilton-Dutoit et al., 1991; Tsai et al., 1996). A clonal population of EBV episomes has been demonstrated in salivary lymphoepithelial carcinoma (Leung et al., 1995). Such clonality suggests by extension cellular clonality and is further evidence for EBV-related oncogenesis (Raab-Traub et al., 1991). In keeping with the above is the ultrastructural finding of enveloped dense bodies, which is consistent with the intracellular presence of the virus, in a lymphoepithelial carcinoma (Christiansen et al., 1995).

The observation that carcinomas associated with EBV are usually of the lymphoepithelial type raises the possibility that the anaplastic "active" appearances of the neoplastic cells may be equivalent to the blastic transformation that occurs in EBV-infected lymphocytes, and that the lymphoid infiltrate may represent a host reaction against the virus-associated antigens expressed on the neoplastic cells (Chan et al., 1994). The intense lymphoid infiltrate has been shown to be primarily of T-cell origin (Christiansen et al., 1995; Weiss et al., 1991).

Like its nasopharyngeal counterpart, lymphoepithelial carcinoma is considered to represent an undifferentiated or poorly differentiated squamous cell carcinoma, with intracytoplasmic tonofilaments and desmosomes identified by electron microscopy. It is significant, that in human keratinocytes, EBV LMP-1 deregulates epithelial growth and inhibits differentiation, with the epithelial cells showing the characteristics of transformation, including loss of contact inhibition, spindling, a tendency to proliferate into multilayer clusters, and decreased cytokeratin expression (Fahraeus et al., 1990). Moreover, there is severe impairment of the cellular response to differentiation signals (Dawson et al., 1990). Thus a role for LMP-1 in a multi-step pathogenetic process of lymphoepithelial carcinoma formation may be inferred from the undifferentiated morphology of the tumor (Leung et al., 1995).

Lymphoepithelial carcinoma (malignant lymphoepithelial lesion) has been noted to resemble, coexist with, and/or follow benign lymphoepithelial lesions. *Benign lymphoepithelial lesion* refers to the presence of metaplastic ductal epithelium, so-called epimyoepithelial islands, in association with a lymphoid proliferation that effaces the acinar architecture (Batsakis, 1983). It is believed that lymphoepithelial carcinoma may arise from the malignant transformation of the epimyoepithelial islands comprising benign lymphoepithelial lesions (Batsakis et al., 1975; Kountakis et al., 1995). A few case reports of documented parotid tumors initially diagnosed as benign lymphoepithelial lesion or lymphoepithelial lesion with atypia, followed temporally by undifferentiated carcinoma with lymphoid stroma, provide the strongest evidence that at least some of the lymphoepithelial carcinomas evolve from a progenitor lesion (Cleary and Batsakis, 1990; Gravanis and Giansanti, 1970). While some authors have noted dysplastic or atypical lymphoepithelial lesions (Gravanis and Giansanti, 1970), detailed characterization (histomorphological, intermediate biomarkers, molecular, etc) of the progression from lymphoepithelial lesion to established lymphoepithelial carcinoma is currently lacking. The pathogenetic relation, if any, between malignant lymphoepithelial lesions and autoimmune disorders that are associated with benign lymphoepithelial lesions has not been addressed (Batsakis, 1983).

While lymphoepithelial lesions may be seen as a reactive change surrounding other salivary gland tumor types, the presence of many areas of epimyoepithelial islands at the periphery of the tumor may prove helpful in reaching the diagnosis of malignant lymphoepithelial lesion, especially when exhibiting an unusual morphology (Christiansen et al., 1995). It may also help determine that the tumor is probably primary, and not a metastatic nasopharyngeal undifferentiated carcinoma, an entity that must be excluded prior to rendering a diagnosis of primary salivary lymphoepithelial carcinoma (Kountakis et al., 1995).

SALIVARY GLAND TUMORS ARISING IN SALIVARY GLAND CYSTS

The epithelial metaplasias and proliferative activity that occur in salivary gland cysts may represent early manifestations of a salivary gland tumor (Seifert, 1996). In an extensive histologic analysis of salivary gland cysts, only two types emerged as likely precursors of salivary gland tumors: salivary duct cysts of parotid gland and mucus retention cysts of minor salivary glands. Characteristic cellular changes were focal epithelial proliferations, with multilayered patterns or plump or papillary projections into the cyst lumen, and epithelial metaplasias (mainly goblet cells, clear reserve cells, squamous cells). Not unexpectedly, the salivary gland tumor types most closely linked to salivary gland cysts, either originating from them or mimicking them grossly and microscopically, are *cystadenomas* and highly differentiated cystic *mucoepidermoid carcinomas*. Despite the frequent occurrence of salivary gland cysts, only few sporadic case reports mention the development of salivary gland tumors in preexisting salivary gland cysts.

TUMOR PROGRESSION OF LOW-GRADE SALIVARY ADENOCARCINOMAS

Transformation or dedifferentiation has been noted to occur in salivary gland tumors generally regarded as low-grade malignancies. Thorough sampling is recommended in a long-standing tumor with a sudden increase in size, or, in recurrent tumors.

Dedifferentiated acinic cell carcinoma has been defined as an aggressive, albeit rare, variant of acinic cell carcinoma (Stanley et al., 1988). Dedifferentiated acinic cell carcinoma is a composite of usual low-grade acinic cell carcinoma and a high-grade, poorly differentiated adenocarcinoma or undifferentiated carcinoma, with no bridging transitional areas (Henley et al., 1997; Stanley et al., 1988). The relative proportion of low-grade and high-grade carcinoma may vary from tumor to tumor. Thus far the few reported cases have been of parotid gland origin. The median age of presentation for dedifferentiated acinic cell carcinoma is higher than that reported for usual acinic cell carcinoma (58 years vs. 44 years). Also, in contrast to low-grade acinic cell carcinoma, dedifferentiated acinic cell carcinoma commonly presents with facial nerve involvement and advanced local disease, comprising both superficial and deep parotid lobes. Vascular and perineural invasion are typically observed in dedifferentiated acinic cell carcinoma. Lymphocytic infiltrates, common in acinic cell carcinoma, may also accompany dedifferentiated acinic cell carcinoma and may be a potential clue to the diagnosis. A single case of undifferentiated spindle cell transformation of a parotid acinic cell carcinoma has been reported (Ferreiro and Kochar, 1994). Dedifferentiation has accompanied local recurrences (Colmenero et al., 1991). The solid and microcystic patterns of acinic cell carcinoma recurred more often, and more commonly showed high-grade, undifferentiated areas (Colmenero et al., 1991).

Dedifferentiation of adenoid cystic carcinoma may occur at initial presentation or upon recurrence (Cheuk et al., 1999). The dedifferentiated component appears as a distinct anaplastic cell population with marked nuclear pleomorphism, distinct nucleoli, frequent mitoses, and coagulative necrosis, displayed in irregularly shaped islands infiltrating a desmoplastic stroma. Sarcomatoid dedifferentiation has also been reported. The dedifferentiated component is distinguished from the solid, high-grade variant of adenoid cystic carcinoma by the total loss of bicellular differentiation and immunophenotypic alteration in the former. Unlike the hyalinized or myxoid stroma accompanying the usual variants of adenoid cystic carcinoma (tubular, cribriform, and solid) with which it may coexist, dedifferentiation is associated with a desmoplastic stroma. The dedifferentiated cells may exhibit a pure epithelial immunophenotype or a myoepithelial immunophenotype in the sarcomatoid component. These findings suggest that the dedifferentiated component arises from the transformation of either the luminal/ductal cells or the myoepithelial cells that compose usual types of adenoid cystic carcinoma. A variant of adenoid cystic carcinoma displaying highly atypical luminal cells, with preserved myoepithelial layer, has been reported and thought to represent incipient

dedifferentiation (Lucas, 1989). Dedifferentiated adenoid cystic carcinoma has followed an accelerated clinical course.

The rare reported cases of *transformation of polymorphous low-grade adenocarcinoma* into a higher grade occurred after a protracted clinical course with multiple recurrences of typical polymorphous low-grade adenocarcinoma (Pelkey and Mills, 1999). Transformation was characterized by loss of architectural variety with predominance of a solid tumor growth pattern with comedonecrosis and cytological progression with nuclear atypia, prominent nucleoli, and higher mitotic rate. Transformation warranted upgrading to at least an intermediate grade lesion. Histologic transformation was associated with an aggressive local tumor growth and multiple recurrences and, thus far, without an increased risk of metastatic disease.

Reports of *transformation of epithelial–myoepithelial carcinomas* have described well-differentiated tumors with typical dual epithelial and myoepithelial components showing progressive cellular atypia to a high-grade component, either an adenocarcinoma or undifferentiated large cell carcinoma (Alos et al., 1999). The presence of a high-grade component confers an increased malignant potential on epithelial–myoepithelial carcinomas. It has also been observed that the presence of nuclear atypia in more than 20% of the tumor is a morphological feature of prognostic value in epithelial–myoepithelial carcinomas.

SALIVARY GLAND TUMORS WITH OSTEOCLAST-LIKE GIANT CELLS

UNDIFFERENTIATED CARCINOMAS WITH OSTEOCLAST-LIKE GIANT CELLS

Salivary gland tumors composed predominantly of mononuclear cells and osteoclast-like giant cells mimicking a giant cell tumor of bone are rare. Once subject to the same controversy as their counterparts in other organs (Donath et al., 1997; Eusebi et al., 1984), they are now believed to represent the phenotypic expression of an advanced stage of tumor progression (Balogh et al.,

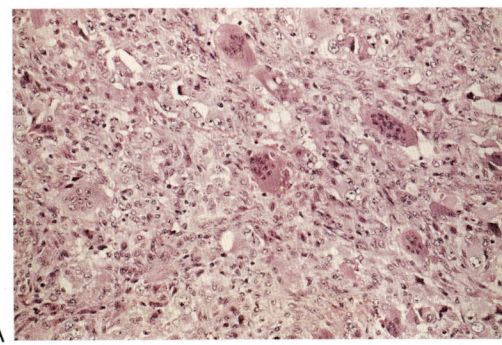 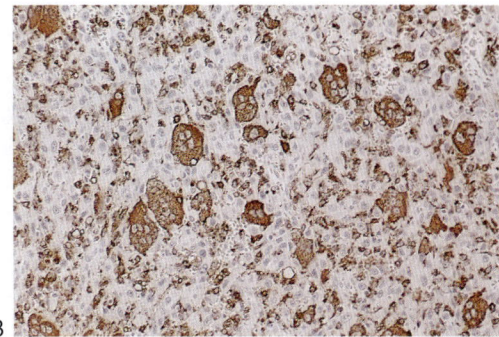

Figure 5–18. *A:* Undifferentiated carcinoma with numerous osteoclast-like giant cells. The epithelial component is difficult to discern with conventional stains. *B:* CD68 immunoperoxidase stain highlights the osteoclast-type giant cells and reveals the presence of a diffuse mononuclear population, also of histiocytic nature.

1985). Although few cases have been reported to date, they are described as aggressive, rapidly metastasizing, and fatal.

The typical histological appearance consists of *multinucleated*, osteoclast-type giant cells rather evenly distributed among mitotically active undifferentiated *mononuclear* cells showing varying degrees of anaplasia (Fig. 5–18A). The osteoclast-type multinucleated giant cells have an eosinophilic to amphophilic cytoplasm and multiple small, ovoid nuclei with convoluted nuclear membranes, dispersed chromatin, and prominent pale eosinophilic nucleoli. The nuclei are one-half to one-third the size of those of the mononuclear cells, and they tend to be centrally placed. The mononuclear cells are large and polygonal, angular, or, less commonly, spindled, with abundant cytoplasm, well-delineated membranes, and large round to ovoid nuclei with coarse chromatin and prominent basophilic nucleoli. Nuclear pleomorphism is variable from tumor to tumor. Multinucleated anaplastic giant cells may coexist. The osteoclast-like giant cells are surrounded by retraction artifact. Some may be pyknotic. The mononuclear cells are disassociated by sinusoidal-like or slit-like spaces containing erythrocytes and hemosiderin.

The osteoclast-type giant cells are reactive in nature and of histiocytic lineage, being immunoreactive to CD68 and leukocyte common antigen. CD68 also unmasks a diffuse population of small mononuclear histiocytes (Fig. 5–18B). The undifferentiated mononuclear cells display an epithelial or myoepithelial phenotype and are the prolif-

erating neoplastic population, as evidenced by frequent mitotic figures and by positivity for Ki-67 proliferating antigen. The formation of osteoclast-like giant cells may result from fusion of mononuclear histiocytes/macrophages attracted to the tumor by growth or chemotactic factors elaborated by the neoplastic epithelial cells (Molberg et al., 1998).

Many of the undifferentiated carcinomas with osteoclast-like giant cells reported to date, as well as those seen by us, have been associated with foci of recognizable salivary carcinoma tumor types, including salivary duct carcinoma ex pleomorphic adenoma, mucoepidermoid carcinoma, acinic cell carcinoma, and myoepithelial carcinoma (Balogh et al., 1985; Nagao et al., 1998C; Figs. 5–19, 5–20 and 5–21). This finding sug-

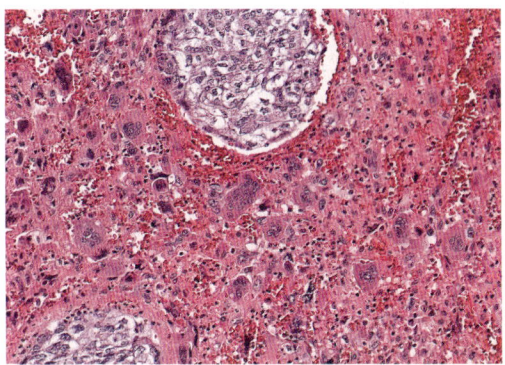

Figure 5–19. Undifferentiated carcinoma with osteoclast-type giant cells associated with foci of high-grade salivary duct carcinoma, the biological precursor.

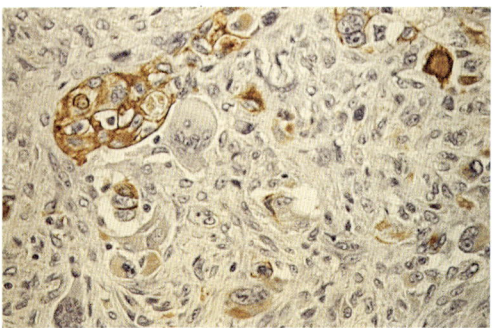

Figure 5–20. Mucoepidermoid carcinoma with osteoclast-like giant cells. The cytokeratin stain highlights the squamous component. The osteoclast-like giant cells are cytokeratin negative.

gests that undifferentiated carcinoma with osteoclast-like giant cells is a convergent pathway of tumor evolution for different histologic tumor types. We found almost uniform p53 nuclear protein overexpression in the mononuclear population, which suggests that p53 alterations may be involved in this late stage of tumor progression. When confronted with this tumor, extensive sampling may be required to identify the precursor tumor(s).

CARCINOSARCOMAS WITH OSTEOCLAST-LIKE GIANT CELLS

In carcinosarcoma, osteoclast-like giant cells occur usually in association with an osteo-

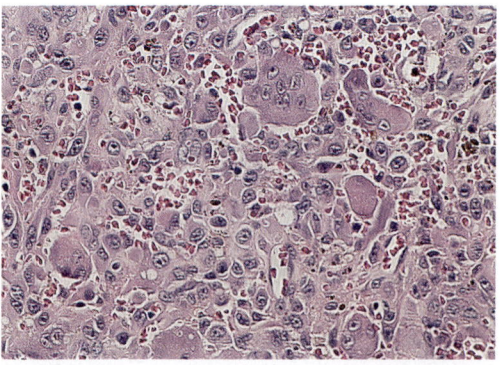

Figure 5–21. Undifferentiated (myoepithelial) carcinoma with osteoclast-type giant cells. The myoepithelial nature of the tumor was evidenced only by immunoreactivity of anaplastic mononuclear cells to calponin and S-100 protein antibodies. No morphologically recognizable component of myoepithelial carcinoma was identified.

sarcoma component (Donath et al., 1997; Grenko et al., 1993). They may be readily found within or in the vicinity of foci of osteoid formation and mineralization but may also be present away from this area amidst the less-differentiated mesenchymal component (Grenko et al., 1993). Although histologically indistinguishable and immunophenotypically similar, it is uncertain whether osteosarcoma-associated osteoclast-like giant cells are ultrastructurally and functionally identical to those associated with undifferentiated carcinoma (Molberg et al., 1998). Osteosarcoma is the second-most common type of sarcomatous component, after chondrosarcoma, encountered in carcinosarcoma ex pleomorphic adenoma or true malignant mixed tumor.

CYTOGENETICS AND MOLECULAR GENETICS

Cytogenetic and molecular studies of salivary gland neoplasms, although still preliminary, show fundamental differences between benign and malignant salivary gland neoplasms. Adenomas are characterized by different types of balanced reciprocal translocations, whereas malignant salivary gland tumors preferentially show deletions (Sandros et al., 1990). Furthermore, it appears that variations at certain chromosomal regions distinguish different neoplastic subtypes.

Approximately 50%–80% of the *pleomorphic adenomas*, the best characterized of the benign salivary gland tumors, display clonal chromosomal abnormalities. It has been demonstrated that pleomorphic adenomas show highly specific rearrangements with preferential involvement of three chromosomal regions: 8q12 (60%), 3p21 (30%), often as t(3;8)(p21;q12), and 12q13-15 (20%) (Bullerdiek et al., 1993; Jin et al., 1998; Mark et al., 1996; Martins et al., 1995; Sandros et al., 1990; Stern et al., 1990). Four cytogenetic subtypes of pleomorphic adenomas are recognized: *(1)* with 8q12 rearrangements (39%); *(2)* with 12q13-15 rearrangements (8%); *(3)* with other sporadic clonal rearrangements (23%); and *(4)* with apparently normal karyotype (30%). This highly specific pattern of chromosome rearrangements with consistent breakpoints at 3p21, 8q12, and 12q13-15 suggests that these chromosomal regions harbor genes that are directly involved in the etiology of these tumors (Geurts et al., 1997b). No correlation was seen between the presence or absence of specific chromosomal alterations and subsequent tumor recurrence or malignant transformation (Mark et al., 1996).

The gene consistently rearranged in adenomas with 12q13-15 involvement is the *HMGIC* gene (Geurts et al., 1997b, 1998), which encodes an architectural transcription factor. *HMGIC* gene is a member of the high mobility group (HMG) protein gene family, which consists of proteins that are heterogeneous, nonhistone components of chromatin. The HMG proteins are not thought to play a direct role in transcriptional activation, but act as so-called architectural transcription factors and participate in the spatial organization of complexes of other transcription factors (Geurts et al., 1997b). The *HMGIC* gene is ubiquitously expressed at readily detectable levels during embryonic development but at relatively low levels in adult tissues (Geurts et al., 1997b). *HMGIC* has also been identified as the gene consistently affected in a variety of other benign mesenchymal tumor types characterized by 12q13-15 (Geurts et al., 1997b). Thus far, two translocation partners have been identified for *HMGIC* in pleomorphic adenomas: the *NFIB* gene, which is the preferential translocation partner, mapped to chromosome 9p24 (Geurts et al., 1998); and the *FHIT* gene, mapped to chromosome 3p14.2. *NFIB* is a member of the human nuclear factor I gene family and has been shown to be involved in the transcriptional regulation of a variety of viral and cellular oncogenes. The *FHIT* gene spans the chromosome 3p14.2 fragile site and is frequently disrupted in tumors (Geurts et al., 1997a). The pathogenetic relevance of the fusion partners remains to be elucidated.

The target gene consistently rearranged in pleomorphic adenomas with chromosome translocations involving 8q12 has been identified and designated *PLAG1* (pleomorphic adenoma gene 1). To date, three translocation partners for *PLAG1* have been identified: *CTNNB1*, the constitutively expressed gene for b catenin; *LIFR*, encoding the receptor for leukemia inhibitory factor; and *SII*, encoding a transcription elongation factor. The b-catenin (*CTNNB1*), a protein with roles in cell–cell adhesion and in the WG/

WNT signaling pathway and specification of cell fate during embryogenesis, is involved in t(3;8) (p21;q12), the most common translocation (Kas et al., 1997; Voz et al., 1998). The *LIFR* gene, mapped to 5p12-p13, encodes the ubiquitously expressed receptor for the leukemia inhibitory factor (LIF), a multifunctional member of the interleukin-6 (IL-6) cytokine family, which is involved in differentiation, survival, and proliferation of a wide variety of fetal and adult cells (Voz et al., 1998). Interestingly, b-catenin and LIFR show several functional similarities, i.e., they are both involved in differentiation, survival, and proliferation of fetal and adult cells (Voz et al., 1998). The novel fusion partner *SII*, previously mapped to 3p21.3-22 (the same region as *CTNNB1*), belongs to the group of RNA polymerase II general elongation factors that are proteins involved in the regulation of the transcription of most if not all eukaryotic protein-coding genes (Åström et al., 1999).

The translocations result in promoter swapping between *PLAG1* and one of the constitutively or ubiquitously expressed translocation partner genes, leading to activation or up-regulation of *PLAG1* gene expression (Åström et al., 1999; Kas et al., 1997; Voz et al., 1998). *PLAG1* is a developmentally regulated zinc finger gene with expression not found in normal salivary glands (Queimado, 1999). It has been established that *PLAG1* possess transcriptional activation capacity, raising the possibility that benign salivary gland tumors may originate because of activation of particular target genes by ectopically overexpressed (activated) *PLAG1*. *PLAG1* activation due to promoter swapping seems to be a crucial event in salivary gland tumorigenesis (Kas et al., 1997). However, it has been shown that *PLAG1* activation is a frequent event irrespective of karyotype, overexpression of *PLAG1* being found in pleomorphic adenomas with normal karyotype and in pleomorphic adenomas with 12q13-15 abnormalities (Åström et al., 1999). *PLAG1* may also be activated by cryptic rearrangements, mutations, or indirect mechanisms. A conserved mechanism of *PLAG1* activation in salivary gland tumors with and without 8q12 aberrations indicates that such activation is a frequent event in these tumors. Recent investigation suggests that *PLAG1* is not exclusively expressed in pleomorphic adenomas and may have an even wider role in salivary gland oncogenesis than was previously thought (Queimado et al., 1999).

Cytogenetic studies of carcinomas ex pleomorphic adenomas have shown widely variable numerical and structural variations suggesting marked heterogeneity, which may reflect their phenotypic differences (El-Naggar et al., 1998). These studies have also identified aberrations in the chromosomal regions 8q and 12q, indicating a close cytogenetic relationship with pleomorphic adenoma (Mark et al., 1996). The superimposed abnormalities are thought to represent events related to tumor progression and are acquired during karyotypic clonal evolution from a preexisting pleomorphic adenoma (El-Naggar et al., 1998). Conversely, malignant salivary gland tumors in which pleomorphic adenoma related translocations are detected among the chromosomal abnormalities are presumed to have arisen from a pleomorphic adenoma, even if the latter component was not identified histopathologically (Bullerdiek et al., 1990).

The karyotypic features of a single metastasizing pleomorphic adenoma differed from the characteristic cytogenetic findings in pleomorphic adenoma by having relatively complex karyotypic changes, including unbalanced translocations, and they also appear to differ from findings in carcinoma ex pleomorphic adenoma. Therefore, different genetic pathways may be involved in the initiation of metastasizing pleomorphic adenoma and carcinoma ex pleomorphic adenoma (Jin et al., 1998).

In studies of *in vitro* life span of cells derived from pleomorphic adenomas, no evidence was found for a longer life span of the cells characterized by chromosomal rearrangements as compared with those with a normal karyotype (Stern et al., 1990), indicating that cells are still under division control. In contrast, pleomorphic adenomas characterized by an unbalanced karyotype showed an exceptionally long lifetime, which suggests that early steps in malignant transformation *in vivo* can be caused by additional unbalanced chromosome aberrations.

Cytogenetic analysis of Warthin's tumor have revealed three distinct categories: *(1)* with normal karyotype; *(2)* with numerical alterations (single chromosome gain or loss) only; and *(3)* with structural alterations only, particularly various reciprocal translocations including a recurrent rearrangement of 6p23 (Mark et al., 1996; Martins et al., 1995; Nordkvist et al., 1994).

Deletion of 6q, loss of chromosome Y, and gain of chromosome 8 are among the most common recurrent deviations found in salivary gland malignancies (Martins et al., 1996; Sandros et al., 1995). Loss of genetic material at 6q is a frequent event in salivary gland carcinomas and occurs in all histological subtypes, including carcinoma ex pleomorphic adenoma (Queimado et al., 1998). Deletions have been localized to two regions, at 6q21-23.3 and at 6q27, supporting the hypothesis that one or more tumor suppressor genes are located in these relatively short regions of 6q, which are relevant to the development of malignant salivary gland tumors.

Polymorphous low-grade adenocarcinoma mostly occurs in intraoral minor salivary glands and does not arise in the major salivary glands, except as the malignant component of carcinoma ex pleomorphic adenoma (Mark et al., 1991). Cytogenetic findings have varied for polymorphous low-grade adenocarcinomas on the basis of its origin from minor or major salivary glands (Dahlenfors et al., 1997). In polymorphous low-grade adenocarcinoma of minor salivary glands, numerical alterations, with simple numerical losses affecting certain chromosomes preferentially (among them the chromosomes Y and 22), and normal karyotypes predominate. Parotid polymorphous low-grade adenocarcinomas ex pleomorphic adenoma are characterized by complicated structural rearrangements and some marker types showing pronounced instability and liability to secondary structural changes. Some of the breakpoints for these markers were close to the region preferentially involved in pleomorphic adenomas, region 12q13-15. This finding suggested that the karyotype of polymorphous low-grade adenocarcinoma resulted from rearrangements (chromosomal progression) superimposed on chromosome 12 deviations present in the preexisting pleomorphic adenoma (Mark et al., 1992). These findings imply a multidirectional genetic pathway in evolution and progression for the same tumor type.

SALIVARY GLAND TUMORS AND RADIATION EXPOSURE

Several independent studies have provided substantial evidence for the causal role of ionizing radiation in salivary gland tumorigenesis. The two main sources of exposure have been the atomic bombings in Hiroshima and Nagasaki, and childhood radiation treatment for benign conditions of the head and neck. In the most recent analysis from the life span study of atomic bomb survivors, a significant dose–response relationship was demonstrated for both benign and malignant tumors. The frequency of mucoepidermoid carcinoma, among the malignant tumors, and of Warthin's tumor, among the benign, was disproportionately high at increasing radiation doses (Land et al., 1996; Saku et al., 1997). Among the second group, one study supported a dose relationship for benign salivary gland tumors, with pleomorphic adenoma being the most common tumor that could be induced by radiation (Schneider et al., 1998). Another study confirmed a dose–response effect for both benign and malignant tumors and a stronger yield of malignant ones, with an excess of mucoepidermoid carcinomas (Modan et al., 1998). Most patients developed tumors in the parotid glands, which were generally within the primary treatment field and therefore received higher doses of radiation (Schneider et al., 1998). Multiple occurrence has also been reported (Katz and Preston-Martin, 1984; Schneider et al., 1998). The mean length of latency period until tumor development was 11 years for malignant tumors and 21.5 years for benign tumors (Modan et al., 1998). These findings dictate a long-term follow-up for patients who have been subject to head and neck radiation, to enable early detection of tumor development.

REFERENCES

Abdulla AK, Mian MY. (1996) Lymphoepithelial carcinoma of salivary glands. *Head Neck* 18:577–581.

Afzelius LE, Cameron WR, Svensson C. (1987) Salivary duct carcinoma clinicopathologic study of 12 cases. *Head Neck Surg* 9:151–156.

Allen CM, Damm D, Neville B, et al. (1994) Necrosis in benign salivary gland neoplasms. Not necessarily a sign of malignant transformation. *Oral Surg Oral Med Oral Pathol* 78:455–461.

Alos L, Cardesa A, Bombi JA, Mallofre C, Cuchi A, Traserra J. (1996) Myoepithelial tumors of salivary glands: a clinicopathologic, immunohistochemical, ultrastructural, and flow-cytometric study. *Semin Diagn Pathol* 13:138–147.

Alos L, Carrillo R, Ramos J, et al. (1999) High-grade carcinoma component in epithelial-myoepithelial carcinoma of salivary glands clinicopathological, immunohistochemical and flow-cytometric study of three cases. *Virchows Arch A Pathol Anat Histopathol* 434:291–299.

Alvarez-Cañas C, Rodilla IG. (1996) True malignant mixed tumor (carcinosarcoma) of the parotid gland. Report of a case with immunohistochemical study. *Oral Surg Oral Med Oral Pathol Oral Radiol Endod* 81:454–458.

Anderson C, Muller R, Piorkowski R, et al. (1992) Intraductal carcinoma of major salivary gland. *Cancer* 69:609–614.

Ardekian L, Manor R, Peled M, Laufer D. (1999) Malignant oncocytoma of the parotid gland: case report and analysis of the literature. *J Oral Maxillofac Surg* 57:325–328.

Åström A-K, Voz ML, Kas K, et al. (1999) Conserved mechanism of *PLAG1* activation in salivary gland tumors with an without chromosome 8q12 abnormalities: identification of *SII* as a new fusion partner gene. *Cancer Res* 59:918–923.

Atula T, Klemi P-J, Donath K, et al. (1993) Basal cell adenocarcinoma of the parotid gland: a case report and review of the literature. *J Laryngol Otol* 107:862–864.

Auclair PL, Ellis GL. (1996) Atypical features in salivary gland mixed tumors: their relationship to malignant transformation. *Mod Pathol* 9:652–657.

Balogh K, Wolbarsht RL. Federman M, O'Hara CJ. (1985) Carcinoma of the parotid gland with osteoclast-like giant cells. *Arch Pathol Lab Med* 109:756–761.

Bankamp DG, Bierhoff E. (1999) Proliferative activity in recurrent and nonrecurrent pleomorphic adenoma of the salivary glands. *Laryngorhinootologie* 78:77–80.

Barfoed C, Graem N, Bretlau P, Rygaard J. (1986) Human pleomorphic adenomas transplanted to nude mice. *Arch Otolaryngol Head Neck Surg* 112:946–948.

Barnes L, Rao U, Krause J, et al. (1994) Salivary duct carcinoma. Part I. A clinicopathologic evaluation and DNA image analysis of 13 cases with review of the literature. *Oral Surg Oral Med Oral Pathol* 78:64–73.

Batsakis JG. (1982) Metastatic patterns of salivary gland neoplasms. *Ann Otol Rhinol Laryngol* 91(4 Pt 1):465–466.

Batsakis JG. (1983) Carcinoma ex lymphoepithelial lesion. *Ann Otol Rhinol Laryngol* 92:657–658.

Batsakis JG. (1987) Carcinoma ex papillary cystadenoma lymphomatosum: malignant Warthin's tumor. *Ann Otol Rhinol Laryngol* 96:234–235.

Batsakis JG, Bernacki EG, Rice DH, Stebler ME. (1975) Malignancy and the benign lymphoepithelial lesion. *Laryngoscope* 85:389–399.

Batsakis JG, Brannon RB. (1981) Dermal analogue tumors of major salivary glands. *J Laryngol Otol* 95:155–164.

Batsakis JG, and El-Naggar AK. (1999) Myoepithelium in salivary and mammary neoplasms is host-friendly. *Adv Anat Pathol* 6:218–226.

Batsakis JS, Luna MA. (1989) Low-grade and high-grade adenocarcinomas of the salivary duct system. *Ann Otol Rhinol Laryngol* 98:162–163.

Batsakis JS, Luna MA. (1991) Basaloid salivary carcinoma. *Ann Otol Rhinol Laryngol* 100:785–787.

Batsakis JS, Luna MA, El-Naggar AK. (1991) Basaloid monomorphic adenomas. *Ann Otol Rhinol Laryngol* 100:687–690.

Bengoechea O, Sánchez F, Larrínaga B, Martínez-Peñuela JM. (1989) Oncocytic adenocarcinoma arising in Warthin's tumor. *Pathol Res Pract* 185:907–911.

Bernacki EG, Batsakis JG, Johns ME. (1974) Basal cell adenoma: distinctive tumor of salivary glands. *Arch Otolaryngol* 88:84B87.

Bocklage T, Feddersen R. (1995) Unusual mesenchymal and mixed tumors of the salivary gland. An immunohistochemical and flow cytometric analysis of three cases. *Arch Pathol Lab Med* 119:69–74.

Bombi JA, Alos L, Rey MJ, Mallofre C, Cuchi A, Trasserra J, Cardesa A. (1996) Myoepithelial carcinoma arising in a benign myoepithelioma, immunohistochemical, ultrastructural, and flow-cytometrical study. *Ultrastruct Pathol* 20:145–154.

Brandwein M, Huvos AG. (1991) Oncocytic tumors of major salivary glands. A study of 68 cases with follow-up of 44 patients. *Am J Surg Pathol* 15:514–528.

Brandwein M, Huvos AG, Dardick I, et al. (1996) Noninvasive and minimally invasive carcinoma ex mixed tumor. A clinicopathologic and ploidy study of 12 patients with major salivary tumors of low (or no?) malignant potential. *Oral Surg Oral Med Oral Pathol Oral Radiol Endod* 81:655–664.

Brandwein MS, Jagirdar J, Patil J, et al. (1990) Salivary duct carcinoma (cribriform salivary carcinoma of excretory ducts) A clinicopathologic and immunohistochemical study of 12 cases. *Cancer* 65:2307–2314.

Buchman C, et al. (1994) Pleomorphic adenoma: effect of tumor spill and inadequate resection on tumor recurrence. *Laryngoscope* 104:1231–1234.

Bullerdiek J, Vollrath M, Wittekind C, et al. (1990) Mucoepidermoid tumor of the parotid gland showing a translocation (3;8)(p21;q12) and a deletion (5) (q22) as sole chromosome abnormalities. *Cancer Genet Cytogenet* 50:161–164.

Bullerdiek J, Wobst G, Meyer-Bolte K, et al. (1993) Cytogenetic subtyping of 220 salivary gland pleomorphic adenomas: correlation to occurrence, histological subtype, and *in vitro* cellular behavior. *Cancer Genet Cytogenet* 65:27–31.

Chan JKC, Yip TTC, Tsang WYW, et al. (1994) Specific association of Epstein-Barr virus with lymphoepithelial carcinoma among tumors and tumor-like lesions of the salivary gland. *Arch Pathol Lab Med* 118:994–997.

Chang A, Harawi SJ. (1992) Oncocytes, oncocytosis, and oncocytic tumors. *Pathol Annu* 27 Pt 1:263–304.

Chen KTK. (1985) Carcinoma arising in monomorphic adenoma of the salivary gland. *Am J Otolaryngol* 6:39–41.

Cheuk W, Chan JKC, Ngan RKC. (1999) Dedifferentiation in adenoid cystic carcinoma of salivary gland. An uncommon complication associated with an accelerated clinical course. *Am J Surg Pathol* 23:465–472.

Christiansen MS, Mourad WA, Hales ML, Oldring DJ. (1995) Spindle cell malignant lymphoepithelial lesion of the parotid gland: clinical, light microscopic, ultrastructural, and *in situ* hybridization findings in one case. *Mod Pathol* 8:711–715.

Clairmont AA, Richardson GS, Hanna DC. (1977) The pseudocapsule of pleomorphic adenomas (benign mixed tumors): the argument against enucleation. *Am J Surg* 134:242–243.

Clark J, Bailey BMW, Eveson JW. (1993) Dysplastic pleomorphic adenoma of the sublingual salivary gland. *Br J Oral Maxillofac Surg* 31:394–395.

Cleary KR, Batsakis JG. (1990) Undifferentiated carcinoma with lymphoid stroma of the major salivary glands. *Ann Otol Rhinol Laryngol* 99:236–238.

Colmenero C, Patron M, Sierra I. (1991) Acinic cell carcinoma of the salivary glands. A review of 20 new cases. *J Craniomaxillofac Surg* 19:260–266.

Colmenero Ruiz C, Patrón Romero M, Martín Pérez M. (1993) Salivary duct carcinoma: a report of nine cases. *J Oral Maxillofac Surg* 51:641–646.

Costa Rosa J, Fonseca I, Félix A, Soares J. (1996) Immunohistochemical study of c-*erb*B-2 expression in carcinoma ex-pleomorphic adenoma. *Histopathology* 28:247–252.

Dahlenfors R, Gertzen H, Wedell B, Mark J. (1997) Cytogenetical observations in a cultured polymorphous low-grade adenocarcinoma originating from the minor salivary glands. *Anticancer Res* 17:105–106.

Damjanov L, Sness EM, Delerme AN. (1983) Squamous cell carcinoma arising in Warthin's tumor of the parotid gland. *Oral Surg Oral Med Oral Pathol* 55:286–290.

Dardick I. (1996) *Color Atlas/Text of Salivary Gland Tumor Pathology.* Igaku-Shoin Medical Publishers, New York.

Dardick I, Thomas MJ, Van Nostrand P. (1989) Myoepithelioma: new concepts of histology and classification: a light and electron microscopic study. *Ultrastruct Pathol* 13;187–224.

Davy CL, Dardick I, Hammond E, et al. (1994) Relationship of clear cell oncocytoma to mitochondrial-rich (typical) oncocytomas of parotid salivary gland. An ultrastructural study. *Oral Surg Oral Med Oral Pathol* 77:469–478.

Dawson CW, Rickinson AB, Young LW. (1990) Epstein-Barr virus latent membrane protein inhibits human epithelial cell differentiation. *Nature* 344:777–780.

de Araujo VC, Calvalho YR, de Araujo NS. (1994) Actin versus vimentin in myoepithelial cells of salivary gland tumors. A comparative study. *Oral Surg Oral Med Oral Pathol* 77:387–391.

Deguchii H, Hamano H, Hayashi Y. (1993) c-myc, ras p21 and p53 expression in pleomorphic adenoma and its malignant form of the human salivary glands. *Acta Pathol Jpn* 43:413–422.

Delgado R, Klimstra D, Albores-Saavedra J. (1996) Low-grade salivary duct carcinoma. *Cancer* 78:958–967.

Delgado R, Vuitch F, Albores-Saavedra J. (1993) Salivary duct carcinoma. *Cancer* 72:1503–1512.

Di Palma S, Guzzo M. (1993) Malignant myoepithelioma of salivary glands: clinicopathological features of ten cases. *Virchows Arch A Pathol Anat Histopathol* 423:389–396.

Di Palma S, Pilottii S, Rilke F. (1991) Malignant myoepithelioma of the parotid gland arising in a pleomorphic adenoma. *Histopathology* 19:273–275.

Donath K, Seifert G, Röser K. (1997) The spectrum of giant cells in tumours of the salivary glands: an analysis of 11 cases. *J Oral Pathol Med* 26:431–436.

Ellis GL. (1988) "Clear cell" oncocytoma of salivary gland. *Hum Pathol* 19:862–867.

Ellis GL, Auclair PL, Gnepp DR. (1991) *Surgical Pathology of the Salivary Glands*, Vol. 25. MMP Series, W.B. Saunders, Philadelphia.

Ellis GL, Wiscovitch JG. (1990) Basal cell adenocarcinomas of the major salivary glands. *Oral Surg Oral Med Oral Pathol* 69:461–469.

El-Naggar AK, Lovell M, Callender DL, et al. (1998) Concurrent cytogenetic, interphase fluorescence *in situ* hybridization and DNA flow cytometric analyses of a carcinoma ex-pleomorphic adenoma of parotid gland. *Cancer Genet Cytogenet* 107:132–136.

Epivationos A, Dimitrakopoulos J, Trigonidis G. (1995) Intraoral salivary duct carcinoma: a clinicopathological study of four cases and review of the literature. *Ann Dent* 54:36–40.

Eusebi V, Martin SA, Govoni E, Rosai J. (1984) Giant cell tumor of major salivary glands: report of three cases, one occurring in association with a malignant mixed tumor. *Am J Clin Pathol* 81:666–675.

Fåhraeus R, Rymo L, Rhim JS, Klein G. (1990) Morphological transformation of human keratinocytes expressing the LMP gene of Epstein-Barr virus. *Nature* 345:447–449.

Félix A, El-Naggar AK, Press MF, et al. (1996) Prognostic significance of biomarkers (c-*erb*B-2, p53, proliferating cell nuclear antigen, and DNA content) in salivary duct carcinoma. *Hum Pathol* 27:561–566.

Félix A, Fonseca I, Soares J. (1993) Oncocytic tumors of salivary gland type: a study with emphasis on nuclear DNA ploidy. *J Surg Oncol* 52:217–222.

Ferrandiz V, Campo E, Bowman E. (1985) Dermal cylindromas (turban tumour) and eccrine spiradenoma in a patient with membranous basal cell adenoma of the parotid gland. *J Cutan Pathol* 12:72–79.

Ferreiro JA, Kochar AS. (1994) Parotid acinic cell carcinoma with undifferentiated spindle cell transformation. *J Laryngol Otol* 108:902–904.

Ferreiro J, Stylopoulos N. (1995) Oncocytic differentiation in salivary gland tumours. *J Laryngol Otol* 109:569–571.

Fliss DM, Rival R, Gullane P, et al. (1992) Pleomorphic adenoma: a preliminary histopathologic comparison between tumors occurring in the deep and superficial lobes of the parotid gland. *Ear Nose Throat J* 71:254–257.

Franquemont DW, Mills SE. (1993) Plasmacytoid monomorphic adenoma of salivary glands. Absence of myogenous differentiation and comparison to spindle cell myoepithelioma. *Am J Surg Pathol* 17:146–153.

Gaffey MJ, Weiss LM. (1992) Association of Epstein-Barr virus with human neoplasia. *Pathol Annu* 27 (Pt 1):55–74.

Gandour-Edwards RF, Donald PJ, Vogt PJ, et al. (1994) Carcinosarcoma (malignant mixed tumor) of the parotid: report of a case with a pure rhabdomyosarcoma component. *Head Neck* 16:379–382.

Garland TA, Innes DJ Jr, Fechner RE. (1984) Salivary duct carcinoma: an analysis of four cases with review of literature. *Am J Clin Pathol* 81:436–441.

Garner SL, Robinson RA, Maves MD, Barnes CH. (1989) Salivary gland carcinosarcoma: true malignant mixed tumor. *Ann Otol Rhinol Laryngol* 98:611–614.

Geurts JMW, Schoenmakers EFPM, Röijer E, et al. (1997a) Expression of reciprocal hybrid transcripts of *HMGIC* and *FHIT* in a pleomorphic adenoma of the parotid gland. *Cancer Res* 57:13–17.

Geurts JMW, Schoenmakers EFPM, Röijer E, et al. (1998) Identification of *NFIB* as recurrent translocation partner gene of *HMGIC* in pleomorphic adenomas. *Oncogene* 16:865–872.

Geurts JMW, Schoenmakers EFPM, Van de Ven WJM. (1997b) Molecular characterization of a complex chromosomal rearrangement in a pleomorphic salivary gland adenoma involving the 3'-UTR of *HMGIC*. *Cancer Genet Cytogenet* 95:198–205.

Gnepp DR. (1983) Sebaceous neoplasms of salivary gland origin: a review. *Pathol Annu* 18(Pt. 1):71–102.

Gnepp DR. (1993) Malignant mixed tumors of the salivary glands: a review. *Pathol Annu* 28:279–328.

Gnepp DR, Brannon R. (1984) Sebaceous neoplasms of salivary gland origin. Report of 21 cases. *Cancer* 53:2155–2170.

Goodisson DW, Buff RGM, Creedon AJ, et al. (1999) A case of metastasizing pleomorphic adenoma. *Oral Surg Oral Med Oral Pathol Oral Radiol Endod* 87:341–345.

Gravanis MB, Giansanti JS. (1970) Malignant histopathologic counterpart of the benign lymphoepithelial lesion. *Cancer* 26:1332–1342.

Grenko RT, Gymryd P, Tytor M, et al. (1995) Salivary duct carcinoma. *Histopathology* 26:261–266.

Grenko RT, Tytor M, Boeryd B. (1993) Giant-cell tumour of the salivary gland with associated carcinosarcoma. *Histopathology* 23:594–595.

Gunduz M, Yamanaka N, Hotomi M, et al. (1999) Squamous cell carcinoma arising in a Warthin's tumor. *Auris Nasus Larynx* 26:355–360.

Hamilton-Dutoit SJ, Hamilton Therkildsen M, H¯jgaard Nielsen N, et al. (1991) Undifferentiated carcinoma of the salivary gland in Greenlandic Eskimos: demonstration of Epstein-Barr virus DNA by *in situ* nucleic acid hybridization. *Hum Pathol* 22:811–815.

Hartwick RWJ, Batsakis JG. (1990) Non-Warthin's tumor oncocytic lesions. *Ann Otol Rhinol Laryngol* 99:674–677.

Headington JT, Batsakis JG, Beals TF, et al. (1977) Membranous basal cell adenoma of parotid gland, dermal cylindromas and trichoepitheliomas: comparative histochemistry and ultrastructure. *Cancer* 39:2460–2469.

Hellquist HB, Karlsson MT, Nilsson C. (1994) Salivary duct carcinoma—a highly aggressive salivary duct gland tumour with overexpression of c-*erb*B-2. *J Pathol* 172:35–44.

Hellquist H, Michaels L. (1986) Malignant mixed tumour. A salivary gland tumour showing both carcinomatous and sarcomatous features. *Virchows Arch A Pathol Anat Histopathol* 409:93–103.

Henley JD, Geary WA, Jackson CL, et al. (1997) Dedifferentiated acinic cell carcinoma of the parotid gland: a distinct rarely described entity. *Hum Pathol* 28:869–873.

Henriksson G, Westrin KM. Carlsoo B, Silfversward C. (1998) Recurrent primary pleomorphic adenomas of salivary gland origin: intrasurgical rupture, histopathologic features, and pseudopodia. *Cancer* 82:617–620.

Herbst EV, Utz W. (1984) Multifocal dermal-type basal cell adenomas of parotid glands with co-existing dermal cylindromas. *Virchows Arch A Pathol Anat Histopathol* 403:95–102.

Herrera-Gayol A, Jothy S. (1999) Adhesion proteins in the biology of breast cancer: contribution of CD44. *Exp Mol Pathol* 66:149–156.

Huang DP, Ng HK, Hoo YH, et al. (1988) Epstein-Barr virus (EBV)–associated undifferentiated carcinoma of the parotid gland. *Histopathology* 13:509–517.

Hui KK, Batsakis JG, Luna MA, et al. (1986) Salivary duct adenocarcinoma: a high-grade malignancy. *J Laryngol Otol* 100:105–114.

Jackson SR, Roland NJ, Clar RW, Jones AS. (1993) Recurrent pleomorphic adenoma. *J Laryngol Otol* 107: 546–549.

Jahan-Parwar B, Huberman RM, Donovan DT, et al. (1999) Oncocytic mucoepidermoid carcinoma of the salivary glands. *Am J Surg Pathol* 23:523–529.

Jin Y, Jin C, Arheden K, et al. (1998) Unbalanced chromosomal rearrangements in a metastasizing salivary gland tumor with benign histology. *Cancer Genet Cytogenet* 102:59–64.

Kamio N. (1996) Coexpression of p53 and c-erbB-2 proteins is associated with histological type, tumour stage, and cell proliferation in malignant salivary gland tumours. *Virchows Arch* 428:75–83.

Kapadia SB, Barnes L. (1998) Expression of androgen receptor, gross cystic disease fluid protein, and CD44 in salivary duct carcinoma. *Mod Pathol* 11:1033–1038.

Katz AD, Preston-Martin S. (1984) Salivary gland tumors and previous radiotherapy to the head or neck. Report of a clinical series. *Am J Surg* 147:345–348.

Kleinsasser O, Klein HJ, Hubner G. (1968) Salivary duct carcinoma. A group of salivary gland tumors analogous to mammary duct carcinoma. *Arch Klin Exp Ohren Nasen Kehlkopfheilkd* 192:100–105.

Klijanienko J, El-Naggar AK, Servois V, et al. (1997) Clinically aggressive metastasizing pleomorphic adenoma: report of two cases. *Head Neck* 19:629–633.

Kotsianti A, Costopoulos J, Morgello S, Papadimitriou C. (1996) Undifferentiated carcinoma of the parotid gland in a white patient: detection of Epstein-Barr virus by *in situ* hybridization. *Hum Pathol* 27:87–90.

Kountakis SE, SooHoo W, Maillard A. (1995) Lymphoepithelial carcinoma of the parotid gland. *Head Neck* 17:445–450.

Kumar RV, Kini L, Bhargava AK, et al. (1993) Salivary duct carcinoma. *J Surg Oncol* 54:193–198.

Kuo T, Hsueh C. (1997) Lymphoepithelioma-like salivary gland carcinoma in Taiwan: a clinicopathological study of nine cases demonstrating a strong association with Epstein-Barr virus. *Histopathology* 31:75–82.

Lam KH, Ho HC, Ho CM, Wei WI. (1994) Multifocal nature of adenolymphoma of the parotid. *Br J Surg* 81:1612–1614.

Land CE, Saku T, Hayashi Y, et al. (1996) Incidence of salivary gland tumors among atomic bomb survivors, 1950–1987. Evaluation of radiation-related risk. *Radiat Res* 146:28–36.

Laskawi R, Schott T, Schroder M. (1998) Recurrent pleomorphic adenomas of the parotid gland: clinical evaluation and long-term follow-up. *Br J Oral Maxillofac Surg* 36:48–51.

Latkovich P, Johnson RL. (1998) Carcinosarcoma of the parotid gland. Report of a case with cytohistologic and immunohistochemical findings. *Arch Pathol Lab Med* 122:743–746.

Leung SY, Chung LP, Yuen ST, et al. (1995) Lymphoepithelial carcinoma of the salivary gland: *in situ* detection of Epstein-Barr virus. *J Clin Pathol* 48:1022–1027.

Lewis JE, McKinney BC, Weiland LH, et al. (1996) Salivary duct carcinoma. Clinicopathologic and immunohistochemical review of 26 cases. *Cancer* 77: 223–230.

Li X, Tsuji T, Wen S. (1997) Detection of numeric abnormalities of chromosome 17 and p53 deletions by fluorescence *in situ* hybridization in pleomorphic adenomas and carcinomas in pleomorphic adenoma. *Cancer* 79:2314–2319.

LiVolsi VA, Perzin KH. (1977) Malignant mixed tumor arising in salivary glands. I. Carcinomas arising in benign mixed tumors: a clinicopathologic study. *Cancer* 39:2209–2230.

Luna MA, Batsakis JG, Ordonez NG, et al. (1987a) Salivary gland adenocarcinomas: a clinicopathologic analysis of three distinctive types. *Semin Diagn Pathol* 4:117–135.

Luna MA, Batsakis JG, Tortoledo ME, del Junco GW. (1989) Carcinomas ex monomorphic adenoma of salivary glands. *J Laryngol Otol* 103:756–759.

Luna MA, Mackay B. (1976) Basal cell adenoma of the parotid gland. Case report with ultrastructural observations. *Cancer* 37:1615–1621.

Luna MA, Tortoledo MME, Allen M. (1987b) Salivary dermal analogue tumors arising in lymph nodes. *Cancer* 59:1165–1169.

Mark HFL, Hanna I, Gnepp DR. (1996) Cytogenetic analysis of salivary gland type tumors. *Oral Surg Oral Med Oral Pathol Oral Radiol Endod* 82:187–192.

Mark J, Dahlenfors R, Stenman G, et al. (1992) Cytogenetical observations in two cases of polymorphous low-grade adenocarcinoma of the salivary glands. *Anticancer Res* 12:1195–1198.

Mark J, Wedell B, Dahlenfors R, Stenman G. (1991) Karyotypic variability and evolutionary characteristics of a polymorphous low-grade adenocarcinoma in the parotid gland. *Cancer Genet Cytogenet* 55:19–29.

Martinez-Barba E, Cortes-Guardiola JA, Minguela-Puras A, et al. (1997) Salivary duct carcinoma: clinicopathological and immunohistochemical studies. *J Craniomaxillofac Surg* 25:328–334.

Martins C, Fonseca I, Félix A, et al. (1995) Benign salivary gland tumors: a cytogenetic study of 21 cases. *J Surg Oncol* 60:232–237.

Martins C, Fonseca I, Roque L, et al. (1996) Malignant salivary gland neoplasms: a cytogenetic study of 19 cases. *Oral Oncol Eur J Cancer* 32B:128–132.

McCluggage WG, Primrose WJ, Toner PG. (1998) Myoepithelial carcinoma (malignant myoepithelioma) of the parotid gland arising in a pleomorphic adenoma. *J Clin Pathol* 51:552–556.

McCluggage G, Sloan J, Cameron S, et al. (1995) Basal cell adenocarcinoma of the submandibular gland. *Oral Surg Oral Med Oral Pathol Oral Radiol Endod* 79:342–350.

McGregor AD, Burgoyne M, Tan KC. (1988) Recurrent pleomorphic salivary adenoma—the relevance of age at first presentation. *Br J Plast Surg* 41:177–181.

Michal M, Skalova A, Simpson RHW, et al. (1996) Clear cell malignant myoepithelioma of the salivary gland. *Histopathology* 28:309–315.

Mini AJ. (1993) Unusual variant of a metastasizing malignant mixed tumor of the parotid gland. *Oral Surg Oral Med Oral Pathol* 76:330–332.

Modan B, Chetrit A, Alfandary E, et al. (1998) Increased risk of salivary gland tumors after low-dose irradiation. *Laryngoscope* 108:1095–1097.

Molberg KH, Heffess C, Delgado R, Albores-Saavedra J. (1998) Undifferentiated carcinoma with osteoclast-like giant cells of the pancreas and periampullary region. *Cancer* 82:1279–1287.

Müller S, Barnes L. (1996) Basal cell adenocarcinoma of the salivary glands. Report of seven cases and review of the literature. *Cancer* 78:2471–2477.

Müller S, Vigneswaran N, Gansler T, et al. (1994) c-*erb*B-2 oncoprotein expression and amplification in pleomorphic adenoma and carcinoma ex pleomorphic adenoma: relationship to prognosis. *Mod Pathol* 7:628–632.

Nagao T, Sugano I, Ishida Y, et al. (1997) Carcinoma in basal cell adenoma of the parotid gland. *Pathol Res Pract* 193:171–178.

Nagao T, Sugano I, Ishida Y, et al. (1998a) Basal cell adenocarcinoma of the salivary glands. Comparison with basal cell adenoma through assessment of cell proliferation, apoptosis, and expression of p53 and bcl-2. *Cancer* 82:439–847.

Nagao T, Sugano I, Ishida Y, et al. (1998b) Mucoepidermoid carcinoma arising in Warthin's tumour of the parotid gland: report of two cases with histopathological, ultrastructural and immunohistochemical studies. *Histopathology* 33:379–386.

Nagao T, Sugano I, Ishida Y, et al. (1998c) Salivary gland malignant myoepithelioma. A clinicopathologic and immunohistochemical study of ten cases. *Cancer* 83:1292–1299.

Natvig K, Soberg R. (1994) Relationship of intraoperative rupture of pleomorphic adenomas to recurrence: an 11–25 year follow-up study. *Head Neck* 16:213–217.

Nordkvist A, Mark J, Dahlenfors R, et al. (1994) Cytogenetic observations in 13 cystadenolymmphomas (Warthin's tumors) *Cancer Genet Cytogenet* 76:129–135.

Ogawa I, Nikai H, Takata T, et al. (1990) The cellular composition of basal cell adenoma of the parotid gland: an immunohistochemical analysis. *Oral Surg Oral Med Oral Pathol* 70:619–626.

Önder T, Tiwarii RM, Van Der Waal I, Snow GB. (1990) Malignant adenolymphoma of the parotid gland: report of carcinomatous transformation. *J Laryngol Otol* 104:656–661.

Palmer TJ, Gleeson MJ, Eveson JW, Cawson RA. (1990) Oncocytic adenomas and oncocytic hyperplasia of salivary glands: a clinicopathological study of 26 cases. *Histopathology* 16:487–493.

Pelkey TJ, Mills SE. (1999) Histologic transformation of polymorphous low-grade adenocarcinoma of salivary gland. *Am J Clin Pathol* 111:785–791.

Phillips PP, Olsen KD. (1995) Recurrent pleomorphic adenoma of the parotid gland: report of 126 cases and a review of the literature. *Ann Otol Rhinol Laryngol* 104:100–104.

Prasad AR, Savera AT, Gown AM, Zarbo RJ. (1999) The myoepithelial immunophenotype in 135 benign and malignant salivary gland tumors other than pleomorphic adenoma. *Arch Pathol Lab Med* 123:801–806.

Queimado L, Lopes C, Du F, et al. (1999) Pleomorphic adenoma gene 1 is expressed in cultured benign and malignant salivary gland tumor cells. *Lab Invest* 79:583–589.

Queimado L, Reis A, Fonseca I, et al. (1998) A refined localization of two deleted regions in chromosome 6q associated with salivary gland carcinomas. *Oncogene* 16:83–88.

Qureshi AB, Gitelis S, Templeton AA, Piasecki PA. (1994) "Benign" metastasizing pleomorphic adenoma. A case report and review of literature. *Clin Orthop* 308:192–198.

Raab-Traub N, Rajadurai P, Flynn K, Lanier AP. (1991) Epstein-Barr virus infection in carcinoma of the salivary gland. *J Virol* 65:7032–7036.

Righi PD, Li Y-Q, Deutsch M, et al. (1994) The role of the p53 gene in the malignant transformation of pleomorphic adenomas of the parotid gland. *Anticancer Res* 14:2253–2258.

Saemundsen AK, Albeck H, Hansen JPH, et al. (1982) Epstein-Barr virus in nasopharyngeal and salivary gland carcinomas of Greenland Eskimos. *Br J Cancer* 46:721–728.

Saku T, Hayashi Y, Takahara O, et al. (1997) Salivary gland tumors among atomic bomb survivors, 1950–1987. *Cancer* 79:1465–1475.

Sampson BA, Jarcho JA, Winters GL. (1998) Metastasizing mixed tumor of the parotid gland: a rare tumor with unusually rapid progression in a cardiac transplant recipient. *Mod Pathol* 11:1142–1145.

Sandros J, Stenman G, Mark J. (1990) Cytogenetic and molecular observations in human and experimental salivary gland tumors. *Cancer Genet Cytogenet* 44:153–167.

Savera AT, Gown AM, Zarbo RJ. (1997) Immunolocalization of three novel smooth muscle-specific proteins in salivary gland pleomorphic adenoma: assessment of the morphogenetic role of myoepithelium. *Mod Pathol* 10:1093–1100.

Saw D, Lau WH, Ho JHC, et al. (1986) Malignant lymphoepithelial lesion of the salivary gland. *Hum Pathol* 17:914–923.

Schmidt KTA, Ma A, Golberg R, Medenica M.. (1991) Multiple adnexal tumors and a parotid basal cell adenoma. *J Am Acad Dermatol* 25(5 Pt 2):960–964.

Schneider AB, Favus MJ, Stachura ME, et al. (1977) Salivary gland neoplasms as a late consequence of head and neck irradiation. *Ann Intern Med* 87:160–164.

Schneider AB, Lubin J, Ron E, et al. (1998) Salivary gland tumors after childhood radiation treatment for benign conditions of the head and neck: dose-response relationships. *Radiat Res* 149:625–630.

Schreibstein JM, Tronic B, Tarlov E, Hybels RL. (1995) Benign metastasizing pleomorphic adenoma. *Otolaryngol Head Neck Surg* 112:612–615.

Seifert G. (1991) *World Health Organization International Histological Classification of Tumours. Histological Typing of Salivary Gland Tumours*, 2nd ed. Springer-Verlag, New York.

Seifert G. (1996) Mucoepidermoid carcinoma in a salivary duct cyst of the parotid gland. *Pathol Res Pract* 192:1211–1217.

Shintaku M, Honda T. (1997) Identification of oncocytic lesions of salivary glands by anti-mitochondrial immunohistochemistry. *Histopathology* 31:408–411.

Simpson RHW, Jones H, Beasley P. (1995) Benign myoepithelioma of the salivary glands: a true entity? *Histopathology* 27:1–9.

Skalova A, Michal M, Ryska A, et al. (1999) Oncocytic myoepithelioma and pleomorphic adenoma of the salivary glands. *Virchows Arch* 434:537–546.

Smith SA. (1976) Radiation-induced salivary gland tumors: report of a case. *Arch Otolaryngol* 102:561–562.

Sørensen M, Baunsgaard P, Frederiksen P, Haahr PA. (1986) Multifocal adenomatous oncocytic hyperplasia of the parotid gland. (Unusual clear cell variant in two female siblings). *Pathol Res Pract* 181: 254–257.

Spiro RH, Huvos AG, Strong EW. (1977) Malignant mixed tumor of salivary origin. A clinicopathologic study of 146 cases. *Cancer* 39:388–396.

Stanley RJ, Weiland LH, Olsen KD, Pearson BW. (1988) Dedifferentiated acinic cell (acinous) carcinoma of the parotid gland. *Otolaryngol Head Neck Surg* 98: 155–161.

Stephen J, Batsakis JG, Luna MA, et al. (1986) True malignant mixed tumors (carcinosarcoma) of salivary glands. *Oral Surg Oral Med Oral Pathol* 61:597–602.

Stern C, Meyer K, Bartnitzke S, et al. (1990) Pleomorphic adenomas with unbalanced chromosomal abnormalities have an increased in vitro lifetime. *Cancer Genet Cytogenet* 46:55–63.

Sternlicht MD, Barsky SH. (1997) The myoepithelial defense: a host defense against cancer. *Med Hypotheses* 48:37–46.

Sugano S, Mukai K, Tsuda H, et al. (1992) Immunohistochemical study of c-*erb*B-2 oncoprotein overexpression in human major salivary gland carcinoma: an indicator of aggressiveness. *Laryngoscope* 102: 923–927.

Suzuki H, Inoue K, Fujioka Y, et al. (1998) Myoepithelial carcinoma with predominance of plasmacytoid cells arising in a pleomorphic adenoma of the parotid gland. *Histopathology* 32:86–87.

Tallini G. (1998) Oncocytic tumours. *Virchows Arch* 433: 5–12.

Taxy JB. (1992) Necrotizing squamous/mucinous metaplasia in oncocytic salivary gland tumors. A potential diagnostic problem. *Am J Clin Pathol* 97:40–45.

Therkildsen MH, Christensen N, Andersen LJ, et al. (1992) Malignant Warthin's tumour: a case study. *Histopathology* 21:167–171.

Thompson LD, Wenig BM, Ellis GL. (1996) Oncocytomas of the submandibular gland. A series of 22 cases and a review of the literature. *Cancer* 78:2281–2287.

Tortoledo ME, Luna MA, Batsakis JG. (1984) Carcinomas ex pleomorphic adenoma and mixed tumors. *Arch Otolaryngol* 110:172–176.

Tsai C-C, Chen C-L, Hsu H-C. (1996) Expression of Epstein-Barr virus in carcinomas of major salivary glands: a strong association with lymphoepithelioma-like carcinoma. *Hum Pathol* 27:258–262.

Viglianii R, Genetta C. (1982) Diffuse hyperplastic oncocytosis of the parotid gland. Case report with histochemical observations. *Virchows Arch A Pathol Anat Histopathol* 397:235–240.

Voz ML, Åström A-K, Kas K, et al. (1998) The recurrent translocation t(5;8)(p13;q12) in pleomorphic adenomas results in upregulation of *PLAG1* gene expression under control of the *LIFR* promoter. *Oncogene* 16:1409–1416.

Weiss LM, Gaffey MJ, Shibata D. (1991) Lymphoepithelioma-like carcinoma and its relationship to Epstein-Barr virus. *Am J Clin Pathol* 96:156–158.

Wenig BM, Hitchcock CK, Ellis GL, Gnepp DR. (1992) Metastasizing mixed tumor of salivary glands. A clinicopathologic and flow cytometric analysis. *Am J Surg Pathol* 16:845–858.

Yamamoto Y, Kishimoto Y, Wistuba II, et al. (1998) DNA analysis at p53 locus in carcinomas arising from pleomorphic adenomas of salivary glands: comparison of molecular study and p53 immunostaining. *Pathol Int* 48:265–272.

Yoshihara T, Shino A, Ishii T, Kawakami M. (1994) Ultrastructural and immunohistochemical study of salivary duct carcinoma of the parotid gland. *Ultrastruct Pathol* 18:553–558.

6

ESOPHAGUS

Donald A. Antonioli

Malignant squamous and glandular tumors of the esophagus are common, with a wide geographic distribution. Because these neoplasms have a poor prognosis when detected at an advanced clinical stage, investigators have focused on the detection of premalignant lesions and early invasive cancers in an attempt to obtain a better outcome. Thus, analysis of incipient squamous and glandular neoplasia is the topic of this chapter.

SQUAMOUS CELL NEOPLASIA

INCIDENCE AND PATHOGENESIS OF CARCINOMA

The incidence of esophageal squamous cell carcinoma exhibits a wide geographic variation. For example, the incidence in the United States and Europe is low (approximately 4 cases per 100,000 population) but is much greater in South Africa, Iran, and parts of Asia. It reaches a rate of 50 per 100,000 among elderly Japanese men and greater than 100 per 100,000 among men and women in parts of northern China (Qui and Yang, 1988; Rubio et al., 1989; Togawa et al., 1994). Even in low-risk countries, the disease is more common in some groups (for example, among Black males in the United States) or in certain areas (i.e., males in northern France) (Jacob et al., 1990; Rubio et al., 1989).

Although certain conditions have been associated with an increased risk of esophageal carcinoma (Table 6–1), they account for only a small minority of cases. As suggested by the geographic variation in incidence, environmental factors play an important role in pathogenesis. Among such factors, dietary deficiencies, carcinogens in foods, and abuse of alcohol and/or tobacco have been primarily implicated (Jacob et al., 1990; Muñoz and Crespi, 1983; Stemmermann et al., 1994). Over the past decade, esophageal infection by human papillomavirus (HPV) has also been implicated in the pathogenesis of these squamous cell carcinomas. In a review of published studies (Polzak et al., 1998), the prevalence of HPV detection in esophageal squamous cell carcinoma and/or in adjacent normal tissue varied from 0% to approximately 60%. The reasons for this wide variation are multiple and include the sensitivity of the methods used for detection (e.g., *in situ* hybridization versus polymerase chain reaction). However, a consensus is emerging that the highest prevalence rates are in countries with the greatest risk for esophageal squamous cancer; in low-risk countries, other factors (such as nutritional deficiencies and ethanol/tobacco abuse) are more significant (Chang et al., 1992; Polzak et al., 1998; Riddell, 1996; Suzek et al., 1996).

Esophageal squamous cell carcinoma is usually advanced at the time of diagnosis, especially in countries with a low prevalence of the disease in which screening protocols are not used. In such cases, extension of tumor into the muscularis propria or adventitia and regional nodal metastases are

Table 6–1. Conditions Associated with an Increased Risk of Esophageal Squamous Cell Carcinoma

---

Familial cases of keratosis palmaris et plantaris (tylosis)

Plummer-Vinson (Paterson-Kelly) syndrome: iron deficiency anemia; ? other nutritional deficiencies; postcricoid dysphagia

Celiac disease

Achalasia

Caustic (lye) ingestion

---

common. As a result, the resectibility rate for advanced carcinoma is only 30%, and the overall 5-year survival remains less than 10% (Ribeiro et al., 1996).

SUPERFICIAL ESOPHAGEAL CARCINOMA

Given the poor outlook for advanced squamous cell carcinoma, various workers (particularly in high-risk populations) have attempted to define and detect earlier stages of the disease. This search has been successful, giving rise to the concept of *superficial esophageal carcinoma*, a lesion with a 5-year survival varying from 55% to 90% in recent series. Potentially curable esophageal squamous cell carcinoma has been given a variety of names, including "superficial esophageal carcinoma," "early esophageal cancer," and "microinvasive squamous cell carcinoma" (Barge et al., 1981; Rubio et al., 1989). In this chapter, the term "superficial esophageal carcinoma" (SEC) is used.

Definition and Prevalence

The precise definition of SEC has varied in different series (Table 6–2). All workers agree that in SEC, the cancer is confined to the mucosa or submucosa (pT1a and pT1b,

Table 6–2. Superficial Esophageal Squamous Carcinoma

A diagnosis of exclusion

Invasion confined to mucosa or submucosa

Lymph node metastases do not exclude a case

No parenchymal metastases

No preoperative induction therapy

Five-year survival: 55% to 90% in various series

---

respectively). However, some authors exclude cases with metastases to lymph nodes, whereas others include them; in some series, the status of resected lymph nodes has not been recorded (Barge et al., 1981; Lewin and Appelman, 1996; Shimazu et al., 1983). Since many reports contain patients with nodal metastases, the following discussion includes patients with positive nodes. Cases with parenchymal metastases are excluded, as are patients with preoperative chemoradiation induction therapy to the esophagus (Rubio et al., 1989). As in the case of early gastric cancer, SEC is a diagnosis of exclusion, based on thorough evaluation of imaging studies such as intracavitary ultrasound or on careful examination of resected specimens (Kato et al., 1990).

The prevalence of SEC as a percentage of resected specimens has increased dramatically over the past several decades, from less than 5% in 1960s and 1970s to approximately 20% in the 1980s. This increase has been attributed to numerous factors: mass screening in high-risk countries, increased use of endoscopy, and use of ancillary mucosal staining techniques (particularly application of iodine solution) to detect and highlight minimally abnormal areas that may, in fact, harbor malignancy (Kato et al., 1990; Lewin and Appelman, 1996; Schmidt et al., 1986).

Clinical Features

Superficial esophageal carcinoma has the same demographic features as advanced esophageal cancer: a predilection for middle-aged males (M:F ratio equals 3–12:1) and, in the West, an association with alcohol and tobacco abuse (Barge et al., 1981; Benasco et al., 1985; Bogomoletz et al., 1989; Froelicher and Miller, 1986; Kato et al., 1990; Schmidt et al., 1986; Shimazu et al., 1983). The age of patients with SEC is, on average, 6 years younger than that of patients with advanced disease. The major complaint is dysphagia, frequently accompanied by pain. Because these tumors are often small, nonconstricting lesions, the dysphagia is considered to be secondary to spasm (Benasco et al., 1985). About 50% of cases are discovered incidentally, either by mass screening or during evaluation of other conditions such as gastritis or peptic ulcer (Kato et al., 1990; Schmidt et al., 1986). Radiology is not especially sensitive at detecting these lesions; even at endoscopy, 40% are misinterpreted grossly as esophagitis or normal mucosa (Barge et al., 1981; Schmidt et al., 1986).

Pathologic Features

The reasons for the frequent difficulty in the clinical detection of SEC can be deduced from a consideration of the pathologic findings. These cancers vary in size from 0.5 cm to 8.0 cm in diameter; however, the majority are small, with an average diameter of less than 3.0 cm. Although there is no uniform classification of their gross appearance, which can vary from polypoid to flat or eroded, a large percentage (40% or more) are flat or slightly depressed lesions with a granular surface that may be difficult to identify or may resemble reflux esophagitis at endoscopy (Barge et al., 1981; Benasco et al., 1985; Kato et al., 1990; Nabeya, 1983; Schmidt et al., 1986; Shimazu et al., 1983). A useful differential diagnostic point is that in patients with SEC, the mucosa distal to the tumor is generally normal, whereas in esophagitis of reflux type, the entire lower esophageal mucosa is abnormal.

Like advanced carcinoma, SEC is located chiefly in the mid- or lower esophagus. SEC is multifocal in approximately 20% of cases and large lesions may be circumferential, but the esophageal wall remains flexible because the lesions are superficial. In surgical specimens, flat or eroded lesions may become more apparent after the application of iodine to the mucosa or after formalin fixation (Barge et al., 1981; Bogomoletz et al., 1989; Froelicher and Miller, 1986; Kato et al., 1990; Nabeya, 1983; Schmidt et al., 1986).

Microscopically, these squamous cell carcinomas vary from well to poorly differentiated. Invasion is often focal. Early invasion can be recognized by an irregular epithelial–stromal interface, frequent development of a desmoplastic response, and the presence of a mononuclear inflammatory infiltrate, often containing lymphoid nodules, at the base of the neoplasm (Benasco et al., 1985; Bogomoletz et al., 1989; Kato et al., 1990; Schmidt et al., 1986; Shimizu et al., 1999; Fig. 6–1). More extensive intramucosal carcinoma consists of sheets and masses of cells in the lamina propria, often associated with surface erosion. In different published series, lesions have been confined to the mu-

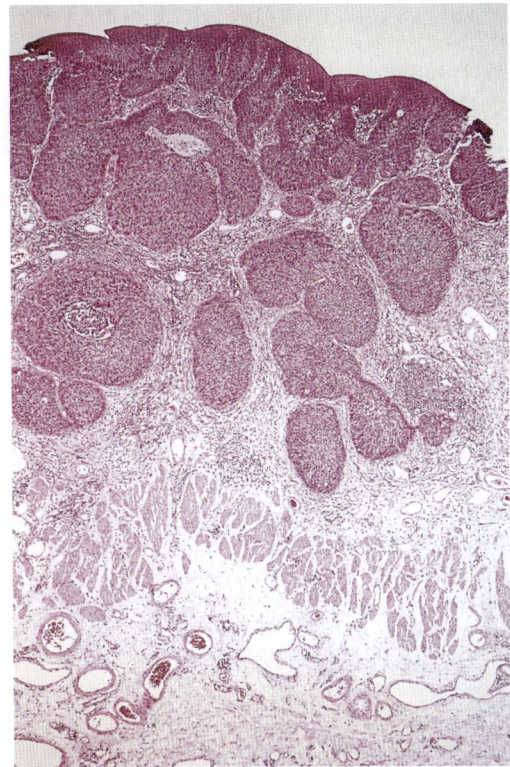

Figure 6–1. Superficial squamous cell carcinoma of the esophagus. Irregular nests of poorly differentiated squamous cells fill the lamina propria, almost to the level of the muscularis mucosae. [Courtesy of Jorge Albores-Saavedra, M.D., University of Texas–Southwestern Medical Center, Dallas, TX.]

cosa in 14% to 65% of cases, with the remainder extending into the submucosa. One reason for the wide range in percentage of intramucosal cancers relates to the fact that some authors include cases of squamous cell carcinoma *in situ* (i.e., carcinoma confined to the epithelium, without lamina propria invasion) in the definition of SEC.

Lymph node metastases are found in up to 50% of patients, more frequently in patients with cancer extending into the submucosa than those with intramucosal neoplasms. Positive nodes may be found away from the esophagus (for example, in the celiac axis), sometimes with sparing of the periesophageal nodes. Postoperative deaths have occurred in 5% to 15% of patients, with 5-year survival rates ranging from 55% to 90% among the remaining cases (Barge et al., 1981; Benasco et al., 1985;

Froelicher and Miller, 1986; Kato et al., 1990; Lewin and Appelman, 1996; Mandard et al., 1984; Nabeya, 1983; Schmidt et al., 1986; Shimazu et al., 1983).

Prognostic Factors

The degree of histologic differentiation of the SEC does not appear to influence either the pathologic stage or survival. The major histologic prognostic factors are depth of invasion, lymphatic space invasion, and lymph nodal status. The results of recent studies suggest that larger lesions and those with an elevated or polypoid (as opposed to a flat or eroded) appearance are the most likely to exhibit these negative prognostic markers (Nagawa et al., 1995; Shimizu et al., 1999).

Depth of invasion correlates with the prevalence of lymphatic invasion and nodal metastases. Lymphatic invasion, identified in fewer than 20% of intramucosal cancers, has been noted in up to 50% of those with submucosal extension. Likewise, nodal metastases have been detected in fewer than 10% of patients with intramucosal cancer in most series, but in 30% to 50% of those with submucosal spread (Bogomoletz et al., 1989; Kato et al., 1990; Lewin and Appelman, 1996; Nagawa et al., 1995; Shimazu et al., 1983; Shimizu et al., 1999). In turn, nodal metastases are a predictor of poor outcome. For example, Kato and colleagues (1990) reported a 5-year survival of 72% for patients with negative lymph nodes but only 39% for those with nodal metastases. Death has been associated with metastases chiefly to bone and liver.

Thus, submucosal spread and nodal metastases significantly decrease survival in SEC. These tumors are biologically more aggressive lesions than early gastric cancer, their counterpart in the stomach, in which 5-year survival rates of 90% or better are consistently recorded regardless of submucosal spread or metastases in perigastric lymph nodes (Froelicher and Miller, 1986). Part of the explanation for this difference is that even superficial esophageal cancers have often spread to distant nodal groups; the disease is systemic at an early stage (Rice, 1999).

Depth of spread and nodal status in SEC cannot, of course, be predicted from routine examination of endoscopically derived mucosal biopsy specimens. However, Sugimachi and associates (1984) have reported that cases of SEC with nodal metastases and re-

current disease typically have a highly aneuploid DNA distribution. DNA analysis of mucosal biopsy specimens may be of value in predicting extensive disease and tailoring preoperative and operative therapy. Similarly, endoscopic ultrasonography is proving to be useful for effective preoperative assessment of tumor extent. Although surgery remains the therapeutic standard for treating SEC, endoscopic ablative or resection procedures have proven to be successful in carefully selected patients who are poor surgical candidates and have no nodal or distant metastases (Gossner et al., 1999; Lightdale, 1999a).

PRECURSOR LESIONS OF ESOPHAGEAL SQUAMOUS CELL CARCINOMA

Despite the improved outlook for early esophageal cancer compared with advanced disease, there has been a search for premalignant lesions significantly associated with SEC, particularly in high-risk populations, in order to treat the pathologic changes before invasion occurs. Putative lesions were first identified in retrospective studies of esophageal resection specimens, and the concepts formulated are being tested in prospective, often controlled, studies. Although a final consensus has not been reached, the delineation of certain lesions as precancerous has been achieved.

Chronic Esophagitis

Chronic esophagitis was originally proposed as a precursor because of its high prevalence in populations at high risk for esophageal cancer. Esophagitis in high-risk areas typically has an onset in childhood, is usually asymptomatic, and may be related to the ingestion of hot and/or coarse foods or to nutritional deficiencies (Guanrei and Songlian, 1987; Jacob et al., 1990; Lewin and Appelman, 1996; Oettlé et al., 1986). Its histologic features, however, are similar to those of active esophagitis in gastroesophageal reflux: basal zone hyperplasia and papillary lengthening with the variable presence of balloon cells, intraepithelial inflammation (neutrophils, eosinophils, and lymphocytes), and, in severe cases, erosion and ulceration (Oettlé et al., 1986; Qui and Yang, 1988; Fig. 6–2). In prospective studies, esophagitis has been identified in biopsies from the major-

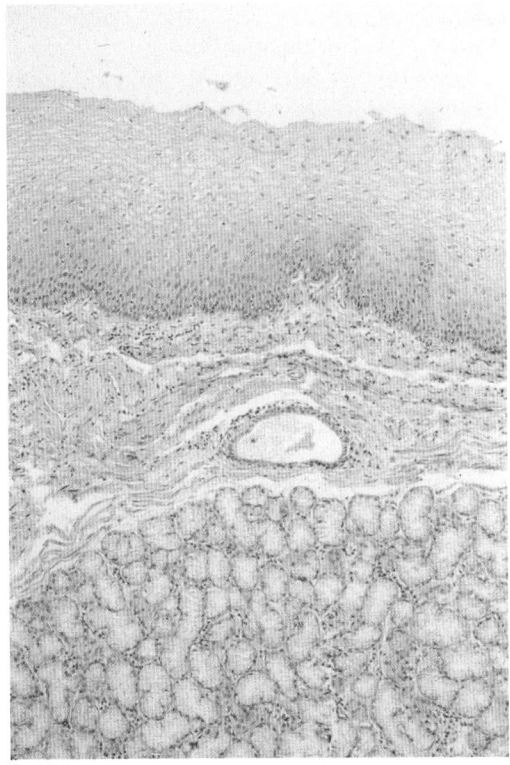

A

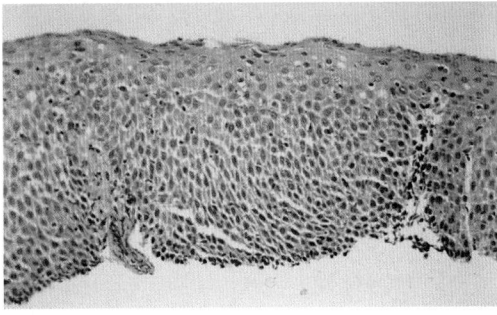

B

Figure 6–2. *A:* Normal esophageal squamous epithelium. The basal zone of small, dark cells is thin; above it, the squamous cells mature by acquiring cytoplasmic glycogen and undergoing nuclear pyknosis. An esophageal mucous gland and its draining duct are visible beneath the epithelium. *B:* Esophagitis. Immature basal-type cells occupy the full thickness of the mucosa; stromal papillae are elongated. Eosinophils and lymphocytes are within the epithelium.

ity (over 70%) of subjects from both high- and low-risk regions of China, although severe changes are more common in high-risk populations. Because of its high prevalence, esophagitis *per se* does not qualify as a pre-

malignant lesion (Guanrei and Songlian, 1987).

Epithelial Dysplasia and Carcinoma *In Situ*

High-grade squamous intraepithelial neoplasia (severe dysplasia and carcinoma *in situ*) appears to be closely related to the development of SEC and advanced carcinoma. This association was first noted in retrospective examination of resected specimens, in which severe dysplasia or carcinoma *in situ* (CIS) was found adjacent to invasive carcinoma in 30% to 100% of cases (Barge et al., 1981; Benasco et al., 1985; Kuwano et al., 1987; Mandard et al., 1984; Ohta et al., 1986; Riddell, 1996; Rubio et al., 1989; Schmidt et al., 1986). Although some workers have thought that CIS represents a secondary intraepithelial spread of invasive carcinoma (Soga et al., 1982), the evidence from experimental and clinical prospective studies supports the concept of dysplasia–CIS as a precursor lesion (see below). Dysplasia and CIS may be multifocal and separate from the invasive tumor; these premalignant processes may encompass a large surface area. They are less often identified in cases of advanced cancer than in those of SEC, presumably because bulky tumor has obliterated the *in situ* precursor, and in patients receiving preoperative radiation therapy (severe dysplasia and CIS noted in approximately 20% of cases, versus more than 60% of those without preoperative treatment), probably because of destruction by the radiation (Benasco et al., 1985; Kuwano et al., 1987; Mandard et al., 1984; Morita et al., 1994; Ohta et al., 1986; Riddell, 1996; Soga et al., 1982).

Pathologic features. At endoscopy, dysplastic lesions (especially moderate and severe grades) as well as early invasive lesions may be recognized as red, friable mucosa or as plaques, nodules, or erosions (Dawsey et al., 1993). The use of toluidine blue or iodine (Lugol's) solution sprayed onto the mucosal surface may aid the endoscopist in defining areas of dysplasia. Since toluidine blue is a vital dye, dysplastic areas stain more intensely blue than the surrounding mucosa because of the greater number of nuclei per unit of area. Conversely, dysplasia stains less intensely or not at all with iodine compared with normal mucosa because of its decreased or absent cytoplasmic component of glycogen (Nakanishi et al., 1998). Although sensitive, these staining techniques are not specific because inflammed and regenerating nondysplastic squamous cells have large nuclei and diminished glycogen (Jacob et al., 1990; Shiozaki et al., 1990).

The cytologic and histologic criteria for dysplasia and CIS are similar to those in the cervix. Increasing degrees of dysplasia, which may be classified as mild, moderate, and severe, are characterized by progressively worsening nuclear abnormalities (increased size, hyperchromasia, chromatin aberrations) and cytoplasmic dedifferentiation. In CIS, nuclei are typically large and hyperchromatic; the cell has inconspicuous cytoplasm and the nuclear-cytoplasmic ratio is high. Abnormal cells are confined to the lowest one-third of the mucosa in mild dysplasia, extend into the middle third in moderate dysplasia, and reach the upper third, but with some surface maturation, in severe dysplasia. Carcinoma *in situ* is characterized by dysplastic cells occupying the full thickness of the epithelium (Fig. 6–3). The dysplastic cells may extend into the ducts and acini of the submucosal glands, but the basement membrane remains intact (Barge et al., 1981; Jacob et al., 1990; Kuwano et al., 1987; Lewin and Appelman, 1996; Rubio et al., 1989; Shu, 1983). Mitoses, rare in mild dysplasia, are frequent at the severe end of the spectrum (Rubio et al., 1989). On occasion, severe dysplasias may exhibit a page-

toid-like spread within the epithelium (Lewin and Appelman, 1996).

Interobserver agreement is suboptimal in distinguishing the four grades of abnormality just described. As a result, alternative classifications have been suggested. One proposal is to include all grades under the heading of *esophageal intraepithelial neoplasia* (analogous to the system used in the lower female genital tract), with subdivisions into low and high grades. Another approach is to use a two-grade system like that for inflammatory bowel disease–associated dysplasia: low-grade (mild to moderate dysplasia) and high-grade (severe dysplasia and CIS) (Lewin and Appelman, 1996; Odze and Antonioli, 1995; Rubio et al., 1989). Whereas low-grade lesions, as a group, are of uncertain significance, high-grade lesions are consistently aneuploid and have a high association with malignancy (Rubio et al., 1989).

Differential diagnosis. It may be difficult to separate cytologic and histologic changes secondary to inflammation and repair from true dysplasia; thus, interobserver variation may be great in the diagnosis of mild and moderate (low-grade) dysplasia (for example, one group's moderate dysplasia may be considered reactive atypia by other workers) (Jacob et al., 1990; Mandard et al., 1984). In injury and repair, cells with enlarged nuclei may extend halfway or more through the epithelial thickness and mitotic activity may

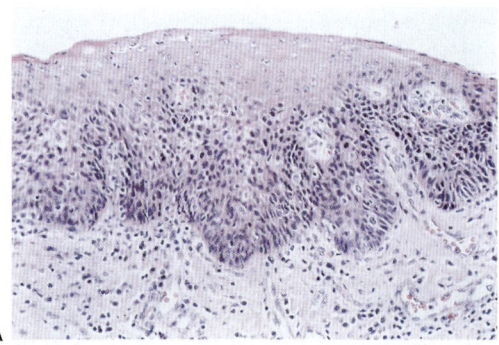 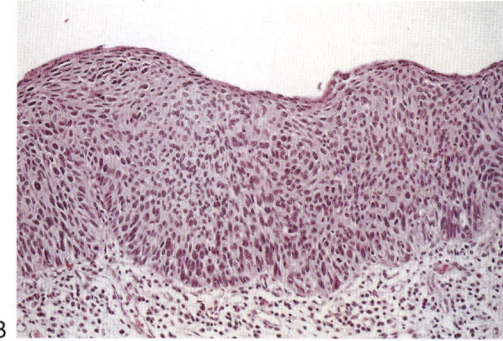

Figure 6–3. *A:* Low-grade (mild) squamous cell dysplasia. The abnormal cells are confined to the lowest third of the epithelium, with maturation above that point. *B:* High-grade (severe dysplasia/carcinoma *in situ*) dysplasia. Undifferentiated basaloid cells occupy the entire thickness of the epithelium. The basement membrane is intact. [Fig. 6-3B courtesy of Jorge Albores-Saavedra, M.D., University of Texas-Southwestern Medical Center, Dallas, TX.]

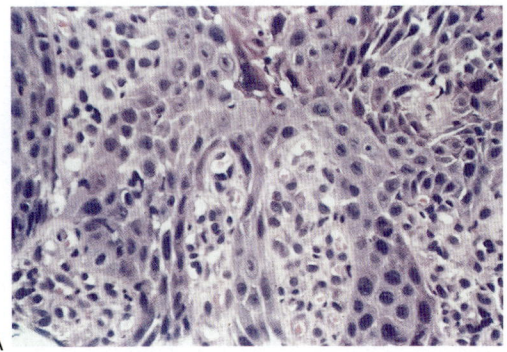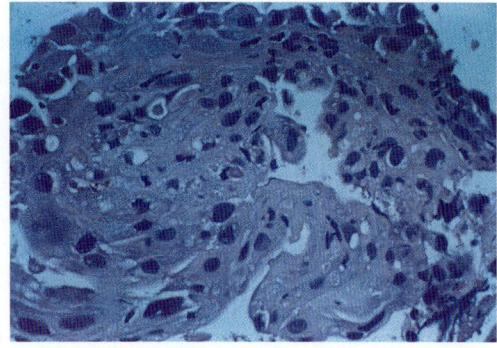

A   B

Figure 6–4. *A:* Reactive atypia in squamous epithelium at the edge of an esophageal ulcer. The immature squamous cells form anastomosing strands in the lamina propria. The interface of epithelium and stroma is smooth. Although enlarged, the epithelial cell nuclei are bland. [Courtesy of Henry D. Appelman, M.D., University of Michigan Medical Center, Ann Arbor, MI]. *B:* Squamous epithelium showing the effects of chemoradiation therapy. Nuclei are pleomorphic, but the nuclear-cytoplasmic ratios are not disturbed. Knowledge of the clinical history will prevent overinterpretation of these changes. [Courtesy of Robert D. Odze, M.D., Brigham and Women's Hospital, Boston, MA.]

be increased. However, the chromatin aberrations typical of dysplasia cannot be clearly identified, and the mitoses have a normal configuration. If marked inflammation is present, the changes should be interpreted with caution (Fig. 6–4A). Equivocal biopsy specimens may be classified as indefinite for dysplasia, with the recommendation for repeat examination after treatment of any associated inflammation.

In a DNA spectrophotometric analysis of esophageal epithelium, Rubio and co-workers (1988) identified two types of dysplasia: one type that had a diploid DNA distribution (which included all of their cases of histologically mild and a few with moderate dysplasia) and a second type with aneuploid DNA distribution (including the remaining cases of moderate and all with severe dysplasia). They suggest that DNA analysis may clarify the nature of histologically mild and moderate forms of dysplasia, many of which may actually be reactive phenomena. The banal nature of many examples of low-grade dysplasia is supported by their lack of aggressive behavior in prospective studies (see later discussion).

Other sources of diagnostic confusion include the effects of radiation and chemotherapy on squamous epithelium (Fig. 6–4B). The spectrum of changes, which can resemble dysplasia, includes multinucleation, nuclear hyperchromasia and pleomorphism, immature regenerative epithelium, and epithelial atrophy with a predominance of basaloid cells (Lewin and Appelman, 1996; Mandard et al., 1984). Appropriate clinical information is required in order not to misinterpret the abnormal epithelium.

In an attempt to clarify the nature of indeterminate lesions (e.g., reactive change versus low-grade dysplasia), DNA content has been evaluted in mucosal biopsy specimens. As noted earlier and confirmed by additional studies, most high-grade dysplasias are aneuploid whereas low-grade dysplasias are typically diploid (Doki et al., 1993; Rubio et al., 1988). Nuclear accumulation of p53 protein (detected by immunohistochemistry or mutational analysis) increases with increasing degrees of dysplasia, but has a low prevalence in low-grade lesions (Bennett et al., 1992; Wang et al., 1993). Thus, these techniques have not proven useful in separating benign reactive change from low-grade dysplasia in cases in which histologic evaluation is inconclusive. Their value in predicting the behavior of dysplastic lesions needs to be determined in prospective studies.

Prevalence and natural history. In geographic areas in which there is a high incidence of esophageal cancer, such as parts of China, dysplasia is common, with an overall prevalence on initial screening varying from 13% to 20% and a significantly higher rate (38%) in high-risk versus low-risk (4%) population subsets. During prospective follow-up in one large study, carcinoma developed in 34% of patients with chronic esophagitis and dysplasia, in contrast to only 4% of patients with chronic esophagitis without dysplasia, thus highlighting the significance of dysplasia as a precursor (Guanrei and Songliang, 1987; Jacob et al., 1990; Qui and Yang, 1988). In prospective cytologic screening studies, the risk of malignancy is, to some extent, related to the degree of dysplasia at entry. Among patients with mild dysplasia initially, only 15% progressed to severe dysplasia after follow-up of 8 years, the mild dysplasia remaining stable or regressing in the remainder. Among patients with severe dysplasia, progression to carcinoma occurred in 30%. About 40% of patients with severe dysplasia showed regression of the cytologic abnormalities over time, a result that emphasizes the variable behavior of and difficulty in categorizing dysplastic lesions (Jacob et al., 1990; Mingxin et al., 1980). Overall, however, severe dysplasia, if followed for 10 years in a high-risk population, is associated with a 2.9× increased risk of esophageal carcinoma compared with controls (Lu et al., 1988).

These findings are corroborated by the results of recent cytologic and histologic studies of patients in the high-risk area of Linxian, China. Compared to patients with no abnormalities on cytologic and histologic screening at entry, those with dysplasia demonstrated a risk of developing malignancy proportional to the degree of severity of dysplasia (Dawsey et al., 1994a,b). Preliminary studies of screening an asymptomatic population of smokers and ethanol abusers in the United States suggest that the yield of significant dysplasia and the rate of progression to cancer are low. Thus, surveillance is probably not cost-effective in low-risk countries (Jacob et al., 1990).

In summary, in high-risk populations, the following pathway for the development of esophageal cancer is proposed (Lewin and Appelman, 1996; Riddell, 1996):

Chronic esophagitis
("Background" condition)
| Carcinogens
| HPV infection (in high-risk populations)
| Nutritional deficiencies
▼ Host factors (genetic, molecular, immune)

Dysplasia/CIS
| Continued effects of host and
▼ environmental factors
Invasive carcinoma

DIAGNOSIS AND MANAGEMENT

As discussed earlier, endoscopy with mucosal staining using toluidine blue or iodine solutions is an effective (but costly) method to detect dysplasia and SEC. However, evaluating cytosmears of esophageal epithelium (obtained by balloon abrasion, sponge, or brush techniques) is a cost-effective screening and surveillance method capable of detecting more than 90% of biopsy-proven malignancies in symptomatic patients, with a false-positive rate of less than 1% in experienced hands (Nabeya, 1983; Shu, 1983). The sensitivity has been less in prospective evaluations of asymptomatic patients, but it is at a level that is still acceptable for screening purposes (Dawsey et al., 1994a; Roth et al., 1997).

Any neoplasm suggested by cytology must be confirmed by endoscopy and biopsy. Multiple biopsy specimens increase the diagnostic yield. In the study by Benasco and colleagues (1985), an average of six biopsy specimens per case was obtained, which yielded a positive result in 77% of the patients ultimately shown to have SEC. A second endoscopic procedure with additional biopsies gave the diagnosis of cancer in the remaining patients.

In terms of managing dysplasia, patients with lesions indefinite for dysplasia should be reevaluated after medical therapy of any confounding inflammation. Patients with high-grade dysplasia should be completely evaluated (endoscopic ultrasonography; imaging studies) to rule out invasive carcinoma. If the latter is ruled out, the high-grade dysplasia must be managed according to the wishes and medical condition of the individual patient. Options include surgical resection and endoscopic ablative techniques (Gossner et al., 1999). Low-grade dysplasia is more problematic since the rate of and time for progression to high-grade dysplasia are as yet unclear. However, continued surveillance is indicated (Odze and Antonioli, 1995; Riddell, 1996).

Table 6–3. Origins of Esophageal
Glandular Neoplasia

Barrett's esophagus (columnar-lined esophagus)

Heterotopic gastric mucosa

Esophageal submucosal mucous glands

Upward extension of primary gastric carcinomas

Metastases from other sites (e.g., lung, breast)

GLANDULAR NEOPLASIA

Glandular dysplasia and carcinoma of the
esophagus can arise from several sites, as
summarized in Table 6–3. Carcinomas arising from submucosal glands are exceedingly
rare, and dysplasia and early (curable) carcinomas in this group are poorly defined
(Odze and Antonioli, 1995). Although extension of proximal gastric carcinoma into
the distal esophagus had previously been
considered the most common source of
glandular neoplasia involving the esophagus, Barrett's esophagus is now recognized
as the origin of most esophageal glandular
dysplasias and adenocarcinomas.

Heterotopic Gastric Mucosa

Located in the upper third of the esophagus
in the cricopharyngeal area, heterotopic gastric mucosa ("inlet patch") consists predominantly of cardiofundic-type gastric
mucosa. The lesions are congenital, arising
secondary to incomplete replacement of the
original esophageal columnar epithelium by
the proximal growth of squamous cells from
the mid-esophagus during fetal development. Commonly identified if the upper
esophagus is serially sectioned at autopsy,
heterotopic gastric mucosa has a clinical
prevalence of 4% at endoscopy in adults
(Christensen and Sternberg, 1987; Jabbari et
al., 1985).

Grossly, the lesions, which are usually single, are variable in size, red and velvety in
appearance, and sharply demarcated from
surrounding squamous epithelium. These islands are lined by surface-foveolar–type gastric mucous cells, whereas the glands in the
lamina propria contain oxyntic, pepsinogen,
endocrine, and mucous cells in variable proportions. Mononuclear inflammatory cells

may be present in the lamina propria, and
foci of intestinal metaplasia are occasionally
seen. Ectopic pancreatic acinar tissue has recently been described within the inlet patch
(Maldonado et al., 1998). The lesions can be
distinguished from Barrett's esophagus by
the presence of squamous epithelium in tissue samples taken distal to the heterotopia
and by the greater prominence of fundic-
type glands (Christensen and Sternberg,
1987; Truong et al., 1986; Van Asche et al.,
1988).

Heterotopic gastric mucosa is usually an
incidental finding at endoscopy, but occasional patients are symptomatic (ulceration,
bleeding, stricture formation), related to
acid-pepsin production within the heterotopia and injury to adjacent tissue (Galen et
al., 1998; Steadman et al., 1988; Truong et
al., 1986; Van Asche et al., 1988). Malignant
transformation is a rare complication, with
13 cases of adenocarcinoma documented in
a recent review (Lauwers et al., 1998). The
cancers, which may be associated with dysplasia in the heterotopia, are variably differentiated and are usually advanced at the
time of clinical detection (Lauwers et al.,
1998). However, recent reports have documented an adenoma and an early adenocarcinoma (carcinoma confined to mucosa
and superficial submucosa) developing in
this type of heterotopia (Mion et al., 1996;
Takagi et al., 1995). Given the rarity of malignant change in this common lesion, no
surveillance of patients with heterotopic gastric mucosa is indicated.

Upward Extension of Gastric Carcinoma

Upward extension of primary carcinomas of
the cardia or fundus is a common reason for
detecting glandular neoplasms in the distal
esophagus. The separation of these cancers
from primary adenocarcinomas arising in
Barrett's esophagus can be difficult, but features favoring an esophageal primary include more than 50% of the tumor located
within the esophagus; presence of Barrett's
epithelium, particularly if dysplastic; and
lack of dysplasia in adjacent gastric epithelium (Haggitt and Dean, 1985; Hamilton et
al., 1988; Smith et al., 1984; Wang et al.,
1986).

BARRETT'S ESOPHAGUS
(COLUMNAR-LINED ESOPHAGUS)

Barrett's esophagus (BE) is an acquired condition in which the esophagus above the lower esophageal sphincter becomes lined for a variable extent by columnar glandular epithelium that resembles gastric and intestinal phenotypes (Spechler and Goyal, 1986). Although it may develop as a consequence of many conditions (such as achalasia and scleroderma) characterized by dysmotility and abnormally increased contact time of luminal contents with the esophageal epithelium, BE most commonly develops as a complication of gastroesophageal reflux disease (GERD) (Smith et al., 1984). In GERD, chronic injury may lead to denudation of the esophageal squamous lining, with repair by glandular metaplastic epithelium in some patients. The precise cell of origin of BE is unknown; however, based on the results of recent ultrastructural and immunohistochemical studies, it most likely is a multipotential stem cell, arising from the basal layer of adjacent squamous epithelium or from cells lining the ducts of esophageal mucous glands, that is capable of expressing several differentiation pathways (Berenson et al., 1993; Boch et al., 1997; Feurle et al., 1990; Levine et al., 1989; Sawhney et al., 1996; Shields et al., 1995).

Definition

The definition of BE in terms of the length of involvement of the esophagus and the histologic features necessary for a definitive diagnosis has undergone significant revision over the past 5 years and is not yet completely clarified. Barrett's esophagus was initially (and arbitrarily) defined as 3 cm or more of columnar mucosa in the distal esophagus. However, the results of recent investigations suggest that any length of esophageal columnar mucosa may represent this entity. Thus, any patient in whom the squamocolumnar junction is above the gastroesophageal junction may have BE, regardless of the distance between these two landmarks. In current practice, BE is divided clinically into long-segment (3 cm or more) and short-segment (less than 3 cm) columnar-lined distal esophagus (Sharma et al., 1998b).

Although a variety of glandular phenotypes may be identified in histologic sections of BE, consensus has emerged that the most diagnostic finding is the presence of goblet mucous cells, classified as "specialized" or "intestinalized" glandular mucosa. By combining these length and histologic criteria, the current clinical working definition of BE is "a change in the esophageal epithelium of any length that can be recognized grossly at endoscopy and is confirmed to have intestinal metaplasia [goblet cells] by biopsy" (Sampliner, 1998).

The pathologist may face several problems when attempting to diagnose BE according to the clinical definition summarized above. Since goblet cells may be few in number or focally distributed, they may not be evident in a single sample; multiple biopsy specimens may be necessary for their identification. An additional factor complicating the histologic diagnosis of BE is that in children, goblet cells may be absent or sparse even in patients with long segments of columnar-lined esophagus. In this population, goblet cells increase in frequency between ages 5 and 29 years when cohorts of patients stratified by age are evaluated (Qualman et al., 1990). Finally, histologic features identical to those of BE may be identified in biopsy specimens of the gastric cardia in patients whose squamocolumnar junction coincides with the gastroesophageal junction (Spechler et al., 1994). If information about the precise site of the biopsy is not available, such specimens are best signed out with a note stating that the findings represent either short-segment BE or intestinal metaplasia of the cardia, depending on the location from which the specimen was obtained. Although even short segments of BE have been associated with the development of dysplasia and adenocarcinoma (Hamilton et al., 1988; Schnell et al., 1992; Sharma et al., 1997), the neoplastic implications of intestinal metaplasia of the cardia are still unclear (Chalasani et al., 1997; Morales et al., 1997; Spechler et al., 1994).

The reader is referred to several recent reviews for a more complete discussion of the controversies concerning the diagnosis of BE (Sampliner, 1998; Sharma et al., 1998b; Spechler and Goyal, 1996).

Prevalence

The clinical prevalence of BE is difficult to determine because of the varied nature of published series (retrospective versus prospective), patient selection, and diagnostic techniques (e.g., radiology versus endoscopy). From data listed in review articles, the prevalence of long-segment BE has varied from 2% to approximately 20% in patients with GERD (Mann et al., 1989; Spechler and Goyal, 1986; Thompson et al., 1983; Winters et al., 1987). Limited prospective data suggest a prevalence of 12% for long-segment BE in patients with persistent reflux (Winters et al., 1987) and 44% in patients with GERD complicated by peptic stricture formation (Spechler et al., 1983). The prevalence of short-segment BE is as yet unclear because of a lack of methodological uniformity among published studies. Prevalence rates have varied from 14% to 36% among patients having upper gastrointestinal endoscopy, with the highest rate being in the study by Nandurkar and colleagues (1997), in which alcian blue staining of biopsy specimens was routinely performed to highlight the presence of goblet cells (Loughney et al., 1998; Nandurkar et al., 1997; Spechler et al., 1994). Given the frequency of GERD (estimated at 10% in the U.S. population), the absolute number of patients with BE is large. However, clinical studies may underestimate the number of people with BE, as evidenced by the results of a recent prospective autopsy study, in which the prevalence of long-segment BE was estimated to be 376 cases per 100,000 population, a rate 15 times greater than clinically detected BE in the same geographic region (Cameron et al., 1990).

Barrett's esophagus typically is first diagnosed in middle age and is more common in White males than in Blacks or females (Caygill et al., 1999). The condition is well documented in children, with a prevalence of 10% in adolescents with histologically proven GERD (Qualman et al., 1990; Spechler and Goyal, 1986). Once established, BE has traditionally been considered an irreversible change in the vast majority of patients (Sampliner et al., 1990; Smith et al., 1984; Thompson et al., 1983).

Pathologic Features

At endoscopy or in resected specimens, BE can be recognized as pink or red, velvety mucosa involving varying lengths of the distal tubular esophagus in either a circumferen-tial or focal tongue-like distribution. The interface with the residual squamous epithelium is usually irregular. On occasion, particularly in children, BE may be difficult to recognize; thus, biopsies are always necessary to confirm the diagnosis.

Microscopically, BE is characterized by a heterogeneous array of cell and gland types recapitulating gastric and intestinal elements. Three types of mucosa may be present: junctional type (resembling normal gastric cardia); atrophic fundic type (resembling gastric corpus and fundus but with a less well-developed glandular architecture than that found in normal stomach); and specialized, or intestinalized, columnar mucosa, which is a mixture of gastric and intestinal types and is currently considered the histologic hallmark of BE (see earlier section on the definition of BE) (Lee, 1984; Sampliner, 1998; Spechler and Goyal, 1996).

Intestinalized columnar epithelium is characterized by a flat or occasionally villiform surface lined by goblet cells and cells with straight lateral borders, whereas the glandular (crypt) portion contains mucous cells and may also contain goblet, Paneth, and endocrine cells (Haggitt, 1994; Thompson et al., 1983; Fig. 6–5). As determined by histochemical, immunohistochemical, and ultrastructural studies, the surface cells with straight lateral borders are hybrids, containing features of both gastric mucous and intestinal absorptive cells, and have been termed "intermediate cells" (Berenson et al.,

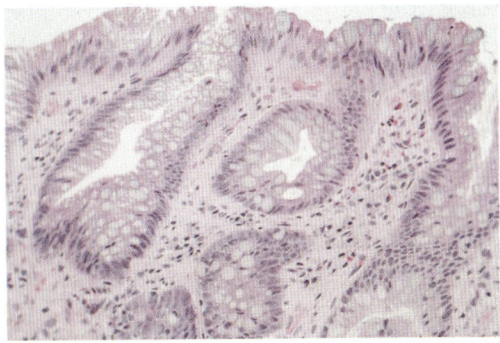

Figure 6–5. Intestinalized columnar-lined esophagus (Barrett's esophagus). The goblet cells have a distended lateral border, blue apical cytoplasm in this hematoxylin and eosin stain, and compressed basal nuclei.

Table 6–4. Barrett's Esophagus: Characteristics of Intermediate Cells in Intestinalized Columnar Epithelium

Apical secretory glycoprotein granules

Production of neutral (gastric-type) and acid (intestinal-type) glycoproteins

Variable apical microvilli, but poorly formed or absent terminal web

Some brush border enzymes

Inability to absorb micellar lipids

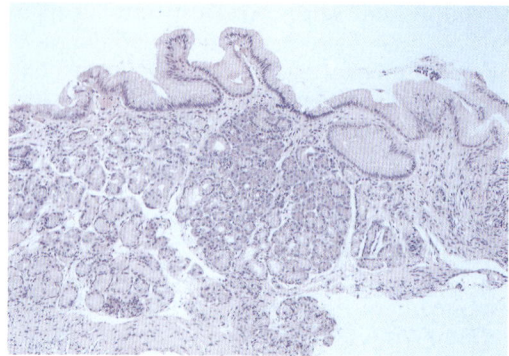

Figure 6–6. Nodule of pancreatic acinar tissue (center of photograph) at the gastroesophageal junction in a patient with Barrett's esophagus. Immunohistochemical stain for lipase was positive in these cells.

1974; Chaves et al., 1999; Levine et al., 1989; Trier, 1970; Zwas et al., 1986; Table 6–4). They may contain neutral or acidic mucins. The various types of mucosae (intestinalized, junctional, and fundic) are typically inter-digitated along the length of the BE segment (Rothery et al., 1986; Thompson et al., 1983).

Intermediate-type cells that stain positively for acidic mucins with alcian blue at pH 2.5 are commonly identified in BE resection specimens (Offner et al., 1996). However, similar cells have been identified in gastric cardia surface-foveolar cells and in the gland neck area in patients without BE and with no symptoms or signs of GERD (Genta et al., 1994; Gottfried et al., 1989). Thus, at the present time, these cells are not considered diagnostic of BE (Haggitt, 1994).

Nodules of ectopic pancreatic acinar tissue have recently been described in BE as well as in the cardia and gastroesophageal junctional area in patients without BE (Doglioni et al., 1993; Krishnamurthy and Dayal, 1995; Fig. 6–6). Rather than representing part of the metaplastic process in BE, this tissue is most likely congenital in origin and, therefore, should not be considered a marker of BE (Wang et al., 1996).

ADENOCARCINOMA IN BARRETT'S ESOPHAGUS

Prevalence and Incidence
The most serious complication of BE is the development of adenocarcinoma (Sanfey et al., 1985). However, the risk of developing this complication is difficult to determine since until recently, most studies have been retrospective, have exhibited a selection bias favoring malignancy, and lacked a denomi-

nator (i.e., the total number of patients with BE in the population containing the patients with carcinoma). In reviewing reports published from 1973 to 1983, Haggitt and Dean (1985) found that the percentage of BE patients who developed cancer varied from 0% to 46.5%. They believe the best available estimate of cancer prevalence is 8% to 10%. However, the risk is much lower if data from retrospective incidence studies are analyzed. In this type of analysis, the rate of cancer developing in cases of BE has varied from 1 case per 175 to 1 case per 441 person-years of follow-up (Cameron et al., 1985; Dent et al., 1991; O'Connor et al., 1999; Spechler et al., 1984). Nevertheless, this rate is still 30 to 40 times greater than the risk of developing esophageal carcinoma in the general population (Spechler and Goyal, 1986).

It should also be noted that the follow-up in these studies is still short; the cumulative risk of developing cancer at 15 or 20 years is unknown. For example, in the report of Spechler and colleagues (1984), the two reported cancers developed after 5.3 and 8 years of follow-up, giving a rate of malignancy of 9% for the 23 patients followed for longer than 5 years. In recent series with prospective endoscopic surveillance, the incidence of carcinoma has varied from 1 case per 55 to 1 case per approximately 200 patient-years of follow-up (Drewitz at al., 1997; Hameeteman et al., 1989; Katz et al., 1998; Ovaska et al., 1989; Robertson et al., 1988; Streitz et al., 1998).

Supporting the importance of BE as a premalignant condition in the United States and Canada is the recent documentation that BE-associated carcinoma comprises an increasingly large proportion of primary esophageal cancer. Traditionally, adenocarcinomas involving the esophagus had been considered rare, and most were thought to be upward extensions of proximal gastric carcinomas. As a result, primary adenocarcinomas constituted less than 8% of all esophageal cancers in most series that analyzed material from the 1970s (Haggitt and Dean, 1985; Hesketh et al., 1989; Mandard et al., 1984; Sons and Borchard, 1984). However, in recent studies using improved methodology and eliminating secondary esophageal involvement by gastric cancer, adenocarcinomas (virtually all associated with BE) now account for 17% to 34% of all primary esophageal malignancies, and 60% to 80% of cancers confined to the lower third of the esophagus (Cameron et al., 1985; Devesa et al., 1998; Hesketh et al., 1989; Levine et al., 1984; Wang et al., 1986).

Demographic Features

As noted above, BE-associated adenocarcinoma has shown a striking increase in incidence in the United States over the past two decades (Devesa et al., 1998). The results of all investigations confirm a marked male predominance (3:1 to 7:1) with a predilection (over 80% of cases) for Whites, the latter finding in sharp contrast to esophageal squamous cell carcinomas, which in the United States occur predominantly in Black men. The mean age of occurrence is in the sixth decade, with dysphagia, pain, and weight loss as the major presenting symptoms (Caygill et al., 1999; Hamilton et al., 1988; Kalish et al., 1984; MacDonald and MacDonald, 1987; Rogers et al., 1986; Sjogren and Johnson, 1983; Thompson et al., 1983; Wang et al., 1986). In general, cancer risk is related to the duration of BE, with smoking and obesity being additional risk factors; however, the risk of malignancy is not necessarily related to the length of BE, with many carcinomas developing in short-segment BE (Devesa et al., 1998; Hamilton et al., 1988; Smith et al., 1984; Weston et al., 1999).

Pathologic Features: Early Esophageal Adenocarcinoma

Until recently, most esophageal adenocarcinomas were detected at a clinically symptomatic, pathologically advanced stage; thus, the 5-year survival for this group has been less than 15% (Fennerty et al., 1989; Haggitt and Dean, 1985; Paraf et al., 1995). However, as a result of patients being enrolled in endoscopic surveillance protocols, a larger number of less advanced cancers are now being recognized and treated (van Sandick et al., 1998; Wright et al., 1996), giving rise to a group of "early" or "superficial" adenocarcinomas in BE that are analogous to the potentially curable superficial squamous cell carcinomas described earlier in the chapter.

Early or superficial adenocarcinoma in BE is defined as cancer confined to the mucosa or submucosa (pT1a and pT1b, respectively), regardless of the status of regional lymph nodes (DeBaecque et al., 1990; Nishimaki et al., 1991). Such cases account for up to 30% of resected BE-associated adenocarcinomas in recent Western series (Paraf et al., 1995). These early cancers vary in size; many are polypoid, but others are flat or depressed lesions that may be difficult to detect at endoscopy (Nishimaki et al., 1991). Therefore, addition of brush cytology, by sampling a large area, may aid in their detection (Antonioli and Wang, 1997). Like advanced cancers, they demonstrate variable degrees of histologic differentiation; however, a majority (60%–70%) are well differentiated and are accompanied by adjacent (or occasionally distant) areas of high-grade dysplasia (Nishimaki et al., 1991; Paraf et al., 1995).

Intramucosal adenocarcinomas contain little lymphatic-vascular invasion and no nodal metastases in most series; in contrast, the cancers with submucosal extension demonstrate vascular invasion in up to 40% of cases and regional nodal metastases in 8% to 18% of patients. These findings explain the differences in 5-year survival: 90% to 100% for intramucosal tumors and 75% to 80% for those with submucosal invasion (Hölscher et al., 1997; Nishimaki et al., 1991; Paraf et al., 1995). These survival figures, which are so much better than those for advanced cancer, are used to support the need for surveillance in BE patients.

Premalignant Lesions in Barrett's Esophagus

Because BE is a premalignant lesion of high prevalence in which carcinomas have often been detected at an advanced stage, there is clinical interest in surveillance of patients to detect dysplasia and the early, potentially curable, carcinomas that can be treated by surgery or, in some cases, by endoscopic ablative therapy. The cost-effectiveness of following all patients with BE is a subject of controversy; therefore, the goal is to define patient subsets at greatest risk for malignant transformation on whom to focus surveillance (Macdonald et al., 1997; Ridell, 1996; van Sandick et al., 1998; Wright et al., 1996).

In the retrospective histologic analysis of resected BE-associated adenocarcinomas, both the presence of intestinalized mucosa and sulfomucin production by the intermediate cells were highly associated with dysplasia and carcinoma (Hamilton et al., 1988; Jass, 1981; Peuchmauer et al., 1984). However, the results of subsequent endoscopic biopsy studies have found both of these findings to be so prevalent (90% for intestinalized epithelium; 40% to 75% for detection of sulfomucins) that they are neither sensitive nor specific for surveillance (Haggitt, 1994; Hamilton and Smith, 1987; Jauregui et al., 1988; Robertson et al., 1988; Rothery et al., 1986; Zwas et al., 1986). The loss of O-acetylated mucins, aberrant expression of sucrase-isomaltese genes, and abnormal expression of blood group antigens (all proposed as markers of heightened dysplasia/cancer risk in BE) need to be validated by prospective studies (Haggitt, 1994). Thus, at the present time, glandular epithelial dysplasia is the best defined premalignant lesion in BE.

Glandular Epithelial Dysplasia

Glandular epithelial dysplasia is defined histologically as unequivocal benign neoplastic change. In retrospective histologic studies of resection specimens, dysplasia has been found adjacent to adenocarcinomas in 50% to 100% of cases. In the majority, the dysplasia was high grade (Haggitt et al., 1978; Haggitt and Dean, 1985; Hamilton and Smith, 1987; Kalish et al., 1984; Lee, 1985; Smith et al., 1984; Spechler and Goyal, 1986; Thompson et al., 1983; Wang et al., 1986).

In biopsy specimens, however, dysplasia as an isolated finding is uncommon, but its presence mandates a careful search for a more serious lesion.

Pathologic features and classification. Dysplasia represents a combination of architectural and cytologic abnormalities that parallel one another in severity for each degree of dysplasia. However, one or the other parameter may predominant in a particular patient. Architectural changes include an exaggerated surface villiform configuration, whereas the glands may show papillary infoldings, irregular shapes, crowding, and cribriform patterns. Cytologic aberrations encompass nuclear enlargement, hyperchromasia, and pleomorphism; stratification of nuclei within the cells; excessively large or abnormal nucleoli; dedifferentiation (i.e., decreased or absent mucin production); and abnormal mitoses (Antonioli and Wang, 1997; Haggitt, 1994; Lewin and Appelman, 1996).

Dysplasia in BE is classified in a manner similar to that used for inflammatory bowel disease (Riddell et al., 1983; Table 6–5). In low-grade dysplasia (LGD), architectural changes are modest, the cells retain the capacity for mucin production, and nuclear stratification is confined to the lower half of the cell. High-grade dysplasia (HGD) (encompassing severe dysplasia as well as carcinoma *in situ*) is characterized by more profound architectural alterations, prominent nuclear abnormalities, markedly diminished or absent mucin production, and stratification of nuclei into the upper half of the cells. A cribriform gland pattern connotes conversion to *in situ* carcinoma (Fig. 6–7). Features that define extension of carcinoma *in situ* into the lamina propria (intramucosal invasive carcinoma) include angulation of glands, single glands or irregular clusters of cells in the lamina propria,

Table 6–5. Classification of Epithelial Dysplasia in Barrett's Esophagus

Negative

Indefinite for dysplasia

Positive
   Low-grade (mild/moderate dysplasia)
   High-grade (severe dysplasia and carcinoma *in situ*)

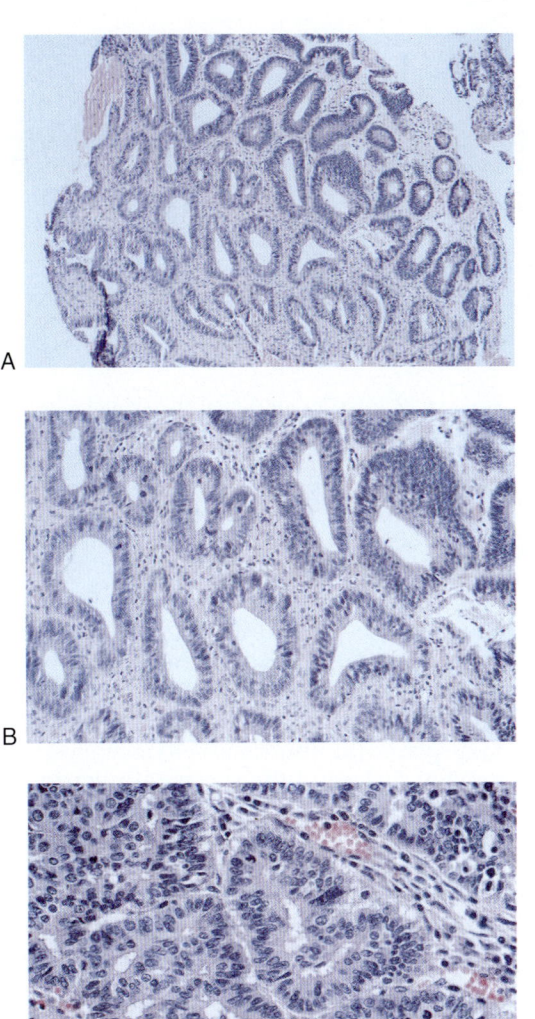

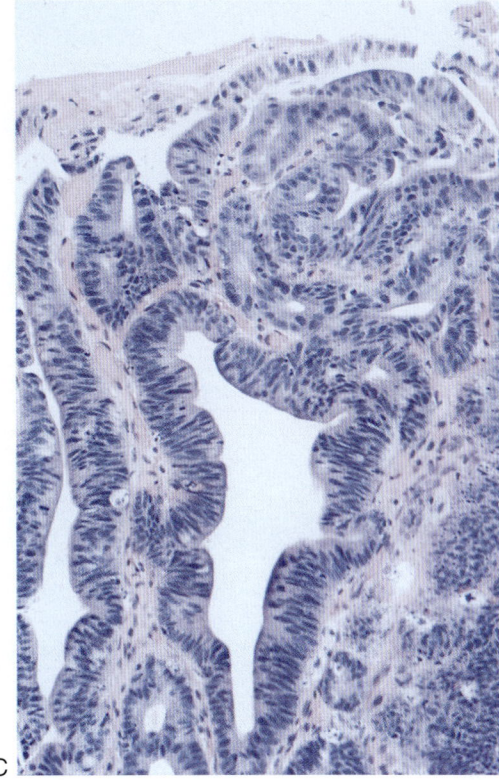

Figure 6–7. Dysplasia in Barrett's esophagus. *A:* Low-grade dysplasia. At low power, there is no architectural distortion and minimal inflammation. *B:* At high power, epithelial cell nuclei are enlarged, hyperchromatic, and focally overlapping. However, they are confined to the basal portion of the cell. *C:* High-grade dysplasia. Compared to low-grade change, the architecture is more complex, nuclei are larger and more hyperchromatic, and the nuclei extend throughout the cellular cytoplasm. *D:* High-grade dysplasia with cribriformed glands.

sheets of cells, and a desmoplastic stromal response (Fig. 6–8; Antonioli and Wang, 1997; Haggitt, 1994; Lewin and Appelman, 1996).

Dysplastic epithelial cells commonly resemble those seen in colonic adenomas, with slim, overlapping, diffusely hyperchromatic nuclei. However, occasional examples are characterized by rounder vesicular nuclei having large nucleoli and aggregated chromatin (Cameron and Carpenter, 1997; Fennerty et al., 1989; Hamilton and Smith, 1987; Lee, 1985; Reid et al., 1988a; Riddell, 1985; Spechler and Goyal, 1986). Dysplasia is most frequently identified in areas of intestinalized mucosa, but this finding is probably due

to the high prevalence of intestinalized mucosa in adults with BE.

Dysplasia in BE may assume a polypoid configuration recognized endoscopically and histologically as a sessile adenoma. These lesions vary in size (0.5 to over 2.0 cm in diameter), are rarely multiple, and typically contain HGD. They should be classified as "polypoid dysplasia," because dysplasia is also usually found in adjacent flat mucosa. Malignant transformation can occur in the polypoid mass (Hamilton and Smith, 1987; Lee, 1986; McDonald et al., 1977; Thompson et al., 1983; Thurberg et al., 1999; Wang et al., 1986).

Biopsy specimens negative for dysplasia

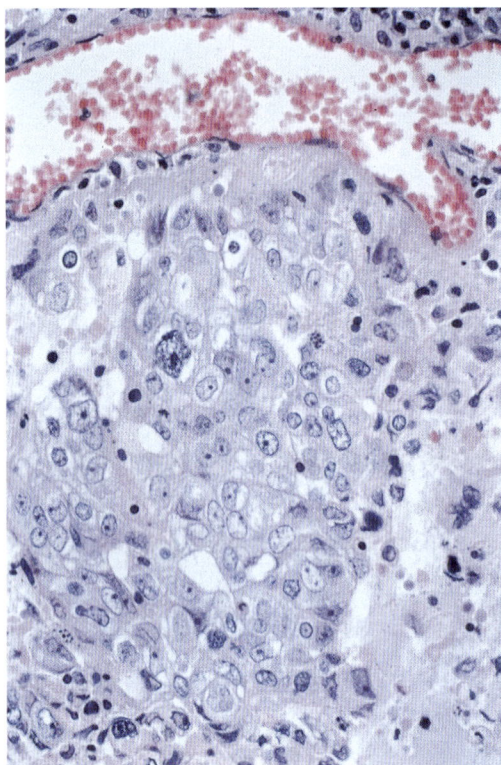

Figure 6–8. Intramucosal invasive adenocarcinoma. A confluent mass of anaplastic cells is present in the lamina propria.

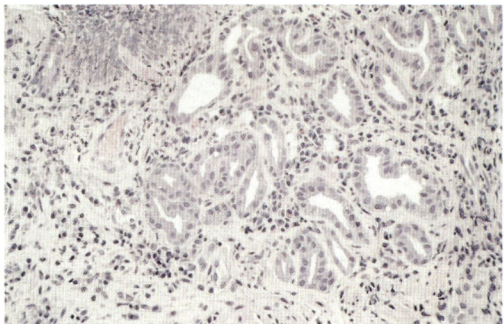

Figure 6–9. Reactive epithelial atypia in glands beneath an erosion in Barrett's esophagus. Although the cells are immature, the nuclei are fairly small and basal in location and do not overlap one another. Awareness of the inflammatory context of the changes should prevent overinterpretation of the findings as dysplasia.

are those that are completely unremarkable or demonstrate reactive cellular changes secondary to inflammation, erosion, ulceration, or regeneration. In reactive change, the architecture is not significantly altered. Epithelial cell nuclei are enlarged, but they are basal in location, do not vary in size, lack chromatin aberrations, and typically contain prominent central nucleoli (Fig. 6–9).

Specimens classified as indefinite for dysplasia should contain features beyond those usually seen in reactive phenomena but insufficient for the diagnosis of true dysplasia. Some degree of architectural distortion is usually present, as well as cellular dedifferentiation and nuclear enlargement and stratification. Mitoses may also be increased in number. However, the nuclear changes lack the degree of chromatin aberrations seen in true dysplasia, and the mitoses have a normal appearance (Fig. 6–10). The presence of active inflammation usually prevents precise categorization of the histologic findings (Reid et al., 1988a). In well-oriented sections, a feature helpful for distinguishing reactive change from dysplasia is the fact that in dysplasia, the abnormal cells extend to the luminal surface of the specimen whereas in reactive change, the abnormalities are confined to the glandular compartment, with evidence of maturation towards the surface.

Although the recognition of HGD is achieved with a high degree of interobserver agreement among experienced gastroin-

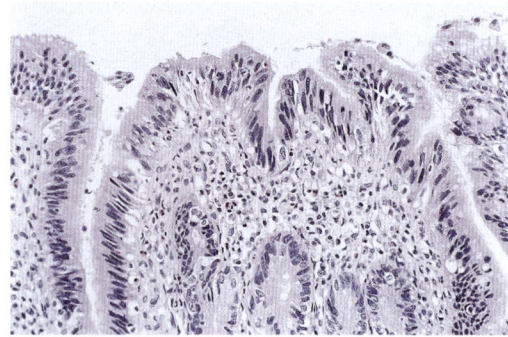

Figure 6–10. Changes indefinite for dysplasia in Barrett's esophagus. Immature cells with enlarged nuclei extend to the luminal surface of the mucosa. However, there is significant inflammation in the lamina propria and focally in the epithelium. Therefore, these findings could be reactive in nature. [Courtesy of Robert D. Odze, M.D., Brigham and Women's Hospital, Boston, MA.]

testinal pathologists, there is a lack of re-producibility for indefinite changes and LGD (Alikhan et al., 1999; Reid, et al., 1988a). This imprecision in defining lesser degrees of abnormality (which may, how-ever, warrant enhanced surveillance) has en-gendered a search for additional methods to distinguish benign reactive from committed neoplastic changes (discussed later).

Natural history. The natural history of dysplasia in BE is unclear because published studies on this topic are few, contain a small number of cases, and vary in design. How-ever, some impressions emerge from analy-sis of recent reports. High-grade dysplasia is closely associated with carcinoma. In pa-tients with HGD on initial screening biopsy who subsequently undergo esophageal re-section, adenocarcinoma has been detected in approximately 35% to 45% of patients (Al-torki et al., 1991; Burke et al., 1991; Hamil-ton and Smith, 1987; Heitmiller et al., 1996; Lee, 1985; Palley et al., 1989; Pera et al., 1992; Reid et al., 1988b; Schmidt et al., 1985). It should be noted that these were not surveillance studies and, therefore, reflect a biased patient population (i.e., dysplasia on first examination). Also, many of the pa-tients had a gross lesion (erosion, ulcer, ir-regular mucosa), although preoperative biopsies did not identify cancer. Residual HGD was found in the remaining patients. However, in some patients HGD may persist for years without clinical or histologic evi-dence of progression (Haggitt et al., 1988; Hameeteman et al., 1989; Lee, 1985; Levine, 1997). Low-grade dysplasia detected in grossly unremarkable BE is apparently not associated with concurrent carcinoma (Lee, 1985); however, if it is detected in associa-tion with a mass or ulcer, the risk of malig-nancy is increased (Ovaska et al., 1989).

In a limited number of prospective stud-ies with 1 to 10 years of follow-up, adeno-carcinoma has developed in up to 20%–25% of patients, often after 5 years of surveillance (Levine, 1997). Serial biopsies in these pa-tients typically document a sequence from LGD to HGD to carcinoma. The rate of tran-sition between these stages is variable, but the diagnosis of cancer is often made shortly (weeks to a few months) after recognition of HGD (Hameeteman et al., 1989; Levine, 1997).

Management. Endoscopic evaluation with multiple biopsies is indicated for patients with BE at first examination, because such speci-mens can detect dysplasia or early carcinoma developing in flat, innocuous-appearing mu-cosa. The addition of brush cytology, by sam-pling a broad mucosal surface area, has been useful in detecting dysplasia and malignancy (Geisinger et al., 1992; Koss et al., 1998; Robey et al., 1988; Wang et al., 1992, 1997), but has been less useful than histology in detecting goblet cells (Wang et al., 1997). Prospective evaluation of brush or balloon esophageal cy-tology is warranted, as it may offer a cost-effective method of surveillance.

The surveillance and management of pa-tients with BE are controversial (Haggitt, 1994; Palley et al., 1989; Riddell, 1996). Al-though some general guidelines are given below and in Table 6–6, the management of dysplasia must be tailored to the needs and medical condition of individual patients.

Patients with normal-appearing BE and biopsies negative for dysplasia can maintain routine follow-up, but changes that are sug-gestive of or positive for dysplasia require ad-ditional intervention. In patients with any gross abnormality (e.g., irregular mucosal surface; stricture; ulcer) at endoscopy, ex-tensive biopsy sampling is required, with fur-ther management based on the results of biopsies (Table 6–6). Given the ominous im-plication of HGD and the significant mor-bidity and possible mortality of esophagec-tomy, the diagnosis of dysplasia should be confirmed by a second pathologist with ex-perience from evaluating large numbers of dysplasia cases (Hameeteman et al., 1989; Palley et al., 1989; Riddell, 1985). As noted earlier, surgery in appropriately selected pa-tients has increased the yield of superficial, potentially curable adenocarcinomas (Falk et al., 1999; Paraf et al., 1995; van Sandick et al., 1998; Wright et al., 1996). In the fu-ture, endoscopic ablative therapy for HGD (and even early carcinoma) may offer suc-cessful conservative management for se-lected patients (van den Boogert, 1999).

Alternative methods for evaluating dys-plasia. At present, dysplasia is the only find-ing in BE that supports the need for enhanced surveillance or more aggressive in-tervention. However, the diagnosis of dys-plasia (particularly LGD) is difficult, and the

Table 6–6. Proposal for Evaluation of Patients with Barrett's Esophagus

Endoscopic Appearance of BE	Mucosal Biopsy Histology	Follow-up
Unremarkable	No dysplasia	Routine surveillance
Unremarkable	Abnormal	
	Indefinite for dysplasia	Treat inflammation; follow-up at shortened interval
	Dysplasia, low-grade[a]	Treat inflammation; follow-up at shortened interval
	Dysplasia, high-grade	Follow-up at reduced intervals; multiple biopsies; consider definitive therapy if high-grade dysplasia persists[b]
Abnormal	No dysplasia	Follow-up at reduced intervals; multiple biopsies
Abnormal	Abnormal	
	Indefinite for dysplasia	Treat inflammation; rapid repeat evaluation; multiple biopsies
	Dysplasia, low or high grade	Rapid repeat evaluation; consider definitive therapy[b]

[a]The diagnosis of dysplasia should be confirmed by a second pathologist who has examined many examples of dysplasia and/or by repeat biopsies.

[b]"Definitive therapy" has traditionally meant resection; however, in the modern era, it may encompass endoscopic ablative therapy in selected patients. (see text for details).

Table constructed from guidelines in Haggitt (1994), Palley et al. (1989), and Riddell (1996). Management must, however, be tailored for each individual patient with Barrett's esophagus.

significance of specimens graded as LGD or indefinite for dysplasia for patient management is unclear. Thus, there is interest in defining objective markers to complement dysplasia in identifying patients at high risk for neoplasia and to identify low-risk populations in whom the frequency of surveillance should be decreased (Garewal et al., 1990). The techniques discussed here, although potentially useful, must be considered investigational at the present time.

Neoplastic transformation in BE progresses through a metaplasia–dysplasia–adenocarcinoma pathway characterized over time by the accumulation of a heterogenous array of genetic abnormalities (Jankowski et al., 1999). Numerous aspects of these molecular biological events are being evaluated to determine their usefulness in predicting outcome for patients with problematic histological findings.

The DNA content of BE mucosal biopsy specimens as determined by flow cytometry has been investigated. In one recent prospective study (mean follow-up: 34 months), patients with no DNA abnormalities on initial evaluation showed no progression, whereas 70% of those with increased G2/tetraploidy or aneuploidy at entry progressed to high-grade dysplasia or adenocarcinoma (Reid et al., 1992). A limitation of this and other flow cytometric studies has been the need for evaluation of large-sized, fresh, and rapidly processed tissue, a set of conditions not amenable for use in routine clinical practice. More recently, flow cytometric DNA analysis of paraffin-embedded archival BE specimens has been performed, with promising initial results (Montgomery et al., 1996). Although there are theoretical and technical limitations to flow cytometry (Ahnen, 1987; Garewal et al., 1990; Giménez et al., 1998) and technical problems with the use of paraffin-embedded tissue (Montgomery et al., 1996), additional prospective studies are needed to determine its usefulness for surveillance in stratifying patients with indefinite–LGD in mucosal biopsies.

Among the many genetic abnormalities being investigated as markers for neoplastic progression in BE, p53 accumulation has been most extensively evaluated (Haggitt,

1994; Jankowski et al., 1999; Ortiz-Hidalgo et al., 1998). The results of initial studies have shown an increasing prevalence of nuclear p53 accumulation with the various steps of the BE metaplasia–dysplasia–adenocarcinoma sequence and suggest that p53 accumulation in LGD may be predictive of progression (Giménez et al., 1998; Giménez et al., 1999; Ramel et al., 1992; Younes et al., 1993). Like DNA analysis, p53 protein expression needs to be examined in large-scale prospective studies to determine its usefulness in triaging patients for surveillance.

Future Directions: Nonsurgical Ablation of Barrett's Esophagus

Given that BE is a highly prevalent premalignant condition and that surgery for its neoplastic complications carries significant morbidity and mortality rates, investigators have recently focused on nonsurgical interventions to remove this columnar mucosa. The rationale is to destroy the glandular mucosa by thermal injury (such as with the KTP laser or argon plasma coagulator) or by photodynamic therapy and simultaneously provide an acid-free environment by suppressing gastric acid production with proton pump inhibitors. The proposed esophageal multipotential stem cells discussed earlier in the chapter may then proliferate and, in the acid-free environment, recreate the native squamous epithelium (Berenson et al., 1993; Biddlestone et al., 1998; Bown, 1998).

In reports published in the last several years, the results suggest that, in fact, regression of BE can be achieved, and dysplasia and early carcinoma treated in patients with major comorbilities, by using ablative therapy (Biddlestone et al., 1998; Gossner et al., 1998; Haag et al., 1999; Overholt et al., 1999; van Laetham et al., 1998). However, the results must still be considered preliminary; several caveats remain. For example, regression of non-neoplastic BE has not been complete in many patients, even those with an endoscopic appearance of renewed squamous mucosa: residual glandular mucosa in the lamina propria, typically beneath a neosquamified surface, has been reported in approximately 25% to 40% of patients when mucosal biopsy specimens are examined (Biddlestone et al., 1998; Lightdale, 1999b; Sharma et al., 1998a; van Laetham et al., 1998), and this residual tissue may harbor or develop dysplasia. In addition, BE may reappear during follow-up despite strict maintainence of acid suppression (van Laetham et al., 1998).

Histologic patterns of squamous replacement after ablative therapy include islands of squamous epithelium within BE, often adjacent to the ducts of submucosal mucous glands; partial or complete squamous metaplasia of BE glands (an appearance similar to that of squamous metaplasia in the cervical transformation zone); and squamification of the mucosal surface with retained glands in the lamina propria (Biddlestone et al., 1998). The long-range significance, in terms of neoplastic risk, of residual BE in the setting of ablative therapy is unknown. Increasing the depth of tissue ablation could reduce the risk of having residual BE; however, tissue damage extending to the deep submucosa or muscularis propria is associated with a high rate of fibrosis and stricture formation (Bown, 1998).

Although promising as a method of managing patients with BE, at the present time ablative therapy should be considered a technique best suited for clinical trials. It also has a role as a therapeutic modality in patients with dysplasia and early cancer who are high-risk surgical candidates (Bown, 1998; Lightdale, 1999b).

REFERENCES

Ahnen DJ. (1987) Flow cytometric analysis of deoxyribonucleic acid content in the gastrointestinal tract: Is aneuploidy more than a new ploy? [Editorial] *Gastroenterology* 93:197–199.

Alikhan M, Rex D, Khan A, et al. (1999) Variable pathologic interpretation of columnar-lined esophagus by general pathologists in community practice. *Gastrointest Endosc* 50:23–26.

Altorki NK, Sunagawa M, Little AG, Skinner DB. (1991) High-grade dysplasia in the columnar-lined esophagus. *Am J Surg* 161:97–99.

Antonioli DA, Wang HH. (1997) Morphology of Barrett's esophagus and Barrett's-associated dysplasia and adenocarcinoma. *Gastroenterol Clin North Am* 26:495–506.

Barge J, Molas G, Maillard, JN, et al. (1981) Superficial oesophageal carcinoma: an oesophageal counterpart of early gastric cancer. *Histopathology* 5:499–510.

Benasco C, Combalia N, Pou JM, Miquel JM. (1985) Superficial esophageal carcinoma: A report of 12 cases. *Gastrointest Endosc* 31:64–67.

Bennett WP, Hollstein MC, Metcalf RA, et al. (1992) p53 mutation and protein accumulation during multistage human esophageal carcinogenesis. *Cancer Res* 52:6092–6097.

Berenson MM, Herbst JJ, Freston JW. (1974) Enzyme and ultrastructural characteristics of esophageal columnar epithelium. *Am J Dig Dis* 19:895–907.

Berenson MM, Johnson TD, Markowitz NR, et al. (1993) Restoration of squamous mucosa after ablation of Barrett's esophageal epithelium. *Gastroenterology* 104:1686–1691.

Biddlestone LR, Barham CP, Wilkinson SP, et al. (1998) The histopathology of treated Barrett's esophagus: squamous reepithelialization after acid suppression and laser and photodynamic therapy. *Am J Surg Pathol* 22:239–245.

Boch JA, Shields HM, Antonioli DA, et al. (1997) Distribution of cytokeratin markers in Barrett's specialized columnar epithelium. *Gastroenterology* 112: 760–765.

Bogomoletz WV, Molas G, Gayet B, Potet F. (1989) Superficial squamous cell carcinoma of the esophagus: A report of 76 cases and review of the literuature. *Am J Surg Pathol* 13:535–546.

Bown SG. (1998) A light at the end of the tunnel. *Gut* 43:737–741.

Burke AP, Sobin LH, Shekitka KM, et al. (1991) Dysplasia of the stomach and Barrett's esophagus. A follow-up study. *Mod Pathol* 4:336–341.

Cameron AJ, Carpenter HA. (1997) Barrett's esophagus, high-grade dysplasia, and early adenocarcinoma: a pathological study. *Am J Gastroenterol* 92: 586–591.

Cameron AJ, Ott BJ, Payne WS. (1985) The incidence of adenocarcinoma in columnar-lined (Barrett's) esophagus. *N Engl J Med* 313:857–859.

Cameron AJ, Zinsmeister AR, Ballard DJ, Carney JA. (1990) Prevalence of columnar-lined (Barrett's) esophagus: comparison of population-based clinical and autopsy findings. *Gastroenterology* 99:918–922.

Caygill CPJ, Reed PI, Johnston BJ, et al. (1999) A single centre's 20 years' experience of columnar-lined (Barrett's) oesophagus diagnosis. *Eur J Gastroenterol Heptaol* 11:1355–1358.

Chalasani N, Wo JM, Hunter JG, et al. (1997) Significance of intestinal metaplasia in different areas of esophagus including esophagogastric junction. *Dig Dis Sci* 42:603–607.

Chang F, Syrjanen S, Wang L, Syrajanen K. (1992) Infectious agents in the etiology of esophageal cancer. *Gastroenterology* 103:1336–1348.

Chaves P, Cardoso P, deAlmeida JCM, et al. (1999) Nongoblet cell population of Barrett's esophagus: an immunohistochemical demonstration of intestinal differentiation. *Hum Pathol* 30:1291–1295.

Christensen WN, Sternberg SS. (1987) Adenocarcinoma of the upper esophagus arising in ectopic gastric mucosa: two case reports and review of the literature. *Am J Surg Pathol* 11:397–402.

Dawsey SM, Lewin KJ, Wang GQ, et al. (1994a) Squamous esophageal histology and subsequent risk of squamous cell carcinoma of the esophagus. A prospective follow-up study from Linxian, China. *Cancer* 74:1686–1692.

Dawsey SM, Wang GQ, Weinstein WM, et al. (1993) Squamous dysplasia and early esophageal cancer in the Linxian region of China: distinctive endoscopic lesions. *Gastroenterology* 105:1333–1340.

Dawsey SM, Yu Y, Taylor PR, et al. (1994b) Esophageal cytology and subsequent risk of esophageal cancer. A prospective follow-up study from Linxian, China. *Acta Cytol* 38:183–192.

DeBaecque C, Patet F, Molas G, et al. (1990) Superficial adenocarcinoma of the esophagus arising in Barrett's mucosa with dysplasia: a clinico-pathological study of 12 patients. *Histopathology* 16:213–220.

Dent J, Bremner CG, Collen MJ, et al. (1991) Working party report to the World Congress of Gastroenterology, Sydney, 1990: Barrett's oesophagus. *J Gastroenterol Hepatol* 6:1–22.

Devesa SS, Blot WJ, Fraumeni JF. (1998) Changing patterns in the incidence of esophageal and gastric carcinoma in the United States. *Cancer* 83:2049–2053.

Doglioni C, Laurino L, Dei Tos AP, et al. (1993) Pancreatic (acinar) metaplasia of the gastric mucosa. *Am J Surg Pathol* 17:1134–1143.

Doki Y, Shiozaki H, Tahara H, et al. (1993) Prognostic value of DNA ploidy in squamous cell carcinoma of the esophagus. *Cancer* 72:1813–1818.

Drewitz D, Sampliner R, Garewal H. (1997) The incidence of adenocarcinoma in Barrett's esophagus: a prospective study of 170 patients followed 4.8 years. *Am J Gastroenterol* 92:212–215.

Falk GW, Rice TW, Goldblum JR, Richter JE. (1999) Jumbo biopsy forceps protocol still misses unsuspected cancer in Barrett's esophagus with high-grade dysplasia. *Gastrointest Endosc* 49:170–176.

Fennerty MB, Sampliner RE, Way D, et al. (1989) Discordance between flow cytometric abnormalities and dysplasia in Barrett's esophagus. *Gastroenterology* 97:815–820.

Feurle GE, Helmstaedter V, Buehring A, et al. (1990) Distinct immunohistochemical findings in columnar epithelium of esophageal inlet patch and of Barrett's esophagus. *Dig Dis Sci* 35:86–92.

Froelicher P, Miller G. (1986) The European experience with esophageal cancer limited to the mucosa and submucosa.*Gastrointest Endosc* 32:88–90.

Galen AR, Katzka DA, Castell DO. (1998) Acid secretion from an esophageal inlet patch demonstrated by ambulatory pH monitoring. *Gastroenterology* 115:1574–1576.

Garewal HS, Sampliner RE, Fennerty MB. (1990) Flow cytometry in Barrett's esophagus: what have we learned so far? *Dig Dis Sci* 36:548–551.

Geisinger KR, Teot LA, Richter JE. (1992) A comparative cytopathologic and histologic study of atypia, dysplasia, and adenocarcinoma in Barrett's esophagus. *Cancer* 69:8–16.

Genta RM, Huberman RM, Graham DY. (1994) The gastric cardia in *Helicobacter pylori* infection. *Hum Pathol* 25:915–919.

Giménez A, deHaro LM, Parilla P, et al. (1999) Immunohistochemical detection of p53 protein could improve the management of some patients with Barrett's esophagus and mild histologic alterations. *Arch Pathol Lab Med* 123:1260–1263.

Giménez A, Minguela A, Parrilla P, et al. (1998) Flow cytometric DNA analysis and p53 protein expression show a good correlation with histologic findings in patients with Barrett's esophagus. *Cancer* 83:641–651.

Gossner L, May A, Sroka R, et al. (1999) Photodynamic destruction of high grade dysplasia and early carcinoma of the esophagus after the oral administration of 5-aminolevulinic acid. *Cancer* 86:1921–1928.

Gossner L, Stolte M, Sroka R, et al. (1998) Photodynamic ablation of high-grade dysplasia and early cancer in Barrett's esophagus by means of 5-aminolevulinic acid. *Gastroenterology* 114:448–455.

Gottfried MR, McClave SA, Boyce HW. (1989) Incomplete intestinal metaplasia in the diagnosis of columnar-lined esophagus (Barrett's esophagus). *Am J Clin Pathol* 92:741–746.

Guanrei Y, Songliang Q. (1987) Endoscopic surveys in high-risk and low-risk populations for esophageal cancer in China with special reference to precursors of esophageal cancer. *Endoscopy* 19:91–95.

Haag S, Nandurkar S, Talley NJ. (1999) Regression of Barrett's esophagus: the role of acid suppression, surgery, and ablative methods. *Gastrointest Endosc* 50:159–164.

Haggitt RC. (1994) Barrett's esophagus, dysplasia, and adenocarcinoma. *Hum Pathol* 25:982–993.

Haggitt RC, Dean PJ. (1985) Adenocarcinoma in Barrett's epithelium. In: *Barrett's Esophagus: Pathophysiology, Diagnosis and Management* (Spechler SJ, Goyal RK, eds.) pp. 153–166. New York, Elsevier.

Haggitt RC, Reid BJ, Rabinovitch PS, Rubin CE. (1988) Barrett's esophagus: correlation between mucin histochemistry, flow cytometry, and histologic diagnosis for predicting increased cancer risk. *Am J Pathol* 131:53–61.

Haggitt RC, Tryzelaar J, Ellis H, Colcher H. (1978) Adenocarcinoma complicating columnar epithelium-lined (Barrett's) esophagus. *Am J Clin Pathol* 70:1–5.

Hameeteman W, Tytgat GNJ, Houthoff HJ, van den Tweel JG. (1989) Barrett's esophagus: development of dysplasia and adenocarcinoma. *Gastroenterology* 96:1249–1256.

Hamilton SR, Smith RRL. (1987) The relationship between columnar epithelial dysplasia and invasive adenocarcinoma arising in Barrett's esophagus. *Am J Clin Pathol* 87:301–312.

Hamilton SR, Smith RRL, Cameron JL. (1988) Prevalence and characteristics of Barrett's esophagus in patients with adenocarcinoma of the esophagus or esophagogastric junction. *Hum Pathol* 19:942–948.

Heitmiller RF, Redmond M, Hamilton SR. (1996) Barrett's esophagus with high grade dysplasia: an indication for prophylactic esophagectomy. *Ann Surg* 224:66–71.

Hesketh PJ, Clapp RW, Doos WG, Spechler SJ. (1989) The increasing frequency of adenocarcinoma of the esophagus. *Cancer* 64:526–530.

Hölscher AH, Bollschweiler E, Schneider PM, Siewert JR. (1997) Early adenocarcinoma in Barrett's oesophagus. *Br J Surg* 84:1470–1473.

Jabbari M, Goresky CA, Lough J, et al. (1985) The inlet patch: heterotopic gastric mucosa in the upper esophagus. *Gastroenterology* 89:352–356.

Jacob P, Kahrilas PJ, Desai T, et al. (1990) Natural history and significance of esophageal squamous cell dysplasia. *Cancer* 65:2731–2739.

Jankowski JA, Wright NA, Meltzer SJ, et al. (1999) Molecular evolution of the metaplasia-dysplasia-adenocarcinoma sequence in the esophagus. *Am J Pathol* 154:965–973.

Jass JR. (1981) Mucin histochemistry of the columnar epithelium of the oesophagus: a retrospective study. *J Clin Pathol* 34:866–870.

Jauregui HO, Davessar K, Hale JH, et al. (1988) Mucin histochemistry of intestinal metaplasia in Barrett's esophagus. *Mod Pathol* 1:188–192.

Kalish RJ, Clancy PE, Orringer MB, Appelman HD. (1984) Clinical, epidemiologic, and morphologic comparison between adenocarcinoma arising in Barrett's esophageal mucosa and in the gastric cardia. *Gastroenterology* 86:461–467.

Kato H, Tachimori Y, Watanabe H, et al. (1990) Superficial esophageal carcinoma: surgical treatment and the results. *Cancer* 66:2319–2323.

Katz D, Rothstein R, Schned A, et al. (1998) The development of dysplasia and adenocarcinoma during endoscopic surveillance of Barrett's esophagus. *Am J Gastroenterol* 93:536–541.

Koss LG, Morgenstern N, Tahir-Kheli N, et al. (1998) Evaluation of esophageal cytology using a neural net-based interactive scanning system. *Am J Clin Pathol* 109:549–557.

Krishnamurthy S, Dayal Y. (1995) Pancreatic metaplasia in Barrett's esophagus: an immunohistochemical study. *Am J Surg Pathol* 19:1172–1180.

Kuwano H, Matsuda H, Matsuoka H, et al. (1987) Intraepithelial carcinoma concomitant with esophageal squamous cell carcinoma. *Cancer* 59:783–787.

Lauwers GY, Scott GV, Vauthey JN. (1998) Adenocarcinoma of the upper esophagus arising in cervical ectopic gastric mucosa: rare evidence of malignant potential of so-called inlet patch. *Dig Dis Sci* 43:901–907.

Lee RG. (1984) Mucins in Barrett's esophagus: a histochemical study. *Am J Clin Pathol* 81:500–503.

Lee RG. (1985) Dysplasia in Barrett's esophagus: a clinical pathologic study of six patients. *Am J Surg Pathol* 9:845–852.

Lee RG. (1986) Adenomas arising in Barrett's esophagus. *Am J Clin Pathol* 83:629–632.

Levine DS. (1997) Management of dysplasia in the columnar-lined esophagus. *Gastroenterol Clin North Am* 26:613–634.

Levine DS, Rubin CE, Reid BJ, Haggitt RC. (1989) Specialized metaplastic columnar epithelium in Barrett's esophagus: a comparative transmission electron microscopic study. *Lab Invest* 60:418–432.

Levine MS, Caroline D, Thompson JJ, et al. (1984) Adenocarcinoma of the esophagus: Relationship to Barrett mucosa. *Radiology* 150:305–309.

Lewin KJ, Appelman HD. (1996) Tumors of the esophagus and stomach. In: *Atlas of Tumor Pathology*, Third Series, Fascicle 18 (Rosai J, ed.). Washington DC, Armed Forces Institute of Pathology.

Lightdale CJ. (1999a) Esophageal cancer. *Am J Gastroenterol* 94:20–29.

Lightdale CJ. (1999b) Ablation therapy for Barrett's esophagus: is it time to choose our weapons? [editorial] *Gastroint Endosc* 49:122–125.

Loughney T, Maydorovitch CL, Wong RKH. (1998) Esophageal manometry and ambulatory 24-hour pH monitoring in patients with short and long segment Barrett's esophagus. *Am J Gastroenterol* 93:916–919.

Lu J-B, Yang W-X, Dong W-Z, Sang J-Y. (1988) A prospective study of esophageal cytological atypia in Linxian county. *Int J Cancer* 41:805–808.

Macdonald CE, Wicks AC, Playford RJ. (1997) Ten years' experience of screening patients with Barrett's oesophagus in a university teaching hospital. *Gut* 41:303–307.

MacDonald WC, MacDonald JB. (1987) Adenocarcinoma of the esophagus and/or gastric cardia. *Cancer* 60:1094–1098.

Maldonado ME, Brady PG, Morgan M. (1998) Pancreatic acinar metaplasia in an inlet patch. *Gastrointest Endosc* 47:545–546.

Mandard AM, Marnay J, Gignoux M, et al. (1984) Cancer of the esophagus and associated lesions: Detailed pathologic study of 100 esophagectomy specimens. *Hum Pathol* 15:660–669.

Mann NS, Tsai ME, Nair PK. (1989) Barrett's esophagus in patients with symptomatic reflux esophagitis. *Am J Gastroenterol* 84:1494–1496.

McDonald GB, Brand DL, Thorning DR. (1977) Multiple adenomatous neoplasms arising in columnar-lined (Barrett's) esophagus. *Gastroenterology* 72: 1317–1321.

Mingxin L, Ping L, Baorong L. (1980) Recent progress in research on esophageal cancer in China. *Adv. Cancer Res* 33:173–249.

Mion F, Lambert R, Partensky M, et al. (1996) High-grade dysplasia in an adenoma of the upper esophagus developing on heterotopic gastric mucosa. *Endoscopy* 28:633–635.

Montgomery EA, Hartmann D-P, Carr NJ, et al. (1996) Barrett esophagus with dysplasia: flow cytometric DNA analysis of routine, paraffin-embedded mucosal biopsies. *Am J Clin Pathol* 106:298–304.

Morales TG, Sampliner RE, Bhattachayya A. (1997) Intestinal metaplasia of the gastric cardia. *Am J Gastroenterol* 92:414–418.

Morita M, Kuwano H, Yasuda M, et al. (1994) The multicentric occurrence of squamous epithelial dysplasia and squamous cell carcinoma. *Cancer* 74:2889–2895.

Muñoz N, Crespi M. (1983) High-risk conditions and precancerous lesions of the oesophagus. In: *Precancerous Lesions of the Gastrointestinal Tract*, (Sherlock P, Morson BC, Barbara L, Veronesi U, eds.) pp. 53–86. New York, Raven Press.

Nabeya K. (1983) Markers of cancer risk in the esophagus and surveillance of high-risk groups. In: *Precancerous Lesions of the Gastrointestinal Tract* (Sherlock P, Morson BC, Barbara L, Veronesi U, eds.) pp. 71–86. New York, Raven Press.

Nagawa H, Kaizaki S, Seto Y, et al. (1995) The relationship of macroscopic shape of superficial esophageal carcinoma to depth of invasion and regional lymph node metastasis. *Cancer* 75:1061–1064.

Nakanishi Y, Ochiai A, Yoshimura K, et al. (1998) The clinicopathologic significance of small areas unstained by Lugol's iodine in the mucosa surrounding resected esophageal carcinoma: an analysis of 147 cases. *Cancer* 82:1454–1459.

Nandurkar S, Talley NJ, Martin CJ, et al. (1997) Short segment Barrett's oesophagus: prevalence, diagnosis and associations. *Gut* 40:710–715.

Nishimaki T, Hölscher AH, Schüler M, et al. (1991) Histopathologic characteristics of early adenocarcinoma in Barrett's esophagus. *Cancer* 68:1731–1736.

O'Connor JB, Falk GW, Richter JE. (1999) The incidence of adenocarcinoma and dysplasia in Barrett's esophagus. *Am J Gastroenterol* 94:2037–2042.

Odze RD, Antonioli DA. (1995) Cancer of the esophagus. In: *Gastrointestinal Cancers: Biology, Diagnosis, and Therapy*. (Rustgi AK, ed). pp. 115–140. New York, Raven Press.

Oettlé GJ, Paterson AC, Leiman G, Segal I. (1986) Esophagitis in a population at risk for esophageal carcinoma. *Cancer* 57:2222–2229.

Offner FA, Lewin KJ, Weinstein WM. (1996) Metaplastic columnar cells in Barrett's esophagus: a common and neglected cell type. *Hum Pathol* 27:885–889.

Ohta H, Nakazawa S, Segawa K, Yoshino J. (1986) Distribution of epithelial dysplasia in the cancerous esophagus. *Scand J Gastroenterol* 21:392–398.

Ortiz-Hidalgo C, DeLa Vega G, Aguirre-Garcia J. (1998) The histopathology and biologic prognostic factors of Barrett's esophagus. *J Clin Gastroenterol* 26:324–333.

Ovaska J, Miettinen M, Kivilaakso E. (1989) Adenocarcinoma arising in Barrett's esophagus. *Dig Dis Sci* 34:1336–1339.

Overholt BF, Panjehpour M, Haydek JM. (1999) Photodynamic therapy for Barrett's esophagus: follow-up in 100 patients. *Gastrointest Endosc* 49:1–7.

Palley SL, Sampliner RE, Garewal HS. (1989) Management of high-grade dysplasia in Barrett's esophagus. *J Clin Gastroenterol* 11:369–372.

Paraf F, Flejou J-F, Pignon J-P, et al. (1995) Surgical pathology of adenocarcinoma arising in Barrett's esophagus: analysis of 67 cases. *Am J Surg Pathol* 19:183–191.

Pera M, Trastek VF, Carpenter HA, et al. (1992) Barrett's esophagus with high-grade dysplasia: an indication for esophagectomy? *Ann Thorac Surg* 54: 199–204.

Peuchmaur M, Potet F, Goldfain D. (1984) Mucin histochemistry of the columnar epithelium of the oesophagus (Barrett's oesophagus): a prospective biopsy study. *J Clin Pathol* 37:607–610.

Polzak M, Cerar A, Seme K. (1998) Human papillomavirus infection in esophageal carcinomas: a study of 121 lesions using multiple broad-spectrum polymerase chain reactions. *Hum Pathol* 29:266–271.

Qualman SJ, Murray RD, McClung J, Lucas J. (1990) Intestinal metaplasia is age related in Barrett's esophagus. *Arch Pathol Lab Med* 114:1236–1240.

Qui S, Yang G. (1988) Precursor lesions of esophageal cancer in high-risk populations in Henan Province, China. *Cancer* 62:551–557.

Rabinovitch PS, Reid BJ, Haggitt RC, et al. (1988) Progression to cancer in Barrett's esophagus is associated with genomic instability. *Lab Invest* 60:65–71.

Ramel S, Reid BJ, Sanchez CA, et al. (1992) Evaluation of p53 protein expression in Barrett's esophagus by two-parameter flow cytometry. *Gastroenterology* 102: 1220–1228.

Reid BJ, Blount PL, Rubin EE, et al. (1992) Predictors of progression to malignancy in Barrett's esophagus: endoscopic, histologic and flow cytometric follow-up of a cohort. *Gastroenterology* 102:1212–1219.

Reid BJ, Haggitt RC, Rubin CE, et al. (1988a) Observer variation in the diagnosis of dysplasia in Barrett's esophagus. *Hum Pathol* 19:166–178.

Reid BJ, Weinstein WM, Lewin KJ, et al. (1988b) Endoscopic biopsy can detect high-grade dysplasia or early adenocarcinoma in Barrett's esophagus without grossly recognizable neoplastic lesions. *Gastroenterology* 94:81–90.

Ribeiro U, Poisner MC, Sofatle-Ribeiro AV, et al. (1996) Risk factors for squamous cell carcinoma of the esophagus. *Br J Surg* 83:1174–1185.

Rice TW. (1999) Superficial oesophageal carcinoma: is there a need for three field lymphadenectomy? *Lancet* 354:792–794.

Riddell RH. (1985) Dysplasia and regression in Barrett's epithelium. In: *Barrett's Esophagus: Pathophysiology, Diagnosis and Management.* (Spechler SJ, Goyal RK, eds.) pp. 143–152. New York, Elsevier.

Riddell RH. (1996) Early detection of neoplasia of the esophagus and gastroesophageal junction. *Am J Gastroenterol* 91:853–863.

Riddell RH, Goldman H, Ransohoff DF, et al. (1983) Dysplasia in inflammatory bowel disease: standardized classification with provisional clinical applications. *Hum Pathol* 14:931–968.

Robertson CS, Mayberry JF, Nicholson DA, et al. (1988) Value of endoscopic surveillance in the detection of neoplastic change in Barrett's oesophagus. *Br J Surg* 75:760–763.

Robey SS, Hamilton SR, Gupta PK, Erozan YS. (1988) Diagnostic value of cytopathology in Barrett's esophagus and associated carcinoma. *Am J Clin Pathol* 89:493–498.

Rogers EL, Goldkind SF, Iseri OA, et al. (1986) Adenocarcinoma of the lower esophagus: a disease primarily of white men with Barrett's esophagus. *J Clin Gastroenterol* 8:613–618.

Roth MJ, Lui S-F, Dawsey SM, et al. (1997) Cytologic detection of esophageal squamous cell carcinoma and precursor lesions using balloon and sponge samples in asymptomatic adults in Linxian, China. *Cancer* 80:2047–2059.

Rothery GA, Patterson JE, Stoddard CL, Day DW. (1986) Histological and histochemical changes in the columnar lined (Barrett's) oesophagus. *Gut* 27:1062–1068.

Rubio CA, Auer GU, Kato Y, Liu F-S. (1988) DNA profiles in dysplasia and carcinoma of the human esophagus. *Anal Quant Cytol Histol* 10:207–210.

Rubio CA, Liu F, Zhao H-Z. (1989) Histological classification of intraepithelial neoplasias and microinvasive squamous carcinoma of the esophagus. *Am J Surg Pathol* 13:685–690.

Sampliner RE. (1998) Practice guidelines on the diagnosis, surveillance and therapy of Barrett's esophagus. *Am J Gastroenterol* 93:1028–1032.

Sampliner RE, Garewal HS, Fennerty MB, Aickin M. (1990) Lack of impact of therapy on extent of Barrett's esophagus in 67 patients. *Dig Dis Sci* 35:93–96.

Sanfey H, Hamilton SR, Smith RRL, Cameron JL. (1985) Carcinoma arising in Barrett's esophagus. *Surg Gynecol Obstet* 161:570–574.

Sawhney RA, Shields HM, Allan CH, et al. (1996) Morphological characterization of the squamocolumnar junction of the esophagus in patients with and without Barrett's esophagus. *Dig Dis Sci* 41:1088–1098.

Schmidt HG, Riddell RH, Wather B, et al. (1985) Dysplasia in Barrett's esophagus. J. *Cancer Res Clin Oncol* 110:145–152.

Schmidt LW, Dean PJ, Wilson RT. (1986) Superficially invasive squamous cell carcinoma of the esophagus. *Cancer* 91:1456–1461.

Schnell T, Sontag S, Chejfec G. (1992) Adenocarcinomas arising in tongues or short segments of Barrett's esophagus. *Dig Dis Sci* 37:137–143.

Sharma P, Morales T, Bhattacharyya A, et al. (1997) Dysplasia in short segment Barrett's esophagus: A prospective 3 year follow-up. *Am J Gastroenterol* 92:2012–2016.

Sharma P, Morales T, Bhattacharyya A. (1998a) Squamous islands in Barrett's esophagus: what lies underneath. *Am J Gastroenterol* 93:332–335.

Sharma P, Morales TG, Sampliner RE. (1998b) Short segment Barrett's esophagus—the need for standardization of the definition and of endoscopic criteria. *Am J Gastroenterol* 93:1033–1036.

Shields HM, Sawhney RA, Zwas F, et al. (1995) Scanning electron microscopy of the human esophagus: application to Barrett's esophagus, a precancerous lesion. *Microsc Res Tech* 31:248–256.

Shimazu H, Kobori O, Shoji M, et al. (1983) Superficial carcinoma of the esophagus. *Gastroenterol Jpn* 18:409–416.

Shimizu Y, Tukagoski H, Oohara M, et al. (1999) Clinicopathologic study of esophageal squamous cell carcinoma confined to the mucosa. *J Clin Gastroenterol* 29:35–38.

Shiozaki H, Tahara H, Kobayashi K, et al. (1990) Endoscopic screening of early esophageal cancer with the Lugol dye method in patients with head and neck cancer. *Cancer* 66:2068–2071.

Shu Y-J. (1983) Cytopathology of the esophagus: an overview of esophageal cytopathology in China. *Acta Cytol* 27:7–17.

Sjogren RW, Johnson LF. (1983) Barrett's esophagus: a review. *Am J Med* 74:313–320.

Smith RRL, Hamilton SR, Boitnott JK, Rogers EL. (1984) The spectrum of carcinoma arising in Barrett's esophagus: a clinicopathologic study of 26 patients. *Am J Surg Pathol* 8:563–573.

Soga J, Tanaka O, Sasaki K, et al. (1982) Superficial spreading carcinoma of the esophagus. *Cancer* 50:1641–1645.

Sons HU, Borchard F. (1984) Esophageal cancer: autopsy findings in 171 cases. *Arch Pathol Lab Med* 108:983–988.

Spechler SJ, Goyal RK. (1986) Barrett's esophagus. *N Engl J Med* 315:362–371.

Spechler SJ, Goyal RK. (1996) The columnar-lined esophagus, intestinal metaplasia, and Norman Barrett. *Gastroenterology* 110:614–621.

Spechler SJ, Robbins AH, Rubins HB, et al. (1984) Adenocarcinoma and Barrett's esophagus: an over-rated risk? *Gastroenterology* 87:927–933.

Spechler SJ, Sperber H, Doos WG, Schimmel EM. (1983) The prevalence of Barrett's esophagus in patients with chronic peptic esophageal stricture. *Dig Dis Sci* 28:769–774.

Spechler SJ, Zeroogian JM, Antonioli DA, et al. (1994) Prevalence of metaplasia at the gastro-oesophageal junction. *Lancet* 344:1533–1536.

Steadman C, Kerlin P, Teague C, Stephenson P. (1988) High esophageal stricture: a complication of "inlet patch" mucosa. *Gastroenterology* 94:521–524.

Stemmermann G, Heffelfinger SC, Noffsinger A, et al. (1994) The molecular biology of esophageal and gastric cancer and their precursors: oncogenes, tumor suppressor genes, and growth factors. *Hum Pathol* 25:968–981.

Streitz JM, Ellis FH, Tilden RL, Erickson RV. (1998) Endoscopic surveillance of Barrett's esophagus: a cost-effective comparison with mammographic surveillance for breast cancer. *Am J Gastroenterol* 93: 911–915.

Sugimachi K, Ide H, Okamura T, et al. (1984) Cytophotometric DNA analysis of mucosal and submucosal cancer of the esophagus. *Cancer* 58:2683–2687.

Suzek L, Noffsinger AE, Hui YZ, Fenoglio-Preiser CM. (1996) Detection of human papillomavirus in esophageal squamous cell carcinoma. *Cancer* 78:704–710.

Takagi A, Ema Y, Horii S, et al. (1995) Early adenocarcinoma arising from ectopic gastric mucosa in the cervical esophagus. *Gastrointest Endosc* 41:167–170.

Thompson JJ, Zinsser KR, Enterline HT. (1983) Barrett's metaplasia and adenocarcinoma of the esophagus and gastroesophageal junction. *Hum Pathol* 14:42–61.

Thurberg BL, Duray PH, Odze RD. (1999) Polypoid dysplasia in Barrett's esophagus: a clinicopathological, immunohistochemical, and molecular study of five cases. *Hum Pathol* 30:745–752.

Togawa K, Jaskiewicz K, Takahashi H, et al. (1994) Human papillomavirus DNA sequences in esophagus squamous cell carcinoma. *Gastroenterology* 107:128–136.

Trier JS. (1970) Morphology of the epithelium of the distal esophagus in patients with midesophageal peptic strictures. *Gastroenterology* 58:444–461.

Truong LD, Stroehlein JR, McKechnie JC. (1986) Gastric heterotopia of the proximal esophagus: A report of four cases detected by endoscopy and review of literature. *Am J Gastroenterol* 81:1162–1166.

Van Asche C, Rahm AE, Goldner F, Crumbaker D. (1988) Columnar mucosa in the proximal esophagus. *Gastrointest Endosc* 34:324–326.

van den Boogert J, van Hillegersberg R, Siersema PD, et al. (1999) Endoscopic ablation therapy for Barrett's esophagus with high-grade dysplasia: a review. *Am J Gastroenterol* 94:1153–1160.

van Laetham J-L, Crener M, Pexy MO, et al. (1998) Eradication of Barrett's mucosa with argon plasma coagulation and acid suppression: immediate and mid-term results. *Gut* 43:747–751.

van Sandick JW, van Lanschot JJB, Tytgat GNJ, et al. (1998) Impact of endoscopic biopsy surveillance of Barrett's oesophagus on pathological stage and clinical outcome of Barrett's carcinoma. *Gut* 43:216–222.

Wang HH, Antonioli DA, Goldman H. (1986) Comparative features of esophageal and gastric adenocarcinomas: recent changes in type and frequency. *Hum Pathol* 17:482–487.

Wang HH, Doria MI, Purohit-Buch S, et al. (1992) Barrett's esophagus: the cytology of dysplasia in comparison to benign and malignant lesions. *Acta Cytol* 36:60–64.

Wang HH, Sovie S, Zeroogian JM, et al. (1997) Value of cytology in detecting intestinal metaplasia and associated dysplasia at the gastroesophageal junction. *Hum Pathol* 28:465–471.

Wang HH, Zeroogian JM, Spechler SJ, et al. (1996) Prevalence and significance of pancreatic acinar metaplasia at the gastroesophageal junction. *Am J Surg Pathol* 20:1507–1510.

Wang LD, Hong JY, Qui SL, et al. (1993) Accumulation of p53 protein in human esophageal precancerous lesions: a possible early marker for carcinogenesis. *Cancer Res* 53:1783–1787.

Weston AP, Badr AS, Hassanein RS. (1999) Prospective multivariate analysis of clinical, endoscopic, and histological factors predictive of the development of Barrett's multifocal high-grade dysplasia or adenocarcinoma. *Am J Gastroenterol* 94:3413–3419.

Winters C, Spurling TJ, Chobanian SJ, et al. (1987) Barrett's esophagus: a prevalent, occult complication of gastroesophageal reflux disease. *Gastroenterology* 92:18–124.

Wright TA, Gray MR, Morris AI, et al. (1996) Cost effectiveness of detecting Barrett's cancer. *Gut* 39:574–579.

Younes M, Lebovitz RM, Lechago LV, Lechago J. (1993) p53 protein accumulation in Barrett's metaplasia, dysplasia, and carcinoma: A follow-up study. *Gastroenterology* 105:1637–1642.

Zwas F, Shields HM, Doos WG, et al. (1986) Scanning electron microscopy of Barrett's epithelium and its correlation with light microscopy and mucin stains. *Gastroenterology* 90:1932–1941.

7

STOMACH

Pelayo Correa and Eiichi Tahara

Recent technologic developments, especially that of flexible endoscopy, have made possible documentation of the initial stages of the gastric neoplastic process in humans. Through this new technology, what has been known for more than a century has been shown in some detail: that there are lesions in the gastric mucosa that can be found years before cancer becomes clinically apparent. This was first documented by Kupfer, who described foci of intestinal epithelium in the gastric mucosa more than a century ago (1883), and was discussed extensively afterward (Jarvi and Lauren, 1951; Michalany, 1959; Schmidt, 1896). It also has been reported that in most cases, intestinal metaplasia appears to be a component of a more basic process, chronic atrophic gastritis, which has been characterized on clinical and pathologic grounds (Correa, 1980; Lambert, 1972; Strickland and Mackay, 1973).

Gastric carcinoma is not a homogeneous disease; rather, it appears to involve two independent etiopathogenic lesions that have, for convenience, been designated "intestinal," or "expansive" and "diffuse," or "infiltrative" (Lauren, 1965; Ming, 1977). Our discussion concentrates on the initial phases of intestinal gastric carcinoma because extensive information is available for this type of carcinoma, unlike the diffuse type, whose initial stages are poorly understood. A few reports describe clusters of poorly organized goblet cells in the gastric epithelium as the initial stage of signet-ring cell (diffuse) carcinoma; this condition has been designated "globoid dysplasia" (Borchard et al., 1979).

It is not clear whether this represents a cancer precursor or foci of carcinoma *in situ* in stomachs that also show invasion of the lamina propia. Contrary to the intestinal type, the great majority of cancers of the diffuse type are not accompanied by precursor lesions in the tumor-free mucosa.

It has been postulated that a continuum of progressive changes precedes clinical gastric carcinoma of the intestinal type (Correa, 1983). The dynamics of the progressive changes of the precursor lesions have been explored in a population at high risk for gastric cancer (Correa, 1990). These lesions are all covered by the term "precursors" but fall into two basic categories: those with mature cellular phenotype and those with immature cellular phenotype. Lesions with a mature cellular phenotype are probably remote from the cancer end point, are highly prevalent in populations at high risk, and probably do not deserve any special surveillance or intervention by clinicians because most will never reach the stage of clinical cancer (Correa, 1982). Cells in precursor lesions with immature phenotype may have reached the stage of irreversibility to normal phenotype, represent a greater threat to the patient, and deserve close clinical surveillance.

PRECURSORS WITH MATURE PHENOTYPE

The major lesions in the mature phenotype category are chronic gastritis, regenerative hyperplasia, atrophy, and intestinal metaplasia. The immature phenotype category corresponds to the dysplasias.

CHRONIC GASTRITIS

Inflammation of the gastric mucosa is probably one of the most frequent clinical syndromes experienced by adults. Ubiquitous irritants such as alcohol, aspirin, and salt are present in most human diets and are frequently abused. *Helicobacter pylori* is the most frequent cause of gastritis (Correa et al., 1989). Acute gastritis in most instances heals completely, but repeated episodes have the potential to induce chronic gastritis. The less advanced form of chronic gastritis is characterized by an infiltrate of mononuclear white blood cells in the superficial layers of the lamina propria (Fig. 7–1). The more advanced forms of chronic gastritis fall into several categories of clinicopathologic lesions, which have been discussed elsewhere (Correa, 1980, 1988). Some forms, such as dif-

fuse antral gastritis (Fig. 7–2), which frequently accompanies duodenal peptic ulcer, appear unrelated to gastric cancer. Other forms such as autoimmune gastritis, which is part of the pernicious anemia syndrome, and multifocal atrophic gastritis are true precursors of gastric carcinoma. The latter displays the same geographic distribution as epidemic gastric cancer and is probably associated with *Helicobacter pylori* infection and the same type of diet (Correa, 1982). An international classification of chronic gastritis and its relationship to the gastric precancerous process has recently been published (Dixon et al., 1996).

REGENERATIVE HYPERPLASIA

The only cells in the normal gastric mucosa with the capacity to replicate are in the glandular necks. Cell loss in any location triggers cell replication in the neck region, and migration followed by differentiation replaces the lost epithelial cells. Migration upward replaces foveolar cells and migration downward replaces glandular cells. Neck cells, therefore, are multipotential and can differentiate either to foveolar or to glandular cells. Gastritis is frequently accompanied by hyperplastic neck cells showing the usual signs of regeneration: large nuclei, hyperchromatism, mitosis, and somewhat irregular lumina. The nuclei of regenerative cells are usually hyperchromatic and round, may overlap, and show frequent mitosis. The background in this situation regularly shows an inflammatory infiltrate and in most cases polymorphonuclear leukocytes participate, indicating "active" acute injury to the mucosa. Occasionally, it is difficult to distinguish regenerative hyperplasia from mild dysplasia.

ATROPHY

The loss of gastric glands characterizes all types of gastritis that are epidemiologically linked to gastric cancer (Correa, 1983). It thus appears to be a critical stage in the process of carcinogenesis. Loss of glands is usually accompanied by neck cell hyperplasia, an apparent attempt to regenerate the missing epithelial cells. Atrophic changes are usually observed in a background of chronic gastritis, but the degree of inflam-

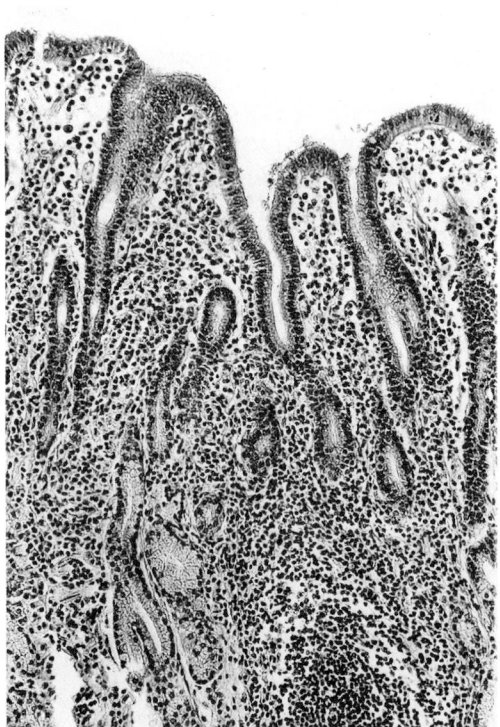

Figure 7–1. Superficial gastritis. Lymphotic and plasma cell infiltrate is in the lamina propria of the upper portion of the mucosa. [From Correa and Tahara, 1993, with permission.]

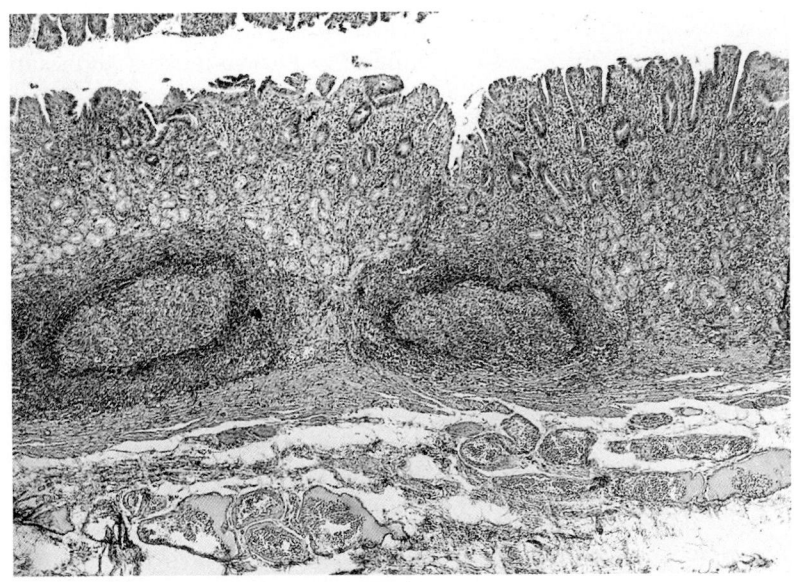

Figure 7–2. Diffuse antral gastritis in patients with duodenal peptic ulcer. Lymphocytic infiltrate involves the full thickness of the mucosa. Prominent lymphoid follicles are apparent, as well as depletion of mucous secretion of the surface epithelium. [From Correa and Tahara, 1993, with permission.]

mation varies from minimal to prominent. These variable degrees of inflammation have inspired classifications that erroneously suggest that chronic atrophic gastritis and gastric atrophy are different lesions. Gastric atrophy consists of gland loss and minimal inflammation and is observed in older individuals with extensive lesions that probably represent the advanced stage of the atrophic gastritis process. Gland regeneration has been observed in atrophic gastritis after cure of *Helicobacter pylori* infection (Garay et al., 1999).

Intestinal Metaplasia

Gastric glands lost in the process of atrophic gastritis are frequently replaced by cells with intestinal phenotypes. It is not clear how this process occurs: old explanations referred to "faulty regenerations" that, in modern terminology, called for the expression of some repressed genes in multipotential cells of the glandular necks. Other investigators interpret the change as a true mutation involving structural changes in the DNA molecule (Sugimura et al., 1982). The faulty *regeneration hypothesis* calls for chronic loss of cells, which could be accomplished by irritants or infectious agents. The *mutation hypothesis* postulates the presence of a mutagenic agent in the environment. The fact that some types of chronic gastritis involving cell

regeneration, such as diffuse antral gastritis, are not associated with an elevated risk of cancer favors the mutation hypothesis (Correa, 1980; Hansson et al., 1996).

Metaplastic glands replace the closely packed tubular glands of the corporal and antral mucosa by crypt-like structures lined by absorptive and goblet cells typical of the intestinal mucosa. Argentaffin and Paneth cells are also present in some intestinalized crypts. Metaplastic glands can also occupy the foveolar region and surface epithelium. Structures resembling both small and large intestinal mucosa have been identified in metaplastic lesions of the gastric mucosa. Some observations suggest that in the initial stages of metaplasia the small intestinal or "complete" type predominates, whereas in the advanced lesions colonic or "incomplete" type crypts, predominantly populated by columnar cells with multiple mucin vacuoles of varying size and without a brush border, are more frequent (incomplete metaplasia) (Heilmann and Hopker, 1979; Jass and Filipe, 1979; Sipponen et al., 1981; Teglbjaerg and Nielsen, 1978).

DYSPLASIA

After many attempts to reach an international classification of dysplasia, a recent proposal brought together by gastrointestinal pathologists from Europe, Asia, and the Americas reached a consensus that reconciles most of the previous semantic misunderstandings (Rugge et al., 2000). The agreement was reached in a final meeting in Padova, Italy in 1998. The Padova International Classification especially addresses differences in nomenclature between Western and Japanese pathology schools. The Western hallmark of malignancy is the stromal invasion. Japanese pathologists pay more attention to cytological aytpia. Table 7–1 displays the categories of the Padova International Classification, which will be addressed below.

1 NEGATIVE FOR DYSPLASIA

This category accounts for a wide spectrum of the histological features, ranging from the normal mucosa to the phenotypes of the atrophic metaplastic or nonmetaplastic gastritis. Foveolar hyperplasia was also inscribed in this category. Such heterogenous histological findings were grouped together on the basis of the lack of any biological evidence suggesting their possible neoplastic or preneoplastic nature.

Table 7–1. Padova International Classification of Gastric Dysplasia and Related Lesions

---

1 Negative for dysplasia

  1.0 Normal

  1.1 Reactive foveolar hyperplasia

  1.3 Intestinal metaplasia

    1.2.1 Intestinal metaplasia, complete type

    1.2.2 Intestinal metaplasia, incomplete type

2 Indefinite for dysplasia

  2.1 Foveolar hyperproliferation

  2.2 Hyperproliferative intestinal metaplasia

3 Dysplasia or noninvasive neoplasia (flat or elevated [synonym adenoma])

  3.1 Low-grade

  3.2 High-grade

    3.2.1 Including suspicious for carcinoma without invasion (intraglandular)

    3.2.2 Including carcinoma without invasion (intraglandular)

4 Suspicious for invasive carcinoma

5 Invasive carcinoma

1.0 Normal Mucosa

The definition of normal mucosa implies its distinction between the antral and oxyntic location. In this case, the mucosal components—namely, foveolae, gland necks, glands, and stroma—are well preserved and keep their positions and proportions intact. Inflammatory infiltration is absent or minimal.

1.1. Reactive Foveolar Hyperplasia

This situation arises when the gastric mucosa is reacting to mitogenic stimuli, which might be of an infectious nature, such as from *Helicobacter pylori;* chemicals, such as bile or nonsteroidal anti-inflammatory drugs (NSAIDs); or regeneration after erosions or ulcerations. The general architecture of the mucosa is well preserved. The foveolae may be elongated and tortuous. The nuclei are enlarged and sometimes hyperchromatic. Mitotic figures may be preset. The nuclear membrane is thin and delicate and multiple small nucleoli may be seen. The Golgi apparatus may be identifiable and mucinous secretion may be decreased or absent. Other changes such as dense inflammatory infiltrate, including polymorphonuclear leukocytes, edema, and vascular dilatation, may be present, reflecting the underlying cause of the hyperproliferative state. In spite of all these changes, which may be very prominent, they have no preneoplastic significance.

1.2. Intestinal Metaplasia

Intestinalization of the gastric mucosa is a well-known reaction to external injury. The most common form of metaplasia replicates rather closely the morphology of the small intestine and is therefore called "complete," "small intestinal–type" or "type I." On hematoxin and eosin (H&E) stain, eosinophilic absorptive enterocytes, with well-defined brush border, alternate with well-formed goblet cells. Special stains reveal that they secrete acid sialo mucin, which stains well with alcian blue at pH 2.5 (Figs. 7–3 and 7–4).

Incomplete metaplasia was originally classified as enterocolic, colonic-type, or type III (Heilmann and Hopker, 1979; Jass and Filippe, 1980). Glands featuring colonic-type metaplasia are more irregular than those showing small intestinal phenotype, their cells lack brush borders and absorptive enterocytes are not easily identifiable. They se-

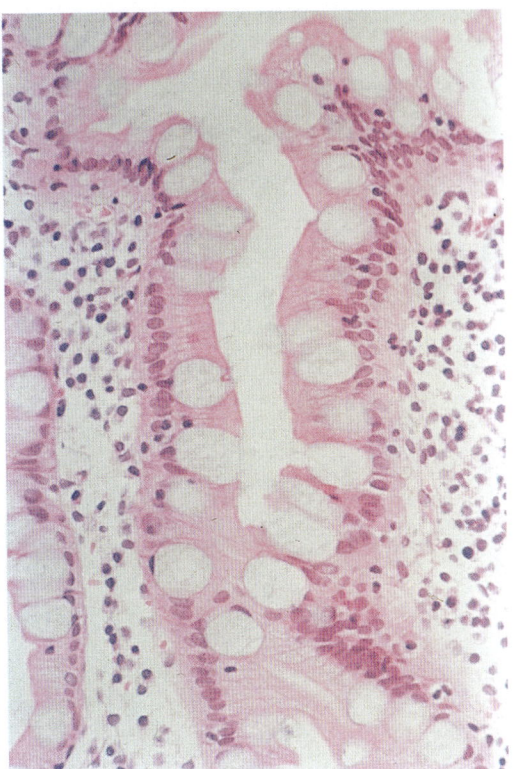

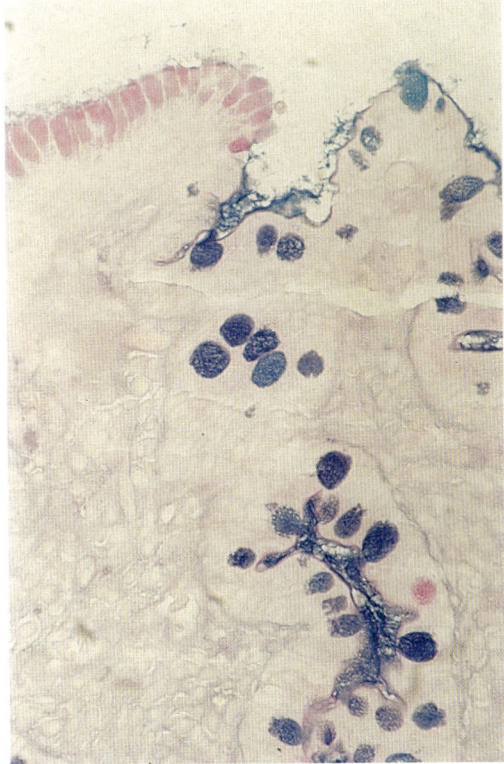

Figure 7–3. Complete metaplasia. Glands are lined by absorptive enterocytes with brush border, alternating with well-formed goblet cells.

Figure 7–4. Complete intestinal metaplasia via high-iron diamine-alcian blue stain. Mucin in goblet cells stains only with alcian blue, pH 2.5, which identifies sialomucins.

crete a mixture of sialo- and sulfomucins, the latter stained dark brown with the high-iron diamine (HID)-alcian blue stain. Foci of complete and incomplete metaplasia frequently coincide. Conventionally, the incomplete classification prevails in such cases. Incomplete-type intestinal metaplasia is frequently found in the vicinity of foci of dysplasia or early carcinomas. While it is generally considered that complete metaplasia does not require special surveillance of patients, incomplete metaplasia may require surveillance of a patient because it increases cancer risk (Filipe et al., 1994; Figs. 7–5 and 7–6).

2 INDEFINITE FOR DYSPLASIA

This category is reserved for cases in which the pathologist is unable to determine whether the lesion being considered represents a neoplastic or nonneoplastic cell (Rid-

dell et al. 1983). This situation may arise because the biopsy material provided is inadequate or because architectural distortion and nuclear atypia are present to the point of creating doubts about the dysplastic nature of the proliferating cells. In such cases, these doubts may be resolved with new, more adequate biopsies or after removing possible sources of cellular hyperproliferation or atypia, such as *Helicobacter pylori* or NSAIDs (Correa et al., 1994; el-Zimaity et al., 1996). In such cases, atypical, tortuous glandular structures are lined by mucus-depleted epithelial cells with large, hyperchromatic nuclei with thickened nuclear membrane and prominent nucleoli. Mitosis may be very prominent.

A similar situation arises in patients with intestinal metaplasia, usually with incomplete components, in which the deep portions of the metaplastic glands are closely

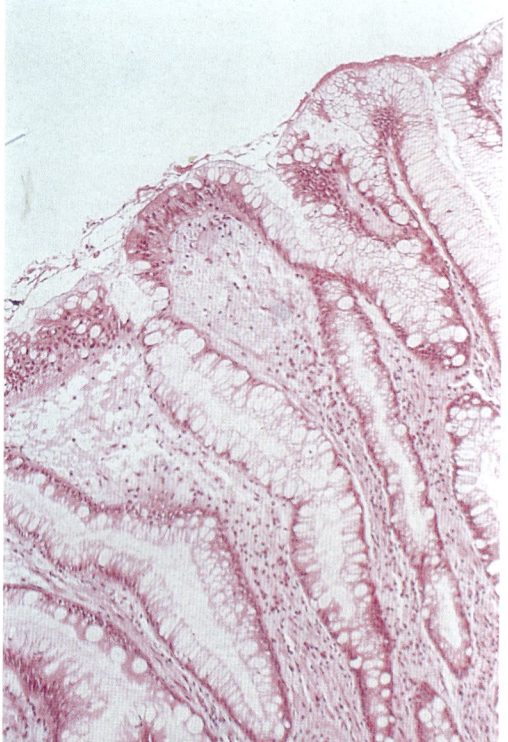

Figure 7–5. Incomplete metaplasia. Glands are lined by goblet cells of different shapes and sizes without brush borders.

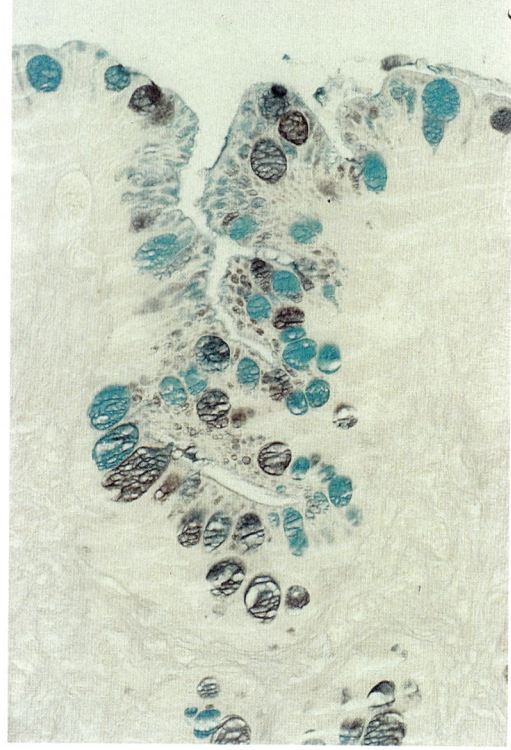

Figure 7–6. Incomplete intestinal metaplasia via high-iron diamine-alcian blue stain. Sialomucins are blue and sulfomucins are dark brown.

packed and lined by large irregular cells with large, hyperchromatic nuclei with frequent mitosis. Some glands show elongated and psuedostratified nuclei. Such lesions have been called "hyperplastic" or "hyperproliferative" or "deep" metaplasia (You et al., 1993). The excessive proliferative activity of such glands contrasts with the normal nuclei, which are basal, small, and normochromatic (Figs. 7–7 to 7–9).

3 DYSPLASIA

The term "dysplasia" has been used in publications referring to gastric precancerous lesions in Japan (Nagayo, 1981) and in Western countries (Morson et al., 1980). It is not part of the official Japanese Classification (Japanese Classification of Gastric Carcinoma (Japanese Research Society for Gastric Cancer) 1995). It was adopted by a World Health Organization (WHO) expert committee and has become more accepted

in recent publications (Morson et al., 1980; Riddell, 1996; Rugge et al., 1994). In this chapter it refers to phenotypically neoplastic epithelium confined to glandular structures inside the basement membrane. When such proliferation forms a discrete macro-

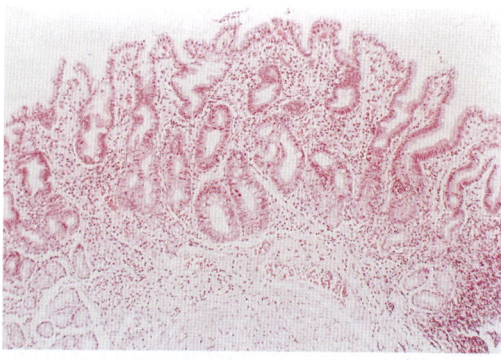

Figure 7–7. Indefinite for dysplasia. Multifocal atrophic gastritis with intestinal metaplasia. The deep glands display hyperproliferation.

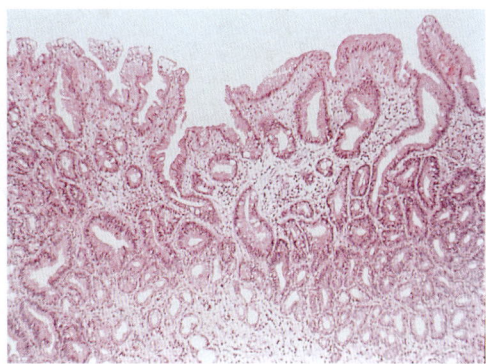

Figure 7–8. Indefinite for dysplasia. Multifocal atrophic gastritis with intestinal metaplasia. The deep metaplastic glands are closely packed and hyperproliferative.

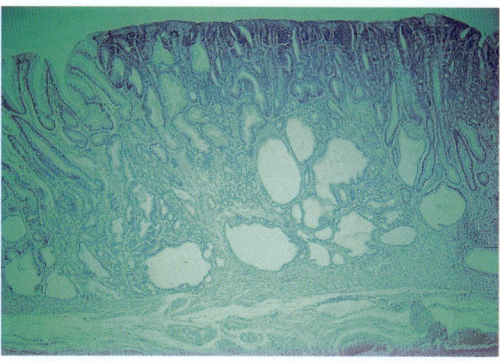

Figure 7–10. Low-grade dysplasia covering the surface (flat mucosa). Cystically dilated glands are in the deep position. Incomplete metaplasia appears on the side.

scopic mass that protrudes into the lumen it is called "adenoma." In both situations it should be divided in two subcategories: low grade and high grade. This dichotomy has been followed for the classification of dysplasia associated with ulcerative colitis, in which case management guidelines have been adopted for each category (Riddell et al., 1983). In general, high-grade dysplasia is equivalent to the carcinoma *in situ* category of squamous epithelia and has therapeutic implications of resection.

Although low-grade gastric dysplasia is not an absolute indicator for resection, the management guidelines are less clear (Weinstein and Goldstein, 1994). In low-grade dysplasia, multiple, small, round glandular structures are identified that resemble adenomatous polyps of the colon. The dysplastic glands are lined by crowded, elongated cells with large, hyperchromatic nuclei, which have been compared with cigar packs. The nuclei are pseudostratified. The secretion of mucins is minimal to none. The dysplastic cells extend

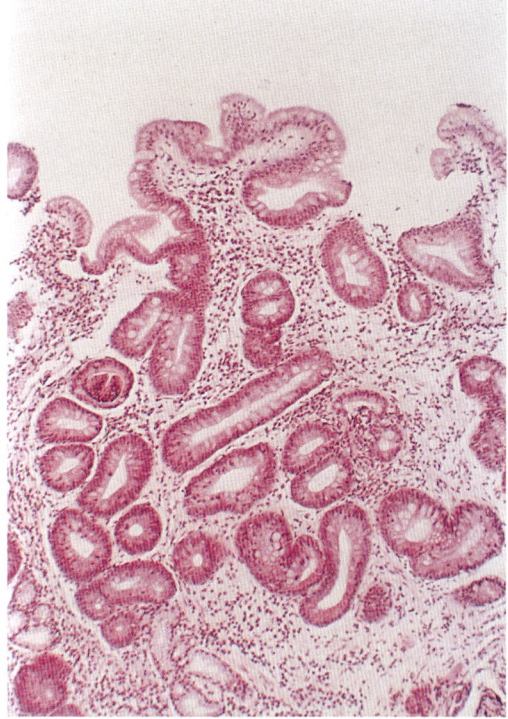

Figure 7–9. Indefinite for dysplasia. Deep metaplastic glands show hyperproliferation.

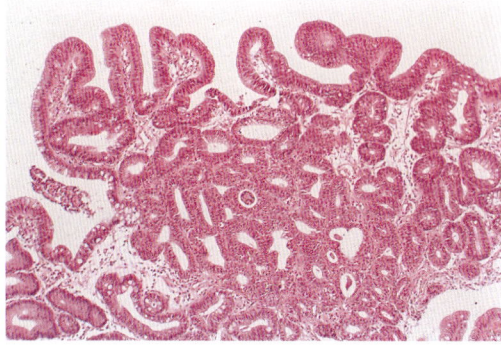

Figure 7–11. Low-grade dysplasia. Closely packed glands have enlarged hyperchromatic nuclei extending to the surface epithelium.

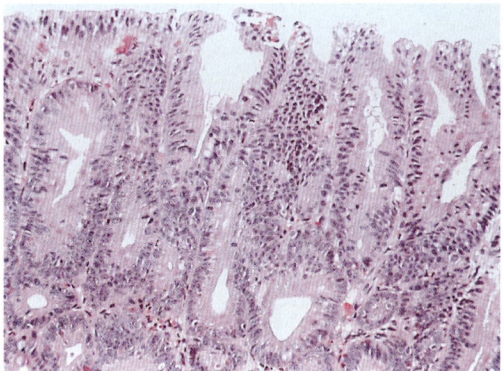

Figure 7–12. Low-grade dysplasia. Closely packed glands are lined by hyperchromatic, elongated nuclei extending to the surface epithelium.

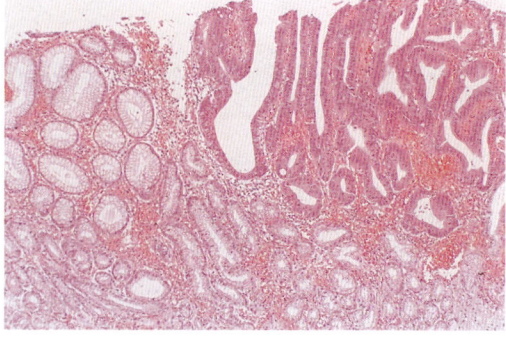

Figure 7–14. High-grade dysplasia. Irregularly shaped glands are lined by enlarged hyperchromatic nuclei extending to the surface. Incomplete metaplasia is on one side.

to the surface epithelium, a feature absent in non-neoplastic proliferations (Figs. 7–10 to 7–13). In high-grade dysplasia, the tubular structures are irregular in shape, with thick membrane and prominent amphophilic nucleoli (Figs. 7–14 to 7–19). No degree of stromal invasion is allowed in this category. For Western pathologists invasion is the hallmark of carcinoma.

4 SUSPICIOUS FOR INVASION

This category recognizes the fact that in some specimens clearly neoplastic epithelium is present but invasion cannot be clearly identified. In Japan it may lead to endoscopic resection, whereas in the West it is an indication for additional biopsies. It is becoming clearer, however, that these require resection of the lesion, since it is not reversible according to the best present knowledge.

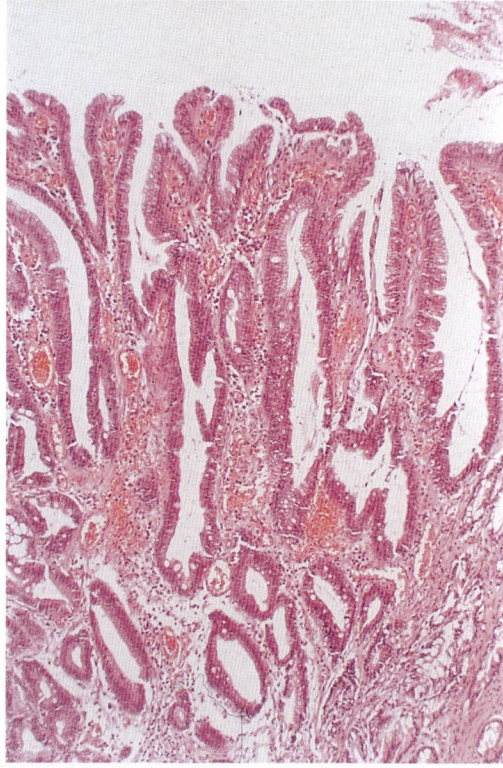

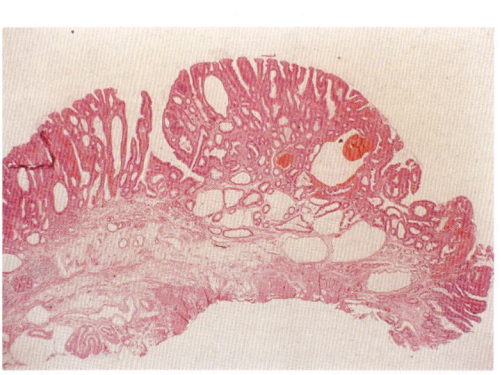

Figure 7–13. Low-grade dysplasia. Polypoid formation projects into the lumen of the stomach.

Figure 7–15. High-grade dysplasia. Irregular glands reach the surface.

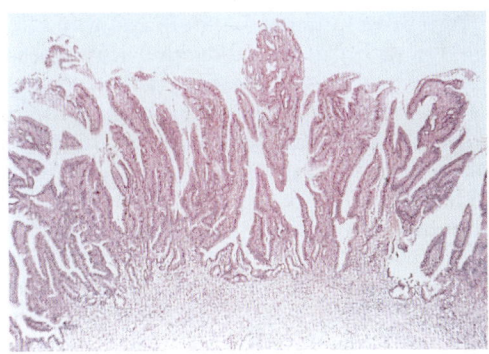

Figure 7–16. High-grade dysplasia. The original mucosa is totally replaced by irregular glands with papillary formations, and there is loss of polarity. The term "carcinoma *in situ*" has occasionally been used for this lesion.

5 INVASIVE CARCINOMA

This category requires no further description. Surgical resection is indicated (Fig. 7–20).

MOLECULAR EVENTS

Recent advances in molecular dissection of preneoplastic and neoplastic lesions of the stomach indicate that an accumulation of genetic and epigenetic alterations in oncogenes, tumor suppressor genes, cell cycle regulators, cell adhesion molecules, and telomere and telomerase as well as genetic instability at several microsatellite foci determines the multistep process of human

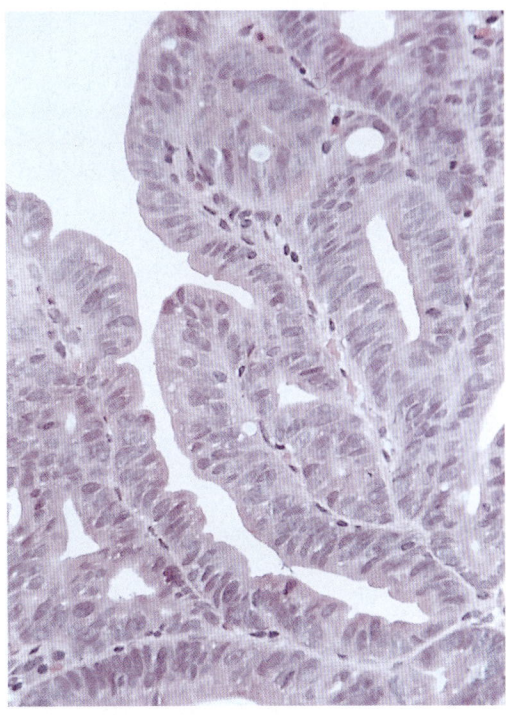

Figure 7–18. High-grade dysplasia showing architectural and cellular atypia.

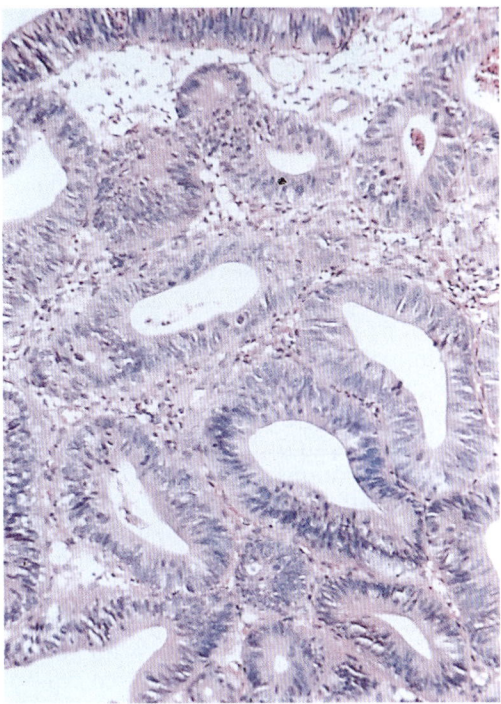

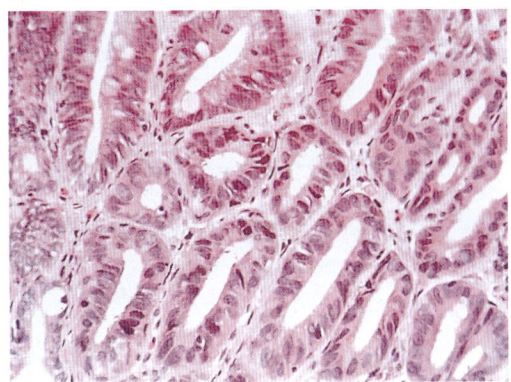

Figure 7–17. High-grade dysplasia. Glands are lined by enlarged, irregular, hyperchromatin nuclei with loss of polarity.

Figure 7–19. High-grade dysplasia showing irregular glandular architecture and dysplastic nuclei.

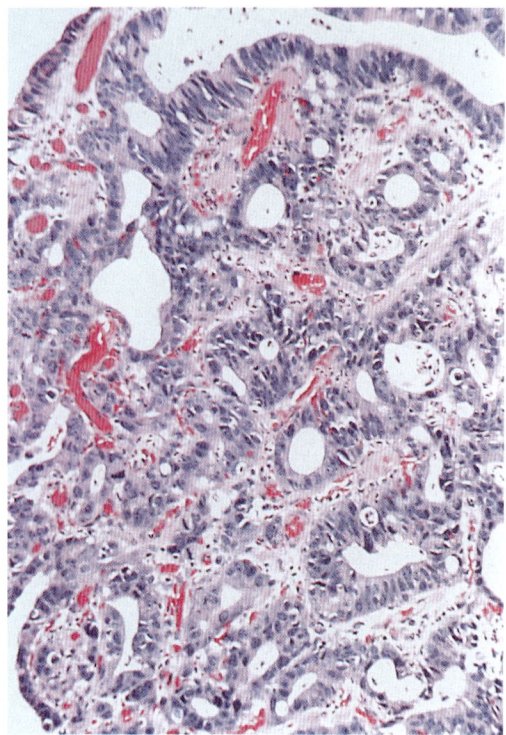

Figure 7–20. Invasive carcinoma. Dysplastic glands invade the stroma.

stomach carcinogenesis. The scenario of mulitple changes found in gastric carcinoma differs depending on the two histological types, which strongly suggests that different genetic pathways exist for well-differentiated or intestinal-type and poorly differentiated or diffuse-type gastric cancers.

Interestingly, at least 30% of incomplete intestinal metaplasia which is associated with hyperplasia of hTERT-expressed stem cells, contain reduced telomere, an altered microsatellite at the DIS191 locus, abnormal CD44 transcripts containing intron 9, DNA hypermethylation at D17S5 locus, PS2 loss, and p53 mutations, followed by abnormal gland formation with dysplasia. All of these epigenetic and genetic alterations are common events in intestinal-type or well-differentiated adenocarcinoma. We propose here a new concept of gastric dysplasia—metaplastic dysplasia—which shares the above molecular events with the intestinal type of gastric carcinoma. Metaplastic dysplasia may be viewed as a bud of intestinal type gastric cancer at genetic and epigenetic levels.

Well-differentiated adenocarcinoma of the stomach can be subdivided into intestinal type and gastric foveolar type according to the phenotypic characteristics of tumor cells. All the cancers with loss of heterozygosity (LOH) of the *p73* gene, which is detected in 30% of gastric cancer, exhibit phenotypes of gastric foveolar epithelium and express PS2. In contrast with a high frequency of p53 mutations in the intestinal type, p53 abnormalities are less common (only 25%) in the foveolar type. Alteration in the *p73* gene may confer the genesis of foveolar-type gastric carcinoma.

EARLY GASTRIC CANCER

Early gastric cancer (EGC) is defined as a carcinoma that is confined to the mucosa (intramucosal cancer) or to the mucosa and submucosa (submucosal cancer) regardless of lymph node metastasis. According to the macroscopic classification of the Japan Society for Gastroenterological Endoscopy (1962), early gastric cancer is divided into three main types as shown in Figure 7–21.

Type I is the protruded type, which may be polypoid, nodular, or villous. *Type II* is the superficial type, which is subdivided into three variants: IIa is the elevated type, which is slightly raised above the surrounding mucosa; *IIb* is the flat type, which shows no obvious alterations macroscopically; and *IIc* is the depressed type, which is slightly de-

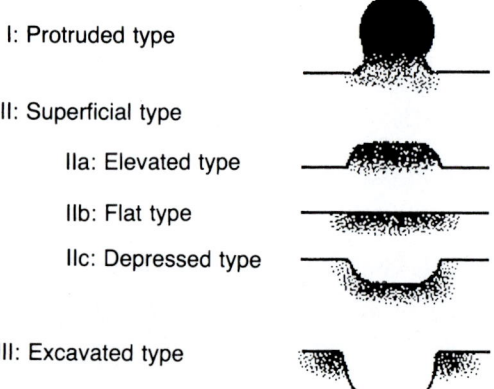

I: Protruded type

II: Superficial type

    IIa: Elevated type

    IIb: Flat type

    IIc: Depressed type

III: Excavated type

Figure 7–21. Schematic representation of the Japanese classification of early gastric cancer.

Table 7–2. Five-Year Survival Rates of Patients with Gastric Carcinoma According to TNM Stage and Periods

TNM stage	1962–71 %	(n)	1972–81 %	(n)	1982–91 %	(n)	Overall %	(n)
Ia	89.0	(420)	92.0	(638)	92.4	(1103)	91.5	(2161)
Ib	80.0	(205)	84.3	(210)	89.8	(266)	84.6	(681)
II	61.7	(280)	72.4	(239)	76.2	(245)	69.2	(764)
IIIa	39.6	(268)	56.4	(234)	58.9	(208)	50.4	(710)
IIIb	27.6	(279)	29.3	(229)	36.5	(189)	30.6	(697)
IV	2.2	(590)	7.7	(428)	7.5	(449)	5.4	(1467)
Total	44.3	(2049)	54.9	(2140)	65.9	(2541)	55.4	(6730)

The figures in parentheses are the number of patients (at the National Cancer Center Hospital, Tokyo) at each stage. TNM, tumor, necrosis, metastasis.

Reprinted with permission from Sasako M, Sano T, Katai H, Maruyama K. (1997) Radical surgery. In: *Gastric Cancer* (Sugimura T, Sasako M, (eds) Oxford Medical Publications, New York.

pressed or associated with superficial erosion. *Type III* is the excavated type, which shows an ulcer of variable depth surrounded by early gastric cancer.

There is ample justification for the special emphasis given to these superficial tumors because survival of patients after gastrectomy is much higher than that observed when the muscularis propria is invaded.

SURVIVAL

A comparison between Japan and other countries concerning the survival rates for patients with gastric cancer has demonstrated that survival rates in Japan are significantly higher than those in other countries. A large proportion of patients with early gastric cancer receive curative resections in Japan.

Five-year survival rates according to depth of invasion are shown in Table 7–2; survival of patients is significantly influenced by depth of tumor invasion. These rates are closely correlated with stage of cancer as well. In the period 1969–73, the 5-year survival rate was 96.4%, 71.8%, 43.8%, and 13.1% for stages I, II, III, IV, respectively (Kinoshita et al., 1993). In the United States the corresponding survival rate for early cancer is approximately 60% (Bringaze et al., 1986). In Japan, EGC accounts for approximately 40% of the cases; in the United States, such tumors account for approximately 4%. This difference is mainly due to the screening programs in Japan.

Type I or protruding type of EGC is most frequently of the intestinal or well-differentiated variety, and is composed of glandular lumina of irregular shape with varying degrees of nuclear abnormalities. This type frequently arises in adenomatous polyps. They may also arise in hyperplastic polyps, although much less frequently.

Type II carcinomas may be of the well-differentiated intestinal type with irregular but well-structured glands. They can also be of the diffuse type, composed of signet ring cells. Variants of type II may be found in the same patients, which contains variants IIa and IIc.

Type III carcinomas tend to be of the intestinal, well-differentiated type, with well-structured, irregularly shaped neoplastic glands.

Early gastric cancer has been further subdivided into strictly mucosal tumors, which have the best prognosis, and tumors involving the submucosa. The latter have in turn been subdivided into two types according to their growth pattern. *Pattern A* (PEN-A) is characterized by expansive growth of a central mass with extensive destruction of the muscularis mucosae. *Pattern B* (PEN-B) refers to multiple, small, finger-like protrusions that penetrate the muscularis mucosae independently without extensive destruction (fenestration) (Kodama et al., 1983; Okabe, 1972). Pattern A tumors in Japanese series accounted for only 10% of the cases but showed a higher incidence of lymph node metastasis, venous invasion, higher ploidy indexes, and clearly poorer prognosis (Kodama et al., 1983).

REFERENCES

Anonymous. (1995) Japanese Classification of Gastric Carcinoma—Japanese Research Society for Gastric Cancer. First English Edition ed. Tokyo: Kanehara & Co., LDT.

Borchard F, Mittelsaedt A, Stux. (1979) Dysplasien in Resektionmagen und Klassificationprobleme verschiedener Dysplasieformen. Verh Dtsch Ges Pathol 63:250–257.

Bringaze WL, Chappus WC, Cohn I, Correa P. (1986) Early gastric cancer. 21-year experience. Ann Surg 204:103–107.

Correa P. (1980) The epidemiology and pathogenesis of chronic gastritis: three etiologic entities. Front Gastroenterol Res 6:98–108.

Correa P. (1982) Precursor of gastric and esophageal cancer. Cancer 50:2554–2565.

Correa P. (1983) The gastric precancerous process. Cancer Surv 2:437–450.

Correa P. (1988) Chronic gastritis: A clinico-pathological classification. Am J Gastroenterol 83:504–509.

Correa P. (1990) Gastric precancerous process in a high-risk population. Cancer Res 50:4731–4740.

Correa P, Muñoz N, Cuello C, et al. (1989) The role of Camplyobacter pylori in: gastroduodenal disease. In: Progress in Surgical Pathology, Vol. X pp. 191–210. (Fenoglio-Preiser C, ed.) Philadelphia, Field & Wood.

Correa P, Ruiz B, Shi TY, Janney A, et al. (1994) Helicobacter pylori and nucleolar organizer regions in the gastric antral mucosa. Am J Clin Pathol 101:656–660.

Correa P, Tahara E. (1993) Stomach. In: Pathology of Incipient Neoplasia, 2nd ed. (Henson DE, Albores-Saavedra J, eds.) pp. 85–103. W.B. Saunders, Philadelphia.

Dixon MF, Genta RM, Yardley YH, Correa P. (1996) Classification and grading of gastritis: the Updated Sydey System. Am J Surg Pathol 20:1161–1181.

el-Zimaity HM, Genta RM, Graham DY. (1996) Histological features do not define NSAID-induced gastritis. Hum Pathol 27:1348–1354.

Garay J, Bravo JC, Ruiz B, et al. (1999) Change in gastric atrophy after long-term intervention. Gastroenterology 116:A168.

Hansson LE, Nyren O, Hsing A, et al. (1996) The risk of stomach cancer in patients with gastric or duodenal ulcer disease. New Engl J Med 335:242–248.

Heilmann KL, Hopker WW. (1979) Loss of differentiation intestinal metaplasia in cancerous stomachs. A comprehensive morphologic study. Pathol Res Pract 164:249–258.

Higgins PJ, Correa P, Cuello C, Lipkin M. (1984) Fetal antigens in the precursor stages of gastric cancer. Oncology 41:73–76.

Jarvi O, Lauren P. (1951) On the role of heterotopias on the intestinal epithelium in the pathogenesis of gastric cancer. Acta Pathol Microbiol Scand 29:26–44.

Jass JR, Filipe MI. (1979) Variants of intestinal metaplasia associated with gastric carcinoma. Histopathology 3:191–199.

Jass JR, Filipe MI. (1980) Sulphomucins of precancerous lesions of the human stomach. Histopathology 4:271–279.

Kita H, Yoshikawa K, Hirota T, et al. (1984) Surgical treatment of early cancer. Jpn J Clin Oncol 14:283–293.

Kodama Y, Inokuchi K, Soejima K, et al. (1983) Growth patterns and prognosis of early gastric carcinoma. Superficially spreading and penetrating growth patterns. Cancer 51:320–326.

Kupfer C. (1883) Festschrift. Arz Verein Munch. p. 7.

Lambert R. (1972) Chronic gastritis. Digestion 7:83–126.

Lauren P. (1965) The two histological main types of gastric carcinoma: diffuse and so-called intestinal-type carcinoma: an attempt at a histoclinical classification. Acta Pathol Microbiol Scand 64:31–49.

Michalany J. (1959) Metaplasia intestinal da mucosa gastrica. Rev Assoc Med Brasil 5:25–36.

Ming SC. (1977) Gastric carcinoma: a pathologic classification. Cancer 39:2475–2485.

Ming SC. (1984) Pathologic features of gastric dysplasias. In: Precancerous Conditions and Lesions of the Stomach (Ming SC, ed.) Praeger, Philadelphia.

Morson BC, Sobin LH, Grundmann E, et al. (1980) Precancerous conditions and epithelial dysplasia in the stomach. J Clin Pathol 33:711–721.

Nagayo T. (1981) Dysplasia of the gastric mucosa and its relation to the precancerous process. Gann 72:813–823.

Okabe H. (1972) Growth of early gastric cancer. In: Early Gastric Cancer (Murakami T, ed.) Gann Monogr Cancer Res 11:67–79.

Riddell RH, Goldman H, Ransohoff DF, et al. (1983) Dysplasia in inflammatory bowel disease: standardized classification with provisional clinical applications. Hum Pathol 14:931–968.

Rugge M, Correa P, Dixon MF, et al. (2000) Gastric dysplasia: the Padova International Classification. Am J Surg Pathol 24:167–176.

Rugge M, Farinati F, Baffa R, et al. (1994) Gastric epithelial dysplasia in the natural history of gastric cancer: a multicenter prospective follow-up study. Interdisciplinary Group on Gastric Epithelial Dysplasia. Gastroenterology 107:1288–1296.

Schmidt A. (1896) Untersuchungen über des mensliche Magenepithel unter normalen und pathologischen Werhältnissen. Virchows Arch Pathol Anat 143:477–508.

Sipponen P, Seppala K, Varis K, et al. (1981) Intestinal metaplasia with colonic type sulfomucins: its association with gastric carcinoma. Acta Pathol Microbiol Scand 88:217–224.

Strickland RC, Mackay IR. (1973) A reappraisal of the nature and significance of chronic atrophic gastritis. Dig Dis 18:426–440.

Sugimura T, Matsukura N, Sato S. (1982) Intestinal metaplasia of the stomach as precancerous stage. In: Host Factors in Human Carcinogenesis (Armstrong B, Bartsch H, eds.) IARC Sci Publ 39:515–530.

Teglbjaerg S, Nielson HO. (1978) Small intestinal type and colonic type intestinal metaplasia of the human stomach. Acta Pathol Microbiol Scand 86:351–355.

Weinstein WM, Goldstein NS. (1994) Gastric dysplasia and its management. Gastroenterology 107:1543–1545.

You WC, Blot WJ, Li JY, et al. (1993) Precancerous gastric lesions in a population at high risk of stomach cancer. Cancer Res 53:1317–1321.

8

SMALL INTESTINE

Carolyn C. Compton

Compared to other parts of the gastrointestinal tract, neoplasia of the small bowel is relatively rare (Thomas and Sobin, 1995). Estimates of the overall incidence of primary small bowel neoplasms have ranged between 1.7% and 6.5% of all gastrointestinal tumors, most of which are malignant epithelial tumors (Norberg and Emas, 1981). The incidence of asymptomatic small bowel neoplasms discovered incidentally at autopsy is only 0.5% (Darling and Welch, 1959). Because small bowel tumors are so uncommon, many textbooks devoted to cancer in general (Osteen, 1996) or to gastrointestinal cancer in particular (Rustgi, 1995) omit discussion of small bowel carcinoma altogether. The reason for the low incidence of neoplasia in this organ, which represents about 75% of the length of the gastrointestinal tract, is unknown. However, it has been hypothesized to be related to the relative sterility of the small bowel, the fluid nature of the luminal contents, the rapid transit time, and the high level of microsomal enzymes (Chow et al., 1996; Lowenfels, 1973; Wattenberg, 1966).

In addition to their rarity, small bowel tumors are relatively inaccessible for study and are, therefore, typically discovered in advanced rather than incipient stages of development (Goel et al., 1976). Tumors of the duodenum and the terminal ileum are within the reach of the regular endoscope, but in the remainder of the small bowel, access to neoplasms is problematic. Neoplasms of the jejunum and most of the ileum can be visualized nonsurgically only by radiologic techniques using contrast material (i.e., a barium swallow with small bowel "follow-through" or a small bowel "enema" [enteroclysis]) or by endoscopic examination using a "long scope" (Donohue, 1994). Radiologic techniques permit neither direct visualization nor histologic examination of neoplastic lesions. Long-scope examination is never performed routinely and rarely performed at all because the endoscope must be carried through the small bowel by peristalsis, a process that may take 12 to 24 hr. Intraoperative endoscopy, with insertion of the endoscope through an incision in the bowel wall, or surgical excision of a small bowel segment provides the only other direct access to the small bowel mucosa. Given these limitations, the understanding of neoplasia of the small intestine is largely limited to (1) adenomas; (2) hamartomas that occur in the context of the Peutz-Jeghers syndrome; (3) dysplasia in Crohn's disease; (4) dysplasia/neoplasia related to other chronic inflammatory or immunologic disorders of the small intestine; and (5) neuroendocrine neoplasms (carcinoid tumors). Crohn's disease, the Peutz-Jeghers syndrome, and carcinoid tumors may also involve the colon and/or stomach, but the small intestine is the most commonly involved organ in these disorders. This chapter reviews these lesions and discusses the diagnostic criteria by which they are recognized, their differential diagnoses, the factors that predict their biologic behavior, and the genetic basis of their initiation and progression, if known.

ADENOMAS AND THE ADENOMA—CARCINOMA SEQUENCE

Sporadic Adenomas

Among the malignant tumors of the small intestine, adenocarcinoma is the most common (Thomas and Sobin, 1995). Adenocarcinomas of the small bowel account for about 1% of all gastrointestinal tract cancer (Lynch et al., 1989). The incidence of small bowel carcinoma is uniform throughout the world (Lynch et al., 1989). There is a slight predominance in males versus females and Blacks versus Whites (Donohue, 1994). Peak incidence occurs during the sixth decade of life. The most frequent site is the duodenum, followed by the jejunum and the ileum (Lien et al., 1988; Lynch et al., 1989). In particular, the proximal duodenum, the proximal jejunum, and the distal ileum appear to be disproportionately affected (Lien et al., 1988). As in the large bowel, most carcinomas arise from preexisting adenomas that occur sporadically (Perzin and Bridge, 1981). However, adenomas of the small intestine also occur in the context of familial adenomatous polyposis (FAP), the hereditary nonpolyposis colon cancer (HNPCC) syndrome, and the variant syndromes that are genetically related to FAP and HNPCC. Patients with these syndromes represent a unique subset of individuals who are known to have an increased risk of small bowel adenomas and carcinomas and may be studied prospectively for small bowel neoplasia. Therefore, more is known about the pathology and the molecular genetics of the adenoma–carcinoma sequence in the hereditary than the sporadic setting.

Many sporadic adenomas of the small bowel are asymptomatic and are discovered incidentally at autopsy or during surgical exploration or endoscopy performed for other reasons (Perzin and Bridge, 1981). The most common symptomatic small bowel adenomas are those that surround the ampulla of Vater and produce biliary obstruction (Perzin and Bridge, 1981; Ulrich et al.,

1987). Elsewhere in the small bowel, adenomas may produce vague symptoms, such as abdominal pain or nausea, or they may present with symptoms of partial or total bowel obstruction, low-grade bleeding and anemia, or gastrointestinal hemorrhage (Norberg and Emas, 1981; Perzin and Bridge, 1981).

Diagnostic Features and Differential Diagnosis

Pathologically, small bowel adenomas closely resemble their colonic counterparts except that they are more often of villous histologic type (Perzin and Bridge, 1981). Macroscopically, small bowel adenomas may be pedunculated or sessile. As in the colon, small adenomas are usually sessile. However, the cells tend to expand horizontally over the villous scaffold of the normal small bowel mucosa and passively acquire villous architecture during the nascent stages of their development. With increasing size, adenomas may either become rounded and elevated on a broad base or stalk or remain sessile and expand horizontally with growth (Fig. 8–1). Whatever the configuration of the adenoma, the borders are usually sharply defined and easily distinguished, both grossly and microscopically, from the surrounding normal mucosa.

Like colonic adenomas, small bowel adenomas may be subclassified into three histologic types: tubular, tubulovillous, or villous. However, defined criteria for subdividing small bowel adenomas into these categories are completely lacking. Some authors have chosen to use a simplified classification system based on the predominant growth pattern (i.e., villous or nonvillous), subdividing small bowel adenomas into "ordinary" and "papillary" types (Perzin and Bridge, 1981). For the sake of consistency, histologic classification of both small bowel and colonic adenomas by the same criteria are suggested (see Chapter 9, Large Intestine). Tubular adenomas consist entirely of tubular structures that invaginate from a flat surface. Tubulovillous adenomas have varying proportions of tubular and villous components but are less than 75% villous in structure. Adenomas with greater than 75% villous components are categorized as villous adenomas.

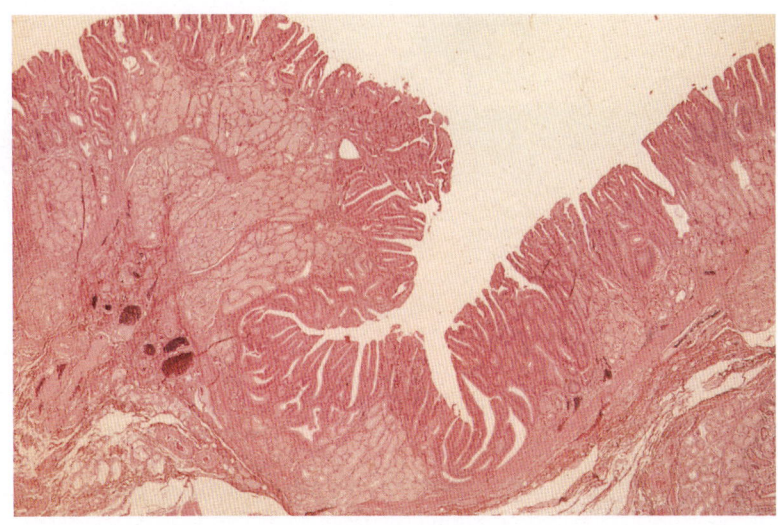

Figure 8–1. Duodenal adenoma showing extensive horizontal growth and villous architecture.

Small bowel adenomas also resemble colonic adenomas cytologically and are composed of epithelial cells with varying degrees of dysplasia ranging to carcinoma *in situ.* The cytologic features that characterize dysplasia include:

- nuclei enlargement (with an increase in the nuclear:cytoplasmic volume ratio)
- nuclear hyperchromasia
- nuclear elongation (typically with the acquisition of a cigar-like shape)
- nuclear relocation farther from the basement membrane
- nuclear crowding and overlapping
- appearance of epithelial stratification
- increased numbers of mitotic figures
- varying amounts of mucin production ranging from abundant to none.

In contrast to the immature cells in the proliferative zone of the normal small bowel mucosal crypts (which they may resemble cytologically), the dysplastic epithelium of the adenoma shows little evidence of maturation. Mitotic figures can be identified throughout the affected mucosa from crypts to villous surface. Evidence of epithelial differentiation is largely limited to mucin production. Paneth cells may be seen within adenomas, but it is unclear whether they are neoplastic or entrapped normal cells.

With increasing degrees of dysplasia, the adenomatous epithelium shows a loss of mucin production and stratification of nuclei into the top halves of the cells. With progression to carcinoma *in situ*, the cells typically acquire more rounded and/or vesicular nuclei with prominent nuclei and display cribiformed growth (Fig. 8–2). In contrast to the colon, however, invasion of the lamina propria is considered to increase the risk of metastasis since the small bowel mucosa is rich in lymphatic vessels. Therefore, in the small bowel, intramucosal carcinoma is staged as an invasive tumor and classified as T1 in the TNM staging system of the American Joint Committee on Cancer and the International Union Against Cancer (Fleming et al., 1997).

The factors that have been shown to be associated with an increased risk of malignancy in small bowel adenomas are similar to those in colonic adenomas. Adenoma size is the primary risk factor. The larger the adenoma, the greater the likelihood that it will contain an invasive carcinoma (Perzin and Bridge, 1981). The average size of adenomas without invasive carcinoma has been found to be 2.7 cm whereas malignant polyps (i.e., adenomas containing invasive carcinoma) average 3.7 cm in size (Perzin and Bridge, 1981). In addition, carcinoma occurs more often in adenomas with a predominantly villous morphology than in adenomas with a predominantly tubular architecture (Perzin and Bridge, 1981).

The differential diagnosis of adenomas is limited. In mucosal biopsies, recently eroded or ulcerated duodenal mucosa showing marked regenerative atypia may be misdiagnosed as adenomatous. Therefore, actively inflamed or ulcerated mucosa should be in-

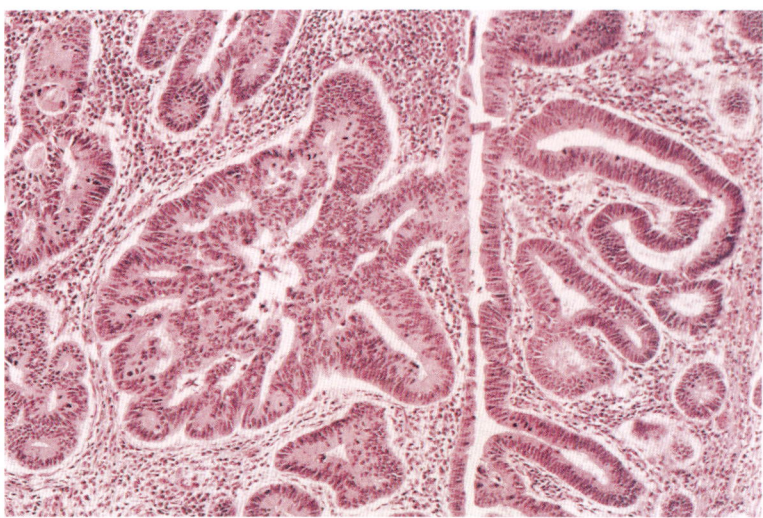

Figure 8–2. Duodenal adenoma showing a focus of cribiformed growth diagnostic of carcinoma *in situ.*

terpreted with caution, and correlation with both the endoscopic appearance of the duodenum and the patient's history (e.g., known peptic ulcer disease) may be helpful. In addition, inflammatory and neoplastic lesions of the ampulla of Vater may be misdiagnosed as duodenal adenomas unless the precise anatomic location of the biopsy is stated by the submitting physician. Intra-ampullary carcinomas arise from preexisting adenomas that are virtually identical to duodenal adenomas histopathologically (Baczako et al., 1985; Talbot et al., 1988). If the lesion is neoplastic (adenomatous or carcinomatous) and is large enough to encompass both the periampullary duodenum as well as the intra-ampullary mucosa, the origin of the process may be impossible to determine. Ultimately, however, this may be a moot point, since tumors of this type are all treated and staged as carcinomas of the ampulla of Vater (Braasch and Camer, 1975; Fleming et al., 1997; Wise et al., 1976).

Polypoid lesions that may mimic adenomas grossly include leiomyomas, lipomas, lymphoid polyps, inflammatory fibroid polyps, and mucosal hamartomas. All but the latter are primarily submucosal lesions and require excision rather than mucosal biopsy for diagnosis. On biopsy, the overlying mucosa may be normal to inflamed or ulcerated but architecturally normal. In contrast, small bowel hamartomas may closely resemble adenomas both grossly and microscopically. When they occur in the context of a hamartomatous polyp syndrome such as the Peutz-Jeghers syndrome or juvenile polyposis, they may develop epithelial dysplasia and become virtually indistinguishable from adenomas. Sporadic hamartomas also may resemble adenomas when eroded or inflamed and showing reactive or regenerative epithelial atypia. In particular, sporadic Peutz-Jeghers polyps with their lobulated gross configuration and papillary microstructure may very closely mimic adenomas even when uninflamed and uneroded.

INHERITED SYNDROMES THAT PREDISPOSE TO SMALL BOWEL ADENOMA FORMATION

Several inherited disorders predispose to small intestinal adenomas and carcinomas: FAP and its variant, Gardner's syndrome, attenuated familial adenomatous polyposis (AFAP), and HNPCC (Lynch and Lynch, 1998). The primary manifestation of all of these syndromes is a marked predisposition to the formation of colorectal adenomas and, ultimately, to the development of colorectal cancer (see Chapter 9, Large Intestine). However, these syndromes are also associated with a significantly increased risk of neoplasia in the small intestine. Neither the gross nor the microscopic features of syndrome-related small bowel neoplasms are distinctive; pathologically, they resemble sporadic neoplasms. In contrast to sporadic tumors of the small bowel, they usually occur in association with synchronous or metachronous malignancies in other organs, particularly the colon (Lynch et al., 1989; Rustgi, 1994).

Familial Adenomatous Polyposis and Its Variants

In *FAP* and its phenotypic variant known as *Gardner's syndrome,* small bowel adenocarcinomas arise in about 2% to 4% of cases (Ryan, 1996). It has been estimated that about 90% of patients with these syndromes develop small intestinal adenomas, most commonly in the duodenum (Ryan, 1996). The syndromes are caused by germline mutations of the adenomatous polyposis coli (APC) gene, typically involving the last exon of the gene (exon 15) (Kinzler and Vogelstein, 1996; Lynch and Lynch, 1998). Other variant forms of FAP, known as *attenuated FAP* because the onset of adenomas and of carcinomas is delayed compared to classical FAP or Gardner's syndrome, are also caused by APC gene mutation, but the mutations are in another region of the gene, usually in exon 1. Gardner's syndrome, classical FAP, and AFAP all predispose to adenoma formation and, ultimately, to carcinoma of the small bowel, but the predisposition is much reduced compared to that in the colon. In all of these syndromes, the most common small bowel manifestations are periampullary duodenal adenomas and periampullary carcinomas (Lynch and Lynch, 1998).

The APC gene is a tumor suppressor gene located on chromosome 5q. It encodes a cytoplasmic protein that is necessary for activation of programmed cell death (apoptosis) and performs an essential role in maintaining cellular growth control in the intestine (Bodmar et al., 1987). As is the case with most tumor suppressor gene mutations, the APC gene mutation is inactivating but recessive. Therefore, it is silent until the other (normal) allele is deleted from the chromosome, a phenomenon known as *loss of heterozygosity* (LOH) at chromosome 5q. With loss of APC gene function in a proliferating cell and subsequent loss of apoptosis among its progeny, a permanent imbalance in cell division over cell death ensues and the epithelium becomes *hyperproliferative.* This is the first step in the multistep process of carcinogenesis along the *tumor suppressor gene pathway* that ultimately involves additional mutations in other tumor suppressor genes and in proto-oncogenes. For colon cancer, the sequence of specific genetic events in the multistep progression from incipient neoplasia through invasive carcinoma has been found to be similar in both inherited and sporadic disease. Although much less is known about the genetic progression of neoplasia in the small bowel in either FAP or sporadic disease, preliminary data suggest that the mechanisms may not be comparable. Specifically, although mutations in K-*ras* and *p53* are common, allelic losses of the APC gene are rare in sporadic small bowel adenomas and carcinomas (Rashid and Hamilton, 1997). This suggests that the molecular alterations underlying tumorigenesis of sporadic small bowel cancers may differ significantly from those of sporadic large bowel cancers and from FAP-related small bowel cancers as well.

Hereditary Nonpolyposis Colon Cancer Syndrome

The other major syndrome of inherited cancer predisposition that poses an increased risk of small bowel neoplasia is the *HNPCC syndrome,* also known as the *Warthin-Lynch syndrome* or *Lynch syndrome* (Lynch and Lynch, 1998; Ponz de Leon, 1996). The number of adenomas that develop in this syndrome is far less compared to that in the FAP syndrome but may be comparable to the amount in the AFAP syndrome. In the HNPCC syndrome, the initiating mutation involves one of the DNA mismatch repair genes (Lynch and Lynch, 1998; Lynch and Smyrk, 1996; Marra and Boland, 1996). Mutation of any one of the genes in the DNA mismatch repair system completely destroys the ability to correct accidental mutations acquired through mistakes in DNA synthesis occurring during mitosis. Abrogation of the function of a DNA repair gene typically requires an inactivating mutation in each allele. In HNPCC, one of these mutations is inherited and the other is acquired. DNA repair-deficient cells accumulate mutations at a very rapid rate, leading to a 1000-fold increase in the frequency of mutations compared to repair-proficient cells (Lynch and Smyrk, 1996). The rapid accumulation of mutations leads to the generation of neoplasms. This mechanism of tumorigenesis is known as the *mutator pathway*, and tumors that arise via this pathway are characterized as *replication error positive*. However, the order of subsequent genetic events by which tumor progression proceeds are not yet fully elucidated.

The HNPCC syndrome predisposes to small bowel carcinoma at a relatively early age, typically a decade earlier than in sporadic disease (Lynch et al., 1989). As in FAP and AFAP, the carcinomas arise from preexisting adenomas (Lynch et al., 1989). It is not yet clear whether the small bowel carcinomas arising in this syndrome have a better prognosis compared to their sporadic or FAP-associated counterparts (Lynch et al., 1989). In one series, about 13% of sporadic small bowel carcinomas were found to be replication error positive (Rashid and Hamilton, 1997).

HAMARTOMAS AND THE DYSPLASIA-CARCINOMA SEQUENCE: THE PEUTZ-JEGHERS SYNDROME

The *Peutz-Jeghers syndrome* (PJS) is an autosomal dominant inherited syndrome of gastrointestinal hamartomas polyposis. In PJS, the mucosal hamartomas are predominantly small intestinal but also occur in the stomach, colon, and rectum, and the entire gastrointestinal tract is at risk for malignancy (Haggitt and Reid, 1986; Lynch and Lynch, 1998). The hamartomatous polyps that characterize PJS are not considered neoplastic, but it is now clear that they may be the precursors of neoplasms. Like all hamartomas, the polyps of PJS are composed of epithelial cells that are cytologically normal and are histologically appropriate for the region of the bowel in which the polyp resides. However, the epithelium may become dysplastic (i.e., neoplastic), and tumor progression through increasing degrees of dysplasia to carcinoma may occur (Haggitt and Reid, 1986; Luk, 1995; Lynch and Lynch, 1998; Perzin and Bridge, 1982).

In addition to intestinal mucosal hamartomas, PJS is characterized by melanin spots resembling freckles on the lips, nose, hands, feet, and the buccal mucosa (Haggitt and Reid, 1986; Luk, 1995). The mucocutaneous pigmentation generally develops in childhood, and the dermal spots may fade with age. Data from polyposis registries indicate that PJS is only about 10% as common as FAP (Luk, 1995). Patients usually present in the third decade with symptoms of small bowel obstruction, rectal bleeding, or the passage of an autoamputated polyp per rectum (Burdick and Prior, 1982). Reports of the prevalence of cancer in patients with PJS have ranged from 2% to 50% (Giardiello et al., 1987; Haggitt and Reid, 1986). It has been estimated that that the relative risk of the development of cancer in patients with PJS is 18-fold greater than that expected in the general population (Giardiello et al., 1987). The risk of cancer begins to increase in the second decade and is not limited to cancers of the gastrointestinal tract. Although duodenal and gastric antral carcinomas are most frequent, PJS-associated malignancies also include other carcinomas of the small intestine and carcinomas of the colon, breast, pancreas, biliary tree, and gallbladder. In addition, a distinctive ovarian tumor known as a sex cord tumor with annular tubules occurs in almost all female patients, and males with PJS may develop Sertoli cell testicular tumors (Luk, 1995; Scully, 1970).

The appearance of Peutz-Jeghers polyps is highly distinctive, both grossly and microscopically. Grossly, they appear highly lobulated and are often described as "hydra-headed." Microscopically, they are composed of highly branched, tightly packed glands with scanty intervening stroma that is rich in smooth muscle (Fig. 8–3). Highly arborized bundles of smooth muscle bundles form the central core of the polyp, and slender fascicles typically extend to the surface of polyp fronds. The glands may show irregular dilatation but do not typically form gross cysts.

Peutz-Jeghers polyps of the small intestine are prone to infarction, possibly related to intestinal intussusception, which they often cause (Shepherd et al., 1987). With healing of an infarcted polyp, benign glandular components may become entrapped within the submucosa, muscularis, and/or subserosa of the subjacent intestinal wall. This phenomenon, known variably as *glandular entrapment*, *epithelial misplacement*, or *pseudoinvasion*, occurs in about 10% of small intestinal Peutz-Jeghers polyps (Shepherd et al., 1987). It

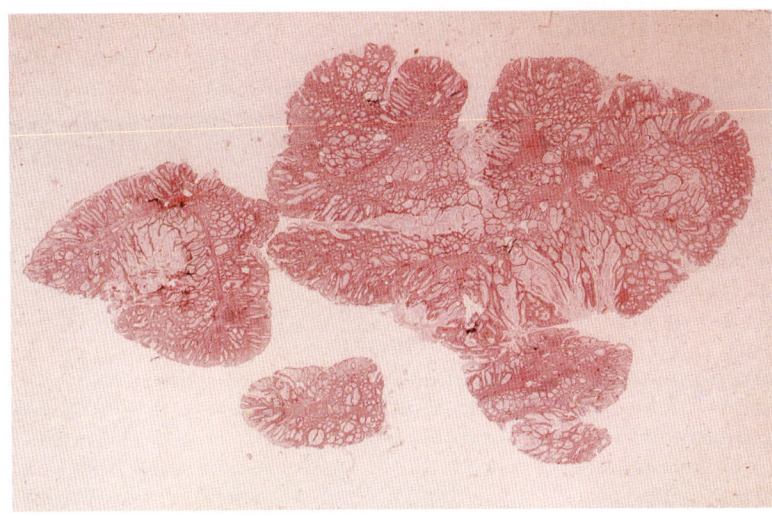

Figure 8–3. Typical Peutz-Jeghers polyp with a lobulated "hydra-headed" that is composed of tightly picked, highly branched glands and bands of smooth muscle.

represents a potential diagnostic pitfall since it may be misinterpreted as invasive carcinoma. It is differentiated from invasive carcinoma by the absence of a desmoplastic reaction to be misplaced glands and by the complete lack of neoplastic features within the glandular epithelium. Inflammation and reactive hyperplasia may be seen, but no dysplastic changes are present (Fig. 8–4). Most of the polyps in which this occurs are larger than 3 cm in diameter, but epithelial misplacement has been reported in polyps as small as 1.6 cm (Shepherd et al., 1987). When glandular entrapment occurs in the subserosa, it may produce cysts that are grossly visible, calcification, and/or hemosiderin deposition related to gland rupture.

True dysplastic change within Peutz-Jeghers polyps produces cytologic findings identical to those of adenomas (see above). When the dysplasia is focal or multifocal and the morphology of the polyp is otherwise characteristic of a Peutz-Jeghers hamartoma, the diagnosis of neoplastic transformation may be relatively straightforward (Perzin and Bridge, 1982; Yaguchi et al., 1982). This is true of most small bowel polyps in which dysplasia has been reported with or without an associated carcinoma (Perzin and Bridge, 1982). If the dysplasia is extensive, differen-

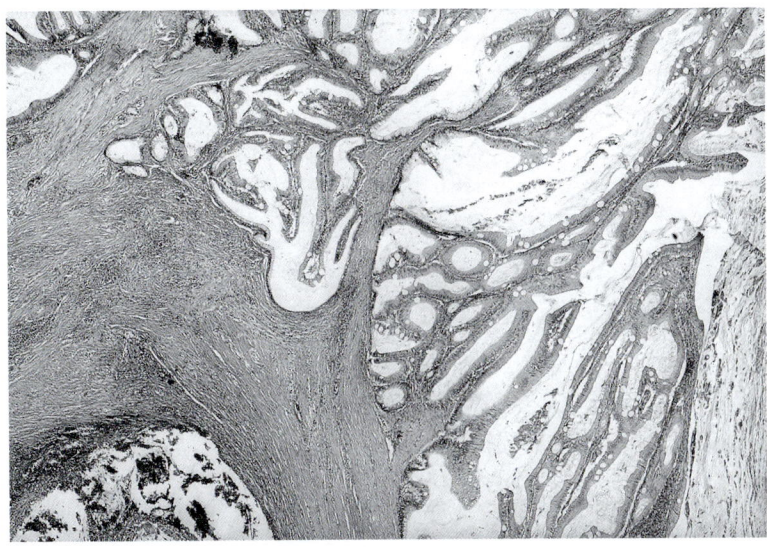

Figure 8–4. Glandular entrapment within the wall of the bowel wall subjacent to an infarcted Peutz-Jeghers polyp shows glands with cytologically normal epithelium and their own scanty lamina propria.

tiation from an adenoma may be difficult on a histologic basis alone. However, since adenomas are rare in the small bowel (see above), polyps with adenomatous features in patients with PJS should be regarded as dysplastic hamartomas until proven otherwise. For any given polyp, the differential diagnosis between a dysplastic hamartoma and an adenoma may be moot, since both are treated in the same fashion. The degree of dysplasia in a Peutz-Jeghers polyp may be graded (e.g., low- or high-grade), and the entire polyp should be examined microscopically for evidence of malignancy. As in small bowel adenomas, *in situ* carcinoma is cured by complete polypectomy, but invasive carcinoma of any extent requires further therapy, usually segmental bowel resection.

The genetic basis of PJS is a germline mutation of the serine/threonine kinase 11 (STK11) gene located on chromosome 19p (Amos et al., 1997; Hemminki et al., 1997; Jenne et al., 1998; Mehenni et al., 1997; Nakagawa et al., 1998). The manifestations of the disease are produced when a defect in the second allele is acquired in a somatic cell (Jenne et al., 1998). At present, the role of this gene in either hamartoma formation or neoplastic transformation of Peutz-Jeghers polyps is not well understood. Somatic mutations in the STK11 gene accompanied by loss of heterozygosity at 19p have been reported in sporadic left-sided colorectal carcinomas and some left-sided adenomas with high-grade dysplasia (Dong et al., 1998). Thus, it is hypothesized that STK11 is a tumor suppressor gene that, even in individuals who do not have PJS, it may play an important role in gastrointestinal carcinogenesis.

CHRONIC ENTERITIS AND INCIPIENT NEOPLASIA: CROHN'S DISEASE AND CELIAC DISEASE

Two chronic inflammatory diseases of the small intestine, *Crohn's disease* and *celiac disease*, are associated with a greatly increased risk of carcinoma. In both of these disorders, carcinomas arise primarily within the chronically inflamed mucosa of the affected segment of bowel in long-standing disease. In Crohn's disease, the precursor lesion is dys-

plasia in flat mucosa identical to that in ulcerative colitis (see chapter 9, Large Intestine). In celiac disease, little is known about the incipient stages of the associated neoplasms.

DYSPLASIA (NEOPLASIA) IN CROHN'S DISEASE

Prevalence, Risk Factors, and Detection

Jejunal carcinoma was the first Crohn's disease–associated small bowel malignancy to be reported (Ginsburg et al., 1956). Since then, the increased risk of small bowel and colonic carcinoma associated with Crohn's disease has been well defined. Estimates of the relative risk of cancer in small bowel Crohn's disease have varied widely, from 6- to 320-fold greater than that of the general population, whereas the risk of cancer in colonic Crohn's disease is estimated to be increased 4- to 20-fold (Greenstein et al., 1980, 1981; Gyde et al., 1980; Michelassi et al., 1993; Shorter, 1983; Weedon et al., 1973). Prevalence of carcinoma in Crohn's disease has been estimated to be 0.13% to 0.60% for small bowel carcinoma and 0.3.4% to 1.8% for colorectal cancer (Korelitz, 1983; Michelassi et al., 1993). In Crohn's disease, the anatomic distribution of small bowel malignancies varies from that of sporadic small bowel cancer in the general population in that the ileum is the most commonly affected site. This corresponds to the anatomic distribution of the inflammatory injury in Crohn's disease (Michelassi et al., 1993; Senay et al., 1989). However, tumors may arise in uninflamed bowel segments and do so more often in Crohn's disease than in ulcerative colitis (Tanaka and Riddell, 1990). In further contrast to sporadic small bowel cancer, carcinoma in Crohn's disease may be multifocal in as many as 20% of cases (Michelassi et al., 1993; Richards et al., 1989).

The average age of diagnosis of small bowel carcinoma is 48 years, and males are affected about three times more often than females even though Crohn's disease itself affects both sexes equally (Michelassi et al., 1993; Tanaka and Riddell, 1990). Duration of disease is an important risk factor (Cooper et al., 1984; Tanaka and Riddell, 1990). The average interval between diagnosis of Crohn's disease and the discovery of carcinoma is about 19 years, but ranges of 0 to 47 years have been reported (Cooper et al., 1984; Michelassi et al., 1993). In some patients, carcinoma may be discovered at the time of presentation with the first attack of ileitis (Cooper et al., 1984). In one series, a significant association between prolonged disease treatment with the immunosuppressive agent 6-mercaptopurine and the development of small bowel cancer has been demonstrated (Lashner, 1992), but this remains to be substantiated. Intestinal bypass surgery also appears to increase the risk of cancer in the bypassed bowel segment (Cooper et al., 1984; Michelassi et al., 1993; Senay et al., 1989).

The poor prognosis that is associated with Crohn's disease–related small bowel carcinoma is directly related to the extreme difficulty in achieving early diagnosis (Michelassi et al., 1993; Senay et al., 1989). Incipient neoplasia of the small bowel cannot be detected radiologically or endoscopically, and there are no biopsy surveillance programs for small intestinal neoplasia in Crohn's disease. Even advanced small bowel malignancies with transmural involvement and intestinal stenosis are often misinterpreted as benign disease (i.e., severe inflammatory involvement) (Cuvelier et al., 1989; Michelassi et al., 1993). Thus, most Crohn's disease–associated cancers are already of advanced stage at the time of diagnosis. In addition, some series of Crohn's

disease–associated small bowel carcinomas have included an exceptionally high proportion of poorly differentiated (high-grade) tumors (Petras et al., 1987).

Diagnostic Features

Dysplastic changes identical to those occurring in the colon in ulcerative colitis characterize the incipient stages of neoplasia in Crohn's disease (Bearzi and Ranaldi, 1985; Cuvelier et al., 1989; Perzin et al., 1984; Petras et al., 1987; Richards et al., 1989; Simpson et al., 1981). All of the cytologic changes that define dysplasia in adenomas (see above), ranging from low-grade (Fig. 8–5) to high-grade (Fig. 8–6) to carcinoma *in situ*, may be seen in mucosal dysplasia in Crohn's disease (Petras et al., 1987; Rubio et al., 1991; Simpson et al., 1981). As in adenomas, the dysplastic nuclei in low-grade dysplasia are confined to the basal halves of the cells and stratify into the luminal halves in high grade dysplasia. Carcinoma *in situ* is recognized either by epithelial cell pleomorphism, vesicular nuclear changes, atypical mitotic figures, intraepithelial apoptosis, and/or cribriform growth. In small bowel resection specimens, these changes are typically seen in the mucosa adjacent to resected carcinomas, but they may also be seen in mucosa remote from an infiltrating carcinoma (Petras et al., 1987; Rubio et al., 1991; Simpson et al., 1981; Tanaka and Riddell, 1990). Overall, the distribution and extent of dysplasia in resection specimens of small bowel

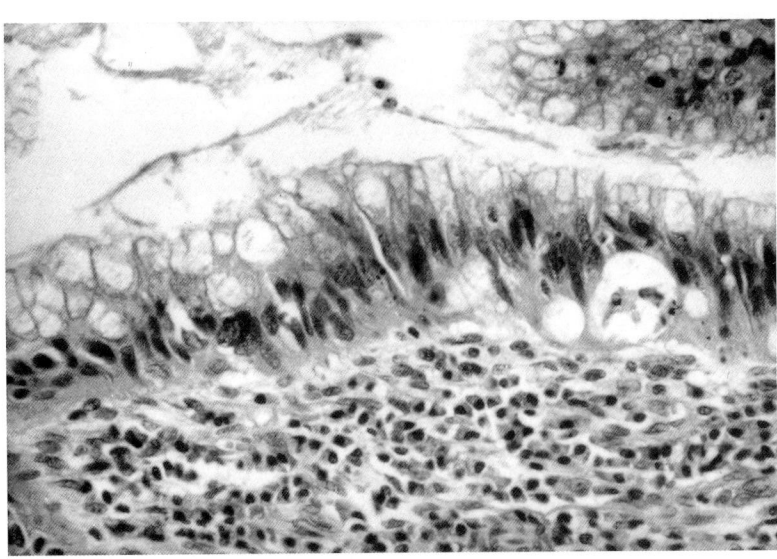

Figure 8–5. Low-grade dysplasia in Crohn's disease showing dysplastic nuclei (and focal apoptotic bodies) confined to the lower half of the epithelium.

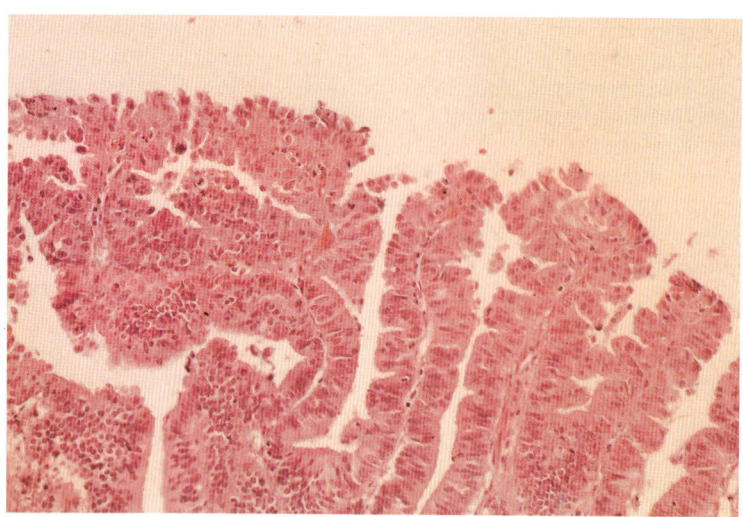

Figure 8–6. High-grade dysplasia in Crohn's disease showing dysplastic nuclei stratifying into the cell apices.

Crohn's disease varies widely from focal to multifocal to diffuse (Fig. 8–7) within a given bowel region (Tanaka and Riddell, 1990).

Genetic Basis of Dysplasia in Crohn's Disease

At present, little is known about the genetic alterations of the dysplasia–carcinoma sequence in Crohn's disease. Preliminary data have suggested that mutations of the *p53* tumor suppressor gene are more common in Crohn's disease–associated cancers than in sporadic small bowel carcinomas but that APC and deleted in colon cancer (DCC) gene mutations are rare in both (Rashid and Hamilton, 1997). Replication error positivity occurs with the same frequency (about 15%) in Crohn's disease–associated cancers and sporadic cancers of the small bowel (Rashid and Hamilton, 1997).

CELIAC DISEASE

Celiac disease is associated with a markedly elevated risk of adenocarcinoma of the small intestinal, primarily the proximal jejunum and the duodenum (Bruno et al., 1997). The relative risk of small bowel cancer among patients with celiac disease has been estimated to be about 80- to 85-fold greater than that

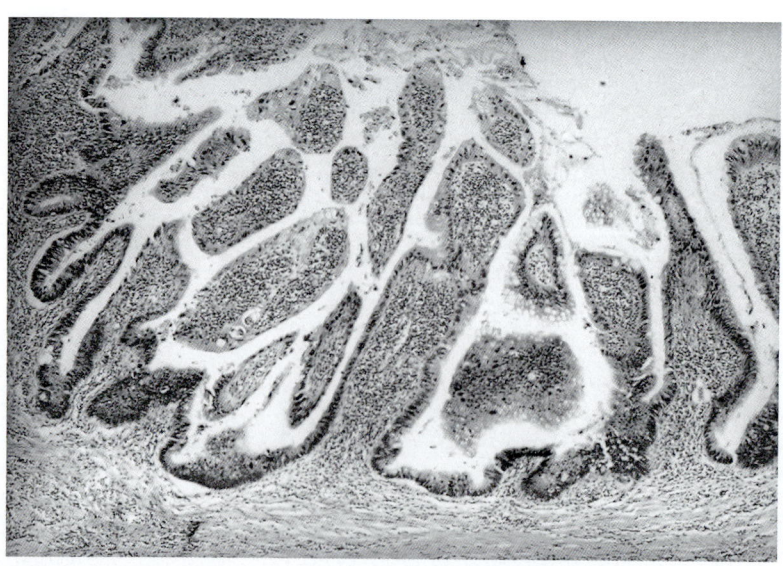

Figure 8–7. Regional dysplasia in Crohn's disease characterized by confluent diffuse epithelial dysplasia.

of the general population (Ryan 1996; Swinson et al., 1983). Thus, the risk of small bowel cancer among patients with celiac disease can be equated with the risk of colon cancer in the general population (Swinson et al., 1983). As in Crohn's disease, the risk of cancer increases with duration of disease, and the cancers occur in younger patients compared to sporadic disease (Bruno et al., 1997). Typically, small bowel cancers arise in patients who have had celiac disease for more than 20 years. Further similarities between celiac disease and Crohn's disease include the increased incidence of multifocal cancers and the difficulty of diagnosing a malignant complication at an early stage. In both disorders, the symptoms of the associated cancers closely resemble those of the diseases themselves, and the diagnosis of carcinoma is typically delayed.

The incipient phases of celiac disease–associated carcinoma have not yet been defined. Dysplastic mucosa that is presumed to represent the precursor of the carcinoma has been identified at the periphery of invasive cancers in celiac disease (Bruno et al., 1997). However, the pathogenetic classification of the dysplasia (i.e., residual adenoma versus dysplasia in flat mucosa) in this setting remains uncertain. In contrast to Crohn's disease, neither diffuse dysplasia nor contiguous fields of dysplasia have been identified. This suggests that either the dysplasia occurring in celiac disease tends to be focal rather than diffuse or the disease predisposes to adenoma formation. The issue remains unresolved at present since documentation of incipient neoplasia in the absence of invasive tumor is lacking. A single case of a benign jejunal adenoma occurring in patient with a 6-year history of celiac disease has appeared in the literature (Fishman et al., 1990), but to date, flat dysplasia in the absence of carcinoma has not been reported.

CARCINOID (NEUROENDOCRINE) TUMORS

Carcinoid tumors encompass a broad histologic spectrum of epithelial neoplasms with neuroendocrine differentiation (Lechago, 1994). Although they may occur anywhere in the gastrointestinal tract (as well as a wide variety of other organs), carcinoid tumors are most frequent in the appendix, rectum, and ileum (Lewin, 1987; Stinner et al., 1996; Zakariai et al., 1975). In some series, the small bowel has been reported as the single most common site of occurrence of carcinoid tumors in the gastrointestinal tract (Gerstle et al., 1995; Marshall and Bodnarchuk, 1993; McDermott et al., 1994). They have been estimated to account for 13% to 34% of all small bowel neoplasms and 17% to 43% of all malignancies of the small bowel (Memon and Nelson, 1997). Thus, they are as common as adenocarcinomas of the small bowel (Barclay and Schapira, 1983; Thomas and Sobin, 1995). Compared to carcinoids in the appendix or rectum, they are more likely to be clinically important because they are associated with more aggressive biologic behavior and shorter survival (Godwin, 1975; Marshall and Bodnarchuk, 1993; Thomas and Sobin, 1995; Zakariai et al., 1975).

Little is known about the incipient stages of carcinoid tumors of the small bowel. In the stomach, endocrine cell hyperplasia has been identified as the precursor to carcinoid tumor formation in the setting of diffuse atrophic gastritis with overproduction of gastrin and resultant ECL-cell hyperplasia (Öberg, 1996). Initially, hyperplasia of neuroendocrine cells is intraepithelial, but with sustained stimulation, stromal penetration occurs. Once the stromal nodules of neuroendocrine cells reach a certain size (usually 150 μm), they are classified as microcarcinoids. Associated neuroendocrine hyperplasia sometimes may be seen with colonic carcinoids developing in the setting of ulcerative colitis, suggesting a field effect (Miller and Summer, 1983). In most other settings, however, associated endocrine cell hyperplasia has not been described, and pathogenetic factors have not been defined. The vast majority of small bowel carcinoids are discovered at an advanced stage because, like other primary small bowel neoplasms, they are extremely difficult to diagnose and localize in their incipient phases of development (Memon and Nelson, 1997).

Given the present limitations of knowledge, all carcinoid tumors of the small bowel must be regarded as potentially malignant, but the biologic behavior of any given carcinoid tumor is difficult to predict. In general, neuroendocrine tumors at opposite ends of the differentiation spectrum tend to behave differently. Specifically, well-differentiated carcinoid tumors tend to behave indolently, and poorly differentiated carcinoids (also called neuroendocrine carcinomas) tend to behave aggressively and to have a poor prognosis (Lewin, 1987). In the absence of metastatic disease, however, there are no absolute criteria by which to judge the malignant (i.e., metastatic) potential of most carcinoid tumors. Furthermore, even in the presence of metastatic disease, most carcinoids are slow growing and are compatible with prolonged survival (Lewin, 1987).

The typical well-differentiated carcinoid tumor is composed of monomorphous, round to polygonal cells with centrally placed nuclei, stippled chromatin and inconspicuous nucleoli. Carcinoid tumors may exhibit a variety of different, but highly characteristic, growth patterns including the formation of (1) solid nests with peripheral pallisading (insular pattern); (2) ribbon-like cords within a highly vascular stroma (trabecular pattern); (3) rosette-like acinar structures (glandular pattern); (4) haphazardly organized solid sheets (undifferentiated pattern); and (5) mixtures of any of these (Johnson et al., 1983; Lewin, 1987; Soga and Tazawa, 1971). The growth pattern tends to correlate with the site of origin in the gut (Memon and Nelson, 1997). Carcinoids of the midgut are predominantly insular in type. Those of the foregut are usually trabecular, and those of the hindgut are mixed. In addition, the growth patterns have been found to correlate with survival (Johnson et al., 1983; Memon and Nelson, 1997). A mixed insular and glandular pattern of growth (the most frequent mixture observed) has the best prognosis of any growth pattern (Johnson et al., 1983), but mixed insular and trabecular growth is also associated with a favorable outcome. Among the pure growth patterns, the insular and trabecular patterns have a better prognosis than the glandular or undifferentiated patterns (Johnson et al., 1983).

Other histopathologic features that have been shown to correlate with an increased risk of metastasis have included tumor size, local extent of tumor, multicentricity, and histologic grade (Burke et al., 1997; Lewin, 1987; Memon and Nelson, 1997). Tumor size is related to the rate of metastasis as follows (Memon and Nelson, 1997):

Size of Carcinoid Tumor	Nodal Metastasis (Incidence)	Liver Metastasis (Incidence)
<1 cm	20%–30%	20%–30%
1–2 cm	60%–80%	20%
>2 cm	>80%	40%–50%

The local extent of tumor is related to tumor size and, therefore, to prognosis. More specifically, however, the overall 5-year survival rate is about 82% for carcinoid tumors confined to the bowel wall and about 52% for tumors that extend to the serosa (McDermott et al., 1994).

The grading of carcinoid tumors is based on cytologic features such as cell shape, size, and nuclear regularity (Lewin, 1987). Well-differentiated carcinoid tumors are of uncertain malignant potential and may be indolent, whereas moderately differentiated tumors have a greater potential for metastasis. Poorly differentiated tumors are highly aggressive and are considered overtly malignant. Well and moderately differentiated carcinoids are usually morphologically distinctive and present little difficulty in diagnosis. Occasionally, however, they may resemble adenocarcinomas, particularly if they produce mucin focally and stain for carcinoembryonic antigen by immunohistochemistry. In these cases, immunostains for chromagranin, neuron-specific enolase, Leu-7, and serotonin, which are all positive in the vast majority of cases, may be useful in establishing the diagnosis (Burke et al., 1997; Martin and Maung, 1987; Nash and Said, 1986). Poorly differentiated neuroendocrine tumors may have either large, pleomorphic cells or small cells with scanty cytoplasm and an "oat cell" morphology. In contrast to well- and moderately differentiated carcinoids, mitotic figures are usually abundant. In addition, poorly differentiated carcinoids usually have an undifferentiated growth pattern (see above), growing in solid, irregular masses, and may resemble poorly differentiated adenocarcinomas. Rarely, poorly differentiated carcinoids may display a spindle cell morphology and mimic a sarcoma. In these cases, immunohistochemistry and/or electron microscopy may be helpful in identifying the tumor as neuroendocrine in type.

The molecular alterations underlying the development of sporadic carcinoid tumors of the bowel are unknown at present.

MISCELLANEOUS CONDITIONS PREDISPOSING TO SMALL BOWEL NEOPLASIA

In a number of iatrogenically created situations, the ileum may be exposed to conditions that ultimately prove tumorigenic. For example, adenocarcinomas are known to occur as late complications of ureteral implantation into the ileum following cystectomy (Meretyk et al., 1987). The development of carcinoma has also been reported to occur in the ileal segments of augmentation cystoplasties (Stone et al., 1987) and in the ileum adjacent to the ileocutaneous junction in long-standing ileostomies (Suarez et al., 1988). Carcinomas arising in these setting are all presumed to progress through increasing degrees of dysplasia in a manner analogous to that of cancers arising in Crohn's disease.

REFERENCES

Amos CI, Bali D, Thiel TJ, et al. (1997) Fine mapping of a genetic locus for Peutz-Jeghers syndrome on chromosome 19p. *Cancer Res* 57:3653–3656.

Baczako K, Buchler M, Beger H, et al. (1985) Morphogenesis and possible precursor lesions of invasive carcinoma of the papillar of Vater: epithelial dysplasia and adenoma. *Hum Pathol* 16:305–310.

Barclay THC, Schapira DV. (1983) Malignant tumors of the small intestine. *Cancer* 51:878–881.

Bearzi I, Ranaldi R. (1985) Small-bowel adenocarcinoma and Crohn's disease: report of a case with differing histogenetic patterns. *Histopathology* 9:343–357.

Bodmar WF, Bailey CJ, Bodmar J, et al. (1987) Localization of the gene for familial adenomatous polyposis on chromosome 5. *Nature* 328:614–616.

Braasch JW, Camer SJ. (1975) Periampullary carcinoma. *Med Clin North Am* 59:309–314.

Bruno CJ, Batts KP, Ahlquist DA. (1997) Evidence against flat dysplasia as a regional field defect in small bowel adenocarcinoma associated with celiac sprue. *Mayo Clin Proc* 72:320–322.

Burdick D, Prior JT. (1982) Peutz-Jeghers syndrome: a clinicopathologic study of a large family with a 27-year follow-up. *Cancer* 50:2139–2146.

Burke AP, Thomas RM, Elsayad AM, et al. (1997) Carcinoids of the jejunum and ileum. An immunohistochemical and clinicopathologic study of 167 cases. *Cancer* 79:1086–1093.

Chow JS, Chen CC, Ahsan H, et al. (1996) A population-based study of the incidence of malignant small bowel tumors: SEER, 1973–1990. *Int J Epidemiol* 25:722–728.

Cooper DJ, Weinstein MA, Korelitz BI. (1984) Complications of Crohn's disease predisposing to dysplasia and cancer of the intestinal tract: considerations of a surveillance program. *J Clin Gastroenterol* 6:217–224.

Cuvelier C, Bekaert E, de Potter C, et al. (1989) Crohn's disease with adenocarcinoma and dysplasia. Macroscopical, histological, and immunohistochemical aspects of two cases. *Am J Surg Pathol* 13:187–1976.

Darling RC, Welch CE. (1959) Tumors of the small intestine. *N Engl J Med* 260:397–408.

Dong SM, Kim KM, Kim SY, et al. (1998) Frequent somatic mutations in serine/threonine kinase 11/Peutz-Jeghers syndrome gene in left-sided colon cancer. *Cancer Res* 58:3787–3790.

Donohue JH. (1994) Malignant tumours of the small bowel. *Surg Oncol* 3:61–68.

Fishman MJ, Jeejeebhoy KN, Gopinath N, et al. (1990) Small intestinal villous adenoma and celiac disease. *Am J Gastroenterol* 85:748–751.

Fleming ID, Cooper JS, Henson DE, et al., eds. (1997) *AJCC Manual for Staging of Cancer*, 5th ed. Lippincott-Raven, Philadelphia.

Gerstle JT, Kauffman GL, Koltun WA. (1995) The incidence, management, and outcome of patients with gastrointestinal carcinoids and second primary malignancies. *J Am Coll Surg* 180:427–432.

Giardiello FM, Welsh SB, Hamilton SR, et al. (1987) Increased risk of cancer in the Peutz-Jeghers Syndrome. *N Engl J Med* 316:1511–1514.

Ginsburg LK, Schneider M, Dreizin DH, et al. (1956) Carcinoma of the jejunum arising in a case of regional enteritis. *Surgery* 39:347–351.

Godwin JD, II. (1975) Carcinoid tumors. *Cancer* 36:560–569.

Goel IP, Didolkar MS, Elias EG. (1976) Primary malignant tumors of the small intestine. *Surg Obstet Gynecol* 143:717–719.

Greenstein AJ, Sacher DB, Smith H, et al. (1980) Patterns of neoplasia in Crohn's disease and ulcerative colitis. *Cancer* 46:403–407.

Greenstein AJ, Sacher DB, Smith H, et al. (1981) A comparison of cancer risk in Crohn's disease and ulcerative colitis. *Cancer* 48:2742–2745.

Gyde SN, Prior P, McCartney JC et al. (1980) Malignancy in Crohn's disease. *Gut* 21:1024–1029.

Haggitt RC, Reid BJ. (1986) Hereditary gastrointestinal polyposis syndromes. *Am J Surg Pathol* 10:871–887.

Hemminki A, Tomlinkson I, Markie D, et al. (1997) Localization of a susceptibility locus for Peutz-Jeghers syndrome to 19p using comparative genomic hybridization and targeted linkage analysis. *Nat Genet* 15:87–90.

Jenne DE, Reimann H, Nezu J-I, et al. (1998) Peutz-Jeghers syndrome is caused by mutations in a novel serine threonine kinase. *Nat Genet* 18:38–43.

Johnson LA, Lavin P, Moertel CG, et al. (1983) Carcinoids: the association of histologic growth pattern and survival. *Cancer* 51:882–889.

Kinzler KW, Vogelstein B (1996) Lessons from hereditary colorectal cancer. *Cell* 87:159–170.

Korelitz BI. (1983) Carcinoma of the intestinal tract in Crohn's disease; results of a survey conducted by the

National Foundation for Ileitis and Colitis. *Am J Gastroenterol* 78:44–46.

Lashner BA. (1992) Risk factors for small bowel cancer in Crohn's disease. *Dig Dis Sci* 37:1179–1184.

Lechago J. (1994) Gastrointestinal neuroendocrine cell proliferations. *Hum Pathol* 25:1114–1122.

Lewin K. (1987) Carcinoid tumors and mixed (composite) glandular-endocrine cell carcinomas. *Am J Surg Pathol* 11(Suppl. 1):71–86.

Lien G-S, Mori M, Enjoji M. (1988) Primary carcinoma of the small intestine. A clinicopathologic and immunohistochemical study. *Cancer* 61:316–323.

Lowenfels AB. (1973) Why are small-bowel tumors so rare? *Lancet* 1:24–25.

Luk GD. (1995) Diagnosis and therapy of hereditary polyposis syndromes. *Gastroenterologist* 3:153–167.

Lynch HT, Lynch JT. (1998) Genetics of colon cancer. *Digestion* 59:481–492.

Lynch HT, Smyrk T. (1996) Hereditary nonpolyposis colorectal cancer (Lynch syndrome): an updated review. *Cancer* 78:1149–1167.

Lynch HT, Smyrk TC, Lynch PM, et al. (1989) Adenocarcinoma of the small bowel in Lynch syndrome II. *Cancer* 64:2178–2183.

Marra G, Boland CR (1996) DNA repair and colorectal cancer. *Gastroenterol Clin North Am* 25:755–772.

Marshall JB, Bodnarchuk G. (1993) Carcinoid tumors of the gut. Our experience over three decades and review of the literature. *J Clin Gastroenterol* 16:123–129.

Martin JME, Maung RT. (1987) Differential immunohistochemical reactions of carcinoid tumors. *Hum Pathol.* 18:941–945.

McDermott EWM, Guduric B, and Brennan MF. (1994) Prognostic variables in patients with gastrointestinal carcinoid tumors. *Br J Surg* 81:1007–1009.

Mehenni H, Blouin J-L, Radhakrishna U, et al. (1997) Peutz-Jeghers syndrome: confirmation of linkage to chromosome 19p13.3 and identification of a potential second locus, on 19q13.4. *Am J Hum Genet* 61:1327–1334.

Memon MA, Nelson H. (1997) Gastrointestinal carcinoid tumors. Current management strategies. *Dis Colon Rectum* 40:1101–1118.

Meretyk S, Landau EH, Okon E, et al. (1987) Adenocarcinoma in an ileal conduit: a late recurrence of urothelial adenocarcinoma. *Cancer* 71:677–685.

Michelassi F, Testa G, Pomidor WJ, et al. (1993) Adenocarcinoma complicating Crohn's disease. *Dis Colon Rectum* 36:654–661.

Miller RR, Summer HW. (1983) Argyrophil cell hyperplasia and an atypical carcinoid in chronic ulcerative colitis. *Cancer* 50:2920–2925.

Nakagawa H, Koyama K, Tanaka T, et al. (1998) Localization of the gene responsible for Peutz-Jeghers syndrome within a 6-cM region of chromosome 19p13.3. *Hum Genet* 102:203–206.

Nash SV, Said JW. (1986) Gastrointestinal neuroendocrine tumors. A histochemical and immunohistochemical study of epithelial (keratin proteins, carcinoembryonic antigen) and neuroendocrine (neuron-specific enolase, bombesin, and chromogranin) markers of foregut, midgut, and hindgut tumors. *Am J Clin Pathol* 86:415–422.

Norberg K-A, Emas S. (1981) Primary tumors of the small intestine. *Am J Surg* 142:569–573.

Öberg K. (1996) Neuroendocrine gastrointestinal tumors. *Ann Oncol* 7:453–463.

Osteen RT. (1996) *Cancer Manual*, 9th ed. American Cancer Society, Framingham, MA.

Perzin KH, Bridge MF. (1981) Adenomas of the small intestine: a clinicopathologic review of 51 cases and a study of their relationship to carcinoma. *Cancer* 48:799–819.

Perzin KH, Bridge MF. (1982) Adenomatous and carcinomatous changes in hamartomatous polyps of the small intestine (Peutz-Jeghers syndrome): report of a case and review of the literature. *Cancer* 49:971–983.

Perzin KH, Peterson M, Castiglione CL, et al. (1984) Intramucosal carcinoma of the small intestine arising in regional enteritis (Crohn's disease). Report of a case studied for carcinoembryonic antigen and review of the literature. *Cancer* 54:151–162.

Petras RE, Mir-Madjlessi SH, Farmer RG. (1987) Crohn's disease and intestinal carcinoma. A report of 11 cases with emphasis on associated epithelial dysplasia. *Gastroenterology* 93:1307–1304.

Ponz de Leon M. (1996) Descriptive epidemiology of hereditary nonpolyposis colorectal cancer. *Tumori* 82:102–106.

Rashid A, Hamilton SR. (1997) Genetic alterations in sporadic and Crohn's-associated adenocarcinomas of the small intestine. *Gastroenterology* 113:127–135.

Richards ME, Rickert RR, Nance FC. (1989) Crohn's disease–associated carcinoma. A poorly recognized complication of inflammatory bowel disease. *Ann Surg* 209:764–773.

Rubio CA, Befritz R, Poppen B, et al. (1991) Crohn's disease and adenocarcinoma of the intestinal tract. Report of four cases. *Dis Colon Rectum* 34:174–180.

Rustgi AK. (1994) Hereditary gastrointestinal polyposis and nonpolyposis syndromes. *N Engl J Med* 331:1694–1702.

Rustgi AK. (1995) *Gastrointestinal Cancers. Biology, Prognosis, and Therapy.* Lippincott-Raven, Philadelphia.

Ryan JC. (1996) Premalignant conditions of the small intestine. *Semin Gastrointest Dis* 7:88–93.

Scully RE. (1970) Sex cord tumor with annular tubules: a distinctive ovarian tumor of the Peutz-Jeghers syndrome. *Cancer* 25:1107–1121.

Senay E, Sachar DB, Keohane M, et al. (1989) Small bowel carcinoma in Crohn's disease. Distinguishing features and risk factors. *Cancer* 63:360–363.

Shepherd NA, Bussey HJR, Jass JR. (1987) Epithelial misplacement in Peutz-Jeghers polyps. A diagnostic pitfall. *Am J Surg Pathol* 11:743–749.

Shorter RG. (1983) Risks of intestinal cancer in Crohn's disease. *Dis Colon Rectum* 26:686–689.

Simpson S, Traube J, Riddell RH. (1981) The histologic appearance of dysplasia (precancerous change) in Crohn's disease of the small and large intestine. *Gastroenterology* 81:492–501.

Soga J, Tazawa K. (1971) Pathologic analysis of carcinoids. Histologic reevaluation of 62 cases. *Cancer* 28:990–998.

Stinner B, Kisker O, Zielke A, et al. (1996) Surgical management of carcinoid tumors of the small bowel, appendix, colon, and rectum. *World J Surg* 20:183–188.

Stone AR, Davies N, Stephenson TP. (1987) Carcinoma associated with augmentation cystoplasty. *Br J Urol* 138:859–860.

Suarez V, Alexander-Williams J, O'Conner HJ, et al. (1988) Carcinoma developing in ileostomies after 25 or more years. *Gastroenterology* 95:205–208.

Swinson CM, Slavin G, Coles EC, et al. (1983) Coeliac disease and malignancy. *Lancet* 1:111–115.

Talbot IC, Neoptolemos JP, Shaw DE, et al. (1988) The histopathology and staging of carcinoma of the ampulla of Vater. *Histopathology* 12:155–165.

Tanaka M, Riddell RH. (1990) The pathological diagnosis and differential diagnosis of Crohn's disease. *Hepatogastroenterology* 37:18–31.

Thomas RM, Sobin LH. (1995) Gastrointestinal cancer. *Cancer* 75(Suppl.):154–170.

Ulich TR, Kollin M, Simmons GE, et al. (1987) Adenomyoma of the papilla of Vater. *Arch Pathol Lab Med* 111:388–390.

Wattenberg LW. (1966) Carcinogenic-detoxifying mechanisms in the gastrointestinal tract. *Gastroenterology* 51:932–935.

Weedon DD, Shorter RG, Ilstrup DM, et al. (1973) Crohn's disease and cancer. *N Engl J Med* 289: 1099–1103.

Wise L, Pizzimbono C, Dehner LP. (1976) Periampullary cancer. A cliniopathologic study of sixty-two patients. *Am J Surg* 131:141–148.

Yaguchi T, Wen-Ying L, Hasegawa K, et al. (1982) Peutz-Jeghers polyp with several foci of glandular dysplasia. Report of a case. *Dis Colon Rectum* 25:592–596.

Zakariai YM, Quan SHQ, Hadju SI. (1975) Carcinoid tumors of the gastrointestinal tract. *Cancer* 35:588–591.

9

LARGE INTESTINE

Carolyn C. Compton

Colon cancer is the second leading cause of cancer deaths in the United States and affects both sexes in equal proportion. In the Western world, overall, about 5% of the population will be diagnosed with colorectal cancer in their lifetime, and this figure may be expected to increase with increased life expectancy (Kinzler and Vogelstein, 1998). The vast majority of colon cancers arise from preexisting benign tumors known as adenomas that are very common, macroscopically visible, and readily obtainable. Through the fibro-optic colonoscope, adenomas anywhere in the colon are accessible, can be removed easily, and are routinely excised during standard patient care. The abundance and ready availability of adenomas at various stages of development and progression towards malignancy have proven enormously advantageous for the study of incipient neoplasia in the colon. These advantages have set the colon apart from other epithelial systems that are either technically difficult to access and/or are characterized by carcinogenetic progression that does not involve the formation of a benign precursor tumor. More is now known about the nascent phases of neoplasia in the colon than in any other epithelial system in the body, and colon cancer has become the paradigm for multistep carcinogenesis.

The cytologic changes that precede malignant transformation are defined as *dysplasia*, and, by analogy, epithelial dysplasia is considered the *sine qua non* of incipient neo-plasia in the colon. In the colon, dysplasia is generally regarded as an irreversible change that is unequivocally neoplastic and is the precursor lesion of all malignant tumors. In general, the dysplastic cells that constitute incipient neoplasia of the colon manifest themselves in two different ways that are, in general, distinct and nonoverlapping. Most commonly, as described above, the dysplastic cells are grouped together into discrete, well-defined tumorous lesions (adenomas) that are sharply defined against the histologically normal mucosa in which they arise. Less commonly, the dysplastic cells are more diffusely and irregularly distributed within flat colonic mucosa. This form of dysplasia occurs in chronic inflammatory states that predispose to colonic neoplasia such as chronic ulcerative colitis. Although less common than adenoma formation, it is more problematic because it cannot be seen macroscopically and may be mimicked microscopically by reactive or regenerative epithelial changes in inflamed mucosa. Intraepithelial dysplasia may also occur in hamartomatous polyps in inherited hamartomatous polyposis syndromes such as familial juvenile polyposis and the Peutz-Jeghers syndrome.

This chapter reviews the types of dysplastic lesions that constitute incipient neoplasia in the colon; the diagnostic criteria by which they are recognized; the differential diagnosis of these lesions; the factors that influence and predict their biologic behavior; the genetic basis of their initiation and progression; and the role of the pathologist in the diagnosis and management of these lesions.

COLONIC ADENOMAS AND THE ADENOMA–CARCINOMA SEQUENCE

PREVALENCE, RISK FACTORS, AND DETECTION

The vast majority of colon cancers arise from sporadic adenomas in individuals who do not have an inherited colon cancer syndrome. Nevertheless, many cases once considered sporadic may fit into a pattern of hereditary predisposition. On the one hand, likelihood analyses and prospective studies have suggested a familial susceptibility to both adenomas and colon cancer for first-degree relatives of individuals with either adenomas or colon cancer (Bazzoli et al., 1995; Bonelli et al., 1988; Burt et al., 1991; Lovett, 1976; Winawer et al., 1996). On the other hand, very few adenomas or carcinomas are found in asymptomatic individuals screened for the sole indication of a positive family history (Grossman and Milos, 1988; Rozen and Ron, 1989). Thus, no firm guidelines have been established for screening individuals on the basis of a positive family history alone.

The true prevalence of adenomas among asymptomatic individuals is difficult to determine. Prevalence rates in autopsy series vary by geographic location. In countries with high rates of colon cancer, such as the United States, the prevalence of adenomas is 30%–40%, whereas in low-risk locales, adenomas are found at autopsy in less than 12% of cases (Itzkowitz, 1996). In all populations, the formation of adenomas is age-related in that the incidence rises sharply at age 40 and, in high-risk locales, as great as 50%–65% of the population over 65 years of age harbor adenomas (Rickert et al., 1979). Increasing age is also associated with a higher incidence of adenomas that are multiple, larger, severely dysplastic, and right-sided (Eide and Stalsberg, 1978; Johannsen et al., 1989; O'Brien et al., 1990; Rickert et al., 1979; Williams et al., 1982). Lifestyle risk factors for both adenomas and carcinomas of the colon include diets that are high in fat, high in red meat, low in fiber from vegetables, fruits, and grains, and low in folate and/or methionine. Lifestyle risk factors for adenomas include high alcohol intake, cigarette smoking, and low physical activity (Itzkowitz, 1996).

Most colonic adenomas are asymptomatic and are discovered incidentally. Tests for occult fecal blood are insensitive because adenomas smaller than 1.5–2.0 cm rarely bleed (Ahlquist et al., 1993; McRae and St. John, 1982). Endoscopy is the most sensitive screening procedure, but it is not specific since there are no macroscopic or endoscopic features that reliably distinguish adenomas from other types of polyps (Itzkowitz, 1996). Total colonoscopy is the most powerful tool available for adenoma detection and treatment, but the cost, labor intensity, and risk are prohibitive for a screening procedure (Papatheodoridis et al., 1996). More limited examinations are used for screening because most adenomas are located in the rectosigmoid (O'Brien et al., 1990) and the presence of rectosigmoid adenomas is associated with an in increased prevalence of synchronous adenomas more proximally (Papatheodoridis et al., 1996). With rigid sigmoidoscopy, the prevalence of polyps in individuals over the age of 40 is 7%, and most, but not all, of these polyps are adenomas. With the flexible sigmoidoscope, the prevalence rate is 10%–15%. If the index polyp is a hyperplastic polyp, the chance of finding an adenoma or carcinoma in the rest of the colon is about 10%, which is identical to the risk of finding a proximal neoplasm when no rectosigmoid polyps are found on initial screening (Zauber and Winawer, 1997). Therefore, full colonoscopy is not recommended. If the index polyp is an adenoma, full colonoscopy may be recommended because synchronous proximal neoplasms are found in more than 20% of patients with rectosigmoid adenomas (Papatheodoridis et al., 1996). In addition, follow-up endoscopies are recommended because 30%–50% of patients develop metachronous adenomas at 2–3 years after endoscopic polypectomy of an index adenoma (Hixson et al., 1994; Winawer et al., 1993b). The number and size of the index adenoma(s) have also proven to be independent risk factors for metachronous adenomas in some studies (Triantafyllou et al., 1997; Winawer et al., 1993b).

The mere presence of an adenoma does not invariably increase the risk for cancer, however, and other predictive factors have been sought. Factors that have shown to be associated with increased risk of synchronous and metachronous advanced adenomas and/or carcinomas proximal to the rectosigmoid include *(1)* the number of index adenomas; *(2)* the size of the index adenoma; and *(3)* the histologic characteristics of the adenoma, such as villous structures or high-grade dysplasia (Grassi et al., 1997; Meijer et al., 1998; Papatheodoridis et al., 1996; Triantafyllou et al., 1997). Therefore, meticulous pathologic evaluation and reporting of adenomas is essential in identifying patients at risk and determining their clinical management.

NATURAL HISTORY

The natural history of adenomas has been difficult to determine precisely. Follow-up studies of unresected adenomas are few and most lack histologic confirmation. Furthermore, the widespread practice of endoscopic polypectomy alters the natural history of adenomas. Radiologic studies have shown that only half of colorectal polyps smaller than 5 mm enlarge to 5 mm over a 2-year period and that a 5-mm polyp requires 2 to 3 years to reach 1 cm in size (Carroll and Klein, 1980; Hoff et al., 1986; Itzkowitz, 1996). It has since been proven that 60% of "small" (defined as ≤8 mm in diameter) colorectal polyps are, in fact, neoplastic and that the great majority (90%) of these neoplasms are tubular adenomas (Tsai and Lu, 1995). Index polyps that are 1 cm in size take about 2 to 5 years to develop carcinoma, and the cumulative risk of cancer at sites of index polyps measuring ≥1 cm has been found to be 2.5%, 8%, and 24% at 5, 10, and 20 years, respectively (Kim and Lance, 1997; Stryker et al., 1987). Studies on histologically proven adenomas have shown a 5- to 10- or 15-year progression to malignancy (Muto et al.,1975; Sherlock and Winawer, 1984) and have estimated that the overall chance of finding carcinoma in an adenoma is 5% (Sherlock and Winawer, 1984). Thus, it seems that only a small proportion of adenomas ever completes the multistep process

of transformation to carcinoma and that the adenoma–carcinoma developmental sequence is relatively slow. In general, the older the adenoma and the larger its size, the more likely it is to contain a malignant clone. Thus, the seminal studies on the pathobiology of adenomas as well as those on the genetic events underlying the adenoma–carcinoma sequence have both been carried out on adenomas stratified by size.

More recently, studies have focused on the smallest adenomas and their microscopic precursors in an attempt to better define and understand the earliest phases of the neoplastic process. Polyps less than 5 mm in size, sometimes called *diminutive polyps*, are common at endoscopy and prove to be adenomatous in about 40%–60% of cases (Church et al., 1988; Gottlieb et al., 1984; Granqvist et al., 1979; Tedesco et al., 1982; Waye et al., 1988). Diminutive adenomas rarely contain villous components, high-grade dysplasia, or cancer. When measured during a 2-year study period, they have evidenced little to no growth (Hoff et al., 1986). Therefore, it has been suggested that they may be safely treated by fulguration without prior biopsy, as long as they do not represent the index polyp of a screening endoscopy (Itzkowitz 1996).

There is mounting evidence that the precursors of adenomas are microscopic dysplastic lesions called *aberrant crypt foci* (ACF) (di Gregorio et al., 1997; Sui et al., 1997; Takayama et al., 1998). These lesions are not visible to the naked eye or by standard fibro-optic magnification. However, they can be visualized at endoscopy by vital staining with methylene blue and appear as groups of glands with compressed lumens and thick, darkly stained epithelial linings (Takayama et al., 1998). Not all ACF identified by this method are dysplastic, and those with a serrated luminal outline are usually hyperplastic rather than dysplastic (di Gregorio et al., 1997; Takayama et al., 1998). Only the dysplastic type of ACF is believed to be neoplastic. Two lines of evidence support this belief. First, the prevalence of dysplastic ACF is significantly increased in patients with adenomas or carcinomas compared to normal individuals (Takayama et al., 1998). Second, hyperplastic ACF harbor K-*ras* mutations, whereas dysplastic ACF exhibit mutations of the adenomatous polyposis coli gene (see

Molecular Pathogenesis of Incipient Neoplasia below; Carethers, 1996). Further study is required to document and define the events in the development of adenomas from dysplastic ACF and to ascertain the nature of the relationship, if any, between nondysplastic and dysplastic ACF in the colon.

Diagnostic Features

Macroscopic Appearance and Differential Diagnosis

Adenomas are composed primarily, if not entirely, of gland-forming dysplastic epithelium. The glands of an adenoma are usually architecturally atypical and structurally complex. The borders of adenomas are sharply defined and easily distinguished, both grossly and microscopically, from the surrounding normal mucosa. The growth patterns and subsequent macroscopic configurations of adenomas vary from slightly depressed or flat to slightly raised, sessile, or pedunculated (Fenoglio-Preiser and Pascal, 1982; Yao et al., 1994). Small adenomas are usually sessile. With increasing size, adenomas may become rounded and elevated in a broad base or project into the lumen on a stalk of normal mucosa of varying length. However, some adenomas remain sessile and expand horizontally with growth. The adenomatous mucosa is typically deeper in color compared to the surrounding normal mucosa because of increased vascularity with congestion or hemorrhage in the lamina propria, and has a courser, more granular surface and/or a finely nodular texture. Nevertheless, microscopic examination is required for definitive diagnosis of an adenoma since adenomas cannot be reliably differentiated from other histologic types of polyps by gross appearance alone. Other types of polyps that may resemble adenomas grossly include hyperplastic polyps, mucosal prolapse polyps, lipomas, and hamartomatous polyps (see below).

The single most important macroscopic feature of an adenoma is its size. Increasing size is directly associated with an increasing probability of villous architecture, high-grade dysplasia, and/or carcinoma (see Microscopic Appearance and Differential Diagnosis below; Grassi et al., 1997; Muto et

al., 1975). Significantly, index adenomas found on rectosigmoid endoscopic screening that are greater than 1 cm in size and/or villous and/or severely dysplastic are associated with an increased risk of synchronous advanced neoplasms (adenomas or carcinomas) in the proximal colon (Grassi et al., 1997; Papatheodoridis et al., 1996).

Microscopic Appearance and Differential Diagnosis

Histologic type. The normal colonic mucosa has a flat surface, and the glands are straight sided and narrow, with a tubular configuration. The glands are evenly spaced within a moderately abundant intervening stroma, and their bases directly abut the underlying linearly arrayed muscularis mucosae. In contrast, the mucosa of adenomas shows a variety of architectural deviations that may include any or all of the following features:

- glandular elongation, branching, budding, and/or papillary infolding
- reduction of interglandular stroma,
- splaying of the muscularis mucosae between gland bases
- projection of frond-like villous folds from the surface (Fig. 9–1).

The latter feature is a variable that has important prognostic associations and is the basis for the subclassification of adenomas into three types (i.e., tubular, tubulovillous, and villous) according to the proportion of villous components present. Although this histologic subclassification is well accepted and has long been widely employed, it lacks universally accepted criteria for the subdivisions. Seminal pathologic studies lacked defined criteria for subclassification, and subsequently, a number of different quantitative schemas appeared in the literature. The significance of subclassifying adenomas by architectural type is related to the association between villous architecture and an increased risk of epithelial dysplasia and carcinoma (Muto et al., 1975; O'Brien et al., 1990). Although cancer risk increases with size for all adenomas, both tubulovillous and villous adenomas have been shown to have a higher frequency of invasive carcinoma than tubular adenomas even after correction for size (Muto et al., 1975).

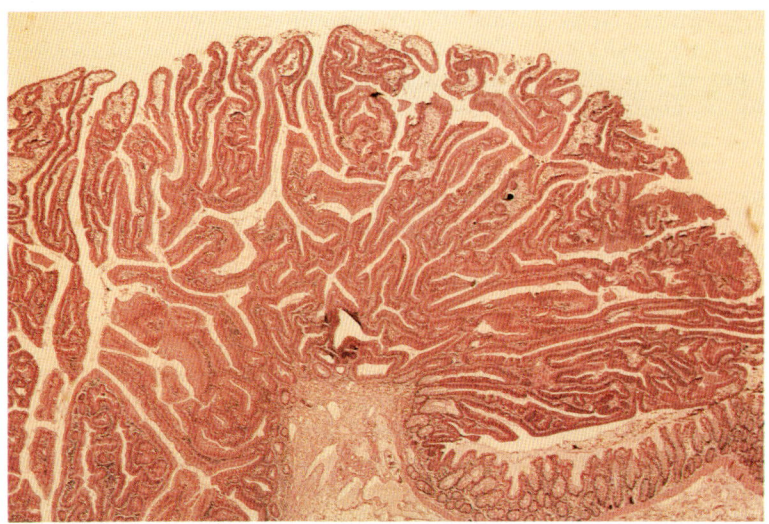

Figure 9–1. Villous adenoma consisting of villiform fronds of dysplastic mucosa sharply demarcated from the surrounding normal colonic mucosa (bottom right).

In general, tubular adenomas are characterized by a complete lack or a limited display of villous components (Fig. 9–2). They consist predominantly or entirely of tubular structures that invaginate from a flat surface. Tubulovillous adenomas are intermediate between tubular and villous, but substantial disagreement has existed among authors as to the proportions of villous components allowable in this category. Likewise, the suggested proportion of villous components required for classification of an adenoma as villous in type has varied. The World Health Organization classification allows for up to 25% villous components in the tubular adenoma category and reserves the villous category for adenomas that are at least 80%

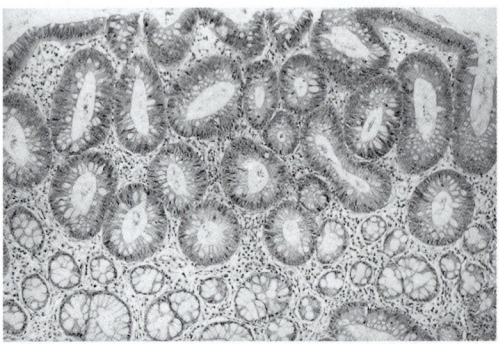

Figure 9–2. Minute tubular adenoma with a flat surface and dysplastic epithelium lining superficial aspects of glands.

villous in structure (Jass and Sobin, 1989). However, the National Polyp Study Classification restricted the tubular category to adenomas with a purely tubular structure and subclassified villous components by quartiles (i.e., villous A = 1%–25% villous; villous B = 26%–75% villous; villous C = 76%–99% villous, and villous D = 100% villous), rejecting the traditional categories. The National Polyp Study also defined villous components more precisely as adjacent crypts or folia of adenomatous (dysplastic) epithelium that, without branching, were elongated to a minimum of twice the length of a normal crypt (O'Brien et al., 1990). That study, which included nearly 4000 adenomas, demonstrated that the risk of finding high-grade dysplasia (intraepithelial carcinoma) in an adenoma was directly proportional to the extent of the villous components but that the risk was identical for villous C and villous D adenomas (O'Brien et al., 1990). Furthermore, only 2.2% of the 2375 purely tubular adenomas (70% of all the adenomas examined) in this study were shown to contain high-grade dysplasia. In contrast, villous A adenomas, a category that would be included in the "tubular adenoma" classification of the World Health Organization, showed a five-fold greater frequency of high-grade dysplasia than adenomas with purely tubular morphology. Based on these data, it is recommended that any adenoma with greater than 75% villous composition be classified as a villous adenoma and that the tubular adenoma category be restricted to adenomas without villous components.

The differential diagnosis of adenomas principally includes hyperplastic polyps, mucosal prolapse polyps, and hamartomatous polyps. Generally, hyperplastic polyps are easily distinguished from adenomas and are recognized by the expansion of the proliferative zone at the bases of the glands and the retention and crowding of mucin-filled differentiated cells at the apices of the glands (Fig. 9–3). Thus, the cells at the gland bases appear immature and those at the gland apices appear "hypermature" (Fig. 9–4). This appearance contrasts with that of small adenomas, since the immature cells are apically located and the cells at the gland bases are often normal in appearance (Fig. 9–2). However, hyperplastic polyps may be misinterpreted as adenomas when the retained cells at the tops of the glands and

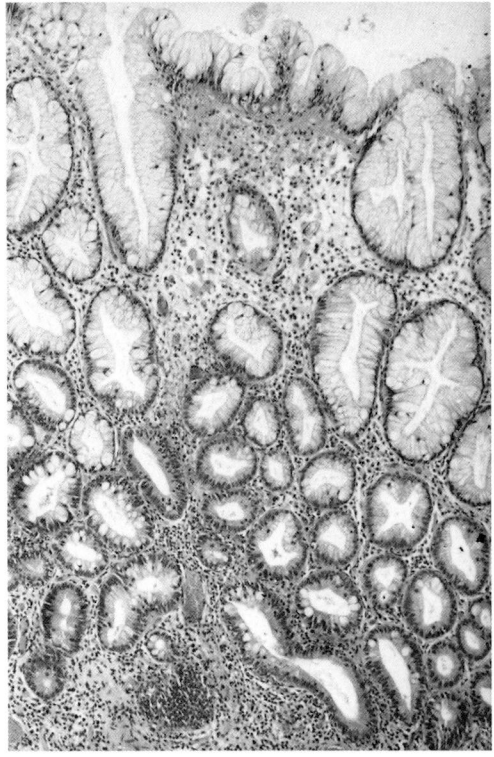

Figure 9–3. Hyperplastic polyp showing typical expansion of the proliferative zone at the gland bases (immature-appearing cells with enlarged nuclei) and crowded, mucin-bloated "hypermature" goblet cells at the gland apices.

polyp surface contain little mucin and lack the typical, highly saw-toothed configuration. Because the nuclei are crowded and slightly tufted, these lesions may resemble small adenomas (Fig. 9–5). Helpful distinguishing features include the smaller size and compact, evenly distributed chromatin of the superficial cells of the hyperplastic polyp and the complete lack of mitotic activity.

The differential diagnosis of adenomas and hyperplastic polyps is further complicated by the occurrence of compound or mixed adenomatous-hyperplastic polyps and serrated adenomas. Both of these variants are classified as adenomas and are regarded as having the same potential for malignant transformation. Mixed polyps contain both hyperplastic and adenomatous foci within the polyp head (Fig. 9–6); the foci are histologically distinct and topographically separate (Longacre and Fenoglio-Preiser, 1990). In contrast, serrated adenomas are composed of adenomatous (dysplastic) epithelium, but the cells often contain abundant mucin and form highly tufted glands that closely resemble the saw-toothed configuration of hyperplastic polyps (Fig. 9–7). Specific microscopic features that are helpful in differentiating serrated adenomas from hyperplastic polyps include the following (Torlakovic and Snover, 1996):

• dilatation of crypts that is predominantly basal
• presence of horizontally oriented crypts
• large areas without endocrine cells
• nuclear atypia that includes enlargement, hyperchromasia, and prominent nucleoli (Fig. 9–7)
• focal mucin overproduction (resembling mucinous cystadenomas of the appendix; see below)
• extension of the proliferation zone (and mitotic figures) into the middle or upper portion of the gland and the presence of numerous goblet cells at the base
• frequent (focal or diffuse) eosinophilia of the cytoplasm.

Both serrated adenomas and true hyperplastic polyps have been reported to occur in the setting of polyposis syndromes (i.e., more than 50–100 polyps) without familial incidence. However, only serrated adenomatous polyposis is associated with an ap-

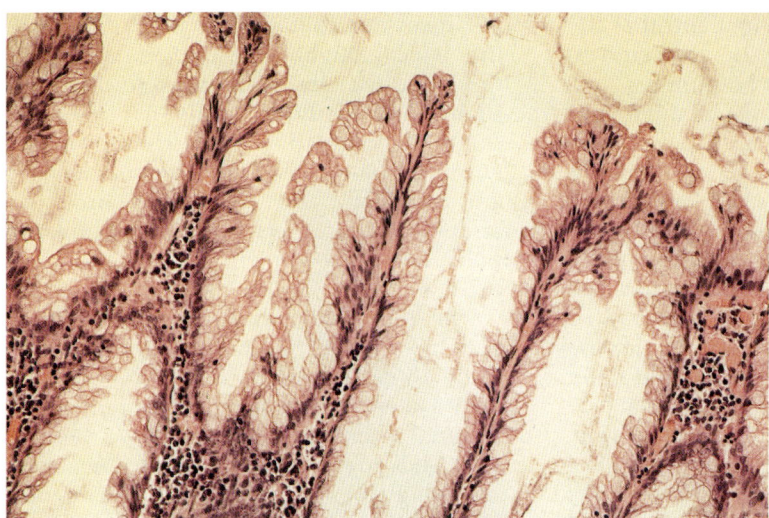

Figure 9–4. Surface of a hyperplastic polyp showing "hypermature" goblet cells with small, crowded nuclei creating epithelial tufts.

parent predisposition to the development of colorectal carcinoma (Torlakovic and Snover, 1996; Williams et al., 1980).

Mucosal prolapse polyps may also be confused with adenomas, especially when stalked (Fig. 9–8). They may have highly abnormal glandular architecture, show considerable reactive cytologic atypia, and typically show splaying of the muscularis mucosa between the glands (Figs. 9–9 and 9–10). These lesions, the result of intermittent ischemia and secondary inflammation of mucosal folds that have prolapsed into the lumen, are known by a number of generic or descriptive names such as *inflammatory pseudopolyps*, "*fibrin cap*" or "*inflammatory cap*"

polyps, or *inflammatory myoglandular polyps.* They are common in specific settings such as colonic diverticular disease or the solitary rectal ulcer syndrome. When they occur at the anorectal dentate line, they may contain squamous epithelium and have been called *inflammatory cloacagenic polyps.* As some of the synonyms for these lesions imply, mucosal prolapse polyps are frequently eroded at the surface (Fig. 9–11) and typically show significant inflammation of the stroma and glands. The stroma may also contain hemosiderin deposits or show significant neovascularization in response to hemorrhage and ulceration, respectively. These features may also be seen in adenomas (see below). Fea-

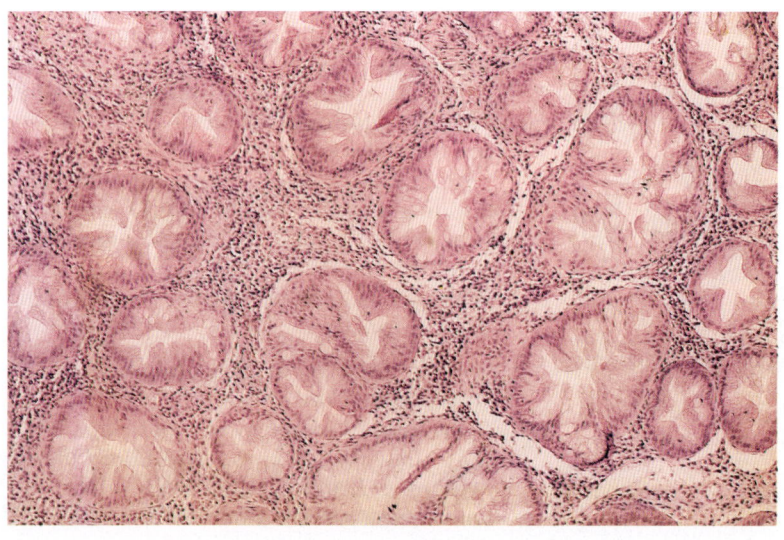

Figure 9–5. Hyperplastic polyp showing elongation and pseudostratification of nuclei that somewhat resemble the changes seen in adenomas with low-grade dysplasia.

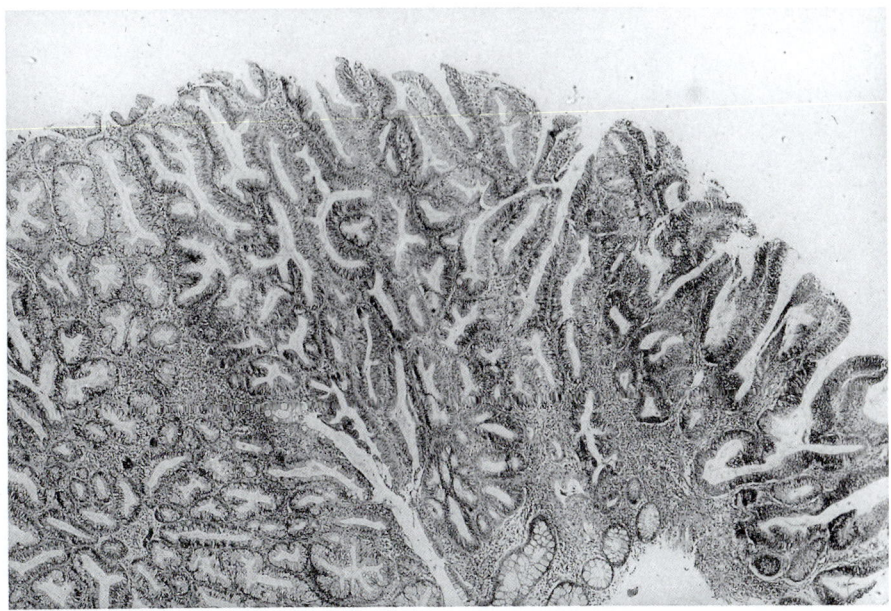

Figure 9–6. Mixed adenomatous-hyperplastic polyp with distinct foci of villiform dysplastic epithelium (far right) and hyperplastic epithelium without dysplasia (top left).

tures that help to differentiate mucosal prolapse polyps from adenomas include the lack of significant nuclear pleomorphism or crowding and the fibrosis of the lamina propria that accompanies the muscular splaying (a change sometimes called *fibromuscular replacement of the lamina propria*). Ultimately, however, the reactive atypia of the epithelium must be distinguished from true dysplasia.

Finally, hamartomatous polyps that occur in inherited hamartomatous polyposis syndromes such as familial juvenile polyposis or the Peutz-Jeghers syndrome may undergo neoplastic transformation and develop dysplastic changes in the epithelium (see below). The dysplasia may be focal, multifocal or diffuse, and when widespread, the polyp may be difficult to distinguish from an adenoma. Knowledge of the clinical setting, comparison with other polyps from the patient, or both may be helpful. Fundamen-

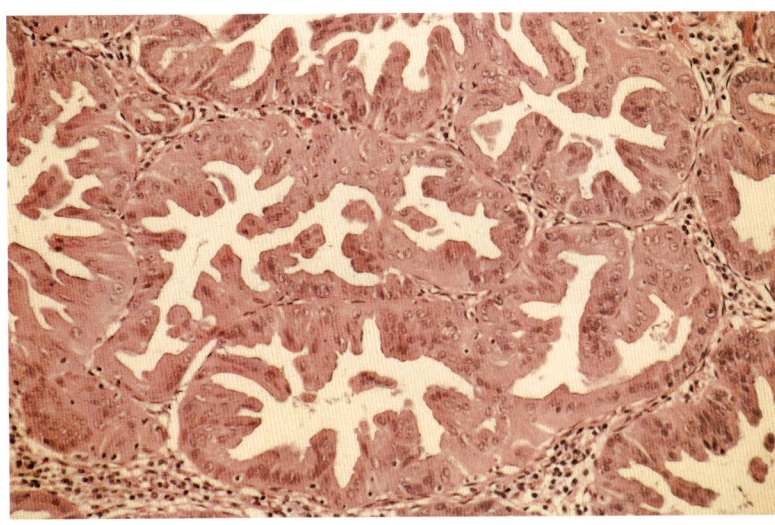

Figure 9–7. Serrated adenoma showing tufted (saw-toothed) epithelial configuration that resembles that seen in hyperplastic polyps but is composed entirely of dysplastic cells.

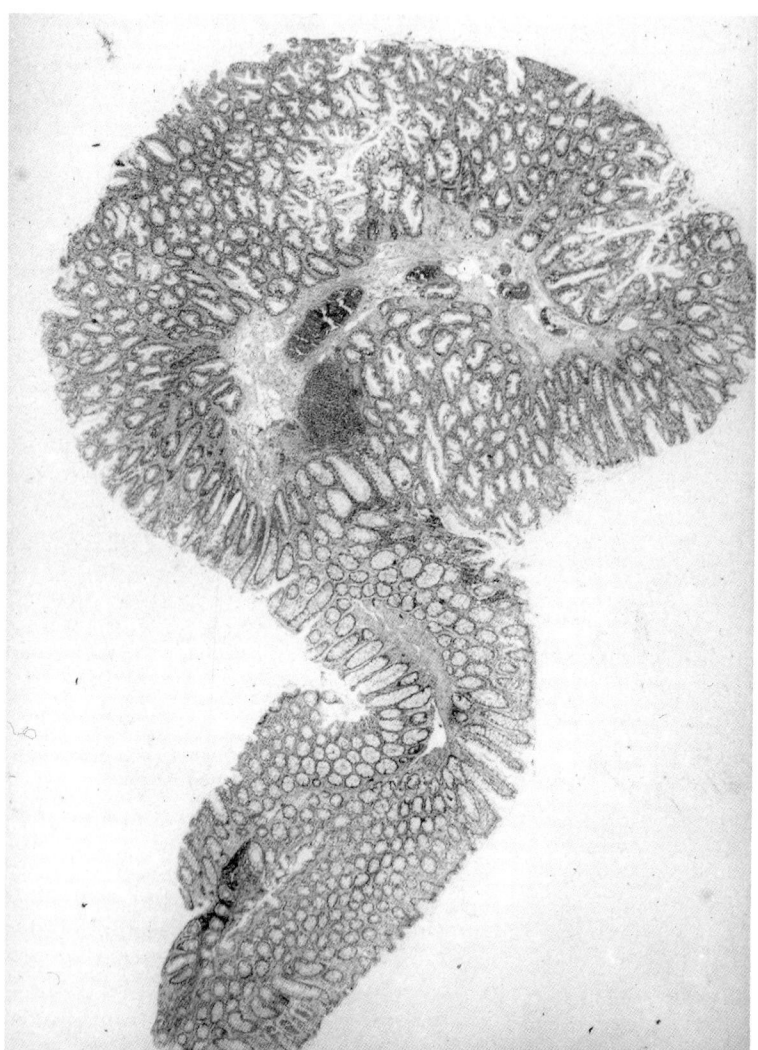

Figure 9–8. Stalked mucosal prolapse polyp that was mistaken clinically for an adenoma.

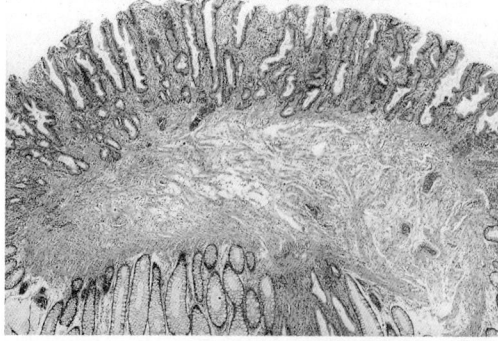

Figure 9–9. Mucosal prolapse polyp showing elongation (reactive/reparative hyperplasia) of glands with abnormal architecture and replacement of the normal lamina propria by fibromuscular stroma.

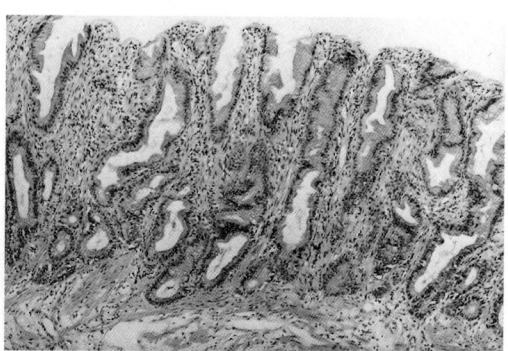

Figure 9–10. Mucosal prolapse polyp with hyperplastic (nondysplastic) glands and fibromuscular replacement of the lamina propria.

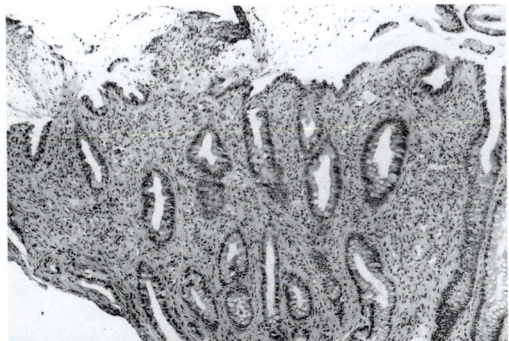

Figure 9–11. Mucosal prolapse polyp with surface erosion, reactive epithelial atypia, and dense fibromuscular stroma.

tally, however, dysplasia in a hamartoma changes the status of the polyp to that of a neoplasm and must be regarded as a premalignant change.

Degree of dysplasia. In normal colonic mucosa, the surface and glands are lined by a single layer of glandular cells (i.e., mucin-filled goblet cells and colonic absorptive cells) with small, basally located nuclei. Mitotic figures in small numbers may be seen in the basal third of the gland known as the *proliferative zone* (zone of cell division). In response to injury with increased rate of cell loss at the surface, the proliferative zone may expand temporarily to encompass a greater proportion of the gland but neither encompasses the full height of the gland nor extends over the mucosal surface. In contrast, the cells that comprise the epithelium of adenomas show a loss of normal differentiated cytologic features and loss of growth controls that normally limit cell proliferation to the bases of the glands. Thus, adenomatous epithelium is characterized by an array of abnormal (dysplastic) cytologic features and an abnormal expansion of the proliferative zone into the top half of the glands (Fig. 9–12). The abnormal cytologic features that define dysplasia include:

- nuclei enlargement (with an increase in the nuclear/cytoplasmic volume ratio)
- nuclear hyperchromasia
- nuclear elongation (typically with the acquisition of a cigar-like shape)
- nuclear relocation farther from the basement membrane

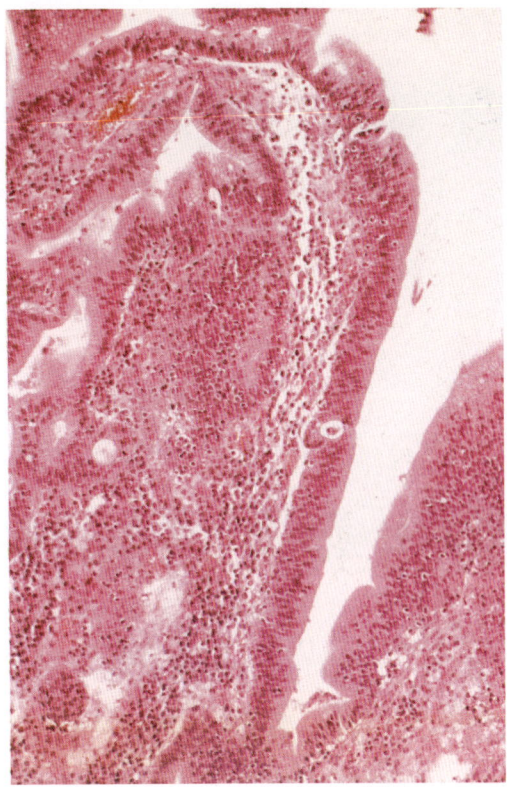

Figure 9–12. A gland opening onto the surface of a colonic adenoma showing epithelium characteristically hyperchromatic pseudostratified, crowded nuclei and loss of cytoplasmic mucin. Nuclei are largely confined to the bottom halves of the cells (low-grade dysplasia).

- nuclei crowding and overlapping
- appearance of epithelial stratification, an illusion created by both nuclear crowding and variation in nuclear location within the cytoplasm of adjacent cells (although all cells maintain contact with the underlying basement membrane)
- increased numbers of mitotic figures.

With increasing severity of dysplasia (Fig. 9–13), the above features may be exaggerated as well as accompanied by the following:

- decreased cytoplasmic mucin content
- increasing nuclear pleomorphism
- loss of nuclear polarity
- atypical mitotic figures
- expansion of the proliferative zone onto the mucosal surface.

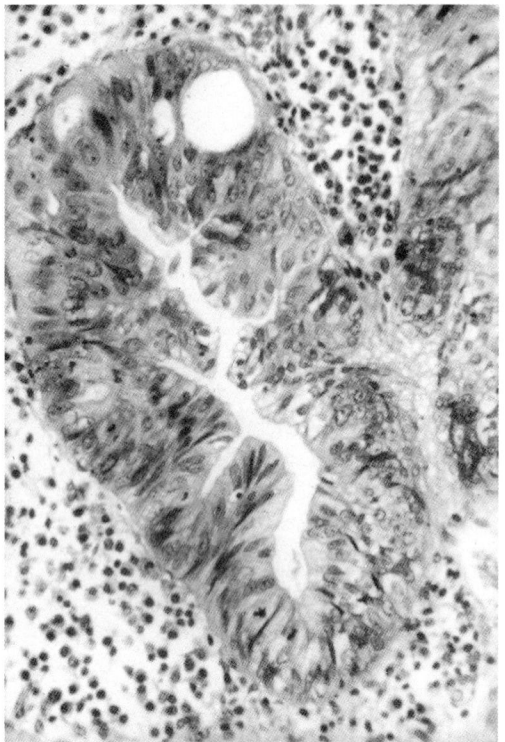

Figure 9–13. High-grade dysplasia of the epithelium in a colonic adenoma is characterized by stratification of dysplastic nuclei into the top halves of the cells.

The importance of assessing the degree of dysplasia in index adenomas has been underscored by recent studies. It has been shown that severe (high-grade) dysplasia in an index polyp found at screening sigmoidoscopy is associated with an increased risk of synchronous and metachronous advanced adenomas and/or carcinomas proximal to the rectosigmoid (Grassi et al., 1997; Meijer et al, 1998; Papatheodoridis et al., 1996; Triantafyllou et al., 1997). Therefore, the pathologist's assessment of the degree of dysplasia in an index adenoma may determine the course of medical follow-up. For example, when severe dysplasia (or worse) is diagnosed, full colonoscopy may be indicated. In grading dysplasia, the extent and severity of all of the dysplastic features listed above are assessed. In particular, however, increasing degrees of nuclear crowding and increased nuclear size have been shown to be associated with an increased risk of metach-

ronous colorectal cancer in retrospective case–control studies using morphometric techniques to assess dysplastic features (Meijer et al., 1998).

The degree of dysplasia in an adenoma may be graded by a two-tiered (low grade and high grade) or a three-tiered (i.e., mild, moderate, severe dysplasia) grading system. However, it has been shown that there is a high degree of interobserver variability among pathologists in differentiating between moderate and severe dysplasia when a three-tiered grading system is used (Demers et al., 1990). In order to increase the ease and reproducibility of grading, a two-tiered grading system like the one used for the assessment of dysplasia in inflammatory bowel disease may be justified. In general, high-grade dysplasia can be readily differentiated from low-grade dysplasia by the degree of nuclear pseudostratification present. High-grade dysplasia is recognized by pseudostratification of the nuclei into the top halves of the cells and/or loss of polarization (Fig. 9–13). In low-grade dysplasia, the nuclei are generally polarized (oriented perpendicular to the basement membrane of the gland) and located in the basal halves of the cells (Fig. 9–12).

Besides predicting metachronous carcinomas, increasing severity of dysplasia also increases the probability of finding invasive carcinoma within a given adenoma (Muto et al., 1975). Therefore, adenomas containing high-grade dysplasia should be examined in their entirety for invasive carcinoma, if possible. Although carcinoma usually develops in a sequential fashion through increasing grades of dysplasia, this progression is not always apparent. In some instances, carcinoma may be found in adenomas displaying only low-grade dysplasia.

With progression of high-grade dysplasia to intraepithelial carcinoma, additional cytologic abnormalities are acquired, such as:

• further nuclear enlargement with the acquisition of prominent nucleoli and a cleared, vesicular appearance
• nuclear chromatin that is irregularly clumped and densely hyperchromatic
• intraepithelial necrosis (apoptosis).

In addition, the epithelial cells may demonstrate the ability to proliferate without the necessity of stromal contact, forming cribi-formed glandular structures, solid growths, or epithelial tufts. This phase of malignant progression is known as "intraepithelial carcinoma" and is the equivalent of carcinoma *in situ* in the traditional sense of the term. That is, despite the malignant phenotype displayed by the cells, they remain localized above their respective glandular basement membranes and evidence no stromal invasion. Like all other carcinoma *in situ*, intraepithelial carcinoma has no potential for metastasis.

Once malignant cells breech the basement membrane and invade the lamina propria of the adenoma, the term *intramucosal carcinoma* is applicable (Fig. 9–14). Because the mucosa of the colon (and adenomas) lacks lymphatic vessels, malignant cells invading into the lamina propria, up to and including the muscularis mucosae, have no possibility of metastasizing to regional lymph nodes and little, if any, access to the systemic circulation via venous invasion. Because of this unique anatomic feature of the mucosa, the colon represents the only epithelial system in the body in which a stromally invasive carcinoma has no associated risk of metastasis and is, therefore, categorized as carcinoma *in situ* (i.e., pTis) by the TNM staging system of the American Joint Committee on Cancer and the International Union Against Cancer (Fleming et al., 1997).

Pathologic Reporting and the Role of the Pathologist in Management of Patients with Adenomas

Adenomas Without Malignant Features

Complete removal of an adenoma constitutes definitive therapy since it perforce prevents the development of a cancer from that lesion. Thus, the net epidemiologic effect of the practice of endoscopic polypectomy is a reduction in the incidence of colonic cancer in screened populations (Winawer et al., 1993). If adenomas are too large to remove endoscopically, they are usually biopsied to confirm the diagnosis and screen for malignant transformation and are then removed by surgical resection, if possible. Because excision of an adenoma is both diagnostic and therapeutic, polypectomy is attempted, whenever feasible, in patients undergoing colonoscopy for any reason. Minute adenomas usually are removed by grasp forceps. Pedonculated adenomas are ensnared and severed through their stalk. Broad-based adenomas are often elevated by submucosal saline injection and then removed in the same fashion. Sessile adenomas or broad-based adenomas that are too large to ensnare may be removed in a piecemeal fashion, yielding a fragmented specimen for pathologic examination.

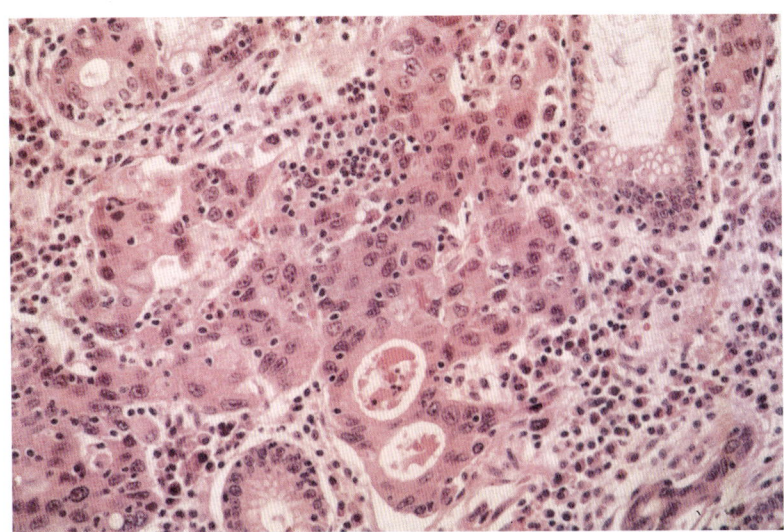

Figure 9–14. Intramucosal carcinoma in an adenoma showing a haphazard proliferation of malignant cells within the lamina propria.

The pathologic report of an adenoma should include the size (usually assessed grossly), the histologic subtype (or the presence or absence of villous features), and an assessment of completeness of excision, if possible. When the adenoma is minute, crushed at the edges by the endoscopic forceps, cauterized, or oriented randomly on embedding, it may be impossible to determine completeness of excision. When received in fragments, assessment for completeness of excision is usually precluded because the resection margins cannot be definitively identified. However, should one of the fragments consist of stalk-shaped normal mucosa with a cauterized base, this may be reported as evidence suggestive of complete excision. When the adenoma has a well-defined base or stalk (which may be inked for identification and orientation at embedding and microscopic examination) and is transected coronally through the polyp head, completeness of excision usually can be confidently assessed. The presence of adenomatous epithelium at the lateral edges of a broad-based polyp indicates incomplete excision.

Adenomas with Malignant Epithelium (Intraepithelial Carcinoma or Intramucosal Carcinoma)

The importance of reporting intraepithelial or intramucosal malignancy within an adenoma relates primarily to the association of "advanced" histologic features in rectosigmoid polyps with increased risk of synchronous and metachronous adenomas and carcinomas of the more proximal colon (Grassi et al., 1997; Meijer et al., 1998; Papatheodoridis et al., 1996).

Adenomas with Carinoma Invading into the Submucosa (Malignant Polyps)

Adenomas containing carcinoma that invades through the muscularis mucosae into the submucosa are termed *malignant polyps* regardless of the overall proportion of the adenoma that is replaced by cancer. Thus, they encompass both polypoid carcinomas in which the entire polyp head is replaced by carcinoma and adenomas with focal car-

cinoma. By definition, malignant polyps exclude adenomas containing intraepithelial carcinoma or intramucosal carcinoma because these polyps possess no biological potential for metastasis, as discussed above. Polyps of this type represent approximately 5% of all adenomas (Itzkowitz, 1996; Sherlock and Winawer, 1984), and the chance that any given adenoma will contain an invasive carcinoma increases with polyp size. Thus, the incidence of invasive carcinoma in adenomas of any histologic type that are greater than 2 cm in size ranges from 35% to 53% (Muto et al., 1975), with villous adenomas having a higher incidence than tubular adenomas of equal size.

Malignant polyps constitute a form of "early colorectal carcinoma" that may be cured by endoscopic polypectomy (Jass, 1995; Morson et al., 1984; Wolff and Shinya, 1975). However, following polypectomy alone, the incidence of an unfavorable outcome (i.e., lymph node metastasis or local recurrence of residual carcinoma) for malignant polyps varies from about 10% to 20% (Cooper et al., 1995; Wilcox et al., 1986). The histopathologic evaluation of malignant polyps removed endoscopically is critical in determining which patients are at risk for adverse outcome, and the findings directly affect the clinical management of the patient (Jass, 1995). Histopathologic parameters that have been shown to significantly increase the risk of adverse outcome include the following (Cooper, 1988; Cooper, et al., 1998; Cranley et al., 1986; Haggitt et al., 1985; Kyzer et al., 1992; Lipper et al., 1983; Muller et al., 1989; Volk et al., 1995):

• carcinoma of high histologic grade (i.e., poorly differentiated or undifferentiated)
• carcinoma at or close to (≤1 mm from) the resection margin of the adenoma
• the presence of submucosal small vessel (lymphatic or venular vessel) involvement.

In the presence of one or more of these features, the estimated risk of an adverse outcome following polypectomy alone is estimated to be about 10%–25% (Cooper, 1983; Coverlizza et al., 1989; Nivatvongs and Goldberg, 1978; Nivatvongs et al., 1991; Wilcox et al., 1986). Therefore, if one or more of these high-risk features are found on pathologic examination of resected polyp, further

therapy may be required. Optimal management is decided on an individual case basis
(Wilcox and Beck, 1987), but segmental resection of the involved colonic segment, local excision (e.g., transanal disk excision for
a low rectal lesion), or radiation therapy may
be considered. In the absence of high-risk
features, the chance of adverse outcome is
extremely small, and polypectomy is considered curative.

It is noteworthy that in the pathologic assessment of malignant polyps for high-risk
features, interobserver variability is greatest
in relation to lymphatic invasion (Cooper et
al., 1995, 1998). This feature may be difficult to assess in some cases and may ultimately be judged as being indeterminate.
Definitive diagnosis of lymphatic or venular
invasion is dependent upon finding carcinoma cells within an endothelial-lined space
(Cooper et al., 1998). Contraction artifact in
the tissue, tumor-induced stromal sclerosis,
or mucinous differentiation of the tumor
may all complicate the evaluation of vessel
invasion. Examination of additional tissue
levels of the specimen, review by a second
observer, and/or immunohistochemical
staining for endothelial markers (e.g., *Ulex
europaeus* lectin binding or factor VII or
CD34 immunostaining) may or may not help
to resolve the dilemma (Cooper et al., 1998).
In published cases in which the malignant
polyps have lacked definitive evidence of
high-risk features but the patients have gone
on to die of their disease, lymphatic invasion
was judged (on blinded review) as indeterminate because of a lack of interobserver
agreement (Cooper et al., 1995).

A potential diagnostic pitfall in the assessment of adenoma for cancer is the misinterpretation of glandular entrapment
(also known as *pseudoinvasion* or *misplaced
adenomatous glands*) for invasive carcinoma.
Glandular entrapment occurs in 2.5%–10%
of adenomas. Thus, the frequency is comparable to the incidence of invasive cancer
(about 5% of adenomas contain intramucosal carcinoma). It occurs in pedunculated
polyps that twist on their stalks and undergo
ischemic necrosis and ulceration of the
polyp head. With repair, adenomatous epithelium becomes entrapped in the base of
the ulcer and resembles invasive tumor in
the submucosa of the polyp head or stalk
(Fig. 9–15). However, pseudoinvasion can

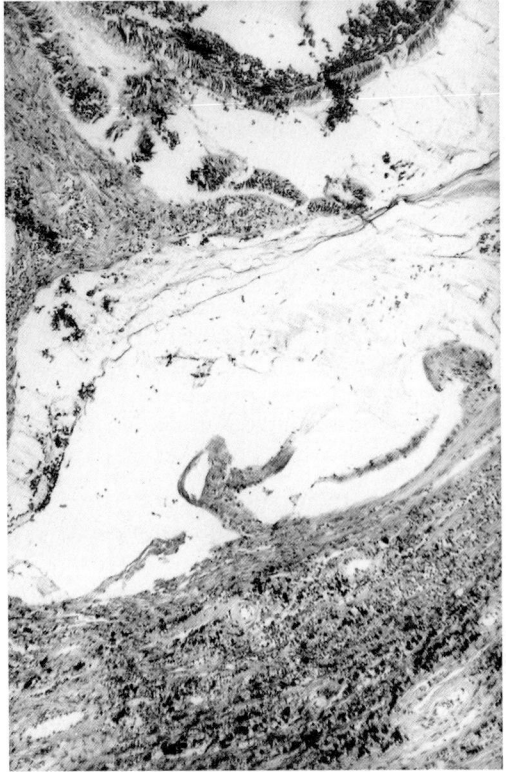

Figure 9–15. Glandular entrapment in submucosa of the head of adenoma shows benign cytologic features of tumor epithelium floating in
extracellular mucin pools and marked hemosiderin deposition (bottom) in the stroma marking the site of tissue infarction.

usually be differentiated from invasive carcinoma by the following (Cooper et al., 1998):

• the benign, adenomatous appearance
of the entrapped mucosa
• the rounded contours of the entrapped
glandular islands
• marked dilatation of the entrapped
glands
• the lack of intraepithelial carcinoma in
the overlying mucosa
• the presence of lamina propria surrounding the entrapped glands
• the presence of hemosiderin and gran-
ulation tissue (secondary to ischemia and ulceration).

The diagnosis of glandular entrapment
may be difficult in some circumstances, however. A fibroblastic stromal reaction may
be induced by the hemosiderin (Fig. 9–15),

and the resultant appearance may closely resemble that of a desmoplastic response to invasive carcinoma. Isolated mucin pools resembling those produced by mucinous carcinoma may occur, and detached, deteriorating adenomatous epithelium within them may appear relatively atypical. Rarely, both true invasive carcinoma and pseudoinvasive glandular entrapment may occur in the same adenoma. For all of these reasons, it sometimes may be impossible to definitively exclude the possibility of invasive carcinoma. However, if the adenoma is completely excised, the problem is academic because polypectomy is curative.

Genetic Basis of Adenoma Formation, Progression, and Malignant Transformation: Inherited and Sporadic Disease

Molecular Pathogenesis of Incipient Neoplasia

The understanding of molecular and histopathologic events occurring during the incipient phases of colorectal cancer development has specifically been enabled because several types of hereditary colon cancer syndromes exist as pathogenic models. In these syndromes, the risk of developing colonic adenomas is essentially 100%, and the adenomas are always multiple. Depending on the syndrome or its variant, the number of adenomas may vary greatly, from a few to myriad (Leppert et al., 1990). In all of these syndromes, however, the risk developing carcinoma is dramatically increased compared to the general population. Molecular studies of these syndromes have revealed that initiation of the neoplastic process is related to the mutation of a single key gene in a colonic epithelial stem cell (Kinzler and Vogelstein, 1998). With cell division, the mutation is passed on to the progeny of the mutated stem cell. Additional mutations are then acquired in a cumulative manner in the progeny of the initiated cells. As the neoplastic process progresses, subclones with mutations that confer the greatest growth advantage come to dominate the process (Kinzler and Vogelstein, 1998). Early in the process, the genetically abnormal cells also undergo cytologic changes by which they can be recognizable morphologically. The cytopathologic changes progress through stages of increasing severity as mutations are accumulated and, in a proportion of cases, a full malignant phenotype develops.

In most colon cancers, the initiating mutation involves the *adenomatous polyposis coli* (APC) tumor suppressor gene, which performs an essential role in maintaining cellular growth control. In familial polyposis coli (FAP), the mutation is inherited through the germline, and in most sporadic colon cancer, it is an acquired mutation in a somatic cell. Additional genetic events then occur, most often in the following order: *(1)* activation of the K-*ras* oncogene; *(2)* inactivation of the *p53* tumor suppressor gene; and *(3)* inactivation of the DCC (deleted in colon cancer) tumor suppressor gene on chromosome 18q (Kinzler and Vogelstein, 1998). This genetic pathway of colorectal tumorigenesis has been termed the *tumor suppressor pathway.*

In the hereditary nonpolyposis colon cancer (HNPCC) syndrome and in about 15%–20% of sporadic colon cancer, the initiating mutation involves one of the genes involved in the molecular system that detects and repairs the random mutations that occur with DNA synthesis during cell replication. This genetic pathway has been termed the *mutator pathway,* because the inability to repair DNA replication errors produces a hypermutable phenotype. Additional mutations leading to tumor formation are then rapidly acquired, but the type and order of acquisition of these mutations are not yet clear and may differ from the tumor suppressor pathway (Watne, 1997). In the hereditary colon cancer syndromes, it is clear that the cancer risk associated with these mutations is linked to epithelial site or organ specificity. Even though all cells contain the inherited mutation in these syndromes, the risk of neoplasia is increased in only a few specific organs, the colon being primary among them. At present, the reasons for this are not understood.

The major classes of genetic events pertinent to colorectal tumorigenesis via the tumor suppressor pathway and the relationship of these events to specific phases of adenoma formation are reviewed below.

Tumor Suppressor Genes and Adenoma Formation

As a class, tumor suppressor genes encode proteins that restrict cell growth and maintain normal differentiation. Mutations of tumor suppressor genes are characteristically inactivating, but they are also typically recessive. Biologically, therefore, tumor suppressor gene mutations are silent unless both alleles are inactivated. In sporadic colon cancers, the mechanism by which this usually occurs is as follows: one allele undergoes an inactivating mutation and the other (normal) allele is deleted from the chromosome. The exact mechanism of allelic loss is unknown but may be related to genomic instability due to asymmetric distribution of chromosomal material. Allelic loss (also known as *loss of heterozygosity* or LOH) is a common event in colorectal neoplasia, congruent with this mechanism of gene inactivation. In some instances, however, inactivation of the second allele of a tumor suppressor gene occurs through other mechanisms such as mutation or dimerization and inactivation of the protein product of the normal allele with the abnormal protein from the mutated allele.

The APC tumor suppressor gene is located on chromosome 5q (Bodmar et al., 1987). It encodes a cytoplasmic protein that is necessary for activation of programmed cell death (apoptosis) of colonic glandular epithelial cells moving from the proliferative zone at the gland bases to the zone of differentiation in the luminal half of the gland. The balance of cell proliferation and apoptosis within colonic glands maintains homeostasis in the normal mucosa. With loss of APC gene function in a proliferating cell and subsequent loss of apoptosis among its progeny, a permanent imbalance in cell division over cell death ensues and the epithelium becomes "hyperproliferative." Therefore, the APC gene has become known as the "gatekeeper" of colonic epithelial proliferation, and hyperproliferation caused by inactivation of the APC gene is thought to be the seminal (initiating) event in most colorectal neoplasia (Carethers, 1996; Kinzler and Vogelstein, 1996). In sporadic disease, APC mutation is present in about 60%–65% of all adenomas (small and large) and carcinomas (Carethers, 1996).

The *p53* tumor suppressor gene (named for its 53 kD protein product) is located on the short arm of chromosome 17 (17p131.1) (Kinzler and Vogelstein, 1998). It encodes a nuclear protein that activates expression of other genes and is therefore considered to be a transcription factor. Most of the genes activated by *p53* are involved in growth inhibition of abnormal cells (i.e., halting division and inducing apoptosis in cells with damaged DNA). Thus, it is an important regulator of normal cell growth. Inactivation of this gene appears to occur late in adenoma development. It is uncommon in small adenomas but is found with increasing frequency in adenomas of increasing size and malignant potential. Correspondingly, LOH at 17 (i.e., loss of the second [normal] p53 allele) is tightly associated with malignant transformation of adenomas. Thus, loss of *p53* function is believed to be the event that most commonly mediates carcinoma development within an adenoma (Carethers, 1996). Mutation of the *p53* gene can be demonstrated by immunohistochemical as well as molecular methods. Mutant p53 protein, although biologically inactive, is overexpressed in colorectal tumors and is more stable than its normal counterpart. Thus, mutant p53 protein accumulates in tumor cell nuclei and can be detected by immunohistochemical methods. It has been demonstrated that reintroduction of a normal, functioning *p53* gene into a tumor cell results in death of the cell. Therefore, *p53* is a focus of interest as a potential candidate for gene therapy in colorectal carcinoma.

The DCC tumor suppressor gene is located on the long arm of chromosome 18 (18q), a segment that is frequently missing in colorectal cancers. One copy of chromosome 18q is lost (LOH at 18q) in about 47% of large adenomas with foci of carcinoma and in about 73% of colorectal carcinomas, but in less advanced adenomas, loss occurs less frequently (Vogelstein et al., 1988). In metastatic disease, LOH at 18q is found in 80% of tumors. The gene encodes a transmembrane protein that is constitutively expressed in normal colonic mucosa. Although its function has not been fully defined, it is known to have structural similarities to known cell adhesion molecules. Thus, the DCC gene is thought to be involved in cell–cell adhesion and cell–matrix interactions, functions that may play a role in preventing tumor growth, invasion, and metastasis. In the adenoma–carcinoma sequence, allelic loss of DCC usually occurs after LOH of the APC gene and mutation of the K-*ras* protooncogene. Loss of the second

DCC allele is rare, and no mutations of the second allele have yet been reported. Apparently, loss of one allele (i.e., a 50% reduction in gene dose) is sufficient to produce the observed biologic effect (Kinzler and Vogelstein, 1998).

Oncogenes and Adenoma Formation

Oncogenes are mutated versions of normal cellular genes (proto-oncogenes) that encode proteins involved in stimulating or otherwise abetting cell division. The proto-oncogene known K-*ras* encodes a cytoplasmic relay protein that helps carry stimulatory signals from the plasma membrane to the nucleus. In contrast to mutated tumor suppressor genes that abrogate normal growth inhibitory feedback signals from other cells, oncogenes cause direct overstimulation of the growth machinery of the cell. Characteristically, the mutation of a proto-oncogene is dominant over the normal allele and is associated with aberrantly increased activity of the protein product (Carethers, 1996). Thus, neither loss nor mutation of the second (normal) allele is required for the oncogene to cause excessive and inappropriate growth stimulation of the affected cell. Molecular genetic studies have shown that mutations of the K-*ras* proto-oncogene (located on chromosome 12p) are common in medium-sized and large adenomas as well as in colorectal carcinomas but are rarely found in small adenomas (Kinzler and Vogelstein, 1998). Therefore, the *Ras* oncogene is thought to play a role in the growth of adenomas, but it is not clear whether it is an essential component of tumor development. It is not essential for malignant transformation of adenomas. Other classes of oncogenes that may contribute to the progression of colonic neoplasia include those that encode *(1)* growth factors or receptors for growth factors (e.g., *HER-2/neu*); *(2)* nuclear transcription factors that activate growth-promoting genes (e.g., *myc*); *(3)* proteins known as cyclins, which stimulate cell cycling (e.g., *Bcl*-1); and *(4)* antagonists of cell suicide (apoptosis) or growth suppressor proteins (e.g., *MDM*2) (Kinzler and Vogelstein, 1998).

Inherited Colon Cancer Syndromes

Familial adenomatous polyposis and its variants. *Familial adenomatous polyposis* (FAP)

is an autosomal dominant disease affecting about 1 in 7000 individuals. In FAP and its variant known as *Gardner's syndrome,* as well as some cases of Turcot's syndrome, the germline mutation is in the APC gene (Kinzler and Vogelstein, 1996; Lynch and Lynch, 1998). The APC mutation is present in all somatic cells, but in FAP, only 1 in 10 million colonic epithelial stem cells gives rise to an adenoma (Kinzler and Vogelstein, 1996). Although allelic loss in any single colonic epithelial cell produces hyperproliferation, additional mutations, as outlined above, are required for tumorigenesis. The hallmark of all of these syndromes is florid colonic adenomatosis (adenomas numbering >100) (Figs. 9–16 and 9–17). Individual adenomas are identical in appearance to sporadic adenomas (Fig. 9–18). In Gardner's syndrome, extracolonic manifestations, such as osteomas of the skull, mandibular cysts, adrenal adenomas, and intra-abdominal desmoid tumors, also occur. In Turcot's syndrome, colonic adenomatosis is accompanied by central nervous system tumors.

In these syndromes, affected individuals develop hundreds to thousands of colonic adenomas during the second and third decades of life, and the risk of colorectal neoplasia at a young age is greatly increased. Although an individual FAP adenoma is no more likely to progress to carcinoma than a sporadic adenoma, the sheer number of adenomas increases the risk of carcinoma to a virtual certainty, and prophylactic colectomies are routinely performed in affected individuals. Although the APC mutation is present in all cells in the FAP syndrome, only the colon, small intestine, stomach, thyroid,

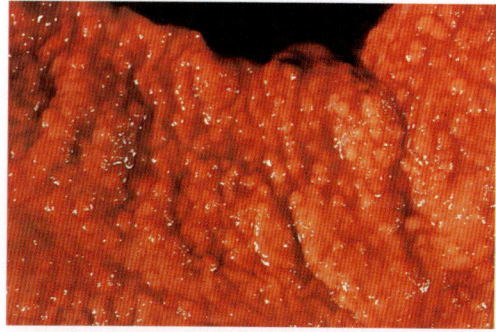

Figure 9–16. Familial adenomatous polyposis showing myriad small adenomas covering the colonic mucosal surface.

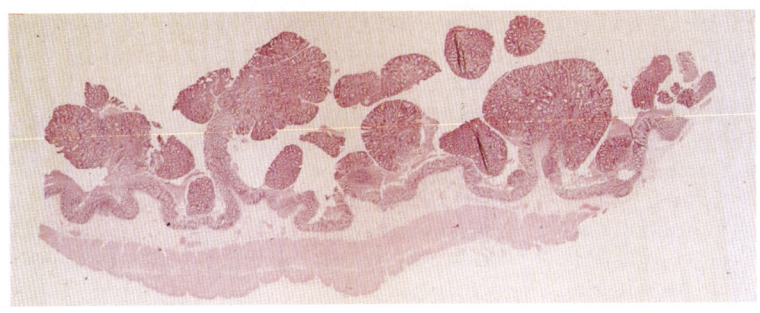

Figure 9–17. Familial adenomatous polyposis showing numerous tubular adenomas of similar size.

and brain appear to be predisposed to development of carcinoma.

The location of the mutation within the APC gene appears to determine the disease phenotype to a large degree (O'Sullivan et al., 1998). The APC gene has 15 coding exons. It is a very large gene, and most of its length resides in exon 15, which holds the distinction of being the largest known human exon (O'Sullivan et al., 1998). Although more than 300 different mutations of the APC gene have been described, the vast majority are chain-terminating mutations that occur in the 5′ end of exon 15 and produce a phenotype of profuse polyposis as seen in classical FAP (Giardiello et al., 1997; O'Sullivan et al., 1998). However, variant forms of FAP with a phenotype of relatively sparse polyposis are linked to unusual mutations of the APC gene, including those in the extreme 5′ region of the gene before codon 158, those within exon 9, and those at the 3′ distal end of the gene in exon 15 (O'Sullivan et al., 1998; Soravia et al., 1998). In these variant forms, the onset of adenomas and of carcinomas is delayed, and the ultimate number of colonic adenomas is consequently greatly reduced (i.e., fewer than 100). Thus, these variants have become known as *attenuated FAP*. In the first reports of attenuated FAP, it was noted that the adenomas tended to be flat rather than polypoid and preferentially distributed in the proximal colon. In attenuated FAP, the risk of colorectal cancer is less than in FAP, and while the risk is still significant, prophylactic colectomy is not recommended for all gene carriers.

Almost all mutations of the APC gene result in a truncated gene product, the detection of which forms that basis for a screening test for FAP known as the in vitro *synthetic protein assay* (Kinzler and Vogelstein, 1996; Powell et al., 1993). In this test, the APC transcript is amplified by the reverse-transcription polymerase chain reaction (PCR) technique, and transcription and translation of the PCR product is performed *in vitro*. Electrophoresis of the resultant product reveals truncated proteins when mutations exist. The test identifies about 85% of individuals with FAP (Kinzler and Vogelstein, 1996). The test is falsely negative in the remaining 15% because of inactivation of the

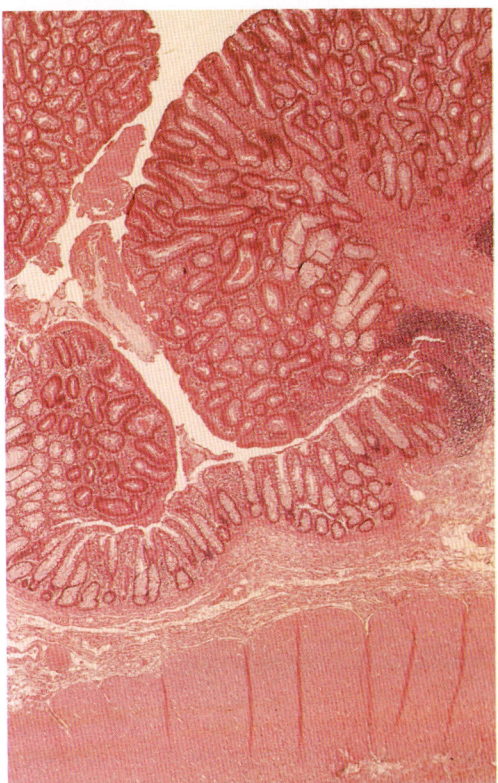

Figure 9–18. Adenomas in familial adenomatous polyposis are identical in histologic appearance to sporadic adenomas, may be stalked or sessile, and are typically tubular in configuration when small.

gene product. Currently, indications for the use of this test as a screening procedure include the following:

• confirmation of a clinical diagnosis when a phenotype of FAP or Gardner's syndrome is identified in any individual
• diagnosis or exclusion of potentially affected family members of a cohort with FAP or Gardner's syndrome (i.e., presymptomatic testing)
• diagnosis or exclusion of a variant form of FAP if 20 or more adenomas are present endoscopically.

Hereditary nonpolyposis colon cancer. The *HNPCC syndrome*, also known as the *Warthin-Lynch syndrome* or *Lynch syndrome*, is an autosomal dominant disorder that has been estimated to account for up to 5%–6% of all colorectal cancer (Ponz de Leon, 1996). The number of adenomas that develop in this syndrome is far less then in the FAP syndrome but may be comparable to that in the attenuated FAP syndrome. In the HNPCC syndrome, some cases of Turcot's syndrome, the Muir-Torre syndrome, and an estimated 15%–20% of sporadic colon cancers, the initiating mutation involves one of the DNA mismatch repair genes (Lynch and Lynch, 1998; Lynch and Smyrk, 1996; Marra and Boland, 1996).

Mutation of any one of the genes in the DNA mismatch repair system completely destroys the ability to correct replication error–derived mutations, but abrogation of gene function typically requires an inactivating mutation in each allele. In HNPCC, one of these mutations is inherited, and the other is acquired. DNA repair–deficient cells accumulate mutations at a very rapid rate, leading to a 1000-fold increase in the frequency of mutations compared to repair-proficient cells (Lynch and Smyrk, 1996). The two most commonly inherited mutations in the HNPCC syndrome are those of genes known as *hMSH-2* (involved in the recognition of deformities in the DNA double helix created by nucleotide base mismatches) and *hMLH-1* (involved in strand resynthesis and ligation). Each of these mutations represents just under half of all HNPCC (Kim, 1997; Lynch and Lynch, 1998). The subsequent genetic events by which tumor progression proceeds are not yet fully

elucidated. Genes involved in growth control may become mutated in both alleles (obviating the requirement for the LOH that typifies the tumor suppressor pathway). However, DNA mispairings occur most often in repetitive sequences of DNA known as *microsatellites*, and mutations at these sequences (producing what is known as *microsatellite instability*) are the hallmark of tumors with defective DNA mismatch repair (i.e., replication error–positive tumors) (Marra and Boland, 1996). As a consequence of this phenomenon, genes with microsatellite sequences within the genome (e.g., transforming growth factor-β receptor gene and the insulin-like growth factor receptor gene) appear to be uniquely and preferentially affected by defective DNA mismatch repair mechanisms (Kim, 1997; Marra and Boland, 1996).

Compared to tumors generated via the tumor suppressor gene pathway, tumors generated via the mutator pathway exhibit several distinctive pathologic features. For example, the adenomas tend to undergo malignant transformation sooner (i.e., at a smaller size) and the cancers tend to be predominantly right sided, poorly differentiated, and locally aggressive, with early invasion (Lynch and Smyrk, 1996; Messerini et al., 1996). Nevertheless, the cancers are associated with a better prognosis when stage-matched to other colorectal malignancies (Lynch and Lynch, 1998; Lynch and Smyrk, 1996). This apparent paradox is thought to be related to the hypermutable phenotype, which initially accelerates the adenoma–carcinoma sequence but ultimately inactivates genes required for such complex tumor activities as metastasis.

HAMARTOMATOUS POLYPOSIS AND THE DYSLASIA–CARCINOMA SEQUENCE

The *familial juvenile polyposis (FJP) syndrome* and the *Peutz-Jeghers syndrome (PJS)* are autosomal dominant inherited syndromes of gastrointestinal hamartomatous polyposis that are both associated with an increased risk of colorectal carcinoma. In FJP, variant expressions of the disease may produce mucosal hamartomas that are mostly colorectal, mostly gastric, or diffusely distributed throughout the gastrointestinal tract (Luk, 1995). Overall, however, colorectal hamartomas occur in 98% of FJP cases, and the increased risk of malignant tumors in this syndrome is associated primarily with colorectal cancer (Desai et al., 1995; Luk, 1995; Lynch and Lynch, 1998). The risk of gastric carcinoma is also increased. In PJS, the mucosal hamartomas are predominantly small intestinal. Therefore, PJS is discussed more fully in chapter 8 on the small intestine. However, hamartomas also occur in the stomach, colon, and rectum in PJS, and the entire gastrointestinal tract is at increased risk for carcinoma (Haggitt and Reid, 1986; Lynch and Lynch, 1998).

The hamartomatous polyps that characterize FJP and PJS are morphologically distinctive, but they share the following characteristics:

• the epithelial cells of the polyp mucosa are cytologically normal and are histologically appropriate for the region of the bowel in which the polyp resides
• the glandular architecture of the polyp mucosa is abnormally complex.

In either syndrome, the polyp epithelium may become dysplastic (i.e., neoplastic), and tumor progression through increasing degrees of dysplasia to carcinoma may occur (Dajani and Kamal, 1984; Giardiello et al.,

1987; Haggitt and Reid, 1986; Järvinen and Franssila, 1984; Lipper et al., 1981; Luk, 1995; Lynch and Lynch, 1998; O'Riordain et al., 1991; Perzin and Bridge, 1982; Rustgi, 1995). In both of these syndromes, patients are often managed by periodic colonoscopy and polypectomy. Careful examination for neoplastic changes within the resected hamartomas is essential. The degree of dysplasia may be graded as low or high grade, and if feasible, the entire polyp should be examined microscopically for evidence of carcinoma. As in adenomas of the colon, intraepithelial and intramucosal carcinoma is cured by complete polypectomy, but invasion of the submucosa may require further therapy if the cancer is poorly differentiated, vasoinvasive, or present at the polypectomy margin.

FAMILIAL JUVENILE POLYPOSIS

Juvenile polyps have a highly distinctive gross and microscopic appearance. They are usually bulbous in shape with a smooth rounded surface and cherry red in color (Haggitt and Reid, 1986; Luk, 1995). They are seldom bigger than 3 cm and usually average 1–1.5 cm in greatest dimension (Haggitt and Reid, 1986). When transected, cystically dilated spaces filled with mucinous fluid are typically evident within the polyp head (Fig. 9–19). On microscopic examination, the cysts are seen to correspond to haphazardly arranged, massively dilated glands

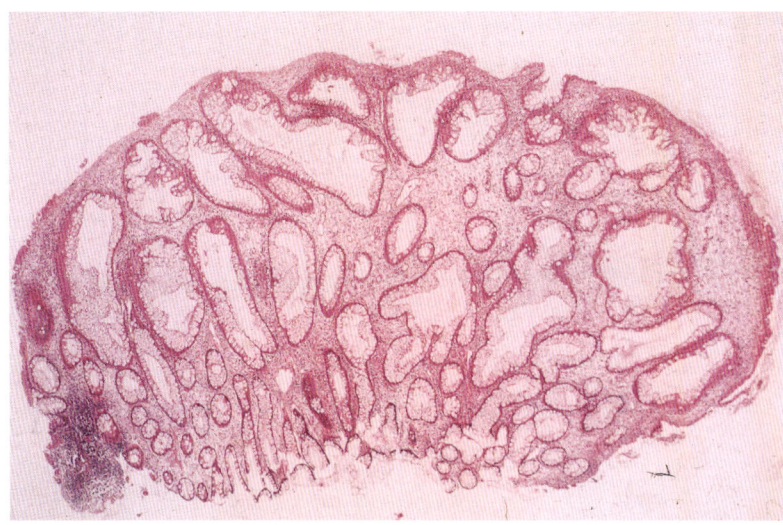

Figure 9–19. A typical juvenile polyp shows a smooth surface and widely separated, architecturally distorted, and cystically dilated glands.

lined by mucin-producing epithelium of the type that is native to the mucosa of origin (Fig. 9–20). The glands may show regenerative atypia or hyperplastic changes if the polyp is eroded and/or inflamed, but the epithelium lacks dysplastic features. The stroma is characteristically abundant and widely separates the glands (Fig. 9–20). It is often edematous, congested, and inflamed, and in contrast to the stroma of Peutz-Jeghers hamartomas, it lacks smooth muscle.

Juvenile polyps occur most often as solitary sporadic lesions in children, and in this setting, they are not associated with an increased risk of gastrointestinal (i.e., colorectal) carcinoma (Nugent et al., 1993). Once the polyp is removed or undergoes autoamputation, additional metachronous polyps rarely form, and any potential risk that might be associated with the index polyp is perforce eliminated. In the FJP syndrome, more than 10 juvenile polyps, often dozens to hundreds, are produced (McColl et al., 1964). Although a family history of polyposis was once thought to be a *sine qua non* of FJP, sporadic (nonfamilial) cases are known to occur and are thought to be related to spontaneous rather than inherited mutations in the germline (Haggitt and Reid, 1986). The risk of malignancy in the colon and rectum and, to a lesser degree, in the stomach is increased because of the typical preponderance of polyps in those sites in both the sporadic and familial cases. Overall, it has been estimated that about 9% of

FJP patients develop carcinoma of the colon (Haggitt and Reid, 1986). Premalignant adenomatous dysplasia may occur in any juvenile polyp in the setting of FJP (Fig. 9–21), and therefore, complete removal and careful pathologic examination for dysplasia and carcinoma are recommended (Haggitt and Reid, 1986; Luk, 1995). For FJP patients with large numbers of colorectal polyps that cannot be adequately managed by endoscopic polypectomy, prophylactic colectomy may be considered (Haggitt and Reid, 1986; Luk, 1995).

Polyps that have been interpreted as true colonic adenomas have been reported to occur synchronously with juvenile polyps in adult patients with FJP (O'Riordan et al., 1991; Rustgi, 1995). Often, in this setting, the juvenile polyps show focal epithelial dysplasia (O'Riordan et al., 1991). Thus, the genesis of these "adenomas" is unclear, and the possibility that they represent diffuse adenomatous dysplasia of preexisting hamartomas has not been excluded. The occurrence of both focal epithelial dysplasia and focal villous architecture in the hamartomas of FJP has been shown to be related to polyp size and may be seen in any FJP hamartoma greater than 1 cm in dimension (Subramony et al., 1994). It has also been shown that here is a very high incidence of focal epithelial dysplasia in the colonic hamartomas of FJP patients in the pediatric age-group, suggesting that adenomatous dysplasia is frequently an early event in this

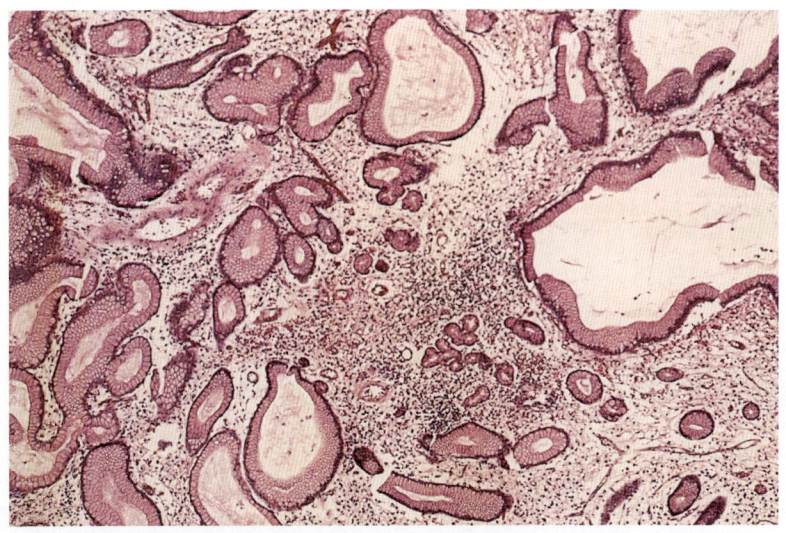

Figure 9–20. The typically edematous, mildly inflamed stroma devoid of smooth muscle and dilated glands lined by cytologically normal goblet cells of a juvenile polyp are shown.

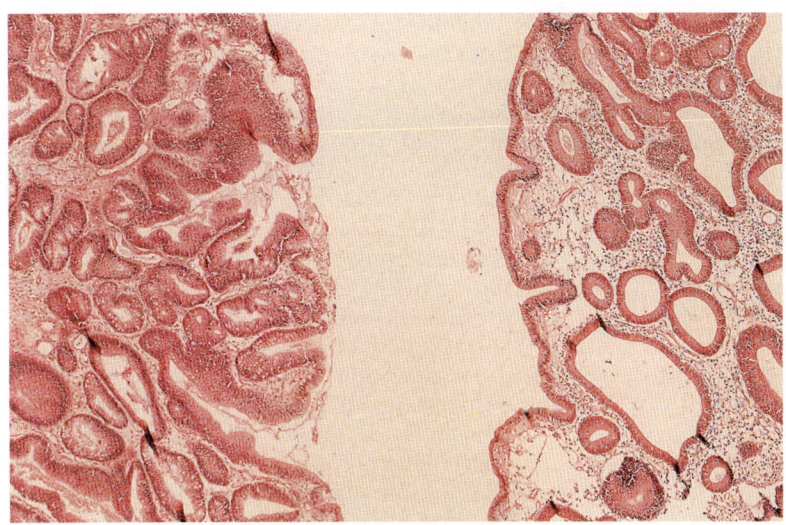

Figure 9–21. Adenomatous dysplasia is seen in one of two polyps (left) from a patient with familial juvenile polyposis.

syndrome (Vaiphei and Thapa, 1997). Thus, with time, dysplastic epithelium may predominate in some hamartomas with the resultant histologic appearance becoming indistinguishable from that of an adenoma. Genetic analysis may help to resolve this issue.

The underlying genetic defect in FJP is a germline mutation in the gene *SMAD4* (also known as *DPC4*) located on chromosome 18q (Howe et al., 1998a, 1998b). This gene encodes a cytoplasmic protein that is a critical mediator in the signaling pathway for transforming growth factor *β*. The mutation leads to the production of a truncated protein that lacks sequences needed for normal function (Howe et al., 1998b). With the development of dysplasia, additional genetic alterations are acquired. Some of the dysplasia-associated molecular changes that have been defined in FJP include the products of the following genes (in decreasing order of incidence): *p21*, APC, and *p53* (Kim et al., 1997; Wu et al., 1997). In contrast to adenomas, mutations in the K-*ras* proto-oncogene do not appear to be related to the evolution of dysplasia in FJP (Wu et al., 1997).

Peutz-Jeghers Syndrome

In PJS, the hamartomas appear highly lobulated and are often stalked, resembling adenomas endoscopically. Microscopically, they are composed of highly branched, tightly packed glands with scanty intervening stroma that contains prominent smooth muscle fascicles that course between glands and typically extend to the polyp surface. When the colonic hamartomas of PJS undergo dysplastic and/or carcinomatous change, especially when the dysplasia is extensive, differentiation from an adenoma may be extremely difficult. Furthermore, it has been reported that both adenomas and hamartomas may apparently occur synchronously in the colon of patients with PJS (Hood and Krush, 1983; Rustgi, 1995). For any given polyp, the differential diagnosis between a dysplastic PJS hamartoma and an adenoma may be moot, since both are treated in the same fashion.

The genetic basis of PJS is a germline mutation in the serine/threonine kinase 11 (*STK11*) gene located on chromosome 19p (Amos et al., 1997; Hemminki et al., 1997; Jenne et al., 1998; Mehenni et al., 1997; Nakagawa et al., 1998). The manifestations of the disease are produced when a defect in the second allele is acquired in a somatic cell (Jenne et al., 1998). At present, the role of this gene either in hamartoma formation or in neoplastic transformation of Peutz-Jeghers polyps is not well understood. However, somatic mutations in the *STK11* gene accompanied by loss of heterozygosity at 19p have been reported in sporadic left-sided colorectal carcinomas and some left-sided adenomas with high-grade dysplasia (but not in early adenomas) (Dong et al., 1998). Thus, it is hypothesized that *STK11* is a tumor suppressor gene that, even in individuals who do not have PJS, it may play an important role in gastrointestinal carcinogenesis.

INFLAMMATORY BOWEL DISEASE AND THE DYSPLASIA–CARCINOMA SEQUENCE

PREVALENCE, RISK FACTORS, AND DETECTION

Colon cancers that arise from dysplasia in flat epithelium usually develop in a background of long-standing chronic colitis. In the United States, inflammatory bowel disease (chronic ulcerative colitis in particular) is the major example of this phenomenon. Crohn's disease is also associated with an increased risk of colorectal and small bowel cancer developing via this mechanism and is discussed in chapters 8 on the small intestine. In other areas of the world, schistosomal colitis or other chronic colidites of infectious etiology also exemplify this process. Carcinoma arising in a background of ulcerative colitis (UC) represents less than 1% of all colorectal cancer in the United States. However, it is an important problem because the disease affects young individuals and is associated with decreased survival that is related directly to death from colon cancer and not from other medical conditions (Ekbom, 1998). Colorectal cancer accounts for about 15% of all deaths in UC (Lashner, 1992). The risk of colon cancer in UC is most strongly related to the anatomic extent of the disease and to disease duration. Thus, proctitis alone poses no greater risk of colon cancer than that in the general population, whereas disease of the left colon increases the risk but less so than pancolitis (Snapper et al., 1998). The risk of malignant transformation first becomes significant when the total duration of the colitis reaches 8 to 10 years and thereafter increases steadily with increasing duration of disease at the rate of 0.5%–2.0% per year (Greenstein et al., 1979; Lennard-Jones et al., 1990). For pancolitis of 30 years duration, the cumulative risk of colorectal cancer is 30% (Snapper et al., 1998). The risk of colorectal cancer is also increased in the subset of patients with onset of colitis before age 15 or with primary sclerosing cholangitis (Marchesa et al., 1997; Riddell, 1998).

The diagnosis of dysplasia, the earliest recognizable stage of incipient neoplasia in the setting of chronic colitis, identifies those individuals who are at risk for colon cancer and is analogous to the identification of an index adenoma in individuals without colitis. However, it is far more difficult to recognize, both grossly and microscopically. Surveillance requires multiple biopsies that are typically acquired at random 5 to 10 sites at different levels of the colon (Bernstein, 1998) and is recommended for patients with extensive colitis beginning at 8 years after first diagnosis of their disease. Even at this time point, as many as 10% of patients may already have dysplasia or carcinoma (Bernstein, 1998; Bernstein et al., 1994; Connell et al., 1994; Ransohoff et al., 1985). If the initial endoscopy findings are negative for dysplasia, only about 3% of patients will ultimately develop neoplasia when followed over time (Bernstein et al., 1994; Connell et al., 1994). However, the absence of dysplasia on surveillance does not assure the absence of carcinoma risk, since dysplasia may be missed because of sampling error. It has been estimated that a set of 10 surveillance biopsies samples only 0.05% of the colonic surface (Rosenstock et al., 1985). Thus, patients may present with carcinoma within 1 to 2 years of their last negative surveillance colonoscopy, presumably because dysplasia has been missed (Collins et al., 1987; Connell et al., 1994; Ransohoff et al., 1985). When dysplasia is present, it has been estimated that 64 biopsies are required to achieve a 95% certainty of finding the highest grade of dysplasia (Rubin et al., 1992). Additional problems associated with surveillance colonoscopy in UC are related to the inherent difficulties in assessing dysplasia microscopically (see Diagnostic Features, Microscopic Appearance, and Differential Diagnosis below). Despite the limitations of surveillance colonoscopy, it is the only available alternative to prophylactic colectomy as an approach to reducing the risk of colorectal cancer. The goal of surveillance is to detect incipient neoplasia in its earliest phases so that interventional colectomy can be performed at a curable stage of disease (Snapper et al., 1998).

Diagnostic Features

Macroscopic Appearance and Differential Diagnosis

When widespread and well advanced, dysplasia may be visible endoscopically as plaques or nodules that have a finely villous or furry appearance. More often, dysplasia is macroscopically indistinguishable from the adjacent nondysplastic mucosa. Furthermore, it is often multifocal, poorly circumscribed, and irregular or patchy in distribution. Grossly apparent lesions or masses that are found at biopsy to have dysplastic mucosa are highly clinically significant since they have a strong association with underlying carcinoma. The chance that a dysplasia-associated lesion or mass (DALM) harbors an underlying cancer is 40% if the dysplasia is low grade and 60% of the dysplasia is high grade (Blackstone et al., 1981; Rosenstock et al., 1985; Snapper et al., 1998). Therefore, the diagnosis of a DALM is an indication for colectomy (Snapper et al., 1998). For this reason, it is important to differentiate DALMs from coincidental adenomas, which can be managed by polypectomy alone (Medlicott et al., 1997; Suzuki et al., 1998; Torres et al., 1998).

The following features, representing a mixture of clinical, macroscopic, and microscopic findings, may help to distinguish adenomas from DALMs (Suzuki et al., 1998; Torres et al., 1998):

Clinical
- occurrence in individuals over 50 years of age
- occurrence in a background of inactive disease
- shorter duration of disease (median 5 years for adenoma vs. 11 years for DALM)
- disease limited to the distal colon or rectum

Macroscopic
- lesion size less than 1.0 cm

Microscopic
- no increased mononuclear inflammation in the lamina propria
- no villous architectural components
- only dysplastic crypts present (versus admixture of normal and dysplastic crypts in DALM).

Microscopic Appearance and Differential Diagnosis

All endoscopic surveillance biopsies require evaluation for dysplasia, which is classified as being absent, present, or indefinite (Riddell et al., 1983). Mucosa that is negative for dysplasia encompasses both typical quiescent colitis with architectural glandular distortion but no significant epithelial atypia and active or resolving colitis with reactive or regenerative epithelial atypia. Mucosa that is unequivocally positive for dysplasia (i.e., neoplastic) is subcategorized as low-grade or high-grade. Epithelial atypia that is indefinite for dysplasia either (1) exceeds the degree expected in quiescent disease but does not quite meet the diagnostic threshold for dysplasia, or (2) closely resembles dysplasia but cannot be definitively differentiated from an exuberant regenerative reaction in active disease. In these settings, the cytologic atypia is neither definitively negative nor definitively positive for dysplasia.

All of the cytologic changes that define dysplasia in adenomas may be seen in mucosal dysplasia in UC. Thus, the diagnosis of dysplasia is most confidently made in flat mucosa that is uninflamed and has the cytologic features of an adenoma. When viewed at low magnification, dysplastic mucosa may show architectural alterations that resemble the glandular arrangement of adenomas with excessive budding of crypts and gland crowding (Riddell et al., 1983). This low-power appearance contrasts with the gland atrophy typical of uncomplicated UC. Alternatively, the surface of dysplastic mucosa may have a villous appearance. Although none of these architectural changes are diagnostic of dysplasia, they may be helpful in localizing foci of dysplasia when scanning the tissue. Ultimately, the diagnostic criteria for dysplasia are cytologic, not architectural.

As in adenomas, the dysplastic nuclei in dysplasia of low grade are confined to the basal halves of the cells and stratify into the luminal halves in high-grade dysplasia (Riddell et al., 1983). High-grade dysplasia also encompasses the changes of carcinoma *in situ*. Other histologic variants of dysplasia may be seen, but all are graded according to these same criteria. The histologic variants of dysplasia include the following (Riddell et al., 1983):

• dysplasia with "incomplete maturation" of crypts but no glandular architectural changes (immature mucin-depleted cells with tall, hyperchromatic, basally located nuclei that display little stratification or pleomorphism fill the glands and extend to the mucosal surface)

• dysplasia with clear cell change (cells with either hyperchromatic or vesicular dysplastic nuclei, stratification, and crowding show a nonmucinous clear cell change of the cytoplasm)

• dysplasia with dystrophic goblet cell predominance (goblet cells that are pseudostratified and show loss of polarity [appear upside down] predominate in the dysplastic epithelium)

• dysplasia with serrated crypts (dysplastic cells demonstrate nuclear tufting resembling that seen in serrated adenomas).

Mucosa that is indefinite for dysplasia encompasses a spectrum of cytologic changes that cannot be definitively categorized as negative or positive for dysplasia. This category is used most often in the setting of active inflammation or ulceration in which the features of injured and/or regenerating epithelial cells simulate those of dysplastic cells but cannot be confidently assessed as neoplastic (Fig. 9–22). In most cases, active inflammation precludes definitive assessment for dysplasia, and in this setting, it is prudent to classify cytologic changes resembling dysplasia as indefinite unless overt architectural changes of carcinoma *in situ* are seen. When the suspicion of dysplasia is high despite the presence of inflammation, the indefinite category may be further qualified as "probably positive." Alternatively, if the cytologic changes are judged to be excessive but most likely reactive, the indefinite category may be qualified as "probably negative." In some cases, the biologic significance of the atypia is unknown and may be qualified as such. In any case, a diagnosis of indefinite for dys-

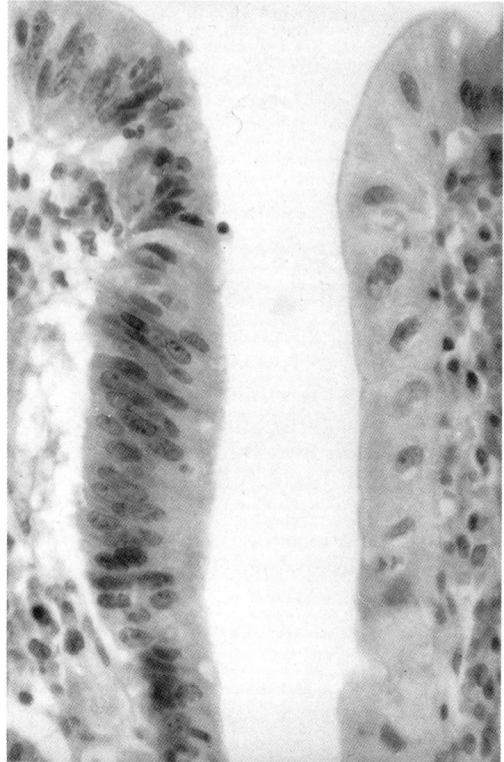

Figure 9–22. Epithelial atypia indefinite for low-grade dysplasia in ulcerative colitis shows nuclear changes that resemble dysplasia but are seen in the setting of active inflammation (neutrophils are present in the epithelium, seen at upper left) and re-epithelialization of an adjacent ulcer (typical regenerative atypia of epithelium, seen at left).

plasia is an indication of uncertainty on the part of the pathologist and is, at the least, an indication for further assessment of the status of the mucosa.

Interobserver variability in the pathologic assessment of dysplasia is one of the most difficult problems associated with surveillance colonoscopy. Even among experts, interobserver variability exists in both the diagnosis of dysplasia and the determination of grade. Reported ranges of interobserver variability vary from 42% to 99% (Bernstein, 1998; Lashner and Shapiro, 1998; Melville et al., 1989; Riddell et al., 1983; Snapper et al., 1998). Interobserver variability is greatest in the diagnosis of low-grade dysplasia, an increasingly critical diagnosis for the patient management algorithm. To reduce the chance of unnecessary colectomy for a false-positive diagnosis of dysplasia, all determinations of dysplasia should be confirmed by two independent pathologists and ideally should be made in the absence of active colitis.

Despite the problems associated with pathologic interpretation of surveillance biopsies, no supplemental aids for diagnosing or grading dysplasia or otherwise predicting cancer risk from tissue markers have proven superior. The classes of cell markers that have been investigated for this purpose include mucins, lectin-binding sites, oncofetal and other tumor antigens, oncogenes, tumor suppressor genes, DNA repair genes, cell proliferation–associated markers, global DNA hypomethylation, and aneuploidy (Lashner and Shapiro, 1998; Levin, 1992; Riddell, 1995, 1998). Some of these hold promise as supplemental markers for neoplastic progression, but none has proven sensitive or specific enough to supplant light microscopy as the gold standard for cancer risk assessment and patient management.

Role of the Pathologist in Clinical Management of Dysplasia

Assessment of endoscopic surveillance biopsies for dysplasia is central to the clinical management of patients with long-standing UC. The treatment algorithm is summarized below.

High-Grade Dysplasia

When high-grade dysplasia is found on colonoscopic surveillance, carcinoma is found in 40%–50% of patients undergoing subsequent colectomy (Bernstein et al., 1994; Ransohoff et al., 1985). Another third of patients with high-grade dysplasia eventually will be found to have cancer (Lashner and Shapiro, 1998). Thus, there is general agreement that high-grade dysplasia, confirmed by a second pathologist who is experienced in inflammatory bowel disease, is an indication for colectomy (Lashner and Shapiro, 1998; Snapper et al., 1998).

Low-Grade Dysplasia

In the past, low-grade dysplasia was widely regarded as an indication for more frequent surveillance rather than colectomy. How-
ever, more recent studies have shown that in as many as 20% of cases with low-grade dysplasia, cancer may already be present (Bernstein et al., 1994; Riddell, 1995; Snapper et al., 1998). Furthermore, patients with low-grade dysplasia progress to high-grade dysplasia or a DALM in 16%–54% of cases (Bernstein, 1998; Connell et al., 1994). Thus, there is an increasing trend to recommend colectomy for low-grade dysplasia (Bernstein, 1998; Snapper et al., 1998).

Dysplasia-Associated Lesion or Mass

As stated above, any degree of dysplasia in association with a visible lesion or mass that is not clearly an adenoma is an indication for colectomy.

Indefinite for Dysplasia

Among patients with a diagnosis of indefinite for dysplasia, about 20%–30% will ultimately progress to high-grade dysplasia, DALM, or carcinoma (Bernstein et al., 1994). Overall, it has been estimated that an individual patient with a diagnosis of indefinite for dysplasia has a 9% likelihood of developing cancer (Axon, 1998). Thus, this diagnosis is an indication for close follow-up with repeat endoscopy at 2 months and an increased number of biopsies or, if the reason for the indefinite diagnosis is related to disease activity, aggressive treatment of the inflammation and repeat biopsy within 6 months is recommended (Bernstein, 1998).

Genetic Basis of Dysplasia in Inflammatory Bowel

Much less is known about the genetic progression of neoplasia via the dysplasia–carcinoma sequence than that of the adenoma–carcinoma sequence, but significant differences have been noted in preliminary studies. In UC, marked chromosomal abnormalities occur early in the neoplastic process and are a prominent feature of both nondysplastic epithelium and preinvasive neoplasia (Willenbucher et al., 1997). The observation that microsatellite instability is frequent in nondysplastic mucosa in UC suggests the possibility that mutator pathway mechanisms may underlie the acquisition of these chromosomal abnormalities (Brentnall et al., 1996; Riddell, 1998). It is also possible that neoplastic progression in UC differs from either of the two major pathways defined for the adenoma–carcinoma sequence. With continual cell injury and repair in the setting of UC, the expression of genes that exert negative control over the cell cycle (e.g., tumor suppressor genes) would be suppressed, whereas expression of growth-promoting genes would be upregulated. Therefore, these genes may be disproportionately susceptible to genetic damage (Fogt et al., 1998). Genetic alterations that have been documented in both dysplasia and carcinoma in UC include LOH of the chromosomal segments encoding the APC, DCC, *p53*, and *p16* genes (Fogt et al., 1998; Lashner and Shapiro, 1998). Allelic deletions of DCC, *p53*, and *p16* as well as K-*ras* mutations have also been documented in nondysplastic epithelium in UC (Fogt et al., 1998; Willenbucher et al., 1997). In the adenoma–carcinoma sequence, histologically normal epithelium rarely shows these genetic alterations, even in the mutator pathway. Furthermore, certain genetic alterations, like allelic deletion of DCC, occur as late rather than early events. Allelic deletion of the APC gene does not seem to play a major role in the early stages of cancer development in UC, whereas allelic deletion of *p16* (a rare event in adenoma formation) does (Benhattar and Saraga., 1995; Fogt et al., 1998; Tarmin et al., 1995).

THE VERMIFORM APPENDIX

The current understanding of appendiceal epithelial neoplasia is limited because of the overall rarity of noncarcinoid appendiceal tumors and the incidental manner by which most are discovered. Adenomas of the appendix are seen only about half as often as appendiceal malignancies (Carr et al., 1995) and are only found in about 0.2% of appendices (Deans and Spence, 1995). Most appendiceal carcinomas are believed to arise from adenomas that progress through the adenoma–carcinoma sequence described above for the colorectum. However, dysplasia may occur as an early neoplastic lesion in the mucosa of an appendix involved by UC in long-standing pancolitis as discussed above in reference to the colon. In addition, some adenocarcinomas of the appendix appear to evolve from goblet cell carcinoid tumors of the appendix, which often lack an epithelial precursor lesion in the overlying mucosa.

ADENOMAS

Benign noncarcinoid appendiceal tumors are categorized by the World Health Organization as either adenomas or mucinous cystadenomas. The adenoma group includes localized, nodular, or polypoid lesions that include the same morphologic subtypes as their colorectal counterparts (Appelman, 1990; Carr et al., 1995). Among these colonic-type lesions, tubular adenomas occur more often than tubulovillous (Fig. 9–23) or villous adenomas (Appelman, 1990). Colonic-type adenomas are made up of immature hyperchromatic epithelial cells with little goblet cell differentiation (Carr et al., 1995). As in the colorectum, mixed adenomatous-hyperplastic polyps and adenomas with serrated appearance of the glands (i.e., serrated adenomas) also occur and are classified as adenomas. Cystadenomas are characterized by diffuse adenomatous mucosa that often encircles the appendiceal lumen and affects much of its length. They are by far more common than localized adenomas.

Two types of dysplastic epithelium, both of which are mucin-rich, may be seen in appendiceal adenomas. The more common of the two consists of tall columnar cells with an abundance of fine apical mucin granules that resemble gastric foveolar cells. The less common type is composed predominantly of goblet cells. The epithelium of these adenomas may form villous projections into the appendiceal lumen or be compressed against the distended wall to form a flattened to undulating or tufted surface. Neuroendocrine cells also may be included in the epithelium of these tumors. Other variable features include ulceration, fibrosis of the appendiceal wall, dissecting mucin lakes, and appendiceal rupture. Complete excision is usually curative for appendiceal adenomas, even those with transmural mucin dissection. Simple appendectomy is typically adequate for adenomas of the appendiceal tip, but right hemicolectomy may be required for appendiceal adenomas that extend to the appendiceal origin and cannot be completely excised by simple appendiceal

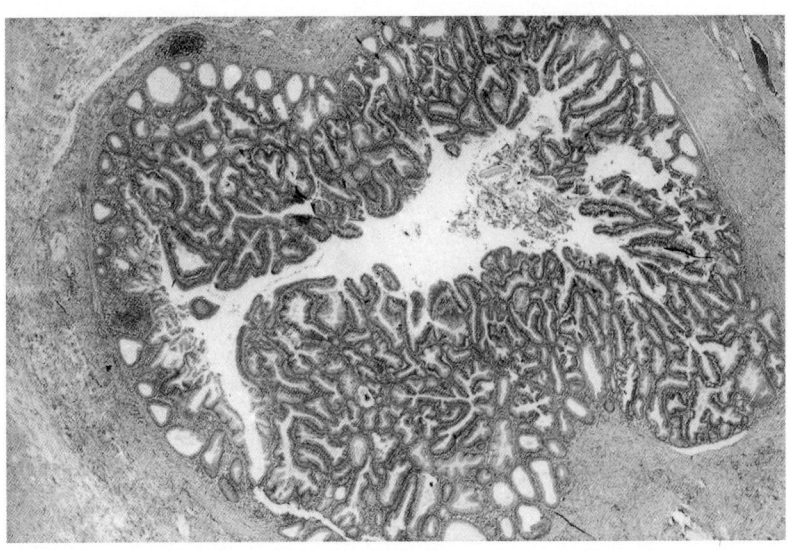

Figure 9–23. Tubulovillous colonic-type adenoma of the appendix is sessile and nearly circumferential.

amputation (Deans and Spence, 1995). Rupture of a mucinous cystadenoma may cause pseudomyxoma peritonei, but in contrast to pseudomyxoma peritonei caused by a malignant tumor, it may be self-limited (Higa et al., 1973). It has been noted that synchronous or metachronous neoplasms elsewhere in the colon occur in almost 25% of patients with appendiceal adenomas (Wolff and Ahmed, 1976). Therefore, the diagnosis of an appendiceal adenoma is itself an indication for follow-up screening of the colon for additional neoplasms.

MUCINOUS TUMORS OF UNCERTAIN MALIGNANT POTENTIAL (BORDERLINE TUMORS)

A subset of mucinous cystic neoplasms of the appendix may be difficult to classify as benign or malignant by histologic criteria and are termed *borderline tumors*. These tumors pose a diagnostic challenge for the pathologist because cytologic criteria are not helpful in differentiating them from adenomas or well differentiated mucinous carcinomas. They are composed of mucinous epithelium with little cytologic atypia or mitotic activity. However, they have expansile growth and push deeply into the underlying tissues, causing compression atrophy and diffuse fibrosis. They are distinguished from mucinous cystadenocarcinomas solely on the basis of their lack of clear-cut invasion (Carr et al., 1995). They show no evidence of in-

filtrative growth into underlying tissues, single cell invasion, or associated desmoplasia, which is typically amphophilic and contrasts with the native stroma. However, borderline tumors often produce acellular pools of mucin within the appendiceal wall or outside the appendix, and in some cases, epithelial cells with the same cytologic characteristics as the main tumor can be identified in the mucin pools. Some of these tumors may represent well-differentiated carcinomas with pushing rather than infiltrative invasion, and some may be adenomas with diverticulum-like tongues of epithelium projection. As a group, however, these tumors seem to be low grade and lack the potential to metastasize. They may recur locally, particularly if treated by appendectomy alone or if coexistent with an ovarian neoplasm of similar type (Carr et al., 1995).

When benign or borderline mucinous tumors of the vermiform appendix and ovary coexist with pseudomyxoma peritonei, the site of origin of the tumor may be difficult to determine. In almost all cases, however, the ovary and peritoneum are secondarily involved by the appendiceal tumor, and, on immunohistochemistry, the tumor cells do not stain for cytokeratin 7, which is an intermediate filament expressed in virtually all ovarian epithelial tumors and rarely expressed in colonic tumors (Guerri et al., 1997; Ronnett et al., 1995; Young et al., 1991). In the setting of pseudomyxoma peritonei associated with a benign or borderline appendiceal mucinous tumor, the cells contained within the peritoneal mucin pools require careful evaluation. Mucin pools containing scant mucinous epithelium with little cytologic atypia or mitotic activity are associated with a significantly better prognosis than mucin pools containing cells that show the architectural and cytologic features of carcinoma (Ronnett et al., 1995).

GOBLET CELL CARCINOID (ADENOCARCINOID) TUMORS

Goblet cell carcinoid tumors of the appendix (also known as *adenocarcinoid, mucinous carcinoid,* and *crypt cell* carcinoma) are tumors composed of cells that demonstrate dual differentiation properties, making both mucin and neuroendocrine secretary granules (Abt and Carter, 1976). Generically, they are classified as *amphicrine tumors* (i.e., characterized by cells that show synchronous endocrine and nonendocrine differentitation) (Chejfec et al., 1985). They most often occur in the appendiceal tip and less frequently in the middle or base of the appendix. They are virtually unique to the appendix, but tumors of this type may very rarely occur in the duodenum, perimapullary region, ileum, colon, or stomach (Burke and Lee, 1990; Höffler et al., 1984; Jones et al., 1989; Lewin, 1987). Grossly, they may appear yellow to gray-white, soft or gelatinous. However, they sometimes invade the appendix diffusely without forming a discrete nodule and may be inapparent on gross.

Microscopically, they are characterized by small nests or glands of goblet-type cells that closely resemble signet ring cells. The individual glands are separated by smooth muscle or stroma (Burke et al., 1990). The tumor cells are filled with periodic acid-Schiff (PAS)–positive and Alcian blue–positive mucin and also stain positively for carcinoembryonic antigen (CEA) on immunohistochemistry. Neuroendocrine differentiation can be demonstrated on argyrophil staining or immunohistochemical staining for chromogranin or serotonin, but the proportion of cells that are positively stained by these methods is typically low (Burke et al., 1990; Lewin, 1987). Paneth cells also may be observed in these lesions. Often the tumors have no obvious origin from the overlying epithelium but invade the submucosa, wall,

and subserosa of the appendix. The mitotic index varies from 0 to 7 (average of 1) mitoses per 10 high-power fields (Burke et al., 1990). Extracellular mucin pools may be present, but the cells within them typically display central lumina resembling normal appendiceal crypts. No cribiformed glands, glandular fusion, or solid sheets of cells should be seen. Nor should solid groups of cells without lumina be found within mucin lakes. These features, along with a mitotic index that exceeds 7 mitoses per 10 high-power fields, indicate that the tumor should be classified as a mixed carcinoid-adenocarcinoma. In contrast to colonic adenocarcinomas, pure goblet cell carcinoids do not show K-*ras* mutations (Ramnani et al, 1999).

The biologic behavior of goblet cell carcinoid tumors is generally more aggressive than that of true appendiceal carcinoid tumors (Anderson et al., 1991; Berardi et al., 1988; Butler et al., 1994; Edmonds et al., 1984; Subbuswamy et al., 1974; Warkel et al., 1978). However, when small and confined to the appendix, they are generally cured by complete excision (i.e., simple appendectomy with a negative margin). Right hemicolectomy is indicated for tumors that are large or have spread beyond the appendiceal wall. It is essential to differentiate goblet cell carcinoid tumors from true signet-ring cell carcinomas and from mixed carcinoid-adenocarcinoma. Both signet-ring cell carcinomas and mixed carcinoid-adenocarcinoma behave as adenocarcinomas and must be graded, staged, and treated accordingly. Cases of combined goblet cell carcinoid and mucinous cystadenoma of the appendix have also been reported (Al-Talib et al., 1995). In combination tumors of this type, both components of the tumor require careful evaluation for aggressive features that would justify classification of the tumor as a malignant or a borderline lesion.

REFERENCES

Abt AB, Carter SL. (1976) Goblet cell carcinoid of the appendix. *Arch Pathol Lab Med* 100:301–306.

Ahlquist DA, Wieand HS, Moertel CG, et al. (1993) Accuracy of fecal occult blood screening for colorectal neoplasia. *JAMA* 269:1262–1267.

Al-Talib RK, Mason CH, Theaker JM. (1995) Combined goblet cell carcinoid and mucinous cystadenoma of the appendix. *Arch Pathol* 48:869–870.

Amos CI, Bali D, Thiel TJ, et al. (1997) Fine mapping of a genetic locus for Peutz-Jeghers syndrome on chromosome 19p. *Cancer Res* 57:3653–3656.

Anderson NH, Somerville JE, Johnston CF, et al. (1991) Appendiceal goblet cell carcinoids: a clinicopathological and immunohistochemical study. *Histopathology* 18:61–65.

Appelman HD. (1990) Epithelial neoplasia of the appendix. In: *Pathology of the Colon, Small Intestine, and Anus* (Norris, HT, ed.) pp. 233–265. Churchill-Livingstone, New York.

Axon T. (1998) Management of dysplasia in ulcerative colitis: Is prophylactic colectomy the preferred strategy? *J Gastrointest Surg* 2:322–324.

Bazzoli F, Rossi S, Sottili S, et al. (1995) The risk of adenomatous polyps in asymptomatic first-degree relatives of persons with colon cancer. *Gastroenterology* 109:783–788.

Benhattar J, Saraga E. (1995) Molecular genetics of dysplasia in ulcerative colitis. *Eur J Cancer* 31A:1171–1173.

Berardi RS, Lee SS, Chen HP. (1988) Goblet cell carcinoids of the appendix. *Surg Gynecol Obstet* 167:81–86.

Bernstein CN. (1998) How do we assess the value of surveillance techniques in ulcerative colitis? *J Gastrointest Surg* 2:318–321.

Bernstein CN, Shanahan F, Weinstein WM. (1994) Are we telling patents the truth about surveillance colonoscopy in ulcerative colitis? *Lancet* 343:71–74.

Blackstone MO, Riddell RH, Rogers BH, et al. (1981) Dysplasia-associated lesion or mass (DALM) detected by colonoscopy in long-standing ulcerative colitis. *Gastroenterology* 80:366–374.

Bodmar WF, Bailey CJ, Bodmar J, et al. (1987) Localization of the gene for familial adenomatous polyposis on chromosome 5. *Nature* 328:614–616.

Bonelli L, Martines H, Conio M, et al. (1988) Family history of colorectal cancer as a risk factor for benign and malignant tumours of the large bowel. A case–control study. *Int J Cancer* 41:513–517.

Brentnall TA, Crispin DA, Bronner MP, et al. (1996) Microsatellite instability in nonneoplastic mucosa from patients with ulcerative colitis. *Cancer Res* 56:1237–1240.

Burke AP, Lee YK. (1990) Adenocarcinoid (goblet cell carcinoid) of the duodenum presenting as a gastric outlet obstruction. *Hum Pathol* 21:238–239.

Burke AP, Sobin LH, Fedespiel BH, et al. (1990) Goblet cell carcinoids and related tumors of the vermiform appendix. *Am J Clin Pathol* 94:27–35.

Burt RW, Albright L, Samowitz W, et al. (1991) Risk of adenomatous polyps in first-degree relatives of individuals with adenomas. *Gastroenterology* 100:A352.

Butler JA, Houshiar A, Lin F, et al. (1994) Goblet cell carcinoid of the appendix. *Am J Surg* 168:685–687.

Carethers JM. (1996) The cellular and molecular pathogenesis of colorectal cancer. *Gastroenterol Clin North Am* 25:737–745.

Carr NJ, McCarthy WF, Sobin LH. (1995) Epithelial noncarcinoid tumors and tumor-like lesions of the appendix. *Cancer* 75:757–768.

Carroll RA, Klein M. (1980) How often should patients be sigmoidoscoped? A mathematical perspective. *Prev Med* 9:741–746.

Chejfec G, Capella C, Solcia E, et al. (1985) Amphicrine cell dysplasias and neoplasms. *Cancer* 56:2683–2689.

Church JM, Fazio VW, Jones IT. (1988) Small colorectal polyps: are they worth testing? *Dis Colon Rectum* 31:50–53.

Collins R, Feldman M, Fordtran J. (1987) Colon cancer, dysplasia, and surveillance in patients with ulcerative colitis. A critical review. *N Engl J Med* 316:1654–1658.

Connell WR, Lennard-Jones JE, Williams CB, et al. (1994) Factors affecting the outcome of endoscopic surveillance for cancer in ulcerative colitis. *Gastroenterology* 107:934–944.

Cooper HS. (1983) Surgical pathology of endoscopically removed malignant polyps of the colon and rectum. *Am J Surg Path* 7:613–623.

Cooper HS. (1988) The role of the pathologist in the management of patients with endoscopically removed malignant colorectal polyps. *Pathol Annu* 23:25–43.

Cooper HS, Deppisch LM, Gourley WK, et al. (1995) Endoscopically removed malignant colorectal polyps: Clinicopathologic correlations. *Gastroenterology* 108:1657–1665.

Cooper HS, Deppisch LM, Kahn EI, et al. (1998) Pathology of the malignant colorectal polyp. *Hum Pathol* 29:15–26.

Coverlizza S, Risio M, Ferrari A, et al. (1989) Colorectal adenomas containing invasive carcinoma: pathologic assessment of lymph node metastatic potential. *Cancer* 64:1937–1947.

Cranley JP, Petras RE, Carey WD, et al. (1986) When is endoscopic polypectomy adequate therapy for colonic polyps containing invasive carcinoma? *Gastroenterology* 91:419–427.

Dajani YF, Kamal MF. (1984) Colorectal juvenile polyps: an epidemiological and histopathological study of 144 cases in Jordanians. *Histopathology* 8:765–779.

Deans GT, Spence RAJ. (1995) Neoplastic lesions of the appendix. *Br J Surg* 82:299–306.

Demers RY, Neale AV, Budev H, et al. (1990) Pathologist agreement in the interpretation of colorectal polyps. *Am J Gastroenterol* 85:417–421.

Desai DC, Neal KF, Talbot IC, et al. (1995) Juvenile polyposis. *Br J Surg* 82:14–17.

Di Gregorio C, Losi L, Fante R, et al. (1997) Histology of aberrant crypt foci in the human colon. *Histopathology* 30:328–334.

Dong SM, Kim KM, Kim SY, et al. (1998) Frequent somatic mutations in serine/threonine kinase 11/Peutz-Jeghers syndrome gene in left-sided colon cancer. *Cancer Res* 58:3787–3790.

Edmonds P, Merino MJ, Li Volsi VA, et al. (1984) Adenocarcinoid (mucinous carcinoid) of the appendix. *Gastroenterology* 86:302–309.

Eide TJ, Stalsberg H. (1978) Polyps of the large intestine in northern Norway. *Cancer* 42:2839–2848.

Ekbom A. (1998) Risk of cancer in ulcerative colitis. *J Gastrointest Surg* 2:312–313.

Fenoglio-Preiser CM, Pascal RR. (1982) Colorectal adenomas and cancer. Pathologic relationships. *Cancer* 50:2601–2608.

Fleming ID, Cooper JS, Henson DE, et al., eds. (1997) *AJCC Manual for Staging of Cancer*, 5th ed, Lippincott-Raven, Philadelphia.

Fogt F, Vortmeyer AO, Goldman H, et al. (1998) Comparison of genetic alterations in colonic adenoma and ulcerative colitis-associated dysplasia and carcinoma. *Hum Pathol* 29:131–136.

Giardiello FM, Brensinger JD, Luce MC, et al. (1997) Phenotypic expression of disease in families that have mutations in the 5' region of the adenomatous polyposis coli gene. *Ann Intern Med* 126:514–519.

Giardiello FM, Welsh SB, Hamilton SR, et al. (1987) Increased risk of cancer in the Peutz-Jeghers Syndrome. *N Engl J Med* 316:1511–1514.

Gottlieb LL, Winawer SJ, Sternberg S, et al. (1984) National polyp study (NPS). The diminutive colonic polyp. *Gastrointest Endosc* 30:143.

Grangvist S, Gabrielsson N, Sundelin P. (1979) Diminutive colonic polyps, clinical significance and management. *Endoscopy* 11:36–42.

Grassi A, Casale V, Fracasso P, et al. (1997) Medium-large polyps of the colon: a contribution for their clinical profile and a proper surveillance. *J Exp Clin Cancer Res* 16:313–319.

Greenstein AJ, Sachar DB, Smith H, et al. (1979) Cancer in universal and left-sided ulcerative colitis. *Gastroenterology* 77:290–294.

Grossman S, Milas M. (1988) Colonoscopic screening of persons with suspected risk factors for colon cancer. *Gastroenterology* 94:395–400.

Guerrieri C, Frandlund B, Fristedt S, et al. (1997) Mucinous tumors of the vermiform appendix and ovary, and pseudomyxoma peritonei: histologic implications of cytokeratin 7 expression. *Hum Pathol* 28:1039–1045.

Haggitt RC, Glotzbach RE, Soffer EE, et al. (1985) Prognostic factors in colorectal carcinomas arising in adenomas: implications for lesions removed by endoscopic polypectomy. *Gastroenterology* 89:328–336.

Haggitt RC, Reid BJ. (1986) Hereditary gastrointestinal polyposis syndromes. *Am J Surg Pathol* 10:871–887.

Hemminki A, Tomlinkson I, Markie D, et al. (1997) Localization of a susceptibility locus for Peutz-Jeghers syndrome to 19p using comparative genomic hybridization and targeted linkage analysis. *Nat Genet* 15:87–90.

Higa E, Rosai J, Pizzimbono CA, et al. (1973) Mucosal hyperplasia, mucinous cystadenoma and mucinous cystadenocarcinoma of the appendix. A re-evaluation of the appendiceal "mucocele". *Cancer* 32:1525–1544.

Hixson LJ, Fennerty MB, Sampliner RE, et al. (1994) Two-year incidence of colon adenomas developing after tandem colonoscopy. *Am J Gastroenterol* 89:687–691.

Hoff G, Foerster A, Van MH. (1986) Epidemiology of polyps in the rectum and colon: recovery and evaluation of unresected polyps 2 years after detection. *Scand J Gastroenterol* 21:853–862.

Höffler H, Kloppel G, Heitz PU. (1984) Combined production of mucus, amines and peptides by goblet-cell carcinoids of the appendix and ileum. *Pathol Res Pract* 178:555–561.

Hood AB, Krush AJ. (1983) Clinical and dermatologic aspects of the hereditary intestinal polyposes. *Dis Colon Rectum* 26:546–548.

Howe JR, Ringold JC, Summers RW, et al. (1998a) A gene for familial juvenile polyposis maps to chromosome 18q21.1. *Am J Hum Genet* 62:1129–1136.

Howe JR, Roth S, Ringold JC, et al. (1998b) Mutations in the SMAD4/DPC4 gene in juvenile polyposis. *Science* 280:1086–1088.

Itzkowitz SH. (1996) Gastrointestinal adenomatous polyps. *Semin Gastrointest Dis* 7:105–116.

Järvinen H, Franssila KO. (1984) Familial juvenile polyposis coli; increased risk of colorectal cancer. *Gut* 25:792–800.

Jass JR. (1995) Malignant colorectal polyps. *Gastroenterology* 109:2034–2035.

Jass JR, Sobin LH, eds. (1989) *World Health Organization: Histologic Typing of Intestinal Tumours*, 2nd ed. Springer-Verlag, New York.

Jenne DE, Reimann H, Nezu J-I, et al. (1998) Peutz-Jeghers syndrome is caused by mutations in a novel serine threonine kinase. *Nat Genet* 18:38–43.

Johannsen LGK, Momsen O, Jacobsen NO. (1989) Polyps of the large intestine in Aarhus, Denmark. An autopsy study. *Gastroenterology* 24:799–806.

Jones MA, Griffith LM, West BA. (1989) Adenocarcinoid tumor of the periampullary region: A novel duodenal neoplasm presenting as biliary tract obstruction. *Hum Pathol* 20:198–200.

Kim EC, Lance P. (1997) Colorectal polyps and their relationship to cancer. *Gastroenterol Clin North Am* 26:1–17.

Kim YS. (1997) Molecular genetic of colorectal cancer. *Digestion* 58(Suppl. 1):65–68.

Kim JC, Roh SA, Yu CS, et al. (1997) Familial juvenile polyposis coli with APC gene mutation. *Am J Gastroenterol* 92:1913–1915.

Kinzler KW, Vogelstein B. (1996) Lessons from hereditary colorectal cancer. *Cell* 87:159–170.

Kinzler KW, Vogelstein B. (1998) Colorectal tumors. In: *The Genetic Basis of Human Cancer* (Vogelstein B, Kinzler KW, eds.) pp. 565–587. McGraw-Hill, New York.

Kyzer S, Begin LR, Gordan PH, et al. (1992) The care of patients with colorectal polyps that contain invasive adenocarcinoma. *Cancer* 70:2044–2050.

Lashner BA. (1992) Recommendations for colorectal cancer screening in ulcerative colitis: a review of research from a single university-based surveillance program. *Am J Gastroenterol* 87:168–175.

Lashner BA, Shapiro BD. (1998) Biology of cancer in ulcerative colitis. *J Gastrointest Surg* 2:307–311.

Lennard-Jones JE, Melville DM, Morson BC, et al. (1990) Precancer and cancer in extensive ulcerative colitis: findings among 401 patients over 22 years. *Gut* 31:800–806.

Leppert M, Burt R, Hughes JP, et al. (1990) Genetic analysis of an inherited predisposition to colon cancer in a family with a variable number of adenomatous polyps. *N Engl J Med* 322:904–908.

Levin B. (1992) Ulcerative colitis and colon cancer: Biology and surveillance. *J Cell Biochem* 16G(Suppl.): 47–50.

Lewin K. (1987) Carcinoid tumors and mixed (composite) glandular-endocrine cell carcinomas. *Am J Surg Pathol* 11(Suppl. 1):71–86.

Lipper S, Kahn LB, Ackerman LV. (1983) The significance of microscopic invasive cancer in endoscopically removed polyps of the large bowel. A clinicopathologic study of 51 cases. *Cancer* 52:1691–1699.

Lipper S, Kahn LB, Sandler RS, et al. (1981) Multiple juvenile polyposis: a study of the pathogenesis of juvenile polyps and their relationship to colonic adenomas. *Hum Pathol* 12:804–813.

Longacre TA, Fenoglio-Preiser CM. (1990) Mixed hyperplastic adenomatous polyps/serrated adenomas. A distinct form of colorectal neoplasia. *Am J Surg Pathol* 14:524–537.

Lovett E. (1976) Family studies in cancer of the colon and rectum. *Br J Surg* 63:13–18.

Luk GD. (1995) Diagnosis and therapy of hereditary polyposis syndromes. *Gastroenterologist* 3:153–167.

Lynch HT, Lynch JT. (1998) Genetics of colon cancer. *Digestion* 59:481–492.

Lynch HT, Smyrk T. (1996) Hereditary nonpolyposis colorectal cancer (lynch syndrome). An updated review. *Cancer* 78:1149–1167.

Marchesa P, Lashner BA, Lavery IC, et al. (1997) The risk of cancer and dysplasia among ulcerative colitis patients with primary sclerosing cholangitis. *Am J Gastroenterol* 92:1285–1288.

Marra G, Boland CR. (1996) DNA repair and colorectal cancer. Gastroenterol Clin North Am 25:755–772.

McColl I, Bussey HJR, Veale AMO, et al. (1964) Juvenile polyposis coli. *Proc R Soc Med* 57:896–897.

McRae FA, St. John DJ. (1982) Relationship between patterns of bleeding and Hemoccult sensitivity in patients with colorectal cancers or adenomas. *Gastroenterology* 82:891–898.

Medlicott SAC, Jewell LD, Price L, et al. (1997) Conservative management of small adenomata in ulcerative colitis. *Am J Gastroenterol* 92:2094–2098.

Mehenni H, Blouin J-L, Radhakrishna U, et al. (1997) Peutz-Jeghers syndrome: confirmation of linkage to chromosome 19p13.3 and identification of a potential second locus, on 19q13.4. *Am J Hum Genet* 61:1327–1334.

Meijer GA, Baak JPA, Talbot IC, et al. (1998) Predicting the risk of metachronous colorectal cancer in patients with rectosigmoid adenomas using quantitative pathological features. A case–control study. *J Pathol* 184:63–70.

Melville DM, Jass JR, Morson BC, et al. (1989) Observer study of the grading of dysplasia in ulcerative colitis: comparison with clinical outcome. *Hum Pathol* 20:1008–1014.

Messerini L, Mori S, Zampi G. (1996) Pathologic features of hereditary non-polyposis colorectal cancer. *Tumori* 82:114–116.

Morson BC, Whiteway JE, Jones EA, et al. (1984) Histopathology and prognosis of malignant colorectal polyps treated by endoscopic polypectomy. *Gut* 25:437–444.

Muller S, Chesner IM, Egan MJ, et al. (1989) Significance of venous and lymphatic invasion in malignant polyps of the colon and rectum. *Gut* 30:1385–1391.

Muto T, Bussey HJR, Morson BC. (1975) The evolution of cancer of the colon and rectum. *Cancer* 36:2251–2270.

Nakagawa H, Koyama K, Tanaka T, et al. (1998) Localization of the gene responsible for Peutz-Jeghers syndrome within a 6-cM region of chromosome 19p13.3. *Hum Genet* 102:203–206.

Nivatvongs S, Goldberg SM. (1978) Management of patients who have polyps containing invasive carcinoma removed via colonoscope. *Dis Colon Rectum* 21:8–11.

Nivatvongs S, Rojanasakul A, Reiman HM, et al. (1991) The risk of lymph node metastasis in colorectal polyps with invasive adenocarcinoma. *Dis Colon Rectum* 34:323–328.

Nugent KP, Talbot IC, Hodgson SV, et al. (1993) Solitary juvenile polyps: not a marker for subsequent malignancy. *Gastroenterology* 105:698–700.

O'Brien MJ, Winawer SJ, Zauber AG, et al, and The National Polyp Study Workgroup. (1990) The National Polyp Study. Patient and polyp characteristics associated with high-grade dysplasia in colorectal adenomas. *Gastroenterology* 98:371–379.

O'Riordain DS, O'Dwyer PJ, Cullen AF, et al. (1991) Familial juvenile polyposis coli and colorectal cancer. *Cancer* 68:889–892.

O'Sullivan MJ, McCarthy TV, Doyle CT. (1998) Familial adenomatous polyposis. From bedside to benchside. *Am J Clin Pathol* 109:521:526.

Papatheodoridis GV, Triantafyllou K, Tzouvala M, et al. (1996) Characteristics of rectosigmoid adenomas as predictors of synchronous advanced proximal colon neoplasms. *Am J Gastroenterol* 91:1809–1813.

Perzin KH, Bridge MF. (1982) Adenomatous and carcinomatous changes in hamartomatous polyps of the small intestine (Peutz-Jeghers syndrome). Report of a case and review of literature. *Cancer* 49:971–983.

Ponz de Leon M. (1996) Descriptive epidemiology of hereditary nonpolyposis colorectal cancer. *Tumori* 82:102–106.

Powell SM, Petersen GM, Krush AJ, et al. (1993) Molecular diagnosis of familial adenomatous polyposis. *N Engl J Med* 329:1982–1987.

Ramnani DM, Wistuba II, Behrens C, Gazdar AF, Sobin LH, Albores-Saavedra J. (1999) K-ras and p53 mutations in the pathogenesis of classical and goblet cell carcinoids of the appendix. *Cancer* 86:14–21.

Ranchod M, Lewin KJ, Dorfman RF. (1978) Lymphoid hyperplasia of the gastrointestinal tract. A study of 26 cases and review of the literature. *Am J Surg Pathol* 2:383–400.

Ransohoff DF, Riddell RH, Levin B. (1985) Ulcerative colitis and colonic cancer: problems in assessing the diagnostic usefulness of mucosal dysplasia. *Dis Colon Rectum* 28:383–388.

Rashid A, Hamilton SR. (1997) Genetic alterations in sporadic and Crohn's-associated adenocarcinomas of the small intestine. *Gastroenterology* 113:127–135.

Richards WO, Webb WA, Morris SJ, et al. (1987) Patient management after endoscopic removal of the cancerous colon adenoma. *Ann Surg* 205:665–672.

Rickert RR, Auerbach O, Garfinkel L, et al. (1979) Adenomatous lesions of the large bowel. An autopsy study. *Cancer* 43:1847–1857.

Riddell RH. (1995) Implications of a diagnosis of dysplasia in ulcerative colitis. *J Gastroenterology* 30(Suppl VIII):25–29.

Riddell RH. (1998) How reliable/valid is dysplasia in identifying at-risk patients with ulcerative colitis? *J Gastrointest Surg* 2:314–317.

Riddell RH, Goldman H, Ransohoff DE, et al. (1983) Dysplasia in inflammatory bowel disease: standardized classification with provisional clinical applications. *Hum Pathol* 14:931–968.

Ronnett BM, Zahn CM, Kurman RJ, et al. (1995) Disseminated peritoneal adenomucinosis and peritoneal mucinous carcinomatosis. *Am J Surg Pathol* 19:1390–1408.

Rosenstock E, Farmer RG, Petras R, et al. (1985) Surveillance for colonic carcinoma in ulcerative colitis. *Gastroenterology* 99:1021–1031.

Rozen P, Ron E. (1989) Cost analysis of screening methodology for family members of colorectal cancer patients. *Am J Gastroenterol* 84:1548–1551.

Rubin CE, Haggitt RC, Burmer GC, et al. (1992) DNA aneuploidy in colonic biopsies predicts future development of dysplasia in ulcerative colitis. *Gastroenterology* 103:1611–1620.

Rustgi AK. (1995) *Gastrointestinal Cancers. Biology, Prognosis, and Therapy.* Lippincott-Raven, Philadelphia.

Sherlock P, Winawer SJ. (1984) Are there markers for the risk of colorectal cancer? *N Engl J Med* 311:118–119.

Siu I, Pretlow TG, Amini SB, et al. (1997) Identification of dysplasia in human colonic aberrant crypt foci. *Am J Pathol* 150:1805–1813.

Snapper SB, Syngal S, Friedman LS. (1998) Ulcerative colitis and colon cancer: more controversy and clarity. *Dig Dis* 16:81–87.

Soravia C, Berk T, Madlensky L, et al. (1998) Genotype-phenotype correlations in attenuated adenomatous polyposis coli. *Am J Hum Genet* 62:1290–1301.

Stryker SJ, Wolff BG, Culp CE, et al. (1987) Natural history of untreated colonic polyps. *Gastroenterology* 93:1009–1013.

Subbuswamy SG, Gibbs NM, Ross CF, et al. (1974) Goblet cell carcinoid of the appendix. *Cancer* 34:338–344.

Subramony C, Scott-Conner CE, Skelton D, et al. (1994) Familial juvenile polyposis. Study of a kindred: evolution of polyps and relationship to gastrointestinal carcinoma. *Am J Clin Pathol* 102:91–7.

Suzuki K, Muto T, Shinozaki M, et al. (1998) Differential diagnosis of dysplasia-associated lesion or mass and coincidental adenoma in ulcerative colitis. *Dis Colon Rectum* 41:322–327.

Takayama T, Katsuki S, Takahashi Y, et al. (1998) Aberrant crypt foci of the colon as precursors of adenoma and carcinoma. *N Engl J Med* 339:1277–1284.

Tarmin L, Yin J, Harpaz N, et al. (1995) Adenomatous polyposis coli gene mutations in ulcerative colitis associated dysplasias and cancers versus sporadic colon neoplasms. *Cancer Res* 55:2035–2038.

Tedesco FJ, Hendrix JC, Pickens CA, et al. (1982) Diminutive polyps: histopathology, spatial distribution, and clinical significance. *Gastrointest Endosc* 28:1–5.

Torlakovic E, Snover DC. (1996). Serrated adenomatous polyposis in humans. *Gastroenterology* 110:748–755.

Torres C, Antonioli D, Odze RD. (1998) Polypoid dysplasia and adenomas in inflammatory bowel disease. A clinical, pathologic, and follow-up study of 89 polyps from 59 patients. *Am J Surg Pathol* 22:275–284.

Triantafyllou K, Papatheodoridis GV, Paspatis GA, et al. (1997) Predictors of the early development of advanced metachronous colon adenomas. *Hepatogastroenterology* 44:533–538.

Tsai CJ, Lu DK. (1995) Small colorectal polyps: histopathology and clinical significance. *Am J Gastroenterol* 90:988–994.

Vaiphei K, Thapa BR. (1997) Juvenile polyposis (coli)—high incidence of dysplastic epithelium. *J Pediatr Surg* 32:1287–1290.

Vogelstein B, Fearon ER, Hamilton SR, et al. (1988) Genetic alterations during colorectal-tumor development. *N Engl J Med* 319:525–532.

Volk EE, Goldblum JR, Petras RE, et al. (1995) Management and outcome of patients with invasive carcinoma arising in colorectal polyps. *Gastroenterology* 109:1801–1807.

Warkel RL, Cooper PH, Helwig EB. (1978) Adenocarcinoid: a mucin-producing tumor of the appendix. A study of 39 cases. *Cancer* 42:2781–2793.

Watne AL. (1997) Colon polyps. *J Surg Oncol* 66:207–214.

Waye JD, Lewis BS, Frankel A, et al. (1988) Small colon polyps. *Am J Gastroenterol* 83:120–122.

Wilcox GM, Anderson PB, Colaccio TA. (1986) Early invasive carcinoma in colonic polyps: a review of the literature with emphasis on the assessment of the risk of metastasis. *Cancer* 57:160–171.

Wilcox GM, Beck JR. (1987) Early invasive cancer in adenomatous colonic polyps ("malignant polyps"). Evaluation of the therapeutic options by decision analysis. *Gastroenterology* 92:1159–1168.

Willenbucher RF, Zelman SJ, Ferrell LD, et al. (1997) Chromosomal alterations in ulcerative colitis-related neoplastic progression. *Gastroenterology* 113:791–801.

Williams AR, Balasooriya BA, Day DW. (1982) Polyps and cancer of the large bowel: a necropsy study in Liverpool. *Gut* 23:835–842.

Williams GT, Artheur JF, Bussey HJR, et al. (1980) Metaplastic polyps and polyposis of the colorectum. *Histopathology* 4:155–170.

Winawer SJ, Zauber AG, Gerdes H, et al. (1996) Risk of colorectal cancer in the families of patients with adenomatous polyps. *N Engl J Med* 334:82–87.

Winawer SJ, Zauber AG, Ho MN, et al. (1993a) Prevention of colorectal cancer by colonoscopic polypectomy. *N Engl J Med* 329:1977–1981.

Winawer SJ, Zauber AG, O'Brien MJ, et al. (1993b) Randomized comparison of surveillance intervals after colonoscopic removal of newly diagnosed adenomatous polyps: the National Polyp Study Workshop. *N Engl J Med* 328:901–906.

Wolff M, Ahmed N. (1976) Epithelial neoplasms of the vermiform appendix (exclusive of carcinoid). II. Cystadenomas, papillary adenomas, and adenomatous polyps of the appendix. *Cancer* 37:2511–2522.

Wolff WI, Shinya H. (1975) Definitive treatment of "malignant" polyps of the colon. *Ann Surg* 182:516–525.

Wu TT, Rezai B, Rashid A, et al. (1997) Genetic alterations and epithelial dysplasia in juvenile polyposis syndrome and sporadic juvenile polyps. *Am J Pathol* 150:939–947.

Yao T, Tada S, Tsuneyoshi M. (1994) Colorectal counterpart of gastric depressed adenoma. A comparison with flat and polypoid adenomas with special reference to the development of pericryptal fibroblasts. *Am J Surg Pathol.* 18:559–568.

Young RH, Gilks CB, Scully RE. (1991) Mucinous tumors of the appendix associated with mucinous tumors of the ovary and pseudomyxoma peritonei. *Am J Surg Pathol* 15:415–429.

Zauber AG, Winawer SJ. (1997) Initial management and follow-up surveillance of patients with colorectal adenomas. *Gastroenterol Clin North Am* 26:85–101.

10

ANUS

ROBERT R. RICKERT

Neoplasms of the anal region are uncommon, accounting for only 2–4% of distal large bowel cancers (Rickert, 1998). Most are variants of squamous cell carcinoma (Williams and Talbot, 1994). Despite its infrequency, anal cancer has recently generated increasing interest and attention. This is due mainly to a significant increase in incidence during the past several decades as well as a rapidly expanding body of information relating to epidemiology, risk factors and etiology (Frisch et al., 1993, 1997; Melbye et al., 1994).

An understanding of both incipient and fully developed anal neoplasia requires knowledge of the rather complex gross and microscopic anatomy of this region. Tumor classifications and the multiplicity of microscopic patterns of squamous neoplasia arising in this region are confusing and often complicated by an inadequate appreciation of the regional anatomy.

In this chapter, the gross and microscopic anatomy of the anal region will be reviewed, followed by a detailed discussion of squamous neoplasia, with emphasis on epidemiological and etiological factors, and the early stages of the neoplastic process. Later, less common tumors including adenocarcinoma, Paget's disease, basal cell carcinoma, and malignant melanoma will be considered.

ANATOMY OF THE ANAL REGION

The anal canal is structurally complex. Descriptions of the anatomy have often been confusing (Fenger, 1988). Defined surgically, the anal canal extends from the upper to the lower borders of the internal sphincter muscle and measures 3 to 4 cm in length (Fig. 10–1). Superiorly the anal canal is in continuity with the rectum and inferiorly with the perianal skin. The *anatomic anal canal* may be defined as beginning at the dentate line and extending distally to the *anal verge*, which is the site where the walls of the anal canal are in contact at rest. In terms of our understanding of the histogenesis of anal cancer, this definition is inadequate since most anal canal neoplasms arise outside of this so-called anatomic anal canal. The most important and reliable gross anatomic landmark is the *dentate (pectinate) line*, located roughly at the midpoint of the surgical anal canal. This circumferential line is formed by the anal valves located at the bases of the anal columns. The dentate line represents the site of the fetal anal membrane at the junction of endodermal (cloaca) and ectodermal (protoderm) components of the anal canal.

The type of epithelial lining within the anal canal varies. The mucosa lining the canal distal to the dentate line is of stratified squamous type without hair or other cutaneous appendages. This portion of the canal is known also as the *pecten*. Distally, the anal canal ends at the anal verge, the site at which the squamous mucosa merges with true perianal skin with its accompanying hair follicles, sweat glands, and apocrine glands.

The dentate line roughly corresponds to the junction of squamous and rectal-type

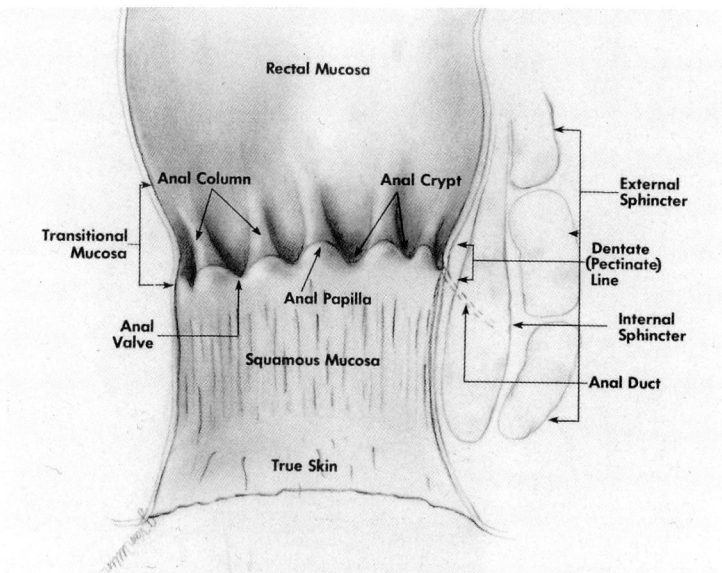

Figure 10–1. Diagram of normal anatomy of the anal region. [From Rickert, 1998, with permission].

columnar epithelium. This interface is not abrupt, but rather there is an intervening zone of characteristic epithelium known as the *anal transitional zone,* or ATZ (Fig. 10–2). The ATZ is important in the presumed histogenesis of the most common anal neoplasms. This zone has been well defined and described, and microscopically varies from an epithelium somewhat reminiscent of the urothelium lining the lower urinary tract to one that is stratified squamous, columnar, cuboidal, or a combination of all of these (Fenger, 1988, 1991). The most typical pattern is an epithelium consisting of rows of cells of columnar to cuboidal shape often with mucus-secreting cells on the surface. Islands of colorectal columnar epithelium or nonkeratinizing squamous epithelium are frequently noted in the ATZ. The upper border of this zone merges with the glandular mucosa of the lower rectum.

An understanding of the microscopic features of the region permits a zonal anatomic definition based on the type of lining epithelium (Fenger, 1991). This practical approach, which recognizes three zones, is helpful in understanding the patterns of neoplasia arising in the region. The upper zone is known as the *colorectal zone* and is lined by mucosa indistinguishable from that in the rectum. Distal to this is the ATZ with the characteristic mucosa just described,

which in turn merges distally with the *squamous zone,* which lies between the dentate line and true perianal skin. When classifying anal cancers, yet another traditional but confusing definition designates the entire nonappendage-bearing squamous zone as the *anal margin* and limits the term anal canal to that portion from the dentate line proximally to the junction with rectal mucosa.

The tumor size distant metastasis (TNM) staging system conveniently incorporates the histological/zonal approach, thereby not contributing to further confusion. The TNM system defines the *anal canal* as extending from the rectum to the perianal skin and lined by the mucous membrane overlying the internal anal sphincter (Fleming et al., 1997). This definition includes the dentate line, the AZT epithelium, and the nonappendage bearing squamous mucosa extending distally to the junction with true perianal skin. In the TNM system the *anal margin* is defined as the junction of the hair-bearing skin and the mucous membrane of the anal canal, or more distal.

Other anatomic structures of the region that may be important to our understanding of anal neoplasia are the *anal ducts* or *glands* that open into the anal crypts. These are branching tubular structures lined by AZT-type epithelium. They often extend distally for a short distance before penetrating into

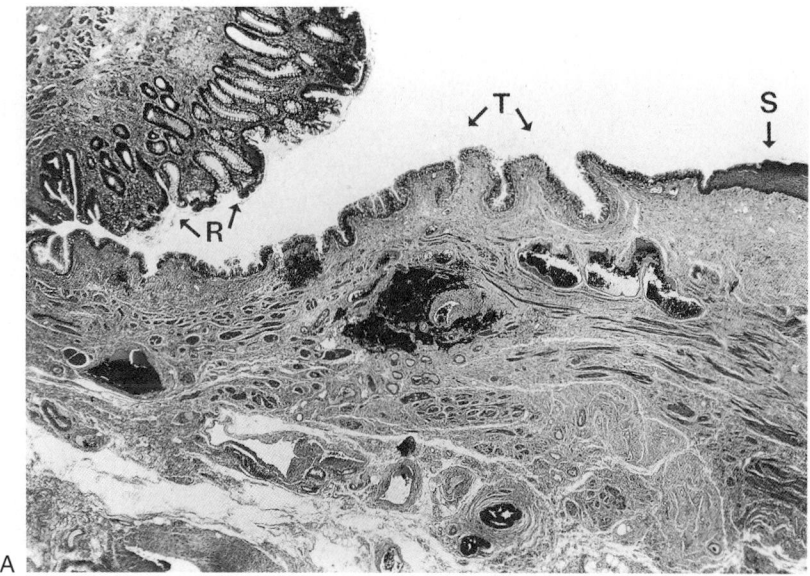

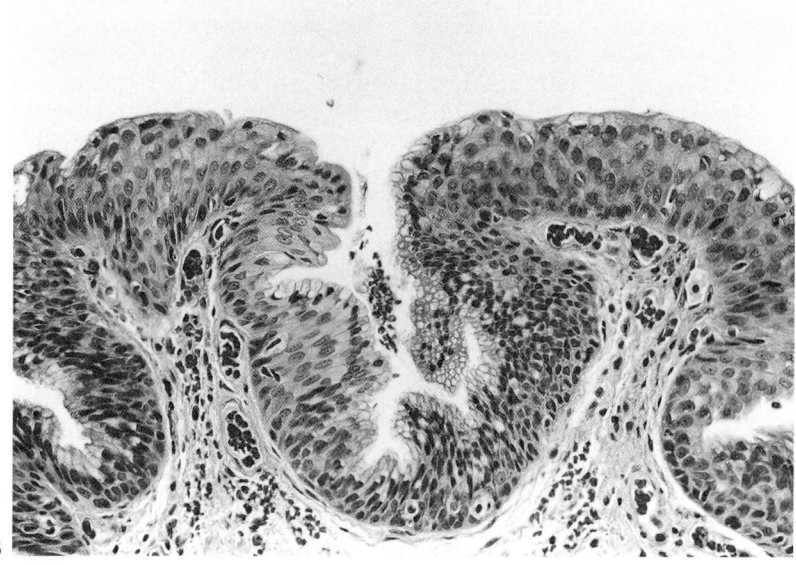

Figure 10–2. *A:* Scanning-power photomicrograph of normal anal transitional zone. Rectal mucosa (R) is on left, transitional mucosa is in broad central region (T) and stratified squamous anal mucosa (S) is on right. *B:* Higher-power photomicrograph of transitional mucosa showing rows of cuboidal to columnar cells with occasional mucus-secreting cells on surface. [From Rickert, 1998, with permission.]

and sometimes through the internal sphincter muscle. Occasionally, the anal ducts may be seen to extend proximally beneath the rectal mucosa. The anal canal epithelium has also been shown to contain endocrine cells and melanocytes (Clemmensen and Fenger, 1991; Fenger and Lyon, 1982).

SQUAMOUS NEOPLASIA OF THE ANAL REGION

EPIDEMIOLOGY, RISK FACTORS, AND ETIOLOGY

During the past several decades there has been a significant increase in the incidence of squamous (epidermoid) neoplasia of the anus (Frisch et al., 1993, 1997; Goldman et al., 1989; Melbye et al., 1994). First demonstrated in Sweden and Denmark, the trend has also been documented in the United States. The increase in incidence has been shown especially in women, has been greater in Blacks than in Whites, and in those living in metropolitan rather than in rural areas. It has been suggested that changes in sexual behavior, including promiscuity among young people, might contribute to the incidence of anal cancer (Frisch et al., 1993; Melbye and Biggar, 1992). Beginning in the late 1970s, a pattern of factors suggesting an increased risk for anal cancer began to emerge (Cooper et al., 1979; Daling et al., 1982, 1987, 1992; Frisch et al., 1997; Holly et al., 1989; Holmes et al., 1988; Peters and Mack, 1983; Scholefield et al., 1990). Included in this risk profile are homosexual contact; a history of genital warts, especially in homosexual men; a history of other sexually transmitted diseases including gonorrhea, herpes simplex virus type 2 infection, lymphogranuloma venereum, syphilis, and chlamydia; receptive anal intercourse; unmarried status (especially never-married men); a large number of sexual partners; young age at time of first sexual intercourse; a history of other squamous genital neoplasms; and cigarette smoking.

In a recent population-based, case–control study in Denmark and Sweden, Frisch and associates reported by multivariate analysis several consistent and statistically significant associations between patterns of sexual promiscuity and risk of anal cancer in both women and men (Frisch et al., 1997). In women there was a strong positive correlation between the lifetime number of sexual partners and anal cancer. Furthermore, women who first had sexual intercourse at or before age 16 were at higher risk than those who first had intercourse after age 20. Women who had anal intercourse before age 30 were also at higher risk but apparently not if anal intercourse first occurred after age 30. The lifetime number of anal-sex partners also correlated with increased risk. Previous studies had suggested that, unlike men, women engaging in anal intercourse were not at increased risk (Daling et al., 1987; Holly et al., 1989). Women who reported a history of anogenital warts were at increased risk, even more so when the warts were specifically designated as anal. There was also a positive, though less strong, correlation with a history of gonorrhea and trichomoniasis. Prior cervical neoplasia was also associated with increased risk of anal cancer. Women with anal cancer also reported more sexual promiscuity among their partners, and their partners were more likely to have a history of a sexually transmitted disease than were the controls. This study also demonstrated positive correlations between indicators of sexual promiscuity and risk of anal cancer among men. Included were the lifetime number of female sex partners and sex with prostitutes. Unmarried men were also at increased risk, especially those without a current female partner and those never having had heterosexual intercourse. Fifteen percent of male patients in the study with anal cancer reported homosexual contact but no controls reported a homosexual experience. Like the women, male patients with anal cancer were also more likely than controls to have had a history of venereal disease, especially anal warts. Other sexually transmitted diseases with a positive but less strong correlation with risk of anal cancer among men were gonorrhea, herpes, syphilis, and hepatitis.

What clearly emerges from these studies is an epidemiologic and risk factor profile that is remarkably similar to that for squamous neoplasia of the genital tract. The reported studies suggest that a sexually transmitted infection is causally related to anal squamous cancer and that members of the human papillomavirus (HPV) family are the most likely etiologic candidates. Epidemiologic studies have demonstrated a strong relationship between HPV and cervical neoplasia, which is independent of other risk factors and has been consistent in several countries (Bosch et al., 1995). More than 70 types of HPV have been defined on the basis of DNA homology (Zurhausen and Devilliers, 1994). More than 30 of these are known to infect the anogenital region. There is a correlation between the viral type isolated from a lesion and its malignant potential. So-called low-risk types, notably HPV 6 and 11, are found most frequently in anogenital warts and may be associated with low-grade dysplasia. More oncogenic or higher risk virus types include HPV types 16,

18, 31, 33, 35, 45, 51, 52, and 56. Among these the highest risk group includes types 16, 18, and 45 (Franco, 1996). These are found predominantly in association with high-grade dysplasias and in invasive carcinoma. Studies have indicated that the types of HPV etiologically linked to cervical neoplasia are also causally related to anal cancer (Duggan et al., 1991; Franco, 1996; Frisch et al., 1997; Higgins et al., 1991; Noffsinger et al., 1992; Palmer et al., 1989; Scholefield et al., 1990, 1991; Shroyer et al., 1995; Zaki et al., 1992). Several conclusions may be drawn from these studies: the proportion of anal cancer specimens with demonstrated HPV DNA has varied among studies but most of the variation appears to be related to the sensitivity of the detection techniques, ranging from 17% to 50% using *in situ* hybridization to up to more than 80% with polymerase chain reaction (PCR); HPV detection rates are higher in women than in men; there is a clear predominance of HPV type 16; the prevalence of HPV in anal squamous cancer is unrelated to the presence or absence of a basaloid pattern; HPV-positive anal cancers tend to occur at a younger age than HPV-negative tumors; and identification of HPV is similar in incipient (pre- or noninvasive) and in invasive anal neoplasia. These etiologic relationships will be further discussed in the section on precursor lesions.

Other studies have further documented the parallel between squamous neoplasia of the female genital tract, especially the cervix, and anal cancer. A case–control study in Denmark demonstrated that patients with anal cancer were more likely than patients with colon, stomach, or vulvar cancer to have had a previous diagnosis of cervical intraepithelial neoplasia (CIN) or invasive cervical cancer (Melbye and Sprogel, 1991). These authors concluded that the strong association between anal cancer and preinvasive/invasive cervical cancer suggested that they share common risk factors. Similar findings have been reported by Dixon and co-workers (1991). A study of the incidence of second primary cancers occurring after cervical and anal cancer using tumor registry data provided additional support for common factors such as HPV infection and cigarette smoking in the etiology of cervical and anal cancer (Rabkin et al., 1992). This study also demonstrated increased relative risks for subsequent lung and prostate cancer in patients with anal cancer. In another study of multiple primary cancers occurring before and after anal cancer, there was an excess of previous cancer of the vulva/vagina and cervix, and lymphoma/leukemia (Frisch et al., 1994). Subsequent cancers were also in excess, particularly of lung, bladder, breast, vulva/vagina, and small intestine. The data suggested a multifactorial etiology for anal cancer in which both an infectious agent and smoking might be involved. The association with hematologic malignancy suggested that immunodeficiency may also be important.

Cigarette smoking is associated with an increased risk of anal cancer in both men and women (Daling et al., 1987, 1992; Holly et al., 1989; Holmes et al., 1988). It has been suggested that smoking has a late stage or promotional effect in the etiology of anogenital cancer. Current smokers and lifetime heavy smokers seem to account for most of the excess risk regardless of gender or sexual orientation. These studies again support an epidemiologic parallel between risk factors for anal and cervical cancer.

Recent studies have demonstrated an association between human immunodeficiency virus (HIV)-induced immunodeficiency and anal cancer and its precursors Palefsky, 1994; (Melbye et al., 1994; Palefsky, 1990; Unger et al., 1997). This again suggests an etiologic parallel with HPV-associated cervical neoplasia in HIV-infected persons. It has been suggested that the presence of high-risk HPV types and multiple HPV types within low-grade lesions may explain the increased risk of neoplastic progression in HIV-infected patients (Unger et al., 1997). It has been demonstrated that the incidence of anal cancer among homosexual men now exceeds the incidence of cervical cancer in women (Palefsky et al., 1998b). Furthermore, HIV-positive homosexual men may be at even higher risk than HIV-negative men. It should be further noted that the increased risk of anal cancer in immunosuppressed individuals is not limited to HIV-infected patients. Immunosuppressed transplant patients have a 100-fold increased incidence of anogenital carcinoma compared to the immunocompetent population (Penn, 1986).

A variety of other factors appears to correlate with an increased risk of anal cancer.

Geography, especially areas of extreme poverty such as parts of Brazil and India, is associated with an increased risk of squamous cancer of the anal margin (Fenger, 1991). Crohn's disease, when associated with fistulae, is associated with an increased risk of both squamous carcinoma and adenocarcinoma (Chaikhouni et al., 1981; Church et al., 1985; Daley and Madrazo, 1980; Preston et al., 1983; Slater et al., 1984). The relationship between other inflammatory disorders involving the anal region and the risk of anal cancer has also been investigated. In a study that focused on the etiologic relationship between anal cancer and the HPV responsible for anal warts, Holly and associates raised the possibility that constant irritation, chronic inflammation, and the accompanying repeated epithelial regeneration present in noninfectious conditions might increase risk (Holly et al., 1989). Frisch and co-workers recently reexamined the association between benign anal lesions such as hemorrhoids and fistulae, and subsequent anal cancer (Frisch et al., 1994). Four types of benign lesions were considered: fissure, fistula, perianal and/or perirectal abscess, and hemorrhoids. Their results showed a strong temporal relationship between the diagnosis of benign anal lesions and the diagnosis of anal cancer, with a high relative risk of anal cancer occurring during the first year after hospitalization for benign lesions. However, there was a rapid decline in the relative risk in subsequent years, an observation that is not compatible with the concept of causality. Although the study did not exclude a moderate increase in anal cancer risk in patients with a benign anal lesion, it was felt that the lesions probably represented the initial symptoms of an undetected anal cancer.

PATHOLOGY OF ANAL SQUAMOUS CARCINOMA

Most anal cancers are variants of squamous cell carcinoma. The multiplicity of microscopic patterns expressed by the tumors reflects the diverse histology of anal canal mucosa, particularly that of the ATZ. Consequently, numerous terms have emerged to describe these variants, including basaloid, transitional, nonkeratinizing and keratinizing squamous cell, cloacogenic, and mu-

coepidermoid carcinoma. The subject of anal squamous cancer has been made unnecessarily complicated by focusing too much attention on the diverse histologic patterns. Before specifically addressing precursor lesions and early squamous cancer, it is appropriate to consider the pathology of fully developed anal cancer. The least complicated approach is to distinguish between tumors arising above and below the dentate line (Rickert, 1998).

SQUAMOUS CARCINOMA ARISING ABOVE THE DENTATE LINE

Tumors that arise grossly above or mainly above the dentate line are sometimes classified as neoplasms of the anal canal proper. They arise mostly from the mucosa of the ATZ and include those tumors often referred to as *cloacogenic carcinoma*. Because large tumors arising at this site may obliterate normal anatomic landmarks, they may be confused grossly with adenocarcinomas arising from the distal rectum. Tumors arising from this portion of the upper anal canal are more frequent than tumors developing in the more distal canal and are more common in women than in men (Boman et al., 1984; Dougherty and Evans, 1985; Clark et al., 1986; Greenall et al., 1985; Singh et al., 1981). Invasive cancer of the anus commonly presents clinically with combinations of bleeding, anal pain, change in bowel habit, sensation of a mass, and pruritis.

Reflecting their probable origin from AZT epithelium, carcinomas arising above the dentate line often show a variety of histologic patterns. The most common is squamous cell carcinoma similar to that arising in the more distal anal canal (pecten) (Fig. 10–3). Keratinization is usually not a prominent feature. Others may have a basaloid (transitional or cloacogenic) pattern. A confusing profusion of terms has evolved to designate these so-called cloacogenic tumors, sometimes as synonyms and sometimes to define specific subtypes including squamous carcinoma of basaloid or transitional type and mucoepidermoid carcinoma (squamous carcinoma with mucinous microcysts). While there may remain some controversy over whether basaloid or cloacogenic carcinoma exists as a specific tumor type, most experts support the position that they are variants of

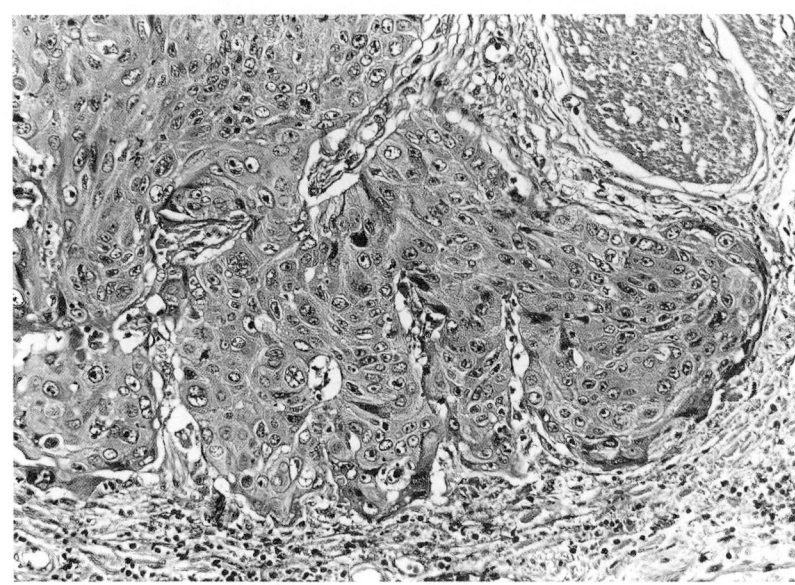

Figure 10–3. Typical moderately differentiated squamous carcinoma arising from anal transitional zone.

squamous carcinoma, the variety of patterns simply reflecting the diversity of their source epithelium. The low-power microscopic view commonly shows an irregular, angulated, branching trabecular pattern (Fig. 10–4). Zones of central necrosis within the neoplastic trabeculae are frequently seen. One or another of the previously enumerated histologic subtypes may dominate, but foci of squamous differentiation are observed in most cases (Fig. 10–5; Rickert, 1998). The typical basaloid or transitional pattern is characterized by nests or trabeculae of small cells without obvious intercellular bridges. Some reserve the term *basaloid* for tumors with recognizable palisading of tumor cells at the periphery of the nests. The pattern formerly designated as mucoepidermoid is now more commonly referred to as *squamous carcinoma with mucinous microcysts.* Perhaps the least common histologic pattern is one that is vaguely reminiscent of adenoid cystic carcinoma of salivary gland. These uncommon patterns usually comprise only a small

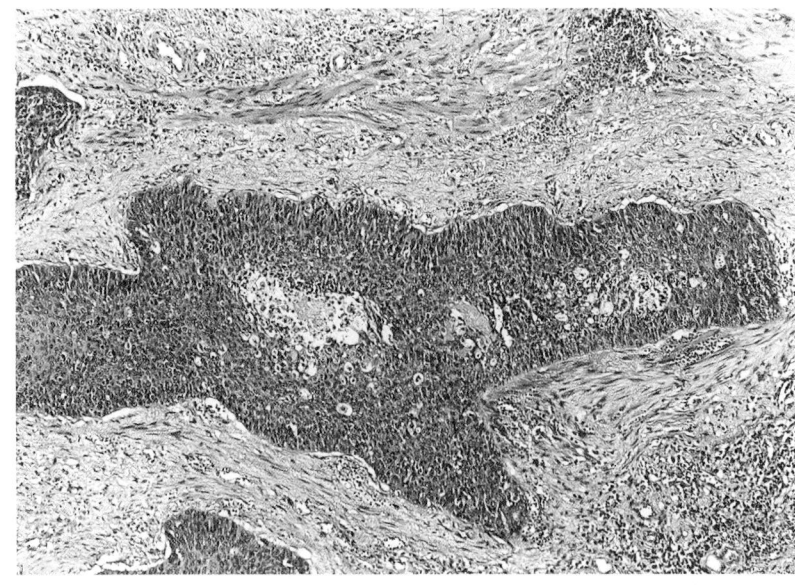

Figure 10–4. Low-power photomicrograph showing typical branching trabecular pattern of basaloid (cloacogenic) variant of anal squamous carcinoma. Note small foci of central necrosis.

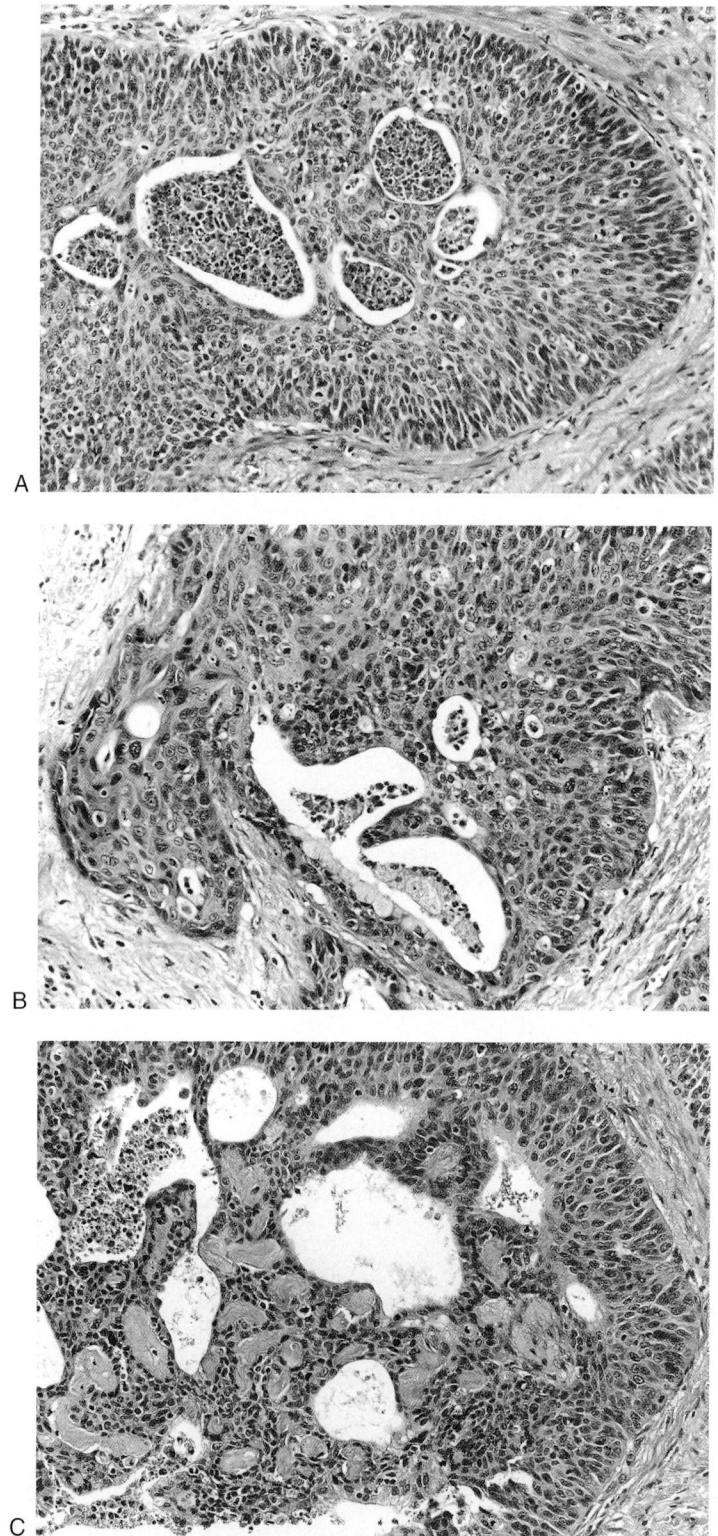

Figure 10–5. Variety of patterns in basaloid squamous carcinoma. *A:* Typical basaloid pattern. Note peripheral palisading of nuclei, focal necrosis, and absence of intercellular bridges. *B:* Microscopic field showing basaloid pattern (right), mucinous microcyst, (lower center), and nonkeratinizing squamous pattern (left). *C:* So-called adenoid cystic pattern with microcysts and hyalinized fibrous trabeculae.

portion of the total tumor. As will be discussed later, the mucosa adjacent to invasive anal carcinoma often shows areas of dysplasia of varying severity including carcinoma *in situ* (anal canal intraepithelial neoplasia, ACIN or AIN).

Tumors showing both the typical basaloid histologic pattern and the several variants described may also arise from anal duct epithelium. This is not surprising because the ATZ and anal ducts share a common embryologic origin.

SQUAMOUS CARCINOMA ARISING BELOW THE DENTATE LINE

Carcinomas arising below the dentate line originate in the nonkeratinized squamous epithelium of the pecten. In some classifications these tumors are designated as tumors of the anal margin. Unlike their counterpart arising at or above the dentate line, these tumors are more common in men than in women. These more distal lesions are more often associated with other coexisting conditions, such as fistulae, fissures, and hemorrhoids, than are tumors arising in the more proximal canal.

Carcinomas arising below the dentate line are usually pure squamous carcinoma of ordinary type (Fig. 10–6). Rarely, tumors arising at this site may have basaloid (cloacogenic) features. There is a tendency toward greater degrees of differentiation and keratinization in the most distal of these lesions (anal margin). Just as in the case of tumors

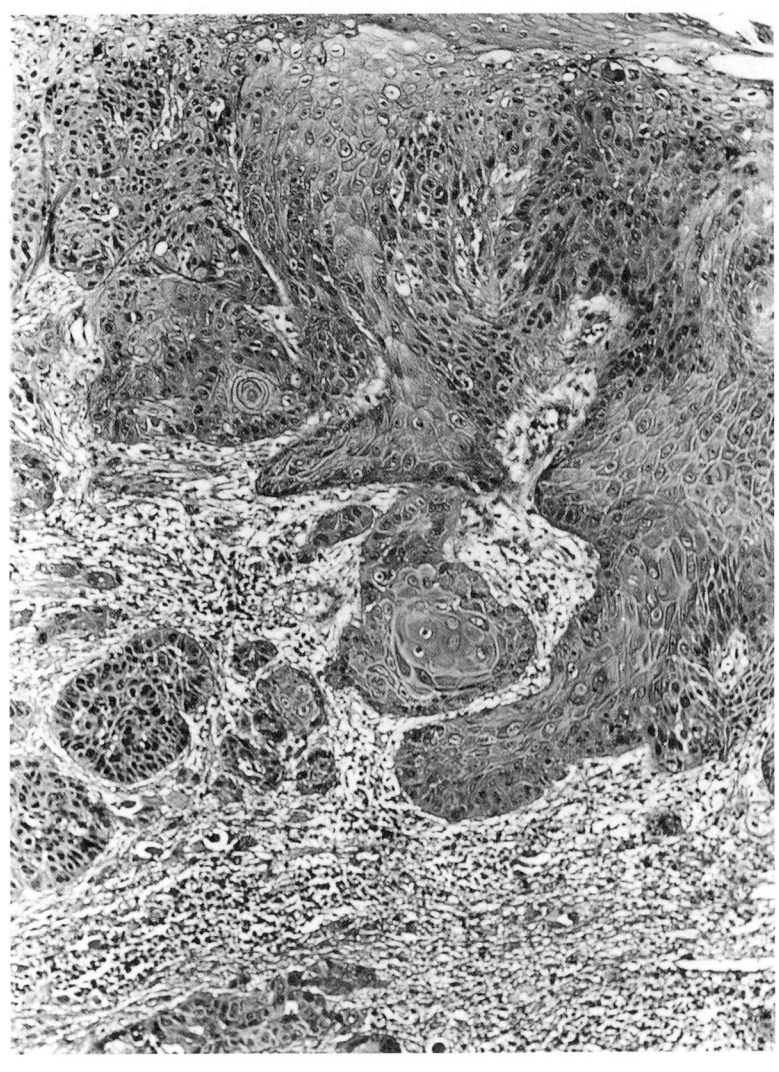

Figure 10–6. Typical pattern of well to moderately differentiated squamous carcinoma arising in distal anal canal near anal margin.

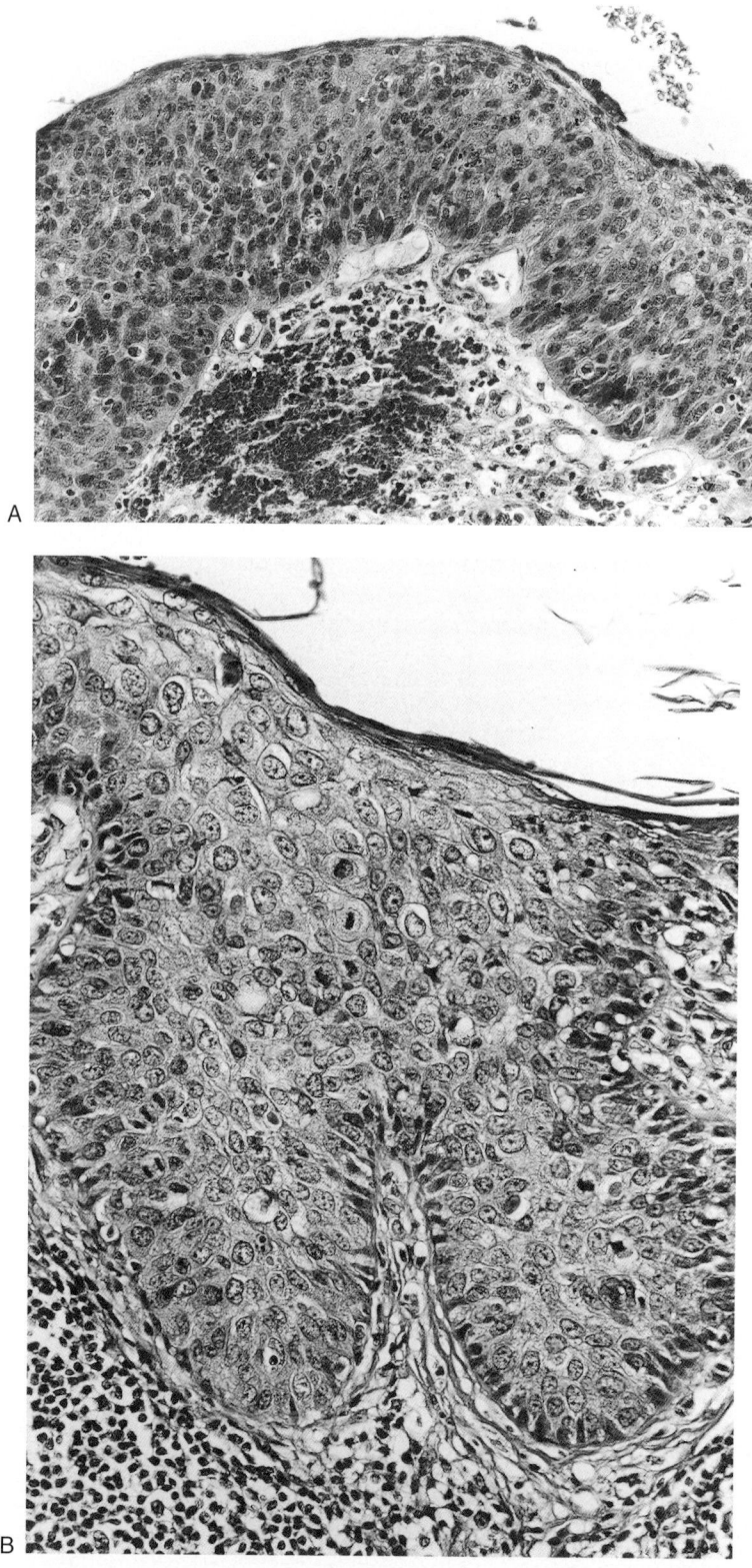

Figure 10–7. *A:* Basaloid pattern of high-grade anal intraepithelial neoplasia (AIN) noted adjacent to an invasive basaloid (cloacogenic) carcinoma. *B:* AIN noted at edge of an invasive carcinoma with nonkeratinizing squamous pattern.

arising high in the anal canal, these more distal and more typically squamous carcinomas are often associated with intraepithelial neoplasia in the adjacent mucosa.

PRECURSOR LESIONS AND ANAL INTRAEPITHELIAL NEOPLASIA

As noted earlier, varying degrees of dysplasia, including changes at a histologic level of carcinoma *in situ*, are commonly observed in mucosa adjacent to invasive anal cancers, whether arising above or below the dentate line. These changes may also be observed in the contiguous anal ducts. The histologic pattern of intraepithelial neoplasia frequently corresponds to that of the adjacent invasive component ranging from basaloid to typical squamous types (Fig. 10–7). Occasionally a single tumor may have a typical basaloid intraepithelial pattern in its more proximal aspect with a more squamous appearance in the distal zone. Consistent with the analogy with neoplastic lesions arising from squamous mucosa of other sites, Fenger proposed the term *anal intraepithelial neoplasia* or *anal canal intraepithelial neoplasia* (AIN or ACIN) (Fenger, 1990; Fenger and Nielsen, 1986b). Changes of this type have been identified next to invasive cancers in more than 80% of cases (Fenger and Nielsen 1986a). The severity of changes varies from low grade to high grade (grades I–III). The designation *AIN I* corresponds to mild dys-plasia, *AIN II* to moderate dysplasia, and *AIN III* to severe dysplasia and carcinoma *in situ*. High-grade AIN in most classifications includes AIN II and III. Just as with other examples of incipient/preinvasive neoplastic lesions, studies of interobserver variation among experts in the grading of AIN has demonstrated only moderate agreement (Carter et al., 1994).

Support for AIN as a precursor of invasive squamous cancer of the anus is similar to that applicable to the uterine cervix. The evidence includes close histologic similarity, appearance at a younger average age than its invasive counterpart, and frequent occurrence adjacent to invasive cancer. Most cervical squamous cancer is believed to arise from high-grade squamous intraepithelial lesions (HSIL). Direct evidence demonstrating progression from high-grade AIN to invasive anal cancer remains more elusive. However, the close similarities with cervical cancer and its precursor and the high incidence of anal cancer in populations with high rates of AIN suggest that high-grade AIN is a precursor. It has been known for many years that AIN may be occasionally observed in anal tissues excised for a variety of benign conditions (Fenger and Nielsen, 1981; Foust et al., 1991). The prevalence of these changes in the so-called general population, based on their identification in minor anal surgical specimens, is probably between 2 to 3 per thousand (Fig. 10–8).

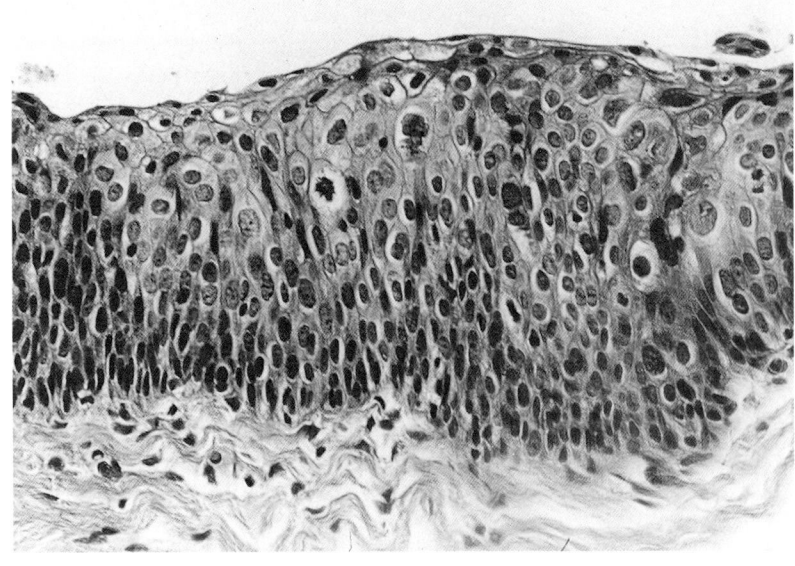

Figure 10–8. Incidental focus of high-grade anal intraepithelial neoplasia in a "routine" hemorrhoidectomy specimen from a middle aged woman.

However, in a population that included a high proportion of young homosexual men, changes of AIN were noted in 4.4% of specimens (Nash et al., 1986). Similar high-grade changes had been reported earlier in condylomata acuminata (anal warts) and/or the adjacent anal mucosa from seven homosexual men (Croxson et al., 1984). Since these early reports, many investigators have studied the various relationships between AIN and other factors, including anal condylomata, sexual orientation, and infection with the human immunodeficiency virus.

Condyloma acuminatum (common genital wart) is a well-known sexually transmitted lesion caused by members of the HPV family. Typically, condylomata are soft, fleshy, papillomatous growths, often occurring as multiple lesions (Fig. 10–9). Lesions generally involve the penis and anus of men and in women are most common on the vulva, vaginal introitus, perineum, anus, and cervix. In the anal region, lesions are most common in the perianal skin, but anal canal involvement

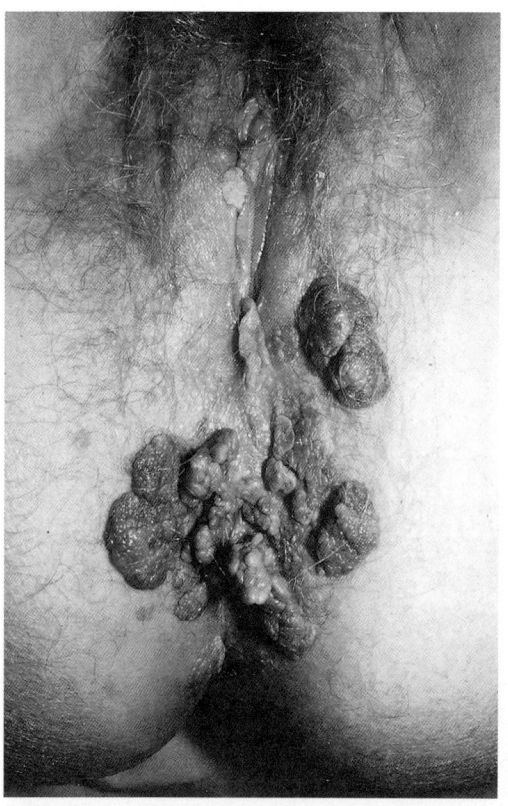

Figure 10–9. Clinical appearance of multiple perianal and perineal condylomata acuminata.

is also common. Histologically the condyloma acuminatum is a papillomatous growth with marked acanthosis and orderly maturation of the squamous epithelium (Fig. 10–10). The surface usually shows areas of parakeratosis and/or hyperkeratosis. Characteristically, some of the squamous cells near the surface have a clear zone of cytoplasm surrounding variably hyperchromatic nuclei that may be enlarged or shrunken. This "koilocytotic" change is a microscopic hallmark of HPV infection. Types 6 and 11 of HPV are the most common viral types associated with the typical grossly papillomatous condyloma. As noted earlier, the so-called oncogenic HPV types, notably 16 and 18, are more likely to be associated with high-grade dysplastic lesions, many of which are flat or grossly invisible. It has already been clearly established that a history of anogenital warts is associated with an increased risk of anal squamous cancer. The actual malignant potential of the condylomatous lesion itself is less clear. High-grade intraepithelial neoplasia has occasionally been reported in anal condylomata (Croxon et al., 1984; Metcalf and Dean, 1995; Fig. 10–11). Of particular interest in the Croxon report is the observation that five of their nine patients (including two who were added after the report had been accepted for publication) had developed acquired immunodeficiency syndrome (AIDS). It is important to distinguish these dysplastic changes in a condyloma from the bizarre atypia occurring after topical application of podophyllum resin. Several cases of invasive squamous carcinoma arising in anal condylomata have also been described (Ejeckman et al., 1983; Kovi et al., 1974).

As noted earlier, the incidence rate for anal cancer among men with a history of anal-receptive intercourse is now several times higher than the current rate of cervical cancer in women in the United States. A relationship between anal cancer and infection with various members of the HPV family is also well established. In recent years, several studies have explored the complex relationship between anal squamous intraepithelial neoplasia (AIN), anal HPV infection, and HIV infection. It has been demonstrated that both AIN and anal HPV infection are more common in HIV-positive homosexual men than in HIV-negative homosexual men

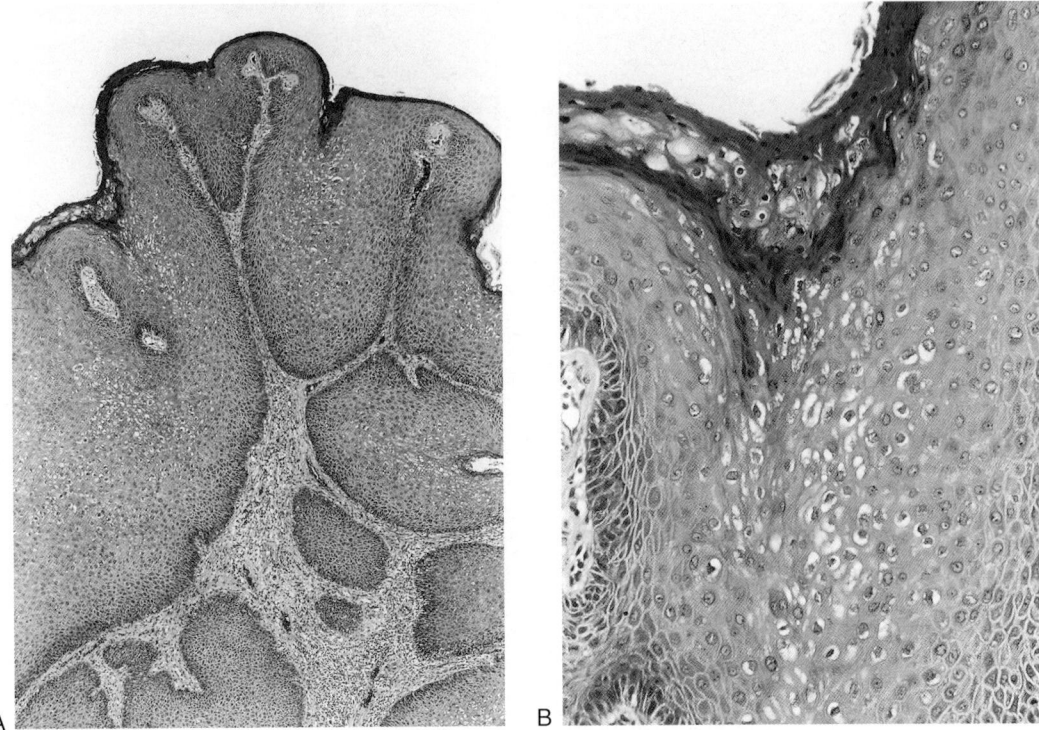

Figure 10–10. *A:* Scanning-power photomicrograph showing typical architecture of condyloma acuminatum. *B:* Higher-power photomicrograph showing characteristic cytoplasmic clearing of koilocytotic change.

(Critchlow et al., 1992; Kiviat et al., 1993; Melbye et al., 1990). Using PCR techniques, Kiviat and co-workers demonstrated anal HPV DNA in 92% and 78% of HIV-seropositive and HIV-seronegative homosexual men, respectively (Kiviat et al., 1993). These studies raised the further possibility that HIV-positive homosexual men may be at even higher risk of developing anal cancer than HIV-negative homosexual men. In fact, a 1994 study by Melbye and associates working with the AIDS/Cancer Working Group demonstrated a strikingly increased (84 times) risk of anal cancer among patients with AIDS (Melbye et al., 1994). A study by Critchlow and co-workers addressed the risk of developing high-grade AIN in relation to HIV infection and immunosuppression, after controlling for the effects of HPV infection (Critchlow et al., 1995). Among men with no baseline lesions, 15.2% of HIV-positive men and 5.4% of HIV-negative men developed high-grade AIN during the follow-up period, which averaged 21 months. The HIV-induced immunosuppression remained an independent predictor of high-grade AIN after adjusting for type and level of detection of HPV. Infection with HIV predicted risk of high-grade AIN after adjustment for number of positive HPV tests. Unger and associates recently studied the relationship between HPV type in anal epithelial lesions and HIV infection (Unger et al., 1997). They demonstrated that for all lesions (condylomas, anal intraepithelial neoplasia, and invasive carcinoma), the presence of high-risk HPV and multiple HPV types was strongly associated with HIV infection. Their findings suggested that the presence of high-risk HPV types and multiple types within low-grade lesions may explain the increased risk of neoplastic progression in HIV-positive patients. The high prevalence of anal HPV infection was recently confirmed in a study of 346 HIV-positive and 262 HIV-negative homosexual and bisexual men (Palefsky et al., 1998a). Using PCR techniques they demonstrated HPV DNA in 93% of HIV-positive and 61% of HIV-negative men studied. The HPV type 16 was the most common, with multiple types demonstrated in 73% of HIV-positive

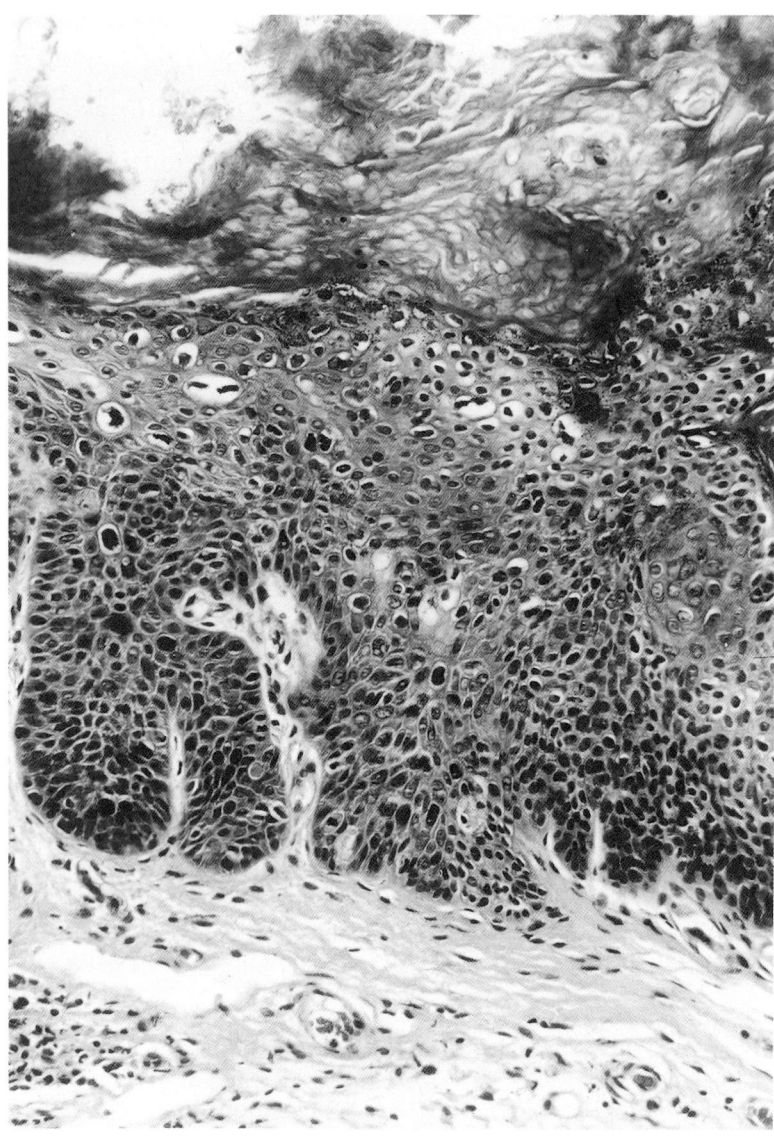

Figure 10–11. Area of high-grade squamous intraepithelial neoplasia in an otherwise typical condyloma from an HIV-positive homosexual man.

and 23% of HIV-negative subjects. Lower CD4 cell levels were associated with higher levels of more oncogenic HPV types, suggesting increased replication of higher-risk HPV types with more advanced immunosuppression. The same group of investigators in another study demonstrated that, among these same men, those who were HIV positive were more likely to develop high-grade AIN (Palefsky et al., 1998b). Life-table estimates of the 4-year incidence of high-grade AIN was 49% among HIV-positive and 17% among HIV-negative men. Furthermore, HIV-positive men with lower baseline CD4

counts and persistent infection with one or more HPV types were more likely to develop high-grade AIN.

While the natural history of anal squamous intraepithelial lesions remains uncertain, the numerous studies described above and the striking epidemiologic and etiologic analogy with cervical neoplasia certainly suggest that invasive anal cancer may be preceded by high-grade anal squamous intraepithelial lesions. In the cervix it is generally acknowledged that high-grade squamous intraepithelial lesions (HSIL) represent the identifiable precursor to invasive squamous carcinoma. Because of the close morphological similarities between cervical HSIL and high-grade AIN as well as the shared strong association with HPV infection, high-grade AIN very likely represents the precursor to invasive anal squamous carcinoma. An additional interesting anatomic parallel between cervical and anal neoplasia is the presence of a transformation zone in each where squamous and columnar epithelium meet and where precursor lesions have been identified.

Since the population at highest risk for anal squamous carcinoma has now been identified, there has been increasing interest in the past several years in the potential utility of screening to detect these possible precursor lesions. Although not yet proven, it is possible that the identification and treatment of high-grade AIN may prevent the development of invasive squamous carcinoma. Surawicz and associates reported their findings on the diagnostic roles of exfoliative cytology, anoscopy, and colposcopic-directed biopsies in the detection of dysplastic lesions and HPV infection in homosexual men (Surawicz et al., 1993). Ninety of 512 homosexual men studied were found to have gross anal abnormalities, which were then subsequently biopsied. Seventy-eight (80%) of these patients had an HPV-associated abnormality on biopsy that was either discrete warts, circumferential warts or rings, or flat white lesions. The gross endoscopic appearance did not correlate with either HIV status, degree of dysplasia (AIN), or HPV type. Cytologic dysplasia was detected in 6% of these patients and 24% of these had high-grade lesions, which were especially likely in the flat white lesions. Of interest was the cytologic detection of dysplasia in 15% of the subjects without grossly recognized lesions. By biopsy, 72 (92%) of subjects with a gross abnormality had histologic dysplasia, which was high grade in 29%. While there was no association between high-grade lesions and HIV seropositivity, among those who were seropositive, high-grade dysplasia was more common in immunosupressed subjects. In a subsequent report, Surawicz and associates reported seven men with histologic evidence of high-grade dysplasia in whom no anoscopic abnormality was noted at the time of biopsy (Surawicz et al., 1995). These abnormalities were detected during routine anal cytologic screening. All men had HPV

type 16 detected at some point. In a follow-up period of 2.5 years after histologic confirmation, none of the patients had developed invasive anal carcinoma. This study indicates that visible lesions need not be present for high-grade AIN to exist. It further suggests that anal cytology may be effective in screening for AIN, although its use in this setting has certainly not been validated as it has in the cervix. Sherman and co-workers investigated the optimal cytologic method for detecting AIN (Sherman et al., 1995). They compared the quality and diagnostic findings in 117 conventionally prepared smears and 191 fluid-based preparations using the CYTYC Thin-Prep method. The smears, which were taken from homosexual or bisexual men, were evaluated according to the Bethesda System used in evaluation of cervical-vaginal cytology (National Cancer Institute Workshop, 1991). Thin-prep smears were satisfactory for evaluation twice as often as conventional smears and detected nearly eight times as many squamous intraepithelial lesions (4.5% of 117 conventional vs. 33.6% of 199 thin-prep smears).

In an effort to evaluate the colposcopic appearance of anal squamous intraepithelial lesions, Jay and co-workers studied 385 biopsied anal lesions (Jay et al., 1997). The colposcopic characteristics (color, contour, surface, and vascular patterns) of these lesions were described and correlated with the histologic findings. Sixty-seven percent of biopsies showed low-grade squamous intraepithelial lesions (LSIL) and 26% showed HSIL. Their findings suggested that the colposcopic appearance of different grades of anal squamous intraepithelial lesions was similar to that described for the cervix and that incorporation of colposcopy into the assessment of anal disease in high-risk patients might aid in distinguishing anal low-grade lesions from high-grade lesions.

Because HIV-infected homosexual and bisexual men are at high risk for HPV-related anal neoplasia and invasive anal squamous cell carcinoma, and because anal cytology may represent a potential screening method, Goldie and co-workers recently studied the clinical benefit and cost-effectiveness of screening for AIN (Goldie et al., 1999). This study utilized a hypothetical cohort of homosexual and bisexual HIV-positive men living in the United States and a statistical model to measure life expectancy, quality-adjusted life expectancy, quality-adjusted years of life saved, lifetime costs, and incremental cost-effective ratio. The authors concluded that screening HIV-positive homosexual and bisexual men with anal cytology was associated with substantial clinical benefit. Regardless of when screening began, the cost-effectiveness of either yearly or biennial screening was comparable to that of other accepted preventive measures in clinical medicine.

Because of the uncertainty of the natural history of anal squamous intraepithelial lesions, optimal approaches to management are also uncertain. In a study of 19 cases of high-grade squamous intraepithelial neoplasia identified in routinely excised hemorrhoidal tissue, there was no evidence of progression or recurrence during a mean follow-up interval of 6 years (Foust et al., 1991).

In Fenger's original group of patients with AIN, 4 of 19 cases recurred but none evolved to invasive cancer over the 5-year period of follow up (Fenger and Nielsen, 1986b). Scholefield and co-workers reported on the management of 70 patients with anal squamous intraepithelial neoplasia (Scholefield et al., 1994). Forty-three patients had low-grade lesions (defined for their study as AIN I and II) and were not further treated. Twenty-seven patients had high-grade lesions (AIN III). Many of the lesions detected in both groups involved both anal canal and perianal skin. Very few involved only anal canal. The authors' policy was to excise high grade lesions (AIN III). Eight patients with treated AIN III developed additional foci of high-grade lesions, but the authors were unable to distinguish between residual and recurrent disease. Eight invasive cancers were associated with AIN III lesions, five in perianal skin and three in the lower anal canal. In four of the patients invasion was not suspected clinically but was detected only on microscopic examination. A further two patients were clinically suspected to have invasive lesions, and invasion in a background of AIN III was confirmed microscopically. While this study did not permit conclusions regarding the natural history of high-grade AIN, the authors recommended surgical excision of high-grade lesions. Because of the suspicion that high-grade AIN may undergo malignant change, others have also suggested treatment with local excision (Carter, 1993; Carter et al., 1994). However, at the present time no generally agreed-upon guidelines exist for the management of patients with anal intraepithelial neoplasia, reflecting the current state of uncertainty about the natural history of these lesions.

Perianal Squamous Neoplasia

Invasive squamous cell carcinoma of the perianal skin, like carcinomas of the distal anal canal and anal margin, are typically pure squamous cell lesions with varying degrees of keratinization. Precursor lesions analogous to those discussed above in the anal canal exist in the perianal region as well.

Bowen's disease is a clinicopathologic variant of *in situ* squamous cell carcinoma of skin that rarely involves the anal region (Scoma and Levy, 1975; Strauss and Fazio, 1979). When there is anal involvement, it is typically at the anal margin or perianal skin, but incidental discovery in hemorrhoidal tissues may also occur (Beck et al., 1988; Sarmiento et al., 1997). Bowen's disease is typically seen clinically as discrete, red plaques with a scaly or fissured surface (Rickert et al., 1977; Fig. 10–12). Patients may report symptomatic itchy and burning. Histologically, Bowen's disease is an intraepithelial squamous carcinoma characterized by marked disorganization with many large, atypical squamous cells and striking loss of normal polarity with disordered maturation (Fig. 10–13). Atypical mitotic figures are frequently noted. The process may extend microscopically to involve the epithelium of the cutaneous appendages. Invasive squamous carcinoma may develop in 5% to 10% of lesions of Bowen's disease. Despite a tendency for recurrence in inadequately treated patients, wide local excision is the treatment of choice. Since the initial description of Bowen's disease, it has been suggested that there is a significant risk of subsequent development of internal malignancies. However, more recent reviews have concluded that patients with Bowen's disease are not at increased risk to develop internal malignancy (Arbesman and Ransohoff, 1987). Furthermore, the two largest series of Bowen's disease specifically involving the pe-

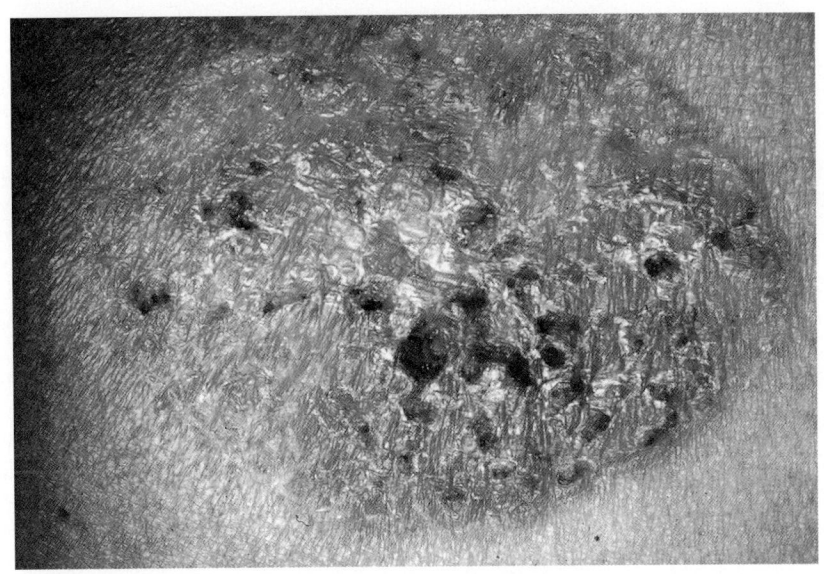

Figure 10–12. Typical slightly raised and scaly plaque of Bowen's disease.

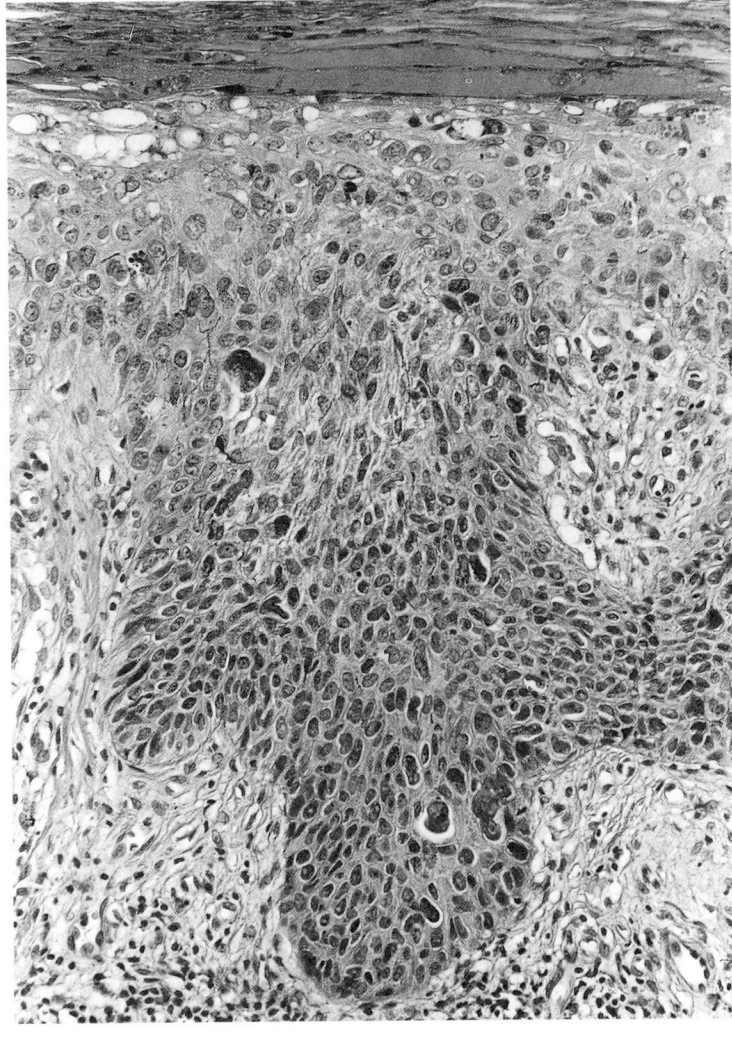

Figure 10–13. Perianal Bowen's disease (*in situ* squamous carcinoma) showing marked cellular anaplasia and disordered maturation.

223

rianal region as well as a survey study failed to demonstrate a significant relationship with internal malignancies (Beck et al., 1988; Marfing et al., 1987; Sarmiento et al., 1997).

Bowenoid papulosis is a condition histologically very similar if not identical to Bowen's disease that was initially described on the genitalia of young adults (Ulbright et al., 1982; Wade et al., 1978). The process may also involve the anus. Clinically the lesions appear as multiple small, pigmented papules. Efforts to separate these lesions histologically from classic Bowen's disease have focused on their more orderly maturation of keratinocytes, greater nuclear uniformity, lack of involvement of cutaneous appendages, and milder cellular anaplasia. However, many feel that these histologic distinctions are not consistent or reproducible enough for reliable separation of the two processes. In addition to their presentation as multiple small papular rather than single larger, plaque-like lesions, bowenoid papulosis has a tendency to regress spontaneously. However, cases of typical bowenoid papulosis have been observed to progress to both Bowen's disease and invasive squamous cell carcinoma (Bergeron et al., 1987; DeVillez and Stevens, 1980; Rudlinger and Buchmann, 1989). It is also of interest that HPV type 16 has been identified in lesions of bowenoid papulosis, further supporting the position that this disorder should be included in the spectrum of intraepithelial neoplasia (Bergeron et al., 1987; Gross et al., 1985; Rudlinger and Buchmann, 1989.). Patients with these bowenoid lesions also often have typical condylomata acuminata. It has been recently recommended that "bowenoid papulosis" be abandoned as a histologic term, reserving the designation only for cases with characteristic clinical features (Prat, 1991).

Verrucous carcinoma is a very well–differentiated variant of squamous cell carcinoma best known in the upper aerodigestive tract (Kraus and Perez-Mesa, 1966). Involvement of the anal region occasionally does occur, usually in the perianal skin (Bogomoletz et al., 1985; Gingrass et al., 1978; Zemstov et al., 1992). The tumors are characterized clinically by a bulky, warty appearance. Most are single lesions. Microscopically these are extremely well–differentiated squamous carcinomas with generally minimal cellular anaplasia. While they invade into the underlying stroma, they do so with pushing rather than infiltrating margins (Fig. 10–14).

Giant condyloma acuminatum (Buschke-Loewenstein's tumor) was described initially as a tumor of the penis, but rare examples have been reported from the anorectal area as well (Alexander and Kaminsky, 1979; Elliot et al., 1979; Wells et al., 1988). This lesion shares many gross and histologic features with verrucous squamous cell carcinoma, and many believe that they represent the same neoplastic process (Elliot et al., 1979; Prioleau et al., 1980). It is likely that examples of invasive squamous carcinomas reportedly arising within a giant condyloma represent low-grade squamous carcinomas from their inception. Bogomoletz and associates have suggested that, while verrucous carcinoma and giant condyloma acuminatum should be considered separate entities, they are parts of a continuous spectrum that also includes simple condylomata acuminata (Bogomoletz et al., 1985). Regardless of how one chooses to classify these two lesions, it is important to remember that they do not metastasize, and complete local excision is the treatment of choice.

ADENOCARCINOMA OF THE ANUS

Adenocarcinoma of the anal region may arise from a variety of sources of glandular epithelium. Included are the colorectal mucosa proximal to the ATZ or occuring as small islands within it, the mucus-secreting cells of the ATZ, anal ducts (glands), and perianal apocrine glands.

The most common variant of adenocarcinoma in the region is that arising from colorectal mucosa, either in the low rectum with extension into anal canal or from islands of colorectal epithelium in the ATZ (Fig. 10–15). These tumors are grossly and microscopically identical to typical colorectal adenocarcinomas and are so classified. Except for very small or early lesions, it may be difficult to determine the precise site of origin. Their precursor lesions are the same as for more proximal colorectal adenocarcinomas and include various types of adenomas and precancerous dysplasia arising in

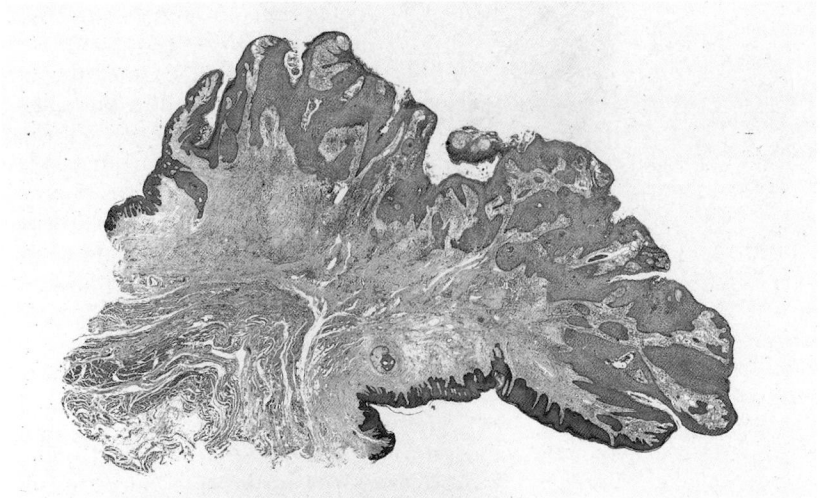

A

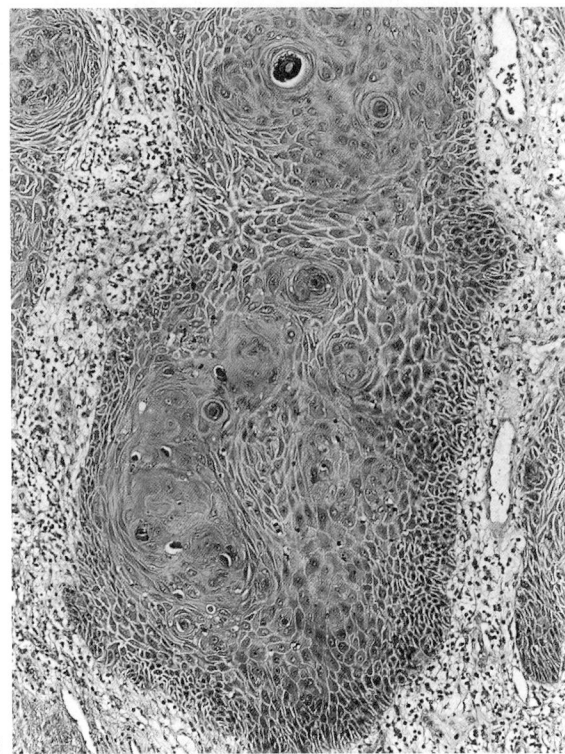

B

Figure 10–14. *A:* Scanning-power photomicrograph of a perianal verrucous squamous carcinoma. Note pushing margins of infiltration. *B:* Higher-power photomicrograph of same lesion showing only minimal cellular anaplasia.

chronic inflammatory bowel disease. These relationships are discussed elsewhere.

As noted earlier, typical squamous cell carcinomas of the basaloid type arising within the anal canal may contain foci of mucus-secreting columnar cells that may form small cysts. This pattern was formerly often referred to as *mucoepidermoid carcinoma*, but is now usually designated as *squamous* (or basaloid) *carcinoma with mucinous microcysts.*

The histogenesis and classification of other variants of anal adenocarcinoma are more problematic (Tarazi and Nelson, 1994). The anal ducts and/or anal glands have been suggested as the likely sources of these rare neoplasms (Fenger, 1991; Jensen

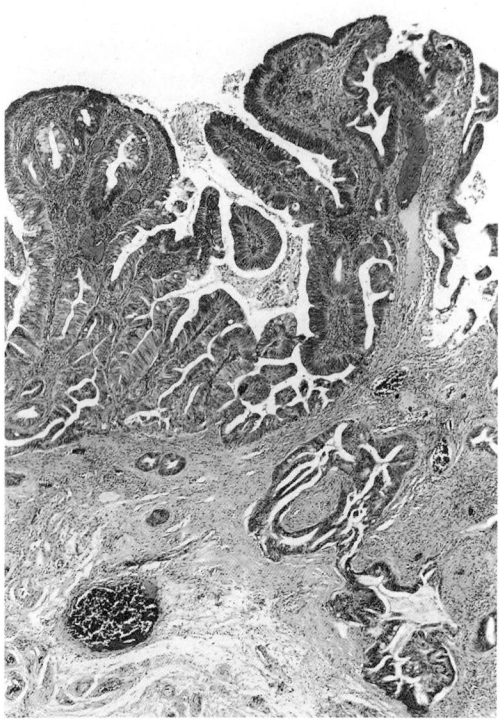

Figure 10–15. Scanning-power photomicrograph of superficially invasive, well-differentiated adenocarcinoma arising at the base of a villous adenoma. The entire lesion was confined to the anal canal.

et al., 1988; Lee et al., 1981; Zaren et al., 1983). However, proof of origin within anal glands/ducts established by meeting strict criteria including location of tumors at sites of anal glands, exclusion of other sources of columnar mucosa, transition from dysplastic anal gland epithelium, as well as characteristic histologic features, is extremely difficult to establish (Behan and Burnett, 1996; Fenger and Morson, 1989). Typical symptoms include pain, rectal bleeding, and the presence of a perianal mass (Abel et al., 1993). Many patients also have an associated fistula.

The common association of anal adenocarcinoma with fistulae presents further problems with classification. Such cases have been designated as perianal mucinous adenocarcinoma or adenocarcinoma in an anal fistula. Most of these are mucinous ("colloid") adenocarcinomas. They typically show little or no involvement of the overlying mucosa. Microscopically, these mucinous adenocarcinomas may be cystic or may have a significant component of signet ring cells (Fig. 10–16). The histogenesis of these tumors has been and remains controversial (Fenger, 1991; Jones and Morson, 1984; Onerheim, 1988; Prioleau et al., 1977; Tarazi and Nelson 1994). There is often a long antecedent history of anal mass, fistulae, and abscesses. Some have suggested origin within anal glands/ducts, but, as noted ear-

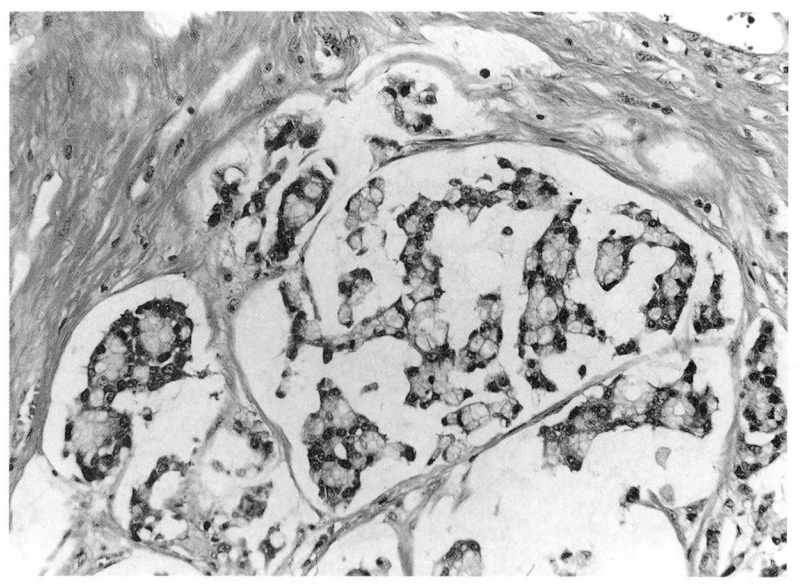

Figure 10–16. Poorly differentiated adenocarcinoma located in the deep perirectal, anal, and perianal soft tissue in a patient with a long-standing anal fistula. Origin of the tumor could not be traced histologically to colorectal mucosa.

lier, this is difficult to prove. Histologically, cases generally accepted as anal gland adenocarcinoma have a small acinar or tubular pattern. An additional incompletely resolved question is whether the fistulae precede or follow the development of the tumor. In some cases, development within a track lined by colorectal mucosa has been documented, suggesting a hindgut duplication (Jones and Morson, 1984). In several cases, the mucosa near the adenocarcinoma has shown dysplastic (adenomatous) changes similar to those associated with ordinary colorectal adenocarcinoma. Of additional interest is the quite favorable prognosis following excision of the rectum in these cases. Because of their frequent position deep within the perianal tissues, diagnosis is often delayed. It is important, therefore, to microscopically evaluate tissue from fistulae and to be suspicious of cases with a mass, induration, anal stenosis, or mucinous discharge.

A recent report has evaluated anal adenocarcinomas for HPV DNA and compared the results with adenocarcinomas of the colorectum (Koulos et al., 1991). The authors identified HPV type 18 DNA in two of six cases of anal adenocarcinoma, and HPV type-16 DNA was identified in each of two cases of anal squamous carcinoma, one of which also contained HPV type 18. No HPV-associated DNA was identified in any of seven cases of colorectal adenocarcinoma or in three colorectal adenomas. The association of HPV type 18 with anal adenocarcinoma is similar to that noted with adenocarcinomas of the cervix.

PERIANAL EXTRAMAMMARY PAGET'S DISEASE

The histogenesis and certain clinical aspects of extramammary Paget's disease are controversial. It has long been known that mammary Paget's disease is virtually always associated with an underlying ductal carcinoma of the breast. This constant association with an underlying carcinoma does not pertain in extramammary Paget's disease.

The most common sites of involvement in extramammary Paget's disease are the vulva and neighboring perineal skin. Less common sites are the axilla, and the scrotum and penis in men. Involvement of perianal skin

alone is distinctly unusual. The usual clinical presentation of extramammary Paget's disease, irrespective of site, is an erythematous patch or plaque that may be scaly, eroded, or sometimes ulcerated (Jones et al., 1979; Fig. 10–17). Pruritis is the most common symptom. Microscopically, Paget's disease is characterized by the presence of large, atypical cells with vesicular nuclei, often large nucleoli, and abundant pale granular or vacuolated cytoplasm (Fig. 10–18). The Paget's cells may be distributed as single cells or nests within the epidermis as well as the cutaneous appendages. Paget's cells are usually more numerous in the basal region and intraepidermal acinar structures may occur. The overlying epidermis may be hyperplastic with hyperkeratosis and parakeratosis.

The two most controversial areas of discussion in extramammary Paget's disease relate to the histogenesis of the neoplastic cells themselves and the association of the disorder with other regional neoplasms. It is generally agreed that the Paget's cell is a neoplastic secretory (glandular) cell. The presence of cytoplasmic acid mucopolysaccharide has been known for a long time and may be demonstrated with a variety of stains for mucosubstances. The use of immunohistochemistry has also made important contributions to our understanding. Paget's cells are typically positive for low-molecular-weight cytokeratins and carcinoembryonic antigen (CEA) (Nagle et al., 1985). Immunohistochemical demonstration of gross cystic disease fluid protein (GCDFP) supported the most prevalent view that Paget's cells are of apocrine derivation (Mazoujian et al., 1984).

As noted earlier, extramammary Paget's disease does not share with the breast counterpart a constant association with underlying malignancy. Even more fascinating is the consistent observation that an association with underlying malignancy in extramammary Paget's disease varies with the site of involvement. For example, vulvar Paget's disease is only infrequently associated with an underlying cancer. In contrast, perianal Paget's disease is much more likely to be associated with an internal cancer, usually a rectal adenocarcinoma. However, many examples of perianal Paget's disease remain confined to the epidermis and cutaneous ap-

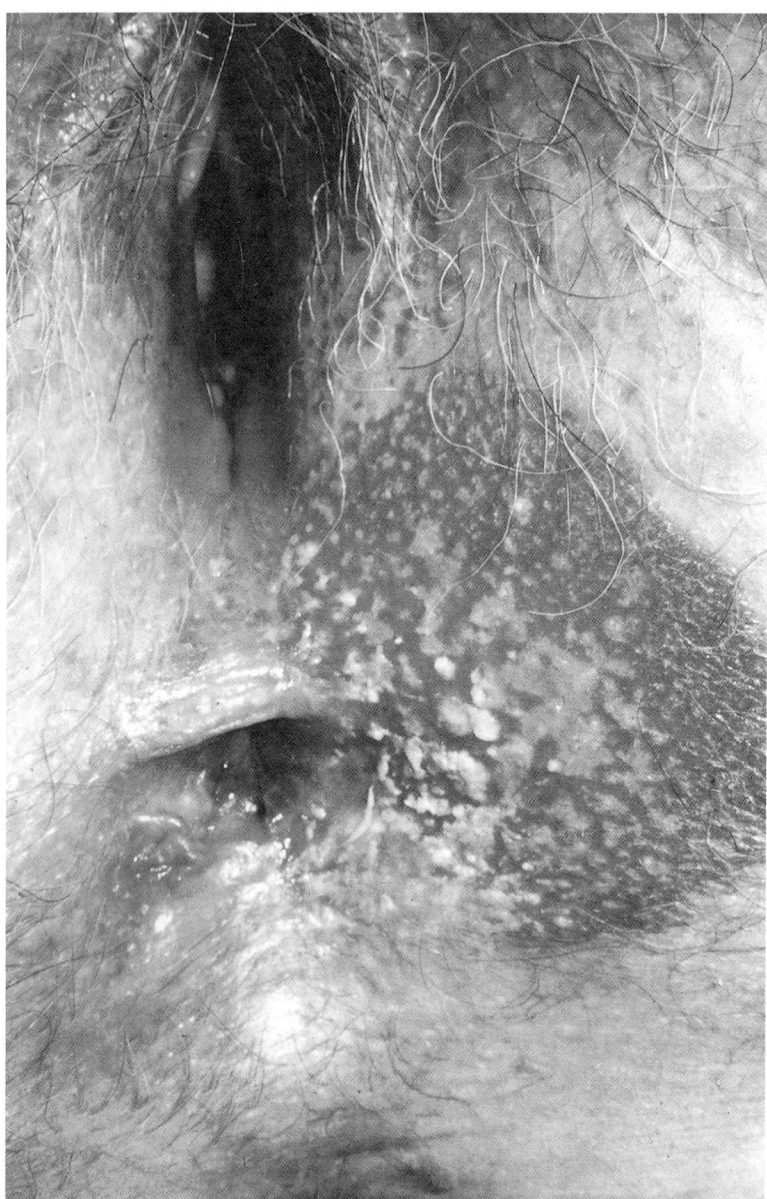

Figure 10–17. Clinical appearance of an erythematous, slightly scaly plaque of extramammary Paget's disease involving perianal and perineal skin.

pendages just as in the vulva. These observations have led several authors to suggest that perianal Paget's disease may represent two disorders and that immunohistochemical staining profiles and histologic features may contribute to their separation (Armitage et al., 1989; Goldblum and Hart, 1998). One type appears to be of endodermal derivation, often with intraepithelial glandular structures, "dirty necrosis" like that seen in the glands in colorectal adenocarcinoma, numerous signet ring cells, pos-

itive staining for CK 20, and a negative reaction for GCDFP-15. These cases are quite likely to be associated with synchronous or metachronous rectal adenocarcinoma. The other type appears to be a primary cutaneous intraepithelial neoplasm of probable apocrine sweat gland origin and is not associated with an underlying rectal adenocarcinoma. These cases histologically lack intraepidermal gland formation and intraluminal "dirty necrosis." Immunohistochemical reaction for GCDFP-15 in this variant is posi-

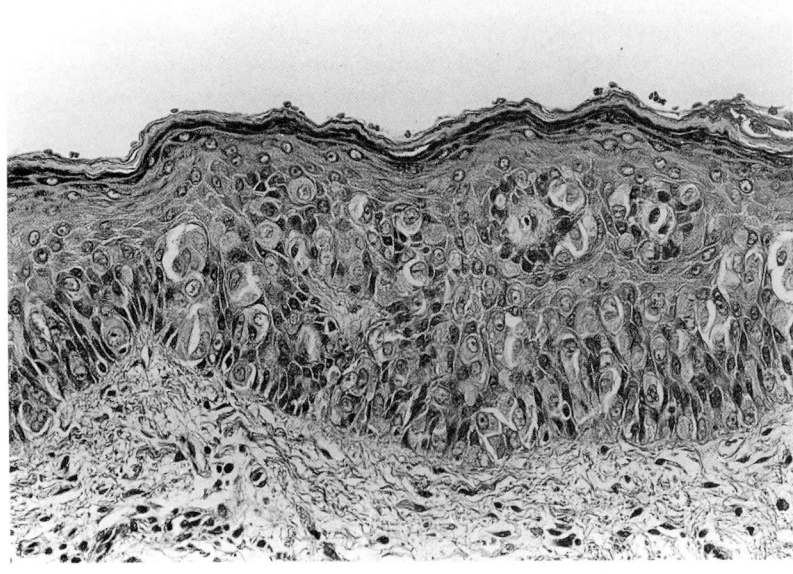

Figure 10–18. Extramammary Paget's disease of perianal skin. Characteristic atypical cells with pale granular cytoplasm and vesicular nuclei with prominent nucleoli are present singly and in small nests within the epidermis.

tive and for CK 20 it is negative (Goldblum and Hart, 1998).

SMALL CELL CARCINOMA

These rare anaplastic tumors of neuroendocrine origin occasionally arise in the distal rectum and may extend into the upper anal canal (Fig. 10–19). They resemble small cell anaplastic carcinomas from other sites (Burke et al., 1991; Wick et al., 1987). They are highly aggressive neoplasms with a propensity to early dissemination, especially to liver. When the anal canal is involved, they must be distinguished from poorly differentiated basaloid squamous carcinomas. Demonstration of neuroendocrine differentiation may require immunohistochemical or ultrastructural studies. Origin within the anal canal proper is a theoretical possibility since neuroendocrine cells may be present in anal canal epithelium (Fenger and Lyon, 1982).

BASAL CELL CARCINOMA

Basal cell carcinoma rarely occurs in the perianal skin. It is histologically and clinically similar to basal cell carcinoma of other cutaneous sites (Nielsen and Jensen, 1981; White et al., 1984). The lesion usually pre-

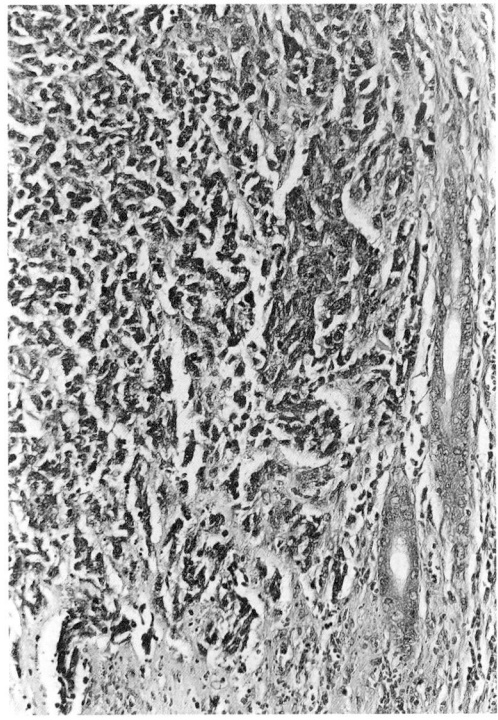

Figure 10–19. High-power photomicrograph of a small cell carcinoma presenting as a large, bulky mass involving distal rectum and extending into anal canal. Note sheets of discohesive, anaplastic tumor cells. Neuroendocrine differentiation was confirmed with immunohistochemistry and electron microscopy.

sents as an ulcerated nodule similar to that occurring elsewhere on the skin. These rare tumors must be distinguished from basaloid (cloacogenic) squamous carcinomas of the anal canal because of the distinctly more aggressive behavior and different therapy of the latter. Usually this is not difficult. Basal cell carcinoma tends to be less anaplastic, has more pronounced peripheral palisading, and frequently its origin can be traced to the basal cell zone of the epidermis (Fig. 10–20). Occasionally the distinction may be very difficult. A recent report describes several immunohistochemical differences between these two neoplasms (Alvarez-Canas et al., 1996). Basaloid carcinomas of the anal canal were positive for a variety of cytokeratin markers as well as for CEA, epithelial membrane antigen (EMA), and Ulex europaeus (UEA 1). In contrast, all cases of basal cell carcinoma were negative for these markers but were positive with Ber-EP4, a monoclonal antibody that has been used to distinguish basal cell carcinoma from cutaneous squamous cell carcinoma.

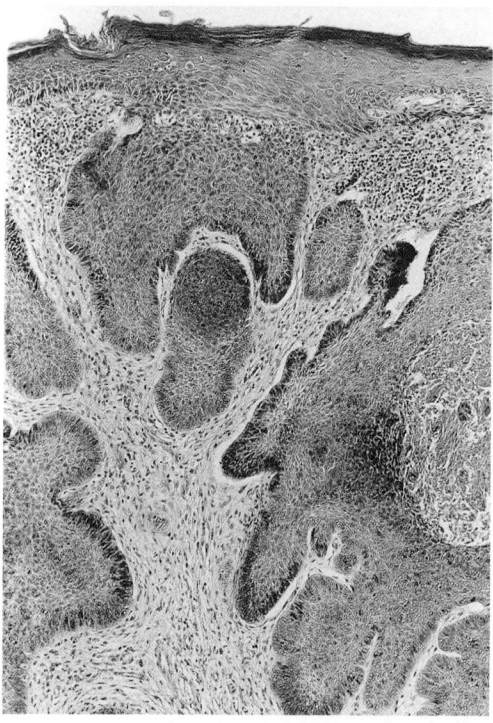

Figure 10–20. Basal cell carcinoma arising in perianal skin. Origin can be traced to basal zone of epidermis. Note prominent palisading of cells at the periphery.

MALIGNANT MELANOMA

Malignant melanoma of the anal canal is a rare but virulent disease with a poor prognosis (Ross et al., 1990). Despite the rarity of anal involvement, this is the third most common site of malignant melanoma after skin and eye and the most common primary site in the gastrointestinal tract. It is a disease of middle age with a roughly equal gender distribution. Patients usually present with bleeding, which may be associated with a mass, pain, or change in bowel habit.

By the time of diagnosis, the average lesion is 3 to 4 cm in diameter (Brady et al., 1995; Mills and Cooper, 1983). The typical gross lesion is a polypoid mass that may be smooth or ulcerated, and about two-thirds are pigmented. When the site of origin can be determined with precision, it is usually at the dentate line or neighboring transitional zone. As noted earlier, melanocytes have been identified in the anal transitional zone (Clemmensen and Fenger, 1991; Fenger and Lyon, 1982). The tumor often grows into the lower rectum where clinical confusion with primary rectal adenocarcinoma can occur, particularly with nonpigmented lesions.

The microscopic appearance of anal malignant melanoma is similar to that arising in skin (Fig. 10–21). There may be evidence of intramucosal junctional involvement at the edge of an invasive lesion. This often consists of a proliferation of single atypical melanocytes in an acral-lentiginous pattern similar to other primary melanomas arising in mucous membranes. When melanin pigment is absent and no adjacent junctional activity is observed, distinction from poorly differentiated carcinoma or Paget's disease may be difficult. Immunohistochemical identification of S-100 protein or melanoma antigen HMB-45 may aid in establishing a diagnosis of melanoma. The immunohistochemical features of anal carcinoma and Paget's disease have been previously addressed.

The 5-year survival rate of primary malignant melanoma is very poor, ranging from 6% to 15% in most series. Common metastatic sites are lymph nodes, liver, and lung. The likelihood of diagnosing this tumor in an early, intraepithelial (*in situ*) stage is very small. However, occasional tumors have been discovered during routine pathologic

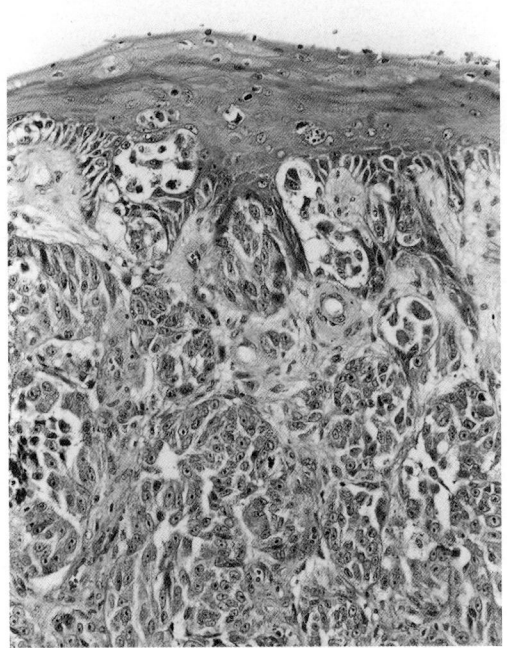

Figure 10–21. Deeply invasive malignant melanoma arising in upper anal canal of a middle-aged man. Note lentiginous junctional component in squamous epithelium overlying the invasive tumor.

examination of hemorrhoidal specimens. In one series three of seven such cases survived for 5 or more years (Brady et al., 1995).

STAGING OF ANAL CANAL CANCER

Staging of anal cancer under the TNM system utilizes two different systems (Fleming et al., 1997). One of these covers carcinomas of the anal canal proper (excluding malignant melanoma), and the other is for carcinomas arising at the anal margin. As noted earlier, this system defines the anal margin as the junction of hair-bearing skin and the mucous membrane of the anal canal, or more distal. Cancers arising at the anal margin are staged according to the system used for skin.

Carcinomas arising in the anal canal are staged according to size and extent of the primary tumor (Table 10–1). Staging of invasive tumors is dependent largely on clinical examination. Pathologists rarely have an

opportunity to examine resection specimens of anal canal carcinoma because of the dramatic changes in therapy during the past 20 years (Beck and Karulf, 1994; Grabenbauer et al., 1998). Combination chemotherapy and radiation therapy (chemoradiation) has become the standard management strategy for squamous carcinoma of the anal canal, with abdominoperineal resection reserved usually for nonresponding and recurrent tumors. The results of chemoradiation are quite impressive and anal function is also preserved.

The most important prognostic indicators are depth of invasion and extent of spread of tumor. Specific histologic type is less important, although some have suggested that squamous variants with mucinous microcysts or a pseudoadenomatoid pattern may behave more aggressively. Histologic differentiation may also be important, but probably not independent of stage. Location is important because pure squamous cell tumors

Table 10–1. Staging of Cancer of Anal Canal: American Joint Committee on Cancer (AJCC) TNM Components

Primary tumor (T)

TX	Primary tumor cannot be assessed
T0	No evidence of primary tumor
Tis	Carcinoma *in situ*
T1	Tumor 2 cm or less in greatest dimension
T2	Tumor more than 2 cm but not more than 5 cm in greatest dimension
T3	Tumor more than 5 cm in greatest dimension
T4	Tumor of any size invades adjacent organ(s), e.g., vagina, urethra, bladder (involvement of the sphincter muscle(s) alone is not classified as T4)

Regional lymph nodes (N)

NX	Regional lymph nodes cannot be assessed
N0	No regional lymph node metastasis
N1	Metastasis in perirectal lymph node(s)
N2	Metastasis in unilateral internal iliac and/or inguinal lymph node(s)
N3	Metastasis in perirectal and inguinal lymph nodes and/or bilateral internal iliac and/or inguinal lymph nodes

Distant metastasis (M)

MX	Distant metastasis cannot be assessed
M0	No distant metastasis
M1	Distant metastasis

From Fleming et al., 1997, with permission.

of the distal anal canal or anal margin, especially if small and superficial, are amenable to local excision. The role of DNA ploidy analysis is controversial, but it has been suggested that it may be an independent predictor of prognosis in anal carcinoma (Shepard et al., 1990).

REFERENCES

Abel ME, Chiu YSY, Volpe PE. (1993) Adenocarcinoma of the anal glands: results of a survey. *Dis Colon Rectum* 36:383–387.

Alexander RM, Kaminsky DB. (1979) Giant condyloma acuminatum (Buschke-Loewenstein tumor) of the anus: case report and review of the literature. *Dis Colon Rectum* 22:561–565.

Alvarez-Canas MC, Fernandez FA, Rodilla IG, Val-Bernal JF. (1996) Perianal basal cell carcinoma: a comparative histologic, immunohistochemical, and flow cytometric study with basaloid carcinoma of the anus. *Am J Dermatopathol* 18:371–379.

Arbesman H, Ransohoff DF. (1987) Is Bowen's disease a predictor for the development of internal malignancy? A methodological critique of the literature. *JAMA* 257:516–518.

Armitage NC, Jass JR, Richard PI, Thompson JPS, Phillips RKS. (1989) Paget's disease of the anus: a clinicopathologic study. *Br J Surg* 76:60–63.

Beck DE, Fazio VW, Jagelman DG, Lavery IC. (1988) Perianal Bowen's disease. *Dis Colon Rectum* 31:419–422.

Beck DE, Karulf RE. (1994) Combination therapy for epidermoid carcinoma of the anal canal. *Dis Colon Rectum* 37:1118–1125.

Behan WMH, Burnett RA. (1996) Adenocarcinoma of the anal glands. *J Clin Pathol* 49:1009–1011.

Bergeron C, Naghashfar Z, Canaan C, Shah K, Fu Y, Ferenczy A. (1987) Human papillomavirus type 16 in intraepithelial neoplasia (bowenoid papulosis) and coexistent invasive carcinoma of the vulva. *Int J Gynecol Pathol* 6:1–11.

Bogomoletz WV, Potet F, Molas G. (1985) Condylomata acuminata, giant condyloma acuminatum (Buschke-Loewenstein tumour) and verrucous squamous carcinoma of the perianal and anorectal region: a continuous precancerous spectrum? *Histopathology* 9:1155–1169.

Boman BM, Moertel CG, O'Connell MJ, Scott M, Weiland LH, Beart RW, Gunderson LL, Spencer RJ. (1984) Carcinoma of the anal canal: a clinical and pathologic study of 188 cases. *Cancer* 54:114–125.

Bosch FX, Manos MM, Muñoz N, Sherman M, Jansen AM, Peto J, Schiffman MH, Moreno V, Kurman R, Shah KV. (1995) Prevalence of human papillomavirus in cervical cancer: a world wide perspective. *J Natl Cancer Inst* 87:796–802.

Brady MS, Kavolius JP, Quan SHQ. (1995) Anorectal melanoma: a 64 year experience at Memorial Sloan-Kettering Cancer Center. *Dis Colon Rectum* 38:146–151.

Burke AB, Shekitka KM, Sobin L. (1991) Small cell carcinoma of the large intestine. *Am J Clin Pathol* 95:315–321.

Carter PS. (1993) Anal cancer: current perspectives. *Dig Dis* 11:239–251.

Carter PS, Sheffield JP, Shepherd N, Melcher DH, Jenkins D, Ewings D, Talbot I, Northover JMA. (1994) Interobserver variation in the reporting of the histopathological grading of anal intraepithelial neoplasia. *J Clin Pathol* 47:1032–1034.

Chaikhouni A, Regueyra FI, Stevens JR. (1981) Adenocarcinoma in perianal fistulas of Crohn's disease. *Dis Colon Rectum* 24:639–643.

Church JM, Weakley FL, Fazio VW, Sebek BA, Achkar E, Carwell M. (1985) The relationship between fistulas in Crohn's disease and associated carcinoma. *Dis Colon Rectum* 28:361–366.

Clark J, Petrilli N, Herrera L, Mittelman A. (1986) Epidermoid carcinoma of the anal canal. *Cancer* 57:400–406.

Clemmensen OJ, Fenger C. (1991) Melanocytes in the anal canal epithelium. *Histopathology* 18:237–241.

Cooper HS, Patchefsky AS, Marks G. (1979) Cloacogenic carcinoma of the anorectum in homosexual men: an observation of four cases. *Dis Colon Rectum* 22:557–558.

Critchlow CW, Holmes KK, Wood R, Krueger L, Dunphy C, Vernon DA, Daling JR, Kiviat NB. (1992) Association of human immunodeficiency virus and anal human papillomavirus infection among homosexual men. *Arch Intern Med* 152:1673–1676.

Critchlow CW, Surawicz CM, Holmes KK, Kuypers J, Daling JR, Hawes SE, Goldbaum GM, Sayer J, Hurt C, Dunphy C, Kiviat NB. (1995) Prospective study of high grade anal squamous intraepithelial neoplasia in a cohort of homosexual men: influence of HIV infection, immunosuppression and human papillomavirus infection. *AIDS* 9:1255–1262.

Croxon T, Chabon AB, Rorat E, Barash IM. (1984) Intraepithelial carcinoma of the anus in homosexual men. *Dis Colon Rectum* 27:325–330.

Daley JJ, Madrazo A. (1980) Anal Crohn's disease with carcinoma in situ. *Dig Dis Sci* 25:464–466.

Daling JR, Sherman KJ, Hislop TG, Maden C, Mandelson MT, Beckmann AM, Weiss NS. (1992) Cigarette smoking and the risk of anogenital cancer. *Am J Epidemiol* 135:180–189.

Daling JR, Weiss NS, Hislop TG, Maden C, Coates RJ, Sherman KJ, Ashley RL, Beagrie M, Ryan JA, Corey. (1987) Sexual practices, sexually transmitted diseases, and the incidence of anal cancer. *N Engl J Med* 317:973–977.

Daling JR, Weiss NS, Klopfenstein LL, Cochran LE, Chow WH, Daifuku R. (1982) Correlates of homosexual behavior and the incidence of anal cancer. *JAMA* 247:1988–1990.

DeVillez RL, Stevens CS. (1980) Bowenoid papulosis of the genitalia: a case progressing to Bowen's disease. *J Am Acad Dermatol* 3:149–152.

Dixon AR, Pringle JH, Holmes JT, Watkin DFL. (1991) Cervical intraepithelial neoplasia and squamous cell carcinoma of the anus in sexually active women. *Postgrad Med J* 67:557–559.

Dougherty BG, Evans HL. (1985) Carcinoma of the anal canal: a study of 79 cases. *Am J Clin Pathol* 83:159–164.

Duggan MA, Boras VF, Inou M, McGregor SE. (1991) Human papillomavirus DNA in anal carcinomas: comparison of *in situ* and dot blot hybridization. *Am J Clin Pathol* 96:318–325.

Ejeckman GC, Idikio HA, Nayak V, Gardiner JP. (1983) Malignant transformation of condyloma acuminatum. *Can J Surg* 26:170–173.

Elliot MS, Werner ID, Immelman EJ, Harrison AC. (1979) Giant condyloma (Buschke-Loewenstein tumor) of the anorectum. *Dis Colon Rectum* 22:497–500.

Fenger C. (1988) Histology of the anal canal. *Am J Surg Pathol* 12:41–55.

Fenger C. (1990) Intra-epithelial neoplasia in the anal canal and peri-anal area. *Curr Top Pathol* 81:91–102.

Fenger C. (1991) Anal neoplasia and its precursors: facts and controversies. *Semin Diagn Pathol* 8:190–201.

Fenger C, Lyon H. (1982) Endocrine cells and melanin-containing cells in the anal canal epithelium. *Histochem J* 14:631–639.

Fenger C, Morson BC. (1989) Anal duct carcinoma: letter to the editor. *Dis Colon Rectum* 32:355–357.

Fenger C, Nielsen V. (1986a) Precancerous changes in the anal canal epithelium in resection specimens. *Acta Pathol Microbiol Immunol Scand [A]* 94:63–69

Fenger C, Nielsen VT. (1981) Dysplastic changes in the anal canal epithelium in minor surgical specimens. *Acta Pathol Microbiol Scand* 89:463–465.

Fenger C, Nielsen VT. (1986b) Intraepithelial neoplasia of the anal canal: The appearance and relation to genital neoplasia. *Acta Pathol Microbiol Immunol Scand [A]* 94:343–349.

Fleming ID, Cooper JS, Henson DE, Hutter RVP, Kennedy BJ, Murphy GP, O'Sullivan B, Sobin LH, Yarbro JW. (1997) Anal Canal. In: *AJCC Cancer Staging Manual*, 5th ed., pp. 91–93. Lippincott-Raven, Philadelphia.

Foust RL, Dean PJ, Stoler MH, Moinuddin SM. (1991) Intraepithelial neoplasia of the anal canal in hemorrhoidal tissue: a study of 19 cases. *Hum Pathol* 22:528–534.

Franco ELF. (1996) Epidemiology of anogenital warts and cancer. *Obstet Gynecol Clin North Am* 23:597–623.

Frisch M, Glimelius B, Vanden Brule AJC, Wohlfahrt J, Meijer CJLM, Walboomers JMM, Goldman S, Svensson C, Adami H-O, Melbye M. (1997) Sexually transmitted infection as a cause of anal cancer. *N Engl J Med* 337:1350–1358.

Frisch M, Melbye M, Moller H. (1993) Trends in incidence of anal cancer in Denmark. *BMJ* 306:419–426.

Frisch M, Olsen JH, Bautz A, Melbye A, Melbye M. (1994) Benign anal lesions and the risk of anal cancer. *N Engl J Med* 331:300–302.

Frisch M, Olsen JH, Melbye M. (1994) Malignancies that occur before and after anal cancer: clues to their etiology. *Am J Epidemiol* 140:12–19.

Gingrass PJ, Burbrick MP, Hitchcock CR, Strom RL. (1978) Anorectal verrucose squamous carcinoma: report of two cases. *Dis Colon Rectum* 21:120–122.

Goldblum JR, Hart WR. (1998) Perianal Paget's disease: a histologic and immunohistochemical study of 11 cases with and without associated rectal adenocarcinoma. *Am J Surg Pathol* 22:170–179.

Goldie SJ, Kuntz KM, Weinstein MC, Freedberg KA, Welton ML, Palefsky JM. (1999) The clinical effectiveness and cost-effectiveness of screening for anal squamous intraepithelial lesions in homosexual and bisexual HIV-positive men. *JAMA* 281:1822–1829.

Goldman S, Gilimelius B, Nilsson B, Pahlman L. (1989) Incidence of anal epidermoid carcinoma in Sweden. *Acta Chir Scand* 155:191–197.

Grabenbauer GG, Matzel KE, Schneider IHF, Meyer M, Wittekind C, Matche B, Hoheberger W, Sauer R. (1998) Sphincter preservation with chemoradiation in anal canal carcinoma: abdominoperineal resection in selected cases? *Dis Colon Rectum* 41:441–450.

Greenall MJ, Quan SHQ, DeCosse JJ. (1985) Epidermoid cancer of the anus. *Br J Surg* (Suppl) 72:S97–S103.

Gross G, Hagedorn M, Ikenberg H, Rufli T, Dahlet C, Grosshans E, Gissmann L. (1985) Bowenoid papulosis: presence of human papillomavirus (HPV) structural antigens and of HPV 16–related DNA sequences. *Arch Dermatol* 121:858–863.

Higgins GD, Uzelin DM, Phillips GE, Pieterse AS, Burrell CJ. (1991) Differing characteristics of human papillomavirus RNA-positive and RNA-negative anal carcinomas. *Cancer* 68:561–567.

Holly EA, Whittemore AS, Aston DA, Ahn DK, Nickoloff BJ, Kristiansen JJ (1989) Anal cancer incidence: genital warts, anal fissure or fistula, hemorrhoids, and smoking. *J Natl Cancer Inst* 81:1726–1731.

Holmes F, Borek D, Owen-Kummer M, Hassanein R, Fishback J, Behbehni A, Baker A, Holmes G. (1988) Anal cancer in women. *Gastroenterology* 95:107–111.

Jay N, Berry JM, Hogeboom CJ, Holly EA, Darragh TM, Palefsky JM. (1997) Colposcopic appearance of anal squamous intraepithelial lesions: relationship to histopathology. *Dis Colon Rectum* 40:919–928.

Jensen SL, Shokouh-Amiri MH, Hagen K, Harling H, Nielsen OV. (1988) Adenocarcinoma of the anal ducts: a series of 21 cases. *Dis Colon Rectum* 31:268–272.

Jones EA, Morson BC. (1984) Mucinous adenocarcinoma in anorectal fistulae. *Histopathology* 8:279–292.

Jones RE Jr, Austin C, Ackerman AB. (1979) Extramammary Paget's disease: a critical reexamination. *Am J Dermatopathol* 1:101–132.

Kiviat NB, Critchlow CW, Holmes KK, Kuypers J, Sayer J, Dunphy C, Surawicz C, Kirby P, Wood R, Daling JR. (1993) Association of anal dysplasia and human papillomavirus with immunosupression and HIV infection among homosexual men. *AIDS* 7:43–49.

Koulos J, Symmans F, Chumas J, Nuovo G. (1991) Human papillomavirus detection in adenocarcinoma of the anus. *Mod Pathol* 4:58–61.

Kovi J, Tillman L, Lee SM. (1974) Malignant transformation of condyloma acuminatum: a light microscopic and ultrastructural study. *Am J Clin Pathol* 61:702–710.

Kraus FT, Perez-Mesa C. (1966) Verrucous carcinoma: clinical and pathologic study of 105 cases involving oral cavity, larynx and genitalia. *Cancer* 19:26–38.

Lee SH, Zucker M, Sato T. (1981) Primary adenocarcinoma of an anal gland with secondary perianal fistulas. *Hum Pathol* 12:1034–1037.

Marfing TE, Abel ME, Gallagher DM. (1987) Perianal Bowen's disease and associated malignancies: results of a survey. *Dis Colon Rectum* 30:782–785.

Mazoujian G, Pinkus GS, Haagensen DE Jr. (1984) Extramammary Paget's disease—evidence for an apocrine origin: an immunoperoxidase study of gross cystic disease fluid protein-15, carcinoembryonic antigen, and keratin proteins. *Am J Surg Pathol* 8:43–50.

Melbye M, Biggar RJ. (1992) Interactions between persons at risk for AIDS and the general population in Denmark. *Am J Epidemiol* 135:593–602.

Melbye M, Cote TR, Kessler L, Gail M, Biggar RJ, the AIDS/Cancer Working Group (1994) High incidence of anal cancer among AIDS patients. *Lancet* 343:636–639.

Melbye M, Palefsky J, Gonzales J, Ryder LP, Nielsen H, Bergmann O, Pindborg J, Biggar RJ. (1990) Immune status as a determinant of human papillomavirus detection and its association with anal epithelial abnormalities. *Int J Cancer* 46:203–206.

Melbye M, Rabkin C, Frisch M, Biggar RJ. (1994) Changing patterns of anal cancer incidence in the United States, 1940–1989. *Am J Epidemiol* 139:772–780.

Melbye M, Sprogel P. (1991) Aetiological parallel between anal cancer and cervical cancer. *Lancet* 338:657–659.

Metcalf AM, Dean T. (1995) Risk of dysplasia in anal condyloma. *Surgery* 118:724–726.

Nagle RB, Lucas DO, McDaniel KM, Clark VA, Schmalzel GM. (1985) New evidence linking mammary and extramammary Paget cells to a common cell phenotype. *Am J Clin Pathol* 83:431–438.

Nash G, Allen W, Nash S. (1986) Atypical lesions of the anal mucosa in homosexual men. *JAMA* 256:873–876.

National Cancer Institute Workshop (1991) The revised Bethesda System for reporting cervical/vaginal cytologic diagnosis: report of the 1991 Bethesda Workshop. *JAMA* 267:1892.

Nielsen OV, Jensen SL. (1981) Basal cell carcinoma of the anus. *Br J Surg* 68:856–857.

Noffsinger A, Witte D, Fenoglio-Preiser CM. (1992) The relationship of human papillomaviruses to anorectal neoplasia. *Cancer* 70:1276–1287.

Onerheim RM. (1988) A case of perianal mucinous adenocarcinoma arising in a fistula-in-ano: a clue to early pathologic diagnosis. *Am J Clin Pathol* 89:809–812.

Palefsky JM. (1994) Anal human papillomavirus infection and anal cancer in HIV-positive individuals: an emerging problem. *AIDS* 8:283–295.

Palefsky JM, Gonzales J, Greenblatt RM, Ahn DK, Hollander H. (1990) Anal intraepithelial neoplasia and anal papillomavirus infection among homosexual males with group IV HIV disease. *JAMA* 263:2911–2916.

Palefsky JM, Holly EA, Ralston ML, Jay N. (1998a) Prevalence and risk factors for human papillomavirus infection of the anal canal in human immunodeficiency virus (HIV)-positive and HIV-negative homosexual men. *J Infect Dis* 177:361–367.

Palefsky JM, Holly EA, Ralston ML, Jay N, Berry JM, Darragh TM. (1998b) High incidence of anal high-grade squamous intra-epithelial lesions among HIV-positive and HIV-negative homosexual and bisexual men. *AIDS* 12:495–503.

Palmer JG, Scholefield JH, Coates PJ, Shepherd MB, Jass JR, Crawford LV, Northover JMA. (1989) Anal cancer and human papillomaviruses. *Dis Colon Rectum* 32:1016–1022.

Penn I. (1986) Cancers of the anogenital region in renal transplant recipients: analysis of 65 cases. *Cancer* 58:611–616.

Peters RK, Mack TM. (1983) Patterns of anal carcinoma by gender and marital status in Los Angeles County. *Br J Cancer* 48:629–636.

Prat J. (1991) Pathology of vulvar intraepithelial lesions and early invasive carcinoma. *Hum Pathol* 22:877–883.

Preston DM, Fiona EF, Lennard-Jones JE, Hawley PR. (1983) Carcinoma of the anus in Crohn's disease. *Br J Surg* 70:346–347.

Prioleau PG, Allen MS, Roberts T. (1977) Perianal mucinous adenocarcinoma. *Cancer* 39:1295–1299.

Prioleau PG, Santa Cruz DJ, Meyer JS, Bauer WC. (1980) Verrucous carcinoma: a light and electron microscopic, autoradiographic, and immunofluorescence study. *Cancer* 45:2849–2857.

Rabkin CS, Biggar RJ, Melbye M, Curtis RE. (1992) Second primary cancers following anal and cervical carcinoma: evidence of shared etiologic factors. *Am J Epidemiol* 136:54–58.

Rickert RR. (1998) Disorders of the anal region. In: *Pathology of the Gastrointestinal Tract*, 2nd ed. (Ming S-C, Goldman H, eds.) pp. 925–947. Williams and Wilkins, Baltimore.

Rickert RR, Brodkin RH, Hutter RVP. (1977) Bowen's disease. *A Cancer J Clin* 27:160–166.

Ross M, Pezzi C, Pezzi T, Meurer D, Hickey R, Balch C. (1990) Patterns of failure in anorectal melanoma: a guide to surgical therapy. *Arch Surg* 125:313–316.

Rudlinger R, Buchmann P. (1989) HPV 16 positive bowenoid papulosis and squamous-cell carcinoma of the anus in an HIV-positive man. *Dis Colon Rectum* 32:1042–1045.

Sarmiento JM, Wolff BG, Burgart LJ, Frizell FA, Ilstrup DM. (1997) Perianal Bowen's disease: associated tumors, human papillomavirus, surgery, and other controversies. *Dis Colon Rectum* 40:912–918.

Scholefield JH, Kerr IB, Shepherd NA, Miller KJ, Bloomfield R, Northover JMA. (1991) Human papillomavirus 16 DNA in anal cancers from six different countries. *Gut* 32:674–676.

Scholefield JH, McIntyre P, Palmer JG, Coates PJ, Shepherd NA, Northover JMA. (1990) DNA hybridization of routinely processed tissue for detecting HPV DNA in anal squamous cell carcinomas over 40 years. *J Clin Pathol* 43:133–136.

Scholefield JH, Ogunbiyi OA, Smith JHF, Rogers K, Sharp F. (1994) Treatment of anal intraepithelial neoplasia. *Br J Surg* 81:1238–1240.

Scholefield JH, Thornton Jones H, Cuzick J, Northover JMA. (1990) Anal cancer and marital status. *Br J Cancer* 62:286–288.

Scoma JA, Levy EI. (1975) Bowen's disease of the anus: report of two cases. *Dis Colon Rectum* 18:137–140.

Shepherd NA, Scholefield JH, Love SB, England J, Northover JMA. (1990) Prognostic factors in anal squamous carcinoma: a multivariate analysis of clinical, pathological and flow cytometric parameters in 235 cases. *Histopathology* 16:545–555.

Sherman ME, Friedman HB, Busseniers AE, Kelly WF, Carner TC, Saah AJ. (1995) Cytologic diagnosis of anal intraepithelial neoplasia using smears and CYTYC Thin-Preps. *Mod Pathol* 8:270–274.

Shroyer KR, Brookes CG, Markham NE, Shroyer AL. (1995) Detection of human papillomavirus in anorectal squamous cell carcinoma: correlation with basaloid pattern of differentiation. *Am J Clin Pathol* 104:299–305.

Singh R, Nime F, Mittelman A. (1981) Malignant epithelial tumors of the anal canal. *Cancer* 48:411–415.

Slater G, Greenstein A, Aufses AH Jr. (1984) Anal carcinoma in patients with Crohn's disease. *Ann Surg* 199:348–350.

Strauss RJ, Fazio VW. (1979) Bowen's disease of the anal and perianal area: a report and analysis of twelve cases. *Am J Surg* 137:231–234.

Surawicz CM, Critchlow C, Sayer J, Hurt C, Hawes S,

Kirby P, Goldbaum G, Kiviat N. (1995) High grade anal dysplasia in visually normal mucosa in homosexual men: seven cases. *Am J Gastroenterol* 90: 1776–1778.

Surawicz CM, Kirby P, Critchlow C, Sayer J, Dunphy C, Kiviat N. (1993) Anal dysplasia in homosexual men: role of anoscopy and biopsy. *Gastroenterology* 105: 658–666.

Tarazi R, Nelson RL. (1994) Anal adenocarcinoma: a comprehensive review. *Semin Surg Oncol* 10:235–240.

Ulbright TM, Stehman FB, Roth LM, Ehrlich CE, Ransburg RC. (1982) Bowenoid dysplasia of the vulva. *Cancer* 50:2910–2919.

Unger ER, Vernon SD, Lee DR, Miller DL, Sharma S, Clancy KA, Hart CE, Reeves WC. (1997) Human papillomavirus type in anal epithelial lesions is influenced by human immunodeficiency virus. *Arch Pathol Lab Med* 121:820–824.

Wade TR, Kopf AW, Ackerman AB. (1976) Bowenoid papulosis of the penis. *Cancer* 42:1890–1893.

Wells M, Robertson S, Lewis F, Dixon MF. (1988) Squamous carcinoma arising in a giant peri-anal condyloma associated with human papillomavirus types 6 and 11. *Histopathology* 12:319–323.

White WB, Schneiderman H, Sayre JT. (1984) Basal cell carcinoma of the anus: clinical and pathological distinction from cloacogenic carcinoma. *J Clin Gastroenterol* 6:441–446.

Wick MR, Weatherby RP, Weiland LH. (1987) Small cell neuroendocrine carcinoma of the colon and rectum. *Hum Pathol* 18:9–21.

Williams GR, Talbot IC. (1994) Anal carcinoma—a histological review. *Histopathology* 25:507–516.

Zaki SR, Judd R, Coffield LM, Greer P, Rolston F, Evatt BL. (1992) Human papillomavirus infection and anal carcinoma: retrospective analysis by in situ hybridization and the polymerase chain reaction. *Am J Pathol* 140:1345–1355.

Zaren HA, Delone FX, Lerner HJ. (1983) Carcinoma of the anal gland: case report and review of the literature. *J Surg Oncol* 23:250–254.

Zemtsov A, Koss W, Dixon L, Tyring S, Rady P. (1992) Anal verrucous carcinoma associated with human papilloma virus type II: magnetic resonance imaging and flow cytometry evaluation. *Arch Dermatol* 128:564–565.

Zurhausen H, Devilliers EM. (1994) Human papillomaviruses. *Annu Rev Microbiol* 48:427–447.

11

LIVER

Kamal G. Ishak

INCIPIENT NEOPLASIA OF HEPATOCELLULAR CARCINOMA

This section deals with lesions that are suspected precursors of hepatocellular carcinoma (HCC) in humans and that have some correlations with precancerous lesions in experimental animals. Diseases that precede and are considered to predispose patients to both benign and malignant hepatocellular liver tumors are listed in Table 11–1; only benign tumors that can undergo malignant change are discussed here. The major precancerous lesions to be described arise mainly, though not exclusively, in the cirrhotic liver, the major risk factor for HCC. They include dysplastic foci, dysplastic nodules, iron-free foci in genetic hemochromatosis, foci of altered hepatocytes, and proliferation of hepatic stem cells. The terminology for dysplastic foci and nodules that is used in this chapter follows that proposed by the International Working Party (1995).

PRECANCEROUS BENIGN HEPATOCELLULAR TUMORS

Hepatocellular Adenoma

Hepatocellular adenoma (HCA) is composed of a sheet-like pattern of cells showing hepatocellular differentiation. The cells are larger and paler than normal liver cells and may contain more glycogen and fat. There is little variation in size and shape and the nuclear/cytoplasmic (N/C) ratio is normal. Canaliculi are present between tumor cells and may contain bile. Recent and old hemorrhages are frequently seen. Malignant transformation is rare, since most HCA are resected when discovered. However, there are a few well-documented cases of HCC arising in unresected solitary or multiple adenomas (liver adenomatosis) (Ferrell et al., 1993; Foster and Bergman, 1994; Ishak, 1979; Janes et al., 1993; Soe et al., 1992). A case on file at Armed Forces Institute of Pathology (AFIP) is illustrated in Figs. 11–1 to 11–3. One report documents development of HCC at the site of a HCA that had regressed 5 years after discontinuation of oral contraceptive use (Galassi et al., 1995). Whether all HCCs reported in women who had used contraceptive steroids develop in a preexisting HCA is not established. There is evidence from case–control studies, however, suggesting an etiologic relationship between HCC and use of contraceptive steroids, particularly use for more than 8 years (Soe et al., 1992; Tavani et al. 1993); thus, some cases must develop through that sequence.

Hepatocellular carcinomas, some of which are presumed to have arisen in adenomas, have also been reported in patients on anabolic steroids and the glycogenoses, particularly glycogenosis type I. In order to link anabolic steroids with HCC, cases have to meet rigid criteria, including an elevated serum α-fetoprotein level, unequivocal histopathology, and/or distant metastases. Of the 10 cases studied (Edmondson et al., 1977; Heffelfinger et al., 1987; Ishak, 1979; Le Bail et al., 1992; Mokrohisky et al., 1977;

Table 11–1. Diseases Preceding Hepatocellular Carcinoma

Diseases	Cirrhosis	Associated Conditions and Comments
Hereditary diseases		
Porphyria cutanea tarda	+	Alcoholic liver disease; chronic hepatitis C or B; hemosiderosis
Acute intermittent porphyria	−	—
Variegate porphyria	−	—
Glycogenosis type I	−	Associated or preexisting hepatocellular adenomas
Glycogenosis type III	−	Associated or preexisting hepatocellular adenomas
Hypercitrullinemia	−	—
Hereditary fructose intolerance	−	Steatosis, periportal fibrosis
Hereditary tyrosinemia	+	Dysplastic nodules, liver cell dysplasia (large, small)
α-1-antitrypsin deficiency	+	Characteristic PAS-positive globules
Genetic hemochromatosis	+	Marked hemosiderosis; iron-free foci
Wilson's disease	+	Copper accumulation (unless treated), steatosis, glycogen nuclei, Mallory's bodies
Ataxia telangiectasia	−	—
Progressive intrahepatic cholestasis (Byler's)	+	Chronic cholestasis
Arteriohepatic dysplasia	−	Ductopenia; chronic cholestasis
Chronic hepatitis	+	Chronic hepatitis C; chronic hepatitis B (±aflatoxin exposure); autoimmune hepatitis
Alcoholic liver disease	+	—
Cirrhosis	+	Miscellaneous etiologies
Chronic cholestatic diseases	+	Primary biliary cirrhosis; extrahepatic biliary atresia
Drug use	−	Anabolic or contraceptive steroids; azathioprine
Toxin exposure	−	Aflatoxin
Thorotrast accumulation	−	Latent period >12 years
Benign hepatocellular tumors	−	
Hepatocellular adenoma		Rare
Focal nodular hyperplasia		Very rare
Nodular regenerative hyperplasia		Very rare

−, not present; +, present.

[Modified from Ishak, 1991.]

Mueller et al., 1995; Raoul et al., 1987; Thysell et al., 1986; Westaby et al., 1983), 1 had documented "postnecrotic" cirrhosis (Raoul et al., 1987) that could have been the underlying etiologic condition for the malignancy. Another tumor was the fibrolamellar variant of HCC (Le Bail et al., 1992). There are at least seven cases of HCC reported in the literature that are related to glycogenosis type Ia (Ishak, 1991). Two unpublished examples are on file at AFIP. None of the patients had an underlying cirrhosis.

Nodular Regenerative Hyperplasia

This condition is characterized by generally small nodules of regeneration composed of two cell–thick plates surrounded by compressed reticulin fibers. There is atrophy of intervening parenchyma but no fibrosis. Occlusive vascular lesions, typically of veins in portal areas, may be demonstrable in some cases. Liver cell dysplasia (large cell change) has been observed in 24% of cases in one series (Stromeyer and Ishak, 1981) and 42% in another series (Colina et al., 1989) of nodular regenerative hyperplasia (NRH). In a series of 804 cases of HCC in North America studied by Nzeako et al. (1996), 342 were found to arise in a noncirrhotic liver; 13 of those livers had NRH (6.7%). Seventeen of the patients (73.9%) with NRH had liver cell dysplasia, and 16 (69.6%) had portal venous invasion by the carcinoma. Liver cell dysplasia occurred in a significantly greater proportion of patients with NRH than in those

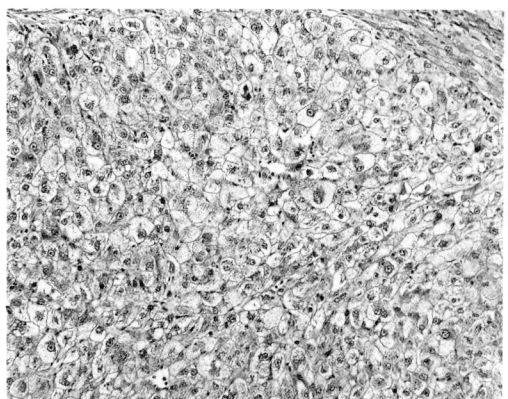

Figure 11–1. Hepatocellular adenoma. The cells appear to be growing in a sheet and have an abundant cytoplasm and a normal nuclear/cytoplasmic ratio (H&E, ×150).

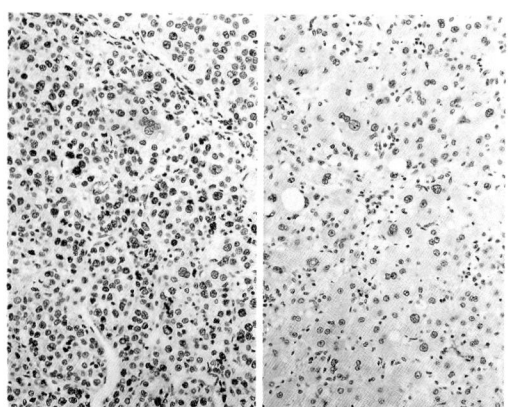

Figure 11–3. Same case as in Figure 11–1. A large number of cells of the hepatocellular carcinoma component (*left*) express Ki-67 compared to cells of the hepatocellular adenoma component (*right*) of the same tumor.

without ($P < 0.01$), but there were no significant differences between groups with regard to portal venous invasion. Nzeako et al. (1996) concluded that the temporal relation between HCC and NRH is probably determined in each case by the interaction of multiple pathogenetic factors. Among patients with HCC, factors other than portal vein obstruction by tumor invasion, for example, chemotherapy and/or radiotherapy, could play a role in the pathogenesis of NRH.

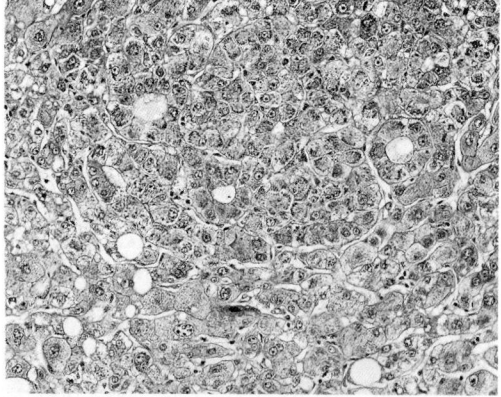

Figure 11–2. Same case as in Figure 11–1, showing an hepatocellular adenoma (HCA) with transition to hepatocellular carcinoma (HCC). The upper half of the field shows HCC with pseudoglands and cells with a high nuclear/cytoplasmic (N/C) ratio. Cells of the HCA (lower half of field) have a normal N/C ratio (H&E, ×200).

Focal Nodular Hyperplasia

This pseudoneoplasm is a hyperplastic response to a spider-like arterial malformation. It is usually occurs singly, but multiple lesions have been reported. The lesion has a central stellate scar and is subdivided into smaller nodulas by fibrous septa connected to that scar. Thick-walled arterial vessels are present in the fibrous scars and septa. Proliferation of ductules occurs at the interface of the hyperplastic hepatic parenchymal component and the septa, and features of chronic cholestasis (cholate stasis and copper storage) are common. Malignant transformation is very rare; there are only 2 such cases in over 800 cases of focal nodular hyperplasia (FNH) on file at AFIP (Figs. 11–4 to 11–6). The suggestion of Vecchio et al. (1984) that the fibrolamellar variant of HCC arises from FNH has not been corroborated by other investigators. Moreover, FNH may be associated with other hepatic neoplasms such as cavernous hemangioma. A FNH adjacent to a fibrolamellar carcinoma has been reported by Saul et al. (1987) and Saxena et al. (1994). In both case reports the authors suggested that the hyperplastic foci in the vicinity of the fibrolamellar carcinoma may be an epiphenomenon due to an abnormal blood supply, possibly derived from the tumor vasculature. The expression of the neurotensin gene by fibrolamellar carcinoma but not by FNH is considered to be further evidence against the suggestion that the lat-

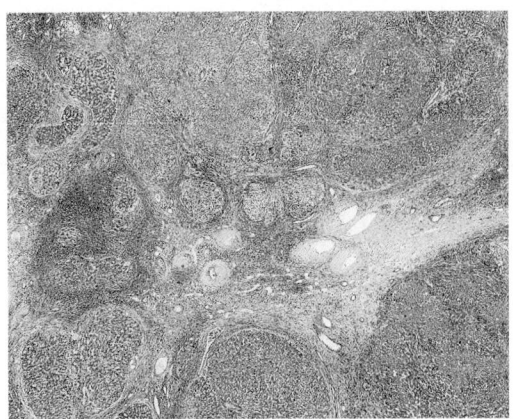

Figure 11–4. Focal nodular hyperplasia exhibiting a central scar and septa (H&E, ×20).

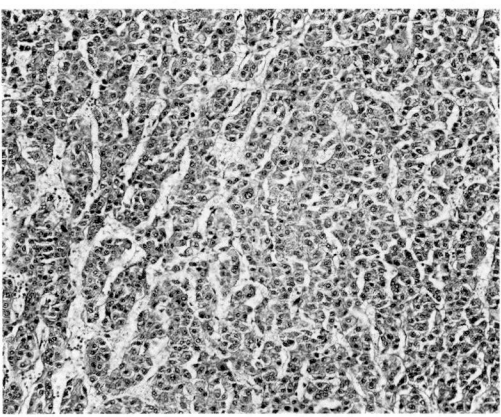

Figure 11–6. Focal nodular hyperplasia; same case as in Figures 11–4 and 11–5 with area of trabecular hepatocellular carcinoma (H&E, ×150).

ter lesion is a precursor of the former (Ehrenfried et al., 1994).

PUTATIVE PRECANCEROUS HEPATOCELLULAR LESIONS

Dysplastic Foci

The term *liver cell dysplasia* (LCD) was first coined by Anthony et al. (1973) to describe a change characterized by cellular enlargement, nuclear pleomorphism, and multinucleation of liver cells occurring in groups or occupying whole cirrhotic nodules (Figs. 11–7 and 11–8). The change was found in only 1% of patients with normal livers, in

6.9% of patients with cirrhosis, and in 64.5% of patients with cirrhosis and HCC. There was a strong correlation between LCD and hepatitis B surface antigen (HBsAg) seropositivity. Anthony et al. (1973) concluded that the presence of LCD identified a group of patients at high risk for development of HCC, and that such patients should be followed by serial α-fetoprotein determinations. A long-term prospective study by Borzio et al. (1996) has confirmed that LCD in patients with cirrhosis is independently associated with an increased risk of HCC, a view supported by the more recent studies of Ganne-Carrie et al. (1996) and Le Bail et al. (1997). Age over 60 and HBsAg positivity

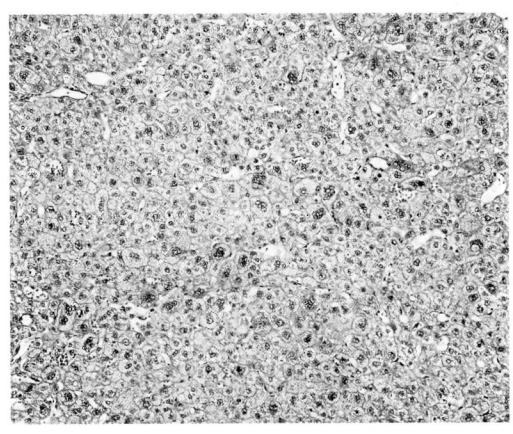

Figure 11–5. Focal nodular hyperplasia showing a focus of large cell change (dysplasia). (H&E, ×75).

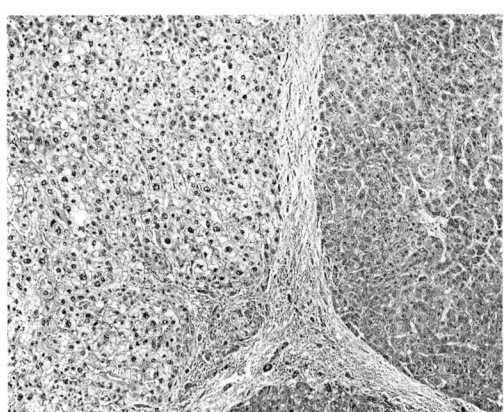

Figure 11–7. Large cell change (dysplasia). Cirrhotic nodule (*left*) is composed of larger cells and nuclei than the nodule on the right (H&E, ×75).

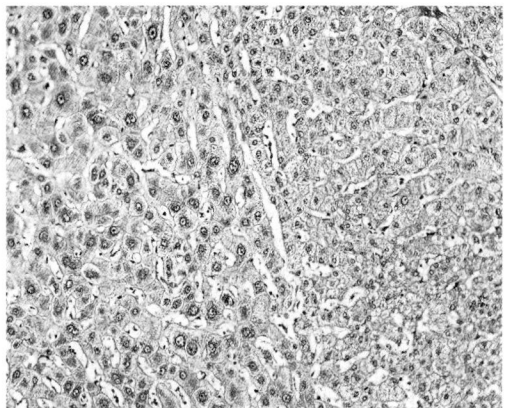

Figure 11–8. Large cell change (dysplasia). Focus (*left*) is composed of large cells with large, hyperchromatic nuclei, but the nuclear/cytoplasmic ratio is normal (H&E, ×100).

have also been found to be independent risk factors by one group of investigators (Borzio et al., 1996). The association of LCD with HCC has been confirmed in many (Akagi et al., 1984; Nakanuma et al., 1985; Nakashima et al., 1983; Omata et al., 1992; Orsatti et al., 1993) but not all (Chen et al, 1984; Henmi et al., 1985) studies.

Whereas LCD was originally linked to hepatitis B infection, it was later reported in 42.5% of cases of non-A, non-B hepatitis, being most often associated with cirrhosis (Lefkowitch and Apfelbaum, 1987). Indeed, it is a change that can occur in cirrhosis of diverse etiology, although about half the cases are found in cirrhosis associated with viral hepatitis (Lefkowitch and Apfelbaum, 1987).

In the report of Anthony et al. (1973), the N/C ratio of the dysplastic liver cells was considered normal. A morphometric study by Watanabe et al. (1983) supported that view. However, in a subsequent study, Roncalli et al. (1988) found an increased N/C ratio of cells in LCD. Several flow-cytometric studies have failed to support the precancerous nature of LCD (Henmi et al., 1985; Kagawa et al., 1984; Rubin et al., 1994). On the other hand, Thomas et al. (1992) and An et al. (1997) found that LCD contains DNA aneuploid cells, thus supporting its role in the evolution of HCC. In the study of An et al. (1997), 92% of dysplastic cases were aneuploid compared to 60% of HCC cases. Ad-

ditional support for the preneoplastic nature of LCD comes from the study of Terris et al. (1997), who found numerical chromosomal abberations in five cases (but in only one of three cases of small cell dysplasia).

Several groups of investigators have attempted to identify histochemical and immunohistochemical differences between hepatocytes in LCD and non-neoplastic liver cells. Omata et al. (1992), using immunohistochemical methods, found that dysplastic cells did not harbor HBsAg any more frequently than nondysplastic cells. Roncalli et al. (1985) were also unable to detect HBsAg or HBcAg in dysplastic liver cells. In another study, Roncalli et al. (1986) found no differences in the immunohistochemical expression of carcinoembryonic antigen (CEA), α-1 antitrypsin, and α-fetoprotein between normal and dysplastic hepatocytes. One histochemical study has shown a pattern of enzyme deviation in HCC that could not be demonstrated in hepatitis B–positive or dysplastic liver cells (Uchida et al., 1981). Cells of HCC gave an intensely positive reaction for γ-glutamyl transpeptidase activity but were deficient in glucose-6-phosphatase, alkaline phosphatase, and nonspecific esterase activities. Cohen and De Rosa (1994) found expression of p53 in 48% of their cases of HCC, but in only 3% of LCD. Zhao and colleagues (1994) noted expression of bcl-2 protein in 5 of 37 (13.5%) hepatocellular carcinomas but not in LCD. In addition to lack of a morphologic transition from LCD to HCC, Lee at al. (1997) found that LCD hepatocytes had a low proliferation rate (Ki-67 and PCNA) but a greater degree of apoptosis than normal hepatocytes. They proposed that LCD derives from derangements of the hepatocyte's normal process of polyploidization, a view suggested earlier by Kagawa et al. (1984). Such derangements, possibly caused by chronic inflammation-induced DNA damage, could yield a population of enlarged liver cells with nuclear atypia and pleomorphism, frequent binucleation, and minimal proliferation. According to that hypothesis, LCD could be a habitual feature of cirrhosis and a regular accompaniment of HCC, but would not represent a direct malignant precursor.

Watanabe et al. (1983) have expanded the original definition of LCD to include a

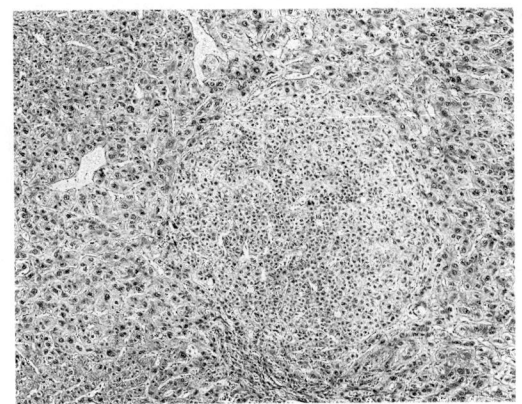

Figure 11–9. Small cell change (dysplasia) showing ill-defined focus of small cells with a high nuclear/cytoplasmic (N/C) ratio (H&E, ×75).

"small cell" variant. *Small cell dysplasia* (small cell change) is characterized by an increased N/C ratio, in contrast to *large cell dysplasia* (large cell change), which has a normal N/C ratio (Figs. 11–9 and 11–10). The small dysplastic cells have a N/C ratio of between that of liver cancer cells and normal hepatocytes. Also, multinucleation and large nucleoli are characteristic of large cell dysplasia but not small cell dysplasia. The small dysplastic cells have more of a tendency to form small, round foci than large dysplastic cells (Fig. 11–9). On the basis of their morphologic and morphometric studies, Watanabe et al. (1983) believe that small cell dysplasia, rather than large cell dysplasia, is the precancerous lesion in humans.

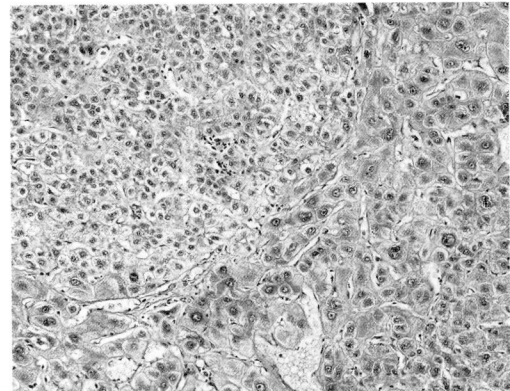

Figure 11–10. Higher magnification of Figure 11–9. Small cells with a high N/C ratio (top, left) are surrounded by large dysplastic cells (H&E, ×150).

Dysplastic Nodules

Adenomatous hyperplasia is a term that has been used for nodular lesions in the cirrhotic liver that are considered premalignant by many investigators (Arakawa et al., 1986a; Eguchi et al., 1992; Ferrell et al., 1992; Le Bail et al., 1995; Nakanuma et al., 1993; Sakamoto et al., 1991; Takayama et al., 1990; Theise, 1995; Theise et al., 1992; Wada et al., 1988; Yamashita, 1996). The nodules vary from small foci a few millimeters in size to larger nodules 10 mm or more in diameter; the latter have been termed *macroregenerative nodules* by some authors. As mentioned earlier, the preferred terminology is *dysplastic nodules* (International Working Party, 1995). Their reported incidence in cirrhotic livers has varied from 14% to 25% (Wada et al., 1988). They are found in cirrhosis associated with viral hepatitis B or C, but also in cirrhosis of other etiologies, e.g., primary biliary cirrhosis (Terada et al., 1989b). Dysplastic nodules are usually less than 15 mm in diameter, have a soft texture, and often bulge from the cut surface (Fig. 11–11). They may be paler than the rest of the liver and can be bile stained; necrosis and hemorrhage are not present. The surrounding liver is usually but not invariably cirrhotic (Theise et al., 1993). Dysplastic nodules have been further subclassified into low- and high-grade types (International Working Group, 1995).

Low-grade dysplastic nodules

These are composed of liver cells that are minimally abnormal and are arranged in two cell–thick plates (Figs. 11–12 and 11–13). Portal areas are present. The N/C ratio is normal or slightly increased. Nuclear atypia is minimal and there are no mitoses. Steatosis and Mallory bodies may be seen (Nakanuma and Ohta, 1985; Terada et al., 1988, 1989a; Fig. 11–14). Dysplastic foci and large cell type may be present.

High-grade dysplastic nodules

These are characterized by one or more additional features—plates more than two cells thick with areas of pseudogland formation, cytoplasmic basophilia, high N/C ratio, nuclear hyperchromasia, irregular nuclear contour, rare mitoses, and resistance to iron accumulation (Figs. 11–15 and 11–16). There

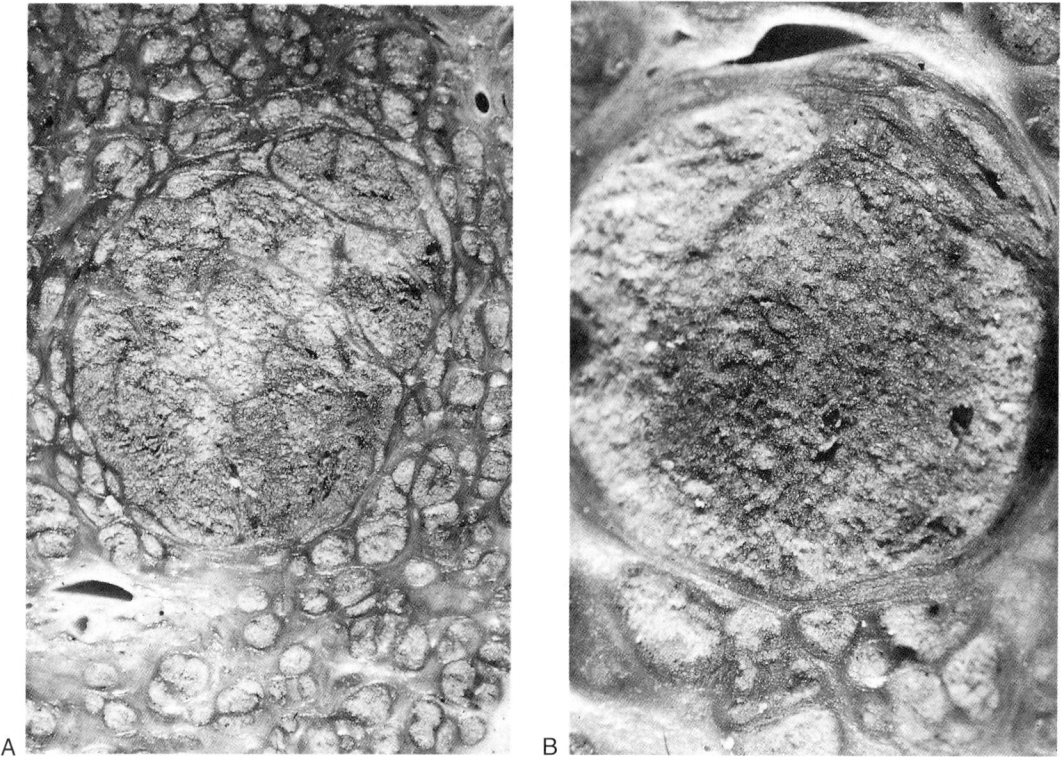

Figure 11–11. *A,B:* Sections of two dysplastic nodules from the same liver. Note the large size of the nodules in comparison to the surrounding cirrhotic nodules.

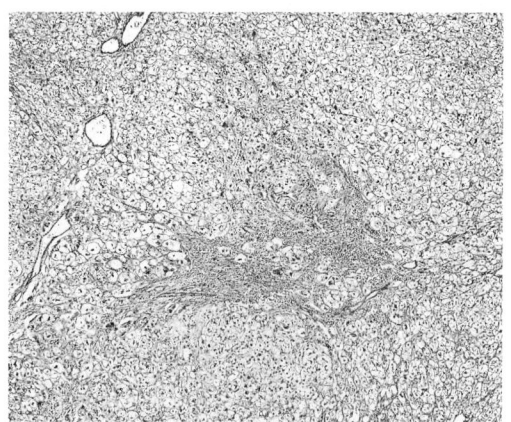

Figure 11–12. Dysplastic nodule, low grade. The nodule contains part of a septum with inflammatory cells. The constituent cells are fairly uniform in size (H&E, ×55).

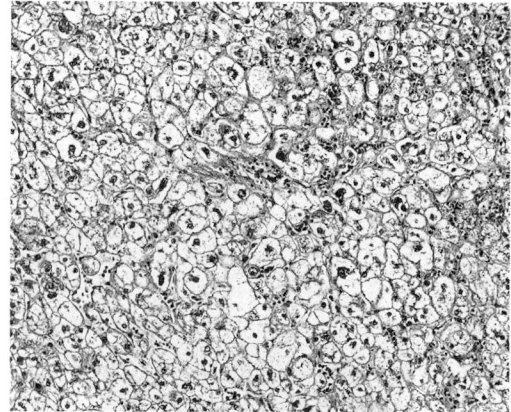

Figure 11–13. Dysplastic nodule, low grade; same case as in Figure 11–12. There is only slight variation in size of cells and nuclei. Note the unpaired arteries (H&E, ×215).

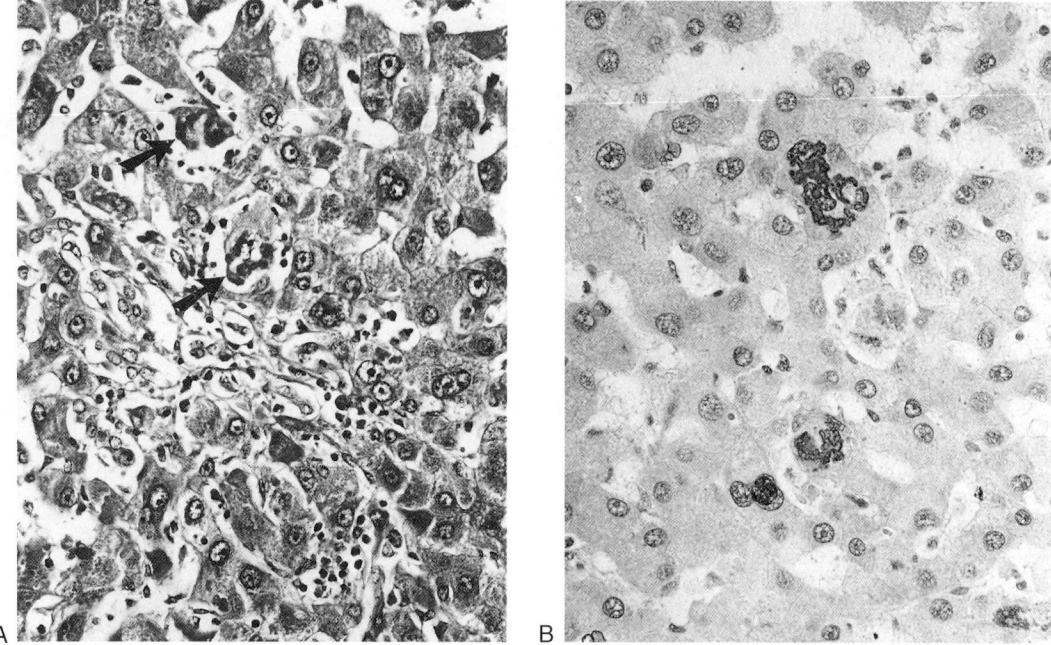

Figure 11–14. Dysplastic nodule, low grade. *A:* Mallory bodies are indicated by arrows (H&E, ×300). *B:* Mallory bodies are decorated by antiubiquitin antibodies (×400).

is no invasion of stroma or portal areas in the nodule. These features may be confined to one or more foci within the nodule, giving the appearance of subpopulations (subcomponents, or "nodule-in-nodule" formation)

(Figs. 11–17 and 11–18). The differences between low-grade and high-grade dysplastic nodules are listed in Table 11–2; they include some features that are referenced but not discussed further here.

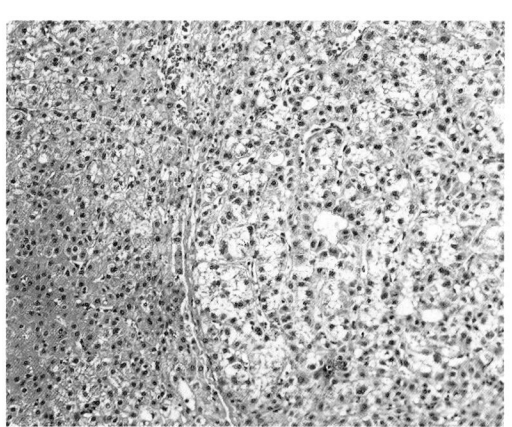

Figure 11–15. Dysplastic nodule, high grade. There is small cell change (left) and pseudogland formation (right). (H&E, ×150).

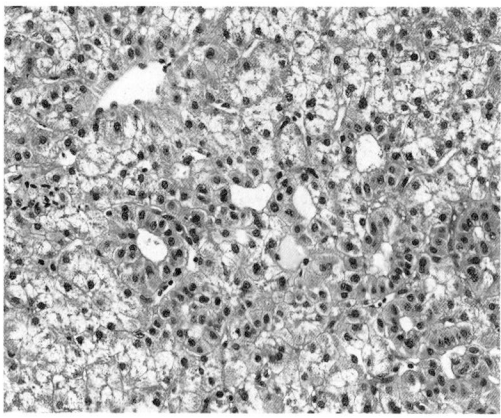

Figure 11–16. Dysplastic nodule, high grade; same case as in Figure 11–15. There are several pseudoglands, and the cells have a high nuclear/cytoplasmic ratio (H&E, ×240).

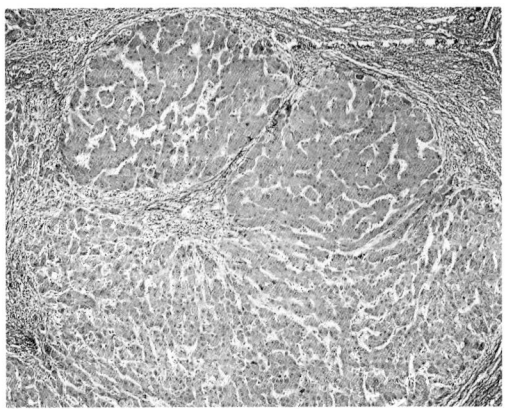

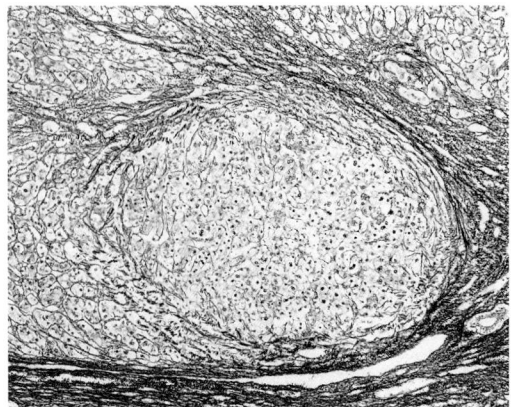

Figure 11–17. "Nodule-in-nodule" formation. Two small nodules are present in the larger nodule (H&E, ×160).

Figure 11–18. "Nodule-in-nodule" formation. The small nodule is demarcated from the larger nodule by compressed reticulin fibers (Manuel reticulin stain, ×30).

High-grade dysplastic nodules and hepatocellular carcinoma

There is general agreement that high-grade dysplastic nodules can evolve into HCC. According to a study by Eguchi et al. (1992), approximately 40% of cases of adenomatous hyperplasia undergo malignant change. These investigators found that the mean size of adenomatous hyperplasia containing cancerous foci (15.8 ± 2.2 mm) was significantly larger than that of adenomatous hyperplasia (10.1 ± 2.6 mm). In another study, all nodules larger than 1.5 cm in diameter were found to be HCC (Sakamoto et al., 1991). In that study it was found that a degree of cellularity more than twice that of a regenerative nodule was an indicator of HCC.

Malignant transformation of adenomatous hyperplasia has been documented in a follow-up study by Takayama et al. (1990), who followed patients for 1 to 5 years after biopsy-proven diagnosis of adenomatous hyperplasia. Criteria for diagnosis were a doubling of nodular volume and changes in imaging studies. Between 6 and 50 months after biopsy, 9 of 18 nodules met criteria for malignant transformation; histological proof of HCC was obtained later in 7 of the 9 nodules. Another study by Lencioni et al. (1994) showed malignant transformation in 68% of adenomatous hyperplasia in up to 31 months follow-up by serial ultrasound examination and biopsies.

Morphologic criteria favoring malignancy include distinct trabeculae or plates more than two cells thick, focal absence of reticulin fibers, marked nuclear atypia, a high N/C ratio, moderate or marked mitotic activity, and invasion of portal areas or the stroma (Kondo et al., 1994; Le Bail et al., 1995; Nakano et al., 1990; Figs. 11–19 to 11–21). Differences in the number and distribution of unpaired arteries and the expression of CD 34 (capillarization) have been found among cirrhotic nodules, dysplastic nodules, and HCC (Park et al., 1998). Thus, unpaired arteries are more numerous and the expression of CD34 is greater in HCC than in dysplastic nodules, but the practical utility of these differences in a given needle biopsy specimen is questionable. The proliferative activity of hepatocellular nodules (using the proliferation markers PCNA and Ki67) was recently studied by Tiniakos and Brunt (1999), who found that dysplastic nodules (in contrast to regenerative nodules) are usually highly proliferative and may represent an early stage of hepatocarcinogenesis. The study was based on the evaluation of the proliferative activity of 45 hepatocellular nodules from 17 liver explants from adults.

Readers interested in further discussion of the relation between dysplastic nodules and HCC are referred to several excellent reviews (Ferrell et al., 1992, 1993; Hytiroglou

Table 11–2. Comparison of Low-Grade and High-Grade Dysplastic Nodules

Criterion	Low-Grade Nodule	High-Grade Nodule
Synonyms	Adenomatous hyperplasia Macroregenerative nodule, ordinary Macroregenerative, type I	Adenomatous hyperplasia, atypical Macroregenerative nodule, atypical Macroregenerative nodule, type II
Portal areas	Present	Present or absent
Plates	Two cells thick	Two cells thick
Pseudoglands	Absent	Absent or present (focally)
"Nodule-in-nodule" change	Absent or present	Present or absent
Reticulin network	Present	Present or focally absent
Unpaired arteries (Park et al., 1998)	Present, few	Present, many
Steatosis (Terada et al., 1988)	Present or absent	Present or absent
Mallory bodies (Nakanuma et al., 1985; Terada et al., 1989a)	Present or absent	Present or absent
Stainable Cu/Cu-binding protein (Ueda et al., 1993)	Present, uneven	?
Stainable iron (Terada and Nakanuma, 1989)	Present or absent	Absent in iron-free foci in genetic hemochromatosis (Deugnier et al., 1993)
Liver cell atypia	Minimal or absent	Present, focal (cyoplasmic basophilia, high N/C ratio, hyperchromasia, moderate mitoses, nuclear irregularities, other)
Clear cell change	Absent	Present or absent
Dysplastic foci	Large cell, present or absent	Large or small cell, present or absent
Proliferative activity (Le Bail et al., 1997; Yamashita, 1996)	Normal	Increased
ABH blood group antigens (Terada and Nakanuma, 1991)	Minimal expression	Marked expression
Alpha fetoprotein (Theise et al., 1995)	Not expressed	Present or absent
Aneuploidy (Orsatti et al., 1993)	6.2%	58.3%
Clonality	Monoclonal or polyclonal (Paradis et al., 1998)	Polyclonal (Piao et al., 1997); monoclonal (An et al., 1997); monoclonal or polyclonal (Paradis et al., 1998)

and Theise, 1998; Nakanuma et al., 1993; Theise, 1995).

Hepatic Iron-Free Foci

Hepatic iron-free foci (IFF) are foci and nodules of hepatocytes found in genetic hemochromatosis that contain much less iron than the surrounding parenchyma (Deugnier et al., 1993; Fig. 11–22). They may occur singly or multiply, and are found in livers with fibrosis or cirrhosis. The foci typically develop near portal areas, and silver stains may reveal an expanding lesion. In a study by Deugnier et al. (1993), 12 patients with IFF were followed for 0.9 to 15 years (7 ± 6 years), and HCC developed in six (50%) of these patients, compared to 2 (8%) from a control group of 24 patients without IFF, matched according to age, sex, degree of fibrosis, liver iron content and duration of follow-up. The mean number of IFF (per IFF-positive specimen) was 3.2 ± 2.1. Ten patients had dysplastic foci (half large and half small cell types), but no correlation was found between the type of dysplastic focus and the subsequent development of HCC (Deugnier et al., 1993). Proliferative cell nuclear antigen was positive in 75% of IFF and

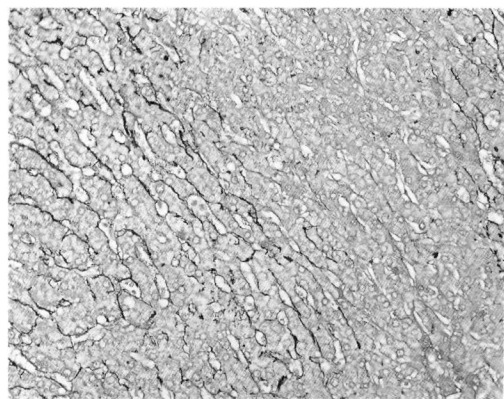

Figure 11–19. Dysplastic nodule, high grade. Note focal absence of reticulin fibers (Manuel's reticulin stain, ×200).

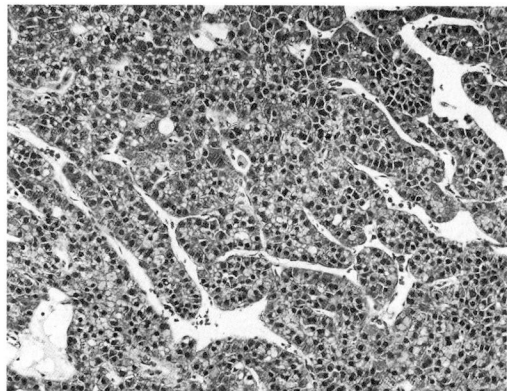

Figure 11–21. Hepatocellular carcinoma. Higher magnification of Figure 11–20 showing classical trabecular pattern (H&E, ×200).

in 24% ± 21% of hepatocyte nuclei in IFF. This study has clearly demonstrated the preneoplastic nature of IFF. The authors recommend that the finding of IFF in a liver biopsy specimen from a patient with genetic hemochromatosis should lead to regular screening for HCC.

Foci of Altered Hepatocytes

Foci of altered hepatocytes (FAH) are preneoplastic lesions identified in various animal models of hepatocarcinogenesis (Bannasch and Zerban, 1997). Their occurrence and significance in the human liver was recently investigated by Su et al. (1997), who studied 163 explanted and resected human livers with or without HCC. Foci of altered hepa-

tocytes, including glycogen-storing foci, mixed cell foci, and basophilic foci, were found in 84 of 111 (75.7%) cirrhotic livers, demonstrating a higher incidence in livers with HCC (29 of 32, or 90.6%) than in those without HCC (55 of 79, or 44.3%). The *glycogen-storing foci* were typically periportal and consisted of 'clear' cells larger than normal hepatocytes; their cytoplasm was full of glycogen (± fat) and the nuclei were small (Fig. 11–23). The *mixed cell foci* consisted of an admixture of clear cells and amphophilic (or less often, basophilic) cells.

Foci of altered hepatocytes were observed by Su et al. (1997) more frequently (78.7%) in HCC-free cirrhosis associated with hepatitis B or C or chronic alcohol abuse (high-

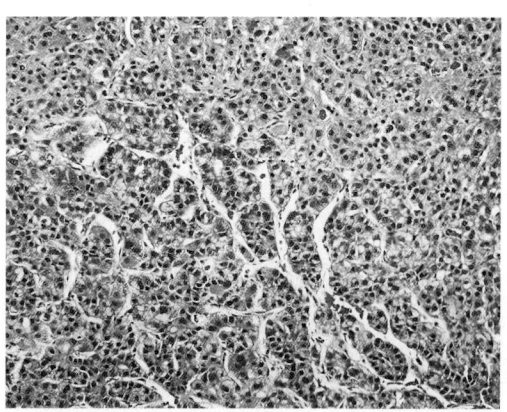

Figure 11–20. Hepatocellular carcinoma in a high-grade dysplastic nodule. Note distinct microtrabeculae (H&E, ×150).

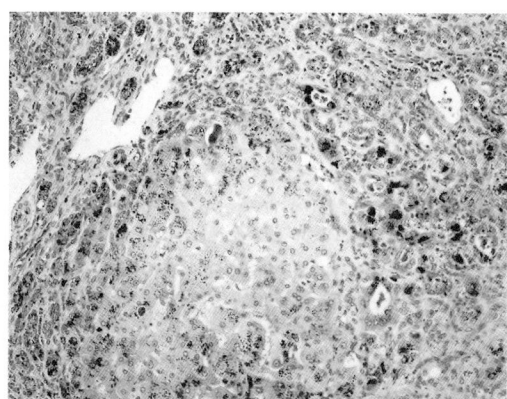

Figure 11–22. Iron-free focus in cirrhotic liver of patient with genetic hemochromatosis (Mallory stain for iron, ×150).

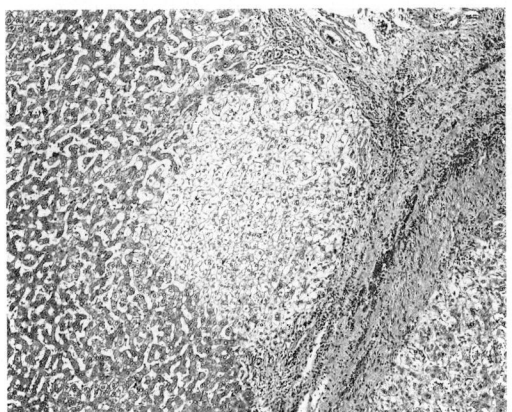

Figure 11–23. Glycogen-rich focus adjacent to a portal area (H&E, ×30).

risk groups) than in cirrhosis due to other causes (50%). Mixed cell foci, predominantly in cirrhotic livers of the high-risk group, were more proliferative, larger, and more often involved in the formation of *nodules* of altered hepatocytes (39.3%) than were glycogen-storing foci (8.5%). The results of this study suggest that FAH are preneoplastic lesions, the mixed cell foci being more advanced than the glycogen-storing foci. Oncocytic and amphophilic cell foci were also observed, but their significance remains to be clarified. Two types of small cell change, "diffuse" and "intrafocal," were identified, but only the intrafocal change was related to increased proliferative activity (PCNA) and a more frequent nodular change of the affected focus of altered hepatocytes, thus suggesting a close association with progression from the altered focus to HCC. The findings are of considerable interest to students of hepatocarcinogenesis but await confirmation by other investigators. One recent study of the proliferative activity of hepatocellular nodules showed that lesions characterized by bile-stained hepatocytes, eosinophilic clear cell change, and large cell change (dysplasia) have low proliferation rates and may not be significant for the development of malignancy (Tiniakos and Brunt, 1999).

Liver Stem Cells

The traditional view of the pathogenesis of experimentally induced liver cancer is the development, after months or years of exposure to a carcinogen, of FAH (basophilic, amphophilic, acidophilic, or "mixed" foci) that then evolve into nodules (hyperplastic, preneoplastic, or neoplastic). These nodules show progressive morphologic or enzymatic changes that antedate the development of liver cancer. The number of nodules progressively decreases such that, at the time when unequivocal carcinoma develops, only one to three "persistent nodules" remain (Bannasch and Zerban, 1997; Farber, 1992). The sequence of foci to nodules to HCC implies "dedifferentiation" of mature hepatocytes. Since the early 1970s, however, it has been known that hepatocarcinogens can stimulate the proliferation of bile duct–like cells (initially termed *oval cells*) in experimental animals. These cells were subsequently found to express liver cell markers (albumin and α-fetoprotein); the antigenic and enzymatic characteristics of these cells are compared to those of hepatocytes and bile duct cells in Table 11–3. They are derived from "bipolar" liver stem cells (LSC) and can differentiate into normal duct cells or hepatocytes. According to Sell (1994), they can also migrate into persistent nodules to give rise to HCC. Cells thought to be oval cells have been identified in human hepatitis B virus (HBV)-associated HCC (Hsia et al., 1992, 1994), although this awaits independent confirmation; the expression of transforming growth factor-α (TGF-α) and HBV markers in these oval cells has been suggested as a possible mechanism of hepatocarcinogenesis (Hsia et al., 1994). The origin and characteristics of LSC and their role in normal development of the liver, regeneration and hepatocarcinogenesis are detailed in numerous reviews (Divan et al., 1992; Farber, 1992; Fausto et al., 1992; Grisham, 1995; Grisham and Coleman, 1996; Marceau et al., 1992; Sell and Dunsford, 1989; Sell, 1993, 1994, 1998; Thorgeirrson, 1993). The LSC may derive from a *transition duct cell* or from a small, nondescript *periportal cell*. There is also evidence for the existence of a *precursor hepatobiliary stem cell* along the biliary tract, and even a *gastrointestinal-determined stem cell* retained in the bile ducts (Sell, 1994). In considering the cellular origin and differentiation of liver neoplasia, Sell (1994) postulates that mutations causing arrest at the stem cell level of dif-

Table 11–3. Markers of Putative Liver Stem Cells (Oval Cells)

Marker	Liver Cells	Duct Cells	Oval Cells
Albumin	+	−	+
α-fetoprotein	−	−	+
OV-6[a]	−	+	+
Cytokeratin 19	−	+	+
Enzymes			
ATPase	+	−	−
γ-glutamyl transpeptidase	−	+	+
β-glucouronidase	+	−	−
Epoxide hydrolase	+	−	−
Glucose-6-phosphatase	+	±	±
Phase I metabolizing enzymes	+	−	−
Phase II metabolizing enzymes	+	+	+
Isoenzymes			
Aldolase	B	A	A, B, C
Pyruvate kinase	L	K	K, K–L
Hematopoietic stem cell markers[a]			
C-kit	−	+	+
CD33	−	+	+
CD34	−	+	+

[a]After Blakolmer et al. (1995).

[Table modified from Sell, 1998.]

ferentiation result in hepatoblastoma; arrest at the transition duct cell level results in mixed hepatocellular and cholangiocarcinoma, arrest at the liver cell level results in hepatocellular carcinoma, and arrest at the bile duct cell level results in cholangiocarcinoma.

It should be clear from the preceding discussions that much remains to be resolved in the field of hepatocellular preneoplasia in humans. For instance, what is the relationship between the currently accepted putative precancerous lesions in humans (dysplastic foci, small cell type; dysplastic nodules, low and high grade; iron-free foci in hemochromatosis) and the liver stem cell? Are the so-called foci and nodules of altered hepatocytes described in human livers (Su et al., 1997) comparable to similarly named lesions in experimental hepatocarcinogenesis? Are the foci of altered hepatocytes in the human liver the result of dedifferentiation, and does a liver stem cell play a role in the subsequent development of HCC?

INCIPIENT NEOPLASIA OF INTRAHEPATIC CHOLANGIOCARCINOMA

Diseases associated with intrahepatic cholangiocarcinoma (ICC) and preceding it, often by many years, are listed in Table 11–4. Benign cholangiocellular tumors that may undergo malignant change are considered first, followed by a discussion of preneoplastic lesions of the intrahepatic bile ducts.

PRECANCEROUS BENIGN CHOLANGIOCELLULAR TUMORS

Solitary Bile Duct Cyst

Malignant tumors, usually adenocarcinomas (Kasai et al., 1977; Kashima et al., 1988), may rarely develop in these cysts. Other malignancies reported to arise in solitary cysts include carcinosarcoma (Terada et al., 1994a), squamous cell carcinoma (Bloustein and Silverberg, 1976; Pliskin et al., 1992; Figs. 11–24

Table 11–4. Diseases Preceding Intrahepatic Cholangiocarcioma

Disease	Comments
Fibrocystic diseases	
Congenital hepatic fibrosis	
von Meyenburg complexes and autosomal dominant polycystic disease	
Caroli's disease	
Inherited metabolic diseases	
Genetic hemochromatosis	Hepatocellular carcinoma more common; usually arises in cirrhotic stage
α-1 antitrypsin deficiency	Hepatocellular carcinoma more common; usually arises in cirrhotic stage
Extrahepatic biliary atresia	
Inflammatory bowel disease	Extrahepatic bile duct carcinoma more common
Chronic cholestatic disease Primary sclerosing cholangitis Primary biliary cirrhosis	
Gallstones	
Recurrent pyogenic ("oriental") cholangitis	Mainly in Southeast Asia
Intrahepatic lithiasis	Mainly in Japan
Parasitic disease Clonorchiasis Opisthorchiasis	Nitrosamines may play a synergistic role
Chronic hepatitis C virus infection	
Thorotrast accumulation ± fibrosis	Latent period over 14 years
Drug use	Contraceptive or anabolic steroids
Occupational exposure	Heavy metal industry; nonelectric machinery industry; asbestos-related work (e.g., ship building)
Benign cholangiocellular tumors	
Solitary (unilocular) cyst	Adenocarcinoma or squamous carcinoma
Peribiliary gland hamartoma (bile duct adenoma)	
Hepatobiliary cystadenoma	
Biliary papillomatosis	

and 11–25), and carcinoid tumor (Ueyama et al., 1992).

Peribiliary Gland Hamartoma (Bile Duct Adenoma)

Follow-up studies of patients with this lesion have confirmed its benign nature (Allaire et al., 1988; Govindrajan and Peters, 1984). There are, however, several cases that appear to have undergone malignant change (Foucar et al., 1979; Hasebe et al., 1995; Tsui et al., 1993). The case of Tsui et al. (1993) exhibited unusual histologic features that included a complex tubulocystic biliary epithelial component set in an abundant fibroblastic stromal background. Also, the glandular element was non–mucin secreting and contained bile concretions. These features prompted the authors (Tsui et al., 1993) to designate their tumor *biliary adenofibroma* (Tsui et al., 1993).

Hepatobiliary Cystadenoma

Foci of atypia (enlargement of cells, multilayering, hyperchromasia, and loss of polarity) were reported in 7 of the 52 cases (13.5%) studied by Devaney et al. (1994). The development of malignancy is a recognized complication of mucinous hepatobiliary cystadenoma (Akwari et al., 1990; Devaney et al., 1994; Ishak et al., 1977; Woods, 1981). In such an event, the base-

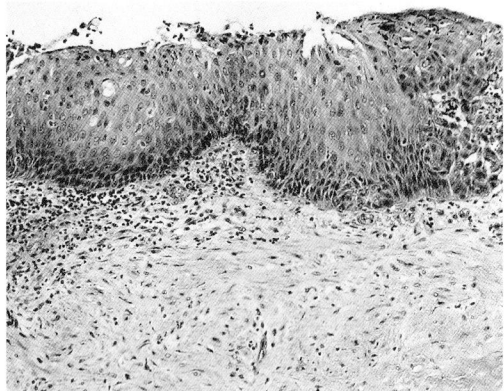

Figure 11–24. Squamous carcinoma that arose in a unilocular (solitary) cyst (H&E, ×90).

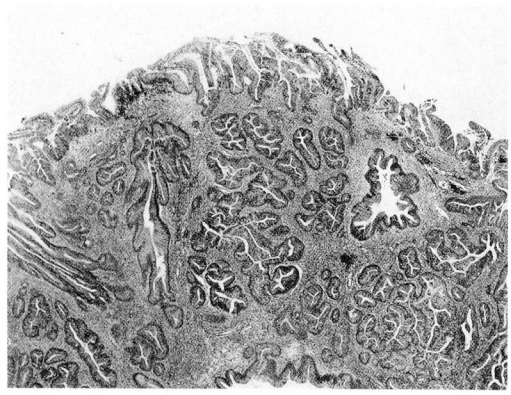

Figure 11–26. Hepatobiliary cystadenocarcinoma. The entire thickness of this locule is infiltrated by a moderately differentiated adenocarcinoma (H&E, ×150).

ment membrane is breached and there is invasion of the underlying stroma. Other features of malignancy, such as loss of polarity, back-to-back glands, nuclear pleomorphism and hyperchromasia, and increased mitotic activity, are used to distinguish cystadenocarcinoma from cystadenoma (Figs. 11–26 to 11–28).

Biliary Papillomatosis

The affected bile ducts in this condition are variably dilated and partially or completely filled with papillary excrescences, composed of columnar epithelial cells supported by delicate fibrovascular stalks (Fig. 11–29). The epithelium of the ducts between the papillary lesions may be ulcerated and in-

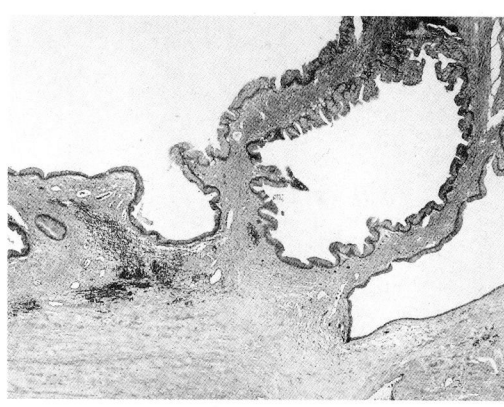

Figure 11–27. Hepatobiliary cystadenocarcinoma. Several locules from the same case illustrated in Figure 11–26 are lined by benign cuboidal to columnar epithelium (H&E, ×40).

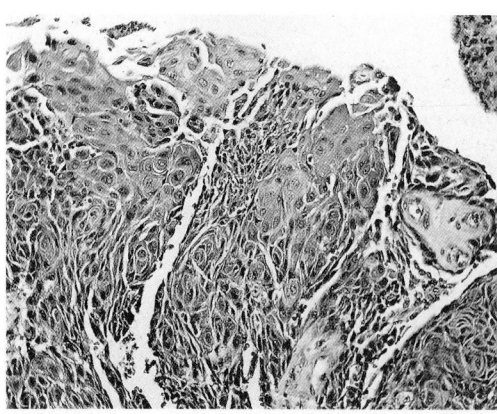

Figure 11–25. Higher magnification of squamous carcinoma illustrated in Figure 11–24 (H&E, ×130).

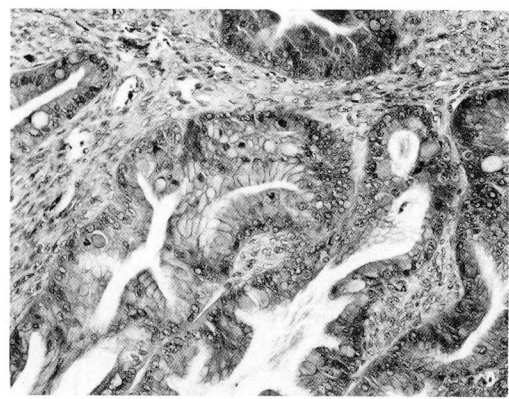

Figure 11–28. Hepatobiliary cystadenocarcinoma. This high-power view demonstrates numerous mitoses (H&E, ×200).

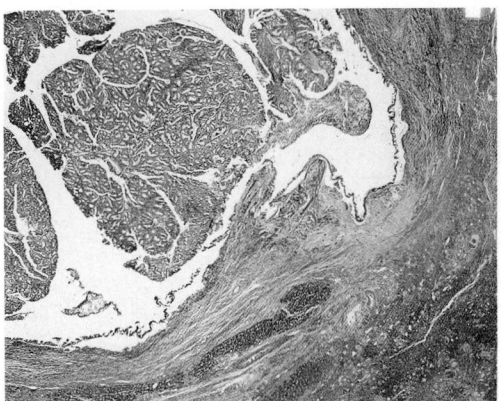

Figure 11–29. Biliary papillomatosis. The dilated intrahepatic bile duct is filled with papillary epithelial formations (H&E, ×15).

volved by acute and chronic inflammation. The lumen of the ducts often contain inspissated mucin, blood, or tumor debris. Malignant transformation (to an intraductal papillary adenocarcinoma) is characterized by marked cellular atypia, loss of polarity, hyperchromasia, numerous mitoses, and invasion beyond the confines of the ducts (Figs. 11–30 and 11–31). Discontinuities of the epithelial basement membrane in the three cases of Padfield et al. (1988) (evaluated by the use of anti-laminin antibodies) led to the conclusion that biliary papillomatosis should be considered a low-grade malignancy. In the review of Gigot et al. (1989), 57% of cases of biliary papillomatosis were benign

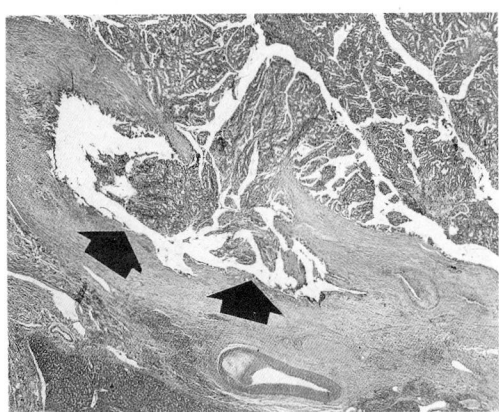

Figure 11–30. Biliary papillomatosis. The tumor has broken through the bile duct and extends into the surrounding fibrous tissue (arrowheads). (H&E, ×15).

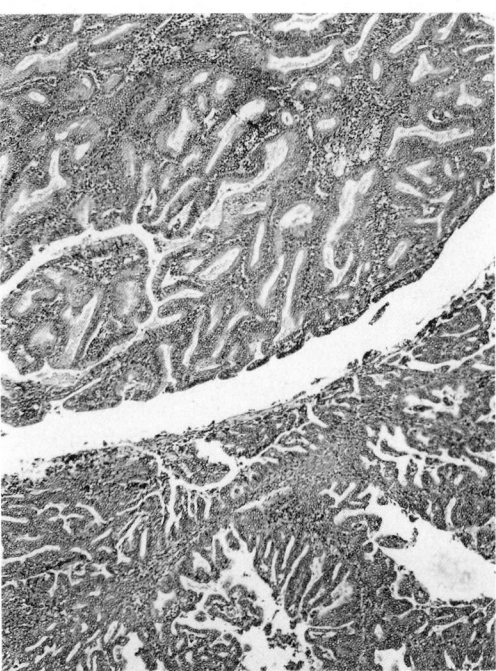

Figure 11–31. Biliary papillomatosis. Intraductal part of the tumor (*top*) and the extension beyond the duct (*bottom*). (H&E, ×150)

and 43% were malignant, either from first detection or secondarily.

PRECANCEROUS LESIONS OF INTRAHEPATIC CHOLANGIOCARCINOMA

Morphologic and cell kinetic studies by Terada et al. (1992) have shown that in hepatolithiasis, carcinogenesis in bile duct epithelial cells progresses in a multistep manner, through hyperplasia, dysplasia, noninvasive adenocarcinoma, and invasive carcinoma. Celli and Que (1998) have proposed that all diseases that predispose to cholangiocarcinoma are characterized by chronic inflammation and cholestasis, in particular, exposure to hydrophobic bile acids, such as glycoursodeoxycholic acid. This can predispose biliary epithelium to oncogenic mutations and progression to malignancy that is due, in part, to failure to activate apoptosis and delete cells with genetic damage (see below).

Mutations of oncogenes and tumor suppressor genes are one mechanism for the development and progression of ICC. *p53* mutations in ICC have been reported by several groups of investigators (Choi et al., 1993; Ohashi et al., 1995; Terada et al., 1994b). In the series of Terada et al. (1994b) 22% of ICC cases in Japan had *p53* mutations; however, in a U.S. study, only 1 in 9 cases of ICC expressed p53 antigen (Choi et al., 1993). The expression of a variety of oncogenes was studied in a series of 63 cases of ICC by Voravud et al. (1989); 95% of the tumors expressed p62 c-*myc*, 75% expressed p21 c-*ras*, and 73% expressed p10 c-*erb* B-2. The expression of c-*myc* and c-*ras*, but not of c-*erb* B-2, correlated directly with tumor differentiation. More recently, Terada and colleagues (1998) found aberrant expression of c-*erb* B-2 protein in 70% of 47 cholangiocarcinomas, as well as in noncancerous biliary proliferative lesions, such as hepatolithiasis. Conflicting results, however, have been reported by Collier et al. (1992), who could not detect c-*erb* B-2 expression in 10 cases of ICC. It is worth noting that overexpression of c-*neu* (the rat proto-oncogene homologue of c-*erb* B-2) is a prominent feature of the furan rat model of cholangiocarcinoma and its precursor lesions (Sirica et al., 1997). In addition to the study of Voravud et al. (1989) *ras* gene mutations were found in 50% of cases of Tada et al. (1992) and 88.6% of the cases of Nonomura et al. (1997).

An alternative mechanism of carcinogenesis involving dysregulation or inhibition of apoptosis has been suggested by Harnois and co-investigators (1997). They compared Bcl-2 expression in two human cell lines—nonmalignant cholangiocytes and cells of a human cholangiocarcinoma cell line. Bcl-2 expression was 15-fold greater in malignant than in nonmalignant cholangiocytes. They concluded that resistance to apoptosis is a characteristic of cholangiocarcinoma cells; it appears to be mediated, in part, by overexpression of Bcl-2. Celli and Que (1998) have further suggested that dysregulation of Bcl-2 expression may also lead to loss of the tumor suppressor gene *p53*.

Precancerous histopathologic lesions of the intrahepatic bile ducts in humans are not as well characterized as those antedating HCC. According to our material at AFIP, precancerous lesions are rarely seen in ICC in the United States. However, several diseases in Southeast Asia that are associated with

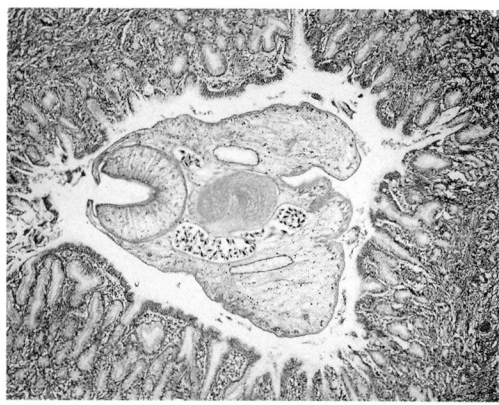

Figure 11–32. "Adenomatous hyperplasia" of a bile duct containing a cross-section of an adult *Clonorchis sinesis*. The change is due to proliferation of peribiliary seromucous glands (H&E, ×60).

presence of intrahepatic stones or parasites are accompanied by metaplastic or dysplastic lesions considered to be precancerous. In one study of hepatolithiasis (intrahepatic lithiasis), chronic proliferative cholangitis, characterized by proliferation of glandular elements within the thickened duct walls and also in the periductal connective tissue, was thought to progress to atypical epithelial hyperplasia and then to ICC (Nakanuma et al., 1985). Later, the same group of investigators described atypical and papillary hyperplasia of the peribiliary glands as precursor lesions of ICC (Terada and

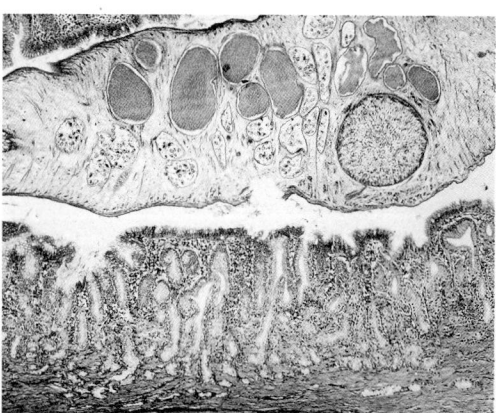

Figure 11–33. "Adenomatous hyperplasia". Segment of duct containing the parasite from the same case illustrated in Figure 11–32 (H&E, ×60).

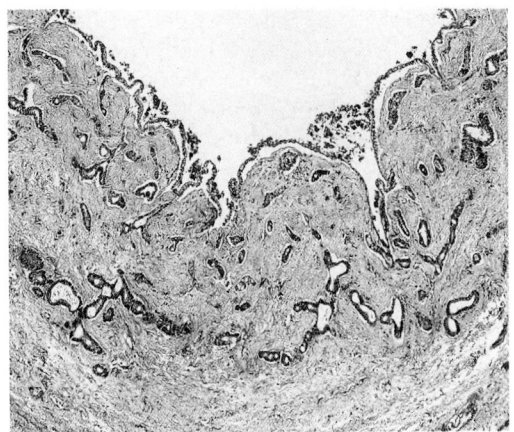

Figure 11–34. Chronic proliferative cholangitis due to proliferation of tubuloalveolar glands in the wall of the bile duct. This patient was also infected with *Clonorchis sinesis* (worm not shown). (H&E, ×75).

Nakanuma, 1990). The atypical epithelial cells showed stronger immunoreactivities to CEA, carbohydrate antigen 19–9, and DU-PAN-2 than cells of normal peribiliary glands. In another study of intrahepatic lithi-

asis, Kurumaya et al. (1990) described intestinal metaplastic lesions in the intrahepatic bile ducts and suggested that they could be precursors of ICC. The metaplastic lesions included goblet cell and Paneth cell metaplasia; endocrine cells were present in more than half of the metaplastic lesions. The duct lesions in livers infected with *Clonorchis sinensis* and *Opisthorchis viverrini* are similar to those of intrahepatic lithiasis. They appear to involve both the intramural and extramural glandular elements of the normal intrahepatic bile ducts (mucous and seromucous glands) and in intrahepatic lithiasis, as described by Terada et al. (1987, 1988). Thus, in many cases there is proliferation of mucous glands in the duct wall (so-called adenomatous hyperplasia) (Figs. 11–32 and 11–33). In other cases there is proliferation of periductal branched tubuloalveolar seromucous glands, a change that corresponds to the chronic proliferative cholangitis originally described by Nakanuma et al. (1985) (Fig. 11–34). An ICC that arose in a liver infected with *Clonorchis sinensis* infection is illustrated in Figure 11–35.

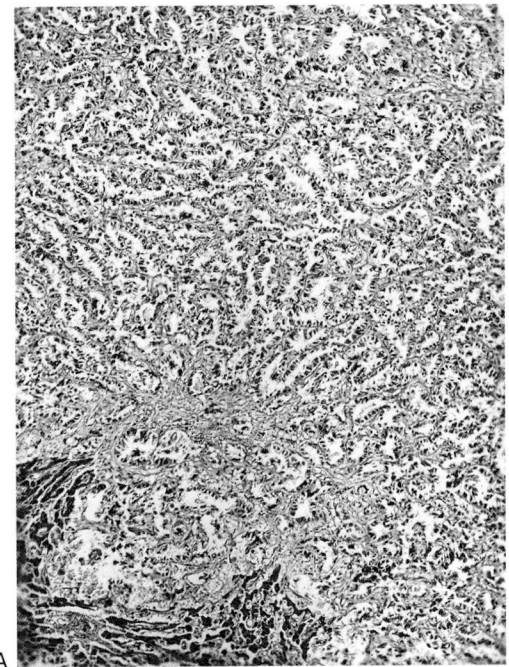
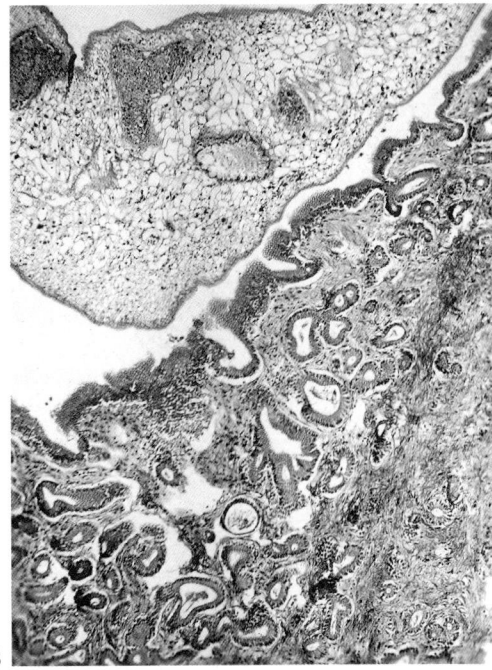

A   B

Figure 11–35. Intrahepatic cholangiocarcinoma that arose in liver of patient infected with *Clonorchis sinensis* (*A*). The duct containing the parasite (*B*) shows chronic proliferative cholangitis with malignant change and invasion of the underlying stroma (H&E, ×70).

INCIPIENT NEOPLASIA OF ANGIOSARCOMA AND OTHER SARCOMAS

PRECANCEROUS BENIGN MESENCHYMAL TUMORS

Infantile Hemangioendothelioma

There is convincing evidence that at least some of the hepatic angiosarcomas arise in a preexisting infantile hemangioendothelioma (Falk et al., 1981; Ishak et al., 1999; Noronha and Gonzalez-Crussi, 1984; Strate et al., 1984; Weinberg and Finegold, 1993). Three small series of pediatric angiosarcomas (Falk et al., 1981; Selby et al., 1992; Weinberg and Finegold, 1993), as well as a number of case reports, have been published (Adam et al., 1972; Alt et al., 1985; Kauffman and Stout, 1961; Ross, 1932; Strate et al., 1984). We now consider the type-2 infantile hemangioendothelioma of the liver of Dehner and Ishak (1971) to be an angiosarcoma. In addition to the histopathologic features of adult angiosarcoma (Fig. 11–36), the pediatric cases have a "Kaposiform," spindle-cell component similar to that of Kaposiform hemangioendothelioma of soft tissues (Ekfors et al. 1993; Fukunaga et al., 1996; Niedt et al., 1989; Sukerberg et al., 1993; Tsang and Chan, 1991). Such Kaposiform areas are often lobulated and are composed of spindle cells arranged in bundles, with scattered slit-like, vascular spaces lined by flat endothelial cells (Fig. 11–37). A whorl-like arrangement of cells, the so-called

glomeruloid foci (Sukerberg et al., 1993), is also seen (Fig. 11–38). Like Kaposi's sarcoma, the spindle cells express CD31 and CD34 but not von Willebrand factor. Mitotic figures vary from a few to many (Fig. 11–37).

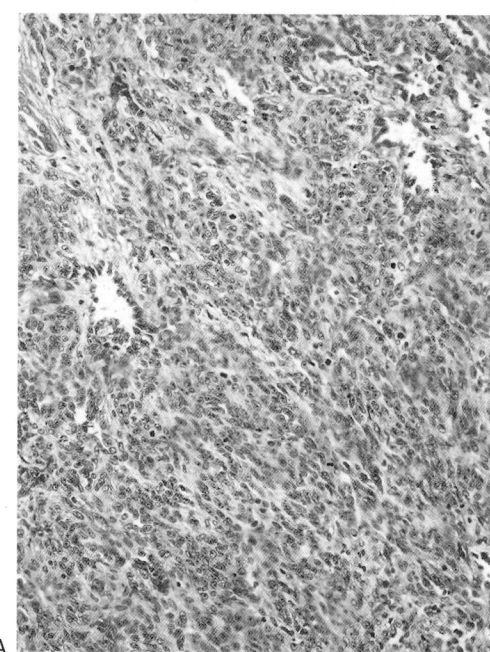

A

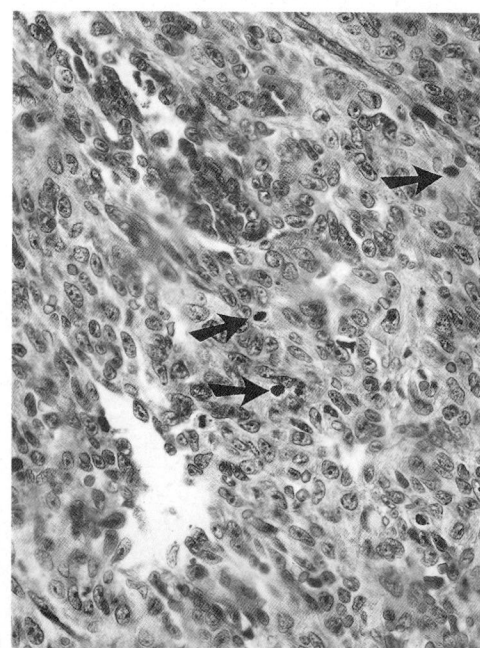

B

Figure 11–37. Kaposiform angiosarcoma. Spindle cell area is shown at medium (*A*) (H&E, ×75) and high power (*B*) (H&E, ×450) magnification. Note mitotic figures (arrows) in B.

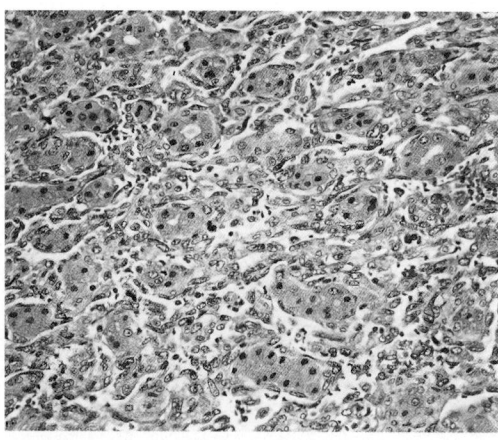

Figure 11–36. Kaposiform angiosarcoma showing sinusoidal infiltration by malignant endothelial cells (H&E, ×250).

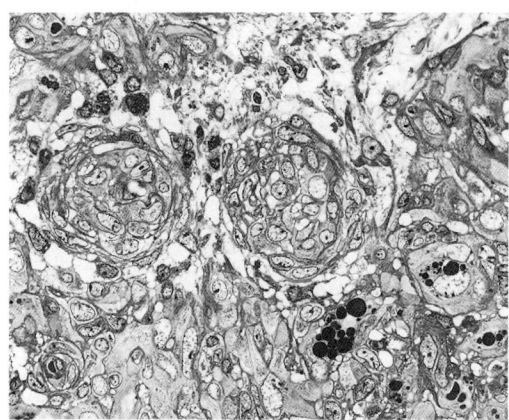

Figure 11–38. Kaposiform angiosarcoma. Two glomeruloid foci. Note globules in right lower corner (Touidine blue stain of 1 μm Epon-embedded section, ×450).

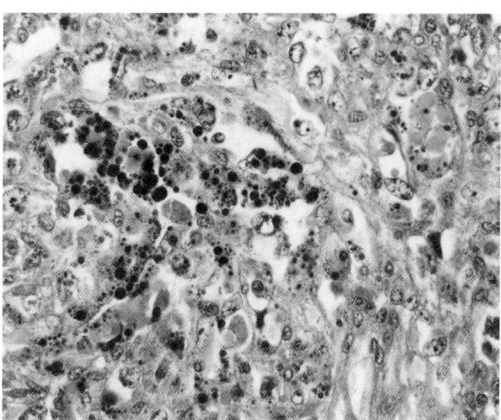

Figure 11–40. Kaposiform angiosarcoma. Intracellular globules (black) are of varied size (PAS after diastase digestion).

Reticulin fibers surround the vascular channels (Fig. 11–39) and many perithelial cells express α-smooth muscle actin. Another feature of the Kaposiform areas is the presence of numerous variably sized, eosinophilic (hyaline) globules in the cytoplasm of the spindle cells and occasionally, extracellularly (Fig. 11–38). These globules are PAS positive and resist diastase digestion (Fig. 11–40). The cytoplasm of the spindle cells expresses α_1-antitrypsin and α_1-antichymotrypsin, but the globules do not. Kaposiform hemangioendothelioma of the retroperitoneum occurs in infancy and childhood (median, 2 years; range, 5 months to 19 years) (Sukerberg et al., 1993).

The pediatric angiosarcomas of the liver (with Kaposiform features) studied by Selby et al. (1992) at AFIP occurred between the ages of 18 months and 7 years (mean 3.7 years). The retroperitoneal (but thus far not the hepatic) tumors have sometimes been associated with locally aggressive disease, lymphangiomatosis, and the Kasabach-Merritt syndrome (consumption coagulopathy) (Sukerberg et al., 1993). Distant metastases have not been reported with the retroperitoneal tumors but have been noted in several of the hepatic cases (Selby et al., 1992). Vascular invasion is present in some of the tumors (Fig. 11–41). Most of the children with angiosarcoma of the liver have died

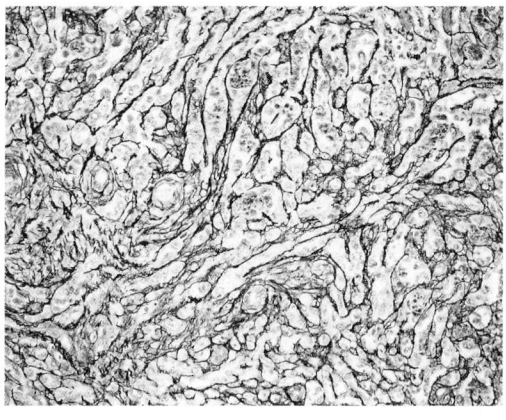

Figure 11–39. Kaposiform angiosarcoma. A well-developed reticulin network surrounds the tumor cells (Manuel reticulin stain, ×160).

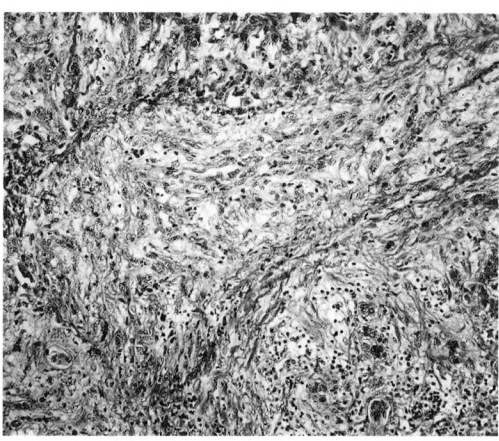

Figure 11–41. Kaposiform angiosarcoma with invasion of a terminal hepatic venule (H&E, ×160).

within 2 years; the mean survival in the AFIP series was 10 months (Selby et al., 1992). Therapy, consisting of surgery, radiotherapy, chemotherapy, or combinations thereof, has been ineffective.

The pediatric angiosarcomas resemble the adult angiosarcomas in their morphology and behavior, but have some morphologic "Kaposiform" features that are distinctive. Such tumors, whether they arise in childhood, adolescence, or early adulthood, can be termed *Kaposiform angiosarcoma*. As noted earlier, some of these cases are clearly traceable to an underlying infantile hemangioendothelioma (Fig. 11–42). The etiology of these tumors remains undetermined, but one of the cases of Falk et al. (1981) had been heavily exposed to arsenic, a recognized cause of adult angiosarcoma of adults (Ishak et al., 1999) or children (Salgado et al., 1995).

Mesenchymal Hamartoma

De Chadarevian and colleagues (1994) reported on a 12-year-old girl who developed an embryonal sarcoma in conjunction with a mesenchymal hamartoma, and they raised the possibility of a histogenetic relationship between the two tumors. However, in over 200 mesenchymal hamartomas on file at AFIP, no malignant features have been identified, and none of the surgically resected cases has shown recurrence or metastases.

Solitary Fibrous Tumor

Most of the cases of solitary fibrous tumor of the liver reported in the literature or on file at AFIP have behaved in a benign fashion (Moran et al., 1998). However, some of these tumors can be highly cellular and display histopathologic features judged to be malignant. These include foci of necrosis, prominent cellular atypia, and mitotic activity in the range of 2–4 mitoses per high-power field (Figs. 11–43 and 11–44). In a series of 10 cases of solitary fibrous tumors (extrahepatic), Yokoi et al. (1998) found that malignant transformation may be associated with loss of expression of CD34 and with *p53* mutation. Comparative genomic hybridization studies have been useful in the evaluation of malignant transformation of solitary fibrous tumors (Kottke-Marchant et al., 1989). Thus, DNA copy number changes (mostly chromosomal gains) were found in tumors larger than 10 cm, including all tumors with more than 4 mitoses per 10 high-power fields.

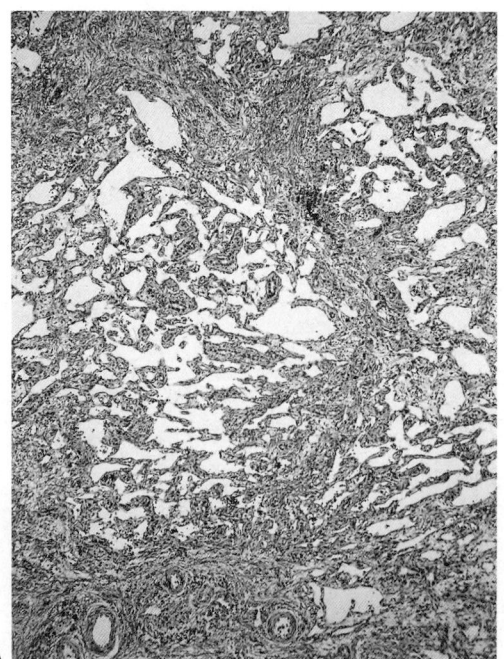
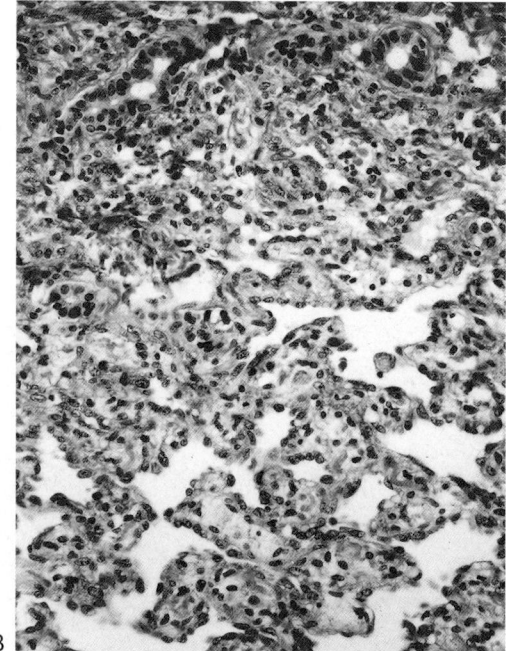

A   B

Figure 11–42. Kaposiform angiosarcoma; same case as in Figure 11–41 showing area of infantile hemangioendothelioma at low (*A*) (×60) and high power (*B*) (×250) magnification (H&E).

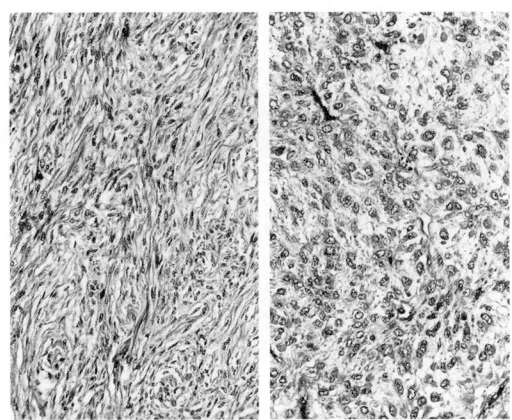

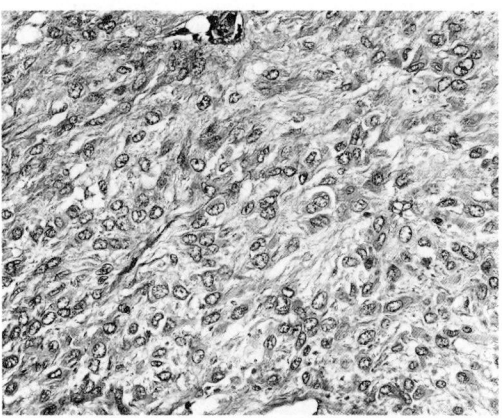

Figure 11–43. Solitary fibrous tumor. A typical benign area shows fascicles of elongated spindle cells (*left*) and a much more cellular area with larger nuclei and less cytoplasm (*right*) in the same tumor (H&E, ×200).

Figure 11–44. Solitary fibrous tumor. Through high-power magnification of an area of the same tumor shown in Figure 11–43 (right) the tumor is judged to be malignant (H&E, ×300).

Precancerous Lesions of Angiosarcoma

Diseases and etiologic factors that precede angiosarcoma of the liver are listed in Table 11–5. A precursor stage in the development of angiosarcoma that has been observed in cases etiologically related to vinyl chloride, Thorotrast, and arsenic (Berk et al., 1976; Falk et al, 1981; Popper et al., 1978, 1980; Tamburro et al., 1984; Thomas et al., 1975) is characterized by foci of simultaneous activation of both hepatocytes and sinusoidal lining cells, with associated lesions in the sinusoids and perisinusoidal spaces. In my experience, the most striking, possibly precancerous lesion is sinusoidal ectasia with hypertrophy of lining cells that have large,

Table 11–5. Diseases and Etiologic Factors Preceding Angiosarcoma of the Liver

Diseases or Etiology	Circumstances of Exposure	Latent period years
Thorotrast	Used as contrast medium for radiographic studies	15–60
Radium	Radium needle implanted for treatment of breast carcinoma (1 case)	3
External radiation	Atomic bomb explosion, Hiroshima (1 case)	36
Vinyl chloride	Industrial exposure during manufacture of polyvinyl chloride; exposure to sprays containing vinyl chloride as propellant	9–35
Arsenical compounds	Insecticide for spraying of vineyards; medicinal use of Fowler's solution; dioxidiaminoarsenobenzol for treatment of syphilis; high levels of arsenic in drinking water	6–46
Copper sulfate	Used for spraying vineyards (1 case)	35
Pesticides	Farmers exposed to organophosphorus, and organochlorine containing pesticides	14
Iron	Genetic hemochromatosis in cirrhotic stage	?
Androgenic/anabolic steroids	Treatment of Fanconi's anemia and other disorders	2–35
Contraceptive steroids	Birth control (1 case)	10
Diethylstilbestrol	Treatment of prostatic cancer (1 case)	13
Phenelzine	Depression (1 case)	6
Benign vascular tumors Infantile hemangioendothelioma		?

Table after Ishak et al., 1999.

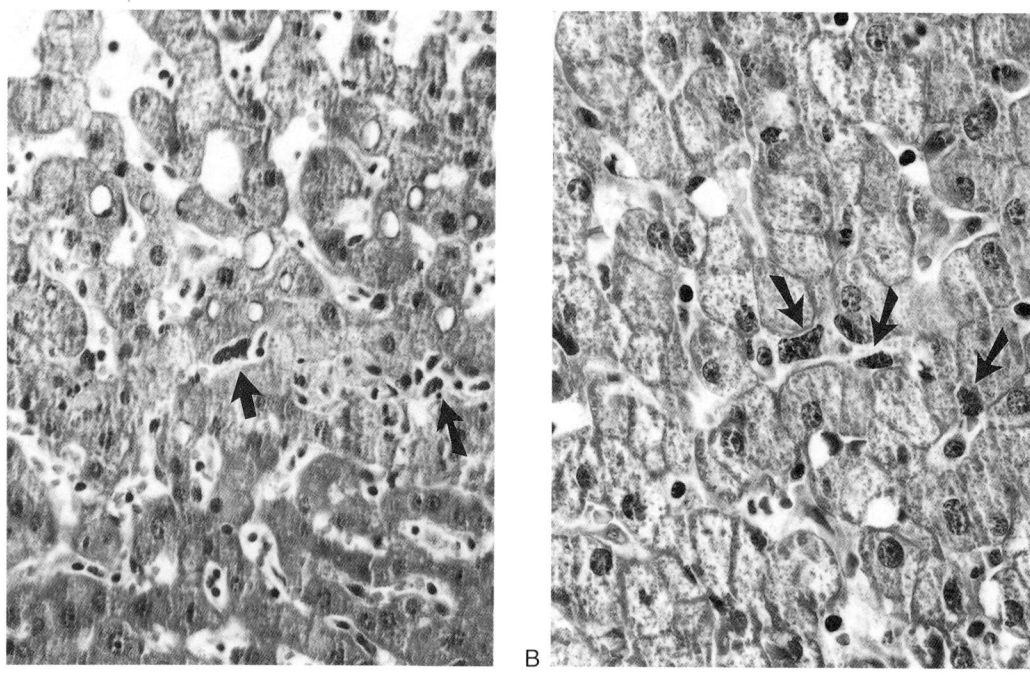

Figure 11–45. *A,B:* Possible precursor lesion of angiosarcoma in a patient with a history of long-term exposure to vinyl chloride. Sinusoidal ectasia is evident and the lining cells (arrowheads) have large, irregular, and hyperchromatic nuclei (H&E, ×630).

irregular, and hyperchromatic nuclei (Fig. 11–45). In vinyl chloride–associated cases, the lesions in humans are quite comparable to those induced experimentally in rodents (Popper et al., 1980). Additional light microscopic and ultrastructural studies of hepatic lesions in workers exposed to vinyl chloride (but who did not have angiosarcoma) have been reported (Gedigk et al., 1975; Schattenberg et al., 1977).

The opinions and assertions contained herein are the private views of the author and are not to be construed as official or as representing the views of the Department of the Army or the Department of Defense.

REFERENCES

Adam YG, Huvos AG, Hadju SI. (1972) Malignant vascular tumors of liver. *Ann Surg* 175:325–383.

Akagi G, Furuya K, Kanamura A, et al. (1984) Liver cell dysplasia and hepatitis B surface antigen in liver cirrhosis and hepatocellular carcinoma. *Cancer* 54: 315–318.

Akwari OE, Tucker A, Seigler HF, Itani KMF. (1990) Hepatobiliary cystademona with mesenchymal stroma. *Ann Surg* 211:18–27.

Allaire GS, Rabin L, Ishak KG, Sesterhenn IA. (1988) Bile duct adenoma. A study of 152 cases. *Am J Surg Pathol* 12:708–715.

Alt B, Hafez GR, Trigg M, et al. (1985) Angiosarcoma of the liver and spleen in an infant. *Pediatr Pathol* 4:331–339.

An CST, Petrovic LM, Reyter I, et al. (1997) The application of image analysis and neural network technology to the study of large-cell liver-cell dysplasia and hepatocellular carcinoma. *Hepatology* 25:1224–1231.

Anthony PP, Vogel CL, Barker LF. (1973) Liver cell dysplasia: a premalignant condition. *J Clin Pathol* 26: 217–223.

Arakawa M, Kage M, Sugihara S, et al. (1986a) Emergence of malignant lesions within an adenomatous hyperplastic nodule in a cirrhotic liver. Observations in five cases. *Gastroenterology* 91:198–208.

Bannasch P, Zerban H. (1997) Experimental chemical hepatocarcinogenesis. In: *Liver Cancer* (Okuda K, Tabor E, eds.) pp. 213–253. Churchill Livingstone, New York.

Berk PD, Martin JF, Young RS. (1976) Vinyl chloride–associated liver disease. *Ann Intern Med* 84:717–731.

Blakolmer K, Jaskiewicz K, Dunsford HA, Robson SC. (1995) Hematopoietic stem cell markers are expressed by ductal plate and bile duct cells in developing human liver. *Hepatology* 21:1510–1516.

Bloustein PA, Silverberg SG. (1976) Squamous cell carcinoma originating in a hepatic cyst: Case report with a review of the hepatic cyst-carcinoma association. *Cancer* 38:2002–2005.

Borzio M, Bruno S, Roncalli M, et al. (1996) Liver cells dysplasia is a major factor for risk hepatocellular carcinoma in cirrhosis: a preliminary report: a prospective study. *Gastroenterology* 108:812–818.

Celli A, Que FG. (1998) Dysregulation of apoptosis in the cholangiopathies and cholangiocarcinoma. *Semin Liver Dis* 18:177–185.

Chen M, Gerber MA, Thung SN, et al. (1984) Morphometric studies of hepatocytes containing hepatitis B surface antigen. *Am J Pathol* 114:217–221.

Choi SW, Hytiroglou P, Geller SA, et al. (1993) The expression of p53 malignant epithelial tumors of the liver: an immunohistochemical study. *Liver* 13:172–176.

Cohen C, DeRosa PB. (1994) Immunohistochemical p53 in hepatocellular carcinoma and liver cell dysplasia. *Mod Pathol* 7:536–539.

Colina F, Alberti N, Solis JA, Martinez-Tello FJ. (1989) Diffuse nodular regenerative hyperplasia of the liver. *Gastroenterology* 9:253–265.

Collier JD, Guo K, Mathew J, et al. (1992) C-erbB-2 oncogene expression in hepatocellular carcinoma and cholangiocarcinoma. *J Hepatol* 14:377–380.

de Chadarevian JP, Powel BR, Ferber EN, Weintraub WH. (1994) Undifferentiated (embryonal) sarcoma arising in conjunction with mesenchymal hamartoma of the liver. *Mod Pathol* 7:490–493.

Dehner LP, Ishak KG. (1971) Vascular tumors of the liver in infants and children: a study of 30 cases and review of the literature. *Arch Pathol* 92:101–111.

Deugnier YM, Charalambous P, Le Quilleuc D, et al. (1993) Preneoplastic significance of hepatic iron-free foci in genetic hemochromatosis: a study of 185 patients. *Hepatology* 18:1363–1369.

Devaney K, Goodman ZD, Ishak KG. (1994) Hepatobiliary cystadenoma and cystadenocarcinoma—a light microscopic and immunohistochemical study of 70 patients. *Am J Surg Pathol* 18:1078–1091.

Divan BA, Ward JM, Rice JM. (1992) Origin and pathology of hepatoblastoma in mice. In: *The Role of Cell Types in Hepatocarcinogenesis* (Sirica AE, ed.) pp. 71–120. CRC Press, Boca Raton.

Edmondson HA, Reynolds TB, Henderson B, Benton B. (1977) Regression of liver cell adenomas associated with oral contraceptives. *Ann Intern Med* 86:180–182.

Eguchi A, Nakashima O, Okudaira S, et al. (1992) Adenomatous hyperplasia in the vicinity of small hepatocellular carcinoma. *Hepatology* 15:843–848.

Ehrenfried JA, Zhou Z, Thompson JC, et al. (1994) Expression of the neurotensin gene in fetal human liver and fibrolamellar carcinoma. *Ann Surg* 220:484–491.

Ekfors TO, Kujari H, Herva R. (1993) Kaposi-like infantile hemangioendothelioma. *Am J Surg Pathol* 16:314–317.

Falk H, Herbert J, Crowley S, et al. (1981) Epidemiology of hepatic angiosarcoma in the United States: 1964–1974. *Environ Health Perspect* 41:107–113.

Falk H, Herbert JT, Edmonds L, et al. (1981) Review of four cases of childhood hepatic angiosarcoma—elevated environmental arsenic exposure in one case. *Cancer* 47:382–391.

Farber E. (1992) On cells of origin of liver cell cancer. In: *The Role of Cell Types in Hepatocarcinogenesis* (Sirica AE, (ed.) pp. 1–28. CRC Press, Boca Raton.

Farrell GC, Joshua DE, Uren RF. (1975) Androgen-induced hepatoma. *Lancet* 1:430–432.

Fausto N, Lemire JM, Shiojiri N. (1992) Oval cells in liver carcinogenesis. In: *The Role of Cell Types in Hepatocarcinogenesis* (Sirica AE, ed.) pp. 89–108. CRC Press, Boca Raton.

Ferrell LD. (1993) Hepatocellular carcinoma arising in a focus of multilobular adenoma: A case report. *Am J Surg Pathol* 17:524–529.

Ferrell LD, Crawford JM, Dhillon AP, et al. (1993) Proposal for standardized criteria for the diagnosis of benign, borderline, and malignant hepatocellular lesions arising in chronic advanced liver disease. *Am J Surg Pathol* 17:1113–1123.

Ferrell LD, Wright T, Lake J, et al. (1992) Incidence and diagnostic features of macroregenerative nodules vs. small hepatocellular carcinoma in cirrhotic livers. *Hepatology* 16:1372–1381.

Foster JH, Berman MM. (1994) The malignant transformation of liver cell adenomas. *Arch Surg* 129:712–717.

Fukunaga M, Ushigome S, Ishikawa E. (1996) Kaposiform hemangioendothelioma associated with Kasabach-Merritt syndrome. *Histopathology* 28:281–284.

Furuya K, Nakamura M, Yamamoto, et al. (1988) Macroregenerative nodule of the liver. A clinicopathologic study of 345 autopsy cases of chronic liver disease. *Cancer* 61:99–105.

Foucar E, Kaplan LR, Gold JH, et al. (1979) Well-differentiated peripheral cholangiocarcinoma with an unusual clinical course. *Gastroenterology* 77:347–353.

Galassi A, Pasquinelli G, Guerini A. (1995) Benign myxoid hepatocellular tumor: a variant of liver cell adenoma. *Liver* 15:233–235.

Ganne-Carrie N, Chastang C, Chapel F, et al. (1996) Predictive score for the development of hepatocellular carcinoma and additional value of liver large cell dysplasia in Western patients with cirrhosis. *Hepatology* 23:112–118.

Gedigk P, Muller R, Bechtelsheimer H. (1975) Morphology of liver damage among polyvinyl chloride production workers: a report of 51 cases. *Ann NY Acad Sci* 245:278–285.

Gigot JF, Geubel A, Haot J, et al. (1989) Papillamatose des voies biliares. *Acta Endoscop* 19:345–366.

Govindrajan S, Peters RL. (1984) The bile duct adenoma. A lesion distinct from Meyenburg complex. *Arch Pathol Lab Med* 108:922–924.

Grisham JW. (1995) Hepatic epithelial stem-like cells. *Verh Dtsch Ges Pathol* 79:47–54.

Grisham JW, Coleman WB. (1996) Neoformation of liver epithelial cells; progenitor cells, stem cells, and phenotypic transitions. *Gastroenterology* 110:1311–1313.

Harnois DM, Que FG, Celli A, et al. (1997) Bcl-2 is overexpressed and alters the threshold for apoptosis in a cholangiocarcinoma cell line. *Hepatology* 26:884–890.

Hasebe T, Sakamoto M, Mukai K, et al. (1995) Cholangiocarcinoma arising in bile duct adenoma with focal area of bile duct hamartoma. *Virchows Arch* 426:209–213.

Heffelfinger S, Irani DR, Finegold MJ. (1987) "Alcoholic hepatitis" in a hepatic adenoma. *Hum Pathol* 18:751–754.

Henmi A, Uchida T, Shikata T. (1985) Karyometric analysis of liver cell dysplasia and hepatocellular carcinoma. Evidence against precancerous nature of liver cell dysplasia. *Cancer* 55:2594–2599.

Hsia CC, Evarts RP, Nakatsukasa H, et al. (1992) Occurrence of oval-type cells in hepatitis B virus-associated human hepatocarcinogenesis. *Hepatology* 16:1327–1333.

Hsia CC, Thorgeirsson SS, Tabor E. (1994) Expression of hepatitis B surface and core antigens and transforming growth factor-α in "oval cells" of the liver in patients with hepatocellular carcinoma. *J Med Viral* 43:216–221.

Hytiroglou P, Theise ND. (1998) Differential diagnosis of hepatocellular nodular lesions. *Semin Diagn Pathol* 15:285–299.

International Working Party. (1995) Terminology of nodular hepatocellular lesions. *Hepatology* 22:983–993.

Ishak KG. (1979) Hepatic neoplasms associated with contraceptive and anabolic steroids. In: *Carcinogenic Hormones* (Lingeman CH, ed.) pp. 73–128. Springer-Verlag, Berlin.

Ishak KG. (1991) Hepatocellular carcinoma associated with the inherited metabolic diseases. In: *Etiology, Pathology and Treatment of Hepatocellular Carcinoma in North America*, Tabor E, Di Biseglie AM, Purcell RH, eds.) pp. 91–103. Gulf Publishing Co, Houston.

Ishak KG, Goodman ZG, Stocker JJ. (1999) Tumors of the liver. In: *Atlas of Tumor Pathology*, Third Series. Armed Forces Institute of Pathology, Washington, DC, (in press).

Ishak KG, Willis GW, Cummins SD, Bullock AA. (1977) Biliary cystadenoma and cystadenocarcinoma: report of 14 cases and review of the literature. *Cancer* 29:322–338.

Janes CH, McGill DB, Ludwig J, Krom RAF. (1993) Liver cell adenoma at the age of 3 years and transplantation 19 years later after development of carcinoma. A case report. *Hepatology* 17:583–585.

Kagawa K, Deguchi T, Tomimasu H, et al. (1984) Feulgen-DNA cytofluorimetry of the liver cell dysplasia LCD) in the liver cirrhosis. *Jpn J Gastroenterol* 81:82–91.

Kasai Y, Sasaki E, Tamaki A, et al. (1977) Carcinoma arising in the cyst of the liver—report of three cases. *Jpn J Surg* 7:65–71.

Kashima S, Asanuma Y, Niwa M, Koyama K. (1988) A case of true hepatic cyst with malignant change. *Acta Hepatol Jpn* 29:1265–1268.

Kauffman SL, Stout AP. (1961) Malignant hemangioendothelioma in infants and children. *Cancer* 6:1186–1196.

Kondo F, Ebara M, Sugiura N, et al. (1990) Histological features and clinical course of large regenerative nodules: evaluation of their precancerous potentiality. *Hepatology* 12:592–598.

Kondo F, Kondo Y, Nagato Y, et al. (1994) Interstitial tumor cell invasion in small hepatocellular carcinoma: evaluation in microscopic and low magnification views. *J Gastroenterol Hepatol* 9:604–612.

Kottke-Marchant K, Hart W, Broughan T. (1989) Localized fibrous tumor (localized fibrous mesothelioma) of the liver. *Cancer* 64:1096–1102.

Kurumaya H, Terada T, Nakanuma Y. (1990) 'Metaplastic lesions' in intrahepatic bile ducts in hepatolithiasis: a histochemical and immunohistochemical study. *J Gastroenterol Hepatol* 5:530–536.

Le Bail B, Belleannée G, Bernard P-H, et al. (1995) Adenomatous hyperplasia in cirrhotic liver: histological evaluation, cellular density, and proliferative activity of 35 macronodular lesions in the cirrhotic explants of 10 adult French patients. *Hum Pathol* 26:897–906.

Le Bail B, Bernard P-H, Carles J, et al. (1997) Prevalence of liver cell dysplasia and association with HCC

in a series of 100 cirrhotic liver explants. *J Hepatol* 27:835–842.

Le Bail B, Jouhanole H, Deugnier Y, et al. (1992) Liver adenomatosis with granulomas in two patients on long-term oral contraceptives. *Am J Surg Pathol* 16:982–987.

Lee R, Tsamandas AC, Demetris AJ. (1997) Large cell change (liver cell dysplasia) and hepatocellular carcinoma in cirrhosis: matched case–control study, pathological analysis, and pathogenetic hypothesis. *Hepatology* 26:1415–1422.

Lefkowitch JH, Apfelbaum TF. (1987) Liver cell dysplasia and hepatocellular carcinoma in non-A, non-B hepatitis. *Arch Pathol Lab Med* 111:170–173.

Lencioni R, Caramella P, Bartolizzi C, DiCoscio G. (1994) Long-term follow-up study of adenomatous hyperplasia in liver cirrhosis. *Ital J Gastroenterol* 26:163–168.

Marceau N, Blouin M-J, Noël M, Török N, Loranger A. (1992) The role of bipotential progenitor cells in liver ontogenesis and neoplasia. In: *The Role of Cell Types in Hepatocarcinogenesis* (Sirica AE, ed.) pp. 121–149. CRC Press, Boca Raton.

Mokrohisky ST, Ambruso DR, Hathaway WE. (1977) Fulminant hepatic neoplasia after androgen therapy. *Lancet* 296:1411–1412.

Moran CA, Ishak KG, Goodman ZG. (1998) Solitary fibrous tumor of the liver: a clinicopathologic and immunohistochemical study of nine cases. *Ann Diagn Pathol* 2:19–24.

Mueller J, Keeffe EB, Esquivel CO. (1995) Liver transplantation for treatment of giant hepatocellular adenomas. *Liver Transplant Surg* 1:99–102.

Nakano M, Saito A, Takasaki K, et al. (1990) A histopathology study of early hepatocellular carcinoma: portal tract invasion and progression to advanced hepatocellular carcinoma. *Acta Pathol Jpn* 31:754–762.

Nakanuma Y, Ohta G. (1985) Is Mallory body formation a preneoplastic change? A study of 101 cases of liver bearing hepatocellular carcinoma and 82 cases of cirrhosis. *Cancer* 55:2400–2404.

Nakanuma Y, Terada T, Tanaka Y, Ohta G. (1985) Are hepatolithiasis and cholangiocarcinoma aetiologically related? *Virchows Arch A Pathol Anat Histopathol* 406:45–58.

Nakanuma Y, Terada T, Ueda K, et al. (1993) Adenomatous hyperplasia of the liver as a precancerous lesion. *Liver* 13:1–9.

Nakashima T, Okuda K, Kojiro M, et al. (1983) Pathology of hepatocellular carcinoma in Japan: 232 consecutive cases autopsied in ten years. *Cancer* 151:863–877.

Niedt GW, Greco MA, Blanc WA, Knowles DM II. (1989) Hemangioma with Kaposi's sarcoma-like features: report of two cases. *Pediatr Pathol* 9:567–575.

Nonomura A, Ohta G, Hayashi M, et al. (1997) Immunohistochemical localization of ras p21 and carcinoembryonic antigens (CEA) in cholangiocarcinoma. *Liver* 7:142–148.

Noronha R, Gonzalez-Crussi F. (1984) Hepatic angiosarcoma in childhood: a case report and review of the literature. *Am J Surg Pathol* 8:863–871.

Nzeako UC, Goodman ZD, Ishak KG. (1996) Hepatocellular carcinoma and nodular regenerative hyperplasia: possible pathogenetic relationship. *Am J Gastroenterol* 91:879–884.

Ohashi K, Nakajima Y, Kanchiro H, et al. (1995) Ki-ras mutations and p53 protein expressions in intrahepatic cholangiocarcinamas: relation to gross tumor morphology. *Gastroenterology* 109:1612–1617.

Omata M, Mori J, Yokosuka O, et al. (1992) Hepatitis B virus antigens in liver tissue in hepatocellular carcinoma and advanced chronic liver disease—relationship to liver cell dysplasia. *Liver* 2:125–132.

Orsatti G, Theise ND, Thung SN, Paronetto F. (1993) DNA image cytometric analysis of macroregenerative nodules (adenomatous hyperplasia) of the liver: evidence in support of their preneoplastic nature. *Hepatology* 17:621–627.

Padfield CJH, Ansell ID, Furness PN. (1988) Mucinous biliary papillomatosis: a tumour in need of widerecognition. *Histopathology* 13:687–694.

Paradis V, Laurnedeau I, Vidaud M, et al. (1998) Clonal analysis of macronodules in cirrhosis. *Hepatology* 28:953–958.

Park YN, Yang C-P, Fernandez GJ, et al. (1998) Neoangiogenesis and sinusoidal "capillarization" in dysplastic nodules of the liver. *Am J Surg Pathol* 22:656–662.

Parker P, Burr I, Slonim A, et al. (1981) Regression of hepatic adenomas in type Ia glycogen storage disease with dietary therapy. *Gastroenterology* 81:534–536.

Piao Z, Park YN, Kim H, Park C. (1997) Clonality of large regenerative nodules in liver cirrhosis. *Liver* 17:251–256.

Pliskin A, Cualing H, Stenger RJ. (1992) Primary squamous cell carcinoma originating in congenital cysts of the liver. *Arch Pathol Lab Med* 166:105–107.

Popper H, Maltoni C, Selikoff IJ. (1980) Vinyl chloride–induced hepatic lesions in man and rodents. A comparison. *Liver* 1:7–20.

Popper H, Thomas LB, Telles NC, et al. (1978) Development of hepatic angiosarcoma induced by vinyl chloride, Thorotrast and arsenic: comparison with cases of unknown etiology. *Am J Pathol* 92:349–376.

Raoul JL, Darnault P, Deugnier Y, et al. (1987) L'adénome du foie chez l'homme: étude d'un cas et revue de la littérature. *Semin Hop Paris* 63:487–490.

Roncalli M, Borzio M, de Biagi G, et al. (1985) Liver cell dysplasia and hepatocellular carcinoma: a histological and immunohistochemical study. *Histopathology* 9:209–221.

Roncalli M, Borzio M, de Biagi G, et al. (1986) Liver cell dysplasia in cirrhosis. A serologic and immunohistochemical study. *Cancer* 57:1515–1521.

Roncalli M, Borzio M, Tombesi MV, et al. (1988) A morphometric study of liver cell dysplasia. *Hum Pathol* 19:471–474.

Ross JM. (1932) A case illustrating the effects of prolonged action of radium. *J Pathol Bacteriol* 35:899–912.

Rubin EM, De Rose PB, Cohen C. (1994) Comparative image cytometric DNA ploidy of liver cell dysplasia and hepatocellular carcinoma. *Mod Pathol* 7:677–680.

Sakamoto M, Hirohashi S, Shimosato Y. (1991) Early stages of multistep hepatocarcinogenesis: Adenomatous hyperplasia and early hepatocellular carcinoma. *Hum Pathol* 22:172–178.

Salgado M, Sans M, Forns X, et al. (1995) Angiosarcoma hepatica: presentacion de un caso asociado al tratamiento con sales de arsenico y revision de la literatura. *Gastroenterol Hepatol* 18:132–135.

Saul SH, Titelbaum DS, Gansler TS, et al. (1987) The fibrolamellar variant of hepatocellular carcinoma: its association with focal nodular hyperplasia. *Cancer* 60:3049–3055.

Saxena R, Humphreys S, Williams R, Portmann B. (1994): Nodular hyperplasia surrounding fibrolamellar carcinoma: a zone of arterialized hepatic parenchyma. *Histopathology* 25:275–278.

Schattenberg PJ, Totovic V, Gedigk P, Marsteller HJ. (1977) Die Ultrastruktur der Leberschadigung bei der chronischen Vinylchlorid-Intoxikation. *Virchows Arch Pathol Anat Histopathol* 373:233–247.

Selby DM, Stocker JT, Ishak KG. (1992) Angiosarcoma of the liver in childhood: A clinicopathologic and follow-up study in 10 cases. *Pediatr Pathol* 12:485–498.

Sell S. (1994) Liver stem cells. *Mod Pathol* 7:105–112.

Sell S. (1993) The role of determined stem-cells in the cellular lineage of hepatocellular carcinoma. *Int J Dev Biol* 37:189–201.

Sell S. (1998) Comparison of liver progenitor cells in human atypical ductular reactions with those seen in experimental models of liver injury. *Hepatology* 27:317–331.

Sell S, Dunsford HA. (1989) Evidence for the stem cell origin of hepatocellular carcinoma and cholangiocarcinoma. *Am J Pathol* 134:1347–1363.

Sirica A, Radaeva S, Caran N. (1997) NEU overexpression in the furan rat model of cholangiocarcinogenesis compared with biliary ductal cell hyperplasia. *Am J Pathol* 151:1685–1694.

Soe KL, Soe M, Gluud C. (1992) Liver pathology associated with the use of the anabolic-androgenic steroids. *Liver* 12:73–79.

Strate SM, Rutledge JC, Weinberg AG. (1984) Delayed development of angiosarcoma in multinodular infantile hepatic hemangioendothelioma. *Arch Pathol Lab Med* 106:943–944.

Stromeyer FW, Ishak KG. (1981) Nodular transformation (nodular regenerative hyperplasia) of the liver. A clinicopathologic study of 30 cases. *Hum Pathol* 12:60–71.

Su Q, Benner A, Hofmann WJ, et al. (1997) Human hepatic preneoplasia: phenotypes and proliferation kinetics of foci and nodules of altered hepatocytes and their relationship to liver cell dysplasia. *Virchows Arch* 431:391–406.

Sukerberg LR, Nickoloff BJ, Weiss SW. (1993) Kaposiform hemangioendothelioma of infancy and childhood: an aggressive neoplasm associated with Kasabach-Merritt syndrome and lymphangiomatosis. *Am J Surg Pathol* 17:321–328.

Tada M, Omata M, Ohto M. (1992) High incidence of ras gene mutation in intrahepatic cholangiocarcinoma. *Cancer* 69:1115–1118.

Takayama T, Makuuchi M, Hirohashi S, et al. (1990) Malignant transformation of adenomatous hyperplasia to hepatocellular carcinoma. *Lancet* 336:1150–1153.

Tamburro CH, Makk L, Popper H. (1984) Early hepatic histologic alterations among chemical (vinyl monomer) workers. *Hepatology* 4:413–418.

Tavani A, Negri E, Parazzini F, et al. (1993) Female hormone utilization and risk of hepatocellular carcinoma. *Br J Cancer* 67:635–637.

Terada T, Ashida K, Endo K, et al. (1998) C-erb B-2 protein is expressed in hepatolithiasis and cholangiocarcinoma. *Histopathology* 33:325–232.

Terada T, Hoso M, Nakanuma Y. (1989a) Mallory body clustering in adenomatous hyperplasia in human cirrhotic livers: report of four cases. *Hum Pathol* 20: 886–890.

Terada T, Kurumaya H, Nakanuma Y, et al. (1989b) Macroregenerative nodules of the liver in primary biliary cirrhosis: report of two autopsies. *Am J Gastroenterol* 84:418–421.

Terada T, Nakanuma Y. (1988) Morphological examination of intrahepatic bile ducts in hepatolithiasis. *Virchows Arch A Pathol Anat Histopathol* 413:167–176.

Terada T, Nakanuma Y. (1989) Survey of iron-accumulative macroregenerative nodules in cirrhotic livers. *Hepatology* 10:851–854.

Terada T, Nakanuma Y. (1990) Pathological observations of intrahepatic peribiliary glands in 1,000 consecutive autopsy livers. II. Possible source of cholangiocarcinoma. *Hepatology* 12:92–97.

Terada T, Nakanuma Y. (1991) Expression of ABH blood group antigens, receptors of Ulex europaeus' agglutinin 1, and factor VIII-related antigen on sinusoidal endothelial cells in adenomatous hyperplasia in human cirrhotic liver. *Hum Pathol* 22:486–493.

Terada T, Nakanuma Y, Hoso M, et al. (1988) Fatty macroregenerative nodule in non-steatotic liver cirrhosis. A morphologic study. *Virchows Arch A Pathol Anat Histopathol* 415:131–136.

Terada T, Nakanuma Y, Ohta G. (1987) Glandular elements around the intrahepatic bile ducts in man: their morphology and distribution in normal livers. *Liver* 7:1–8.

Terada T, Nakanuma Y, Ohta T, Nagakawa T. (1992) Histological features and interphase nucleolar organizer regions in hyperplastic, dysplastic and neoplastic epithelium of intrahepatic bile ducts in hepatolithiasis. *Histopathology* 21:233–240.

Terada T, Notsumata K, Nakanuma Y. (1994a) Biliary carcinosarcoma arising in nonparasitic cyst of the liver. *Virchows Arch* 424:331–335.

Terada T, Shimizu K, Izumi R, Nakanuma Y. (1994b) p53 expression in formalin-fixed, paraffin-embedded archival specimens of intrahepatic cholangiocarcinoma: retrieval of p53 antigenicity by microwave oven heating of tissue sections. *Mod Pathol* 7: 249–252.

Terris B, Ingster O, Rubbia L, et al. (1997) Interphase cytogenetic analysis reveals numerical chromosome aberrations in large liver cell dysplasia. *J Hepatol* 27:313–319.

Theise ND. (1995) Macroregenerative (dysplastic) nodules and hepatocarcinogenesis: Theoretical and clinical considerations. *Semin Liver Dis* 15:360–371.

Theise ND, Fiel IM, Hytiroglou P, et al. (1995) Macroregenerative nodules in cirrhosis are not associated with elevated serum or stainable tissue alpha-fetoprotein. *Liver* 15:30–34.

Theise ND, Lapook JD, Thung SN. (1993) A macroregenerative nodule containing multiple foci of hepatocellular carcinoma in a noncirrhotic liver. *Hepatology* 17:993–996.

Theise ND, Schwartz M, Miller C, Thung SN. (1992) Macroregenerative nodules and hepatocellular carcinoma in forty-four sequential adult liver explants with cirrhosis. *Hepatology* 16:949–955.

Thomas RM, Berman JJ, Yetter RA, et al. (1992) Liver cell dysplasia: a DNA aneuploid lesion with distinct morphologic features. *Hum Pathol* 23:496–503.

Thomas LB, Popper H, Berk PD, et al. (1975) Vinylchloride induced liver disease. From idiopathic portal hypertension (Banti's syndrome) to angiosarcomas. *N Engl J Med* 292:17–22.

Thorgeirrson SS. (1993) Hepatic stem cells. *Am J Pathol* 142:1331–1333.

Thysell H, Ingvar C, Gustafson T, Holmin T. (1986) Systemic reactive amyloidosis caused by hepatocellular adenoma: a case report. *J Hepatol* 2:450–457.

Tiniakos DG, Brunt EM. (1999) Proliferating cell nuclear antigen and Ki-67 labeling in hepatocellular nodules: a comparative study. *Liver* 19:58–68.

Tsang WYW, Chan JKC. (1991) Kaposi-like infantile hemangioendothelioma: a distinctive vascular neoplasm of the retroperitoneum. *Am J Surg Pathol* 15: 982–989.

Tsui WMS, Loo KT, Chow LTC, Tse CCH. (1993) Biliary adenofibroma: a heretofore unrecognized benign biliary tumor of the liver. *Am J Surg Pathol* 17: 186–192.

Uchida T, Miyata H, Shikata T. (1981) Human hepatocellular carcinoma and putative precancerous disorders. Their enzyme histochemical study. *Arch Pathol Lab Med* 105:180–186.

Ueda K, Matsui O, Nakanuma Y, et al. (1993) Deposition of copper and copper-binding protein (CBP) in adenomatous hyperplasia of the liver: relevance to magnetic resonance imaging. *Int Hepatol Commun* 1:326–330.

Ueyama T, Ding J, Hashimoto H, et al. (1992) Carcinoid tumor arising in the wall of a congenital bile duct cyst. *Arch Pathol Lab Med* 116:291–293.

Vecchio FM, Fabiano A, Ghirlanda G, et al. (1984) Fibrolamellar carcinoma of the liver: the malignant counterpart of focal nodular hyperplasia with oncocytic change. *Am J Clin Pathol* 81:521–526.

Voravud N, Foster CS, Gilbertson JA, et al. (1989) Oncogene expression in cholangiocarcinoma and in normal hepatic development. *Hum Pathol* 20:1163–1168.

Wada K, Kondo F, Kondo Y. (1988) Large regenerative nodules and dysplastic nodules in cirrhotic livers: a histopathologic study. *Hepatology* 8:1684–1688.

Watanabe S, Okita K, Harada T, et al. (1983) Morphologic studies of the liver cell dysplasia. *Cancer* 51: 2197–2205.

Weinberg AG, Finegold MJ. (1993) Primary hepatic tumors of childhood. *Hum Pathol* 14:512–537.

Westaby D, Portmann B, Williams R. (1983) Androgen related primary hepatic tumors in non-Fanconi patients. *Cancer* 51:1947–1983.

Woods GL. (1981) Biliary cystadenocarcinoma: case report of hepatic malignancy originating in benign cystadenoma. *Cancer* 47:2936–2940.

Yamashita A. (1996) Comparison of the proliferative capacity of adenomatous hyperplasia and well differentiated hepatocellular carcinoma. *J Gastroenterol* 31:373–378.

Yokoi T, Tsuzuki T, Yatabe Y, et al. (1998) Solitary fibrous tumour: significance of p53 and CD34 immunoreactivity in its malignant transformation. *Histopathology* 423–432.

Zhao M, Zhang N-X, Economou M, et al. (1994) Immunohistochemical detection of bcl-2 protein in liver cell lesions: bcl-2 protein is expressed in hepatocellular carcinomas but not in liver cell dysplasia. *Histopathology* 25:237–245.

12

GALLBLADDER, EXTRAHEPATIC BILE DUCTS, AND AMPULLA OF VATER

Jorge Albores-Saavedra and Donald Earl Henson

Carcinoma of the gallbladder is a major cause of death among the populations of many countries (Albores-Saavedra et al., 2000). In the general population of the United States, where the mortality rate is considered low, this cancer is responsible for 3,400 deaths per year (Gremlee et al., 2000). For many years, the early changes in the development of invasive carcinoma of the gallbladder were virtually unknown. Two reasons can explain the late recognition of these changes: *(1)* invasive carcinoma of the gallbladder is uncommon in many countries, consequently, few pathologists have had the opportunity to study the precursor lesions; and *(2)* although foci of dysplasia and carcinoma *in situ* are found adjacent to most invasive carcinomas of the gallbladder, multiple sections are needed for identification. In some cases, however, despite extensive sampling, dysplasia and carcinoma *in situ* cannot be identified because they have been obliterated by the invasive carcinomas of the gallbladder. In recent years, a study of multiple sections of gallbladders excised for cholelithiasis, examination of the mucosa adjacent to invasive carcinomas, and cytologic studies of bile obtained from cholecystectomy specimens have allowed the characterization of dysplasia and carcinoma *in situ* (Albores-Saavedra et al., 1980; Alonso de Ruiz et al., 1982; Laitio, 1983a; Laitio, 1983b,c). Moreover, the histologic criteria for the diagnosis of epithelial atypia secondary to repair, which is often seen in acute and chronic cholecystitis, have been established. Differentiation of this atypia from true dysplasia and carcinoma *in situ*, once thought to be quite difficult, is now possible (Albores-Saavedra et al., 1984).

Carcinoma of the gallbladder is often associated with the presence of stones, a correlation first observed over 100 years ago. Despite the association of gallbladder cancer with a preexisting benign disease, early diagnosis of the cancer is difficult. Many cases are not suspected clinically and are first discovered during exploratory laparotomy. Most of the *in situ* carcinomas are incidentally found in gallbladders removed for lithiasis. We should emphasize that for early diagnosis, dysplasia and carcinoma *in situ* can be recognized by cytologic examination of bile collected by gallbladder puncture, a procedure that is not hazardous. Complications are minimal and usually resolve with conservative management (Ropertz and Wagner, 1976). Correct preoperative diagnosis and treatment of these precursor lesions not only prevent progression but also may reduce the incidence of invasive carcinoma.

DYSPLASIA AND CARCINOMA *IN SITU* OF THE GALLBLADDER

The frequency of dysplasia and carcinoma *in situ* of the gallbladder reflects that of invasive carcinoma. In countries in which carcinoma of the gallbladder is endemic, the prevalence of dysplasia and carcinoma *in situ* is higher than in countries in which this tumor is sporadic. Studies from different countries have shown that the incidence of high-grade dysplasia or carcinoma *in situ* in gallbladders with lithiasis has varied from 0.5% to 3% (Ojeda, 1985). This variation in the incidence of dysplasia and carcinoma *in situ* is also attributable to other factors, such as lack of uniformity in morphologic criteria applied for these lesions and sampling methods. Gallbladder dysplasia has also been reported in patients with familial adenomatous polyposis (Nugent 1994).

Dysplasia and carcinoma *in situ* are usually not recognized on macroscopic examination because they often occur in association with chronic cholecystitis. Grossly, no distinctive features will alert the pathologist to the presence of these two lesions. The mucosa may appear granular, nodular, plaque-like, or trabeculated. The papillary type of dysplasia or carcinoma *in situ* usually appears as a small, cauliflower-like excrescence that projects into the lumen and can be recognized on close inspection. However, in most cases of dysplasia and carcinoma *in situ*, the gallbladder shows only a thickened and indurated wall, the result of chronic inflammation and fibrosis.

Microscopically, two types of dysplasia and carcinoma *in situ* are recognized: papillary and flat, the latter being more common. The papillary type is characterized by short fibrovascular stalks that are covered by dysplastic or neoplastic cells.

Dysplasia and carcinoma *in situ* usually begin on the surface epithelium and subsequently extend downward into the Rokitansky-Aschoff sinuses and into metaplastic pyloric glands (Yamaguchi, 1992; Yamamoto, 1989). Columnar, cuboidal, and elongated cells with variable degrees of nuclear atypia, loss of polarity, and occasional mitotic figures characterize dysplasia. The dysplastic cells are usually arranged in a single layer. However, because of cellular proliferation and nuclear crowding, pseudostratification often occurs (Figs. 12–1, 12–2, and 12–3). Later, dysplastic cells may extend into epithelial invaginations and even into metaplastic antral-type glands (Fig. 12–4) or may grow outward and cover small fibrovascular stalks that protrude into the lumen. The

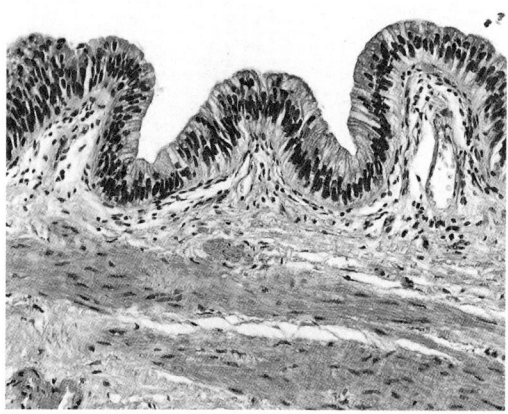

Figure 12–1. Mild (low-grade) dysplasia. The enlarged, elongated, mildly hyperchromatic nuclei are pseudostratified and some are not basally located.

large nuclei of dysplastic cells may be round, oval, or fusiform, with one or two nucleoli that are more prominent than those of normal cells. The cytoplasm usually stains eosinophilic and contains nonsulfated acid and neutral mucin. Goblet cells are found in one-third of cases. An abrupt transition between normal-appearing columnar cells and dysplastic epithelium is seen in nearly all cases, which is an important clue for the differential diagnosis of dysplasia. In general, the cell population of dysplasia is homogeneous, unlike the heterogeneous cell population of the epithelial atypia of repair.

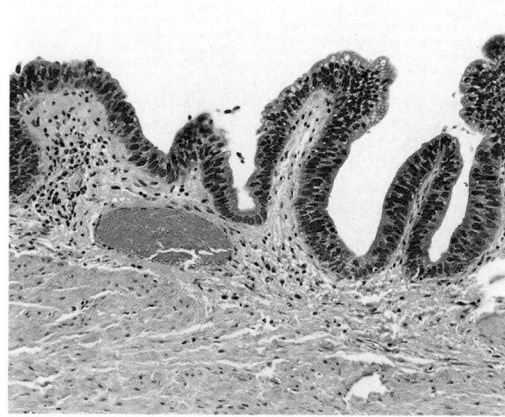

Figure 12–2. Severe (high-grade) dysplasia. The columnar cells show elongated, hyperchromatic, and pseudostratified nuclei.

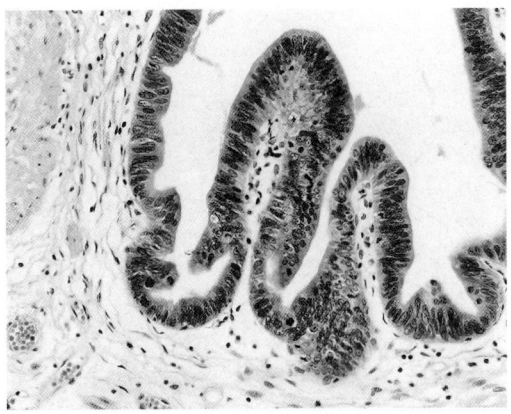

Figure 12–3. High-grade dysplasia. The surface epithelium shows nuclear enlargement and hyperchromatism.

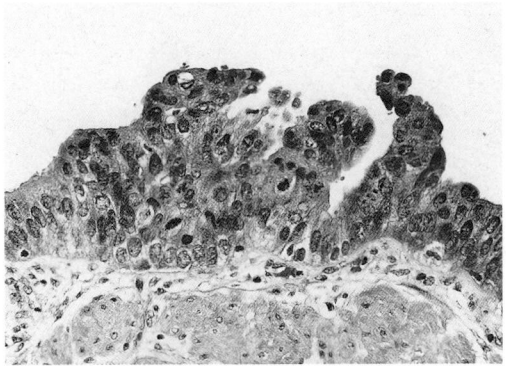

Figure 12–5. Carcinoma *in situ.* The epithelial lining is highly atypical. The cells are pseudostratified and have large, bizarre, hyperchromatic nuclei, some with prominent nucleoli. Mitotic figures are present.

In many cases, the dysplastic lesions are continuous with areas of carcinoma *in situ,* although normal-appearing epithelium may separate the two. Widespread involvement of the mucosa by dysplasia and *in situ* carcinoma often occurs. For this reason, we have suggested that some, if not most, invasive carcinomas of the gallbladder arise from a field change within the epithelium (Albores-Saavedra et al., 2000).

Cells from carcinoma *in situ* have all the cytologic features of malignancy. Because of the excessive cellular proliferation, mitotic figures are more common and nuclear crowding and pseudostratification are more prominent in cases of carcinoma *in situ* than in cases of dysplasia (Figs. 12–5 and 12–6).

Neoplastic cells first appear along the surface epithelium and later spread into the epithelial invaginations and antral-type metaplastic glands. In the late stages of carcinoma *in situ,* the histologic picture is that of back-to-back glands located in the lamina propria but often connected with the surface epithelium. However, not all *in situ* carcinomas exhibit this type of growth pattern.

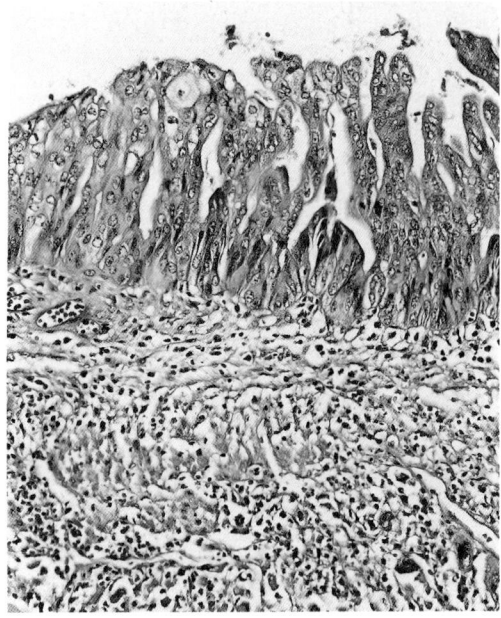

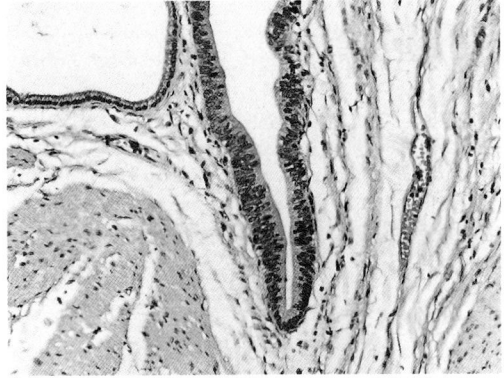

Figure 12–4. Highly dysplastic cells extend into an epithelial invagination (Rokitansky-Aschoff sinus).

Figure 12–6. Carcinoma *in situ.* The normal lining epithelium is replaced by carcinoma cells that are stratified and form micropapillary structures.

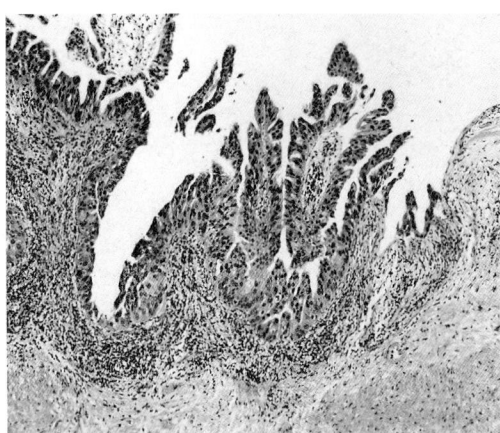

Figure 12–7. This *in situ* papillary carcinoma shows a dense lymphocytic infiltrate in the lamina propria.

Some show distinctive papillary features with small fibrovascular stalks lined by neoplastic cells (Figs. 12–7 and 12–8). Not infrequently, a combination of these growth patterns is seen.

UNUSUAL HISTOLOGIC VARIANTS OF CARCINOMA IN SITU

An *in situ* carcinoma composed of goblet cells, columnar cells, Paneth's cells, and endocrine cells has been described. The endocrine cells are argyrophil and chromogranin positive (Fig. 12–9; Albores-Saavedra et al., 2000). It is assumed that this lesion represents the *in situ* phase of the tumor des-

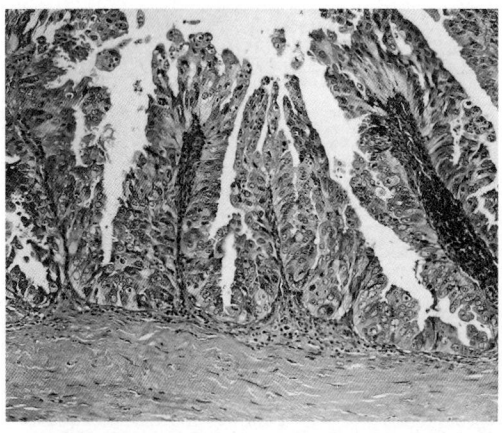

Figure 12–8. Papillary carcinoma *in situ*. Papillary structures are lined by neoplastic cells with vesicular nuclei and prominent nucleoli.

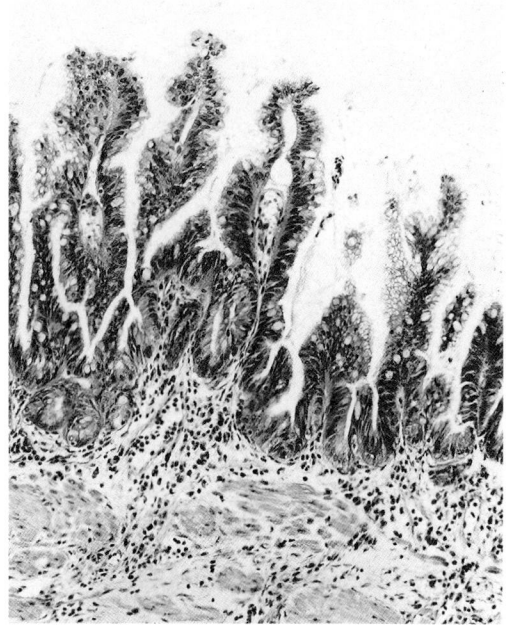

Figure 12–9. Intestinal-type carcinoma *in situ*. This papillary *in situ* carcinoma is composed of columnar cells, and goblet and Paneth cells, the latter of which are difficult to recognize at this low power. Endocrine cells were demonstrated with silver stains.

ignated *intestinal-type adenocarcinoma*, because both the infiltrating and the intraepithelial forms have the same cell population (Albores-Saavedra et al., 1986a, 2000). Goblet cells may also be a component of the ordinary type of carcinoma *in situ*. Their presence is regarded as an example of intestinal differentiation occurring within the neoplastic epithelium.

Another type of *in situ* intestinal carcinoma is composed of cells closely resembling those of colonic carcinomas at the light and electron microscopic levels. The neoplastic columnar cells extend into the epithelial invaginations and the antral-type glands. This tumor also has scattered endocrine cells, most of which contain serotonin. These cells can be demonstrated with the Grimelius or immunoperoxidase techniques.

Two examples of signet-ring cell carcinoma confined to the surface epithelium and to the epithelial invaginations of the gallbladder have been reported (Albores-Saavedra et al., 1996; Figs. 12–10 and 12–11).

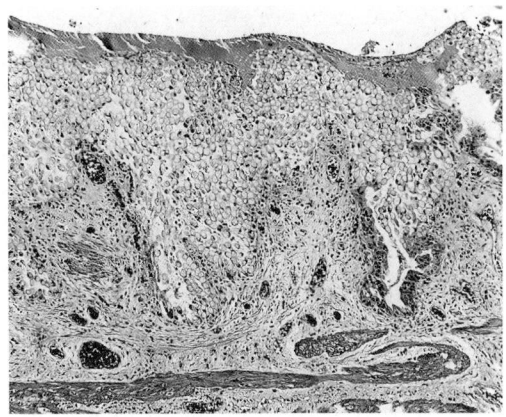

Figure 12–10. Signet-ring cell carcinoma *in situ.* The neoplastic cells are confined to the mucosa.

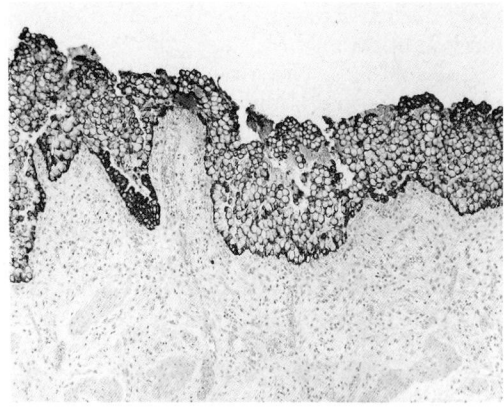

Figure 12–12. Neoplastic signet ring cells show cytokeratin reactivity. Similar reactivity was obtained with CEA.

The signet ring cells showed reactivity for cytokeratin and carcinoembryonic antigen (CEA) (Fig. 12–12). Despite examination of multiple sections, stromal invasion was not found. These *in situ* signet-ring cell carcinomas represented incidental findings in cholecystectomy specimens and were cytologically similar to those reported in the stomach. This unusual form of carcinoma *in situ* should be distinguished from epithelial cells that acquire signet-ring cell morphology when desquamated within the lumen of dilated metaplastic pyloric glands in cases of chronic cholecystitis. These CEA-negative cells are often poorly preserved, lack nuclear atypia, and appear floating with other de-

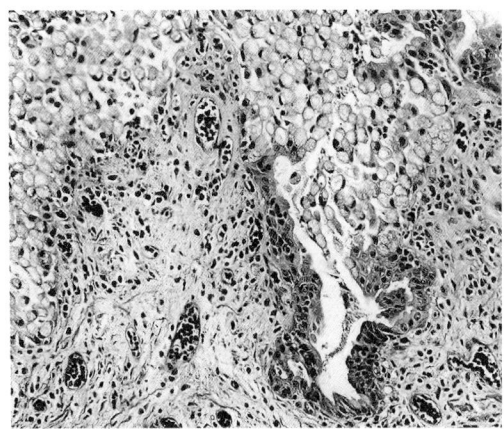

Figure 12–11. Signet-ring cell carcinoma *in situ* with detail of neoplastic signet ring cells extending into an epithelial invagination.

generating epithelial and inflammatory cells. Likewise, mucin-containing histiocytes (muciphages) that are occasionally seen in mucoceles of the gallbladder may simulate signet-ring cell carcinoma *in situ.* These muciphages however, are cytokeratin and CEA negative.

The mucosa adjacent to pure squamous cell carcinomas of the gallbladder often shows areas of squamous metaplasia, dysplasia, and carcinoma *in situ* (Albores-Saavedra et al., 2000). It seems, therefore, that these squamous cell carcinomas, which are unusual in the gallbladder, undergo the same pathologic changes in their development as those arising in other sites (Albores-Saavedra et al., 1991).

The morphological type of *in situ* carcinoma does not always correspond with that of the invasive carcinoma. For example, we have seen conventional adenocarcinoma *in situ* in the mucosa adjacent to invasive squamous cell carcinomas, small cell carcinomas, and undifferentiated carcinomas of spindle and giant cell type.

The wall of the gallbladder with dysplasia or carcinoma *in situ* usually shows variable inflammatory changes. As expected, the most common type of inflammatory response is chronic, with a predominance of lymphocytes and plasma cells, although xanthogranulomatous inflammation or even an acute inflammatory reaction may be present. In some cases, lymphoid follicles with germinal centers may even be seen in the lamina propria and muscle layer. Reactive epithelial atypia is discussed under differential diagnosis.

If dysplasia or carcinoma *in situ* is found, multiple sections should be examined to exclude invasive cancer. Cholecystectomy is a curative surgical procedure for patients with *in situ* carcinoma or with carcinoma extending into the lamina propria.

DIFFERENTIAL DIAGNOSIS

The differential diagnosis between severe dysplasia and carcinoma *in situ* is difficult and often impossible in many cases. This is not important because the two lesions, which vary only in degree histologically, are closely related biologically. However, differentiation of dysplasia or carcinoma *in situ* from the epithelial atypia of repair is of great clinical significance because the last lesion does not progress to carcinoma. The atypia of repair consists of a heterogeneous cell population in which columnar mucus-secreting cells, low cuboidal cells, atrophic-appearing epithelium, and pencil-like cells are present. In addition, there is a gradual transition of the cellular abnormalities, in contrast with the abrupt transition seen in dysplasia and carcinoma *in situ*. Finally, the extent of nuclear atypia is usually less pronounced in the epithelial atypia of repair than in dysplasia or in carcinoma *in situ* (Fig. 12–13).

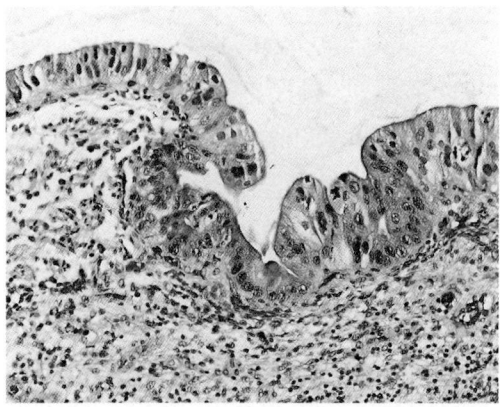

Figure 12–13. Reactive epithelial atypia mimicking dysplasia. The heterogeneity of the cell population and the presence of intraepithelial polymorphonuclear leukocytes are suggestive of reactive atypia.

IMMUNOHISTOCHEMISTRY AND MOLECULAR PATHOLOGY

By immunohistochemical methods it has been shown that dysplasia and carcinoma *in situ* are immunoreactive for polyclonal and monoclonal CEA (Albores-Saavedra et al., 1983) and for the carbohydrate antigen CA19-9 (Yamaguchi and Enjoji, 1988). The reactivity is usually focal and displays a linear pattern along the apical cytoplasmic border. However, faint cytoplasmic staining is also seen mainly with CEA. This oncofetal antigen can also be detected in both the bile and in the serum, but an elevated CEA level is not diagnostic of dysplasia or carcinoma because extrahepatic bile duct obstruction from any cause also leads to a rise. The lack of specificity of CEA limits its use in the diagnosis of early carcinoma of the gallbladder. Recent studies have shown a crucial role of *p53* gene mutations in the early pathogenesis of gallbladder carcinoma. By immunohistochemistry, p53 nuclear staining was found in 32% of dysplasias and in 44% of *in situ* carcinomas (Wistuba et al., 1996). Genetic analysis has shown a high incidence of loss of heterozygosity (LOH) at the *p53* gene, in both dysplasia (58%) and carcinoma *in situ* (85%). Other molecular abnormalities include LOH at 9p and 8p loci and the *18q* gene. These molecular abnormalities are also early events and most likely contributing factors in the pathogenesis of gallbladder carcinoma (Wistuba et al., 1995). However, K-*ras* mutations were not detected in dysplasia or carcinoma *in situ* (Wistuba et al., 1995).

NATURAL HISTORY

Little is known about the natural history of dysplasia and carcinoma *in situ* of the gallbladder. Most of these lesions are diagnosed after cholecystectomy and the entire lesion removed. This is a limiting factor in the study of their rate of progression. Similarly, the proportion of invasive carcinomas that pass through the sequence of dysplasia and carcinoma *in situ* is unknown. However, there is evidence that progression from *in situ* to infiltrating carcinoma does occur. For instance, when *in situ* carcinomas were studied by subserial sections, foci of microinvasion were found in the lamina propria continuous with the overlying carcinoma *in situ* (Albores-Saavedra et al., 1984). Dysplasia and carcinoma *in situ* are seen in the areas of intact mucosa that are found adjacent to nearly all invasive carcinomas. These two changes do not represent lateral neoplastic growth because normal or metaplastic epithelium is often seen between the invasive and the *in situ* carcinomas. Dysplasia and carcinoma *in situ* are most often found in the fundus and body, the areas of the gallbladder from which most carcinomas arise. Finally, patients with dysplasia and carcinoma *in situ* are 5 years younger than those with invasive carcinoma (Albores-Saavedra et al., 1980).

ADENOMAS AS POSSIBLE CANCER PRECURSORS

Adenomas of the gallbladder are uncommon benign neoplasms of glandular epithelium that are usually polypoid and well demarcated. They are found in 0.3% to 0.5% of gallbladders removed for cholelithiasis. According to their growth pattern, adenomas of the gallbladder are divided into three categories: *tubular*, *papillary*, and *tubulopapillary*. Cytologically they are classified as *pyloric gland* type, *intestinal* type, and *biliary* type (Figs. 12–14 and 12–15). The tubular pyloric gland type is the most common adenoma of the gallbladder.

In recent years, the role played by adenomas of the gallbladder as possible precursors to invasive cancer has been investigated. Some authors have claimed that the adenoma–carcinoma sequence is the usual route for the development of invasive carcinomas of the gallbladder. Kosuka and associates (1982), for example, based their conclusion on the fact that they were able to demonstrate the remnants of an adenoma in 15 of 79 invasive carcinomas.

We are inclined to believe, however, that what these authors were describing is only the well-differentiated component of some adenocarcinomas. It is therefore possible that most of these adenomas that allegedly gave rise to malignant tumors were carcinomas from the beginning. Well-differentiated adenocarcinomas, including the papillary

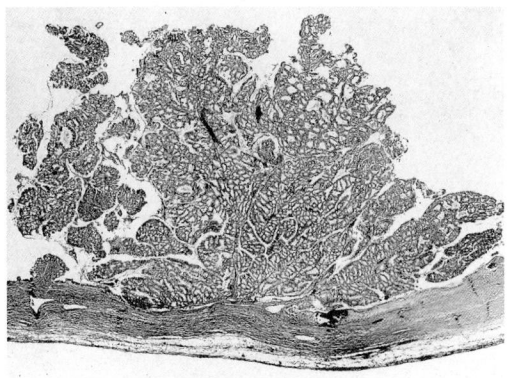

A

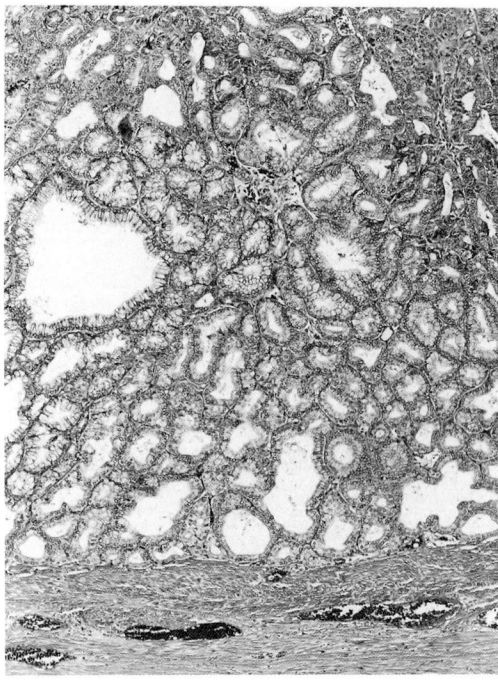

B

Figure 12–14. *A:* Pyloric gland adenoma. Low-power view shows a sessile tubular adenoma of pyloric gland type. *B:* Higher magnification shows closely packed tubular glands, some of which are cystically dilated.

type, usually exhibit a broad morphologic spectrum with areas that may simulate an adenoma or even normal epithelium. Furthermore, hyperplasia of antral-type glands, which often coexists with carcinoma, may easily be confused with the residua of a tubular adenoma. In more than 600 carcinomas of the gallbladder, we were able to find rem-

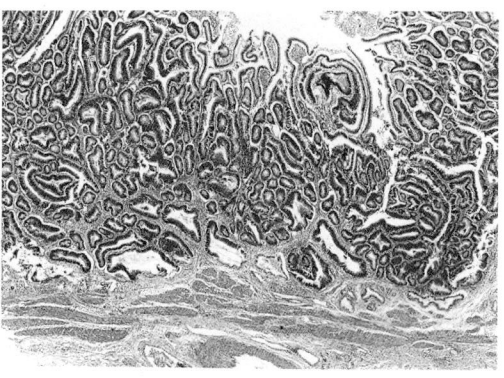

Figure 12–15. Tubular adenoma of intestinal type of the gallbladder. The glands are similar to those of colonic adenomas.

nants of tubular or papillary adenomas in less than 5% of the cases. Intestinal and pyloric gland type adenomas, however, may rarely contain foci of high-grade dysplasia, carcinoma *in situ*, and invasive cancer (Fig. 12–16).

A detailed study of 35 cases of early carcinoma (larger than 5 mm) and 16 microcarcinomas (up to 5 mm in greatest diameter)

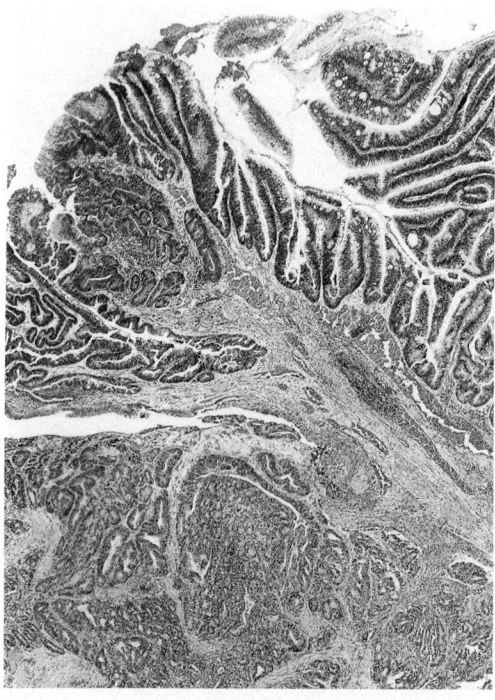

Figure 12–16. Moderately differentiated invasive adenocarcinoma that arose in a papillary adenoma of intestinal type.

of the gallbladder revealed that only 7 (13.7%) arose in adenomas (Kijima et al., 1989). Since most of the carcinomatous changes were confined to the adenomas and did not invade the wall of the gallbladder, they can be regarded as *in situ* carcinomas within adenomas. We have seen only four examples of invasive adenocarcinomas arising in both tubular and papillary adenomas. As in the stomach, dysplasia and carcinoma *in situ* in the nonpolypoid mucosa are the main precancerous lesions in the gallbladder and bile ducts, whereas only a small number of carcinomas appear to arise from preexisting adenomas.

The molecular abnormalities of adenomas of the gallbladder differ from those of carcinomas. Of 16 adenomas, 14 pyloric and 2 intestinal, subjected to genetic analysis, none showed *p53* and *p16* Ink 4/CD k2a mutations, which are the most common and sometimes the only molecular abnormalities in carcinomas. Four of the 16 adenomas (25%) had K-*ras* mutations, which are considered rare and late events in the pathogenesis of carcinomas of the gallbladder (Wistuba et al., 1998). These observations suggest that the molecular pathways involved in the pathogenesis of adenomas and carcinomas are different.

Finally, it would be difficult to accept adenomas as the precursors of most adenocarcinomas of the gallbladder because the latter are more common than the former (Albores-Saavedra and Henson, 1986; Chan, 1988). In all other anatomic sites, the opposite is true: the precursor lesions are more common than the corresponding invasive cancers.

METAPLASIA AND CARCINOMA OF THE GALLBLADDER

It has long been established that carcinomas of the gallbladder are often associated with cholelithiasis and that chronic irritation caused by the presence of stones can induce a variety of metaplastic changes in the mucosa (Laitio, 1985). Consequently, dysplasia and carcinoma of the gallbladder nearly always arise in an abnormal mucosa (Black, 1980). Pyloric-type glands, intestinal cells, and superficial gastric-type epithelium are the metaplastic changes most commonly seen (Fig. 12–17; Laitio, 1985). Other types of metaplastic changes, which are quite rare, include the development of squamous epithelium and fundic-type gastric mucosa. Two or more metaplastic changes may even be seen in the same gallbladder. Because cholelithiasis causes cell proliferation in the epithelium (Putz and Willems, 1978), it has been postulated that it also stimulates the appearance of endodermal stem cells that can differentiate in several directions, thereby giving rise to cells with intestinal, gastric, or squamous phenotypes (Albores-Saavedra et al., 1986b).

These metaplastic changes are first seen on the tips of the mucosal folds, an area that may represent the stem cell zone of the gallbladder epithelium. The metaplastic pyloric and intestinal glands are usually confined to the lamina propria but may extend into the muscular wall and serosa. Moreover, perineural invasion by metaplastic pyloric glands can rarely occur. This lesion can be confused with adenocarcinoma, a mistake that may have serious therapeutic implications.

Because intestinal-type carcinomas of the gallbladder have the same cell population as intestinal metaplasia and both lesions often coexist in the same specimen, it is possible that these tumors originate from the metaplastic intestinal cells (Albores-Saavedra et al., 1988). However, it is possible that the same stem cell that differentiates into cells with mature intestinal phenotypes may become neoplastic, thus eventually giving rise to the intestinal-type carcinomas. Previously, we gave reasons why we consider squamous cell metaplasia to be the precursor to squamous cell carcinoma. Pyloric-type glands may show dysplastic and *in situ* changes that may be independent of those of the surface epithelium.

PROGNOSIS

As in other sites, a continuum of cellular abnormalities occurs in the gallbladder epithelium during neoplastic transformation. At present, the evidence indicates that the neoplastic change begins along the surface epithelium and later extends into the epithelial invaginations or Rokitansky-Aschoff sinuses and pyloric-type metaplastic glands located in the lamina propria. In the gallbladder, *in situ* carcinoma are classified as "TisN0M0". Cancer that has extended into the lamina propria or muscle layer is designated "T1N0M0". Infiltration of the perimuscular connective tissue or serosa, "T2N0M0", occurs later and is of great clinical significance because these layers contain many lymphatic and blood vessels that facilitate metastasis. In addition, the perimuscular connective tissue is so close to the liver that direct extension is almost unavoidable. As expected, carcinoma *in situ* is cured by cholecystectomy alone. Patients with stage TI carcinoma have high survival rates. However, it is important to recognize that a small proportion of these patients will eventually develop lymph node and liver metastases. After the tumor has spread beyond the serosa to adjacent organs—"T3N0M0" or "T4N0M0"—the prognosis is very poor. Survival is usually measured in months (Henson et al., 1992).

The correlation that exists between pathologic stage and survival in cases of gallbladder carcinoma should encourage pathologists to include the information about extent of disease in their reports.

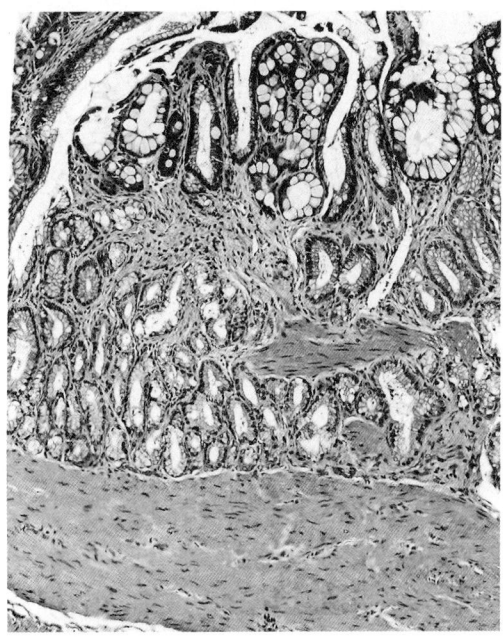

Figure 12–17. Intestinal and pyloric gland metaplasia of the gallbladder.

CANCER DISCOVERED AFTER LAPAROSCOPIC CHOLECYSTECTOMY

Occasionally, invasive carcinoma is found in gallbladders removed by laparoscopic surgery. Not recognized clinically or by imaging techniques, tumor is discovered during pathologic evaluation of the resected specimen. In these cases, the surgeon usually does not request an intraoperative consultation. An alarming consequence is tumor spillage with seeding along the endoscopic tract or intraabdominal dissemination (Fong et al., 1993). Tumor has also implanted in the umbilicus (Baer et al., 1995; Clair et al., 1982; Nally and Preshaw, 1994). Even carcinoma *in situ* can be implanted if the organ is torn during dissection (Wibbenmeyer et al., 1995). Because of these complications, it has been proposed that patients with radiographic gallbladder changes suggestive of carcinoma or with suspicious lesions of malignancy noted during laparoscopic cholecystectomy should undergo an open cholecystectomy (Wibbenmeyer et al., 1995).

Since few patients with carcinoma confined to the gallbladder are correctly diagnosed preoperatively and as laparoscopic cholecystectomy becomes more widely used, pathologists can expect more cases of early gallbladder cancer resected by this surgical procedure. The utility of surgical reexploration following a diagnosis of invasive carcinoma in a laparoscopic cholecystectomy specimen has recently been addressed (Fong et al., 1998). The survival rate of 16 patients with T2 and T3 tumors subjected to subsequent segmental liver resection and portal lymphadenectomy was better than that of patients in whom this surgical procedure was not possible because of tumor dissemination. However, larger series and longer follow-up are needed to determine whether the second surgical procedure improves the survival in these patients.

DYSPLASIA AND CARCINOMA *IN SITU* OF THE EXTRAHEPATIC BILE DUCTS

Morphologic studies concerning the precursor lesions of invasive carcinoma of the extrahepatic bile ducts are almost nonexistent. A large proportion of these tumors are unresectable at the time of diagnosis. In these cases, a small biopsy is usually taken for histologic confirmation. As a rule, the biopsy specimen does not include adjacent noninvolved mucosa. At autopsy, however, these carcinomas, with the possible exception of the papillary type, are quite large and have invaded the adjacent mucosa, obliterating all precursor changes. Another limitation in the study of these lesions is the lack of clinical markers that can be used to identify patients at risk for carcinoma of the extrahepatic bile ducts. These tumors, contrary to those that arise in the gallbladder, are usually not associated with cholelithiasis or choledocholithiasis. In fact, the incidence of cholelithiasis coexisting with carcinoma of the extrahepatic bile ducts is no greater than the expected prevalence of gallstones in the general population. Moreover, there are no known genetic syndromes that increase the risk for cancer of the extrahepatic bile ducts. Occasionally, there are reports of carcinoma of the extrahepatic ductal system occurring in patients with familial polyposis of the colon (Lees and Hermann, 1981). A more significant finding appears to be the association of bile duct carcinoma with ulcerative colitis (Harvath et al., 1989; Ross and Braasch, 1973). Bile duct carcinoma is also a complication of long-standing primary sclerosing cholangitis (Chapman et al., 1981; Wiesner et al., 1985). Dysplastic change have been reported in the bile ducts of patients with primary sclerosing cholangitis (Ludwig et al., 1992). However, until the predisposing factors for extrahepatic bile duct carcinoma are further delineated, a systematic search for the precursor lesions is not practical.

With the wider use of cholangiography, computed tomography, and ultrasonography, an increasing number of relatively small carcinomas of the extrahepatic bile ducts have been found and excised, along with fragments of normal-appearing mucosa. Histologic examination of the latter has revealed cellular abnormalities that have been interpreted as dysplasia or carcinoma *in situ* and that essentially show the same cell composition and architectural changes as similar lesions occurring in the gallbladder (Albores-Saavedra and Henson, 1986; Laitio, 1983a). The dysplastic and neoplastic cells

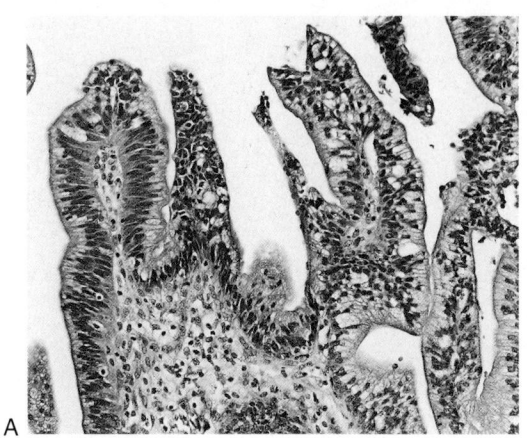
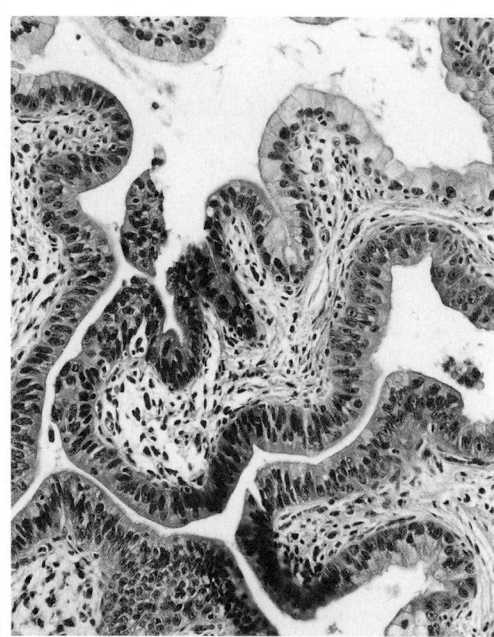

Figure 12–18. Dysplasia of common bile duct. *A:* The dysplastic cells line small papillary structures. *B:* The dysplastic cells extend into the sacculi of Beale.

are first demonstrated on the surface epithelium and subsequently extend downward into the sacculi of Beale and intramural
glands. The neoplastic cells may also project
into the lumen as small papillary structures.
(Figs. 12–18 and 12–19).

In an elegant computer-assisted, three-dimensional reconstruction of the biliary tree
from 12 patients with bile duct carcinoma,
Suzuki et al. (1989) demonstrated multiple

foci of dysplasia in 75% of cases and carcinoma *in situ* in 42%. On the basis of these
findings, the authors concluded that bile
duct carcinomas evolve through a dysplasia–carcinoma *in situ* sequence.

Dysplasia and carcinoma *in situ* may arise
in a background of metaplasia. The most
common metaplastic changes encountered
in the mucosa consist of antral-type glands
and, less frequently, cells that express in-

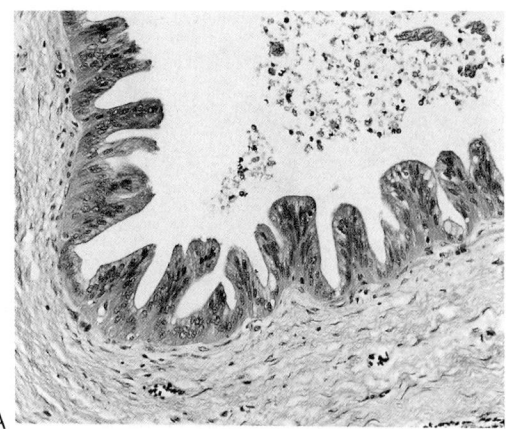
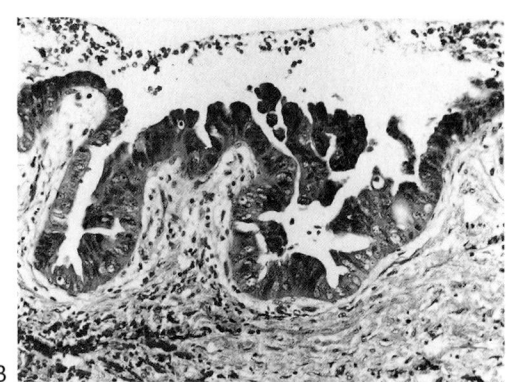

Figure 12–19. Carcinoma *in situ* of common bile duct. *A:* The neoplastic cells form micropapillary structures. *B:* The lining cells show marked nuclear atypia.

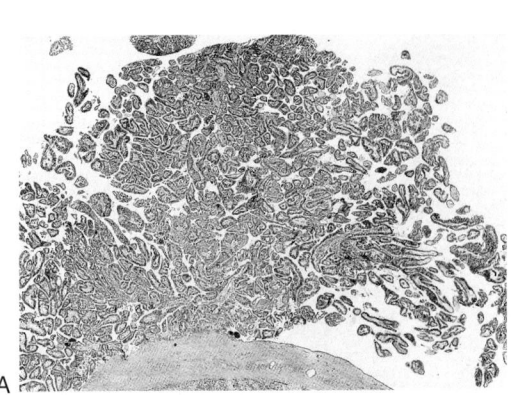
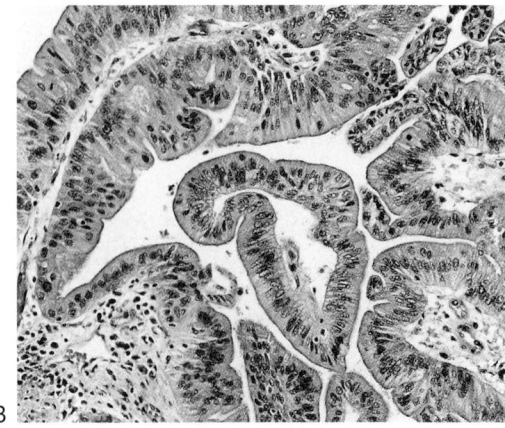

Figure 12–20. *A:* Noninvasive papillary carcinoma of common bile duct. *B:* The papillary structures are lined by columnar biliary-type epithelium.

testinal phenotypes, such as goblet cells and endocrine cells.

In some cases, we have seen carcinoma *in situ* at the margin of resection, which was at a considerable distance from the primary tumor. Residual carcinoma *in situ* at the margins of resection may explain some of the recurrences in the stump of the bile ducts. The mucin and CEA contents of these cells are similar to those described for the gallbladder. Independent foci of carcinoma *in situ* are often seen, which again seems to reflect a multicentric origin for cancers arising in the extrahepatic bile ducts.

Noninvasive or minimally invasive papillary carcinomas of the extrahepatic bile ducts fall into the category of incipient neoplasia because they behave as *in situ* lesions (Albores-Saavedra et al., 2000). We have followed 9 patients, four with noninvasive and five with minimally invasive papillary carcinomas of the common bile duct (Fig. 12–20). All patients except one are alive and symptom-free 1 to 13 years after surgery. One patient died of postoperative complications.

DIFFERENTIAL DIAGNOSIS

Dysplasia and carcinoma *in situ* should be distinguished from reactive atypia, which occurs in a number of situations. If, for instance, a stent has been left in the common bile duct for longer than 2 weeks, reactive atypia is often prominent. Inflammatory diseases, such as primary and secondary sclerosing cholangitis, may also cause atypical reactive changes in the epithelium. Impacted stones are another cause of reactive atypia. In contrast to dysplasia and carcinoma *in situ*, atypical reactive cells are heterogenous; they may be cuboidal or columnar and have a clear or basophilic cytoplasm (Figs. 12–21). The nuclei are usually vesicular and contain prominent nucleoli. Pseudostratification and even pseudocribriform structures are common. A variable number of normal mitotic figures are present. More importantly, atypical reactive cells may extend into the intramural glands, which can cause confusion with invasive cancer. It is advisable to avoid a diagnosis of dysplasia or carcinoma *in situ* in areas with extensive inflammatory changes. In small endoscopic biopsies, the distinction be-

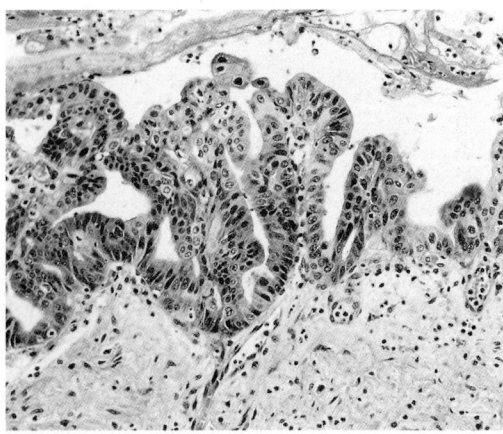

Figure 12–21. Reactive atypia of common bile duct with micropapillary features.

tween reactive atypia and dysplasia or carcinoma *in situ* may be impossible.

THE ADENOMA–CARCINOMA SEQUENCE

In contrast to the ampulla of Vater, where adenomas are considered precursors of a significant proportion of adenocarcinomas, solitary adenomas (tubular or papillary) of the extrahepatic bile ducts do not play a major role in the development of invasive carcinoma. Certainly, most clinical and pathological observations do not support the adenoma–carcinoma sequence. The finding of an "adenomatous residue" by some authors (Kosuka et al., 1984) can be explained, as in the gallbladder, by the broad morphologic spectrum of these tumors, most of which contain a well-differentiated component, as well as by the presence of metaplastic antral-type glands. Further complicating the interpretation is the fact that these glands may even show dysplastic and *in situ* changes. Intestinal-type adenomas rarely show foci of adenocarcinoma *in situ* and some may become invasive (Fig. 12–22).

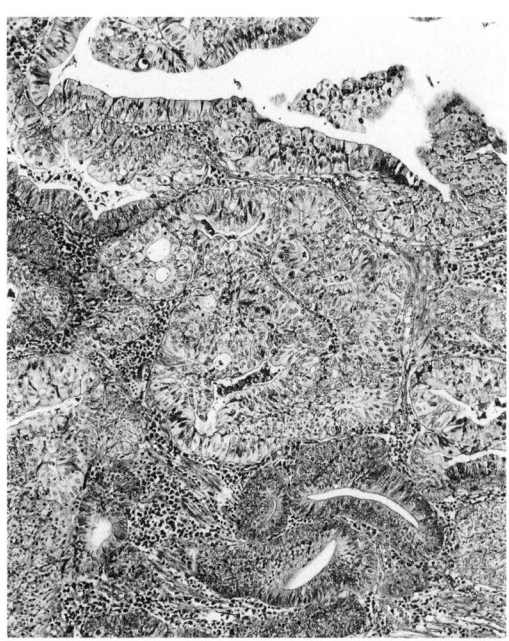

Figure 12–22. Focus of carcinoma *in situ* in a papillary adenoma of intestinal type that arose in the common bile duct. The highly dysplastic glands are closely packed and form small cubiform structures.

CYSTADENOMA AS A CANCER PRECURSOR

Cystadenoma is a rare but distinctive neoplasm of the biliary tree, more often found within the liver or pancreas than in the bile ducts or gallbladder (Albores-Saavedra and Henson, 1986). Occasionally, cystadenomas of the pancreas and extrahepatic bile ducts coexist in the same patient. The cyst wall has three layers: an inner layer of cuboidal or columnar biliary type epithelium which contains mucin, a cellular stroma resembling ovarian stroma, and an outer layer of fibrous tissue. Focal dysplastic changes are seen in the lining epithelieum in about 12% of the tumors, suggesting that progression may occur in some cases. In fact, malignant epithelial transformation has been reported in cystadenomas arising in the liver (Devaney et al., 1994; Ishak et al., 1977; Marsh et al., 1974; Wheeler and Edmonson, 1985), but the malignant potential of the extrahepatic bile duct tumors is unknown.

PAPILLOMATOSIS OF THE EXTRAHEPATIC BILE DUCTS

Papillomatosis is characterized by multiple and complex papillary lesions that may involve extensive areas of the biliary tree, including the gallbladder and intrahepatic bile ducts. Even extension into the pancreatic ducts has been observed. Obvious carcinomatous changes have been reported in some cases (Neumann et al., 1976), and for this reason, papillomatosis is regarded by some as precancerous condition. The possibility, however, that this lesion is a low-grade intraductal papillary carcinoma is supported by the demonstration of benign-appearing epithelium in metastatic deposits. The prognosis of papillomatosis of the extrahepatic bile ducts is poor because complete excision of the multicentric lesions is difficult or impossible. Of 13 patients for whom follow-up is available, the mean survival was 3 years (Hubens et al., 1991).

CARCINOID TUMORS

Carcinoid tumors of the extrahepatic biliary ducts are exceedingly rare. They account for less than 1% of all carcinoid tumors of the gastrointestinal tract. They are often discovered late in their course as a result of biliary obstruction. In contrast to carcinoids of the stomach, little is known about the incipient stages of carcinoids of the extrahepatic bile ducts. Endocrine cell hyperplasia has not been identified in the bile duct mucosa adjacent to carcinoid tumors. Carcinoid tumors of the extrahepatic bile ducts behave as low-grade, indolent malignancies. Tumor size correlates with clinical course. Tumors over 2 cm invade periductal tissues and metastasize more frequently than smaller tumors. Microscopically, these tumors consists of cords and trabeculae of small, uniform neuroendocrine cells separated by fibrous stroma. Gland-like or tubular structures are noted in some carcinoid tumors. Frequently they are immunoreactive for serotonin and a variety of peptide hormones. Some carcinoid tumors are immunoreactive for a single peptide hormone such as gastrin or somatostatin but do not give rise to systemic manifestations.

AMPULLA OF VATER

Tubular and papillary adenomas of intestinal type are the most common cancer precursors in the ampulla of Vater. Papillary adenomas have a greater risk for malignant transformation than tubular adenomas (Stolte and Pscherer, 1996; Yamaguchi and Enjoji, 1991). A significant proportion of ampullary carcinomas arise from preexisting adenomas (Kosuka, et al., 1981; Perzin and Bridge, 1981, Stolte and Pscherer, 1996). Most adenocar-

cinomas that arise from adenomas are well to moderately differentiated and of intestinal type. However, undifferentiated and small cell carcinomas have also been reported (Albores-Saavedra et al., 2000; Lee et al., 1992; Sarker et al., 1992; Figs. 12–23 and 12–24). Since most carcinomas arise from the base of the adenomas, endoscopic biopsy may show only the adenoma. About 25%–50% of ampullary adenomas on biopsy contain carcinomas in the resected specimen (Ryan et al., 1986; Seifert et al., 1992). Foci of adenomas have been detected in 35% to 75% of ampullary carcinomas (Kozuka et al., 1981; Neoptolemos et al, 1988; Stolte and Pscherer, 1996; Yamaguchi and Enjoji, 1991). The time required for an adenoma to become carcinoma is unknown. However, it is likely that neoplastic progression occurs over many years. Noninvasive papillary carcinomas are also precursors of invasive carcinoma.

Ampullary carcinoma that arise from intestinal-type adenomas and show only microinvasion with no lymph node metastasis have an excellent prognosis (Fig. 12–25). Patients with early ampullary carcinoma that extend to the submucosa or to the sphincter of Oddi have an 80% 5-year survival rate (Howe et al., 1998). A significant correlation between tumor size, lymph node status, and survival has been established in patients with ampullary carcinoma.

Although most ampullary carcinomas arise from adenomas, some invasive carcinomas may also arise from a flat precursor (flat dysplasia or carcinoma *in situ*). Severe dysplasia has been observed in the ampullary epithelium in the absence of adenoma.

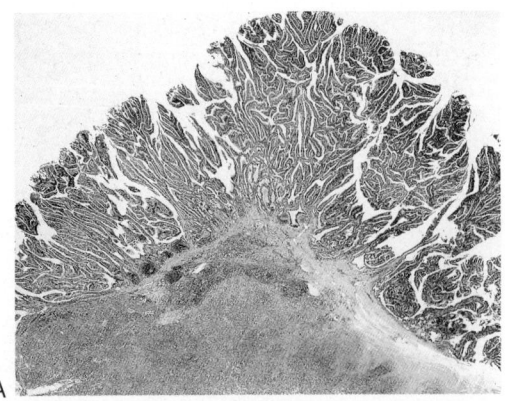
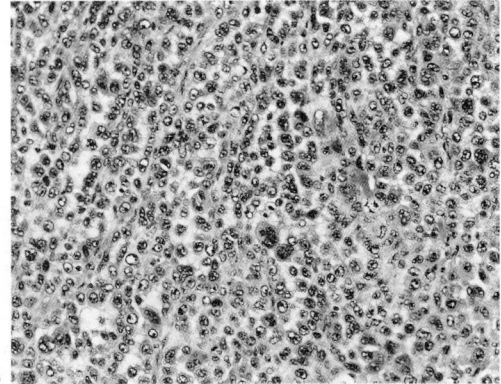

A

B

Figure 12–23. *A:* Undifferentiated carcinoma of the ampulla of Vater arising at the base of a papillary adenoma. *B:* Higher magnification of the undifferentiated carcinoma showing a solid growth pattern.

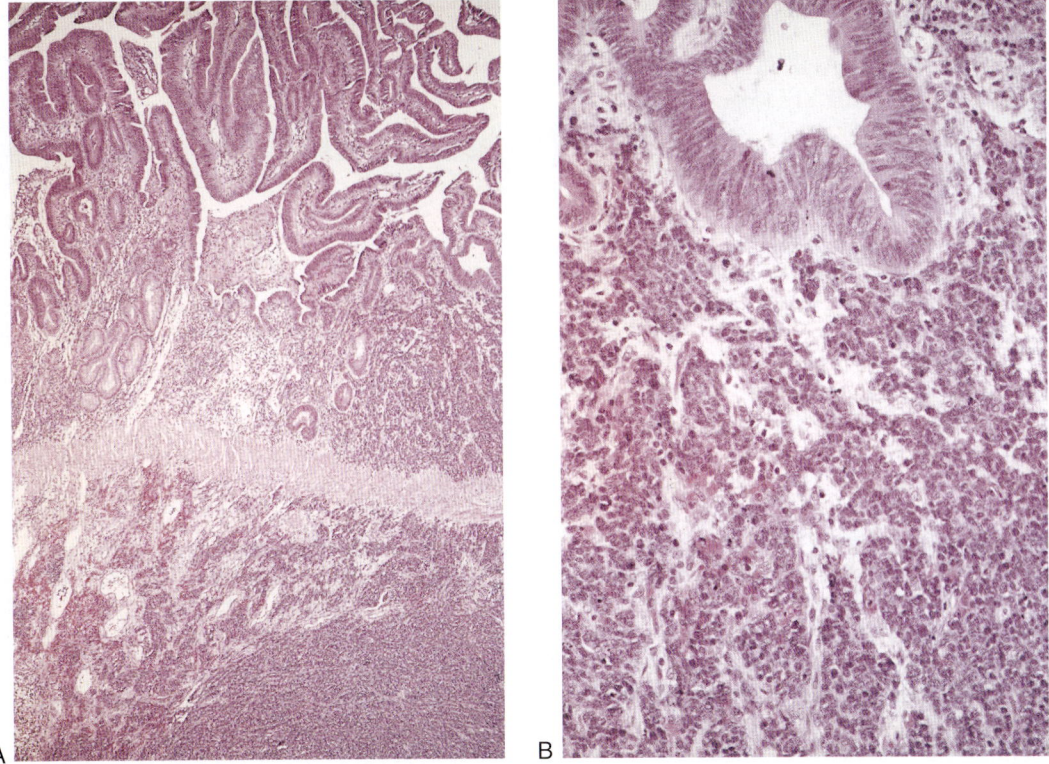

Figure 12–24. *A:* Small cell carcinoma arising at the base of a tubulovillous adenoma. *B:* Higher magnification of tumor shown on A that depicts the adenomatous change and the small cell carcinoma.

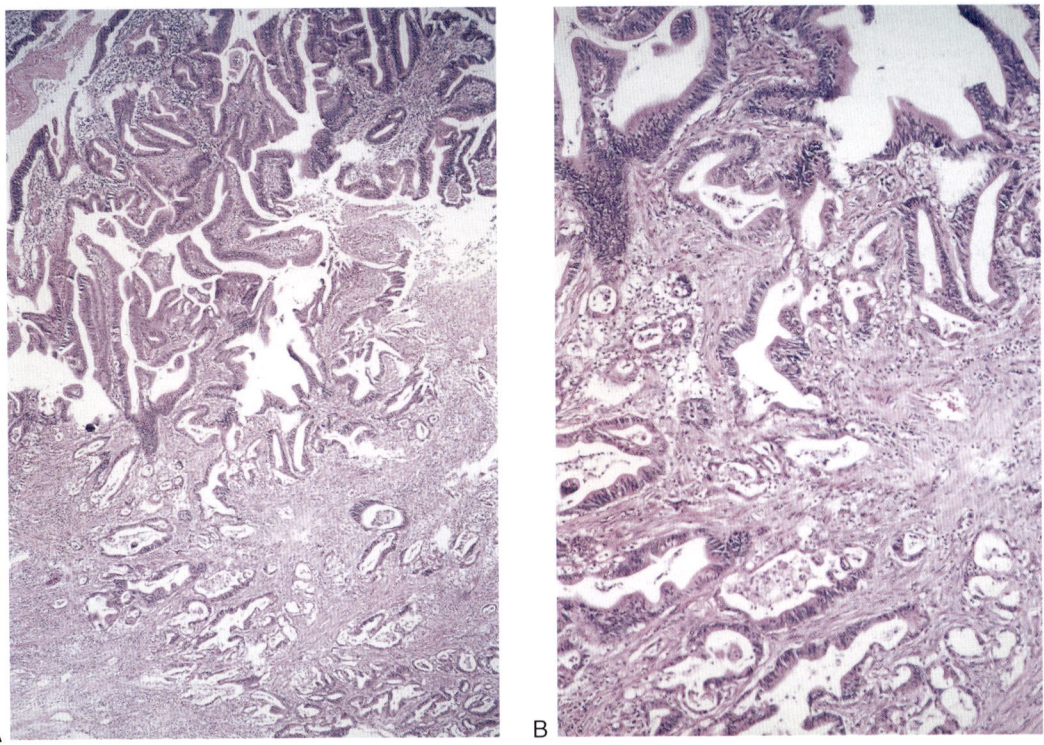

Figure 12–25. *A:* Focus of well-differentiated adenocarcinoma arising at the base of a tubulovillous adenoma. *B:* Detail of the adenocarcinoma.

FAMILIAL ADENOMATOUS POLYPOSIS

Since ampullary adenomas are common in patients with familial adenomatous polyposis (FAP) (or Gardner's syndrome) and are recognized cancer precursors, it is not surprising that ampullary carcinomas are more frequent in patients with polyposis (Kurtz et al., 1987; Noda et al., 1992). The prevalence of ampullary or periampullary adenomas in polyposis patients ranges from 50% to 95% (Alexander et al., 1989; Domizio et al., 1990; Noda et al., 1992; Yao et al., 1977) and the increased risk for carcinoma has been estimated to be 100- to 200-fold (Jagelman et al., 1988; Offerhaus et al., 1992; Pauli et al., 1980), with an estimated lifetime incidence as high as 12% (Alexander et al., 1989). The ampullary carcinomas that arise in patients with FAP occur at a younger age (mean 45–50 years) than in nonpolyposis patients, probably because of earlier detection due to screening endoscopy.

Patients with neurofibromatosis are at risk for a variety of ampullary neoplasms including somatostatin-producing carcinoid tumors, neurofibromas, gangliocytic paragangliomas, and adenocarcinomas (Colarian et al., 1990; Klein et al., 1989; Makhlouf et al., 1999).

MOLECULAR PATHOLOGY

As with extrahepatic bile duct carcinomas, ampullary carcinomas show K-*ras* oncogene and *p53* mutations (Scarpa et al. 1993). K-*ras* mutations appear to be early events in the pathogenesis of these tumors. Approximately 40% of cases show mutations that involve codon 12; codon 13 mutations are present in 10% to 12% of cases (Howe et al., 1997; Watanabe et al., 1994). K-*ras* mutations do not correlate with biologic behavior. The proportion of cases with *p53* mutation varies from 60% to 70% of cases according to different series. Mutations in exons 5, 6, and 7 have been reported. Some authors believe that *p53* mutation is a relatively late event present only or predominantly in invasive carcinomas.

Overexpression of the epidermal growth factor receptor has been shown in 50% of

invasive carcinomas of the ampulla (Resnick et al., 1995).

REFERENCES

Albores-Saavedra J, Alcantara-Vazquez A, Cruz-Ortis H, et al. (1980) The precursor lesions of invasive gallbladder carcinoma. *Cancer* 43:919–927.

Albores-Saavedra J, Henson DE. (1986) Tumors of the Gallbladder and Extrahepatic Bile Ducts. Atlas of Tumor Pathology, Fascicle 22, Second Series. Armed Forces Institute of Pathology, Washington, DC. pp. 44–53.

Albores-Saavedra J, Henson DE, Klimstra D. (2000) Tumors of the Gallbladder and Extrahepatic Bile Ducts and Ampulla of Vater, Fascicle 25, Third Series. Armed Forces Institute of Pathology, Washington, DC.

Albores-Saavedra J, Henson DE, Sobin L. (1991) Histological Typing of Tumours of the Gallbladder and Extrahepatic Bile Ducts. Springer-Verlag, Berlin.

Albores-Saavedra J, Manrique JJ, Angeles-Angeles A, Henson DE. (1984) Carcinoma *in situ* of the gallbladder. A clinicopathologic study of 18 cases. *Am J Surg Pathol* 8:323–333.

Albores-Saavedra J, Molberg K, Henson DE. (1996) Unusual malignant epithelial tumors of the gallbladder. *Semin Diagn Pathol* 13:326–338.

Albores-Saavedra J, Murakata L, Krueger JE, Henson DE. Noninvasive and minimally invasive papillary carcinoma of the extrahepatic bile ducts. *Carcinoma* 2000; In press.

Albores-Saavedra J, Nadji M, Henson DE. (1986a) Intestinal-type adenocarcinoma of the gallbladder. A clinicopathologic and immunocytochemical study of seven cases. *Am J Surg Pathol* 10:19–25.

Albores-Saavedra J, Nadji M, Henson DE, et al. (1986b) Intestinal metaplasia of the gallbladder. *Hum Pathol* 17:614–620.

Albores-Saavedra J, Nadji M, Henson DE, et al. (1988) Enteroendocrine differentiation in carcinomas of the gallbladder and mucinous cystadenocarcinomas of the pancreas. *Pathol Res Pract* 183:169–174.

Albores-Saavedra J, Nadji M, Morales A, Henson DE. (1983) Carcinoembryonic antigen in normal, preneoplastic and neoplastic gallbladder epithelium. *Cancer* 52:1069–1072.

Alexander JR, Andrews JM, Buchi KN, et al. (1989) High prevalence of adenomatous polyps of the duodenal papilla in familial adenomatous polyposis. *Dig Dis Sci* 34:167–170.

Alonso de Ruiz P, Albores-Saavedra J, Henson DE, et al. (1982) Cytopathology of precursor lesions of invasive carcinoma of the gallbladder. *Acta Cytol* 6:144–152.

Baczako K, Buchler M, Beger HG, et al. (1985) Morphogenesis and possible precursor lesions of invasive carcinoma of the papilla of Vater: epithelial dysplasia and adenoma. *Hum Pathol* 16:305–310.

Baer HU, Metzger A, Glattli A, et al. (1995) Subcutaneous periumbilical metastasis of a gallbladder carcinoma after laparoscopic cholecystectomy. *Surg Laparosc Endosc* 5:59–63.

Black WX. (1980) The morphogenesis of gallbladder carcinoma. In: *Progress in Surgical Pathology*, Vol. 2. (Fenoglio CM, Wolff M, eds.) pp. 207–223. Masson Publishing, New York.

Bombi JA, Rives A, Astudillo E, et al. (1984) Polyposis coli associated with adenocarcinoma of the gallbladder. Report of a case. *Cancer* 53:2561–2563.

Chan KW. (1988) Review of 253 cases of significant pathology in 7,910 cholecystectomies in Hong Kong. *Pathology* 20:20–23.

Chapman RWG, Burroughs AD, Bass NM, et al. (1981) Longstanding asymptomatic primary sclerosing cholangitis. *Dig Dis Sci* 26:778–782.

Clair DG, Lautz DB, Brooks DC. (1982) Rapid development of umbilical metastases after laparoscopic cholecystectomy for unsuspected gallbladder carcinoma. *Surgery* 113:355–358.

Colarian J, Pietruk T, LaFave L, et al. (1990) Adenocarcinoma of the ampulla of Vater associated with neurofibromatosis. *J Clin Gastroenterol* 12:118–122.

Davis RI, Sloan JM, Hood JM, Maxwell P. (1988) Carcinoma of the extrahepatic biliary tract: a clinicopathological and immunohistochemical study. *Histopathology* 12:623–631.

Devaney K, Goodman ZD, Ishak KG. (1994) Hepatobiliary cystadenoma and cystadenocarcinoma. A light microscopic and immunohistochemical study of 70 patients. *Am J Surg Pathol* 18:1078–1091.

Domizio P, Talbot IC, Spigelman AD, et al. (1990) Upper gastrointestinal pathology in familial adenomatous polyposis: results from a prospective study of 102 patients. *J Clin Pathol* 43:738–743.

Dowling GP, Kelly JK. (1986) The histogenesis of adenocarcinoma of the gallbladder. *Cancer* 58:1702–1708.

Duarte I, Llanos O, Domke H, Harz C, et al. (1993) Metaplasia and precursor lesions of gallbladder carcinoma. *Cancer* 72:1878–1884.

Fong Y, Brennan MF, Turnbull AT, et al. (1993) Gallbladder cancer discovered during laparoscopic surgery. Potential for iatrogenic tumor dissemination. *Arch Surg* 128:1054–1056.

Fong Y, Heffernan N, Blumgart LH. (1998) Gallbladder cancer discovered during laparoscopic cholecystectomy. *Cancer* 83:423–427.

Gremlee RT, Murray T, Bolden S, et al. Cancer statistics, 2000. *CA Cancer J Clin* 2000; 50:7–33.

Harvath AC, Manley PN, Groll A, et al. (1989) Bile duct carcinoma and biliary tract dysplasia in chronic ulcerative colitis. *Arch Pathol Lab Med* 113:434–436.

Haworth AC, Manley PN, Groll A, et al. (1989) Bile duct carcinoma and biliary tract dysplasia in chronic ulcerative colitis. *Arch Pathol Lab Med* 113:434–436.

Henson DE, Albores-Saavedra J, Corle D. (1992) Carcinoma of the gallbladder: histologic types, stage of disease, grade, and survival rates. *Cancer* 70:1493–1497.

Howe JR, Klimstra DS, Cordon-Cardo C, et al. (1997) K-*ras* mutation in adenomas and carcinomas of the ampulla of Vater. *Clin Cancer Res* 3:129–33.

Howe JR, Klimstra DS, Moccia RD, et al. (1998) Factors predictive of survival in ampullary carcinoma. *Ann Surg* 228:87–94.

Hubens G, Delvaux G, Willems G, et al. (1991) Papillomatosis of the intra- and extrahepatic bile ducts with involvement of the pancreatic duct. *Hepatogastroenterology* 38:413–418.

Ishak KG, Willis GW, Cummins SD, et al. (1977) Biliary cystadenoma and cystadenocarcinoma. *Cancer* 39:322–338.

Jagelman DG, DeCosse JJ, Bussey HJR. (1988) Upper gastrointestinal cancer in familial adenomatous polyposis. *Lancet* 1149–1151.

Kijima H, Watanabe H, Iwafuchi M, et al. (1989) Histogenesis of gallbladder carcinoma from investigation of early carcinoma and microcarcinoma. *Acta Pathol Jpn* 39:235–244.

Klein A, Clemens J, Cameron J. (1989) Periampullary neoplasms in von Recklinghausen's disease. *Surgery* 106:815–819.

Kosuka S, Tsubone M, Hachisuka K. (1984) Evolution of carcinoma in the extrahepatic bile ducts. *Cancer* 54:65–72.

Kosuka S, Tsubone M, Yamaguchi A, et al. (1981) Adenomatous residue in cancerous papilla of Vater. *Gut* 22:1031–1034.

Kosuka S, Tsubone M, Yasui A, et al. (1982) Relation of adenoma to carcinoma in the gallbladder. *Cancer* 50:2226–2234.

Kurtz RC, Sternberg SS, Miller HH, et al. (1987) Upper gastrointestinal neoplasia in familial polyposis. *Dig Dis Sci* 32:459–65.

Laitio M. (1983a) Carcinoma of the extrahepatic bile ducts. A histopathologic study. *Pathol Res Pract* 178:67–72.

Laitio M. (1985) Goblet cells, enterochromaffin cells, superficial gastric-type epithelium and antral-type glands in the gallbladder. *Beitr Pathol* 156:343–358.

Laitio M. (1983b) Histogenesis of epithelial neoplasms of human gallbladder. I. Dysplasia. *Pathol Res Pract* 178:51–56.

Laitio M. (1983c) Histogenesis of epithelial neoplasms of human gallbladder. II. Carcinoma. *Pathol Res Pract* 178:57.

Lee CS, Machet D, Rode J. (1992) Small cell carcinoma of the ampulla of Vater. *Cancer* 70:1502–1504.

Lees CD, Hermann RE. (1981) Familial polyposis coli associated with bile duct cancer. *Am J Surg* 141:378–380.

Ludwig J, Wahlstrom HE, Batts KP, et al. (1992) Papillary bile duct dysplasia in primary sclerosing cholangitis. *Gastroenterology* 102:2134–2138.

Lurie BB, Loewenstein MS, Zamcheck NP. (1975) Elevated carcinoembryonic antigen levels and biliary tract obstruction. *JAMA* 233:326–330.

Makhlouf HR, Burke AP, Sobin LH. (1999) Carcinoid tumors of the ampulla of Vater. A comparison with duodenal carcinoid tumors. *Cancer* 85:1241–1249.

Marsh JL, Dahms B, Longmire WG Jr. (1974) Cystadenoma and cystadenocarcinoma of the biliary system. *Arch Surg* 109:41–43.

Nakajo S, Yamamoto M, Tahara E. (1989) Morphometric analysis of gallbladder adenocarcinoma: discrimination between carcinoma and dysplasia. *Virchows Arch A Anat Pathol Histopathol* 416:133–140.

Nally C, Preshaw RM. (1994) Tumour implantation at umbilicus after laparoscopic cholecystectomy for unsuspected gallbladder carcinoma. *Can J Surg* 37:243–244.

Neoptolemos JP, Talbot IC, Shaw DC, et al. (1988) Long-term survival after resection of ampullary carcinoma is associated independently with tumor grade and a new staging classification that assesses local invasiveness. *Cancer* 61:1403–1407.

Neumann RD, LiVolsi VA, Rosenthal NS, et al. (1976) Adenocarcinoma in biliary papillomatosis. *Gastroenterology* 70:779–782.

Noda Y, Watanabe H, Iida M, et al. (1992) Histologic follow-up of ampullary adenomas in patients with familial adenomatosis coli. *Cancer* 70:1847–1856.

Nugent KP, Spigelman AD, Talbot IC, Phillips RKS. (1994) Gallbladder dysplasia in patients with familial adenomatous polyposis. *Br J Surg* 81:291–292.

Offerhaus GJ, Giardiello FM, Krush AJ, et al. (1992) The risk of upper gastrointestinal cancer in familial adenomatous polyposis. *Gastroenterology* 102:1980–1982.

Ojeda VJ, Shilkin KB, Walters MN-I. (1985) Premalignant epithelial lesions of the gallbladder. A prospective study of 120 cholecystectomy specimens. *Pathology* 17:451–454.

Pauli RM, Pauli ME, Hall JG. (1980) Gardner syndrome and periampullary malignancy. *Am J Med Genet* 6: 205–219.

Perzin KH, Bridge MF. (1981) Adenomas of the small intestine: a clinicopathologic review of 51 cases and a study of their relationship to carcinoma. *Cancer* 48: 799–819.

Putz P, Willems G. (1978) Proliferative changes in the epithelium of the human lithiasic gallbladder. *J Natl Cancer Inst* 60:283–287.

Resnick MB, Gallinger S, Wang HH, Odze RD. (1995) Growth factor expression and proliferation kenetics in periampullary neoplasms in familial adenomatous polyposis. *Cancer* 76:187–194.

Ropertz S, Wagner K. (1976) Die laparaskopische Gallenblasenpunktiontechnik und diagnostische. *Leber Magen Darm* 6:19–24.

Ross AP, Braasch JW. (1973) Ulcerative colitis and carcinoma of the proximal bile ducts. *Gut* 14:94–97.

Ryan DP, Schapiro RH, Warshaw AL. (1986) Villous tumors of the duodenum. *Ann Surg* 203:301–306.

Sarker AB, Hoshidal Y, Akagi S, et al. (1992) An immunohistochemical and ultrastructural study of a case of small-cell neuroendocrine carcinoma in the ampullary region of the duodenum. *Acta Pathol Jpn* 42:529–535.

Scarpa A, Capelli P, Zamboni G, et al. (1993) Neoplasia of the ampulla of Vater. Ki-*ras* and *p53* mutations. *Am J Pathol* 142:1163–1172.

Seifert E, Schulte F, Stolte M. (1992) Adenoma and carcinoma of the duodenum and papilla of Vater: a clinicopathologic study. *Am J Gastroenterol* 87:37–42.

Stolte M, Pscherer C. (1996) Adenoma-carcinoma sequence in the papilla of Vater. *Scand J Gastroenterol* 31:376–382.

Suzuki M, Takahashi T, Ouchi K, et al. (1989) The development and extension of hepatohilar bile duct carcinoma. A three-dimensional tumor mapping in the intrahepatic biliary tree visualized with the aid of a graphics computer system. *Cancer* 64:658–666.

Tatsuta M, Yamamura H, Yamamoto R, et al. (1982) Carcinoembryonic antigen in the bile in patients with pancreatic and biliary cancer. *Cancer* 50:2903–2909.

Watanabe M, Asaka M, Tanaka J, et al. (1994) Point mutations of K-*ras* gene codon 12 in biliary tract tumors. *Gastroenterology* 107:1147–1153.

Wee A, Ludwig J, Coffey RJ Jr, et al. (1985) Hepatobiliary carcinoma associated with primary sclerosing cholangitis and chronic ulcerative colitis. *Hum Pathol* 16:719–726.

Wheeler DA, Edmonson HA. (1985) Cystadenoma with mesenchymal stroma (CMS) in the liver and bile ducts. A clinico-pathologic study of 17 cases, 4 with malignant change. *Cancer* 56:1434–1439.

Wibbenmeyer LA, Wade TP, Chen RC, et al. (1995) Laparoscopic cholecystectomy can disseminate *in situ* carcinoma of the gallbladder. *J Am Coll Surg* 181: 504–510.

Wiesner RH, Ludwig J, LaRusso NF, et al. (1985) Diagnosis and treatment of primary sclerosing cholangitis. *Semin Liver Dis* 5:241–253.

Wistuba II, Gazdar AF, Roa I, Albores-Saavedra J. (1996) p53 protein over-expression in gallbladder carcinoma and its precursor lesions. An immunohistochemical study. *Hum Pathol* 27:360–365.

Wistuba II, Miquel JF, Gazdar AF, Albores-Saavedra J. (1998) Gallbladder adenomas have molecular abnormalities different from those present in gallbladder carcinomas. *Hum Pathol* 30:21–25.

Wistuba II, Sugio K, Hung J, et al. (1995) Allele-specific mutations involved in the pathogenesis of endemic gallbladder carcinoma in Chile. *Cancer Res* 55:2511–2515.

Yamagiwa H. (1987) Dysplasia of gallbladder. Its pathological significance. *Acta Pathol Jpn* 37:747–54.

Yamagiwa H. (1989) Mucosal dysplasia of gallbladder: isolated and adjacent lesions to carcinoma. *Jpn J Cancer Res* 80:238–243.

Yamagiwa H, Tomiyama H. (1986) Intestinal metaplasia-dysplasia-carcinoma sequence of the gallbladder. *Acta Pathol Jpn* 36:989–997.

Yamaguchi K, Enjoji M. (1988) Carcinoma of the gallbladder. A clinicopathology of 103 patients and a new proposed staging. *Cancer* 62:1425–1432.

Yamaguchi K, Enjoji M. (1991) Adenoma of the ampulla of Vater: putative precancerous lesion. *Gut* 32: 1558–1561.

Yamaguchi A, Hachisuka K, Isogai M, et al. (1992) Carcinoma *in situ* of the gallbladder with superficial extension into the Rokitansky-Aschoff sinuses and mucous glands. *Gastroenterol Jpn* 27:765–772.

Yamamoto M, Nakajo S, Tahara E. (1989) Dysplasia of the gallbladder. Its histogenesis and correlation to gallbladder adenocarcinoma. *Pathol Res Pract* 185: 454–460.

Yao T, Iida M, Ohsato K, et al. (1977) Duodenal lesions in familial polyposis of the colon. *Gastroenterology* 73:1086–1092.

13

EXOCRINE PANCREAS

ROBB E. WILENTZ, JORGE ALBORES-SAAVEDRA, AND RALPH H. HRUBAN

Even though pancreatic cancer makes up only 2% of new cancer cases in the United States, it is the fifth leading cause of cancer death (Parker et al., 1997; Warshaw and Castillo, 1992). This is true for primarily two reasons. First, pancreatic cancer, particularly ductal adenocarcinoma, is extremely virulent (Baylor and Berg, 1973; Beazley and Cohn, 1981; Cubilla and Fitzgerald, 1992; DiGiuseppe et al., 1996; Geer and Brennan, 1993; Gudjonsson, 1987; Nagakawa et al., 1993; Yeo et al., 1995). For example, most "small" pancreatic adenocarcinomas (of less than 2 cm) have already metastasized by the time of diagnosis (Cubilla et al., 1978; Manabe et al., 1988; Tsuchiya et al., 1985, 1986). Second, because it produces few symptoms, pancreatic cancer often goes undetected until after it has spread beyond the gland (Allema et al., 1995; Connolly et al., 1987; DiGiuseppe et al., 1996; Michelassi et al., 1989; Moossa and Levin, 1981; Willett et al., 1993). Although surgical resection can produce survival rates of up to 40%, most patients with pancreatic adenocarcinoma do not present with resectable tumors (Yeo et al., 1995). Recognizing the precursors to invasive carcinoma (and thus patients at risk to develop an invasive cancer) may lead to increased survival (DiGiuseppe et al., 1996; Hruban and Wilentz, 2000; Hruban et al., 1998, 1999; Klimstra et al., 1994; Wilentz and Hruban, 1998; Wilentz et al., 1998a).

There is a variety of distinct types of invasive cancer of the pancreas; precursors to several of these have already been identified and in some cases are now well characterized. For example, *duct lesions* have been shown to be the precursors of invasive ductal adenocarcinomas (DiGiuseppe et al., 1996; Hruban and Wilentz, 2000; Hruban et al., 1998, 1999; Klimstra and Longnecker, 1994; Wilentz and Hruban, 1998; Wilentz et al., 1998a). Benign and borderline *mucinous cystic neoplasms* can develop into invasive mucinous cystadenocarcinomas (Albores-Saavedra et al., 1987; Becker et al., 1965; Compagno and Oertel, 1978; Corbally et al., 1989; Hyde et al., 1984; Katoh et al., 1989; Sachs et al., 1989; Yamaguchi and Enjoi, 1987; Yu and Shetty, 1985). Similarly, benign and borderline *intraductal papillary mucinous neoplasms* (IPMNs) can progress to invasive papillary carcinomas (Conley et al., 1987; Furukawa et al., 1992; Kawarada et al., 1992; Nagai et al., 1995; Nishihara et al., 1993; Obara et al., 1991; Ohta et al., 1992; Payan et al., 1990; Rickaert et al., 1991; Santini et al., 1995; Sessa et al., 1994; Warshaw et al., 1990; Yamada et al., 1991; Yamaguchi and Tanaka, 1991; Yanagisawa et al., 1993a), and *intraductal oncocytic papillary neoplasms* (IOPNs) can develop into invasive oncocytic carcinomas (Adsay et al., 1996).

This chapter will address the clinical characteristics, morphology, and genetics of each of these types of incipient neoplasia. An understanding of early neoplasia in the pancreas will increase and solidify the pathologist's role in advising patient care and predicting patient outcome.

DUCT LESIONS

Duct lesions (also called *duct hyperplasias* and *pancreatic intraepithelial neoplasias*) are the precursors of infiltrating ductal adenocarcinoma. Normal pancreatic ducts contain low cuboidal or flattened cells with amphophilic cytoplasm (Fig. 13–1A). The *sine qua non* of a duct lesion is instead a tall, columnar, mucin-producing epithelium (DiGiuseppe et al., 1996; Hruban and Wilentz, 2000; Hruban et al., 1998, 1999; Klimstra et al., 1994; Wilentz and Hruban, 1998; Wilentz et al., 1998a).

Duct lesions can be subdivided into four categories, each defined by *(1)* the architectural growth pattern and *(2)* the degree of cytologic and architectural atypia (DiGiuseppe et al., 1996; Hruban and Wilentz, 2000; Hruban et al., 1998, 1999; Klimstra et al., 1994; Wilentz and Hruban, 1998; Wilentz et al., 1998a). The epithelium in *flat duct lesions* is flat, and no significant cytologic or architectural atypia is seen. The epithelium in *papillary duct lesions without atypia* has a papillary architecture but lacks cytologic atypia (Fig. 13–1B). *Papillary duct lesions with atypia* are papillary lesions with significant atypia (Fig. 13–1C). We define atypia to include nuclear hyperchromatism, enlargement, and irregularity; loss of nuclear polarity; nucleolar prominence; and papillary complexity. The papillary lesions of *carcinoma in situ* (Fig. 13–1D) may lack fibrovascular cores and have marked atypia with mitoses and cribriforming or bridging structures similar to

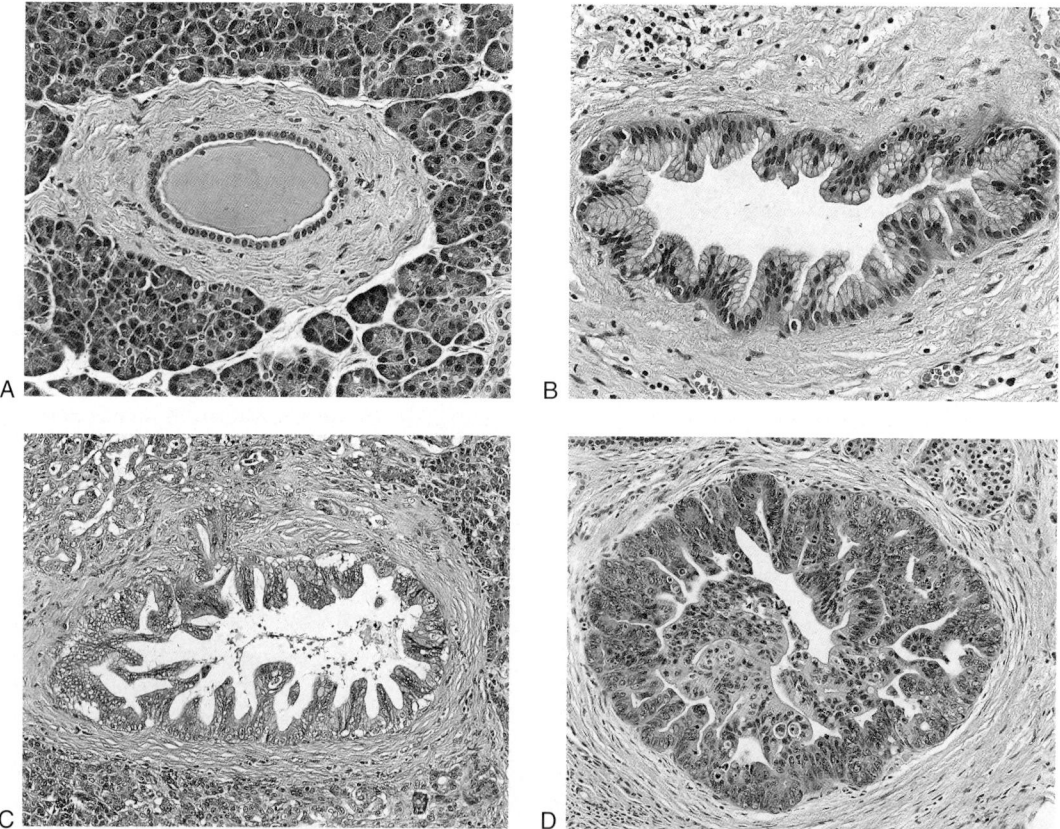

Figure 13–1. Histology of a normal pancreatic duct *(A)* and various duct lesions *(B–D)*. Duct lesions contain tall, columnar, mucinous epithelium, instead of the normally flattened or cuboidal type. In papillary duct lesions without *(B)* and with *(C)* atypia, the epithelium forms papillary infoldings. One judges atypia by nuclear hyperchromatism, irregularity, and enlargement; loss of nuclear polarity; nucleolar prominence; mitoses; and papillary complexity. Some duct lesions even meet the histopathologic criteria (severe atypia, cribriforming structures, and mitoses) for carcinoma *in situ (D)*.

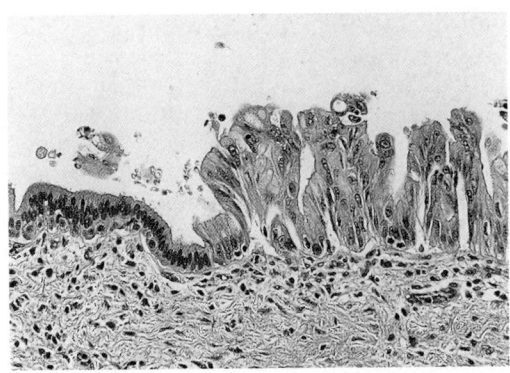

Figure 13–2. Pancreatic duct partially involved by a papillary duct lesion with atypia. Note the tall, columnar, mucinous epithelium of the duct lesion, compared to the cuboidal epithelium of the uninvolved portion of the duct. The nuclei of this duct lesion are atypical; that is, they show irregular contours, contain prominent nucleoli, and have lost their orientation with respect to their basement membrane.

those seen in mammary ductal carcinoma *in situ* (DCIS) (DiGiuseppe et al., 1996; Hruban and Wilentz, 2000; Hruban et al., 1998, 1999; Klimstra, et al. (1994); Wilentz and Hruban, 1998; Wilentz et al., 1998a). Figures 13–1 and 13–2 show examples of a normal pancreatic duct and various duct lesions.

Growing evidence suggests that just as there is progression in the colon from adenoma, to adenoma with high-grade dysplasia, to infiltrating adenocarcinoma, so too is there progression in the pancreas from flat duct lesion, to papillary duct lesion without atypia, to papillary duct lesion with atypia, to carcinoma *in situ,* to infiltrating ductal adenocarcinoma (DiGiuseppe et al., 1996; Fearon and Vogelstein, 1990; Hruban and Wilentz, 2000; Hruban et al., 1998, 2000; Klimstra et al., 1994; Wilentz and Hruban, 1998; Wilentz et al., 1998a). Figure 13–3 illustrates this progression model for pancreatic duct lesions.

The evidence for this model is morphological, clinical, and genetic. For example, morphologically, pancreata with infiltrating ductal adenocarcinomas also frequently contain duct lesions. Cubilla and Fitzgerald (1976) compared the duct changes in 227 pancreata with pancreatic cancer with those in 100 pancreata obtained from age- and sex-matched controls without pancreatic cancer. Papillary duct lesions were three times more common in pancreata from patients with pancreatic cancer than they were in pancreata from patients without pancreatic cancer. Remarkably, they identified atypical papillary duct lesions only in pancreata with infiltrating pancreatic cancer (Cubilla and Fitzgerald, 1976). Kozuka et al. (1979) and Pour et al. (1982) have reported similar findings, and Furukawa et al. (1994), using three-dimensional mapping techniques, have demonstrated a stepwise progression from mild dysplasia to severe dysplasia in pancreatic duct lesions.

Second, there have been several clinical case reports of duct lesions progressing to infiltrating cancer over time. For example,

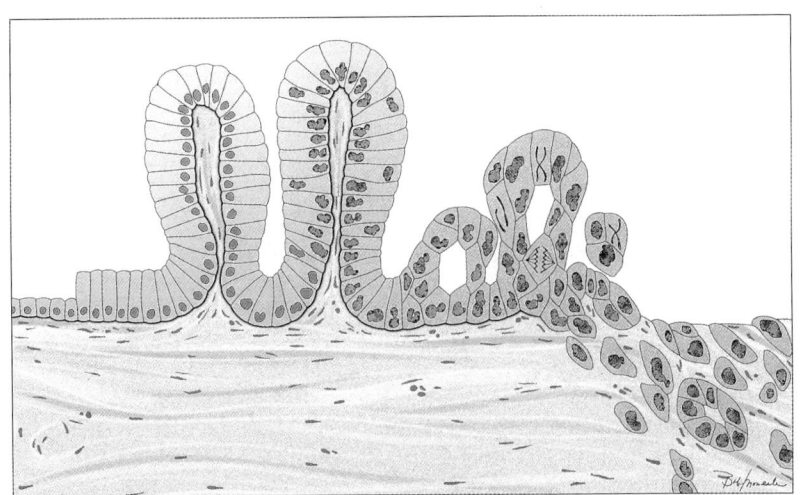

Figure 13–3. Neoplastic progression model for cancer of the pancreas. A duct lesion may "evolve" from flat duct lesion to papillary duct lesion, to papillary duct lesion with atypia, to carcinoma *in situ.* Some carcinomas *in situ* will develop into infiltrating ductal adenocarcinomas. [Artwork by Bob Morreale.]

Brat et al. (1998) reported three patients who developed infiltrating ductal adenocarcinomas 17 months, 9 years, and 10 years after the identification of atypical papillary duct lesions in their pancreata. Brockie et al. (1998) reported two patients with duct lesions that progressed to infiltrating cancers 9 and 29 years after their identification. Since the pancreas is rarely biopsied, duct lesions are not commonly seen *before* the development of an associated invasive carcinoma; therefore, these case reports are critical, because they establish the temporal progression of duct lesions to infiltrating carcinoma.

Third, molecular genetic analysis of duct lesions has demonstrated that they contain some of the same genetic changes seen in infiltrating ductal adenocarcinomas. For example, activating point mutations in codon 12 of the K-*ras* oncogene, present in approximately 90% of infiltrating duct adenocarcinomas, have been demonstrated in duct lesions, most often the atypical ones (Caldas et al., 1994; DiGiuseppe et al., 1994b; Lemoine et al., 1992; Tabata et al., 1993; Tada et al., 1996; Wilentz et al., 1998a; Yanagisawa et al., 1993b). Duct lesions also harbor alterations in tumor-suppressor genes, including *p16, p53, BRCA2,* and *DPC4* (Boschman et al., 1994; DiGiuseppe et al., 1994a; Goggins et al., 2000; Hameed et al., 1994; Moskaluk et al., 1997; Wilentz et al., 1998b). We recently stained 126 duct lesions of varying histologic types for nuclear p16 expression and found that there was a significant, albeit not an absolute, correlation between the severity of the atypia in a duct lesion and loss of nuclear p16 expression (Wilentz et al., 1998b). Similarly, *DPC4* inactivation appears to occur only in more advanced duct lesions (Wilentz et al., 2000).

This morphologic–clinical–genetic model has two important implications. First, it suggests that duct lesions are, in fact, neoplasms. It has therefore been suggested that the terminology for these lesions be changed from "duct lesions" and "hyperplasias" to "pancreatic intraepithelial neoplasias" (Brat et al., 1998; Hruban and Wilentz, 2000; Klimstra and Longnecker, 1994). A summary of the pancreatic intraepithelial neoplasia (PanIN) nomenclature and diagnostic criteria for each grade of PanIN can be found on the World Wide Web. (http://pathology.

jhu.edu/pancreas_panin). Second, this progression model implies that screening for PanINs and early invasive carcinoma should be possible. Indeed, DNA with mutant K-*ras* genes has been detected in stool, duodenal fluid, and pancreatic juice samples obtained from patients with infiltrating pancreatic cancer and/or pancreatic duct lesions (Berthélemy et al., 1995; Brentnall et al., 1995; Caldas et al., 1994; Wilentz et al., 1998a). In fact, Berthélemy et al. (1995) reported two patients without clinical or radiologic evidence of cancer who developed ductal adenocarcinomas 18 and 40 months after K-*ras* mutations were found in samples of their pancreatic juice. These mutant K-*ras* signals presumably originated in DNA shed from PanINs, which only later developed into clinically detectable infiltrating cancer (Berthélemy et al., 1995).

Thus, although the progression of PanINs to carcinoma is not completely understood, duct lesions represent microscopically and genetically recognizable early neoplasms in the pancreas, some of which over time will progress to infiltrating carcinoma. An understanding of these PanINs will provide new tools to identify patients with an early neoplasm *before* they actually develop an unresectable invasive cancer.

MUCINOUS CYSTIC NEOPLASMS

Mucinous cystic neoplasms comprise approximately 1%–2% of all pancreatic tumors (Albores-Saavedra et al., 1987, 1990; Corbally et al., 1989; Hyde et al., 1984; Katoh et al., 1989; Sachs et al., 1998; Yamaguchi and Enjoi, 1987; Yu and Shetty, 1985). They typically present in older women with epigastric pain or an abdominal mass; because these neoplasms are more common in the tail than in the head of the pancreas, obstructive jaundice is rare (Becker et al., 1965; Compagno and Oertel, 1978; Warshaw et al., 1990). Often they are multiloculated, larger than 10 cm, and filled with a tenacious fluid (Becker et al., 1965; Compagno and Oertel, 1978; Warshaw et al., 1990).

Microscopically, the cysts, which do not communicate with the native pancreatic duct system, are lined by tall, mucin-producing, columnar cells. In addition, mucinous cystic neoplasms, but only in women, often have a dense, cellular, intercystic stroma resembling ovarian stroma that shows immunoreactivity for estrogen receptor and inhibin (Ridder et al., 1998). Immunohistochemical staining in most cases demonstrates that the epithelium expresses carcinoembryonic antigen (CEA), carbohydrate antigen (CA) 19-9, cytokeratin, and epithelial membrane antigen (EMA) (Albores-Saavedra et al., 1987; Becker et al., 1965; Compagno et al., 1978; Corbally et al., 1989; Cubilla and Fitzgerald, 1984; Hruban and Wilentz, 2000; Hyde et al., 1984; Katoh et al., 1989; Sachs et al., 1989; Solcia et al., 1997; Warshaw et al., 1990; Yamaguchi and Enjoi, 1987; Yu et al., 1985). Focal endocrine differentiation, including the expression of serotonin, gastrin, and somatostatin, can also be seen in close to 40% of the tumors. Interestingly, the expression of neuroendocrine markers appears to be more common in mucinous cystadenocarcinomas and borderline mucinous cystic tumors than in mucinous cystadenomas (Albores-Saavedra et al., 1998).

Mucinous cystic neoplasms can be histologically categorized, based on the presence or absence of cytological and architectural atypia, into mucinous cystadenomas, borderline mucinous cystic neoplasms, mucinous cystic neoplasms with *in situ* carcinoma, and invasive mucinous cystadenocarcinomas. *Mucinous cystadenomas* contain a single layer of epithelium lacking significant atypia.

In *borderline mucinous cystic neoplasms*, the epithelium may form papillae and complex architectural patterns. The epithelium of *mucinous cystic neoplasms with* in situ *carcinoma* shows significant architectural and cytologic atypia, but no invasive carcinoma is seen. When an invasive carcinoma is present in association with mucinous cystic neoplasms, then the diagnosis of *invasive mucinous cystadenocarcinoma* should be made. It is important to note that a single mucinous cystic neoplasm can show a range of architectural and cytological atypia; as expected, each neoplasm should be classified based on the most atypical areas (Hruban and Wilentz, 2000; Klöppel et al., 1996; Solcia et al., 1997). Figures 13–4 and 13–5 show examples of mucinous cystic neoplasms.

Mucinous cystadenomas, borderline mucinous cystic neoplasms, and mucinous cystic neoplasms with *in situ* carcinoma are forms of early neoplasia because *if untreated* they may develop into invasive mucinous cystadenocarcinomas (Compagno and Oertel, 1978; Cubilla and Fitzgerald, 1984; Hyde et al., 1984; Solcia et al., 1997; Wilentz et al., 1999b). In fact, one can propose a progression model for mucinous cystic neoplasms similar to that for PanINs. We believe that mucinous cystadenomas may progress to borderline mucinous cystic neoplasms, to mucinous cystic neoplasms with carcinoma *in situ*, and to invasive mucinous cystadenocarcinomas.

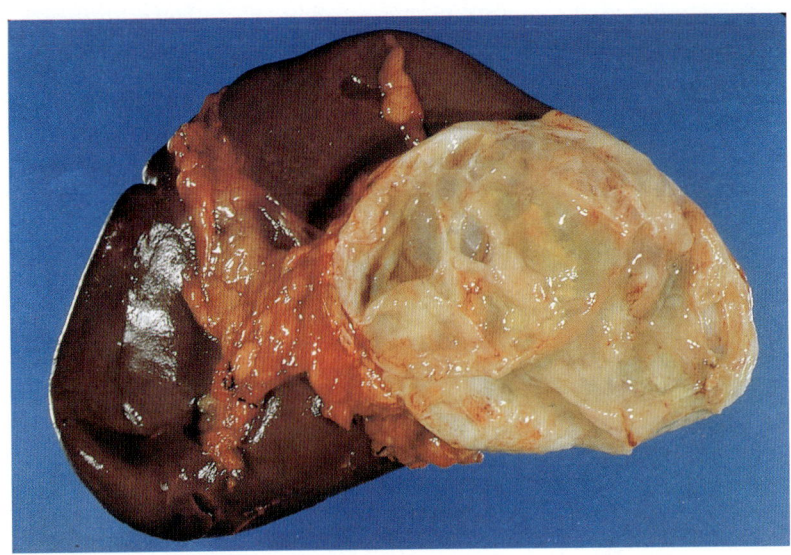

Figure 13–4. Gross appearance of an invasive mucinous cystadenocarcinoma, located in the pancreatic tail, next to the spleen. Note the large cysts filled with a tenacious fluid. Because benign and malignant mucinous cystic neoplasms can have similar gross appearances, each mucinous cystic neoplasm should be completely resected and completely histologically examined to rule out invasive carcinoma.

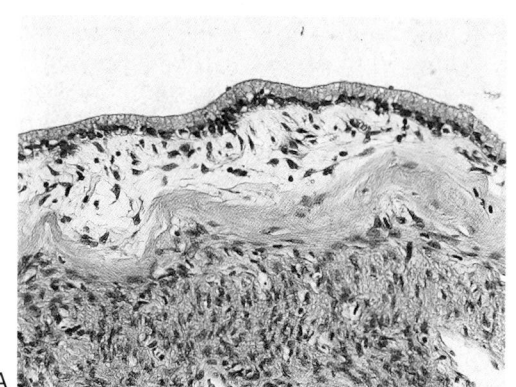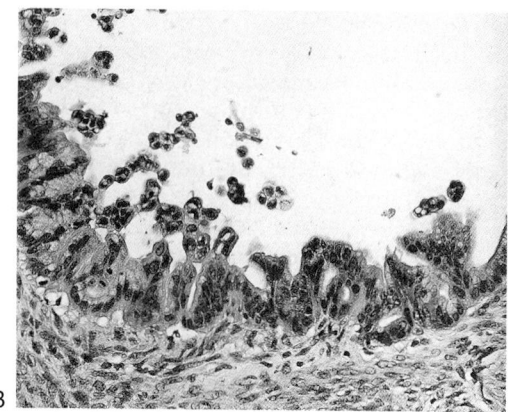

Figure 13–5. Microscopic appearances of a mucinous cystic neoplasm with an *in situ* carcinoma. Some areas of the neoplasm contain tall, columnar, mucinous epithelium with no significant cellular or architectural atypia *(A)*. Other areas show cells with the changes of carcinoma *in situ*, including marked cellular atypia, scattered mitoses, and cribriforming structures *(B)*.

Limited genetic evidence supports such a model, with the more "advanced" mucinous cystic neoplasms tending to show more genetic changes. For example, Flejou et al. (1996) have reported that p53 protein immunoreactivity is common (80%) in mucinous cystadenocarcinomas but absent in benign and borderline cases. In addition, Bartsch et al. (1998) have noted that K-*ras* mutations are more common in invasive mucinous cystadenocarcinomas than in benign mucinous cystic neoplasms.

The ability of some mucinous cystic neoplasms to progress into invasive carcinomas has led to a debate about the prognosis of patients with mucinous cystic neoplasms. While the progression model implies that once completely resected, a mucinous cystic neoplasm can no longer progress, and therefore, a completely resected mucinous cystadenoma, borderline mucinous cystic neoplasm, or mucinous cystic neoplasm with *in situ* carcinoma should follow a benign course, some pathologists have reported that a small minority of completely removed noninvasive mucinous cystic neoplasms can recur and even metastasize (Compagno and Oertel, 1978; Cubilla and Fitzgerald, 1984; Solcia et al., 1997).

We believe that incomplete sampling explains this paradox. We studied 61 mucinous cystic neoplasms and categorized each as mucinous cystadenoma ($n = 27$, 44%), borderline mucinous cystic neoplasm ($n = 5$, 8.2%), mucinous cystic neoplasm with *in situ* carcinoma ($n = 9$, 15%), or invasive mucinous cystadenocarcinoma ($n = 20$, 33%) (Wilentz et al., 1999b). Only those mucinous cystadenomas, borderline mucinous cystic neoplasms, and mucinous cystic neoplasms with *in situ* carcinoma that were completely resected and completely histologically examined were included in the study. Not one of the mucinous cystadenomas, borderline mucinous cystic neoplasms, or mucinous cystic neoplasms with *in situ* carcinoma recurred or metastasized. The 5-year survival for patients with mucinous cystadenomas, borderline mucinous cystic neoplasms, mucinous cystic neoplasms with *in situ* carcinoma, and invasive mucinous cystadenocarcinomas was 83%, 67%, 100%, and 31%, respectively ($p < 0.01$). The three patients who died with noninvasive mucinous cystic neoplasms expired from causes unrelated to their tumors. One tumor, originally showing only benign histology on biopsy, contained foci of invasive carcinoma on complete resection. These data imply that because mucinous cystic neoplasms sometimes harbor only small foci of invasive carcinoma, they should be completely resected and completely submitted for histological examination (Compagno and Oertel, 1978; Hyde et al., 1984; Wilentz et al., 1999b). Failure to do so may result in the miscategorization of a tumor and in the incorrect assertion that even completely removed noninvasive mucinous cystic neoplasms can recur and metastasize.

These data also re-emphasize that although mucinous cystadenocarcinomas are fully malignant tumors, patients with these neoplasms live longer than patients with typical infiltrating ductal adenocarcinomas (Talamini et al., 1992). Indeed, Compagno and Oertel (1978) originally had reported that approximately 50% of patients with completely resected invasive mucinous cystadenocarcinomas lived at least 5 years. More recently, we analyzed the Surveillance, Epidemiology, and End Results (SEER) database of the National Cancer Institute and found that 10-year survival rates are now close to 50% for invasive mucinous cystadenocarcinomas (Wilentz et al., 1999a,b).

Therefore, we believe that just as there is a progression of PanINs to infiltrating ductal adenocarcinoma, so too can mucinous cystic neoplasms progress from adenomas to borderline lesions to carcinomas *in situ* to invasive carcinomas. If completely removed before an invasive carcinoma develops, a mucinous cystic neoplasm will follow a benign course. However, because invasive carcinoma can arise focally within an otherwise benign-appearing mucinous cystic neoplasm, mucinous cystic neoplasms must be histologically examined in their entirety to avoid misclassifying an invasive mucinous cystic neoplasm as an adenoma or borderline tumor.

INTRADUCTAL PAPILLARY MUCINOUS NEOPLASMS

A relatively newly recognized tumor, the *intraductal papillary mucinous neoplasm* (IPMN), also known as *mucinous duct ectasia*, is a clinically and pathologically distinct neoplasm. The tumor usually affects older men and women, and endoscopic examination of these patients typically reveals mucin oozing from the ampulla of Vater (Conley et al., 1987; Furukawa et al., 1992; Kawarada et al., 1992; Morohoshi et al., 1989; Nagai et al., 1995; Nishihara et al., 1993; Obara et al., 1991; Ohta et al., 1992; Payan et al., 1990; Rickaert et al., 1991; Santini et al., 1995; Sessa et al., 1994; Warshaw et al., 1990; Yamada et al., 1991; Yamaguchi and Tanaka, 1991; Yanagisawa et al., 1993a; see Fig. 13–6A).

The IPMNs are villous tumors that grow within the large ducts of the pancreas (Fig. 13–6B). Like duct lesions and mucinous cystic tumors, they contain tall, columnar, mucin-producing cells (Fig. 13–6C). In effect, IPMNs are macroscopic PanINs. The IPMNs can be distinguished from mucinous cystic neoplasms by the absence of ovarian-type stroma in IPMNs and by the prominent connections between the neoplasm and the pancreatic duct system in IPMNs. Nevertheless, like mucinous cystic tumors, IPMNs typically express cytokeratin, EMA, CEA, and CA 19-9 (Compagno and Oertel, 1978; Cubilla and Fitzgerald, 1984; Hruban and Wilentz, 2000; Kench et al., 1997; Nagai et al., 1995; Solcia et al., 1997).

The IPMNs, like the other forms of incipient neoplasia in the pancreas, can show varying degrees of atypia and can progress from adenoma to borderline tumor, to carcinoma *in situ*, to invasive carcinoma. In fact, approximately 25% of IPMNs are associated with an invasive adenocarcinoma (Fig. 13–6D). These invasive cancers may be conventional ductal adenocarcinomas or may show abundant extracellular mucin production (mucinous carcinoma) (Compagno and Oertel, 1978; Cubilla and Fitzgerald, 1984; Hruban and Wilentz, 2000; Solcia et al., 1997).

As one would expect, IPMNs can therefore be categorized in a scheme similar to that for PanINs and mucinous cystic neoplasms. *Intraductal papillary mucinous adenomas* are IPMNs without significant cytologic or architectural atypia. *Borderline* IPMNs show a moderate amount of dysplasia. Finally, *papillary mucinous carcinoma* is the designation given to those tumors in which the intraductal lesion displays significant cytologic and architectural atypia (carcinoma *in situ*) or in which an invasive cancer is identified (Klöppel et al., 1996; Solcia et al., 1997). Like mucinous cystic tumors, IPMNs often show varying degrees of cytologic and architectural atypia. Therefore, IPMNs should be completely resected, submitted, and histologically examined. Figure 13–6 shows an example of an IPMN.

Not surprisingly, recent genetic studies support a progression model for IPMNs. Several groups have reported activating point mutations in codon 12 of the K-*ras* oncogene in approximately 60% of IPMNs, and these

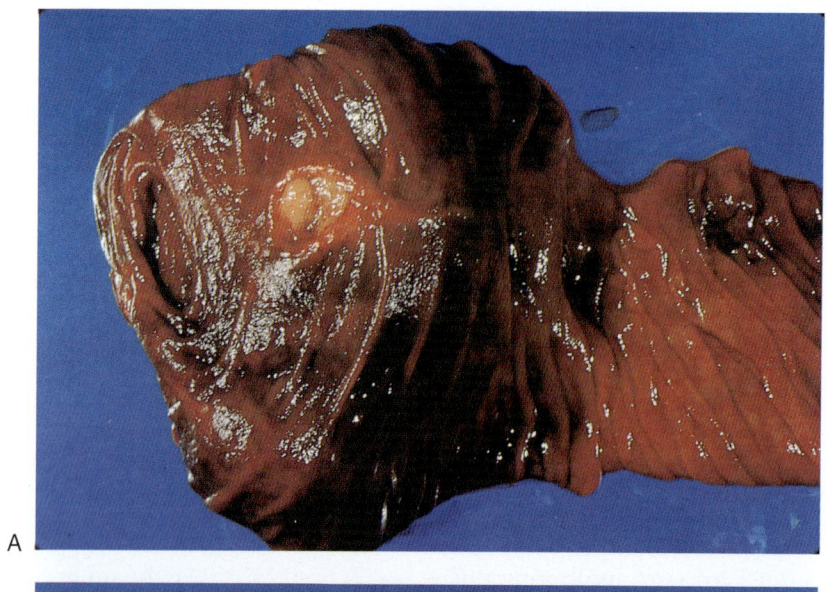

A

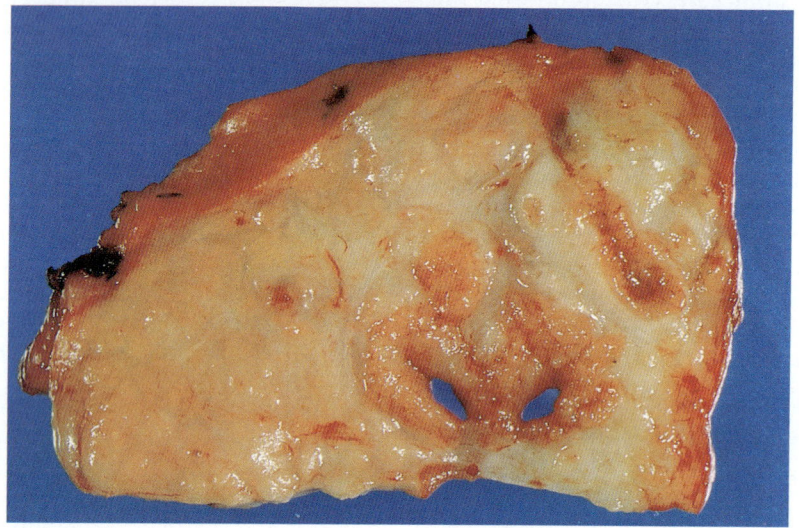

B

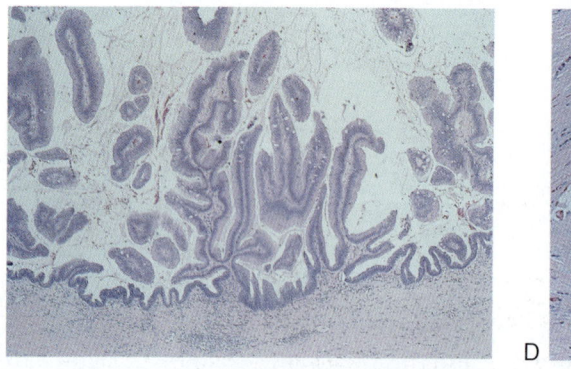

C

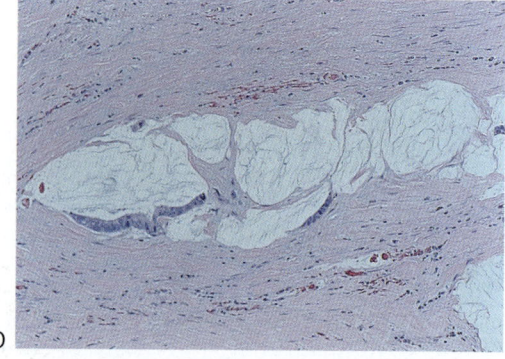

D

Figure 13–6. Gross and microscopic appearances of an intraductal papillary mucinous neoplasm (IPMN) with invasive mucinous adenocarcinoma (papillary mucinous carcinoma). This neoplasm "fills" the large ducts of the pancreas, including the main pancreatic duct, and it even extends out into the ampulla of Vater *(A, B)*. Microscopically, some areas of the tumor contain papillae lined by tall, columnar, mucin-producing cells with moderate dysplasia *(C)*. Other areas show infiltrating mucinous adenocarcinoma *(D)*. Because IPMNs may contain small foci of invasive cancer, each IPMN should be entirely removed and entirely histologically examined.

mutations seem to occur more frequently in the more atypical areas of the IPMNs (Satoh et al., 1993, 1996; Tada et al., 1991; Z'graggen et al., 1997). Fujii et al. (1997) identified allelic loss at 9p in 62%, at 17p in 38%, and at 18q in 38% of the IPMNs that they allelotyped using microsatellite markers. These allelic losses suggest that the *p16* and *p53*, tumor-suppressor genes are inactivated in 40%–60% of IPMNs, and Fujii et al. (1997) found that, like K-*ras* mutations, these allelic losses occurred more frequently in the more atypical areas of the IPMNs. In contrast to ductal adenocarcinomas, the *DPC4* tumor suppressor gene appears to be only very rarely inactivated in IPMNs (Iacobuzio-Donahue et al., 2000).

Just like for mucinous cystic neoplasms, this progression model implies that noninvasive IPMNs follow benign courses. Indeed, current evidence supports this assertion (Nagai et al., 1995; Sessa et al., 1994). In contrast, invasive papillary mucinous carcinomas can recur and metastasize. Sessa et al. have reported metastases in 2 of 13 patients with invasive papillary mucinous carcinomas. Nagai et al. found lymph node metastases in two of five patients with invasive IPMNs. These same two groups reported two deaths at 12 and 28 months and one death at 13 months after resection, respectively (Nagai et al., 1995; Sessa et al., 1994).

INTRADUCTAL ONCOCYTIC PAPILLARY NEOPLASMS

The intraductal oncocytic papillary neoplasm (IOPN) is a rare cousin of the IPMN. First reported in 1996, the IOPN typically presents in men and women in their 60's (Adsay et al., 1996).

The IOPNs have a growth pattern similar to that seen in IPMNs. However, unlike IPMNs and the other forms of incipient neoplasia, these tumors contain primarily eosinophilic, granular cells (oncocytes) that have large, round, vesicular nuclei with prominent nucleoli (see Fig. 13–7.) The tall, columnar, mucin-producing cells seen in the other forms of incipient neoplasia are also scattered throughout the epithelium of the tumor, but they are not the predominant cell type seen. Not surprisingly, electron microscopy of the oncocytic cells shows numerous mitochondria and mucigen granules (Adsay et al., 1996). Immunohistochemical staining reveals the focal expression of CEA and CA 19-9 (Adsay et al., 1996; Morohoshi et al., 1989; Rickaert et al., 1991).

Because most of these tumors contain complex or cribriforming intraductal papillae, they usually meet the pathologic criteria for *in situ* carcinoma. Nevertheless, IOPNs are forms of incipient neoplasia because invasive adenocarcinoma may develop within them. Ten of the 11 cases reported by Adsay et al. (1996) showed areas of carcinoma *in situ*; only 2 of the 11 had invasive carcinoma.

In general, patients with IOPNs have favorable outcomes. Seven of the 11 patients studied by Adsay et al., including 2 with invasive tumors, were alive and free of disease an average of 1 year post-resection. Two patients had died from postoperative complications, and two died 2.5 and 5 years after resection from unrelated causes. One of the

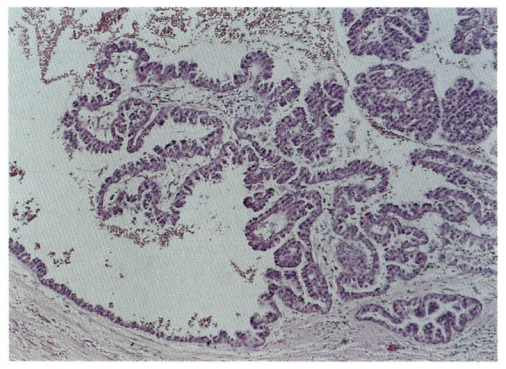
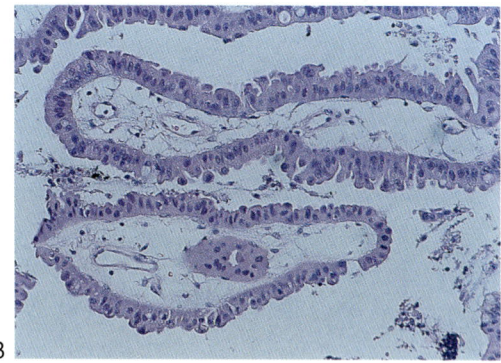

A   B

Figure 13–7. Microscopic appearance of an intraductal oncocytic papillary neoplasm (IOPN). The neoplasm contains plump, eosinophilic, granular cells (oncocytes) with prominent nucleoli *(A, B)*. No invasive carcinoma was seen in this specimen.

patients who died postoperatively had a possible liver metastasis, but no biopsy of the liver lesion was taken. Paradoxically, an invasive component could not be identified in this patient's tumor (Adsay et al., 1996).

Therefore, IOPNs are similar to IPMNs, except that the epithelium in IOPNs is oncocytic, whereas that in IPMNs is mucinous. In both neoplasms, there appears to be a progression from adenoma to borderline tumor, to carcinoma *in situ*, to invasive carcinoma.

PRECURSORS OF OTHER PANCREATIC NEOPLASMS

Over three-fourths of pancreatic neoplasms are ductal adenocarcinoma and its variants (Cubilla et al., 1984; Hruban and Wilentz, 2000; Solcia et al., 1997; Wilentz and Hruban, 1998b). Naturally, therefore, most clinical, morphologic, and genetic studies, including those on neoplastic progression, have focused on this highly aggressive form of cancer. In addition, because of their large size, mucinous cystic neoplasms and intraductal papillary tumors have also been well studied. As molecular techniques are refined and our understanding of the progression of incipient neoplasia of the pancreas grows, attention can be paid to other rare forms of pancreatic cancer (Wenig et al., 1997).

For example, incipient neoplasms have recently been identified in the rare osteoclast-like giant cell tumors of the pancreas (Berendt et al., 1987; Cubilla and Fitzgerald, et al., 1984; Kay and Harrison, 1969; Molberg et al., 1998; Posen, 1981; Robinson et al., 1977; Rosai, 1968; Solcia et al., 1997; Trepeta et al., 1981; Westra et al., 1998). Osteoclast-like giant cell tumors contain sheets of relatively bland mononuclear cells within which are scattered multinucleated giant cells resembling osteoclasts (Fig. 13–8A). In some cases an epithelial component, either a PanINs or a mucinous cystic neoplasm, can also be identified (Fig. 13–8B). Westra and Hruban have shown that the mononuclear cells of osteoclast-like giant cell tumors of the pancreas harbor K-*ras* mutations identical to those seen in the epithelial cells of their associated PanINs and mucinous cystic tumors (Westra et al., 1998). These data indicate that osteoclast-like giant-cell tumors, like invasive ductal adenocarcinomas and invasive mucinous cystadenocarcinomas, may arise from PanINs and mucinous cystic neoplasms. They also imply that osteoclast-like giant-cell tumors are in fact undifferentiated ductal adenocarcinomas with osteoclast-like giant cells (Westra et al., 1998). Figure 13–8 shows an example of an osteoclast-like giant cell tumor with an associated duct lesion with carcinoma *in situ*.

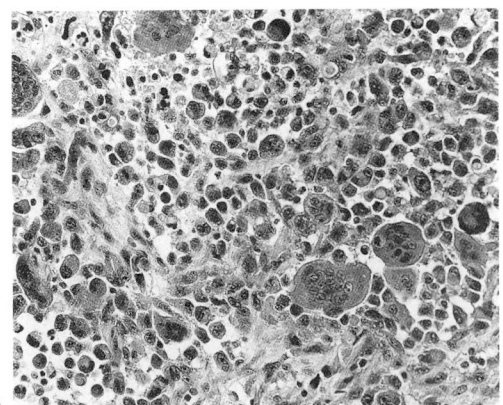 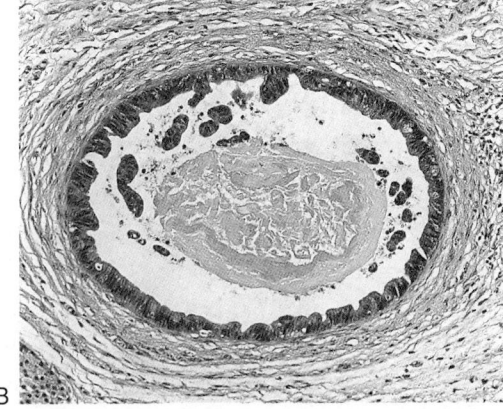

A   B

Figure 13–8. Osteoclast-like giant-cell tumor of the pancreas *(A)* with an associated PanIN showing carcinoma *in situ (B)*. The tumor contains sheets of bland, mononuclear cells within which are scattered multinucleated giant cells resembling osteoclasts. The finding of identical K-*ras* mutations in the PanIN and the tumor supports the hypothesis that the tumor originated from the PanIN and that the tumor is epithelial in origin.

SUMMARY

It has been firmly established that most pancreatic neoplasms arise from histologically recognizable precursors. The three most common precursors to invasive cancer—PanINs, mucinous cystic neoplasms, and intraductal papillary mucinous neoplasms—all contain tall, columnar, mucin-producing cells. In PanINs, these cells line small native pancreatic ductules; in intraductal papillary mucinous neoplasms, they form a villiform mass within large native pancreatic ducts. In contrast, mucinous cystic neoplasms contain *de novo* cysts not connected to the native pancreatic duct system. As molecular techniques are applied to other, rarer pancreatic tumors, we believe that most will be found to have morphologically recognizable precursors.

This research is supported in part (R.E.W. and R.H.H.) by NIH grant P50CA-62924.

REFERENCES

Adsay NV, Adair CF, Heffess CS, Klimstra D. (1996) Intraductal oncocytic papillary neoplasms of the pancreas. *Am J Surg Pathol* 20:980–994.

Albores-Saavedra J, Angeles-Angeles A, Nadji M, Henson DE, Alvarez L. (1987) Mucinous cystadenocarcinoma of the pancreas. Morphologic and immunocytochemical observations. *Am J Surg Pathol* 11:11–20.

Albores-Saavedra J, Gould EW, Angeles-Angeles A, Henson DE. (1990) Cystic tumors of the pancreas. *Pathol Annu* 25(2):19–50.

Albores-Saavedra J, Nadji M, Henson DE, Angeles-Angeles A. (1998) Entero-endocrine cell differentiation in carcinomas of the gallbladder and mucinous cystadenocarcinomas of the pancreas. *Pathol Res Pract* 183:169–175.

Allema JH, Reinders ME, van Gulik TM, Koelemay MJW, Van Leeuwen DJ, de Wit TM, Gouma DJ, Obertop H. (1995) Prognostic factors for survival after pancreaticoduodenectomy for patients with carcinoma of the pancreatic head region. *Cancer* 75:2069–2076.

Bartsch D, Bastian D, Barth P, Schudy A, Nies C, Kisker C, Wagner HJ, Rothmund M. (1998) K-*ras* oncogene mutations indicate malignancy in cystic tumors of the pancreas. *Ann Surg* 228:79–86.

Baylor SM, Berg JW. (1973) Cross-classification and survival characteristics of 5,000 cases of cancer of the pancreas. *J Surg Oncol* 5:335–338.

Beazley RM, Cohn I. (1981) Pancreatic cancer. *CA Cancer J Clin* 31:347–358.

Becker WF, Welsh RA, Pratt HS. (1965) Cystadenoma and cystadenocarcinoma of the pancreas. *Ann Surg* 161:845–863.

Berendt RC, Shnitka TK, Wiens E, Manickavel V, Jewell LD. (1987) The osteoclast-type giant cell tumor of the pancreas. *Arch Pathol Lab Med* 111:43–48.

Berthélemy P, Bouisson M, Escourrou J, Vaysse N, Rumeau JL, Pradayrol L. (1995) Identification of K-*ras* mutations in pancreatic juice in the early diagnosis of pancreatic cancer. *Ann Intern Med* 123:188–191.

Boschman CR, Stryker S, Reddy JK, Rao MS. (1994) Expression of p53 protein in precursor lesions and adenocarcinoma of human pancreas. *Am J Pathol* 145:1291–1295.

Brat DJ, Lillemoe KD, Yeo CJ, Warfield PB, Hruban RH. (1998) Progression of pancreatic intraductal neoplasias (high-grade PanIN) to infiltrating adenocarcinoma of the pancreas. *Am J Surg Pathol* 22:163–169.

Brentnall TA, Chen R, Lee JG, Kimmey MB, Bronner MP, Haggitt RC, Kowdley KV, Hecker LM, Byrd DR. (1995) Microsatellite instability and K-*ras* mutations associated with pancreatic adenocarcinoma and pancreatitis. *Cancer Res* 55:4264–4267.

Brockie E, Anand A, Albores-Saavedra J. (1998) Progression of atypical ductal hyperplasia/carcinoma *in situ* of the pancreas to invasive adenocarcinoma. *Ann Diagn Pathol* 2:286–292.

Caldas C, Hahn SA, Hruban RH, Redston MS, Yeo CJ, Kern SE. (1994) Detection of K-*ras* mutations in the stool of patients with pancreatic adenocarcinoma and pancreatic ductal hyperplasia. *Cancer Res* 54:3568–3573.

Compagno J, Oertel JE. (1978) Mucinous cystic neoplasms of the pancreas with overt and latent malignancy (cystadenocarcinoma and cystadenoma). A clinicopathologic study of 41 cases. *Am J Clin Pathol* 69:573–580.

Conley CR, Scheithauer BW, Weiland LH, van Heerden JA. (1987) Diffuse intraductal papillary adenocarcinoma of the pancreas. *Ann Surg* 205:246–249.

Connolly MM, Dawson PJ, Michelassi F, Moossa AR, Lowenstein F. (1987) Survival in 1001 patients with carcinoma of the pancreas. *Ann Surg* 206:366–373.

Corbally MT, McAnena OJ, Urmacher C, Herman B, Shiu MH. (1989) Pancreatic cystadenoma. A clinicopathologic study. *Arch Surg* 124:1271–1274.

Cubilla AL, Fitzgerald PJ. (1976) Morphological lesions associated with human primary invasive nonendocrine pancreas cancer. *Cancer Res* 36:2690–2698.

Cubilla AL, Fitzgerald PJ. (1984) *Tumors of the Exocrine Pancreas*, 2nd Series Armed Forces Institute of Pathology, Washington, DC.

Cubilla A, Fitzgerald PJ. (1978) Pancreas cancer. I. Duct adenocarcinoma. A clinical-pathologic study of 380 patients. *Pathol Annu* 13 Pt 1:241–289.

Cubilla A, Fortner J, Fitzgerald PJ. (1978) Lymph node involvement in carcinoma of the head of the pancreas area. *Cancer* 41:880–887.

DiGiuseppe JA, Hruban RH, Goodman SN, Polak M, van den Berg FM, Allison DC, Cameron JL, Offerhaus GJA. (1994a) Overexpression of p53 protein in adenocarcinoma of the pancreas. *Am J Clin Pathol* 101:684–688.

DiGiuseppe JA, Hruban RH, Offerhaus GJA, Clement MJ, van den Berg FM, Cameron JL, van Mansfeld ADM. (1994b) Detection of K-*ras* mutations in mucinous pancreatic duct hyperplasia from a patient with a family history of pancreatic carcinoma. *Am J Pathol* 144:889–895.

DiGiuseppe JA, Yeo CJ, Hruban RH. (1996) Molecular biology and the diagnosis and treatment of adenocarcinoma of the pancreas. *Adv Anat Pathol* 3:139–155.

Fearon ER, Vogelstein B. (1990) A genetic model for colorectal tumorigenesis. *Cell* 61:759–767.

Flejou JF, Boulange B, Bernades P, Belghiti J, Henin D. (1996) p53 protein expression and DNA ploidy in cystic tumors of the pancreas. *Pancreas* 13:247–252.

Fujii H, Inagaki M, Kasai S, Miyokawa N, Tokusashi Y, Gabrielson E, Hruban RH. (1997) Genetic progression and heterogeneity in intraductal papillary-mucinous neoplasms of the pancreas. *Am J Pathol* 151:1447–1454.

Furukawa T, Chiba R, Kobari M, Matsuno S, Nagura H, Takahashi T. (1994) Varying grades of epithelial atypia in the pancreatic ducts of humans. Classification based on morphometry and multilvariate analysis and correlated with positive reactions of carcinoembryonic antigen. *Arch Pathol Lab Med* 118: 227–234.

Furukawa T, Takahashi T, Kobari M, Matsuno S. (1992) The mucus-hypersecreting tumor of the pancreas. Development and extension visualized by three-dimensional computerized mapping. *Cancer* 70: 1505–1513.

Geer RJ, Brennan MF. (1993) Prognostic indicators for survival after resection of pancreatic adenocarcinoma. *Am J Surg* 165:68–73.

Goggins M, Hruban RH, Kern SE. The late temporal pattern of BRCA2 inactivation in pancreatic intraductal neoplasia: Evidence and implications. *Am J Pathol* 2000, In press.

Gudjonsson B. (1987) Cancer of the pancreas. 50 years of surgery. *Cancer* 60:2284–2303.

Hameed M, Marrero AM, Conlon KC, Brennan MF, Klimstra DS. (1994) Expression of p53 nucleophosphoprotein in *in situ* pancreatic ductal adenocarcinoma: An immunohistochemical analysis of 100 cases. *Lab Invest* 70:132A.

Hruban RH, Offerhaus GJA, Graves T, Parnes H, Albores-Saavedra J. (1998) Molecular pathology of early pancreatic cancer. In: *Molecular Pathology of Early Cancer* (Scrivastava S, Henson DE, Gazdar A, eds.) pp. 289–299 IOS Press, Amsterdam.

Hruban RH, Wilentz RE. (2000) Pancreas. In: *Modern Surgical Pathology* (Weidner N, Cote RJ, Suster S, Weiss LM, eds.) W.B. Saunders, Philadelphia, In press.

Hruban RH, Wilentz RE, Goggins M, Offerhaus GJA, Yeo CJ, Kern SE. (1999) Pathology of incipient pancreatic cancer. *Ann Oncol* 10 Suppl 4:9–11.

Hyde GL, Davis JB, McMillin RD, McMillin M. (1984) Mucinous cystic neoplasm of the pancreas with latent malignancy. *Am Surg* 50:225–229.

Iacobuzio-Donahue CA, Klimstra DS, Adsay NV, Wilentz RE, Argani P, Sohn TA, Yeo CJ, Kern SE, Hruban RH (2000). DPC-4 protein in expressed in virtually all intraductal papillary mucinous neoplasms of the pancreas. *Am J Pathol,* In press.

Katoh H, Rossi RL, Braasch JW, Munson JL, Shimozawa E, Tanabe T. (1989) Cystadenoma and cystadenocarcinoma of the pancreas. *Hepatogastroenterology* 36:424–430.

Kawarada Y, Yano T, Yamamoto T, Yokoi H, Imai T, Ogura Y, Mizumoto R. (1992) Intraductal mucin-producing tumors of the pancreas. *Am J Gastroenterol* 87:634–638.

Kay S, Harrison JM. (1969) Unusual pleomorphic carcinoma of the pancreas featuring production of osteoid. *Cancer* 23:1158–1162.

Kench JG, Eckstein RP, Smith RC. (1997) Intraductal papillary-mucinous neoplasm of the pancreas: a report of five cases with immunohistochemical findings. *Pathology* 29:7–11.

Klimstra D, Longnecker DS. (1994) K-*ras* mutations in pancreatic ductal proliferative lesions. *Am J Pathol* 145:1547–1550.

Klöppel G, Solcia E, Longnecker DS, et al. (1996) *World Health Organization International Histological Classification of Tumors."* 2nd ed. Springer-Verlag, Berlin.

Kozuka S, Sassa R, Taki T, Masamoto K, Nagasawa S, Saga S, Hasegawa K, Takeuchi M. (1979) Relation of pancreatic duct hyperplasia to carcinoma. *Cancer* 43:1418–1428.

Lemoine NR, Jain S, Hughes CM, Staddon SL, Maillet B, Hall PA, Klöppel G. (1992) Ki-*ras* oncogene activation in preinvasive pancreatic cancer. *Gastroenterology* 102:230–236.

Manabe T, Miyashita T, Ohshio G, Nonaka A, Suzuki T, Endo K, Takahashi M, Tobe T. (1988) Small carcinoma of the pancreas. Clinical and pathologic evaluation of 17 patients. *Cancer* 62:135–141.

Michelassi F, Erroi F, Dawson PJ, Pietrabissa A, Noda S, Handcock M, Block GE. (1989) Experience with 647 consecutive tumors of the duodenum, ampulla, head of the pancreas, and distal common bile duct. *Ann Surg* 210:544–556.

Molberg KH, Heffess C, Albores-Saavedra J. (1998) Undifferentiated carcinoma with osteoclast-like giant cells of the pancreas and periampullary region. *Cancer* 82:1279–1287.

Moossa AR, Levin B. (1981) The diagnosis of "early" pancreatic cancer: The University of Chicago experience. *Cancer* 47:1688–1697.

Morohoshi T, Kanda M, Asanuma K, Klöppel G. (1989) Intraductal papillary neoplasms of the pancreas. A clinicopathologic study of six patients. *Cancer* 64: 1329–1335.

Moskaluk CA, Hruban RH, Kern SE. (1997). *p16* and K-*ras* gene mutations in the intraductal precursors of human pancreatic adenocarcinoma. *Cancer Res* 57:2140–2143.

Nagai E, Ueki T, Chijiiwa K, Tanaka M, Tsuneyoshi M. (1995) Intraductal papillary mucinous neoplasms of the pancreas associated with so-called mucinous ductal ectasia. Histochemical and immunohistochemical analysis of 29 cases. *Am J Surg Pathol* 19: 576–589.

Nagakawa T, Mori K, Nakano T, Kadoya M, Kobayashi H, Akiyama T, Kayahara M, Ohta T, Ueno K, Higashino Y, Konishi I, Miyazaki I. (1993) Perineural invasion of carcinoma of the pancreas and biliary tract. *Br J Surg* 80:619–621.

Nishihara K, Fukuda T, Tsuneyoshi M, Kominami T, Maeda S, Saku M. (1993) Intraductal papillary neoplasm of the pancreas. *Cancer* 72:689–696.

Obara T, Maguchi H, Saitoh Y, Ura H, Koike Y, Kitazawa S, Namiki M. (1991) Mucin producing tumor of the pancreas: a unique clinical entity. *Am J Gastroenterol* 86:1619–1625.

Ohta T, Nagakawa T, Akiyama T, Fukushima W, Ueno K, Miyazaki I, Suzuki M, Matsui O, Terada T, Nakanuma Y, Kanno M, Uogishi M, Sodani H. (1992) The "duct-ectatic" variant of mucinous cystic neoplasm of the pancreas: clinical and radiologic studies of seven cases. *Am J Gastroenterol* 87:300–304.

Parker SL, Tong T, Bolden S, Wingo PA. (1997) Cancer statistics, 1997. *CA Cancer J Clin* 47:5–27.

Payan M, Xerri L, Moncada K, Bastid C, Agostini S, Sastre B, Sahel J, Choux R. (1990) Villous adenoma of the main pancreatic duct: a potentially malignant tumor?. *Am J Gastroenterol* 85:459–463.

Posen JA. (1981) Giant cell tumor of the pancreas of the osteoclastic type associated with a mucous secreting cystadenocarcinoma. *Hum Pathol* 12:944–947.

Pour PM, Sayed S, Sayed G. (1982) Hyperplastic, preneoplastic and neoplastic lesions found in 83 human pancreases. *Am J Clin Pathol* 77:137–152.

Rickaert F, Cremer M, Devière J, Tavares L, Lambilliotte JP, Schröder S, Wurbs D, Klöppel G. (1991) Intraductal mucin-hypersecreting neoplasms of the pancreas. A clinicopathologic study of eight patients. *Gastroenterology* 101:512–519.

Ridder GJ, Maschek H, Flemming P, Nashan B, Klempnauer J. (1998) Ovarian-like stroma in an invasive mucinous cystadenocarcinoma of the pancreas positive for inhibin. A hint concerning its possible pathogenesis. *Virchows Arch A Pathol Anat Histopathol* 432:451–454.

Robinson L, Damjenov I, Brezina P. (1977) Multinucleated giant cell neoplasm of pancreas. Light and electron microscopy features. *Arch Pathol Lab Med* 101:590–593.

Rosai J. (1968) Carcinoma of pancreas simulating giant cell tumor of bone. Electron-microscopic evidence of its acinar cell origin. *Cancer* 22:333–344.

Sachs JR, Deren JJ, Sohn M, Nusbaum M. (1989) Mucinous cystadenoma: pitfalls of differential diagnosis. *Am J Gastroenterol* 84:811–816.

Santini D, Campione O, Salerno A, Gullo L, Mazzoleni G, Leone O, Martinelli G, Marrano D. (1995) Intraductal papillary-mucinous neoplasm of the pancreas. A clinicopathologic entity. *Arch Pathol Lab Med* 119:209–213.

Satoh K, Sawai T, Shimosegawa T, Koizumi M, Yamazaki T, Mochizuki F, Toyota T. (1993) The point mutation of c-Ki-*ras* at codon 12 in carcinoma of the pancreatic head region and in intraductal mucin-hypersecreting neoplasm of the pancreas. *Int J Pancreatol* 14:135–143.

Satoh K, Shimosegawa T, Moriizumi S, Koizumi M, Toyota T. (1996) K-*ras* mutation and p53 protein accumulation in intraductal mucin-hypersecreting neoplasms of the pancreas. *Pancreas* 12:362–368.

Sessa F, Solcia E, Capella C, Bonato M, Scarpa A, Zamboni G, Pellegata NS, Ranzani GN, Rickaert F, Klöppel G. (1994) Intraductal papillary-mucinous tumours represent a distinct group of pancreatic neoplasms: an investigation of tumour cell differentiation and K-*ras*, p53 and c-*erb*B-2 abnormalities in 26 patients. *Virchows Arch A Pathol Anat Histopathol* 425:357–367.

Solcia E, Capella C, Klöppel G. (1997) *Tumors of the Pancreas*, 3rd Series Armed Forces Institute of Pathology, Washington, DC.

Tabata T, Fujimori T, Maeda S, Yamamoto M, Saitoh Y. (1993) The role of *ras* mutation in pancreatic cancer, precancerous lesions, and chronic pancreatitis. *Int J Pancreatol* 14:237–244.

Tada M, Omata M, Ohto M. (1991) *Ras* gene mutations in intraductal papillary neoplasms of the pancreas. Analysis in five cases. *Cancer* 67:634–637.

Tada M, Ohashi M, Shiratori Y, Okudaira T, Komatsu Y, Kawabe T, Yoshida H, Machinami R, Kishi K, Omata M. (1996) Analysis of K-*ras* gene mutation in hyperplastic duct cells of the pancreas without pancreatic disease. *Gastroenterology* 110:227–231.

Talamini MA, Pitt H, Hruban RH, Boitnott JK, Coleman J, Cameron JL. (1992) Spectrum of cystic tumors of the pancreas. *Am J Surg* 163:117–124.

Trepeta RW, Mathur B, Lagin S, LiVolsi V. (1981) Giant cell tumor ("osteoclastoma") of the pancreas: a tumor of epithelial origin. *Cancer* 48:2022–2028.

Tsuchiya R, Noda T, Harada N, Miiyamoto T, Tomioka T, Yamamoto K, Yamaguchi T, Izawa K, Tsunoda T, Yoshino R, Eto T. (1986) Collective review of small carcinomas of the pancreas. *Ann Surg* 203:77–81.

Tsuchiya R, Oribe T, Noda T. (1985) Size of the tumor and other factors influencing prognosis of carcinoma of the head of the pancreas. *Am J Gastroenterol* 80:459–462.

Warshaw AL, Castillo CFD. (1992) Pancreatic carcinoma. *N Engl J Med* 326:455–465.

Warshaw AL, Compton CC, Lewandrowski K, Cardenosa G, Mueller PR. (1990) Cystic tumors of the pancreas. New clinical, radiologic, and pathologic observations in 67 patients. *Ann Surg* 212:432–445.

Wenig BM, Albores-Saavedra J, Buetow PC, Heffess CS. (1997) Pancreatic mucinous cystic neoplasm with sarcomatous stroma: a report of three cases. *Am J Surg Pathol* 21:70–80.

Westra WH, Sturm PJ, Drillenburg P, Choti MA, Klimstra DS, Abores-Saavedra J, Montag A, Offerhaus GJA, Hruban RH. (1998) K-*ras* oncogene mutations in osteoclast-like giant cell tumors of the pancreas and liver: genetic evidence to support origin from the duct epithelium. *Am J Surg Pathol* 22:1247–1254.

Wilentz RE, Chung CH, Sturm PDJ, Musler A, Sohn TA, Offerhaus GJA, Yeo CJ, Hruban RH, Slebos RJC. (1998a) K-*ras* mutations in the duodenal fluid of patients with pancreatic carcinoma. *Cancer* 82:96–103.

Wilentz RE, Geradts J, Maynard R, Offerhaus JA, Kang M, Goggins M, Yeo CJ, Kern SE, Hruban RH. (1998b) Inactivation of the p16 (INK4A) tumor-suppressor gene in pancreatic duct lesions: loss of intranuclear expression. *Cancer Res* 58:4740–4744.

Wilentz RE, Hruban RH. (1998) Pathology of cancer of the pancreas. *Surg Oncol Clin North Am* 7:43–65.

Wilentz RE, Hruban RH, Albores-Saavedra J. (1999a) Prognosis of invasive mucinous cystadenocarcinomas of the pancreas: a study of over 29,000 patients from the SEER database. *Mod Pathol* 12:169A.

Wilentz RE, Albores-Saavedra J, Zahurak M, Talamini MA, Yeo CJ, Cameron JL, Hruban RH. (1999) Pathologic examination accurately predicts prognosis in mucinous cystic neoplasms of the pancreas. *Am J Surg Pathol* 23:1320–1327.

Wilentz RE, Iacobuzio-Donahue CA, Pedram A, McCarthy DM, Parsons JL, Yeo CJ, Kern SE, Hruban RH. (2000) Loss of expression of *DPC4* in pancreatic intraepithelial neoplasia (PanIN): Evidence that *DPC4* inactivation occurs late in neoplastic progression. *Cancer Res*, 60:2002–2006.

Willett CG, Lewandrowski K, Warshaw AL, Efird J, Compton CC. (1993) Resection margins in carcinoma of the head of the pancreas. Implications for radiation therapy. *Ann Surg* 217:144–148.

Yamada M, Kozuka S, Yamao K, Nakazawa S, Naitoh Y, Tsukamoto Y. (1991) Mucin-producing tumor of the pancreas. *Cancer* 68:159–168.

Yamaguchi K, Enjoji M. (1987) Cystic neoplasms of the pancreas. *Gastroenterology* 92:1934–1943.

Yamaguchi K, Tanaka M. (1991) Mucin-hypersecreting tumor of the pancreas with mucin extrusion through an enlarged papilla. *Am J Gastroenterol* 86:835–839.

Yanagisawa A, Ohashi K, Hori M, Takagi K, Kitagawa T, Sugano H, Kato Y. (1993a) Ductectatic-type mucinous cystadenoma and cystadenocarcinoma of the human pancreas: A novel clinicopathological entity. *Jpn J Cancer Res* 84:474–479.

Yanagisawa A, Ohtake K, Ohashi K, Hori M, Kitagawa T, Sugano H, Kato Y. (1993b) Frequent c-Ki-*ras* oncogene activation in mucous cell hyperplasias of pan-creas suffering from chronic inflammation. *Cancer Res* 53:953–956.

Yeo CJ, Cameron JL, Lillemoe KD, Sitzmann JV, Hruban RH, Goodman SN, Dooley WC, Coleman J, Pitt HA. (1995) Pancreaticoduodenectomy for cancer of the head of the pancreas. 201 patients. *Ann Surg* 221: 721–733.

Yu HC, Shetty J. (1985) Mucinous cystic neoplasm of the pancreas with high carcinoembryonic antigen. *Arch Pathol Lab Med* 109:375–377.

Z'graggen K, Rivera JA, Compton CC, Pins M, Werner J, Fernandez-del Castillo C, Rattner DW, Lewandrowski KB, Rustgi AK, Warshaw AL. (1997) Prevalence of ac-tivating K-*ras* mutations in the evolutionary stages of neoplasia in intraductal papillary mucinous tumors of the pancreas. *Ann Surg* 226:491–498.

14

LUNG

WILLIAM D. TRAVIS

Lung cancer is currently the most common cause of cancer incidence and mortality worldwide (Parker et al., 1999). In 1999 it is estimated that lung cancer will account for over 187,000 new cases and over 164,000 cancer deaths in the United States (Landis et al., 1999). Although overall lung cancer incidence for both sexes combined is declining in the United States primarily because of decreases in males that began in the early 1980s (Travis et al., 1996), it continues to increase in women (Wingo et al., 1999). Despite all the efforts at treatment of lung cancer, the 5-year survival has remained between 10% and 15% over the past few decades (Travis et al., 1995). For this reason, there is great interest in early detection of lung cancer by means of a variety of approaches, including fluorescence bronchoscopy (Lam et al., 1998), and in screening of high-risk patients by spiral or helical computed tomography (CT) (Gartenschlager et al., 1998; Itoh et al., 1998). Along with the interest in early diagnosis of lung cancer, clinical trials of chemoprevention based on mechanisms of drug action and dietary modification have been conducted (Boone et al., 1993; Buiatti et al., 1996).

Concepts of pulmonary incipient neoplasia are not as advanced as those in other organ systems such as the cervix, gastrointestinal tract, and bladder. However, there has been considerable evolution in the concepts of incipient neoplasia for lung carcinoma in the past few decades. This is re-flected in the progression of interest from the first World Health Organization (WHO) histologic classification of lung tumors in 1967 in which there was no mention of preinvasive lesions (World Health Organization, 1967; Table 14–1). In the 1981 WHO histologic classification of lung tumors, bronchial squamous dysplasia and carcinoma *in situ* (CIS) were the only preinvasive lesions recognized for lung cancer (World Health Organization, 1981; Table 14–1). Since the 1981 proposal two new lesions have been described: atypical adenomatous hyperplasia (AAH) (Mori et al., 1990) and diffuse idiopathic pulmonary neuroendocrine cell hyperplasia (DIPNECH) (Aguayo et al., 1992; Table 14–1). Because these lesions were recognized as potential precursor lesions for adenocarcinomas and carcinoids, respectively, they were added to the category of preinvasive lesions in the new 1999 *Histologic Typing of Lung and Pleural Tumors* (Travis et al., 1999). In addition, the lesion of malignant mesothelioma *in situ*, has been proposed (Henderson et al., 1998; Whitaker et al., 1992). However, this is a controversial concept that has not been widely accepted.

Another major development in the field of incipient pulmonary neoplasia over the past two decades has been the explosion of molecular data accumulated, which has contributed to our understanding of the genetic events involved in lung carcinogenesis (Brambilla et al., 1998, 1999; Colby et al., 1998; Ikeda et al., 1998; Kitaguchi et al.,

Table 14–1. History of Classification of Preinvasive Lesions by the World Health Organization

1967 WHO Classification[a]	1981 WHO Classification[b]	1999 WHO/IASLC Classification[c]
No category of preinvasive lesions	Squamous dysplasia/carcinoma *in situ*	Squamous dysplaisa/carcinoma *in situ* Atypical adenomatous hyperplasia Diffuse idiopathic pulmonary neuroendocrine cell hyperplasia

[a]From World Health Organization (1967).

[b]From World Health Organization (1981).

[c]From Travis et al., 1999.

1998; Kurasono et al., 1998; Niho et al., 1999; Sozzi et al., 1992; Wistuba et al., 1999).

PREINVASIVE BRONCHIAL SQUAMOUS LESIONS

Bronchial carcinogenesis is conceptualized as a multistep process involving transformation of the normal bronchial mucosa through a continuous spectrum of lesions, including basal cell hyperplasia, squamous metaplasia, dysplasia, and CIS (Auerbach et al., 1957; Becci et al., 1978; Bennett et al., 1993; Brambilla et al., 1998; Carter, 1978; Colby et al., 1995; McDowell et al., 1978; Woolner, 1993). In addition to these epithelial changes, alterations of the extracellular matrix, particularly destruction of the epithelial basement membrane, are critical events in the development of invasion and in the eventual occurrence of metastases (Aznavoorian et al., 1993; Bosman, 1994; Flug and Kopf-Maier, 1995).

In the new 1999 WHO/International Association for the Study of Lung Cancer (IASLC) classification, squamous dysplasia and CIS were grouped together under the term *preinvasive bronchial squamous lesions.* The term *preinvasive* does not necessarily imply that progression to invasion would have to occur. However, these lesions are considered to be potential precursors to squamous cell carcinoma. A variety of bronchial epithelial hyperplasias and metaplasias may occur that are not regarded as preneoplastic, including goblet cell hyperplasia, basal cell (reserve cell) hyperplasia, and squamous metaplasia (Müller and Müller, 1983).

GROSS AND BRONCHOSCOPIC FEATURES

The bronchoscopic and gross features of preinvasive and early squamous lung carcinomas are similar. Preinvasive bronchial squamous lesions may be very difficult to see grossly. In up to 39% of cases of CIS and even 17% of carcinomas with intramucosal invasion, Woolner et al. (1984) found the bronchial mucosa to be grossly normal in surgical resection specimens. Therefore, preinvasive lesions of dysplasia or CIS are easily missed by gross or bronchoscopic inspection and it is difficult to separate CIS from dysplasia or squamous metaplasia without a biopsy. Gross abnormalities of CIS include loss of rugal folds, slightly increased thickness, granularity or nodularity, and papillary or polypoid projections on the bronchial mucosal surface Melamed et al., 1977; Fig. 14–1). Carcinoma *in situ* is often identified on the spur or point of bifurcation of the segmental bronchi (Carter et al., 1976; Nagamoto et al., 1993).

The difficulty in detecting preinvasive squamous lesions by traditional white light bronchoscopy has led to the development of the light-induced fluorescence endoscopy (LIFE) device by Lam and others (1993, 1998). This technique greatly enhances the bronchoscopist's ability to localize small neoplastic lesions, especially intraepithelial lesions (Lam et al., 1998). The sensitivity of detecting dysplastic lesions is increased by about 50% (Lam et al., 1993).

HISTOLOGIC FEATURES

Normal Bronchial Mucosa

The normal airway mucosa consists of pseudostratified ciliated epithelium resting on a thin basement membrane. The epithelial cells consist primarily of ciliated cells, a few goblet cells, and basal cells at the base of the mucosa (Müller and Müller, 1983). Other cells that can be seen include parabasal cells, mostly in the proximal airways, and a few

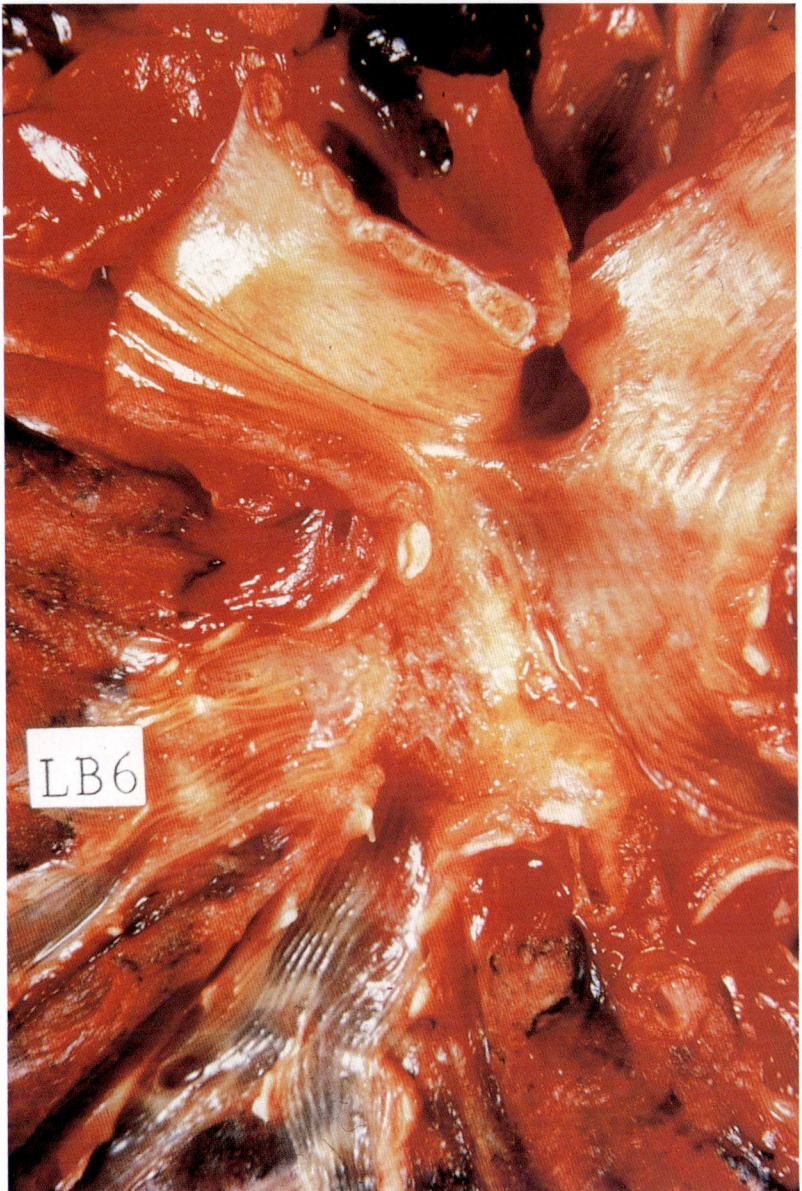

Figure 14–1. Carcinoma *in situ,* gross features. The bronchial mucosa shows loss of rugal folds and focal granularity, which corresponded, to carcinoma *in situ* histologically.

scattered neuroendocrine cells (Lam et al., 1999). Clara cells are limited to the peripheral airways. The epithelial cells are 3–4 layers thick in central bronchi and this number decreases toward the peripheral airways until, in the terminal bronchioles, there is only a single cell layer (Müller and Müller, 1983).

Epithelial Hyperplasia

The major forms of epithelial hyperplasia in the bronchial mucosa consist of basal cell and goblet cell hyperplasia. Neuroendocrine cell hyperplasia may also occur; this is addressed below as a separate topic.

Basal cell hyperplasia. Basal cell hyperplasia consists of an increased number of basal cells forming a layer several cells thick (Fig. 14–2). The overlying ciliated and goblet cells are preserved. The term *reserve cell hyperplasia* has also been used for this lesion. Ciliated cells may be present. Goblet cells are

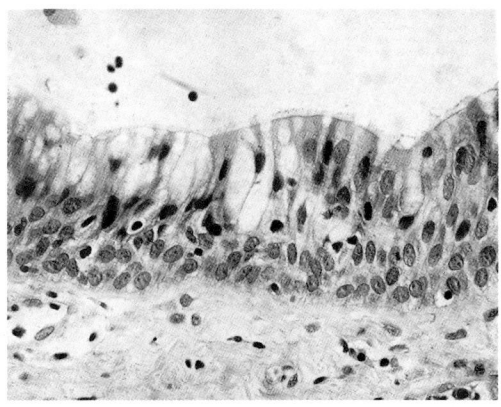

Figure 14–2. Basal cell hyperplasia. There are at least two layers of basal cells at the base of the bronchial epithelium. There are also a few too many goblet cells. Ciliated cells are preserved.

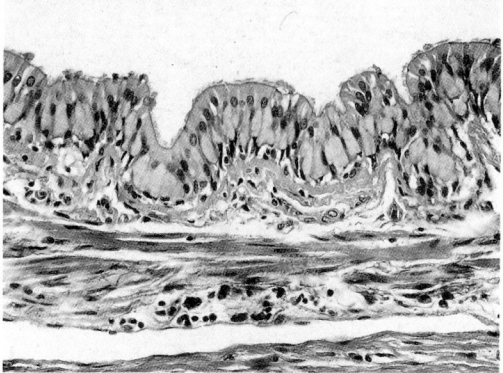

Figure 14–4. Goblet cell hyperplasia. Numerous goblet cells appear in this bronchial mucosa. Ciliated cells are preserved.

usually absent, but occasionally, goblet cell and basal cell hyperplasia may be seen together.

In some cases the basal cells replace almost the entire mucosal surface (Fig. 14–3). The lack of keratinization, the relatively small size of the cells, and the full-thickness mucosal abnormality may result in confusion with severe dysplasia or even CIS. However, these cells show little atypia, no nuclear hyperchromatism or angulation, and pleomorphism or increased mitoses are lacking.

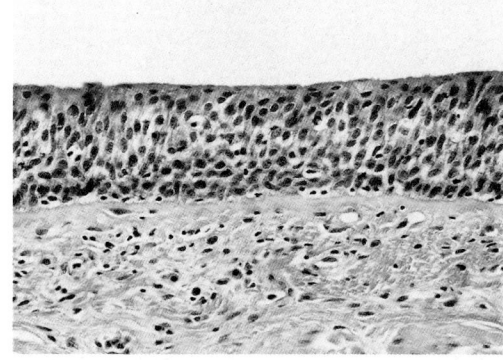

Figure 14–3. Marked basal cell hyperplasia. Nonkeratinizing epithelial cells replace the glandular epithelium but it is not thickened. There is minimal atypia and only slight maturation. The cells are relatively small with only moderate abundant cytoplasm. The nuclei have finely granular chromatin and nucleoli are absent or inconspicuous. Mitoses are absent, and there is minimal nuclear angulation.

The term *immature squamous metaplasia* has occasionally been used for such cases, since some have regarded these cells as representing nonkeratinizing squamous cells.

Goblet cell hyperplasia. In goblet cell hyperplasia the bronchial mucosa contains an increased number of mucus-filled goblet-shaped cells (Fig. 14–4). Cytologic atypia is lacking. Ciliated cells are preserved. Goblet cell hyperplasia may be accompanied by basal cell hyperplasia.

Squamous Metaplasia

In squamous metaplasia, squamous cells replace the pseudostratified and ciliated res-

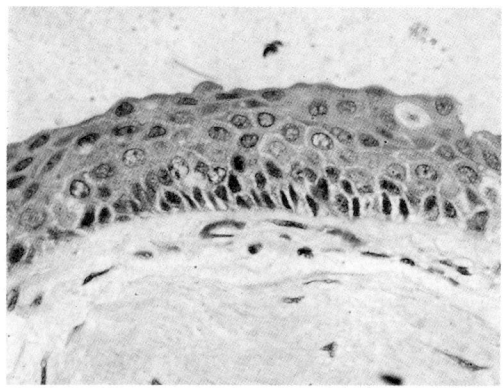

Figure 14–5. Squamous metaplasia. The glandular epithelium is completely replaced by mature squamous cells that show intercellular bridges and maturation at the surface.

piratory epithelium (Fig. 14–5). In contrast to dysplasia and CIS, cytologic atypia is lacking. The cells demonstrate squamous differentiation either by keratinization or intercellular bridges. There is maturation from the basal layer to a layer of surface keratinized cells. The ciliated and goblet cells are lost (Müller and Müller, 1983).

Squamous Dysplasia

Squamous dysplasia may be mild (Fig. 14–6), moderate (Fig. 14–7), or severe (Fig. 14–8); however, each form falls short of the full-thickness involvement that characterizes CIS. The WHO/IASLC criteria for the grades of dysplasia and for CIS are summarized in Table 14–2. While each of the detailed morphologic criteria listed in Table 14–2 may be useful in separating these grades of dysplasia, there is a continuum of morphologic abnormalities and a great deal of overlap between categories. Furthermore, there is a spectrum of morphology within each of the grades of dysplasia/CIS and rarely are all of the criteria listed present in lesions from the various categories. In addition to the relatively small experience of most pathologists with bronchial dysplastic lesions, these difficult morphologic issues are the source of considerable reproducibility problems.

If inflammation is present or if the specimen was obtained after a previous biopsy or therapy, caution should be exercised not to overinterpret reactive atypia (Fig. 14–9). Poor orientation of the mucosa in the his-

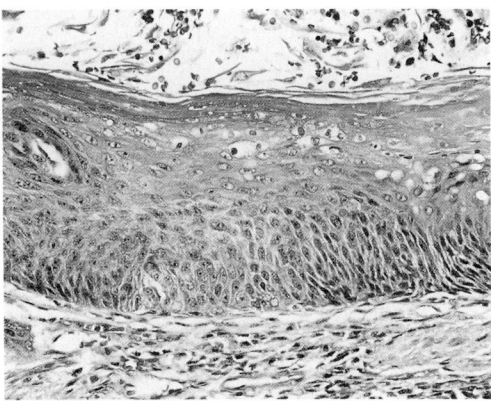

Figure 14–7. Moderate dysplasia. The squamous epithelium shows maturation and keratinization at the surface. However, up to the middle third of the epithelium there is nuclear crowding and hyperchromasia with numerous prominent nucleoli. Nucleoli are visible up to the upper third of the mucosa. Mitoses are lacking.

tologic section due to tangential sectioning may also complicate the interpretation of biopsy specimens.

Micropapillary change. Rarely, the bronchial mucosa associated with squamous metaplastic or dysplastic epithelium may show *micropapillary change*, also called *micropapillomatosis* (Müller and Müller, 1983), which is characterized by papillary projections above the mucosal surface with a fibrovascular core within the papillae (Fig. 14–10A). The epithelium overlying these papillae is usually

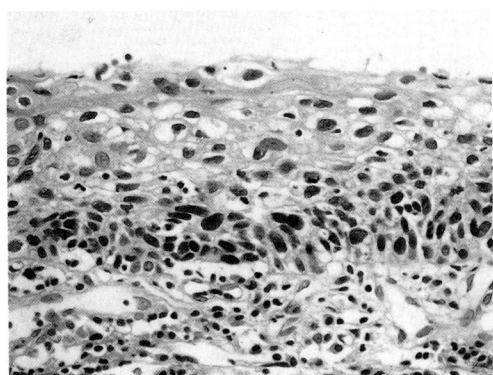

Figure 14–6. Mild dysplasia. The epithelium is squamous with maturation toward the surface and an intermediate layer. There is atypia in the lower third with nuclear hyperchromasia.

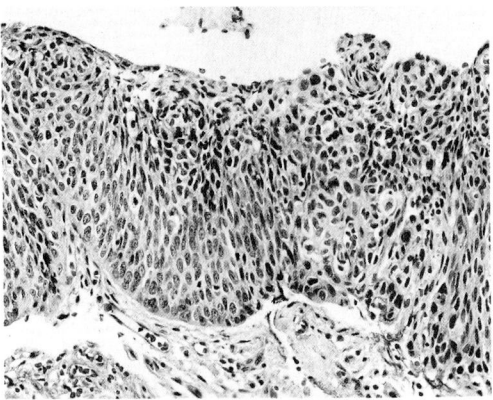

Figure 14–8. Severe dysplasia. The squamous epithelium shows marked cytologic atypia into the upper third of the mucosa with nuclear enlargement and hyperchromasia.

Table 14–2. Microscopic Features of Squamous Dysplasia and Carcinoma in *Situ*

Abnormality	Thickness	Cell Size	Maturation/Orientation	Nuclei
Mild dysplasia	Mildly increased	Mildly increased; Mild anisocytosis, Pleomorphism	Continuous progression of maturation from base to luminal surface; Basilar zone expanded with cellular crowding in lower third; Distinct intermediate (prickle cell) zone present; Superficial flattening of epithelial cells	Mild variation of N/C ratio; Finely granular chromatin; Minimal angulation; Nucleoli inconspicuous or absent; Nuclei vertically oriented in lower third; Mitoses absent or very rare
Moderate dysplasia	Moderately increased	Mild increase in cell size; cells often small; May have moderate anisocytosis, pleomorphism	Partial progression of maturation from base to luminal surface; Basilar zone expanded with cellular crowding in lower two thirds of epithelium; Intermediate zone confined to upper third of epithelium; Superficial flattening of epithelial cells	Moderate variation of N/C ratio; Finely granular chromatin; Angulations, grooves, and lobulations present; Nucleoli inconspicuous or absent; Nuclei vertically oriented in lower two thirds; Mitotic figures present in lower third
Severe dysplasia	Markedly increased	Markedly increased; May have marked anisocytosis, pleomorphism	Little progression of maturation from base to luminal surface; Basilar zone expanded with cellular crowding well into upper third; Intermediate zone greatly attenuated; Superficial flattening of epithelial cells	N/C ratio often high and variable; Chromatin coarse and uneven; Nuclear angulations and folding prominent; Nucleoli frequently present and conspicuous; Nuclei vertically oriented in lower two thirds; Mitotic figures present in lower two thirds
Carcinoma *in situ*	May or may not be increased	May be markedly increased; May have marked anisocytosis, pleomorphism	No progression of maturation from base to luminal surface; epithelium could be inverted with little change in appearance; Basilar zone expanded with cellular crowding throughout epithelium; Intermediate zone absent; Surface flattening confined to the most superficial cells	N/C ratio often high and variable; Chromatin coarse and uneven; Nuclear angulations and folding prominent; Nucleoli may be present or inconspicuous; No consistent orientation of nuclei in relation to epithelial surface; Mitotic figures present through full thickness

Table from Travis et al. (1999), with permission. Contribution by Dr. Wilbur Franklin is gratefully acknowledged.

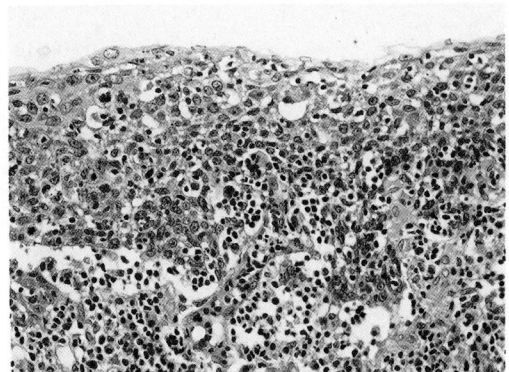

Figure 14–9. Squamous metaplasia with marked chronic inflammation. There is such extensive chronic inflammation involving the mucosa that it is difficult to assess the cytologic features and to classify this lesion as dysplasia.

squamous and is often attenuated, showing only a one- or two-cell layer thickness (Fig. 14–10B). Sometimes the epithelium is denuded or only a few fragmented epithelial cells, usually basal cells, are present. It can be difficult to grade dysplasia and to make a distinction between squamous metaplasia and CIS because of the disorientation of the epithelium associated with micropapillary change.

Carcinoma *in Situ*

In CIS, squamous cells with cytologic features of carcinoma replace the entire thickness of the bronchial epithelium. There is no invasive growth or penetration past the level of the subepithelial basement membrane (Fig. 14–11). Cytologically, the tumor cells may have marked variation in size and shape. The nuclear-to-cytoplasmic (N/C) ratio is increased with frequent nuclear enlargement and hyperchromasia. Nucleoli and nuclear angulation may be prominent. Mitoses may be seen throughout the thickness of the epithelium. In CIS the epithelial cells lose their stratification and orientation. Maturation is lacking, so the mucosa would appear the same if it were inverted, although some flattening of the superficial cells may be seen. The CIS may spread into submucosal glands, but if the basement membrane is intact or if the tumor cells do not spread beyond the border of the glands, this does not represent invasive growth (Fig. 14–12). The basement membrane may be difficult to evaluate in CIS since it is often markedly thinned and breaks may be present. Occasionally, CIS may undermine adjacent mucosa, so cytologically malignant cells are present within benign respiratory epithelial cells. Submucosal chronic inflammation is often present in association with CIS.

Carcinoma *in situ* is found most often in the segmental bronchi and it frequently extends proximally into the lobar bronchi (Carter, 1978; Carter et al., 1976). It is also often associated with an abrupt change to normal bronchial mucosa rather than dysplastic epithelium. This finding has led to some debate as to whether CIS represents in-

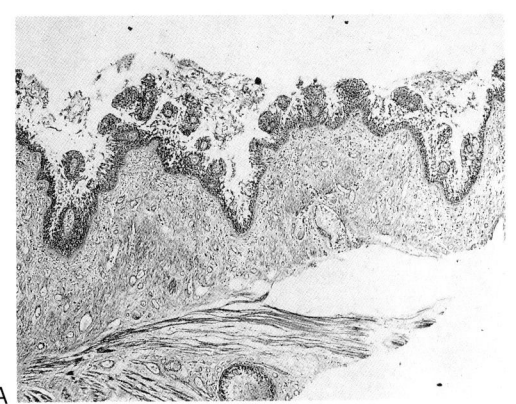
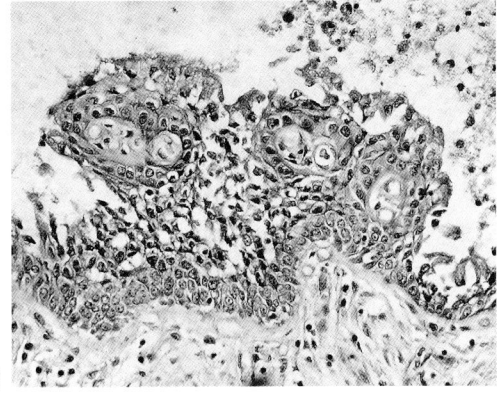

Figure 14–10. Micropapillary change. *A:* The bronchial mucosa shows multiple papillary excrescences protruding from the surface. *B:* The papillae contain vascular cores and are covered by mature squamous cells along the surface. The orientation of the epithelium is distorted because of the papillary configuration.

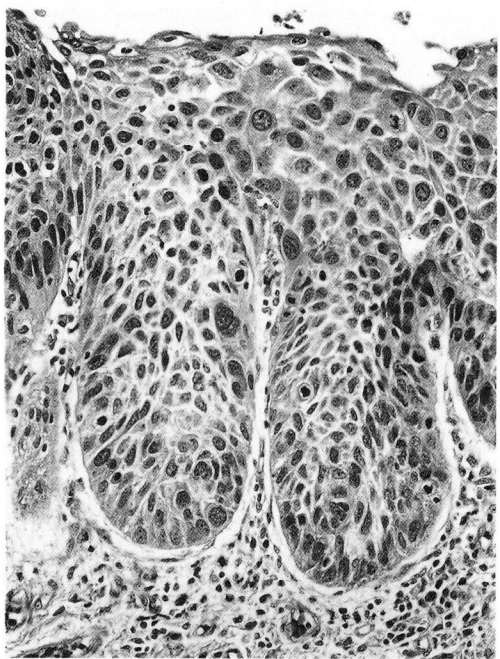

Figure 14–11. Carcinoma *in situ*. The orientation of the epithelium (left) is lost, so the mucosa could be inverted. The cells show marked nuclear hyperchromasia.

the lung (Woolner et al., 1984). This is helpful in patients with a history of a squamous cell carcinoma in another site, such as the upper aerodigestive tract, for the question of whether a lung tumor is primary or metastatic. The presence of CIS is also a criterion favoring the diagnosis of adenosquamous carcinoma rather than high-grade mucoepidermoid carcinoma (Colby et al., 1995). From a clinical viewpoint, if a carcinoma is completely *in situ*, it is not capable of metastasizing (Woolner et al., 1984). The presence of CIS also raises the possibility of multicentricity, future recurrence, and concurrent or subsequent invasive carcinoma (Woolner et al., 1984). Therefore patients diagnosed with severe dysplasia and/or CIS, in the absence of invasive carcinoma, are targets for chemoprevention (Buiatti et al., 1996), and close clinical follow-up.

Microinvasive Squamous Cell Carcinoma

Invasion requires the passage of tumor cells through the basement membrane into the underlying submucosa (Fig. 14–13). However, it can be difficult to identify the base-

tramucosal spread of the carcinoma in some cases rather than a preneoplastic lesion (Carter et al., 1976).

Recognition of CIS has several clinical implications. The presence of an *in situ* component within or adjacent to a tumor supports the view that it arose primarily within

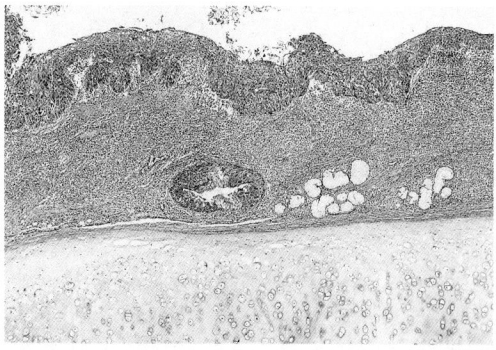

Figure 14–12. Carcinoma *in situ* (CIS) with submucosal gland involvement. The mucosal surface is diffusely involved by CIS. There is extension into the underlying submucosal gland, but this does not qualify as invasive carcinoma.

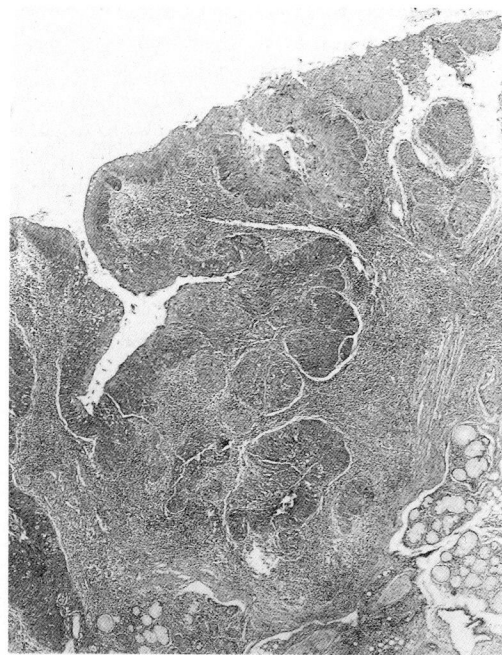

Figure 14–13. Invasive squamous cell carcinoma. There is extensive mucosal involvement by carcinoma *in situ* but there is also a focus of invasion into the underlying submucosa.

Table 14–3. Pathologic Classification of 68 Occult Lung Cancers Resected at Mayo Clinic

Category	Depth of Invasion	Cancers n (%)
1. *In situ* carcinoma	0	23 (34)
2. Intramucosal invasion	<0.10	12 (18)
3. Invasion to bronchial cartilages	0.11–0.30	11 (16)
4. Deep invasion to full thickness of bronchial wall	0.31–0.50	10 (14)
5. Extrabronchial invasion	>0.50	12 (18)
Total		69 (100)

Data adapted from Woolner et al. (1984).

ment membrane in many cases since even before invasive growth occurs, a variety of alterations occur, such as marked thinning and small breaks. Woolner et al. (1984) outlined four different levels of invasive growth in occult lung carcinomas (Table 14–3). In most cases, invasive growth is identified by the presence of carcinoma cells, singly or in clumps, invading the underlying stroma. This identification can be very difficult in small bronchoscopic specimens. In cases where invasion is suspected but not certain, deeper histologic sections may be helpful in resolving the question. If it remains unclear, additional biopsies may be necessary.

Differential Diagnosis

The differential diagnosis for squamous dysplasia and CIS includes atypical squamous metaplasia associated with bronchial inflammation or fibrosis as well as radiation- and/or chemotherapy-induced atypia. In the presence of acute and or chronic inflammation of the airways or a history of previous biopsy or treatment, the threshold for diagnosis of malignancy must be increased.

ROENTGENOGRAPHICALLY OCCULT LUNG CANCER

In the 1970s the National Cancer Institute's randomized controlled trials of screening for early lung cancer drew attention to the problem of roentgenographically "occult" lung cancers that were detected by sputum cytology screening in high-risk patients rather than by chest radiographs (Woolner et al., 1984). Careful analysis of those surgical specimens provided valuable information about the pathology of early squamous cell carcinoma, including the entire spectrum of dysplastic lesions, CIS, and progression to invasion. Woolner et al. (1984) described these specimens in great detail on the basis of serial block sectioning of the entire bronchial tree and developed a pathologic classification of occult lung cancers (Table 14–3). Other studies by Carter (1976, 1978), Melamed (1977), and Nagamoto (1989, 1993) have also analyzed such specimens and have provided valuable information about the pathology of squamous dysplasia and CIS.

Molecular Studies

Molecular studies have demonstrated that lung carcinogenesis is a multistep process with accumulation of genetic changes in the epithelial cells and alterations in the extracellular matrix.

Genetic changes of epithelial cells. Early genetic changes in squamous cell lung carcinogenesis include loss of heterozygosity (LOH) at chromosome regions 3p (including 3p12, 3p14.2 [FHIT gene; Fong et al., 1977; Sozzi et al., 1998], 3p14.1-21.3, 3p21, 3p22-24, 3p25) (Sundaresan et al., 1992), and 9p21 (Wistuba et al., 1999). Recent data indicates that these changes can be found even in histologically normal bronchial mucosa of former cigarette smokers (Wistuba et al., 1997). Loss of heterozygosity of other chromosome regions including 17p13 (*p53* gene), 13q (*RB* gene), and 5q (APC-MCC region) and K-*ras* mutations is detected in later stages (Chung et al., 1995; Wistuba et al., 1999). Brambilla et al. (1998, 1999) showed abnormalities of the p53 transcription pathway (Bcl2, Bax, waf-1) and the RB pathway (rb, p16, cyclin D1) in preinvasive squamous bronchial lesions. Several studies have shown an increasing percentage of cases staining immunohistochemically for p53 with progression through dysplasia, CIS, and invasive carcinoma (Bennett et al., 1993; Orfanidou et al., 1998; Sozzi et al., 1992; Sundaresan et al., 1992; Fig. 14–14). Microdissection techniques have allowed for molecular analysis of specific areas of abnormal mucosa (Fig. 14–15).

Other genetic alterations, such as telomerase (Yashima et al., 1997), aneuploidy, and

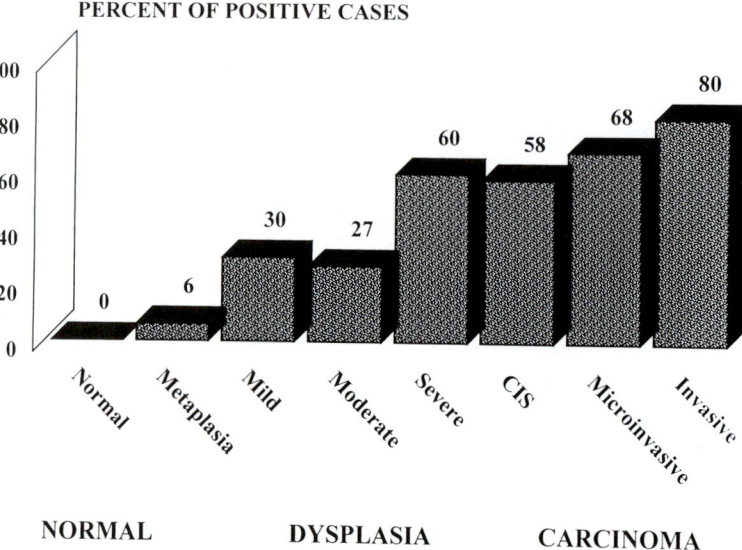

PERCENT OF POSITIVE CASES

NORMAL   DYSPLASIA   CARCINOMA

Figure 14–14. Summary of p53 immunohistochemical staining results in normal bronchial mucosa and preinvasive squamous lesions. Data are from Bennett et al. (1993).

proliferating cell nuclear antigen (PCNA) (Smith et al., 1996), have been correlated with increasing grades of dysplasia or CIS.

Alterations in the extracellular matrix. In contrast to the extensive studies on invasive lung carcinomas (Brown et al., 1993; Garbisa et al., 1992; Grigioni et al., 1987; Momiki et al., 1991; Nakagawa and Yagihashi, 1994; Urbanski et al., 1992; Zucker et al., 1989, 1992), only a few immunohistochemical and/or molecular biology studies have been carried

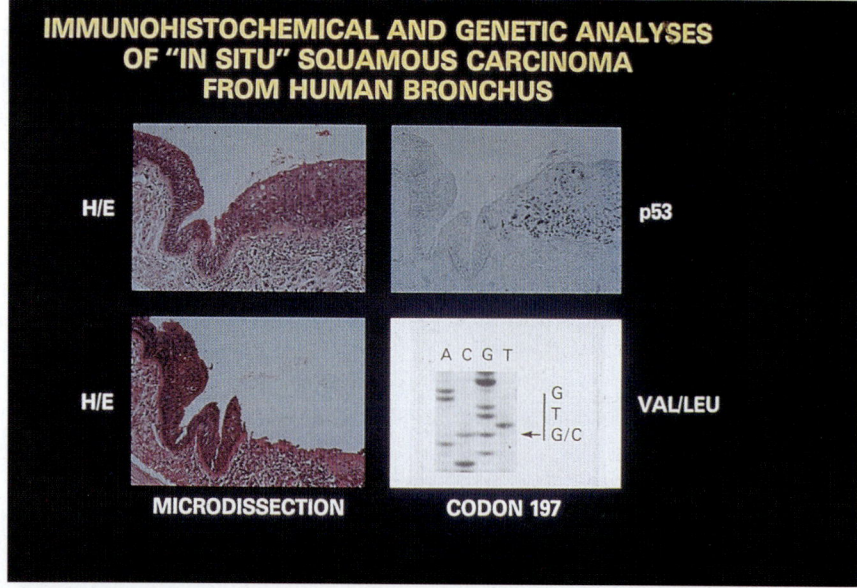

Figure 14–15. Microdissection technique with p53 immunohistochemistry and sequencing of bronchial squamous carcinoma *in situ.* Bronchial mucosa before microdissection (top left), a bronchial mucosa after microdissection (bottom, left), a p53 immunostain showing positive nuclear staining of tumor cells (top right), and a sequencing gel for showing a p53 mutation of codon 197 (bottom right). [Reproduced courtesy of Dr. Curtis C. Harris, from Harris and Holstein, 1993, with permission.]

out on the extracellular matrix or matrix metalloproteinases (MMPs) in preinvasive bronchial lesions (Bolon et al., 1996; Fisseler-Eckhoff et al., 1990; Imai et al., 1988; Müller and Müller, 1983). Fisseler-Eckhoff et al. (1990) found an increasing degree of matrix rearrangement of the basement membrane with increasing severity of epithelial changes in squamous preinvasive bronchial lesions. However, they described basement membrane thickening only with basal cell and goblet cell hyperplasia; Galateau-Salle et al. (1998) also observed this thickening in squamous metaplasia. Through immunohistochemical staining of frozen sections, Bolon et al. (1996) found that stromelysin-1 (MMP-3) was inconsistently expressed in 31% of preinvasive lesions, whereas stromelysin-3 (MMP-11) and urokinase type plasminogen activator were frequently expressed in such lesions. Galateau-Salle et al. (1998) have shown that the epithelial cells in bronchial preinvasive lesions undergo a series of changes in their expression of MMPs and tissue inhibitors of metalloproteinases (TIMPs). This study also suggests that MMP-1, MMP-2, MMP-9, and, to a lesser extent, MMP-3 play important roles in the remodeling of the basement membrane and extracellular matrix associated with progression of bronchial squamous preinvasive lesions. In addition, by means of confocal microscopy, Galateau et al. (1998) demonstrated a progressive decrease in colocalization of TIMP-1 and type IV collagen beginning with dysplasia, which suggests a protective effect of TIMP-1 on basement membranes in early preinvasive lesions that is lost as progression to CIS and invasive carcinoma occurs.

ATYPICAL ADENOMATOUS HYPERPLASIA

Atypical adenomatous hyperplasia (AAH) is a bronchioloalveolar proliferation thought to be a precursor to adenocarcinoma (Naguchi and Shimosato, 1995; Figs. 14–16 to 14–20). These lesions resemble, but fall short of criteria for bronchioloalveolar carcinoma, nonmucinous type (Kitamura et al., 1999; Miller, 1990; Travis et al., 1999). They are seen most often as incidental histologic findings in lung specimens removed for other reasons, commonly, a lung carcinoma.

Cases of multiple AAH and multiple adenocarcinomas provide empirical support for the concept that they are precursor lesions to adenocarcinoma. One patient with the Li-Fraumeni syndrome and multiple lung adenocarcinomas was found to have a single lesion of AAH (Nadav et al., 1998). With improved chest CT techniques, it is possible to identify these lesions radiographically; they appear as a small nodule with ground-glass attenuation simulating a focal lesion of pulmonary interstitial disease (Kushihashi et al., 1994).

A variety of terms have been used for these lesions (Table 14–4), however, the one used most often in the literature and chosen by the WHO/IASLC panel was AAH (Kitamura et al., 1999; Travis et al., 1999). Virtually all studies of AAH have documented these lesions in lung cancer resection specimens (Fig. 14–17). The incidence of AAH varies from 5.7% to 21.4%, depending on extent of the search and the criteria used for the diagnosis (Carey et al., 1992; Miller, 1990; Nakawishi, 1990; Weng et al., 1992). In an

Table 14–4. Atypical Adenomatous Hyperplasia: Other Published Terms

Term	Reference
Atypical adenomatous hyperplasia	Anami et al. (1998); Kitaguchi et al. (1998); Kitamura et al. (1996); Mori et al. (1993, 1996b); Nadav et al. (1998); Nakayama et al. (1990); Suzuki et al. (1997, 1998).
Alveolar atypical hyperplasia	Carey et al. (1992); Miller (1993)
Alveolar cell hyperplasia	Rao and Fraire (1995)
Atypical alveolar hyperplasia	Kerr et al. (1994)
Atypical bronchioloalveolar cell hyperplasia	Weng et al. (1992)
Alveolar epithelial hyperplasia	Nakawishi (1990)
Bronchioloalveolar adenoma	Kushihashi et al. (1994)
Bronchioloalveolar cell adenoma	Miller (1990)
Early stage lesions of bronchioloalveolar carcinoma	Kitamura et al. (1995)

exhaustive study by Weng et al. (1992), the examined lobectomy and pneumonectomy specimens of 165 primary and 45 metastatic tumor cases after processing an average of 51 blocks per specimen. They found AAH in 16.4% of lung cancer resection specimens, with 20% in males and 9.1% in females. In lung specimens resected for metastases, they found AAH in 4.4% of cases, with 4.8% in males and 4% in females.

Lesions of AAH are readily seen grossly in specimens processed in Bouin's fixative, as illustrated by Miller (1990), although they can also be seen in formalin-fixed specimens. This fixative makes the lesions stand out more than formalin fixation. The lesions appear as ill-defined nodules with a lacy architecture and they lack central fibrosis. The size of an AAH lesion is generally less than 5 mm in diameter, although most studies have included a small percentage of cases in which lesions measured up to 10 mm (Miller, 1990; Weng et al., 1992).

Atypical adenomatous hyperplasia frequently presents as multiple lesions. The number of lesions varies depending on how carefully one searches the specimen. In the study by Weng et al. (1992), multiple lesions were found in 6.7% of lung cancer resection specimens and 2% of lung specimens resected for metastases.

Histologically, AAH is a focal lesion in which the involved alveoli and respiratory bronchioles are lined by monotonous, slightly atypical cuboidal to low columnar epithelial cells (Figs. 14–16 and 14–17). At the edges of the lesion there is a gradual transition to the surrounding lung with normal alveolar epithelial cells (Fig. 14–18). The nuclear chromatin is dense, nucleoli are inconspicuous, and cytoplasm is scant (Fig. 14–19). There may be slight thickening of alveolar septa and mild lymphocytic infiltration. Lymphoid aggregates may be present (Fig. 14–16 and 14–17), and eosinophilic intranuclear inclusions may be found (Fig. 14–20). Mitotic figures are rarely seen. The degree of atypia varies from mild to moderate and tends to be greater in larger lesions. Rarely, it may be severe, but in such cases, one must consider the possibility of a bronchioloalveolar carcinoma (Fig. 14–20). Millers (1990) "as a practical matter, . . . it is my policy to view a tumor over 0.5 cm in diameter with marked atypia as a carci-

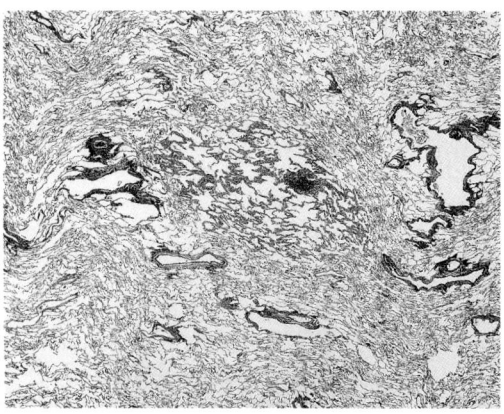

Figure 14–16. Atypical adenomatous hyperplasia. An ill-defined bronchioloalveolar proliferation is situated in a peribronchiolar location. A single lymphoid aggregate is present. [Case contributed by Dr. Masayuki Noguchi, Tsukuba-shi, Ibaraki, Japan.]

noma." However, this does not imply that lesions larger than 0.5 cm that show very little atypia are necessarily malignant.

The differential diagnosis of AAH includes the nonmucinous subtype of bronchioloalveolar carcinoma, type II pneumocyte hyperplasia with interstitial inflammation and/or fibrosis (Fraire and Greenberg, 1973; Meyer and Liebow, 1965; Raeburn and Spencer, 1953; Spencer and Raeburn, 1956), micronodular pneumocyte hyperplasia (Muir et al.,

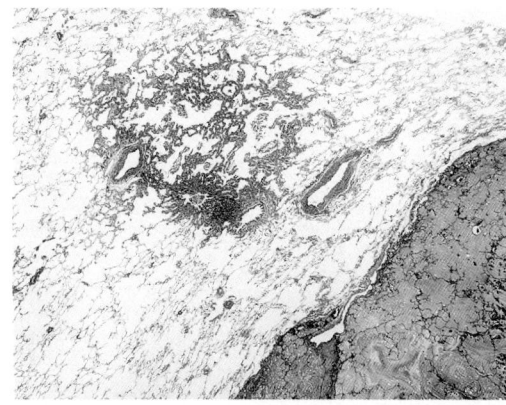

Figure 14–17. Atypical adenomatous hyperplasia. This lesion is situated adjacent to a mucinous adenocarcinoma. It also consists of a peribronchiolar bronchioloalveolar proliferation. A single lymphoid aggregate is present. [Case contributed by Dr. Masayuki Noguchi, Tsukuba-shi, Ibaraki, Japan.]

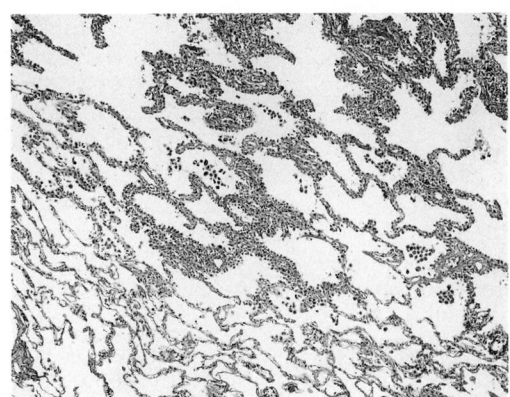

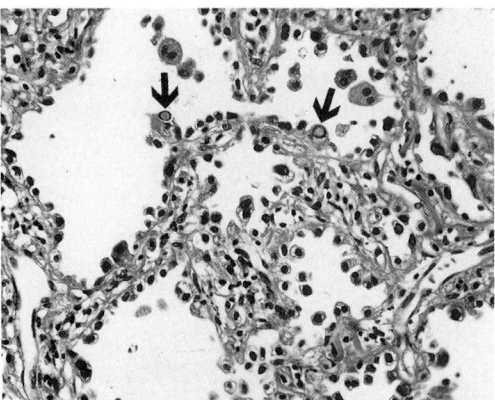

Figure 14–18. Atypical adenomatous hyperplasia. The bronchioloalveolar proliferation shows atypical pneumocytes proliferating along the alveolar walls. The alveolar architecture is preserved. The edge of the lesion (lower left) shows the transition to normal alveolar epithelium. [Case contributed by Dr. Masayuki Noguchi, Tsukuba-shi, Ibaraki, Japan.]

Figure 14–20. Atypical adenomatous hyperplasia. The pneumocytes show mild to moderate atypia. Two pneumocytes show nuclear cytoplasmic inclusions (arrow).

1998), respiratory bronchiolitis (Myers et al., 1987), peribronchiolar fibrosis with peribronchiolar metaplasia (Colby, 1998), and papillary adenoma (Mori et al., 1996a; Sanchez-Jimenez, et al., 1994). There is considerable overlap in the morphologic features of AAH and the nonmucinous variant of bronchioloalveolar carcinoma, especially that consisting mostly of type II pneumocytes

(Mori et al., 1993). Therefore, the distribution of AAH from adenocarcinoma is very difficult and subjective (Kitamura et al., 1999; Ritter, 1999; Travis et al., 1999). Features that favor adenocarcinoma include marked cell crowding and/or overlapping of nuclei, cytologic atypia with nuclear hyperchromasia and/or prominent nucleoli, large size, and loss of alveolar architecture with prominent papillary or invasive growth (Fig. 14–21). A size threshhold of 0.5 cm is a useful measure, but a small percentage of AAH lesions are larger and a small percentage of bronchioloalveolar carcinomas may be smaller. Extensive papillary growth with loss of the

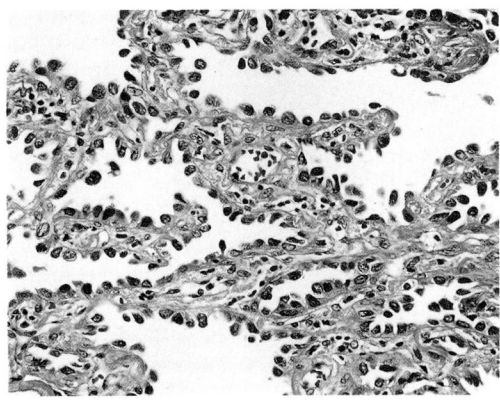

Figure 14–19. Atypical adenomatous hyperplasia. The hyperplastic pneumocytes are uniform with mild to moderate atypia. Gaps appear between the atypical pneumocytes, and there is mild fibrous thickening of the alveolar septa. [Case contributed by Dr. Masayuki Noguchi, Tsukuba-shi, Ibaraki, Japan.]

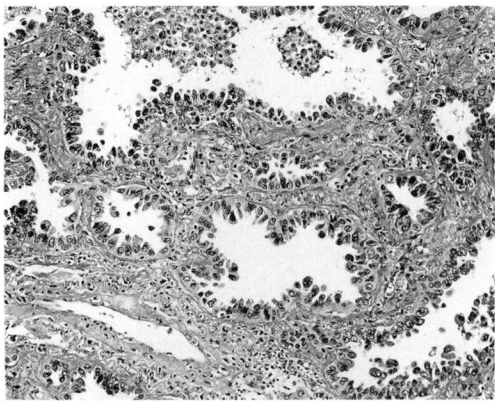

Figure 14–21. Bronchioloalveolar carcinoma. This nonmucinous bronchioloalveolar carcinoma shows greater nuclear crowding and atypia than the lesions of atypical adenomatous hyperplasia.

alveolar architecture would favor a diagnosis of papillary adenocarcinoma, and infiltrative growth would favor that of an invasive adenocarcinoma. Most cases of AAH show only mild interstitial inflammation and/or fibrosis (Kitamura et al., 1999; Travis et al., 1999; Weng et al., 1992). AAH lesions also tend to be more discrete than cases of reactive pneumocyte hyperplasia, where the inflammation and fibrosis often extend beyond the site of the epithelial proliferation. The term *AAH* should not be used for atypical pneumocyte hyperplasia in the setting of diffuse interstitial fibrosis. Micronodular pneumocyte hyperplasia is a rare proliferation of type II pneumocytes that occurs almost exclusively in patients with tuberous sclerosis (Flieder and Travis, 1997; Guinee et al., 1995; Muir et al., 1998). Some of these patients will also have pulmonary lymphangioleiomyomatosis. Distinction from AAH may be difficult. These are small, millimeter-sized lesions that generally lack atypia and they tend to be more sharply circumscribed than AAH without the peripheral lepidic spread merging imperceptibly with the surrounding alveolar pneumocytes. A clinical history would be important to know if the patient has tuberous sclerosis.

Problems with the Concept of Atypical Adenomatous Hyperplasia

There are several problems with the concept of AAH. First, the term implies that there should be a category of nonatypical adenomatous hyperplasia. While the terms *pneumocyte hyperplasia* or *alveolar epithelial hyperplasia* have been used for lesions showing hyperplasia of type II pneumocytes and/or Clara cells, the term *adenomatous hyperplasia* is not used for this lesion. It also can be very difficult to distinguish AAH from the nonmucinous variant of bronchioloalveolar carcinoma (Mori et al., 1993; Ritter, 1999). In fact, a detailed morphometric study by Mori et al. (1993) showed extensive overlap between AAH and the nonmucinous subtype of bronchioloalveolar carcinoma (Kitamura et al., 1999; Mori et al., 1993).

Given the difficulty in separating AAH from BAC, it is not very practical to try to grade AAH or to try to diagnose areas of AAH that are continuous with a lung carcinoma. Grading of AAH has been attempted using various criteria based mostly on the degree of atypia or cell crowding. It is difficult enough to identify a lesion as AAH and to separate it from bronchioloalveolar carcinoma—to add a grading scheme would create further problems in reproducibility and probably result in more bronchioloalveolar carcinomas being called AAH. For these reasons, the new WHO/IASLC classification does not recognize grades of AAH (Travis et al., 1999).

Some investigators have attempted to recognize AAH in continuity with adenocarcinomas (Nakayama et al., 1990). While it is recognized that very bland areas of lepidic growth are seen at the periphery of some lung carcinomas, it is very difficult to distinguish where the carcinoma ends and the AAH pattern begins. Furthermore, if pathologists were required to recognize such areas, undesirable clinical implications could ensue from altering tumor size assessment for staging purposes. Another confusing term that should be avoided is *AAH-like carcinoma* (Kitamura et al., 1995).

The concept of AAH and the new definition of bronchioloalveolar carcinoma by the 1999 WHO/IASLC as an adenocarcinoma with lepidic growth and lacking invasion make it tempting to propose the latter as an adenocarcinoma *in situ* (Travis et al., 1999). This would have some conceptual problems in that bronchioloalveolar carcinomas are often multicentric, especially those of the mucinous subtype, and they can invade extensively along the surface of the alveolar walls, causing lobar consolidation and, ultimately, respiratory death. The WHO/IASLC panel considered this terminology and chose not to adopt it (Travis et al., 1999).

Another problem with the concept of AAH is the uncertain clinical implication of the diagnosis in a patient without a lung carcinoma. Since virtually the entire literature on AAH consists of reports on surgically resected specimens for lung cancer or metastases, little is known about the potential for progression to carcinoma. The paucity of published cases of AAH in patients without carcinoma who subsequently developed lung carcinoma suggests that this risk is very low even with multicentric lesions. One study indicated that the presence of AAH had no bearing on the prognosis for patients with lung cancer (Suzuki et al., 1997). For this reason, patients found to have AAH, even with multicentric lesions, should not receive surgical, radiation, or chemotherapy. In such cases, careful clinical follow-up is warranted to see if the patient subsequently develops a lung carcinoma.

MOLECULAR, IMMUNOHISTOCHEMICAL AND MORPHOMETRIC STUDIES OF ATYPICAL ADENOMATOUS HYPERPLASIA

Atypical adenomatous hyperplasia has been studied with many different special techniques, including molecular (Kitaguchi et al., 1998; Kitamura et al., 1996; Kurasono et al., 1998; Nakayama et al., 1990; Niko et al., 1999; Pueblitz and Hieger, 1997; Yashima et al., 1997), cell proliferation, immunohistochemical (Mori et al., 1996b; Rao and Fraire, 1995), DNA quantification (Nakayama et al., 1990), ultrastructural (Mori et al., 1978), and morphometric (Kodama et al., 1986; Mori et al., 1993) methods.

Studies have shown sufficient different molecular abnormalities to support the concept that AAH represents a preneoplastic and even possibly a neoplastic lesion. Immunohistochemical staining for p53 has been reported in 8%–58% of lesions (Kerr et al., 1994; Kitaguchi et al., 1998; Kitamura et al., 1995; Pueblitz and Hieger, 1997; Slebos et al., 1998). Interestingly, some investigators have reported a greater percentage of cases staining with "higher-grade atypia" (Kerr et al., 1994; Kitamura et al., 1995). As mentioned above, grading of AAH is very difficult and studies of AAH attempting to characterize molecular markers in "high- versus low-grade AAH" probably have data from cases that overlap with bronchioloalveolar carcinomas. So these data need to be interpreted with caution. Kitaguchi et al. (1998) found LOH of chromosomes 3p, 9p, and 17p in 18%, 13%, and 6%, respectively, in the AAH lesions, whereas the corresponding carcinomatous lesions showed LOH of 67%, 50%, and 17%, respectively. Cyclin D1 is highly expressed in AAH but it is lost in adenocarcinomas (Kurasono et al., 1998). K-*ras* codon 12 mutations have been found in 17%–50% of AAH lesions, which suggests that AAH is an early lesion in the development of adenocarcinoma (Cooper et al., 1997; Ohshima et al., 1994; Sugio et al., 1994; Westra et al., 1996).

DIFFUSE IDIOPATHIC PULMONARY NEUROENDOCRINE CELL HYPERPLASIA

Diffuse idiopathic pulmonary neuroendocrine cell hyperplasia (DIPNECH) is a rare condition in which there is widespread proliferation of neuroendocrine cells in the peripheral airways that ranges from neuroendocrine cell hyperplasia to multiple tumorlets. It may present as a form of interstitial lung disease with airway obstruction as it is frequently associated with bronchiolar fibrosis. Since a subset of these patients has one or more carcinoid tumors, DIPNECH is thought to represent a precursor lesion for carcinoid tumors (Travis et al., 1999).

Less than 20 cases of DIPNECH have been reported (Aguayo et al., 1992; Brown et al., 1997; Sheerin et al., 1995; Travis et al., 1999). Aguayo et al. (1992) described this entity, proposing that the neuroendocrine cell proliferation was the primary lesion and that substances such as bombesin produced by the neuroendocrine cells promoted the airway fibrosis. While this concept goes against tradition (Johnson, 1993), it has become generally accepted. Given the possibility that neuroendocrine cells may undergo a primary proliferation when such patients develop carcinoid tumors, it is reasonable to accept that DIPNECH is a preneoplastic lesion for carcinoid tumors.

Neuroendocrine cell hyperplasia and tumorlets are much more commonly seen as a reactive secondary lesion in the setting of airway inflammation and/or fibrosis (Canessa et al., 1997; Pelosi et al., 1992; Ranchod, 1977; Whitwell, 1955). Therefore, most neuroendocrine cell hyperplasias probably do not represent a preneoplastic condition. There is, however, a continuum between tumorlets and carcinoid tumors. Tumorlets are typically incidental histologic findings measuring several millimeters in size. They represent micronodular proliferations of neuroendocrine cells that usually infiltrate beyond the bronchial/bronchiolar wall. Although these features are "invasive," according to a review of the literature, lymph node metastases are very rare when these lesions measure 0.5 cm or less in diameter (D'Agati and Perzin, 1985). But neuroendocrine proliferations reported as tumorlets measuring approximately 1 cm in size have been known to metastasize (Hausman and Weimann, 1967). Recognizing there is a continuum of size and also probably malignant potential in neuroendocrine proliferations, we arbitrarily use the term *carcinoid tumor* for neuroendocrine proliferations measuring greater than 0.5 cm in diameter (Colby et al., 1995; Travis et al., 1999).

Histologically, lung biopsies from patients with DIPNECH show a neuroendocrine cell hyperplasia that can consist of increased numbers of scattered single cells, small nodules (neuroendocrine bodies), or linear proliferations of neuroendocrine cells within the bronchiolar epithelium (Figs. 14–22 to 14–25). Micronodular lesions represent tumorlets and if they are 0.5 cm in size or greater they are called *carcinoid tumors*. The neuroendocrine proliferations and tumorlets may cause airway narrowing and/or obliteration (Figs. 14–22 and 14–23). Sometimes airway obstruction is due to fibrosis. The surrounding lung parenchyma is generally normal. Bronchiolectasis is a common finding.

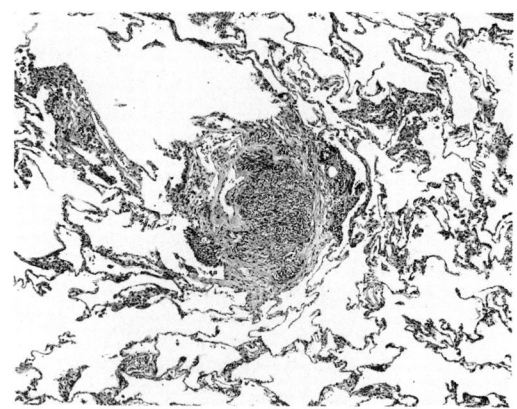

Figure 14–23. Diffuse idiopathic neuroendocrine cell hyperplasia. The bronchiolar lumen is obliterated by a nodular neuroendocrine proliferation. [Case contributed by Anthony A. Gal, Emory University, Atlanta, GA.]

Miller and Müller (1995) found neuroendocrine cell hyperplasia in the mucosa of bronchioles adjacent to 75% of 25 peripheral carcinoid tumours. They also found obliterative bronchiolar fibrosis in 32% of cases. It is not clear whether hyperplastic neuroendocrine cells in this setting represent a local reaction to the tumour or a localized preneoplastic condition.

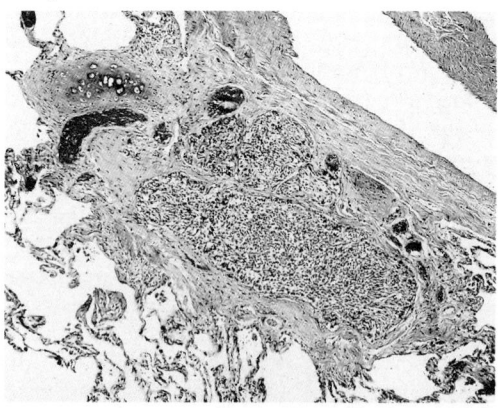

Figure 14–22. Diffuse idiopathic neuroendocrine cell hyperplasia. The bronchial lumen is obliterated by a nodular proliferation of neuroendocrine cells. Bronchial cartilage (upper left) and a large artery (upper right) surround the airway. [Case contributed by Anthony A. Gal, Emory University, Atlanta, GA.]

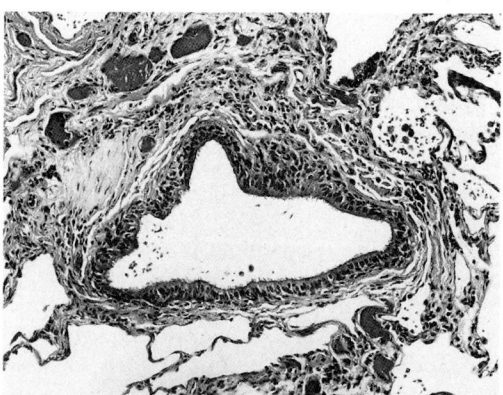

Figure 14–24. Diffuse idiopathic neuroendocrine cell hyperplasia. There is nodular proliferation of neuroendocrine cells along the bronchiolar wall. [Case contributed by Anthony A. Gal, Emory University, Atlanta, GA.]

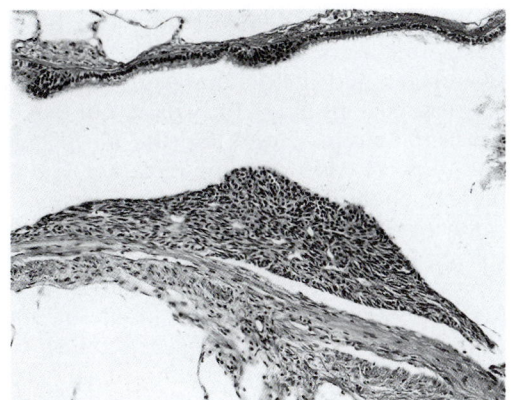

Figure 14–25. Diffuse idiopathic neuroendocrine cell hyperplasia. There are increased numbers of neuroendocrine cells in the bronchiolar epithelium with some nodular aggregates (bottom right–center). Submucosal fibrosis is also apparent (bottom left). [Case contributed by Anthony A. Gal, Emory University, Atlanta, GA.]

ATYPICAL MESOTHELIAL HYPERPLASIA (MALIGNANT MESOTHELIOMA *IN SITU*)

Occasionally, pleural biopsies show such a marked atypical mesothelial proliferation that malignancy is highly suspected (Fig. 14–26). Even in the absence of invasive growth in the biopsy specimen, one is tempted to suggest that the process is ma-

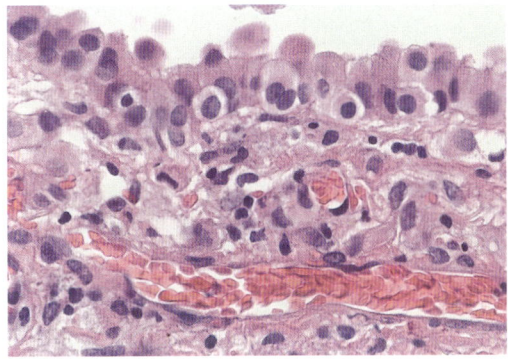

Figure 14–26. Atypical mesothelial proliferation, suspicious for malignancy. This is a malignant mesothelioma growing along the pleural surface. The cells show marked cytologic atypia with binucleation. Elsewhere this tumor showed foci of invasive growth.

lignant. Such cases have led to the concept of malignant mesothelioma *in situ*.

While the concept of malignant mesothelioma *in situ* is appealing, since there must be a preinvasive phase for this neoplasm (Henderson et al., 1998; Whitaker et al., 1992), from the perspective of clinical practice, it is very problematic. The recently formed International Mesothelioma Panel has recommended against use of the term malignant mesothelioma *in situ*. Instead, such lesions should be called *atypical mesothelial hyperplasia*, and if there is a high level of concern for malignancy, one should state "suspicious for malignancy." If possible additional biopsy material should be obtained in such cases in order to identify areas of invasion. One of the problems with the term malignant mesothelioma *in situ* is that surgeons sometimes perform radical surgery, such as extrapleural pneumonectomies for pleural mesotheliomas, and once they hear the words "malignant mesothelioma," they seriously consider this therapeutic approach.

Unlike the preinvasive lesions of the bronchus, bladder, and cervix, one of the fundamental criteria for the diagnosis of malignant mesothelioma *in situ* in the pleura is the documentation of invasive malignancy. Thus, unlike carcinoma *in situ* in these sites, malignant mesothelioma *in situ* cannot be diagnosed without an invasive component. A major problem with mesothelial proliferations is that very atypical reactive lesions may occur that can be easily mistaken for malignant mesothelioma. The presence of invasion or exuberant mass-like proliferation of mesothelial cells in the absence of inflammation is required for the diagnosis of malignant mesothelioma. For these reasons, the new 1999 WHO/IASLC classification did not formally recognize malignant mesothelioma *in situ* as a preinvasive lesion (Travis et al., 1999).

Whitaker proposed the concept of malignant mesothelioma *in situ* in the early 1980s after conducting experimental work in rats (Whitaker et al., 1982, 1992), and subsequently defined this condition on the basis of a series of seven cases in 1992 (Whitaker et al., 1992). The criteria for diagnosis were the following:

(1) A diagnosis of malignant mesothelioma was proven at some stage in the development of the

disease, by cytological or histological means, or by necropsy. *(2)* Up to the time of obtaining the tissue for the study, no gross tumor or tumor mass was present, as judged by observation at open thoracotomy or pleuroscopy, and also no lesions were identified radiologically. The presence of minute spots or sand grains or nondescript focal pleural thickening did not exclude a case. *(3)* Tissue was available for histological assessment. The biopsy material was taken before or at the time that pleuroscopy or thoracotomy demonstrated absence of gross tumor,

Whitaker et al. (1992)

In Whitaker's report, the pleura showed several possible gross features, including normal, slight pleural thickening, or varying numbers of tiny nodules resembling grains of sand. Histologically, these cases showed a variety of patterns, including a flat, single layer of cells, or papillary, tubular, or sheet-like proliferation of cells that was sometimes up to 10–20 cells thick. The flat, single layer of cells sometimes showed a picket fence type of pattern. Inflammation in the subserosal connective tissue was inconspicuous or absent. Cytologically, the cells resembled mesothelial cells with abundant cytoplasm, a large nucleus, and occasional binucleate cells (Fig. 14–26). Several investigators have suggested that positive immunohistochemical staining with epithelial membrane antigen (EMA) and p53 favors a malignant rather than a reactive mesothelial proliferation (Cagle et al., 1994; Dowell et al., 1993;

Henderson et al., 1998; Mayall et al., 1992; Ramael et al., 1992; Whitaker et al., 1992; Wolaski et al., 1998). However, these are controversial findings that have not been consistently reproduced and the use of immunohistochemistry for these markers is not recommended for diagnostic purposes.

Occasionally, metastatic carcinomas involving the pleura will spread along the surface and may mimic atypical mesothelial hyperplasia (malignant mesothelioma *in situ*). However, these tumor cells often show a substantial amount of pleomorphism and they will demonstrate histochemical or immunohistochemical features of a carcinoma with positive stains for mucin or immunohistochemistry for carcinoembryonic antigen (CEA), Leu-M1, B72.3, or BER-EP4 and negative stains for calretinen and CK5/6 (Doglioni et al., 1996; Ordonez, 1998; Riera et al., 1997).

One of the useful contributions of this concept of malignant mesothelioma *in situ* is that it highlights the difficulty in distinguishing atypical reactive mesothelial proliferations from malignant mesothelioma. Features that aid in the differential diagnosis are summarized in Table 14–5. Because of the difficulty in making this distribution, generous sampling of the pleura is frequently needed to make a definitive diagnosis in cases of early malignant mesothelioma. The great danger is the potential for overtreatment such as extrapleural pneumonectomy in the absence of invasive malignant mesothelioma.

Table 14–5. Criteria for Distinguishing Mesothelioma from Reactive Mesothelial Proliferation

	Reactive Mesothelial Proliferation	*Mesothelioma*
True stromal invasion	Not present	Strong evidence of malignancy
Cellularity	Low except under effusion	High except in desmoplastic tumors
Sidedness of cell proliferation	More cellular toward effusion; less cellular away from effusion	Cellularity may be high anywhere
Necrosis	Rare	Uncommon
Capillaries	Often long, with perpendicular orientation toward surface	Inconspicuous in tumor
Cytologic atypia	Benign reactions can be atypical, particularly in the pleural space	Useful when marked, but many mesotheliomas appear relatively monotonous and bland
Mitoses	Common in reactive proliferations	Uncommon in most mesotheliomas
Immunohistochemistry	P53 or EMA may be positive in benign conditions Keratin positive	p53 or EMA may be positive or negative Keratin positive

Modified from Churg and Green (1998), Table 10–11, with permission.

Table 14–6. Other Potential Preneoplastic Conditions for Lung Cancer

Condition	Reference
Interstitial fibrosis	
Localized Fibrosis	
Scar carcinoma	Auerbach et al. (1957)
Tuberculosis	Auerbach et al. (1957); Wu et al. (1995)
Histoplasmosis	
Shrapnel injury	
Diffuse fibrosis	
Idiopathic pulmonary fibrosis	Lee et al. (1996); Nagai et al. (1992); Turner-Warwick et al. (1980)
Interstitial fibrosis with collagen vascular disease	
Scleroderma	Gruber et al. (1992); Peters-Golden et al. (1985); Roumm and Medsger (1985); Winkelmann et al. (1988)
Rheumatoid arthritis	Matteson et al. (1991); Moolten (1973)
Radiation	Lesser et al. (1983); Tokarskaya et al. (1995)
Pneumocoriosis	Chung (1985)
Bronchiectasis	Tonelli (1997)
Squamous papillomatosis	DiLorenzo et al. (1992); Guillou et al. (1991); Harding et al. (1989); Simma et al. (1993)
Cystic lung lesions	
Congenital cystic adenomatoid malformation	Benjamin and Cahill (1991); Ribet et al. (1995)
Intralobar sequestration	Bell-Thomson et al. (1979)
Long-standing lung cysts	Hurley et al. (1985); Prichard et al. (1984)

OTHER CONDITIONS IN WHICH LUNG MALIGNANCIES MAY ARISE

There are a number of other clinical settings in which lung carcinomas may arise. These are summarized in Table 14–6, and few will be specifically addressed below.

The concept of *scar carcinoma* was predicated on the assumption that the scars seen in most lung cancers developed first and provided the setting for the cancer to arise (Auerbach et al., 1979; Friedrich, 1939). However, studies by Shimosato et al. (1980) and others demonstrated that the scars seen in most lung carcinomas were the result of neoplastic growth rather than being the cause (Barsky et al., 1986; Cagle et al., 1985; el-Torky et al., 1985). Nevertheless, there appear to be cases where lung carcinomas arise at the site of preexisting localized fibrosis from a variety of potential causes, including shrapnel injury or granulomatous infections (Dubeau and Fraser, 1984; Richardson et al., 1987; Yoneda, 1990).

Lung carcinomas are also known to occur in the setting of *diffuse interstitial fibrosis.* Lung cancer has been reported in 10%–31% of patients with idiopathic pulmonary fibrosis (Lee et al., 1996; Nagai et al., 1992; Panos et al., 1990; Turner-Warwick et al., 1980). It has also been found in patients with collagen vascular disease who have diffuse interstitial fibrosis, including those with scleroderma (Gruber et al., 1992; Peters-Golden et al., 1985; Roumm and Medsger, 1985; Salvant et al., 1988; Winkelmann et al., 1988) and rheumatoid arthritis (Matteson et al., 1991; Moolten, 1973). Patients with Sjögren's syndrome are at risk for developing pulmonary malignant lymphomas (Capron et al., 1985; Hansen et al., 1985; Strimlan et al., 1976; Zufferey et al., 1995). A variety of pneumoconioses are known to increase the risk for lung cancer, especially asbestosis (Churg, 1985; Mollo et al., 1990).

Patients with juvenile laryngotracheal papillomatosis are also known to develop squamous cell carcinomas (DiLorenzo et al., 1992; Guillou et al., 1991; Helmuth and

Strate, 1987; Lie et al., 1994; Simma et al., 1995). While some of these cases have occurred in the setting of radiation therapy, it is now well documented that this can occur in nonirradiated, nonsmoking patients with juvenile laryngotracheal papillomatosis and infection with human papillomavirus 11 can commonly be demonstrated (Guillou et al., 1991; Helmuth and Strate, 1987; Runckel and Kessler, 1980; Simma et al., 1993; Tsao et al., 1987).

The opinions and assertions contained herein are the private views of the author and are not to be construed as official or as representing the views of the Department of the Army or the Department of Defense.

REFERENCES

Aguayo SM, Miller YE, Waldron JA Jr, et al. (1992) Brief report: idiopathic diffuse hyperplasia of pulmonary neuroendocrine cells and airways disease. *N Engl J Med* 327:1285–1288.

Anami Y, Matsuno Y, Yamada T, et al. (1998) A case of double primary adenocarcinoma of the lung with multiple atypical adenomatous hyperplasia. *Pathol Int* 48:634–640.

Auerbach O, Garfinkel L, Parks VR. (1979) Scar cancer of the lung: increase over a 21 year period. *Cancer* 43:636–642.

Auerbach O, Gere B, Forman JB, et al. (1957) Changes in the bronchial epithelium in relation to smoking and cancer of the lung. *N Engl J Med* 256:97–104.

Aznavoorian S, Murphy AN, Stetler-Stevenson WG, Liotta LA. (1993) Molecular aspects of tumor cell invasion and metastasis. *Cancer* 71:1368–1383.

Barsky SH, Huang SJ, Bhuta S. (1986) The extracellular matrix of pulmonary scar carcinoma is suggestive of a desmoplastic origin. *Am J Pathol* 124:412–419.

Becci PJ, McDowell EM, Trump BF. (1978) The respiratory epithelium. IV. Histogenesis of epidermoid metaplasia and carcinoma *in situ* in the hamster. *J Natl Cancer Inst* 61:577–586.

Bell-Thomson J, Missier P, Sommers SC. (1979) Lung carcinoma arising in bronchopulmonary sequestration. *Cancer* 44:334–339.

Benjamin DR, Cahill JL. (1991) Bronchioloalveolar carcinoma of the lung and congenital cystic adenomatoid malformation. *Am J Clin Pathol* 95:889–892.

Bennett WP, Colby TV, Travis WD, et al. (1993) p53 protein accumulates frequently in early bronchial neoplasia. *Cancer Res* 53:4817–4822.

Bolon I, Brambilla E, Vandenbunder B, et al. (1996) Changes in the expression of matrix proteases and of the transcription factor c-Ets-1 during progression of precancerous bronchial lesions. *Lab Invest* 75:1–13.

Boone CW, Kelloff GJ, Freedman LS. (1993) Intraepithelial and postinvasive neoplasia as a stochastic continuum of clonal evolution, and its relationship to mechanisms of chemopreventive drug action. *J Cell Biochem Suppl* 17G:14–25.

Bosman FT. (1994) The borderline: basement membranes and the transition from premalignant to malignant neoplasia. *Microsc Res Tech* 28:216–225.

Brambilla E, Gazzeri S, Lantuejoul S, et al. (1998) p53 mutant immunophenotype and deregulation of p53 transcription pathway (Bcl2, Bax, and Waf1) in precursor bronchial lesions of lung cancer. *Clin Cancer Res* 4:1609–1618.

Brambilla E, Gazzeri S, Moro D, et al. (1999) Alterations of Rb pathway (Rb-p16INK4-cyclin D1) in preinvasive bronchial lesions. *Clin Cancer Res* 5:243–250.

Brown MJ, English J, Muller NL. (1997) Bronchiolitis obliterans due to neuroendocrine hyperplasia: high-resolution CT—pathologic correlation. *AJR Am J Roentgenol* 168:1561–1562.

Brown PD, Bloxidge RE, Stuart NS, Gatter KC, Carmichael J. (1993) Association between expression of activated 72-kilodalton gelatinase and tumor spread in non-small-cell lung carcinoma. *J Natl Cancer Inst* 85:574–578.

Buiatti E, Geddes M, Arniani S. (1996) Epidemiology of lung cancer. *Ann Ist Super Sanita* 32:133–144.

Cagle PT, Brown RW, Lebovitz RM. (1994) p53 immunostaining in the differentiation of reactive processes from malignancy in pleural biopsy specimens [see comments]. *Hum Pathol* 25:443–448.

Cagle PT, Cohle SD, Greenberg SD. (1985) Natural history of pulmonary scar cancers. Clinical and pathologic implications. *Cancer* 56:2031–2035.

Canessa PA, Santini D, Zanelli M, Capecchi V. (1997) Pulmonary tumourlets and microcarcinoids in bronchiectasis. *Monaldi Arch Chest Dis* 52:138–139.

Capron F, Audouin J, Diebold J, et al. (1985) Pulmonary polymorphic centroblastic type malignant lymphoma in a patient with lymphomatoid granulomatosis, Sjögren syndrome and other manifestations of a dysimmune state. *Pathol Res Pract* 179:656–665.

Carey FA, Wallace WA, Fergusson RJ, Kerr KM, Lamb D. (1992) Alveolar atypical hyperplasia in association with primary pulmonary adenocarcinoma: a clinicopathological study of 10 cases. *Thorax* 47:1041–1043.

Carter D. (1978) Pathology of early squamous cell carcinoma of the lung. *Pathol Annu* 13 Pt 1:131–147.

Carter D, Marsh BR, Baker R, Erozan YS, Frost JK. (1976) Relationships of morphology to clinical presentation in ten cases of early squamous cell carcinoma of the lung. *Cancer* 37:1389–1396.

Chung GT, Sundaresan V, Hasleton P, et al. (1995) Sequential molecular genetic changes in lung cancer development. *Oncogene* 11:2591–2598.

Churg A. (1985) Lung cancer cell type and asbestos exposure. *JAMA* 253:2984–2985.

Churg A, Green FHY. (1998) *Pathology of Occupational Lung Disease*, Williams and Wilkins, Baltimore.

Colby TV. (1998) Bronchiolitis. Pathologic considerations. *Am J Clin Pathol* 109:101–109.

Colby TV, Koss MN, Travis WD. (1995) *Tumors of the Lower Respiratory Tract*, Armed Forces Institute of Pathology Fascicle, Third Series, Armed Forces Institute of Pathology, Washington, DC.

Colby TV, Wistuba II, Gazdar A. (1998) Precursors to pulmonary neoplasia. *Adv Anat Pathol* 5:205–215.

Cooper CA, Carby FA, Bubb VJ, et al. (1997) The pattern of K-ras mutation in pulmonary adenocarcinoma defines a new pathway of tumour development in the human lung. *J Pathol* 181:401–404.

D'Agati VD, Perzin KH. (1985) Carcinoid tumorlets of the lung with metastasis to a peribronchial lymph node. Report of a case and review of the literature. *Cancer* 55:2472–2476.

DiLorenzo TP, Tamsen A, Abramson AL, Steinberg BM. (1992) Human papillomavirus type 6a DNA in the lung carcinoma of a patient with recurrent laryngeal papillomatosis is characterized by a partial duplication. *J Gen Virol* 73:423–428.

Doglioni C, Tos AP, Laurino L, et al. (1996) Calretinin: a novel immunocytochemical marker for mesothelioma. *Am J Surg Pathol* 20:1037–1046.

Dowell S, Derias N, Wilson PO, Lane DP, Hall PA. (1993) Expression of p53 in reactive mesothelium [letter]. *Histopathology* 22:96–97.

Dubeau L, Fraser RS. (1984) Long-term effects of pulmonary shrapnel injury. Report of a case with carcinoma and residual shrapnel tract. *Arch Pathol Lab Med* 108:407–409.

el-Torky M, Giltman LI, Dabbous M. (1985) Collagens in scar carcinoma of the lung. *Am J Pathol* 121:322–326.

Fisseler-Eckhoff A, Prebeg M, Voss B, Müller KM. (1990) Extracellular matrix in preneoplastic lesions and early cancer of the lung. *Pathol Res Pract* 186:95–101.

Flieder DB, Travis WD. (1997) Clear cell "sugar" tumor of the lung: association with lymphangioleiomyomatosis and multifocal micronodular pneumocyte hyperplasia in a patient with tuberous sclerosis. *Am J Surg Pathol* 21:1242–1247.

Flug M, Kopf-Maier P. (1995) The basement membrane and its involvement in carcinoma cell invasion. *Acta Anat (Basel)* 152:69–84.

Fong KM, Biesterveld EJ, Virmani A, et al. (1997) FHIT and FRA3B 3p14.2 allele loss are common in lung cancer and preneoplastic bronchial lesions and are associated with cancer-related FHIT cDNA splicing aberrations. *Cancer Res* 57:2256–2267.

Fraire AE, Greenberg SD (1973) Carcinoma and diffuse interstitial fibrosis of lung. *Cancer* 31:1078–1086.

Friedrich G. (1973) Periphere Lungenkrebse auf dem Boden pleuranaher Narben. *Virchows Arch A Pathol Anat Histopathol* 304:230–247.

Galateau-Salle FB, Luna RE, Horiba K, Sheppard MN, Hayashi T, Fleming MV, Colby TV, Bennett W, Harris CC, Stetler-Stevenson WG, Liotta LA, Ferrans VJ, Travis WD. (1998) Matrix metalloproteinases (MMPs) and tissue inhibitors of metalloproteinases (TIMPs) in bronchial squamous preneoplastic lesions. *Hum Pathol* 31:296–305, 2000.

Garbisa S, Scagliotti G, Masiero L, et al. (1992) Correlation of serum metalloproteinase levels with lung cancer metastasis and response to therapy. *Cancer Res* 52:4548–4549.

Gartenschlager M, Schweden F, Gast K, et al. (1998) Pulmonary nodules: detection with low-dose vs. conventional-dose spiral CT. *Eur Radiol* 8:609–614.

Grigioni WF, Biagini G, Garbisa S, et al. (1987) Immunohistochemical study of basement membrane antigens in bronchioloalveolar carcinoma. *Am J Pathol* 128:217–224.

Gruber BL, Miller F, Kaufman LD. (1992) Simultaneous onset of systemic sclerosis (scleroderma) and lung cancer: a case report and histologic analysis of fibrogenic peptides [letter]. *Am J Med* 92:705–708.

Guillou L, Sahli R, Chaubert P, et al. (1991) Squamous cell carcinoma of the lung in a nonsmoking, nonirradiated patient with juvenile laryngotracheal papillomatosis. Evidence of human papillomavirus-11 DNA in both carcinoma and papillomas. *Am J Surg Pathol* 15:891–898.

Guinee D, Singh R, Azumi N, et al. (1995) Multifocal micronodular pneumocyte hyperplasia: a distinctive pulmonary manifestation of tuberous sclerosis. *Mod Pathol* 8:902–906.

Hording M, Hording U, Daugaard S, Norrild B, Faber V. (1989) Human papilloma virus type 11 in a fatal case of esophageal and bronchial papillomatosis. *Scand J Infect Dis* 21:229–231.

Hansen LA, Prakash UB, Colby TV. (1989) Pulmonary lymphoma in Sjögren's syndrome. *Mayo Clin Proc* 64:920–931.

Harris CC, Hollstein M. (1993) Clinical implications of the *p53* tumor suppressor gene. *N Engl J Med* 329:1318–1327.

Hausman DH, Weimann RB. (1987) Pulmonary tumorlet with hilar lymph node metastasis. Report of a case. *Cancer* 20:1515–1519.

Helmuth RA, Strate RW. (1987) Squamous carcinoma of the lung in a nonirradiated, nonsmoking patient with juvenile laryngotracheal papillomatosis. *Am J Surg Pathol* 11:643–650.

Henderson DW, Shilkin KB, Whitaker D. (1998) Reactive mesothelial hyperplasia vs mesothelioma, including mesothelioma *in situ*: a brief review. *Am J Clin Pathol* 110:397–404.

Hurley P, Corbishley C, Pepper J. (1985) Bronchioloalveolar carcinoma arising in longstanding lung cysts [letter]. *Thorax* 40:960–960.

Ikeda N, MacAulay C, Lam S, et al. (1998) Malignancy associated changes in bronchial epithelial cells and clinical application as a biomarker. *Lung Cancer* 19:161–166.

Imai T, Saito Y, Nagamoto N, et al. (1988) Electron microscopic observations in *in situ* and microinvasive bronchogenic squamous cell carcinoma. *J Pathol* 156:241–249.

Itoh S, Ikeda M, Isomura T, et al. (1998) Screening helical CT for mass screening of lung cancer: application of low-dose and single-breath-hold scanning. *Radiat Med* 16:75–83.

Johnson JE. (1993) Idiopathic hyperplasia of pulmonary neuroendocrine cells [letter]. *N Engl J Med* 328:581–582.

Kerr KM, Carey FA, King G, Lamb D. (1994) Atypical alveolar hyperplasia: relationship with pulmonary adenocarcinoma, p53, and c-erbB-2 expression. *J Pathol* 174:249–256.

Kitaguchi S, Takeshima Y, Nishisaka T, Inai K. (1998) Proliferative activity, p53 expression and loss of heterozygosity on 3p, 9p and 17p in atypical adenomatous hyperplasia of the lung. *Hiroshima J Med Sci* 47:17–25.

Kitamura H, Kameda Y, Ito T, Hayashi H. (1999) Atypical adenomatous hyperplasia of the lung. Implications for the pathogenesis of peripheral lung adenocarcinoma *Am J Clin Pathol* 111:610–622.

Kitamura H, Kameda Y, Nakamura N, et al. (1996) Atypical adenomatous hyperplasia and bronchoalveolar lung carcinoma. Analysis by morphometry and the expressions of p53 and carcinoembryonic antigen. *Am J Surg Pathol* 20:553–562.

Kitamura H, Kameda Y, Nakamura N, et al. (1995) Proliferative potential and p53 overexpression in precursor and early stage lesions of bronchioloalveolar lung carcinoma. *Am J Pathol* 146:876–887.

Kodama T, Biyajima S, Watanabe S, Shimosato Y. (1986) Morphometric study of adenocarcinomas and hyperplastic epithelial lesions in the peripheral lung. *Am J Clin Pathol* 85:146–151.

Kurasono Y, Ito T, Kameda Y, Nakamura N, Kitamura H. (1998) Expression of cyclin D1, retinoblastoma gene protein, and p16 MTS1 protein in atypical adenomatous hyperplasia and adenocarcinoma of the lung. An immunohistochemical analysis. *Virchows Arch A Pathol Anat Histopathol* 432:207–215.

Kushihashi T, Munechika H, Ri K, et al. (1994) Bronchioloalveolar adenoma of the lung: CT-pathologic correlation. *Radiology* 193:789–793.

Lam S, Kennedy T, Unger M, et al. (1998) Localization of bronchial intraepithelial neoplastic lesions by fluorescence bronchoscopy. *Chest* 113:696–702.

Lam S, LeRiche JC, Zheng Y, et al. (1999) Sex-related differences in bronchial epithelial changes associated with tobacco smoking *J Natl Cancer Inst* 91: 691–696.

Lam S, MacAulay C, Hung J, et al. (1993) Detection of dysplasia and carcinoma *in situ* with a lung imaging fluorescence endoscope device. *J Thorac Cardiovasc Surg* 105:1035–1040.

Landis SH, Murray T, Bolden S, Wingo PA. (1999) Cancer statistics, 1999. *CA Cancer J Clin* 49:8–31.

Lee HJ, Im JG, Ahn JM, Yeon KM. (1996) Lung cancer in patients with idiopathic pulmonary fibrosis: CT findings. *J Comput Assist Tomogr* 20:979–982.

Lesser M, Chang JC, Yoo OH, Roswit B. (1983) Bronchioalveolar carcinoma arising in areas previously irradiated for Hodgkin's disease. *South Med J* 76:689–691.

Lie ES, Engh V, Boysen M, et al. (1994) Squamous cell carcinoma of the respiratory tract following laryngeal papillomatosis. *Acta Otolaryngol (Stockh)* 114: 209–212.

Matteson EL, Hickey AR, Maguire L, Tilson HH, Urowitz MB. (1991) Occurrence of neoplasia in patients with rheumatoid arthritis enrolled in a DMARD Registry. Rheumatoid Arthritis Azathioprine Registry Steering Committee. *J Rheumatol* 18: 809–814.

Mayall FG, Goddard H, Gibbs AR. (1992) p53 immunostaining in the distinction between benign and malignant mesothelial proliferations using formalin-fixed paraffin sections. *J Pathol* 168:377–381.

McDowell EM, McLaughlin JS, Merenyl DK, et al. (1978) The respiratory epithelium. V. Histogenesis of lung carcinomas in the human. *J Natl Cancer Inst* 61:587–606.

Melamed MR, Zaman MB, Flehinger BJ, Martini N. (1977) Radiologically occult *in situ* and incipient invasive epidermoid lung cancer: detection by sputum cytology in a survey of asymptomatic cigarette smokers. *Am J Surg Pathol* 1:5–16.

Meyer EC, Liebow AA. (1965) Relationship of interstitial pneumonia, honeycombing, and atypical epithelial proliferation to cancer of the lung. *Cancer* 18:322–351.

Miller RR. (1990) Bronchioloalveolar cell adenomas. *Am J Surg Pathol* 14:904–912.

Miller RR. (1993) Alveolar atypical hyperplasia in association with primary pulmonary adenocarcinoma: a clinicopathological study of 10 cases [letter]. *Thorax* 48:679–680.

Miller RR, Muller NL. (1995) Neuroendocrine cell hyperplasia and obliterative bronchiolitis in patients with peripheral carcinoid tumors. *Am J Surg Pathol* 19:653–658.

Mollo F, Piolatto G, Bellis D, et al. (1990) Asbestos exposure and histologic cell types of lung cancer in surgical and autopsy series. *Int J Cancer* 46:576–580.

Momiki S, Baba M, Caamano J, et al. (1991) *In vivo* and *in vitro* invasiveness of human lung carcinoma cell lines. *Invasion Metastasis* 11:66–75.

Moolten SE. (1973) Scar cancer of lung complicating rheumatoid lung disease. *Mt Sinai J Med* 40:736–743.

Mori M, Chiba R, Takahashi T. (1993) Atypical adenomatous hyperplasia of the lung and its differentiation from adenocarcinoma. Characterization of atypical cells by morphometry and multivariate cluster analysis. *Cancer* 72:2331–2340.

Mori M, Chiba R, Tezuka F, et al. (1996a) Papillary adenoma of type II pneumocytes might have malignant potential. *Virchows Arch A Pathol Anat Histopathol* 428:195–200.

Mori M, Kaji M, Tezuka F, Takahashi T. (1998) Comparative ultrastructural study of atypical adenomatous hyperplasia and adenocarcinoma of the human lung. *Ultrastruct Pathol* 22:459–466.

Mori M, Tezuka F, Chiba R, et al. (1996b) Atypical adenomatous hyperplasia and adenocarcinoma of the human lung. Their heterology in form and analogy in immunohistochemical characteristics. *Cancer* 77: 665–674.

Muir TE, Leslie KO, Popper H, et al. (1998) Micronodular pneumocyte hyperplasia. *Am J Surg Pathol* 22:465–472.

Müller KM, Müller G. (1983) The ultrastructure of preneoplastic changes in the bronchial mucosa. *Curr Top Pathol* 73:233–263.

Myers JL, Veal CF Jr, Shin MS, Katzenstein AL. (1987) Respiratory bronchiolitis causing interstitial lung disease. A clinicopathologic study of six cases. *Am Rev Respir Dis* 135:880–884.

Nadav Y, Pastorino U, Nicholson AG. (1998) Multiple synchronous lung cancers and atypical adenomatous hyperplasia in Li-Fraumeni syndrome. *Histopathology* 33:52–54.

Nagai A, Chiyotani A, Nakadate T, Konno K. (1992) Lung cancer in patients with idiopathic pulmonary fibrosis. *Tohoku J Exp Med* 167:231–237.

Nagamoto N, Saito Y, Sato M, et al. (1993) Clinicopathologic analysis of 19 cases of isolated carcinoma *in situ* of the bronchus. *Am J Surg Pathol* 17:1234–1243.

Nagamoto N, Saito Y, Suda H, et al. (1989) Relationship between length of longitudinal extension and maximal depth of transmural invasion in roentgenographically occult squamous cell carcinoma of the bronchus (nonpolypoid type). *Am J Surg Pathol* 13: 11–20.

Nakagawa H, Yagihashi S. (1994) Expression of type IV collagen and its degrading enzymes in squamous cell carcinoma of lung. *Jpn J Cancer Res* 85:934–938.

Nakanishi K. (1990) Alveolar epithelial hyperplasia and adenocarcinoma of the lung. *Arch Pathol Lab Med* 114:363–368.

Nakayama H, Noguchi M, Tsuchiya R, Kodama T, Shimosato Y. (1990) Clonal growth of atypical adenomatous hyperplasia of the lung: cytofluorometric analysis of nuclear DNA content. *Mod Pathol* 3:314–320.

Niho S, Yokose T, Suzuki K, et al. (1999) Monoclonality of atypical adenomatous hyperplasia of the lung. *Am J Pathol* 154:249–254.

Noguchi M, Shimosato Y. (1995) The development and progression of adenocarcinoma of the lung. *Cancer Treat Res* 72:131–142.

Ohshima S, Shimizu Y, Takahama M. (1994) Detection of c-Ki-ras gene mutation in paraffin sections of adenocarcinoma and atypical bronchioloalveolar cell hyperplasia of human lung. *Virchows Arch A Pathol Anat Histopathol* 424:129–134.

Ordonez NG. (1998) Value of cytokeratin 5/6 immunostaining in distinguishing epithelial mesothelioma of the pleura from lung adenocarcinoma. *Am J Surg Pathol* 22:1215–1221.

Orfanidou D, Kalomenidis J, Rasidakis A, et al. (1998) Immunohistochemical detection of p53 protein in neoplastic, preneoplastic and normal bronchial mucosa specimens obtained during diagnostic bronchoscopy. *Oncol Rep* 5:763–769.

Panos RJ, Mortenson RL, Niccoli SA, King TE Jr. (1990) Clinical deterioration in patients with idiopathic pulmonary fibrosis: causes and assessment. *Am J Med* 88:396–404.

Parkin DM, Pisani P, Ferlay J. (1999) Global cancer statistics. *CA Cancer J Clin* 49:33–64.

Pelosi G, Zancanaro C, Sbabo L, et al. (1992) Development of innumerable neuroendocrine tumorlets in pulmonary lobe scarred by intralobar sequestration. Immunohistochemical and ultrastructural study of an unusual case. *Arch Pathol Lab Med* 116: 1167–1174.

Peters-Golden M, Wise RA, Hochberg M, Stevens MB, Wigley FM. (1985) Incidence of lung cancer in systemic sclerosis. *J Rheumatol* 12:1136–1139.

Prichard MG, Brown PJ, Sterrett GF. (1984) Bronchioloalveolar carcinoma arising in long-standing lung cysts. *Thorax* 39:545–549.

Pueblitz S, Hieger LR. (1997) Expression of p53 and CEA in atypical adenomatous hyperplasia of the lung [letter; comment]. *Am J Surg Pathol* 21:867–868.

Raeburn C, Spencer H. (1953) A study of the origin and development of lung cancer. *Thorax* 8:1–10.

Ramael M, Lemmens G, Eerdekens C, et al. (1992) Immunoreactivity for p53 protein in malignant mesothelioma and non-neoplastic mesothelium. *J Pathol* 168:371–375.

Ranchod M. (1977) The histogenesis and development of pulmonary tumorlets. *Cancer* 39:1135–1145.

Rao SK, Fraire AE. (1995) Alveolar cell hyperplasia in association with adenocarcinoma of lung. *Mod Pathol* 8:165–169.

Ribet ME, Copin MC, Soots JG, Gosselin BH. (1995) Bronchioloalveolar carcinoma and congenital cystic adenomatoid malformation. *Ann Thorac Surg* 60: 1126–1128.

Richardson S, Hirsch A, Ruffie P, Bickel M. (1987) Relationship between tuberculous scar and carcinomas of the lung. *Eur J Radiol* 7:163–164.

Riera JR, Astengo-Osuna C, Longmate JA, Battifora H. (1997) The immunohistochemical diagnostic panel for epithelial mesothelioma: a reevaluation after heat-induced epitope retrieval [see comments]. *Am J Surg Pathol* 21:1409–1419.

Ritter JH. (1999) Pulmonary atypical adenomatous hyperplasia. A histologic lesion in search of usable criteria and clinical significance. *Am J Clin Pathol* 111: 587–589.

Roumm AD, Medsger TA Jr. (1985) Cancer and systemic sclerosis. An epidemiologic study. *Arthritis Rheum* 28: 1336–1340.

Runckel D, Kessler S. (1980) Bronchogenic squamous carcinoma in nonirradiated juvenile laryngotracheal papillomatosis. *Am J Surg Pathol* 4:293–296.

Salvant EE, Carter JM, Armstrong EM, Polk OD Jr, Austin KI. (1988) CREST syndrome: a variant of progressive systemic sclerosis, associated with interstitial pulmonary fibrosis and malignancy. *South Med J* 81:1185–1187.

Sanchez-Jimenez J, Ballester-Martinez A, Lodo-Besse J, et al. (1994) Papillary adenoma of type 2 pneumocytes. *Pediatr Pulmonol* 17:396–400.

Sheerin N, Harrison NK, Sheppard MN, et al. (1995) Obliterative bronchiolitis caused by multiple tumourlets and microcarcinoids successfully treated by single lung transplantation. *Thorax* 50:207–209.

Shimosato Y, Suzuki A, Hashimoto T, et al. (1980) Prognostic implications of fibrotic focus (scar) in small peripheral lung cancers. *Am J Surg Pathol* 4:365–373.

Simma B, Burger R, Uehlinger J, et al. (1993) Squamous-cell carcinoma arising in a non-irradiated child with recurrent respiratory papillomatosis. *Eur J Pediatr* 152:776–778.

Slebos RJ, Baas IO, Clement MJ, et al. (1998) p53 alterations in atypical alveolar hyperplasia of the human lung. *Hum Pathol* 29:801–808.

Smith AL, Hung J, Walker L, et al. (1996) Extensive areas of aneuploidy are present in the respiratory epithelium of lung cancer patients. *Br J Cancer* 73: 203–209.

Sozzi G, Miozzo M, Donghi R, et al. (1992) Deletions of 17p and p53 mutations in preneoplastic lesions of the lung. *Cancer Res* 52:6079–6082.

Sozzi G, Pastorino U, Moiraghi L, et al. (1998) Loss of FHIT function in lung cancer and preinvasive bronchial lesions. *Cancer Res* 58:5032–5037.

Spencer H, Raeburn C. (1956) Pulmonary (bronchiolar) adenomatosis. *J Pathol Bacteriol* 71:145–154.

Strimlan CV, Rosenow EC, Divertie MB, Harrison EG Jr. (1976) Pulmonary manifestations of Sjögren's syndrome. *Chest* 70:354–361.

Sugio K, Kishimoto Y, Virmani AK, Hung JY, Gazdar AF. (1994) K-*ras* mutations are a relatively late event in the pathogenesis of lung carcinomas. *Cancer Res* 54:5811–5815.

Sundaresan V, Ganly P, Hasleton P, et al. (1992) p53 and chromosome 3 abnormalities, characteristic of malignant lung tumours, are detectable in preinvasive lesions of the bronchus. *Oncogene* 7:1989–1997.

Suzuki K, Nagai K, Yoshida J, et al. (1997) The prognosis of resected lung carcinoma associated with atypical adenomatous hyperplasia: a comparison of the prognosis of well-differentiated adenocarcinoma associated with atypical adenomatous hyperplasia and intrapulmonary metastasis. *Cancer* 79: 1521–1526.

Suzuki K, Takahashi K, Yoshida J, et al. (1998) Synchronous double primary lung carcinomas associated with multiple atypical adenomatous hyperplasia. *Lung Cancer* 19:131–139.

Tokarskaya ZB, Okladnikova ND, Belyaeva ZD, Drozhko EG. (1995) The influence of radiation and nonradiation factors on the lung cancer incidence among the workers of the nuclear enterprise Mayak. *Health Phys* 69:356–366.

Tonelli P. (1997) A morphologic study of nodular lung carcinomas and their possible pathogenesis from a cluster of non-obstructive bronchiectasis. *Lung Cancer* 17:135–145.

Travis WD, Colby TV, Corrin B, Shimosato Y, Brambilla E, and collaborators from 14 countries. (1999) *Histological Typing of Lung and Pleural Tumors.* Springer-Verlag, Berlin.

Travis WD, Lubin J, Ries L, Devesa S. (1996) United States lung carcinoma incidence trends: declining for most histologic types among males, increasing among females. *Cancer* 77:2464–2470.

Travis WD, Travis LB, Devesa SS. (1995) Lung cancer [published erratum appears in *Cancer* 1995; 75(12): 2979]. *Cancer* 75:191–202.

Tsao MS, Fraser RS, Howley PM. (1987) Human papillomavirus-11 DNA in a patient with chronic laryngotracheobronchial papillomatosis and metastatic squamous-cell carcinoma of the lung. *N Engl J Med* 317:873–878.

Turner-Warwick M, Lebowitz M, Burrows B, Johnson A. (1980) Cryptogenic fibrosing alveolitis and lung cancer. *Thorax* 35:496–499.

Urbanski SJ, Edwards DR, Maitland A, et al. (1992) Expression of metalloproteinases and their inhibitors in primary pulmonary carcinomas. *Br J Cancer* 66:1188–1194.

Weng SY, Tsuchiya E, Kasuga T, Sugano H. (1992) Incidence of atypical bronchioloalveolar cell hyperplasia of the lung: relation to histological subtypes of lung cancer. *Virchows Arch A Pathol Anat Histopathol* 420:463–471.

Westra WH, Baas IO, Hruban RH, et al. (1996) K-*ras* oncogene activation in atypical alveolar hyperplasias of the human lung. *Cancer Res* 56:2224–2228.

Whitaker D, Henderson DW, Shilkin KB. (1992) The concept of mesothelioma *in situ*: implications for diagnosis and histogenesis. *Semin Diagn Pathol* 9:151–161.

Whitaker D, Papadimitriou JM, Walters MN. (1982) The mesothelium and its reactions: a review. *Crit Rev Toxicol* 10:81–144.

Whitwell F. (1955) Tumourlets of the lung. *J Pathol Bacteriol* 70:529–541.

Wingo PA, Ries LA, Giovino GA, et al. (1999) Annual report to the nation on the status of cancer, 1973–1996, with a special section on lung cancer and tobacco smoking. *J Natl Cancer Inst* 91:675–690.

Winkelmann RK, Flach DB, Unni KK. (1988) Lung cancer and scleroderma. *Arch Dermatol Res* 280 Suppl: S15–S18.

Wistuba II, Behrens C, Milchgrub S, et al. (1999) Sequential molecular abnormalities are involved in the multistage development of squamous cell lung carcinoma. *Oncogene* 18:643–650.

Wistuba II, Lam S, Behrens C, et al. (1997) Molecular damage in the bronchial epithelium of current and former smokers. *J Natl Cancer Inst* 89:1366–1373.

Wolanski KD, Whitaker D, Shilkin KB, Henderson DW. (1998) The use of epithelial membrane antigen and silver-stained nucleolar organizer regions testing in the differential diagnosis of mesothelioma from benign reactive mesothelioses. *Cancer* 82:583–590.

Woolner LB. (1993) Lung. In: *Pathology of Incipient Neoplasia*, 2nd ed. Henson DE, Albores-Saavedra J, eds. pp. 191–221. W.B. Saunders, Philadelphia.

Woolner LB, Fontana RS, Cortese DA, et al. (1984) Roentgenographically occult lung cancer: pathologic findings and frequency of multicentricity during a 10-year period. *Mayo Clin Proc* 59:453–466.

World Health Organization. (1967) *Histological Typing of Lung Tumours.* World Health Organization, Geneva.

World Health Organization. (1981) *Histological Typing of Lung Tumors.* World Health Organization, Geneva.

Wu AH, Fontham ET, Reynolds P, et al. (1995) Previous lung disease and risk of lung cancer among lifetime nonsmoking women in the United States. *Am J Epidemiol* 141:1023–1032.

Yashima K, Litzky LA, Kaiser L, et al. (1997) Telomerase expression in respiratory epithelium during the multistage pathogenesis of lung carcinomas. *Cancer Res* 57:2373–2377.

Yoneda K. (1990) Scar carcinomas of the lung in a histoplasmosis endemic area. *Cancer* 65:164–168.

Zucker S, Lysik RM, Malik M, et al. (1992) Secretion of gelatinases and tissue inhibitors of metalloproteinases by human lung cancer cell lines and revertant cell lines: not an invariant correlation with metastasis. *Int J Cancer* 52:366–371.

Zucker S, Wieman J, Lysik RM, et al. (1989) Gelatin-degrading type IV collagenase isolated from human small cell lung cancer. *Invasion Metastasis* 9:167–181.

Zufferey P, Meyer OC, Grossin M, Kahn MF. (1995) Primary Sjogren's syndrome (SS) and malignant lymphoma. A retrospective cohort study of 55 patients with SS. *Scand J Rheumatol* 24:342–345.

15

BREAST

Ruth A. Lininger and Fattaneh A. Tavassoli

A clinically silent disease, mammary intraepithelial neoplasia is either detected mammographically (most commonly as a result of suspicious microcalcifications), as a mass, nipple discharge, pagetoid involvement of the nipple, or as an incidental finding in biopsies for other clinically evident breast lesions (fibrocystic change, sclerosing adenosis, fibroadenoma, etc.). The median age of women with intraductal hyperplasia (IDH) is 45 years (Tavassoli and Norris, 1990), which is 5 years younger than the median age of women with atypical intraductal hyperplasia (AIDH) (50 years) (Tavassoli and Norris, 1990), and 10 years younger than the average age of presentation of women with ductal carcinoma *in situ* (DCIS) (55 years) (Silverberg and Chitale, 1973; Westbrook and Gallager, 1975).

Prior to the extensive use of screening mammography, about 25% of women who had breast biopsies were found to have IDH, whereas 2% to 5% were found to have an atypical hyperplasia (AH) of either ductal or lobular type (Kodlin et al., 1977; Nielsen et al., 1987; Page and Dupont, 1990; Page et al., 1985). With increased screening and improvements in mammographic techniques, the incidence of AH has increased to 9.8% in a study of 100 consecutive mammographically directed biopsies performed in women presenting with nonpalpable lesions (Rubin et al., 1988). Using autopsy data, the incidence of AIDH was 5.9% in a study of 185 women whose breasts were randomly evaluated at autopsy (Alpers and Wellings,

1985). These incidence changes for AIDH most likely parallel the changes in incidence of DCIS (Ernster et al., 1996). Interestingly, a trend toward an increased number of sections submitted for histologic sampling over the years may also account for a proportion of this observed increase in incidence of these lesions, simply due to increased sampling (Dupont et al., 1993; Page et al., 1985). A smaller percentage of the observed increase in incidence is also likely due to the slight, but progressive, increase in the incidence of breast cancer over the past 30–40 years. Between 1950 and 1979, new cases of breast cancer increased an average of 1% a year, according to the National Cancer Institute's (Surveilance, Epidemiology, and End Results (SEER) program (Newman, 1990), with incidence rates for breast cancer increasing to approximately 4% a year in the United States from 1982 to 1987 (Garfinkel, 1993), followed by a more recent stabilization in annual incidence (Landis et al., 1998).

Among the consults received at the Armed Forces Institute of Pathology (AFIP), a diagnosis of IDH accounted for 22% of all cases of ductal epithelial proliferations in 1970, compared to 28% in 1990. More dramatic, however, are the statistics for AIDH. The frequency of a diagnosis of AIDH nearly tripled between 1970 and 1990 among the consults received at the AFIP during the same interval (AIDH comprised 6% of ductal epithelial lesions diagnosed in 1970 versus 17% in 1990); this paralleled an increase in the frequency of a diagnosis of DCIS at AFIP which more than quadrupled during this same period of time (accounting for 6% of all cases in 1970, compared to 28% in 1990; see Table 15–1). These percentages most likely reflect a combination of the changing incidence of in situ breast lesions in the general population as well as the level of difficulty perceived by contributing pathologists. As attempts are made to detect breast lesions earlier and earlier, accurate identification and classification of pathologic breast lesions become of paramount importance.

This chapter will focus primarily on noninvasive ductal and lobular proliferations of the breast. The terminology, diagnostic criteria, clinical significance, and management, as well as what is currently known about the biology of these lesions, will be discussed. We will also elaborate on the unifying concept of mammary intraepithelial neoplasia, which is the basis of our recently introduced translational classification of epithelial proliferations in the duct system. This new classification may be used either alone or as a working formulation alongside any system preferred by various pathologists to assist in comparison of the types of cases used in any given study. Due to space constraints, a number of other important lesions that may be classified under the spectrum of incipient neoplasia of the breast, including intraductal papillary neoplasms, microglandular adenosis, and sclerosing adenosis will not be addressed in this chapter.

A vast majority of mammary epithelial proliferations, whether ductal or lobular, arise in the terminal duct–lobular unit (TDLU). The distinction between atypical ductal and lobular proliferations is, therefore, based predominantly on the proliferative pattern, rather than on the site of origin of the lesion in the duct versus the lobule. Certain cytologic features are more commonly observed in lobular neoplasia (LN). So many cytologic variants of both LN and DCIS have been described, however, that cytology alone is not adequate for separating the two.

THE UNIFYING CONCEPT OF MAMMARY INTRAEPITHELIAL NEOPLASIA

In 1978, Haagensen proposed the term *lobular neoplasia* for the spectrum of lobular pathologic proliferations, subdivided variably into *atypical lobular hyperplasia* (ALH) and *lobular carcinoma* in situ (LCIS) by most pathologists. More than 10 years later, the suggestion to use the term *mammary intraepithelial neoplasia* (MIN) of ductal and lobular types for "borderline" ductal lesions of the breast was made by Rosai (1991) when he noted significant problems in the reproducibility of diagnosing borderline noninvasive mammary epithelial lesions. Subsequent and more recent reproducibility studies have shown continuous and persistent problems in this area (Palazzo and Hyslop, 1996; Schnitt et al., 1992). To reduce the impact of interobserver variability on patient management, we reintroduced the concept of MIN in 1997. A detailed classification scheme followed with a new approach for classifying intraductal proliferations. We believe that adoption of this new classification will help in the effort to standardize diagnostic criteria while allowing gradual modifications as we better understand the biology and behavior of these lesions. Mammary in-

Table 15–1. Comparison of Distribution of Diagnoses of Ductal Epithelial Lesions of the Breast[a] Rendered at the Armed Forces Institute of Pathology, 1970 and 1990

	IDH n (%)	IDH + FA n (%)	AIDH n (%)	DCIS n (%)	DCIS + MI n (%)	Invasive DC n (%)	Ductal Diagnosis Total n	Ductal/All Breast Diagnosis n (%)
1990	369 (28)	181 (14)	222 (17)	363 (28)	29 (2)	148 (11)	1312	1312/3738 (35)
1970	155 (22)	0 (0)	40 (6)	47 (6)	0 (0)	472 (66)	714	714/1398 (51)

AIDH, atypical intraductal hyperplasia; DC, ductal carcinoma; DCIS, ductal carcinoma *in situ*; DCIS + MI, ductal carcinoma *in situ* with microinvasion; IDH, intraductal hyperplasia; IDH + FA, intraductal hyperplasia with focal atypia.

[a]Includes papillary lesions.

Reprinted from R.A. Lininger and F.A. Tavassoli, Atypical intraductal hyperplasia of the breast, in *Ductal Carcinoma in Situ of the Breast*, ed. M. Silverstein, 1997, with permission from Williams & Wilkins.

traepithelial neoplasia is a general term referring to all noninvasive proliferative lesions in the duct system. These proliferations may assume a ductal growth pattern (ductal intraepithelial neoplasia [DIN]), a lobular architecture (lobular neoplasia [LN]), or a papillary pattern (papillary intraductal neoplasia [PIN]). This chapter will focus on the spectrum of ductal and lobular neoplasia, the major features of which are presented.

DUCTAL INTRAEPITHELIAL NEOPLASIA

Briefly, the DIN classification system subdivides intraductal epithelial proliferations into three major grades: *grade 1 DIN* includes IDH, AIDH, and low grade DCIS; *grade 2 DIN* incorporates all intermediate-grade DCIS lesions; and *grade 3 DIN* consists of all high-grade DCIS lesions (see Table 15–2). Incorporated into this translational system is the simple and practical AFIP DCIS grading approach (Tavassoli, 1988, 1999).

Although Haagensen's proposed terminology "lobular neoplasia" was readily adopted at AFIP, we found the application of this concept to ductal proliferations more complicated. One important reason is the greater variety of cell types and patterns in ductal proliferations. Furthermore, even though the ascending magnitude of the risk associated with IDH, AIDH, and DCIS may suggest otherwise, many observers do not consider IDH in the same morphologic spectrum or in the same league with atypical intraductal hyperplasia and DCIS. The heterogeneous cell population in IDH is totally devoid of recognizable atypia on hematoxylin and eosin (H&E)–stained sections. Sometimes, there is an admixture of epithelial, myoepithelial, and/or metaplastic apocrine cells. When only the epithelial cell population proliferates in IDH, it does not display the uniformity and monotony of the atypical cells proliferating in AIDH or DCIS. In lobular neoplasia, a distinctive cell population proliferates and either displaces or replaces the native epithelial cells, sometimes even dislodging the myoepithelial cells. The spectrum of lobular neoplasia refers to the various extent or degrees of proliferation of the neoplastic cells within the lobules. There is no counterpart for IDH within the spectrum of lobular neoplasia. Therefore, if the term DIN were to be applied to the ductal proliferations, some may argue that it should be exclusive of IDH since there is no justification for including IDH in the same spectrum, because morphologically it also

Table 15–2. Ductal Intraepithelial Neoplasia (Intraductal Hyperplasia, Atypical Intraductal Hyperplasia, and Ductal Carcinoma *In Situ*)

DIN Classification	Current Designation	Pleomorphic Nuclear Atypia	Necrosis	Absolute Risk of Invasion (%)	Molecular Findings	Re-excision, if +/close margin
DIN 1a	IDH	−	− or +	1.9	Clonal[b]/MSI	No
DIN 1b	AIDH	−[a]	−	5.1–12	Clonal/LOH	No
DIN 1c	AIDH, extensive[c] DCIS, grade 1 (crib/micropap)	−[a]	−	10–32	Clonal/LOH	Yes
DIN 2	DCIS, grade 2 (crib/micropap + necrosis or atypia)	− +(+)	+ +	20–75	Clonal/LOH	Yes
DIN 3	DCIS, grade 3 (anaplastic DCIS, +/− necrosis)	+++ +++	+++ −	20–75	Clonal/LOH	Yes

AIDH, atypical intraductal hyperplasia; DCIS, ductal carcinoma *in situ*; crib, cribriform; DIN, ductal intraepithelial neoplasia; IDH, intraductal hyperplasia; LOH, loss of heterozygosity micropap, micropapillary; MSI, microsatellite instability.

[a]No significant pleomorphic nuclear atypia is present, although at least a minor degree of atypia is assumed in all DCIS (as well as AIDH) proliferations.

[b]A few cases of IDH have been shown to be clonal.

[c]Partial involvement of either >20 duct cross sections or similar involvement distributed over 1.5 cm.

Reprinted, with modifications, from F.A. Tavassoli, Ductal carcinoma *in situ*: introduction of the concept of ductal intraepithelial neoplasia. *Mod Pathol* 11:140–154, 1998, with permission from The United States and Canadian Academy of Pathology.

reflects a proliferative process. There are, however, AIDH lesions that start as clusters of uniform cells in an area of IDH while the IDH architecture persists. Furthermore, some atypical cells within IDH are not easily recognizable on examination of H&E–stained sections and have been unmasked only incidentally during special studies with a variety of markers (Tavassoli and Man, 1995). Interestingly, the relative risk (RR) for subsequent invasive carcinoma has been assessed at 1.5–2.0 times that for the general population (Bodian et al., 1993b; McDivitt et al., 1992; Page and Dupont, 1990), which is rather close to the latest RR of 2.4 for AIDH, based on a recent publication from the Nurses' Health Study (Marshall et al., 1997). Considering the possibility of a genetic spectrum as noted earlier, IDH is grouped in the spectrum of DIN with AIDH and low-grade DCIS.

In AIDH, there are at least some clusters of proliferating cells that resemble the cells of low-grade DCIS on H&E sections. The various patterns of AIDH including low-grade lesions designated *clinging carcinoma* by many European pathologists are regarded as DIN 1b. Finally, all proliferations that meet both the qualitative and quantitative criteria for the nonnecrotic low-grade, cribriform, or micropapillary variants of DCIS are designated DIN 1c (see Table 15–2). The rationale for grouping low-grade DCIS with AIDH and IDH in DIN 1 is the observation that the behavior of low-grade DCIS more closely parallels AIDH than intermediate or high-grade DCIS, with regard to the risk for subsequent invasive carcinoma and recurrence (Silverstein et al., 1996). Given the similarity in the behavior of AIDH to low grade DCIS and the marked interobserver variability in the diagnosis of these two lesions, it seems logical that the management should be similar and based on the extent of disease.

The category DIN 2 encompasses intermediate-grade DCIS. Using the AFIP DCIS grading system, this category would include DCIS, grade 2, and would include lesions showing either necrosis but only mild or no cytologic atypia, or lesions showing a moderate degree of cytologic atypia in the absence of necrosis. The category DIN 3 encompasses high-grade DCIS (DCIS, grade 3) and includes DCIS showing significant

(pleomorphic) cytologic atypia regardless of the presence (e.g., comedocarcinoma) or absence of necrosis.

LOBULAR NEOPLASIA

Lobular neoplasia (LN) is a designation used to encompass the entire spectrum of lobular disease ranging from atypical lobular hyperplasia to lobular carcinoma *in situ*. Lobular neoplasia is characterized by a uniform population of generally small and loosely cohesive cells growing in a solid, occlusive fashion, with or without distension of the affected acini, involving one or more terminal duct–lobular units (TDLU), and often showing pagetoid spread into adjacent ducts. To convey the degree of acinar involvement and distension, LN can be graded as LN 1 to 3 (see Table 15–3 and section on lobular neoplasia; Tavassoli, 1999).

MAMMARY INTRAEPITHELIAL NEOPLASIA, NOT OTHERWISE SPECIFIED

There are occasionally epithelial proliferations within TDLUs that are difficult to subclassify as ductal or lobular. There are also lesions that have features of both ductal and lobular growth patterns. A vast majority of these are early lesions composed of uniform cells without significant pleomorphic atypia. For these cases, the designation of MIN 1, 2, or 3, without further subdivision, akin to the three-tiered classification system for LN, has been proposed.

Table 15–3. Classification of Lobular Neoplasia

LN 1		Partial or complete lobular involvement by uniform cells with poorly defined margins, which fill, but do not distend, the acini
LN 2		Cells distend some or all acini; acinar outlines, however, remain distinct and separate, and intervening lobular stroma persists; residual lumens may persist in some acini
LN 3	Type 1	Cells may show increased cytologic atypia; massive acinar distension with nearly confluent acini is present; interacinar stroma is barely evident
	Type 2	Signet ring cell variant; significant acinar distension may not be present with this type

Reprinted, with modifications, from R.A. Lininger and F.A. Tavassoli, Atypical intraductal hyperplasia of the breast, in *Ductal Carcinoma* in Situ *of the Breast*, ed. M.J. Silverstein, 1997, with permission from Williams & Wilkins.

Table 15–4. Morphologic Features to Evaluate in the Differential Diagnosis of Ductal Intraepithelial Neoplasia

Cytologic features
Cellular type and composition
Presence and degree of cytologic atypia

Architectural features
Presence of intraluminal necrosis
Architectural pattern (solid, cribriform, stratified spindle cell, micropapillary)
Size of the lesion
Degree of duct involvement (partial or complete)
Extent of the proliferation

Reprinted, with modifications, from R.A. Lininger and F.A. Tavassoli, Atypical intraductal hyperplasia of the breast, in *Ductal Carcinoma* in Situ *of the Breast*, ed. M.J. Silverstein, 1997, with permission from Williams & Wilkins.

DUCTAL INTRAEPITHELIAL NEOPLASIA (INTRADUCTAL HYPERPLASIA, ATYPICAL INTRADUCTAL HYPERPLASIA, AND DUCTAL CARCINOMA *IN SITU*)

The cytologic and architectural features to evaluate in the differential diagnosis of ductal intraepithelial neoplasia are listed in Table 15–4.

DUCTAL INTRAEPITHELIAL NEOPLASIA, GRADE 1

Grade 1 DIN includes intraductal hyperplasia (DIN 1a), atypical intraductal hyperplasia (DIN 1b), and low-grade DCIS (DIN 1c).

DUCTAL INTRAEPITHELIAL NEOPLASIA 1A (INTRADUCTAL HYPERPLASIA)

Intraductal hyperplasia is present any time the number of cell layers lining a duct exceeds the two layers—a continuous layer of luminal epithelial cells surrounded by an interrupted layer of myoepithelial cells—typical of the normal mammary unit structure. The designation of intraductal hyperplasia is preferred to the less frequently used alternate designations of epitheliosis (Azzopardi, 1979) and papillomatosis (Foote and Stewart, 1945; Haagensen, 1986; McDivitt et al.,

1968). The term epitheliosis is not commonly used in the United States, and it does not convey any information regarding the ductal growth pattern of these lesions; papillomatosis is also inaccurate, as it refers to a specific pattern of proliferation supported by fibrovascular cores.

Morphologic Features of Ductal Intraepithelial Neoplasia 1a

Microscopic assessment of epithelial proliferations in the mammary duct system should include evaluation of the architectural pattern at low magnification, followed by cytologic appraisal at higher magnification. The architectural and cytologic features of DIN 1a (IDH) are listed in Table 15–5.

Intraductal hyperplasia (Figs. 15–1 and 15–2) is characterized by the proliferation of a heterogeneous cell population that may be purely epithelial, or it may have an admixture of epithelial, myoepithelial, and metaplastic apocrine cells. The cells are irregular in outline with indistinct cell margins that frequently overlap; streaming of the cells may be present. The nuclei are variable in appearance and lack a uniform, round contour. The proliferation is often fenestrated, but the secondary lumens are irregular in size and shape, angulated, slit-like, and sometimes peripheral in location. The original duct lumen may persist as a crescent at one side of the duct. Epithelial bridges may

Table 15–5. Morphologic Features of Intraductal Hyperplasia

Cytologic features of intraductal hyperplasia
Admixture of cell types (epithelial cells, with or without myoepithelial and/ or metaplastic apocrine cells)
Variation in the appearance of epithelial cells
Indistinct cell margins and deviation from a round contour
Variation in the appearance of nuclei (angulated, spindled, oval, or round)

Architectural features of intraductal hyperplasia
Irregular and slit-like fenestrations
Peripheral fenestrations
Stretched epithelial bridges
Streaming or spindling of cells
Uneven distribution of nuclei and overlapped nuclei

Reprinted, with modifications, from F.A. Tavassoli, *Pathology of the Breast*, 1999, with permission from Appleton & Lange.

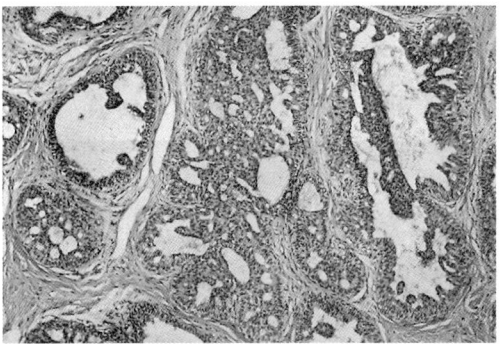

Figure 15–1. Ductal intraepithelial neoplasia, grade 1a (DIN 1a)—intraductal hyperplasia. A focally florid, ordinary intraductal epithelial proliferation forms multiple irregular spaces and peripheral clefts (H&E, low power).

form, but they are stretched with elongation of the cells. Sometimes the proliferation assumes the pattern observed in the hyperplastic ducts of gynecomastia. Foam cells may be present in the lumen of the hyperplastic ducts. Mitotic figures are observed only rarely, and their presence does not influence the ultimate diagnosis. Necrotic debris is also seen on rare occasions in the lumen (Fig. 15–3). It should be emphasized that the presence of luminal necrosis is not diagnostic of DCIS, and the lesion should be interpreted on the basis of the proliferating cell type.

Intraductal hyperplasia may be quite florid or of limited extent and degree. Intraductal hyperplasia may be mild (3 to 4 cell

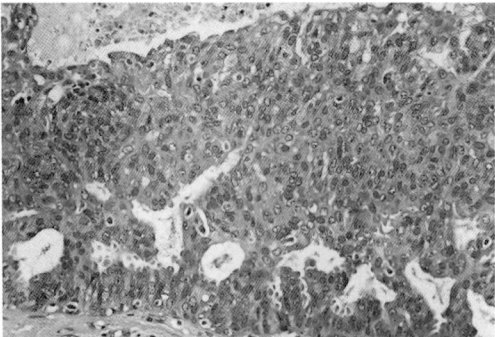

Figure 15–2. Ductal intraepithelial neoplasia, grade 1a (DIN 1a)—intraductal hyperplasia. Proliferation of a heterogenous cell population shows spindling and streaming, with peripheral fenestrations (H&E, high power).

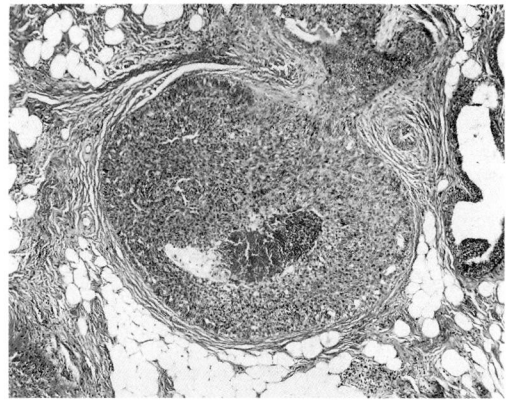

Figure 15–3. Ductal intraepithelial neoplasia, grade 1a (DIN 1a)—intraductal hyperplasia with intraluminal necrosis. Intraluminal necrosis may be observed in ordinary intraductal hyperplasia. In the absence of cytologic and/or architectural atypia, necrosis alone does not alter the designation of an ordinary intraductal epithelial proliferation to that of atypical intraductal hyperplasia (or intraductal carcinoma) (H&E, medium power).

layers above the basement membrane), moderate (tufting and a tendency to cross lumens), or severe (formation of epithelial bridges across the lumen, or filling and distension of the duct). Mild intraductal hyperplasia is so common and relatively inconsequential that it was not included in the AFIP study that compared the follow-up of 117 women with IDH to that of 82 women with AIDH (Tavassoli and Norris, 1990). Also excluded were proliferations composed purely of apocrine cells. In general, for practical purposes, we diagnose IDH when it is present and at least of moderate degree (unless a more atypical intraductal epithelial process is present), and further qualify the IDH as extensive, and/or florid, when applicable. Otherwise, we do not routinely distinguish among grades of IDH (e.g., mild, moderate, and severe or florid IDH).

Clinical Features and Significance of Ductal Intraepithelial Neoplasia 1a

Women with DIN 1a (IDH) may present clinically with either a palpable mass, area of induration, or mammographically suspicious lesion. They range in age from 15 to 83 years with a median of 45 years at presentation.

Women with IDH have a slightly increased relative risk for subsequent development of breast carcinoma that is 1.5 to 2.0 times that of the general population (Bodian et al., 1993b; McDivitt et al., 1992; Page and Dupont, 1990; Table 15–6). Of the 117 women with IDH in Tavassoli and Norris's series (1990), 3 women (2.6%) developed subsequent invasive ductal carcinoma during the (8 year, mean) follow-up interval. The subsequent carcinomas developed 11.8, 14, and 17.5 years after the diagnosis of IDH; two of these were ductal, while one was lobular in type. They all developed in the same breast; two in the same quadrant, and the third in a quadrant below the almost completely excised quadrant harboring the IDH. The degree and/or extent of hyperplasia did not influence the outcome. Bodian et al. (1993b) also noted that fine distinctions among levels of hyperplasia and atypia did not significantly alter risk among affected patients in their study.

Table 15–6. Relative Risk[a] Categories for Invasive Breast Carcinoma Based on Histopathology, Age at Presentation, and Presence or Absence of a Family History of Breast Cancer,[b] Compiled from Studies Since 1985

No increased risk

Mild intraductal hyperplasia (RR 1)

Slightly increased risk

Moderate or florid intraductal hyperplasia (RR 1.5–2×)

Mild to moderately increased risk

Atypical hyperplasia, ductal or lobular (with no family history) (RR 3.2–4.3)

Atypical hyperplasia, ductal or lobular (in a postmenopausal woman) (RR 3.3–6.5)

High risk

Atypical hyperplasia, ductal or lobular (with a family history) (RR 7.2–22)

Atypical hyperplasia, ductal or lobular (in a premenopausal woman) (RR 4.5–12)

Ductal carcinoma *in situ* (RR 8–10)

Lobular carcinoma *in situ* (RR 8–10)

---

[a]These risks should not be interpreted as lifetime risks, since the follow-up intervals ranged widely, from approximately 8 to 17 years.

[b]Family history of breast cancer in a first-degree relative (mother, sister, or daughter).

Reprinted, with modifications, from R.A. Lininger and F.A. Tavassoli, Atypical intraductal hyperplasia of the breast, in *Ductal Carcinoma* in Situ *of the Breast*, ed. M.J. Silverstein, 1997, with permission from Williams & Wilkins.

It is important to note that the reported conclusions of the cancer risk attributed to IDH have been questioned in a study that assessed the reproducibility of a diagnosis of IDH (Bodian et al., 1993a). In this study, Bodian et al. chose 63 cases at random and admixed them twice in a review of 1799 biopsies in a way that was inapparent to the participating pathologists. No disagreements were noted in the diagnosis of DCIS or invasive carcinoma in 5 cases and of lobular neoplasia in 10 cases. There were disagreements in 17 of the remaining 18 cases. The two reviews differed in 9 of the 48 cases (19%) with respect to the presence of hyperplasia. Both reviews agreed on the presence of hyperplasia in 39 cases, but classification of the type of the lesion (ductal versus lobular) differed in 11 cases. Furthermore, 219 of 240 cases (91%) initially interpreted as IDH were confirmed by a second pathologist, but 21 were interpreted as having mild to moderate atypia (Bodian et al., 1993a). Overall, an excellent agreement was achieved for diagnosing carcinoma and lobular neoplasia, good agreement for adenosis and intraductal papilloma, and relatively poor agreement on the levels of hyperplasia and atypia, and whether ducts or lobules were involved. The number of slides available for review also influenced distinction among levels of hyperplasia. Bodian and colleagues concluded that the lack of reliability of precise distinctions among levels and sites of hyperplasia and atypia seem to limit the usefulness of such classifications as guidelines for individual patient care (Bodian et al., 1993a).

Management of Patients with Intraductal Hyperplasia

Because of the low risk for development of subsequent invasive carcinoma associated with IDH (RR 1.5–2.0), follow-up of the patient in the form of annual or biannual examination of the breasts by a physician is generally recommended. Patients need to become aware of the problem and learn breast self-examination. In the absence of other risk factors, mammography every 1 or 2 years for patients between 40 to 49 years of age would be prudent. Annual mammography is advised for women 50 years of age or older.

Special Studies

Immunohistochemical studies have shown that ordinary epithelial hyperplasia is composed of cytokeratin 5/6 positive (progenitor) cells admixed with cytokeratin 8/18/19–positive glandular cells (Bocker, 1997; Bocker et al., 1992, 1997a). In our laboratory, Moinfar et al. (1999) have confirmed that IDH reacts with cytokeratin 18 and 19 as well as high-molecular-weight cytokeratin 34BetaE12. Ordinary intraductal hyperplasia is composed of a mosaic of cells, some of which react only with S-100-α and others that express only S-100-β (Ichihara et al., 1997). Furthermore, estrogen receptor (ER), progesterone receptor (PR), and the bcl-2 protein are expressed in IDH (Siziopikou et al., 1996), but the levels are relatively low compared to the levels found in AIDH and DCIS (Mustonen et al., 1997). No immunoreactivity for p53 protein was observed among 39 examples of IDH in two studies (Tavassoli and Man, 1995; Umekita et al., 1994). IDH characteristically lacks immunoreactivity for c-erbB-2 (Allred et al., 1992, 1994).

Morphometrically, IDH is characterized by the arrangement of groups of oval nuclei pointing toward a certain direction, forming a complex streaming pattern (Ozaki and Kondo, 1995). In contrast, in cribriform carcinoma the nuclear arrangement tends to be multidirectional, possibly because of vertical nuclear arrangement toward acinar lumens (Ozaki and Kondo, 1995).

Genetic alterations in the form of microsatellite instability (MSI) and loss of heterozygosity (LOH) have been studied in a very small number of cases of IDH. No mutations in exons 4–8 of p53 were identified by single-stranded conformational polymorphism (SSCP) among 20 cases of IDH (Done et al., 1998). Detection of allelic imbalance in a small proportion of IDH suggests that some cases of IDH are also clonal (Lakhani et al., 1996), which supports their inclusion in the DIN classification. Clonal chromosome alterations have been noted in two of five cases of IDH and these changes may indicate the presence of continuing genetic instability (Burbano et al., 1996). Kasami et al. (1997) found MSI in one (25%) of five women with IDH; the patient remained free of disease 21 years following her diagnosis of IDH. They concluded that there is no obligate correlation of genetic alterations with subsequent malignancy. The number of cases studied is too small to allow any definitive conclusions, however. Also, structural alterations involving chromosomes 1 and 5 have been reported (Burbano et al., 1996). It is also possible that we don't know which crucial locus or mutation to look for. Furthermore, some genetic and chromosomal alterations may be solely related to proliferation, whereas others may be a reflection of changes that may be potentially life threatening, and invariably associated with invasive carcinoma.

Ductal Intraepithelial Neoplasia 1b (Atypical Intraductal Hyperplasia)

From a historical perspective, AIDH is a relatively recent diagnostic category in breast pathology, which has been plagued by a significant degree of interobserver variability. The introduction of screening mammography resulted in detection of a wide variety of mammary intraductal proliferative lesions, the clinical significance of which was not known and to a great extent remains unknown. At the AFIP, beginning in the mid-1970s, we routinely designated proliferative lesions that were morphologically identical to intraductal carcinoma but limited in quantity (minuscule foci) as AIDH. The major reason for this quantitative approach was the fact that a diagnosis of DCIS was routinely followed by mastectomy and there were no convincing data to suggest that such minuscule low-grade DCIS warranted extensive surgery, particularly considering the fact that some of these lesions were found in women in their early 40's.

Atypical intraductal hyperplasia became better characterized in the 1980s as a result of multiple studies by Page et al. (1985) that eventually established AIDH as a risk factor for invasive breast carcinoma that is intermediate in its magnitude between the risk associated with IDH and that with DCIS. Application of Page et al.'s diagnostic criteria for AIDH has resulted in an unacceptably high level of interobserver variability and low level of consensus as to what constitutes AIDH as well as the magnitude of its clinical significance. Unfortunately, aside from among a relatively small number of individuals at some major academic medical centers, there remains significant variation in the diagnosis of AIDH versus low-grade DCIS at the national and international level, making comparison of results of various studies problematic. More significantly, this variability results in a diagnosis of cancer (DCIS) versus a noncancer (AIDH) and different approaches to management of the patient. Recognition of the kinship of AIDH and low-grade DCIS (which may differ in quantity only) and inclusion of the two in the category of DIN 1 would allow a similar approach to the management of the two that would differ only based on the variable extent/ size of the lesion. The DIN system eliminates the impact of having two different diagnoses (of cancer versus noncancer) for the same lesion.

Definition of Atypical Intraductal Hyperplasia

In simple descriptive terms, AIDH is a lesion that shows some, but not all, of the morphologic features of intraductal carcinoma (Page et al., 1985). This simplified definition does not explain what features of DCIS are shared by AIDH or why it fails to qualify as DCIS. In an attempt to provide a more precise definition of AIDH, Tavassoli and Norris (1990) assessed the architectural and cytologic features of a variety of intraductal proliferations to determine how AIDH could be separated from IDH and DCIS (Table 15–4). Two types of AIDH were defined by Tavassoli and Norris (1990; Table 15–7). One variant of AIDH (AIDH type I) appears

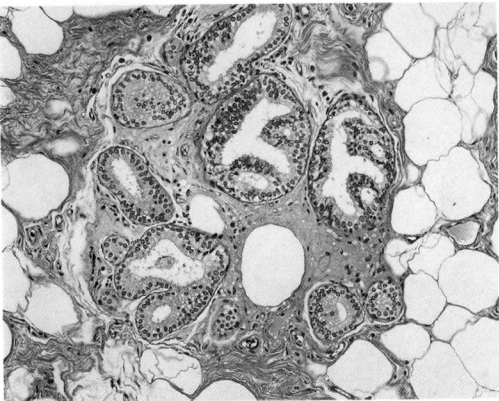

Figure 15–4. Ductal intraepithelial neoplasia, grade 1b (DIN 1b)—atypical intraductal hyperplasia. Several small ducts show a proliferation of uniform cells forming rigid arcades with rounded spaces and incomplete duct involvement, qualifying for atypical intraductal hyperplasia, since some but not all of the features of intraductal carcinoma are present (H&E, ×150).

to evolve from IDH (Figs. 15–4 and 15–5), as it displays some or all of the architectural features of ordinary intraductal hyperplasia but either almost purely comprised of subtly atypical cells simulating those found in low-grade intraductal carcinoma or more frequently shows an admixture of clusters of atypical cells within areas of ordinary hyperplasia. The second variant (AIDH type 2) displays both the architectural and cytologic features of low-grade DCIS but is quantitatively limited (Figs. 15–6 and 15–7). This sec-

Table 15–7. Morphologic Features of Atypical Intraductal Hyperplasia

Cytologic features of atypical intraductal hyperplasia

Monotonous, uniform rounded cell population

Subtle increase in nuclear/cytoplasmic ratio

Equidistant, highly organized or rosette-like nuclear distribution

Rounded nuclei

Hyperchromasia may or may not be present

Architectural features of atypic intraductal hyperplasia

AIDH type 1.	Any of the architectural patterns typical of IDH
AIDH type 2.	Cribriform, micropapillary, stratified spindle cell, or papillary pattern involving either a portion of a single duct or multiple ducts or ductules, of which the aggregate cross- sectional diameter does not exceed 2 mm

Reprinted, with modifications, from F.A. Tavassoli, *Pathology of the Breast*, 1999, with permission from Appleton & Lange.

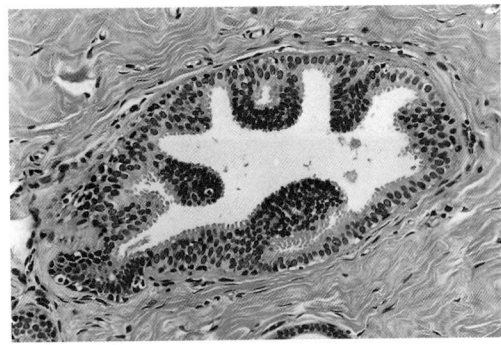

Figure 15–5. Ductal intraepithelial neoplasia, grade 1b (DIN 1b)—atypical intraductal hyperplasia. Several small ducts show a proliferation of uniform cells forming rigid arcades and micropapillae with incomplete duct involvement, qualifying for atypical intraductal hyperplasia (H&E, medium-high power).

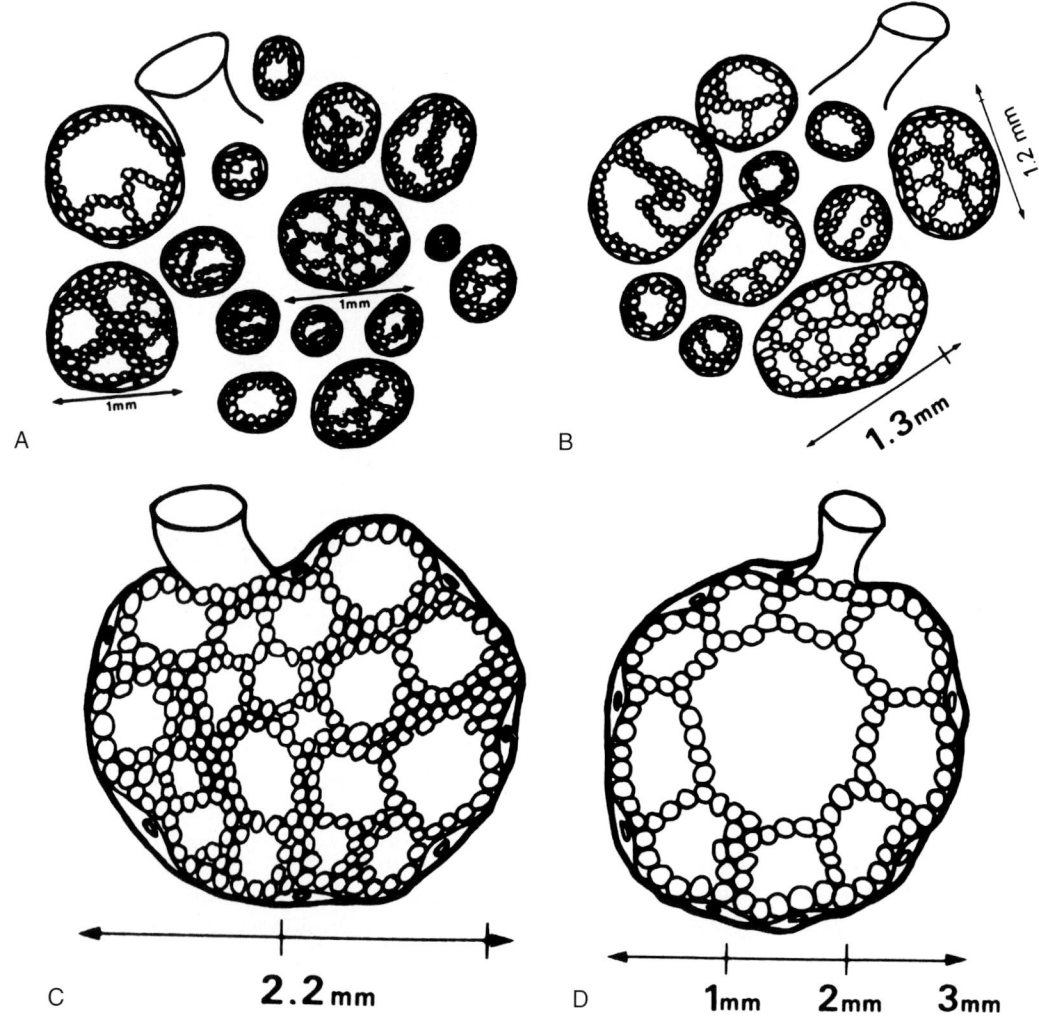

Figure 15–6. *A:* Two ductules in this terminal duct-lobular unit (TDLU) show a complete cribriform arrangement. Together they measure 1.8 mm; this is less than the required 2 mm aggregate diameter for a diagnosis of ductal carcinoma *in situ* (DCIS). Therefore, the proliferation qualifies as atypical intraductal hyperplasia (AIDH) (DIN 1b). *B:* The two ductules here exceed 2 mm in aggregate measurement. Therefore, the changes qualify them as DCIS. *C:* The cribriform proliferation has unfolded the TDLU (lobule), resulting in a ductal transformation of the lobule. The cross section of this structure exceeds 2 mm in diameter, thus the lesion qualifies as DCIS. *D:* Another TDLU is unfolded by the proliferation of a uniform population of cells forming epithelial bridges. The cross-sectional diameter of this structure is over 2 mm, thus the lesion qualifies as DCIS. [Reprinted from Tavassoli FA (1999) *Pathology of the Breast*, with modifications, with permission from Appleton & Lange.]

ond type of AIDH may result from progression of lesions arising in IDH with eventual assumption of both architectural and cytologic features of low-grade DCIS; alternatively, this variant may start de novo and proliferate from the onset with both the cytologic and architectural phenotype of low-grade DCIS. The propensity for subsequent development of infiltrating carcinoma did not differ among the two subtypes of AIDH over the period of follow-up (Tavassoli and Norris, 1990).

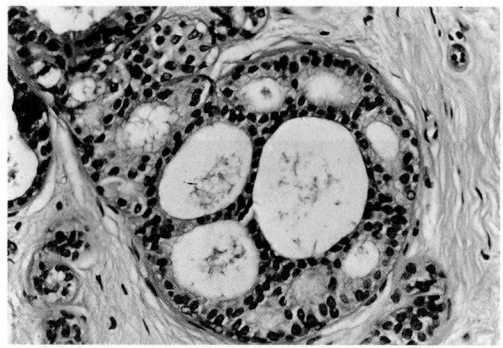

Figure 15–7. Ductal intraepithelial neoplasia, grade 1b (DIN 1b)—atypical intraductal hyperplasia. One small duct contains a proliferation of uniform cells that forms a cribriform pattern with round luminal spaces and moderately rigid bridges, morphologically forming a pattern of intraductal carcinoma that is nonetheless quantitatively limited (the aggregate cross-sectional diameter measures less than 2 mm). Therefore this specimen qualifies as atypical intraductal hyperplasia (2 mm rule) (H&E, medium-high power).

Morphologic Criteria for A Diagnosis of Atypical Intraductal Hyperplasia

Two major characteristics are evaluated during assessment of intraductal proliferations: *(1)* cytology and *(2)* architecture. Based on assessment of these features, lesions are divided into IDH, AIDH, and DCIS. The morphologic features to evaluate in AIDH are summarized in Tables 15–4 and 15–7.

Cytologic features of atypical intraductal hyperplasia. The cytologic appearance is the most important feature in separating AIDH from ordinary intraductal hyperplasia (Tavassoli and Norris, 1990). The proliferating cells in AIDH display the cytologic monotony and uniformity that is characteristic of the non-necrotic, low-grade variants of DCIS; cytologically, the changes qualify as an atypia of a low nuclear grade. The uniform rounded cells show a subtle increase in nuclear-to-cytoplasmic (N/C) ratio, rounded nuclei, and often distinct cell margins (see Table 15–7; Tavassoli and Norris, 1990). The proliferation may display focal aggregation of the uniform cells admixed with ordinary IDH or it may be composed purely of these uniform, subtly atypical cells. The criteria for

AIDH used at the AFIP were derived from a group of cases that specifically excluded apocrine proliferations (Tavassoli and Norris, 1990).

Mitotic activity is not helpful in subdividing the spectrum of intraductal proliferations. Mitotic activity may be quite prominent in ordinary IDH in some young women probably due to endogenous hormonal alterations. In contrast, most cases of AIDH and low-grade DCIS lack any notable mitotic activity. Utilization of a mitotic index could therefore result in overdiagnosis of AIDH and potentially even of DCIS in younger women.

Hyperchromasia is not assessed as a morphologic feature of atypia in the intraductal epithelial proliferations of the breast because tissue preparation and staining can significantly influence the appearance of this feature. For similar reasons, assessment of hyperchromasia is no longer used in grading infiltrating carcinomas either (Elston, 1984; Elston and Ellis, 1991; Elston et al., 1982).

Architectural features of atypical intraductal hyperplasia. A number of architectural features deserve specific comment, including the significance of intraluminal necrosis, tumor size, and presence of an extensive lesion.

Necrosis may be seen in a variety of intraductal proliferations within the breast. Intraluminal necrosis is a feature most commonly associated with higher-grade intraductal lesions. Intraductal papillomas, however, may also show necrosis, generally due to partial infarction secondary to torsion.

If necrosis is found within areas of AIDH that have qualitative features of DCIS but are of limited quantity, the lesion would qualify as DCIS. Presence of necrosis within ordinary IDH, however, does not alter the diagnosis.

The *2 mm aggregate diameter* was introduced arbitrarily after noting in our consultation practice that it was at the level of one or more small ducts or ductules measuring around 2 mm in aggregate cross-sectional diameter that most pathologists felt hesitant to diagnose a lesion as DCIS (Fig. 15–6). In support of this 2 mm requirement are the findings that tumor cells may grow as avascular spheroids up to 2 mm in size *in vivo* (Gimbrone et al., 1972, 1974) and 4 mm *in vitro* (Blood and Zetter, 1990). These sizes appear to be the physical limits of passive diffusion for nutrients and waste products in tumor cell aggregates. Beyond this size, the tumor cells must have the ability to induce angiogenesis for growth, an important feature of malignant proliferations (Weidner, 1995).

Two key points deserve emphasis:

1. The 2 mm size criterion is invoked only in assessing non-necrotic atypical intraductal proliferations with both architectural and cytologic features similar to those of low grade DCIS.
2. Proliferations with high-grade cytology (with or without necrosis) qualify as DCIS, regardless of size or quantity of epithelial proliferation.

The method of measurement of the ductules is illustrated in Figure 15–6. The AIDH begins in the TDLU where the ductules or acini are more or less spherical in shape. The proliferative activity may distort the cross-section to an ovoid or irregular shape. Generally, it is at the level of TDLU involvement that size becomes an issue and the maximum diameter of the structure is measured. The 2 mm rule is applied to longitudinal segments of ducts. When the proliferation extends into the extralobular terminal or major ducts, it is often advanced enough to be recognizable as DCIS and there is no need to resort to this quantitative approach.

To qualify as intraductal carcinoma, Page et al. (1985) required that all features of carcinoma *in situ* be uniformly present throughout two separate spaces. Since even a single space may occasionally assume large proportions, at the AFIP we adhere to the >2 mm quantitative criterion. Some pathologists claim that they do not recognize the need for a size criterion and will diagnose DCIS regardless of quantity when a proliferation qualitatively similar to DCIS is present. It is our firm belief that all practicing pathologists exercise some conscious or subconscious form of quantitation. It would be a rare event to find a pathologist who would diagnose DCIS based on a single cell or a cluster of cells with features of low-grade DCIS admixed with ordinary IDH. If quantity were not an issue, even a single cell with

morphologic features of low-grade DCIS should be designated as such.

For practical purposes, when a diagnosis of AIDH is considered on the basis of size limitation, it is prudent to perform a recut on the worrisome block(s) and determine if the lesion can be demonstrated to be larger and therefore qualify as DCIS with further sampling. When in doubt, as a rule, it is best to favor the more conservative (more benign) diagnosis in borderline cases when distinguishing IDH from AIDH or AIDH from DCIS.

Both IDH and DCIS are frequently rather florid and widespread throughout a biopsy. In comparison, AIDH is usually focal in nature and of limited extent. AIDH is most frequently found either focally in a background of florid IDH, or is present as an isolated lesion. Among mammographically detected lesions, however, we have encountered an occasional case, although still relatively rare, where *extensive duct involvement* by AIDH is present—that is, where numerous ducts within various TDLUs are partially involved by classic cribriform, arcade, or micropapillary growths. We suspect the RR for these lesions is similar to that of low-grade DCIS, due to their extensive proliferative activity. In one case where we suggested re-excision because of florid AIDH and presence of AIDH within 1 mm of the inked margin, the re-excision sample showed unequivocal DCIS. Therefore, we recommend grouping extensive AIDH, defined as AIDH involving >>20 duct cross-sections, with low-grade DCIS as DIN 1c, for management purposes.

Persistence of a *myoepithelial cell layer* around the duct wall does not influence the diagnosis of the intraductal proliferative lesions (IDH, AIDH, and DCIS), since even comedocarcinomas can have a myoepithelial cell layer around the duct that harbors the carcinoma. It is the admixture of cell types within the areas of proliferation that is significant. The absence of a myoepithelial cell layer around a duct with an intraluminal proliferation would favor DCIS but does not necessarily imply invasion since the basement membrane may persist.

Differential Diagnosis of Atypical Intraductal Hyperplasia

The pathologic entities most commonly considered in the differential diagnosis of AIDH

Table 15–8. Morphologic Features of Lobular Neoplasia

Cytology

Generally small, round cells with scant cytoplasm

Cellular homogeneity

Intracytoplasmic vacuolization

More abundant cytoplasm, in higher-grade lesions

Cytologic atypia, in higher-grade lesions

Signet-ring cell differentiation, in higher-grade lesions

Architecture

Cellular discohesion

Pagetoid spread

Lobular expansion, especially in higher-grade lesions

include pure epithelial proliferations such as IDH, low-grade DCIS, and lobular neoplasia. The cytologic, architectural and quantitative criteria discussed help to differentiate among these three entities (Tables 15–5, 15–7, and 15–8, and Fig. 15–6). Treatment may also produce changes that simulated AIDH and DCIS.

Distinction from papillomatosis. We restrict the terms IDH and AIDH to epithelial proliferations lacking a papillary configuration with fibrovascular supportive cores. The term papillomatosis is applied only when papillae and epithelial tufts are supported by fibrovascular cores. Both epithelial and myoepithelial cells are present in the papillary processes of papillomatosis.

Distinction from lobular neoplasia. In contrast to the formation of epithelial mounds, tufts, luminal bridges, multiple secondary lumens, and sieve-like formations characteristic of ductal proliferations, lobular neoplasia forms a solid, occlusive growth pattern (see section on lobular neoplasia). In our consultation practice at the AFIP, ductal hyperplasias and lobular neoplasia coexist in around 10% of the biopsies. The cells forming the two patterns may be identical in appearance, or they may differ morphologically.

Clinical history of radiation therapy or chemotherapy. It is well known that radiation and chemotherapy can induce cytologic alterations in the mammary epithelial cells within ducts and lobules superficially comparable to atypia. When proliferative activity is absent or minimal and history of recent therapy is provided, the lesion is generally interpreted as reflecting radiation or chemotherapy effect. However, when radiation-induced changes are superimposed on an epithelial proliferation, distinction from DCIS becomes very difficult, if not impossible. Fortunately, this scenario does not occur very commonly. Helpful features that would support treatment effect include evidence of similar atypia elsewhere, i.e., in the non-proliferative epithelium or in endothelial cells, and/or presence of sclerosis of vessel walls. With increasing use of radiotherapy for DCIS, this could potentially become a major differential diagnostic problem.

Other Types of Atypical Intraductal Hyperplasia

Atypical intraductal hyperplasia is most commonly composed of ductal epithelial cells of no special type. On occasion, however, it consists of a clear or apocrine cell population. One variant of "clinging carcinoma", the low-grade monomorphous variant, which we designate as AIDH, flat type (DIN 1b), will also be discussed. A variety of other unusual types of AIDH also occur, most of which are not well characterized because of their rarity (Tavassoli, 1999).

Low-grade (monomorphous) "clinging carcinoma" (DIN 1b, flat type). Judging from the illustration of papers from Europe on DCIS, it is clear that some of the lesions interpreted as DCIS, particularly those interpreted as clinging carcinoma by our European colleagues (Eusebi et al., 1994; Holland et al., 1990), would qualify as atypical hyperplasia to many viewers in the U.S, and possibly even IDH by some. Eusebi et al. (1994) evaluated the risk of subsequent invasive carcinoma in women with DCIS. Interestingly, 51% of the cases (41 of 80 cases) included in one study were lesions diagnosed as "clinging carcinoma." Analyzing only for pure clinging carcinomas, the RR was 1.0 (95% confidence interval [CI] 0.2–6.5). Interestingly, even when cases of usual-type DCIS were included in the analysis with cases of clinging carcinoma, an overall RR of only 2.0 was detected (95% CI 1.0–3.6). An earlier study had reported a RR of 3.9 (90% CI 0.7–12.2) associated with clinging carcinoma (Eusebi et al., 1989b). Since the CI ranges included 1 in both studies, however, neither of these risk ratios are considered statistically significant at a 95% level of confidence (Fletcher et al., 1982). In effect, some carcinomas diagnosed in Europe appear to have a lower RR for subsequent development of invasive carcinoma than lesions diagnosed as AIDH (or even IDH) in the U.S. (Dupont et al., 1993; London et al., 1992; Page et al., 1985).

The true biology of clinging carcinoma and its risk for subsequent invasion, however, may not be reflected in the statistical analysis results of these studies, since the limited number of cases most likely accounts for the lack of reported statistical significance of an association. Future studies will need larger numbers of cases with meaningful follow-up intervals to answer this question. Therefore, based on analysis of the available data in the literature, both for routine diagnostic purposes and in the MIN translational classification system, the monomorphous variant of clinging carcinoma is equated to AIDH, flat type (DIN 1b) (Fig. 15–8), until there is compelling evidence to do otherwise. The polymorphous variant of clinging carcinoma, distinguished by the presence of high-grade

cytologic atypia, qualifies as a high-grade DCIS (Fig. 15–9).

Atypical apocrine metaplasia and hyperplasia. Simple apocrine metaplasia, hyperplasia, and adenosis may show cytologic atypia. To qualify as *atypical apocrine metaplasia* (AAM), the nuclei should display at least a three-fold variation in size. Proliferation of these atypical cells or epithelial bridging with partial to complete cribriform growth by uniform cells not exceeding 2 mm would qualify as *atypical apocrine hyperplasia* (AAH) (Figs. 15–10 and 15–11; Tavassoli, 1999). The presence of nucleolar prominence alone does not signify atypia in apocrine cells. Occasionally, mitotic activity is increased. The presence of papillary apocrine cell hyperplasia or tufting is not as worrisome as the finding of epithelial bridges formed by metaplastic apocrine cells. A cribriform arrangement by metaplastic apocrine cells is always worrisome and should be carefully assessed for the possibility of apocrine intraductal carcinoma; the cribriform pattern of intraductal apocrine carcinoma may not be associated with significant cytologic atypia. A majority of apocrine intraductal carcinomas display significant cytologic atypia and necrosis (Tavassoli and Norris, 1994), however, thus facilitating recognition.

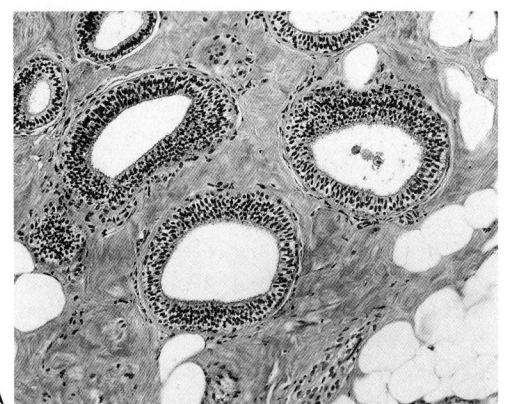
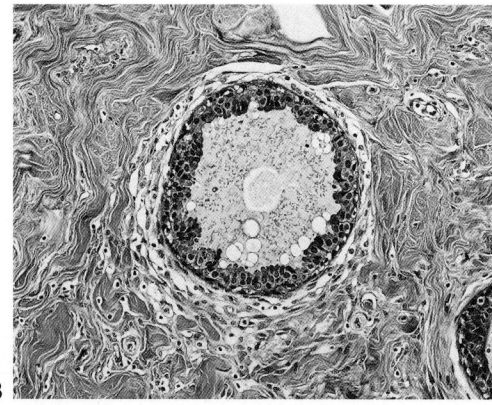

Figure 15–8. *A:* Ductal intraepithelial neoplasia, grade 1b (DIN 1b)—atypical intraductal hyperplasia, stratified spindle cell pattern. Several ducts are lined by a minimally hyperplastic layer of uniform epithelial cells showing cellular stratification, which we interpret as a variant of atypical intraductal hyperplasia (DIN 1b, flat type) in the absence of intraluminal necrosis (H&E, medium power). *B:* Ductal intraepithelial neoplasia, grade 1b (DIN 1b)—atypical intraductal hyperplasia, stratified spindle cell pattern. This is another example of a duct lined by uniform cells forming a stratified spindle cell pattern with focal intraluminal apical cytoplasmic projections. Some pathologists may classify this as the low-grade, monomorphous variant of "clinging carcinoma," but we would interpret it as a variant of atypical intraductal hyperplasia (DIN 1b, flat type) (H&E, medium high power).

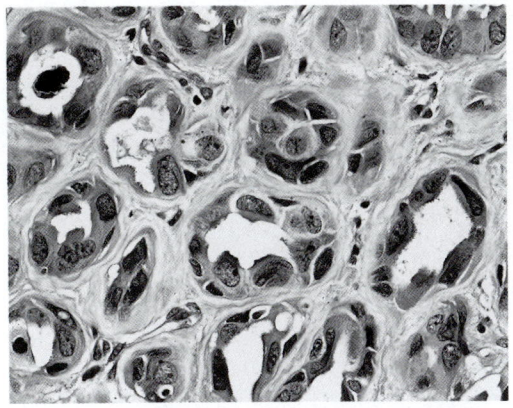

Figure 15–9. Ductal intraepithelial neoplasia, grade 3 (DIN 3, flat type). Polymorphous variant of "clinging carcinoma." This subtype is characterized by a population of cells showing significant cytologic atypia forming a minimally hyperplastic layer of cells that lines a duct. Illustrated here is an example of an adenosis-like pattern (H&E, medium-high power).

Curiously, in the setting of a papilloma, atypia is often apocrine in nature. Atypical apocrine metaplasia may also involve sclerosing adenosis; in such instances it has been termed *atypical apocrine adenosis* (AAA), and is described as a risk factor for the develop-

ment of subsequent invasion with a RR of 5.5 (95% CI, 1.9–16) (Seidman et al., 1996). All subsequent carcinomas developed in women who were over 60 years of age at the time of initial breast biopsy. Among the 11 women over 60 years of age at diagnosis, the RR for invasive carcinoma was 14 (95% CI 4.1–48).

Problems with Reproducibility of a Diagnosis of Atypical Intraductal Hyperplasia and Its Implications

Significant historical, interobserver, and international differences in criteria for diagnosis of AIDH and DCIS exist, which make comparison of more recent studies with those performed 10 or more years ago, as well as comparison among studies using different pathologic criteria and/or originating in different countries, inherently problematic (Lininger and Tavassoli, 1997). This is compounded by the fact that some previous studies that evaluated risk factors, treatment, and prognosis of AIDH and DCIS have not addressed the specific criteria by which the pathologic diagnoses were made. This is a serious flaw with potentially profound implications for the interpretation of the results. Even among studies that have provided diagnostic criteria, the morpho-

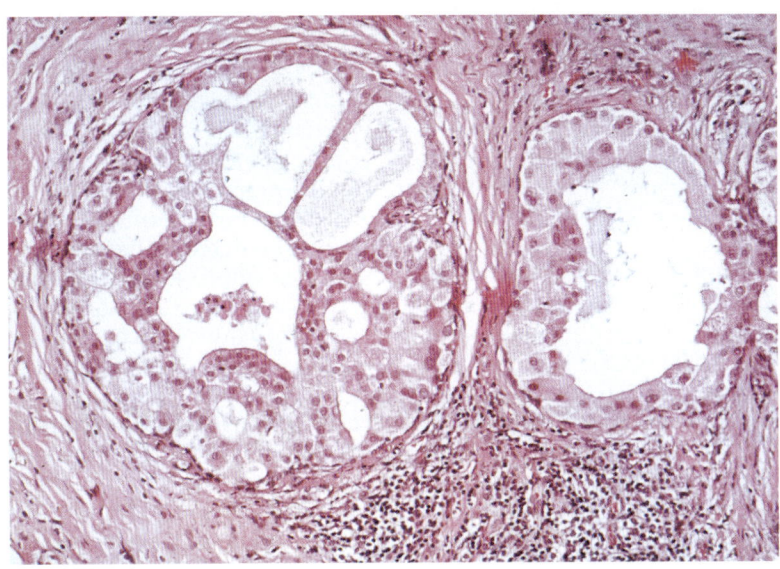

Figure 15–10. Ductal intraepithelial neoplasia, grade 1b (DIN 1b)—atypical apocrine hyperplasia. Intraglandular cribriform architecture can be discerned within one of these two ducts, a feature often associated with atypia when noted within intraductal apocrine lesions (H&E, ×40).

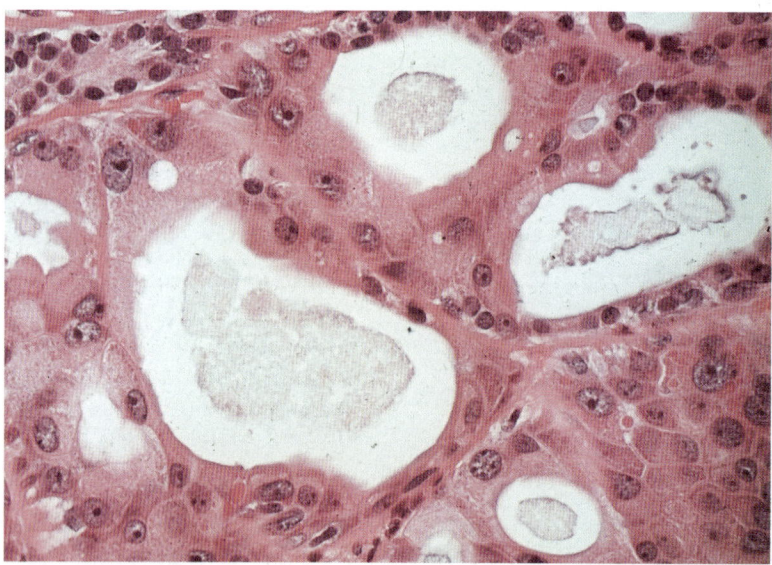

Figure 15–11. Ductal intraepithelial neoplasia, grade 1b (DIN 1b)—atypical apocrine hyperplasia. At this higher power, a threefold variation in nuclear size is noted within the intraductal apocrine hyperplasia, therefore the lesion qualifies as an atypical apocrine hyperplasia. The presence of prominent nucleoli alone is not sufficient for a diagnosis of atypia within an apocrine proliferation (H&E, high power).

logic characteristics of AIDH have necessarily evolved and been refined over time, as additional information has been obtained. For example, cases of florid IDH were classified as AIDH in Page et al.'s initial report in 1978. These cases were subsequently grouped with IDH in the 1985 report by Page et al. There are even problems when the same criteria are applied by different investigators. The RR for AIDH in the study by Page et al. (1985) was found to be 4.3. Applying Page's criteria, a RR of only 2.4 was observed for women with AIDH in the recent Nurses' Health Study (Marshall et al., 1997). This figure is very close to the RR for IDH.

Furthermore, significant trends in methods of detection of breast lesions and sampling of tissue specimens have also evolved over time. Since AIDH is largely a clinically silent disease, major studies defining diagnostic criteria have been based on identification of AIDH in samples removed from women who have had a surgical biopsy because of some other clinical complaint referable to the breast (Page et al., 1985; Tavassoli and Norris, 1990). Even among these biopsied women, the tissues were processed during an era when sampling was far more limited, without assessment of margins, and

often suboptimal by current standards. In more recent studies based on (at least a proportion of) mammographically detected AIDH, a potentially different risk association has emerged, with RRs ranging from 2.4 to 13 (Carter et al., 1988; Dupont et al., 1993; London et al., 1992; Marshall et al., 1997; Palli et al., 1991). Moreover, we have recently encountered occasional cases of extensive AIDH detected mammographically—that is, numerous ducts in multiple sections showing partial cribriform AIDH. We did not have a single case of this type in our study (Tavassoli and Norris, 1990). It is unlikely that extensive AIDH is a new lesion. More probably, it is simply being detected more commonly now because of improved screening methods.

Since a large proportion of the female population does not participate in screening mammography and not all AIDH lesions are picked up by mammography, we can never expect to have absolute information, but we do anticipate a continuous increase in the numbers of biopsies that will be designated as AIDH. It is imperative to reexamine the significance of what we are currently designating as AIDH among these screened women and examine breasts more thoroughly in autopsies to better understand this lesion.

Interobserver variability. The lack of consensus surrounding the diagnosis of "borderline" breast lesions has been identified as a problem for over half a century (Rosen, 1991). More recently, Rosai (1991) reported a similar lack of consensus in the diagnosis of borderline epithelial lesions of the breast. In his paper, 17 slides, each with a specific area circled, were reviewed by a panel of five pathologists. Not a single lesion was interpreted unanimously. All five pathologists agreed that eight lesions were not carcinomas; however, they failed to reach a consensus as to whether the lesions were IDH or AIDH. Reciprocally, all five pathologists agreed that three lesions were not ordinary hyperplasia, but they failed to reach a consensus as to whether the lesion represented AIDH or DCIS. In six lesions, the diagnoses ranged the entire spectrum from IDH to DCIS. Interestingly, a tendency toward benignity or malignancy in diagnosis was noted in two pathologists; one pathologist failed to diagnose IDH in any lesion and one pathologist failed to diagnose DCIS in any lesion. This exercise showed quite clearly that even pathologists with experience in breast pathology have totally different thresholds for recognition of atypia and DCIS.

With the use of standardized criteria, however, interobserver reproducibility has improved and can be further improved. Complete agreement among 6 pathologists was observed in the evaluation of 24 difficult intraductal proliferations in 14 cases (58%); 5 or more pathologists agreed in 17 of the cases (71%); and 4 or more pathologists arrived at the same diagnosis in 22 cases (92%) (Schnitt et al., 1992). There remain, however, significant differences in the threshold for the diagnosis of low-grade intraductal carcinoma.

Relatively poor reproducibility is also reported for the diagnosis of levels of hyperplasia and atypia, and whether a ductal or lobular process was involved, in one study involving a "blinded" retrospective pathology review of benign breast biopsies (Bodian et al., 1993a). A recent study of 31 ductal, lobular, and papillary lesions that included both academic and community pathologists found that only 33% agreed on the diagnosis of cancer in 10 cases (Palazzo and Hyslop, 1996).

Implications of a lack of consensus in the differentiation of atypical intraductal hyperplasia from ductal carcinoma in situ. Interobserver variability in the interpretation of borderline breast lesions has important implications for epidemiological and clinical studies of breast cancer and their conclusions. Clinical trials for determination of the efficacy of conservative treatment in management of DCIS may now involve multiple centers in the U.S. and Europe (Solin et al., 1993). Since the criteria for diagnosis of DCIS vary extensively in different centers across the continents (Bobrow et al., 1994; Eusebi et al., 1994; Holland et al., 1985; London et al., 1992; Ottesen et al., 1992; Page et al., 1985; Schnitt et al., 1992; Tavassoli and Norris, 1990), comparison of the results of these studies is problematic.

Variable interpretation of the same lesion as DCIS versus AIDH has a serious impact not only on a patient's emotional state but also potentially on access to insurance and management of disease, as well as statistics on progression and cure. Standardization of criteria and terminology across the continents is crucial. An analysis of the impact of such differential classification has not been attempted but would be very interesting and important.

Clinical Features and Significance of Atypical Intraductal Hyperplasia

Detection of atypical intraductal hyperplasia. Since the introduction of mammography in the early 1970s and the subsequent increase in breast cancer screening and patient awareness, the detection of lesions interpreted as atypical hyperplasia has increased dramatically, contributing to the increase in incidence. Among biopsies from mammographically screened women, 10% to 17.7% have AIDH (Dupont et al., 1993; Palli et al., 1991; Rubin et al., 1988), compared to only 2.1% of biopsies in the premammography study by Page et al. (1985). A large proportion of reported cases of AIDH are detected incidentally, however. Histologically, calcification is reported in over 50% of cases with AIDH compared to almost 40% of cases of IDH, but it is found in only 14% of cases of fibroadenoma or other benign breast diseases (Carter et al., 1988).

Risk for subsequent invasive carcinoma. The absolute risk of a woman with atypical hyperplasia developing invasive breast carcinoma has ranged from 5.1% to 12.9%, within 8.3 to 21 years of follow-up (Table 15–2; Bodian et al., 1993b; Carter et al., 1988; Dupont and Page, 1985; Eusebi et al., 1989b, 1994; Page et al., 1985, Tavassoli and Norris, 1990). The RR for invasive carcinoma of a diagnosis of AIDH among studies published since 1985 ranges from 2.4 to 22, depending on the age of the patient and presence or absence of a family history of breast cancer (Table 15–6; Lininger and Tavassoli, 1997; Tavassoli, 1999). Of 82 women with AIDH in the AFIP study, 9.8% subsequently developed invasive carcinomas, compared to 2.6% of 117 women with IDH (Tavassoli and Norris, 1990). The average interval to subsequent invasive carcinoma was about 8.3 years for patients with AIDH, and 14.3 years for those with IDH (Page et al., 1985; Tavassoli and Norris, 1990). Therefore, patients with AIDH are not only at greater risk for subsequent development of invasive carcinoma but they are so within a shorter period of time (average interval of 8.2 years) compared to women with IDH (average interval of 14.3 years).

It is also significant that patients with AIDH are at risk for developing invasive carcinoma in the contralateral as well as the ipsilateral breast where the majority arise; furthermore, the subsequent carcinomas may be of either ductal or lobular type. In women with AIDH 25% (Tavassoli and Norris, 1990) to 44% (Page et al., 1985) of subsequent invasive carcinomas occurred in the contralateral breast. Four of the six subsequent carcinomas in the AFIP study, however, were specified as being in the same quadrant of the ipsilateral breast; five of the carcinomas were invasive ductal, while one was invasive lobular in type (Tavassoli and Norris, 1990). None of the patients had any evidence of lobular disease in their previous biopsies, however. Of the subsequent carcinomas in Page's study, 56% were in the ipsilateral breast and 61% were ductal carcinomas of no special type (Page et al., 1985). In this regard, AIDH may be considered a marker of breast cancer risk similar to lobular neoplasia.

Despite the large number of published studies on atypical hyperplasia of the breast, only three studies specifically characterized AIDH (of no specialized type) separate from atypical lobular proliferations of the breast (lobular neoplasia or atypical lobular hyperplasia) (Marshall et al., 1997; Page et al., 1985; Tavassoli and Norris, 1990). Two of these studies reported the subsequent risk of invasive carcinoma specifically for AIDH: Page et al. (1985) reported a RR of 4.3, whereas Marshall et al. (1997), using Page's criteria, reported an odds ratio (OR) of 2.4 for AIDH. All the remaining studies have combined atypical ductal and lobular lesions for purposes of analysis, with the exception of one recent study of atypical apocrine adenosis, an AIDH of specialized type (Seidman et al., 1996). Although Page found that the RR for AIDH was similar to atypical lobular hyperplasia (ALH) (Page et al., 1985), and a subsequent nested case–control study by Dupont et al. (1993), reported similar results obtained for atypical hyperplasia of ductal or lobular types (RR 4.3, CI 1.7–11), with other pathologists applying Page's criteria, Marshall et al. found that ALH was more strongly associated with overall breast cancer risk (OR of 5.3) than AIDH (OR of 2.4), and that ALH was more strongly associated with risk of premenopausal breast cancer (OR of 9.6) than with the risk of postmenopausal breast cancer (OR of 3.7). The risk of breast cancer associated with AIDH in their study did not vary by menopausal status.

Taking into consideration all the studies since 1985 that have assessed the risk of atypical hyperplasia (combining both atypical ductal and lobular types) for subsequent invasive carcinoma (including both cohort and case–control studies), the RR (or OR) range from 1 to 13, depending on the population studied, the reference population used, and the diagnostic criteria for AH/AIDH used (Bodian et al., 1993b; Carter et al., 1988; Dupont and Page, 1985; Dupont et al., 1993; Eusebi et al., 1989b, 1994; London et al., 1992; Marshall et al., 1997; McDivitt et al., 1992; Page et al., 1985; Palli et al., 1991). If older studies published before 1985 are included (including cohort, case–control, and cross-sectional studies) (Alpers and Wellings, 1985; Ashikari et al., 1974; Ashikari et al., 1974; Black et al., 1972; Hutchinson et al., 1980; Karpas et al., 1965; Kern and Brooks, 1969; Kodlin et al., 1977; Moskowitz et al., 1980; Ryan and Coady, 1962; Tellem et al., 1962), the RR are even wider, ranging from 0.5 to 30.6 (Ma and Boyd, 1992). Despite this wide range, the College of American Pathology (CAP) has made no attempt to reevaluate the validity of the RR of 5 for AIDH and ALH adopted by the Consensus Meeting of the Cancer Committee of the College of American Pathologists in 1985 (Hutter et al., 1986).

Clinical Management of Atypical Intraductal Hyperplasia

Most AIDH lesions are adequately treated by excision. Presence of AIDH at or close to (within less than 2 mm) the surgical margins makes no difference in its management. On rare occasions, we have recommended re-excision when an AIDH lesion that is particularly worrisome because of its abundance is at or close to (within 2 mm of) the surgical margin. Adjuvant therapy such as radiation therapy is not advocated for AIDH.

In view of the moderately increased risk for development of subsequent carcinoma associated with AIDH, and the shorter interval to the development of subsequent carcinoma compared to IDH (8.2 years vs. 14.4 years), women with AIDH require closer follow-up. The follow-up regimen recommended includes two to four examinations of both breasts by a physician each year, along with annual mammograms for those over 40 years of age. If a patient with AIDH also has a strong positive family history of breast carcinoma or has dense breast tissue that cannot be adequately followed by mammography, then wide excision or mastectomy may be a legitimate consideration. In practice, the final therapeutic decision is often determined not only by the magnitude of the risk involved but also by assessing the patient's level of understanding of this risk, her reliability in adhering to the follow-up regimen, and her level of anxiety.

Implications of atypical intraductal hyperplasia versus ductal carcinoma in situ in clinical management. The significance of designating a lesion as AIDH, rather than DCIS, is profound, in that it may dramatically alter a woman's treatment. The proportion of cases of DCIS treated by mastectomy fell from 71% to 43.8% between 1983 and 1992, whereas the proportion of cases treated by lumpectomy increased from 25.6% to 53.3% (Ernster et al., 1996). It may be argued that this trend toward the conservative manage-

ment of both AIDH and DCIS may make the distinction between AIDH and DCIS (at least low-grade DCIS) less important, at least for management purposes. Despite the trend toward conservative management of selected DCIS lesions (Ernster et al., 1996), however, a diagnosis of DCIS in 1992 resulted in a mastectomy in 43.8% of patients (10,242 patients) and lumpectomy plus radiation therapy in another 23.3% (5445 patients), based on SEER study data. In contrast, a diagnosis of AIDH usually results in no further treatment. The increasing incidence of DCIS has compensated for the decreasing rates of mastectomy, resulting in an absolute increase in numbers of mastectomies performed for DCIS up until the year 1990. One wonders how many of these mastectomies and radiotherapies could have been prevented if the lesions had been interpreted as AIDH by another reviewer, and what the outcome would have been and at what cost!

Biology of Atypical Intraductal Hyperplasia and Breast Neoplasia

The natural history of AIDH is unclear. Both IDH and DCIS are frequently rather florid and quite widespread throughout a biopsy. In comparison, AIDH is frequently focal in nature and of limited extent. This implies that AIDH is at most generally a transitional stage. The assignment of a quantitative criterion for separating AIDH from low-grade DCIS further suggests that it is considered a more limited extent of low-grade DCIS. The 2 mm quantity suggested by the AFIP appears to have support from the biologic necessity for vascularization to develop prior to further growth of tumor cells beyond a 2 mm cluster size *in vivo* (Gimbrone et al., 1972, 1974). Atypical intraductal hyperplasia is most frequently found either in a background of florid IDH or is present as an isolated lesion. The two forms of AIDH observed and described by Tavassoli and Norris (1990) suggest that whatever induces proliferation of the epithelial cells in the ducts may either induce a malignant (atypical) cell population from the onset or cause a benign cellular proliferation. The continuous proliferative activity and cell division of even the benign cells, however, provides additional opportunities for development of further genetic alterations and a malignant clone to develop at some point. If such a cell type develops, it can progressively displace or replace the benign cell population. A subclone may attain even further genetic alterations and proceed to the eventual development of a recognizable carcinoma and invasion, unless the progression is interrupted by a biopsy. Rare cases of extensive low-grade cribriform DCIS—treated by biopsy alone because of the patient's refusal to undergo additional surgery—have recurred after 15 years in a more limited extent and persisted in an *in situ* phase (Lininger et al., 1998). Such cases suggest that progression to invasive carcinoma is by no means inevitable or universal. Apparently, while some cancer cells have or quickly develop the potential to invade, not all cancer cells have this capability, or they attain it over such a long period of time that it may be considered inconsequential for an elderly patient. Would the finding of a 5 mm low-grade DCIS in an elderly woman, 80 years of age, justify radiation therapy? Interestingly, a recent study on DCIS found five subsequent invasive carcinomas following diagnosis of low-grade DCIS; four of these (80%) occurred in the contralateral breast (Done et al., 1996). This suggests that low-grade DCIS is also a marker for increased risk for subsequent development of carcinoma in either breast, rather than an unequivocal precursor.

Special Studies

At present, there are no special studies that are diagnostically useful in helping to distinguish AIDH from either IDH or DCIS with a high level of specificity, although

there are some interesting studies that may reflect the biology and etiology of these lesions. Recent data in our laboratory have shown that determination of the immuno-profile for the high-molecular-weight cytokeratin antibody cocktail 34BetaE12 is useful in distinguishing between AIDH/DCIS and IDH (Moinfar et al., 1999). Intraductal hyperplasia stains with 34BetaE12, whereas AIDH/DCIS characteristically does not show immunoreactivity (see discussion in Ductal Carcinoma *In Situ* Special Studies section below). However, no true "gold standard" for confirmation of a diagnosis of AIDH exists. Current knowledge of biomarker expression in precursor lesions of the breast cancer is still very limited, although they could be important for improving the prediction of a patient's risk. The most frequently studied markers include estrogen (ER) and progesterone receptor (PR) expression, proliferation rate, ploidy, c-*erb*B-2/*HER*-2/*neu* oncogene expression, and Tp53 tumor suppressor gene expression and mutation (see Table 15–9 for a summary of biomarker expression in AIDH compared to DCIS).

The variation in morphologic appearance and grade of intraductal proliferations ranging from IDH to AIDH to DCIS is associated with variable expression of hormone receptors and molecular markers. The different patterns and morphologies of breast cancer may be explained by different patterns of randomly acquired mutations (Smith et al., 1993). Information on these markers and other recent studies that address AIDH are discussed below, in the context of what is known about DCIS and IDH.

Table 15–9. Biomarker Expression in Atypical Intraductal Hyperplasia and Various Grades of Ductal Carcinoma *In Situ*

Biomarker	AIDH (%)	Grade 1 (Low) (%)	Grade 2 (Intermediate) (%)	Grade 3 (High) (%)
Estrogen receptor	~90–100	80–100	90	20–75
Progesterone receptor	~90–100	80–100	65–80	12–75
Ki67	—	0–22	35–50	70–90
p53	—	0–5	5–35	60–65
c-erbB-2	0	0–10	20–50	70–80

Approximate percentages compiled from a combination of published data.

Reprinted, with modifications, from R.A. Lininger and F.A. Tavassoli, Atypical intraductal hyperplasia of the breast, in *Ductal Carcinoma* in Situ *of the Breast*, ed. M.J. Silverstein, 1997, with permission from Williams & Wilkins.

Clonality. Loss of heterozygosity (LOH) and degrees of LOH or allelic imbalance have been demonstrated at various chromosomal loci in AIDH (Lakhani et al., 1995b), DCIS (Stratton et al., 1995), and LCIS (Lakhani et al., 1995a) microdissected from paraffin-embedded material. Furthermore, allelic imbalance was demonstrated at various chromosomal loci in a proportion of microdissected mammary hyperplasia of usual type, suggesting that a proportion of these lesions are also clonal, neoplastic proliferations (Lakhani et al., 1996).

Hormone receptors. Several immunohistochemical (IHC) studies suggest that most AIDH, as well as IDH and non-comedo DCIS (about 90% of low-grade cribriform and micropapillary DCIS) express high levels of ER and PR (Barnes, 1993; Barnes and Masood, 1990; Jacquemier et al., 1990; Poller et al., 1993b). A majority of high-grade (comedo) DCIS, in contrast, is ER and PR negative (Poller et al., 1993b).

Proliferation index and ploidy status. Proliferation index (S-phase fraction) and ploidy are not well characterized for either AIDH or IDH. In general, however, non-comedo DCIS shows a low proliferation index (over 90% of low grade micropapillary and cribriform DCIS fail to react with Ki-67), whereas it is elevated in comedo DCIS in about 60% of cases (Aasmundstad and Haugen, 1990; Meyer, 1986). Non-comedo DCIS are usually diploid, in contrast to comedo DCIS lesions, which are most frequently aneuploid (Aasmundstad and Haugen, 1990; Killeen and Namiki, 1991).

Oncogenes. Amplification and/or overexpression of c-erbB-2 is reportedly absent in AIDH and IDH, is rare in non-comedo DCIS, but is common in comedo-DCIS (Allred et al., 1992, 1993; Gusterson et al., 1988a,b). Overexpression and/or amplification of epidermal growth factor receptor (EGFR) (Tsutsumi et al., 1990), *ras* (Fromowitz et al., 1987), and c-*myc* (Watson et al., 1993) have also been reported.

Tumor suppressor genes. Mutation and/or overexpression of the tumor suppressor gene *p53* has not been well characterized for precursor lesions such as AIDH, although it has been reported in 40% to 60% of comedo-DCIS and 10% of non-comedo DCIS (over 90% of low-grade micropapillary and cribriform DCIS fail to react with p53) (Davidoff et al., 1991a,b; Poller et al., 1993). Loss of heterozygosity was reported in microdissected tissues of 5 of 9 informative cases of AIDH on chromosome 16q (D16-S413) and in 2 of 8 informative cases on chromosome 17p (D17S796) (Lakhani et al., 1995b).

DUCTAL CARCINOMA *IN SITU* (DIN 1c, DINS 2, AND DIN 3)

Currently regarded as a precursor of invasive carcinoma, ductal carcinoma *in situ* (DCIS) is a biologically and morphologically heterogeneous disease. Defined as a proliferation of epithelial cells with morphologic features of malignancy within the confines of the duct system and without stromal invasion, DCIS reflects a spectrum of lesions composed of a proliferation of cells assuming a variety of cytologic appearances and growth patterns. This spectrum ranges from proliferations with minimal atypia to those with a highly anaplastic cytologic appearance. The extent of the disease varies from a highly localized process confined to one or more adjacent terminal duct–lobular units (TDLUs) to a widespread process that extends from multiple TDLUs to multiple major ducts in one or more segments.

In the context of DIN, the heterogeneous patterns of proliferation currently referred to as DCIS grades I, 2, and 3 fall within the three grades of DIN: DIN 1c, DIN 2, and DIN 3. The diagnostic criteria for DCIS will be discussed.

The 2 mm Quantitative Rule

The AFIP criteria require complete involvement of one or more ductal cross sections by either the cribriform or micropapillary proliferation of a uniform population of cells, the aggregate cross-sectional diameter of which exceeds 2 mm (Tavassoli and Norris, 1990). Lesions displaying partial involvement of duct cross-sections of 2 mm or less in aggregate cross sectional diameter qualify as AIDH (Tavassoli and Norris, 1990). The 2 mm aggregate diameter was introduced at a time when a diagnosis of DCIS invariably led to mastectomy and we felt that such minimal lesions found incidentally in biopsies performed for a variety of benign lesions did not warrant mastectomy. In support of this 2 mm requirement, as discussed previously in the section on AIDH, it has been shown that tumor cells may grow as avascular spheroids of up to 2 mm in size *in vivo* (Gimbrone et al., 1972, 1974) and 4 mm *in vitro* (Blood and Zetter, 1990). These sizes appear to be the physical limits of passive diffusion for nutrients and waste products in tumor cell aggregates. Beyond this size, the tumor cells must have the ability to induce angiogenesis for growth, an important feature of malignant proliferations (Weidner, 1995).

For practical purposes, when a diagnosis of AIDH is considered on the basis of size limitation, it is prudent to perform a recut on the worrisome block(s) and determine if the lesion enlarges on a deeper level and/or further sampling, if the biopsy has been incompletely submitted, to declare itself as DCIS.

Myoepithelial Cell Layer

Persistence of a myoepithelial (ME) cell layer around the duct wall does not influence or alter the diagnosis of DCIS. Even comedocarcinomas can and most often do have a myoepithelial cell layer around the ducts that harbors the carcinoma. This is a feature that is easily recognizable to the trained morphologist and does not even require the utilization of immunostains for enhancement. In case the myoepithelial cells are not readily apparent, immunostains for actin (Bussolati et al., 1980) are superior to those for S-100 protein since the latter is also expressed sporadically among epithelial cells. While the absence of a myoepithelial cell layer around a duct would support a diagnosis of DCIS, it does not necessarily imply invasion since the basement membrane may persist. The absence of a myoepithelial cell layer indicates that a major obstacle to invasion has been removed, however.

Increasing Incidence of Ductal Carcinoma *In Situ*

The overall age-adjusted incidence of DCIS increased from 2.4 per 100,000 women in 1973 to 15.8% per 100,000 women in 1992—more than a fivefold increase (Ernster et al., 1996). While 20 years ago only 3%–5% of all breast cancers diagnosed were DCIS, this percentage has increased to 15%–40% of all breast cancers in screening centers (Ashikari et al., 1971; Lagios et al., 1989; Margolin and Lagios, 1986). As noted earlier in the section on AIDH, there has also been a concurrent increase in the proportion of atypical intraductal hyperplasias diagnosed. This undeniable increase in the number of cases of DCIS and AIDH over the past decade has been predominantly due to the increasing use of screening mammography.

Frequency of Ductal Carcinoma *In Situ* in Autopsy Series

The frequency of DCIS among women with no prior history of breast carcinoma has been assessed in several autopsy series and is important in helping us understand the natural history of DCIS. It ranges from 0.2 to 18.2 (Alpers and Wellings, 1985; Bhathal et al., 1985; Kramer and Rush, 1973; Nielsen et al., 1984, 1987; Wellings and Jensen, 1973). Clearly, some cases of DCIS never detected by mammography may not cause any problems during a woman's lifetime.

Clinical Features

Prior to the widespread application of screening mammography, most ductal carcinomas *in situ* were clinically obvious lesions that presented as a palpable mass, Paget's disease, nipple discharge, or a combination of these findings (Ashikari et al., 1977; Sunshine et al., 1985). In two separate studies, one of which was nationwide (Baker, 1982), 58% and 59% of the DCIS were detected by mammographic calcification (Baker, 1982; Schwartz et al., 1989). When mammography is interpreted as "suspicious calcifications," a carcinoma of predominantly intraductal type is identified in 25% of the specimens (Powell et al., 1983; Schwartz et al., 1980). A high proportion of lesions that are currently biopsied now, secondary to mammographic abnormalities, are minuscule lesions, the biologic and clinical significance of which have never been established. Other patients, however, continue to present with either areas of irregularity or lumpiness in the breast that have been discovered on self-examination by the patient or during routine checkup by a clinician.

Male Ductal Carcinoma *In Situ*

Ductal carcinoma *in situ* also occurs in the male breast (Cutuli et al., 1997; Hittmair et al., 1998). Male breast cancer accounts for approximately 0.5% of all breast cancers (Ewertz et al., 1989), with DCIS accounting for only approximately 5% (2.3 to 17%) of all male breast cancer (Hittmair et al., 1998), the majority of the tumors being invasive. Interestingly, in our review of 94 cases of pure DCIS in the male breast, not a single case of comedo DCIS was identified (Hittmair et al., 1998), which suggests that the absence of the TDLU in the male may play a role in the phenotypes of DCIS encountered. In the male, gynecomastoid hyperplasia may sometimes develop atypia (Tham et al., 1989); if and when it does, then it would qualify as AIDH.

Risk Factors

The risk factors for DCIS are similar to those for invasive breast carcinoma (Kerlikowske et al., 1997). Whether or not a positive family history of breast carcinoma should influence the management of patients with DCIS has also not been established. Cady (1993) estimated that the incidence of subsequent invasive carcinoma among patients with comedo DCIS and a negative family history of breast carcinoma is 2% annually and 40% after 20 years. For women with comedo DCIS and a positive history of breast carcinoma, he estimated a 4% annual incidence of subsequent invasive breast carcinoma and a cumulative risk exceeding 50% at 20 years. This is an issue that should be carefully evaluated as it may help determine the optimum management of women with DCIS. The recent preliminary report that 80% of subsequent invasive carcinomas associated with low-grade DCIS occur in the contralateral breast further supports inclusion of low-grade DCIS in the same group with AIDH and as a marker for breast cancer risk rather than as an obligate precursor (Done et al., 1996).

Frozen Section

Intraoperative frozen section (FS) diagnosis is discouraged since it does not always allow accurate morphologic interpretation (Association of Directors of Anatomic and Surgical Pathology; Fehner RE, 1996). A FS should not be performed when no lesion or mass is identified by macroscopic inspection of the specimen. The accuracy of a FS diagnosis of DCIS is low, mainly because of sampling error (Cheng et al., 1997). Furthermore, the tissue alterations induced by freezing may render the lesion permanently uninterpretable on subsequent paraffin-embedded sections.

The Surgical Pathology Report

The following information should be provided on the pathology report for each lesion once it is determined that it qualifies as DCIS (see Table 15–10): *(1)* type of DCIS (comedo, cribriform, micropapillary, solid, signet-ring cell, apocrine type, etc.); *(2)* overall grade of DCIS (including nuclear grade); *(3)* presence of necrosis; *(4)* extent of DCIS (estimation of size); *(5)* status of the margin (positive, or specify distance from margin); *(6)* presence or absence of microcalcifications; and *(7)* DIN translational classification designation.

Morphologic Subtypes of Ductal Carcinoma *In Situ* and Their Significance

It is important to state which of the specific morphologic patterns of DCIS is present within the diagnosis. For example, it should be noted not only whether the carcinoma is of the comedo, cribriform, micropapillary, papillary, solid "mosaic" (non-comedo), or clinging type (the six most common subtypes) but also whether it displays apocrine, clear cell, signet-ring cell, spindle cell, neuroendocrine, basaloid, squamous, secretory, or lipid-rich differentiation. The importance of recognizing and specifying the pattern and cell type of DCIS is to aid in the further study of pattern and subtype-specific outcomes, as well as to assist the clinician in the selection of appropriate therapy and follow-up for the patient.

Several studies have shown that there is a higher chance of recurrence after conservative treatment with the comedo variant of DCIS than with the cribriform and micropapillary types. In the classic study by Lagios et al. (1989), among DCIS lesions less than 2.5 cm in extent, 19% of those with the comedo pattern recurred after tylectomy, compared to 10% of intermediate-grade DCIS cases showing a generally cribriform

Table 15–10. Features to Specify in Pathologic Report of Ductal Carcinoma *In Situ*

Morphologic pattern (subtype) of DCIS
  Mention all morphologic patterns present in the biopsy
  Specify proportion of different morphologic patterns, when more than one
    pattern is present (eg. when one is the dominant pattern)
DCIS Grade
  Nuclear grade, based on nuclear atypia and variability in size (1–3)
  Classify overall DCIS grade according to the most advanced grade in the biopsy
  Mention various proportion of different DCIS grades, when the lesion is
    composed of more than one grade
Presence of necrosis
  Also mention presence of apoptosis, when prominent
Extent (size)
  Measure, with a linear estimation, the maximal area involved by DCIS
  Mention presence of extensive DCIS (DCIS involving >> 20 duct spaces)
Margin status
  Report presence of DCIS extending to within 2 mm (and possibly up to 10 mm)
    of the margin
Presence or absence of microcalcifications
DIN translational classification designation (DIN 1c, DIN 2, or DIN 3)

DCIS, ductal carcinoma *in situ;* DIN, ductal intraepithelial neoplasia.

pattern with atypia, and none of 33 patients with the low-grade micropapillary DCIS lesions recurred, with an average follow-up interval of 8 years after diagnosis. In general, comedo DCIS recurs more frequently and within a shorter interval than to the cribriform and micropapillary variants. However, as longer follow-up is becoming available on the conservatively treated cases, the frequency of local recurrence for the lower-grade micropapillary and cribriform variants of DCIS is catching up and may actually surpass that of the high-grade comedocarcinoma lesions, according to a recent 15-year status report (Solin et al., 1996) of the multi-institutional study on conservative surgery and radiation therapy for DCIS. In this study, the comedo and high nuclear grade DCIS had a 12% actuarial local recurrence at 5 years that increased to 18% at 10 years; those DCIS lacking both comedonecrosis and high-grade nuclei had a 3% recurrence at 5 years and 15% at 10 years (Solin et al., 1996). High-grade DCIS has traditionally been observed more frequently in association with invasive carcinoma (Moriya and Silverberg, 1995). With longer follow-up intervals of 10 years or more, almost an equal proportion of low-grade and high-grade DCIS recur.

Importantly, the non-necrotic variants of DCIS have come to constitute a high pro-portion of intraductal carcinomas since the widespread use of screening mammography. Micropapillary DCIS is characteristically multifocal and extensive, involving multiple ducts in a wide area, in contrast to cribriform DCIS, which may be quite localized. Intraductal papillary carcinomas characteristically present as a central, usually solitary, lesion involving a major duct. This form of DCIS is uncommonly associated with invasion, and when it is, the invasion is often quite small (microinvasive). The solid pattern of DCIS is often present in association with comedocarcinoma, although not necessarily; the behavior of this subtype has not been studied. Clinging carcinoma (DIN, flat type) presents as the low-grade form (characterized by low-grade cytology, and classified as an AIDH, DIN 1b, or low-grade clinging carcinoma) (Fig. 15–8) and a high-grade form (characterized by high-grade nuclear cytology, and classified as a high-grade DCIS, DIN 2 or 3, or high-grade clinging carcinoma) (Fig. 15–9). These forms have not been studied in sufficient numbers to characterize their risk for subsequent invasive carcinoma; however, recent molecular analysis in our laboratory suggests that they show some of the same genetic alterations as DCIS of more conventional types (see Special Studies) (Moinfar et al., 1999).

Among the less common morphologic patterns of DCIS that may occur, the signet-ring cell variant is important to recognize and specify, since it is well known that the presence of even 20% of this cell type in invasive carcinomas is associated with a more aggressive behavior (Merino and LiVolsi, 1981). Noting the presence of an apocrine cell population is important because this cell population has a hormonal control mechanism that is different from the usual cancer cell types (Tavassoli et al., 1996); apocrine cells, whether benign or malignant, generally do not express ER, PR, or bcl-2, but they do express androgen receptor (AR) in a relatively high proportion of cases. Different forms of treatment that are based on such specific hormonal and molecular characteristics of specific variants (for example anti-androgen therapy for apocrine carcinomas) may some day be offered to women. While generally morphologically distinct, little is known about the other patterns of DCIS—those showing neuroendocrine, spindle cell, clear cell, and squamous differentiation. In addition, some of the rare special types of carcinoma (secretory, lipid-rich, basaloid) also have an *in situ* counterpart; these latter patterns of DCIS are particularly difficult to study because of their exceptional rarity.

When More Than One Pattern of Ductal Carcinoma *In Situ* is Present

Frequently, more than a single pattern or cell type is evident in a given biopsy (Figs. 15–12 and 15–13). The different cell types and patterns sometimes display a gradual transition or they may collide and result in unusual appearances. If a combination of types is present, the various types should be noted in the diagnosis. If a DCIS lesion is predominantly composed of one pattern, with a minor component of a second, especially higher-grade, pattern, an estimate of the relative percentage of each pattern is made. Although we do not know the significance of such admixtures, it is important to have them recorded in case they prove to be of prognostic or therapeutic significance in the future.

Comedo Carcinoma

Comedo carcinoma accounts for up to 67% of cases of DCIS (Bellamy et al., 1993; Fow-

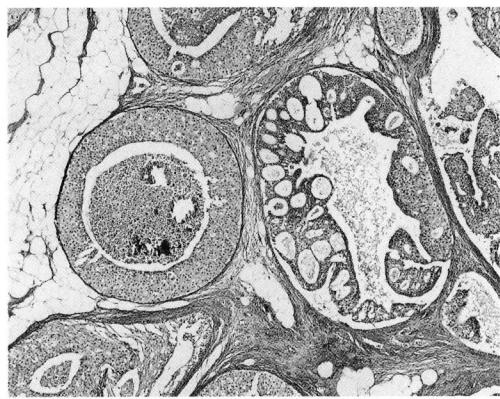

Figure 15–12. Two patterns of ductal intraepithelial neoplasia—ductal carcinoma *in situ* (DCIS), comedo and cribriform patterns, overall grade 3 (DIN 3). This tumor shows two patterns of DCIS; a solid pattern with cytologic atypia and necrosis (comedocarcinoma or DIN 3), and a cribriform pattern with some atypia and intraluminal debris, but no definite necrosis (this pattern alone would be assigned the category DIN 2) (H&E, ×40).

ble et al., 1997; Holland et al., 1990; Poller et al., 1994; Quinn et al., 1997) and is characterized by the presence of cytologic atypia and intraluminal necrosis. Mitotic figures are abundant in some cases and few in others. Sometimes the stroma surrounding the

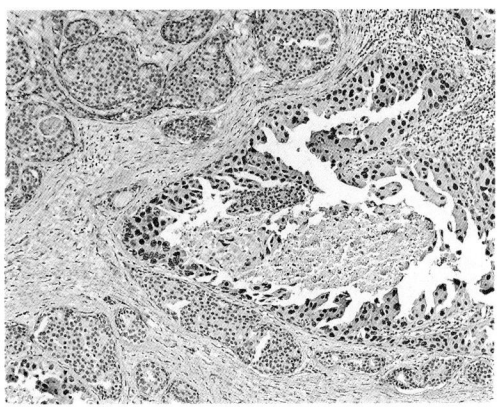

Figure 15–13. Two patterns of ductal intraepithelial neoplasia—ductal carcinoma *in situ* (DCIS). One is high-grade, micropapillary pattern with necrosis that is immunoreactive for p53 (DIN 3), and the second is low-grade, nonnecrotic cribriform pattern that is negative for p53 (and which alone would qualify as DCIS, grade 1 (DIN 1c) (immunostain for p53, ×100).

ducts displays a reactive or desmoplastic appearance, and occasionally a prominent lymphoplasmacytic infiltrate surrounds the ducts. A diagnosis of comedocarcinoma is warranted even if a single small duct shows these classic features. The 2 mm rule only applies to non-necrotic forms of DCIS with low-grade cytologic atypia. Some of the most extensive intraductal carcinomas are of this type, showing the involvement of practically every TDLU in a generous (larger than 5 cm) breast biopsy. The myoepithelial cell layer may be well retained around the ducts in some cases and barely apparent due to attenuation, or absent in others. It is noteworthy that breaks in the basement membrane, even if present, are not detectable on H&E sections.

The necrotic debris in the lumen of comedocarcinoma reflects both apoptotic and oncotic type of necrosis, not infrequently admixed (Figs. 15–12 and 15–13; Malmusi and Ackerman, 1998). Apoptotic necrosis affects scattered cells and is characterized by nuclear shrinkage (pyknosis), nuclear fragmentation (karyorrhexis), cytoplasmic condensation, apoptotic bodies, and lack of an inflammatory infiltrate. Oncotic necrosis affects cells *en masse* and is characterized by karyolysis in concert with swelling of cytoplasm (ballooning). Bodis et al. (1996) concluded that the extensive necrosis in DCIS is likely to represent apoptosis but is independent of p53 regulation. Our preliminary ultrastructural studies, however, suggest that the cellular debris in the lumen of the ducts reflects a combination of the two types of necrosis.

Definition of Intraluminal Necrosis

Intraluminal necrosis is defined as the presence of five or more fragments of intraluminal karyorrhectic debris. The presence of intraluminal necrotic "ghost" cells can also suffice. Careful evaluation to distinguish the intraluminal material from granular intraluminal secretions is necessary. Schwartz et al. (1997) have qualified necrosis as "comedo" in type when it is central and zonal, and which shows a linear pattern if longitudinally sectioned, and as "punctate," when it is nonzonal, and which does not exhibit a linear pattern if longitudinally sectioned.

Cribriform Ductal Carcinoma *In Situ*

The cribriform variant of DCIS is characterized by a proliferation of a population of cells forming uniformly rounded, punched-out spaces with a sieve-like arrangement, epithelial arcades, "Roman bridges," and "cartwheels" (Fig. 15–12). The secondary lumens are generally rounded and often surrounded by low columnar cells with basally located nuclei. The epithelial bridges are rigid. The nuclei are round to ovoid and evenly distributed with minimal, if any, nuclear overlap. Mitotic figures are only rarely observed. Calcification can be prominent within the secondary lumens. This variant has a tremendous range of appearances. The growth pattern sometimes assumes a spoked-wheel appearance, with a central nest of cells connected to the duct wall by numerous epithelial bridges. A relatively solid variant of cribriform DCIS, with rosette-like arrangement of the nuclei as the only sign of early secondary lumen formation, also occurs (Fig. 15–14). Cytologically, some lesions are composed of small, uniform cells with rounded nuclei and sparse cytoplasm. Others are composed of a slightly more atypical cell population with some nuclear variation and small amounts of granular eosinophilic cytoplasm. Intraluminal necrosis may also be present (Fig. 15–15).

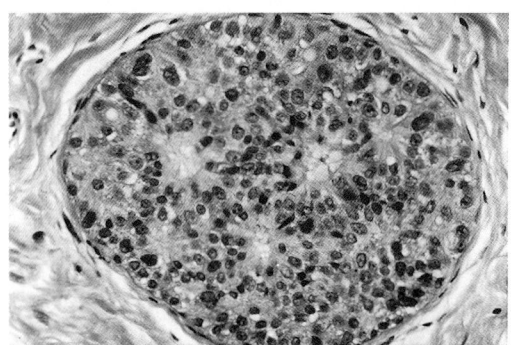

Figure 15–14. Ductal intraepithelial neoplasia, grade 2 (DIN 2)—ductal carcinoma *in situ* (DCIS), grade 2. Focal, significant nuclear atypia (nuclear enlargement and irregularity) within this duct (which shows rosette formation and incipient glandular spaces) qualifies this as DCIS, grade 2. The presence of significant cytologic atypia excludes the quantitative 2 mm size requirement (H&E, high power).

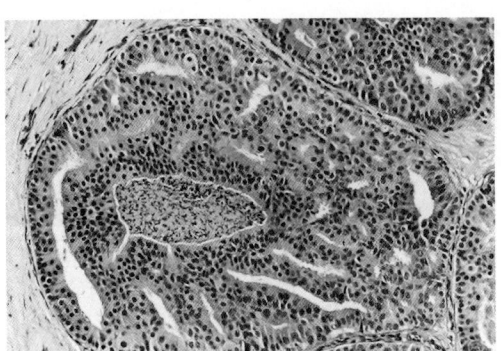

Figure 15–15. Ductal intraepithelial neoplasia, grade 2 (DIN 2)—ductal carcinoma *in situ* (DCIS), grade 2. Intraluminal necrosis within a duct showing uniform cells with grade 1 nuclear atypia (forming a cribriform pattern) elevates the overall grade to DCIS, grade 2. The presence of necrosis excludes the quantitative 2 mm size requirement (H&E, medium-high power).

Micropapillary Ductal Carcinoma *In Situ*

A uniform cell population similar to that described for the cribriform variant but forming epithelial tufts projecting into the lumen proliferates in the micropapillary type (Figs. 15–16 to 15–18). A fibrovascular supportive core is not identified in micropapillary carcinoma and the cells are small and round. The tufts are often regularly distributed around the duct walls. In the interval between the epithelial tufts, two cell layers line

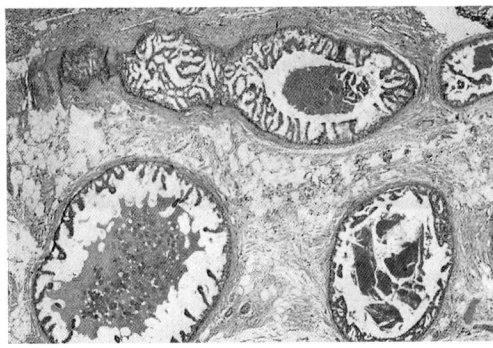

Figure 15–16. Ductal intraepithelial neoplasia, grade 1c (DIN 1c)—ductal carcinoma *in situ* (DCIS), grade 1, micropapillary pattern. Multiple ducts are lined by a monomorphic population of cells forming epithelial tufts or micropapillae (H&E, low power).

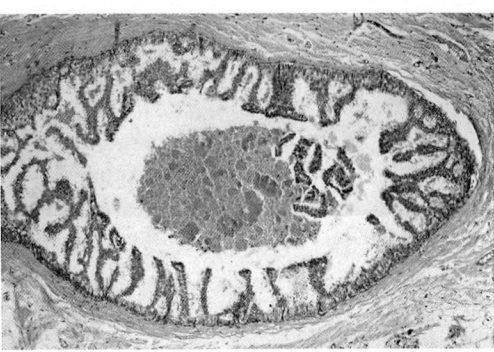

Figure 15–17. Ductal intraepithelial neoplasia, grade 1c (DIN 1c)—ductal carcinoma *in situ* (DCIS), grade 1, micropapillary pattern. Multiple ducts are lined by a monomorphic population of cells forming epithelial tufts or micropapillae, which often show terminal bulbous processes. Intraluminal debris with inflammatory cells and detached papillary tufts are present, but there is no true necrosis by our criteria, (H&E, medium power).

the duct wall; the luminal epithelial cell layer may appear identical to those proliferating within the tufts or it may appear normal. The myoepithelial cell layer is generally unaltered. Occasionally, the neoplastic cells display atypia and even a hobnail appearance.

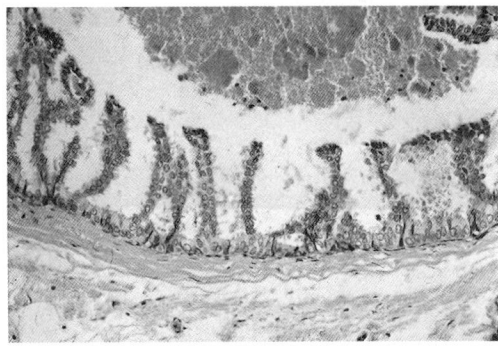

Figure 15–18. Ductal intraepithelial neoplasia, grade 1c (DIN 1c)—ductal carcinoma *in situ* (DCIS), grade 1, micropapillary pattern. Note the absence of fibrovascular cores within these micropapillary projections (a distinguishing feature between papillary and micropapillary lesions). Also note that the micropapillary projections emanate from a single epithelial cell layer, rather than from a hyperplastic epithelial cell layer (the latter being a feature of gynecomastoid hyperplasia) (H&E, high power).

This pattern is one of the most difficult ones to recognize as a carcinoma when present by itself. Micropapillary DCIS is more frequently multifocal and even multicentric, involving multiple quadrants compared to other variants of DCIS (Bellamy et al., 1993).

There are frequent transitional forms of DCIS in which the micropapillary pattern merges with the cribriform variety. Either the cribriform or the micropapillary pattern may occasionally display cytologic atypia. Intraluminal necrosis may sometimes be observed in association with either pattern, even in the absence of cytologic atypia. Occasionally, either pattern may show distension of the ducts or ductules with abundant intraluminal secretory material, which has prompted the designation of *cystic hypersecretory intraductal carcinoma* by some authors (Guerry et al., 1988; Rosen and Scott, 1984). We, however, prefer the designation of DCIS on the basis of its pattern and cytologic features, regardless of the presence or absence of secretory material within the duct lumen(s).

Solid "Mosaic" Ductal Carcinoma *In Situ*

A solid, "mosaic" pattern of intraductal carcinoma composed of large, round to polygonal cells with distinct cell margins is also observed (Fig. 15–19).

Intraductal Apocrine Carcinoma

To qualify as intraductal apocrine carcinoma, the proliferating cells should display abundant granular, eosinophilic cytoplasm, and moderate to severe atypia (Tavassoli and Norris, 1994; Fig. 15–20). Some cells contain coarse intracytoplasmic, eosinophilic granules, whereas others show vacuolization. Intraluminal necrosis is often present. Apical cytoplasmic protrusions are not always evident. Nucleoli are often present in either setting. When necrosis is present, involvement of even a single duct is sufficient for a diagnosis of carcinoma regardless of the duct size. When necrosis is absent, the same quantitative rule used for the cribriform and micropapillary patterns is applied. Because of the high frequency of apocrine metaplasia and hyperplasia in association with fibrocystic changes, it is important to be particularly cautious in the diagnosis of apocrine DCIS. Therefore, very stringent criteria are required to prevent misinterpretation of the common hyperplasia or metaplasia of apocrine cells as malignant and to avoid overdiagnosis of carcinoma. In this regard, prominent nucleoli are also observed in benign apocrine cells and, by themselves, do not indicate atypia or malignancy.

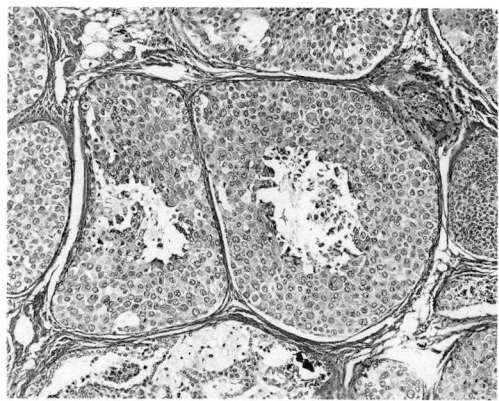

Figure 15–19. Ductal intraepithelial neoplasia, grade 2 (DIN 2)—ductal carcinoma *in situ* (DCIS), grade 2. The presence of focal nuclear atypia (nuclear enlargement and irregularity) within this duct, associated with a small degree of necrosis, qualifies this as DCIS, grade 2 (H&E, ×100).

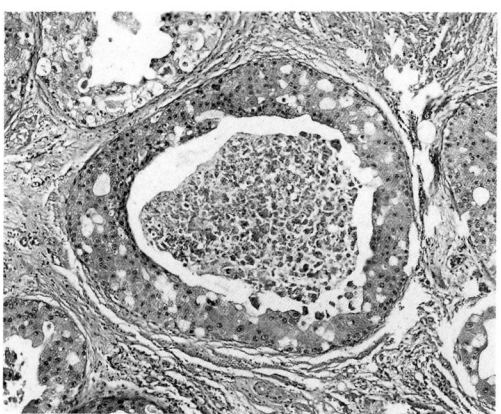

Figure 15–20. Ductal intraepithelial neoplasia, grade 3 (DIN 3)—ductal carcinoma *in situ* (DCIS), apocrine type, with necrosis. The presence of necrosis within this intraductal apocrine proliferation boosts the overall grade to grade 3. Note the variably sized nuclei with prominent nucleoli, in addition to abundant foamy cytoplasm, which are characteristic of intraductal apocrine carcinomas (H&E, ×100).

Other Less Common Variants of Ductal Carcinoma *In Situ*

Rarely, DCIS may assume a clear cell (Fig. 15–21), spindle cell (Figs. 15–22 and 15–23), neuroendocrine (Figs. 15–24 and 15–25), signet-ring cell, or basaloid phenotype. The spindle cell and neuroendocrine variants are immunoreactive with chromogranin and synaptophysin. The spindle cell variant should be distinguished from myoepithelio-sis. Immunostains for cytokeratin, actin, and S-100 are useful in helping to establish the nature of the spindle cells.

Grading Intraductal Carcinoma

There has been an increasing trend toward grading DCIS (Holland et al., 1994; Lagios et al., 1989; Silverstein et al., 1996; Tavassoli, 1998, 1999). We grade all intraductal carci-nomas using a simple approach (Tavassoli, 1998) based on the assessment of cellular (nuclear) atypia and presence of intralumi-nal necrosis (Table 15–2); in our experience, this system is highly reproducible and easy to apply. Using this grading system, DCIS is divided into three grades. Lesions lacking ei-ther nuclear atypia or intraluminal necrosis qualify as grade 1 and correspond to the clas-sic micropapillary and cribriform DCIS. When both atypia and intraluminal necrosis are present or when there is significant nu-clear atypia, the lesion qualifies as grade 3. When either mild to moderate atypia or in-traluminal necrosis is present or a little bit

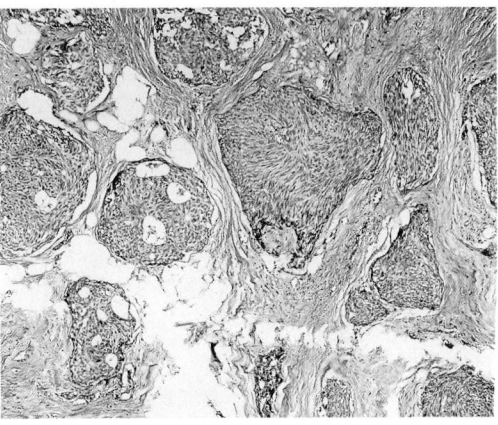

Figure 15–22. Ductal intraepithelial neoplasia, grade 2 (DIN 2)—ductal carcinoma *in situ* (DCIS), spindle cell pattern, grade 2. At low power, these ducts are expanded by a uniform proliferation of spindle cells that show a solid and often streaming pattern within multiple ducts that may be confused with intraductal hyperpla-sia (H&E, ×75).

of both features are present, the lesion qual-ifies as grade 2. We have also provided guide-lines for some special types of DCIS. For example, signet-ring cell DCIS would qual-ify as grade 3 from our understanding of this

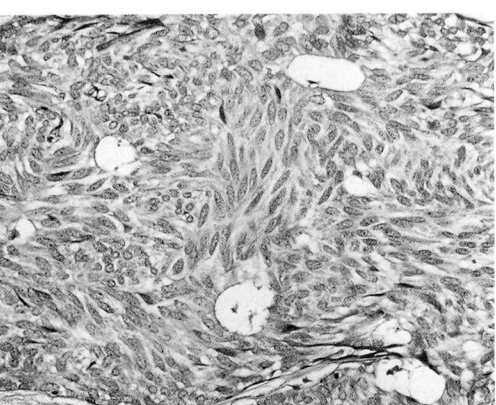

Figure 15–23. Ductal intraepithelial neoplasia, grade 2 (DIN 2)—ductal carcinoma *in situ* (DCIS), spindle cell pattern, grade 2. This high-power view shows a generally solid, uniform pro-liferation of spindle cells with streaming pattern and formation of several secondary lumina. The absence of cellular heterogeneity distinguishes this rare variant from intraductal hyperplasia. Given the unknown clinical behavior, this pattern of DCIS is assigned an intermediate DIN grade of 2 (H&E, ×300).

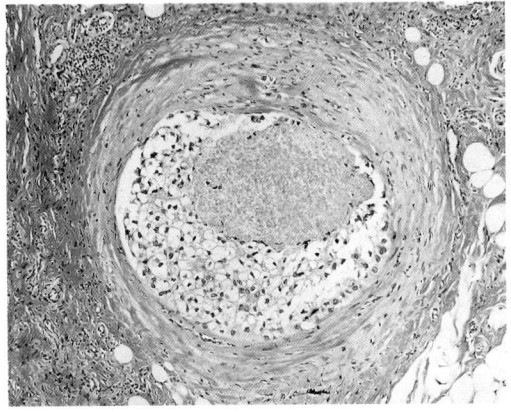

Figure 15–21. Ductal intraepithelial neoplasia, grade 3 (DIN 3)—ductal carcinoma *in situ* (DCIS), clear cell type, grade 3. The clear cells form a solid pattern here with intraluminal necro-sis (necrotic ghost cells) (H&E, ×150).

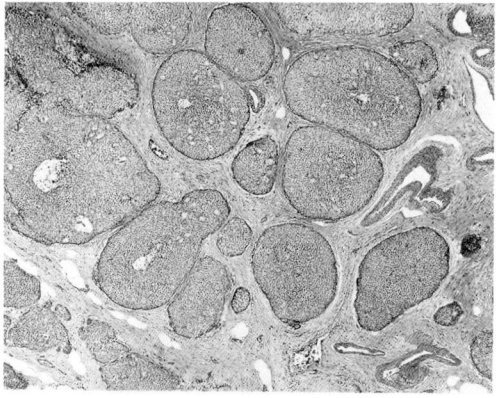

Figure 15–24. Ductal intraepithelial neoplasia, grade 1c (DIN 1c)—ductal carcinoma *in situ* (DCIS), grade 1, with neuroendocrine differentiation. Multiple ducts are expanded by a generally solid proliferation of cells which, upon careful evaluation at this low power, show formation of multiple rosettes. (H&E, ×40).

cell population's association with aggressive behavior among the invasive carcinomas. The DCIS should be classified according to the most advanced grade identifiable in the sample, with comments on the various proportions of different grades throughout the biopsy (Tables 15–10 and 15–11).

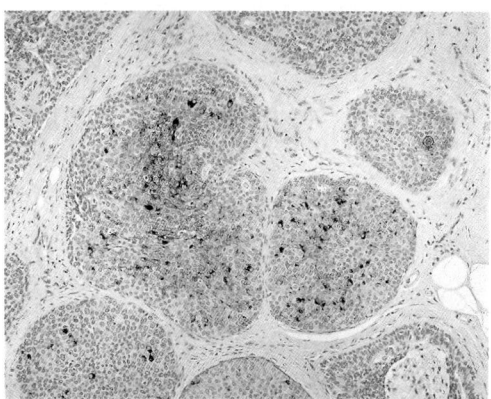

Figure 15–25. Ductal intraepithelial neoplasia, grade 1c (DIN 1c)—ductal carcinoma *in situ* (DCIS), grade 1, with neuroendocrine differentiation. Both a growth pattern of a recognized carcinoid tumor and immunoperoxidase confirmation of neuroendocrine differentiation are required for the above diagnosis. In addition to rosette formation, this case shows scattered cells strongly immunoreactive for chromogranin, supporting the above diagnosis (immunostain for chromogranin, ×120).

This three-tiered approach has been adopted with minor modifications in two recent studies (Scott et al., 1997; Silverstein et al., 1995b). More recently, a comparison of five grading systems by 23 European pathologists in the European Commission Working Group on Breast Screening Pathology found that only two features—necrosis and nuclear atypia—were the most robust histologic features to assess (Sloane et al., 1998). These studies have basically confirmed the validity of our three-tiered grading system, which we first proposed for use in 1992.

In another comparison of several available modern classifications of DCIS, Douglas-Jones et al. (1996) found disagreements that most frequently involved assessment of architecture and least commonly involved the assessment of necrosis. These were precisely the basis for the simple and reproducible AFIP grading system (Tavassoli, 1999), which they failed to test. Another study found significantly less heterogeneity in the nuclear grade of DCIS compared to the prominent architectural heterogeneity characteristic of most cases of DCIS (Harrison et al., 1996).

The significance of grading DCIS is to further characterize the DCIS lesion in order to most accurately determine a patient's risk for recurrence and to assist in designing appropriate treatment as well as post-treatment follow-up regimens. Importantly, the nuclear grade of DCIS correlates with the grade of the invasive carcinoma (Goldstein and Murphy, 1996). Criteria for grading DCIS using the AFIP approach are summarized in Table 15–11.

Extent (Size) of Intraductal Carcinoma

It is often not quite clear what is implied by the size of DCIS. Various measurements may be of importance, such as *(1)* the gross, and questionably meaningful, linear measurement encompassing maximally distant DCIS foci within a biopsy, or on a single slide; *(2)* the extension of DCIS from its site of origin in the TDLU into the terminal and major duct; *(3)* the degree of duct distension by DCIS; *(4)* the number or relative percent involvement of acini in one or more TDLUs; and *(5)* the volume of tumor cells. Whether we should use a combination of some and possibly all of these aspects has not been well studied. For practical purposes, the mea-

Table 15–11. Grading Ductal Carcinoma *In Situ*—the AFIP Approach

Low-grade (grade 1) ductal carcinoma in situ (DIN 1c)

Intraductal carcinomas composed of a uniform population of cells showing mild cytologic atypia and lacking necrosis
  Most intraductal carcinomas showing a cribriform and/or micropapillary pattern

Extensive AIDH, defined as AIDH involving numerous ($\gg 20$) ductal cross-sections

Moderate-grade (grade 2) ductal carcinoma in situ (DIN 2)

Intraductal carcinomas showing both mild-to-moderate cytologic atypia as well as intraluminal necrosis
  Solid, cribriform or micropapillary patterns with central necrosis

Intraductal carcinomas which display moderate cytologic atypia, but which lack intraluminal necrosis

Rare variants of DCIS (e.g., clear cell, basaloid), with or without necrosis

DCIS showing an admixture of two uniform cell types, with or without necrosis.

High-grade (grade 3) ductal carcinoma in situ (DIN 3)

Intraductal carcinomas displaying significant (severe) cytologic atypia

Intraductal carcinomas displaying moderate to severe cytologic atypia and necrosis
  Comedocarcinoma
  Many intraductal apocrine carcinomas, including all those with necrosis

Intraductal carcinoma, signet ring cell type

AIDH, atypical intraductal neoplasia; DCIS, ductal carcinoma *in situ*; DIN, ductal intraepithelial neoplasia.

surement of DCIS provided in pathology reports is most frequently the linear measurement described in point 1 and is often estimated from a less than optimally sampled specimen.

The extent of DCIS represents a major component of a recently proposed Van Nuys Prognostic Index (VNPI) (Silverstein et al., 1996), and its assessment has been required as part of routine evaluation of DCIS for management purposes. In obtaining the size component of the VNPI, it has been suggested that measurements be obtained after the sample is serially sectioned at 2–3 mm intervals. The tissue sections are arranged and processed in sequence. The size of the lesion is based on direct measurement from the slide (for smaller lesions) or estimation of the distribution of the lesions in a sequential series of slides.

The combination of systematic orientation, sectioning, and processing of biopsy specimens toward the nipple is probably the best way to determine the true extent of DCIS along its natural route of progression and its distribution in multiple TDLUs (King, 1994). It has been shown that DCIS begins in the TDLU and extends along the duct system, whether associated with or without an invasive component (Ohtaki et al.,

1995; Ohuchi et al., 1994). Furthermore, it has been noted that DCIS lesions that have extended some distance toward the nipple are more likely to develop subsequent recurrences or invasive carcinoma than those confined to the TDLU (Ohuchi et al., 1994).

Extensive Atypical Intraductal Hyperplasia

For the purposes of the MIN translational classification system, we have designated lesions morphologically qualifying as extensive AIDH, defined as presence of AIDH of the partial cribriform or micropapillary types involving numerous (i.e., more than 20) ductal cross sections, as DIN 1c, since we feel the extensiveness of such proliferations warrants management as a low-grade DCIS.

Assessment of Margins

A margin is clearly positive when tumor is bisected at the time of resection or when tumor is covered by the ink painted over the resection margin. When the DCIS has not been cut through, the distance between the edge of the DCIS closest to the resection margin is conveyed in mm (i.e., DCIS extends to within 1 mm of the inked margin or to within 2 mm of the inked margin). It is also important to note whether the proximity is focal (specify which margin) and what proportion of the DCIS is in the proximity of the margin. Since 43% of samples with negative margins in one study (defined as the presence of 1 mm or more uninvolved tissue between the tumor and inked margin) show residual DCIS on re-excision (Silverstein et al., 1994), determination of margin status is of prognostic importance. In the VNPI, extension of DCIS to within 10 mm of the margin is indicated and assessed (Silverstein et al., 1996).

Microcalcifications

Because a substantial number of breast biopsies are performed following detection of microcalcifications on mammography, it is the responsibility of the pathologist to correlate and confirm the presence and amount of microcalcifications in the slides with the level of suspicion expressed by the mammographer and the pattern and quantity evident on specimen mammograms. The presence of microcalcifications should be noted in the list of diagnoses. Microcalcifications may be granular or laminar. Laminar and granular calcifications that have a core of mucosubstances are found mainly in low- and intermediate-grade DCIS; granular calcifications with a core of nuclear debris are seen most frequently in intermediate- and poorly differentiated DCIS (Foschini et al., 1996).

Van Nuys Prognostic Index

In an effort to stratify the heterogenous population of DCIS (Smart et al., 1978) into categories with different outcomes and amenable to different management approaches, the Van Nuys Prognostic Index (VNPI) has been introduced (Silverstein et al., 1996). The VNPI, an attempt to pathologically stage DCIS, scores three features and adds the results to arrive at a final score. The three features include tumor size (1 = small tumors of 15 mm or less; 2 = 16–40 mm; 3 = 41 mm or more), the degree of tumor free margin (1 = 10 mm or more; 2 = 1–9 mm; 3 = less than 1 mm), and DCIS grade (3 = nuclear grade 3; 2 = nuclear grade 1 or 2 with comedo necrosis; and 1 = nuclear grade 1 without comedo necrosis). Only 2% of those patients ($n = 101$) with a VNPI of 3–4 developed local recurrence, compared to 19% of those ($n = 209$) with a score of 5–7 and 57% of those ($n = 23$) with a score of 8–9. Recommendations for treatment are made on the basis of the VNPI score. At the AFIP, we do not use the VNPI score.

Interobserver Variability in the Diagnosis and Grading of Ductal Carcinoma *In Situ*

As previously discussed in the section on AIDH, distinction of AIDH from low-grade DCIS remains one of the most difficult problems in breast pathology because of the magnitude of interobserver variability. Significant differences remain in the threshold for the diagnosis of low-grade DCIS even among experts in breast pathology. Sloane et al. (1998) reported on the consistency achieved by 23 European pathologists in categorizing DCIS using five different classifications. They concluded that the most useful grading systems were those that used the histologic features of nuclear atypia (high and low grade) and presence or absence of necrosis.

Differential Diagnosis

In many cases, the diagnosis of intraductal carcinoma is relatively simple and straightforward. Increasingly, however, the distinction from IDH and AIDH at one extreme and from invasive carcinoma at the other is problematic.

With the increasing use of needle localization, aspiration, and biopsy procedures, dislodgement of tumor cells has become a common occurrence. The dislodgement of DCIS tumor cells into the surrounding stroma (Tavassoli and Pestaner, 1995) often mimics, and may be confused with, microinvasive carcinoma (Silver and Tavassoli, 1998; Solin et al., 1992). Sometimes it is difficult to determine if there is stromal invasion, particularly in cases of extensive comedocarcinoma. Often such areas are characterized by blurring of the normally sharp epithelial-stromal interface in association with an altered stroma (e.g., stroma that is edematous and/or desmoplastic), which frequently shows an inflammatory response, compared to the periductal stroma surrounding normal ducts elsewhere in the biopsy. Since our routine diagnosis is based on evaluation of H&E–stained sections, unless there is unequivocal evidence of invasion, it is best to designate the lesion as *in situ*. Such lesions deserve careful evaluation of sometimes numerous levels of the areas of concern before designating the changes as either *in situ* or invasive carcinoma.

Intraductal carcinoma involving sclerosing adenosis (Giri et al., 1989; Ichihara and Aomaya, 1994; Rasbridge and Millis, 1995) sometimes poses a diagnostic problem and may be misinterpreted as an invasive carcinoma. The presence of a surrounding well-defined PAS-positive basement membrane and/or myoepithelial cells around the proliferating tubules usually helps to distinguish DCIS involving sclerosing adenosis from invasive carcinoma (Eusebi et al., 1989a). Immunostains for actin may be helpful in demonstrating the myoepithelial cell layer in this and other difficult situations.

It is also worth noting that, although relatively infrequent, patterns morphologically identical to those we recognize as DCIS are occasionally seen in lymph node metastases. These, however, are not thought to represent DCIS but rather metastatic carcinoma mimicking DCIS.

Distinction of low-grade DCIS from AIDH remains a major problem (See section on Differential Diagnosis of AIDH). There is no agreement on the optimum approach to resolving this problem; we have found the ductal intraepithelial neoplasia concept helpful, however, in resolving this critical issue.

Intraductal carcinoma confined to lobules (Fechner, 1971) sometimes poses as a diagnostic problem and may be misinterpreted as lobular neoplasia. The cells of ductal carcinoma involving lobules are generally more pleomorphic and larger than the cells of lobular neoplasia. Even when the cells are small and uniform, the formation of rosette-like arrangement of the nuclei, multiple secondary lumen formation, and distinct, cohesive cell margins support a ductal process.

Bilaterality

The incidence of bilaterality for DCIS varies from 2.2% to 22% (Ashikari et al., 1971; Ciatto et al., 1990; Fechner, 1971; Griffin and Frazee, 1993; Lagios et al., 1982; Millis and Thynne, 1975; Ringberg et al., 1982; Schuh et al., 1986; Silverstein et al., 1988; Stratton et al., 1995; Urban, 1969; Ward et al., 1992; Webber et al., 1981; Westbrook and Gallager, 1975). Up to 22% of 217 women with DCIS in one breast had either invasive or *in situ* carcinoma in the opposite breast (Ward et al., 1992).

Multicentricity and Multifocality

The frequency of multicentricity ranges from 12% to 45.5% but has been noted to be as high as 64% to 80% (Anastassiades et al., 1993; Carter and Smith, 1977; Lagios et al., 1989; Moriya and Silverberg, 1994; Rosen et al., 1979; Schwartz et al., 1980) in patients with DCIS treated by mastectomy. The definition of multicentricity is not uniform in the various studies, however, and this may account for the wide range of frequency noted. Some use the terms "multifocal" and "multicentric" interchangeably; in the AFIP criteria, however, these forms are considered as two different measures of tumor distribution. A vast majority of DCIS is multifocal (defined as presence of tumor involving more than one focus, or in the case of DCIS, involvement of more than one duct cross section); in contrast, however, a much smaller number of DCIS are multicentric (defined as presence of tumor involving different quadrants—non-contiguous areas, or presence of foci of DCIS separated by 5 cm of uninvolved breast tissue). Among subtypes of DCIS in one study, the comedo variant was noted to be more frequently (24/26) monocentric and confined to one quadrant, whereas the micropapillary variant was more often (10/14) multicentric, involving multiple quadrants (Bellamy et al., 1993).

Using a variety of markers (B72.3, CEA, p53, c-erbB-2, and DF3), Dawson et al. (1995) concluded that multifocal breast cancer may result from either intramammary spread of a single primary tumor or multiple synchronous primary tumors. Interestingly, analysis of clonality by X-chromosome inactivation has shown that most invasive carcinomas are multifocal rather than multicentric (Noguchi et al., 1994a,b). Analysis of eight separate foci of DCIS from one woman's biopsy by the same technique concluded that DCIS is also monoclonal, implying that a single cancer spreads through the ducts (Noguchi et al., 1994a).

Occult Invasive Carcinoma and Axillary Lymph Node Metastasis in Ductal Carcinoma *In Situ*

The frequency of occult invasive carcinoma in the mastectomy specimens of women with DCIS ranges from 6% to 21%, among different reports (Carter and Smith, 1977; Lagios et al., 1982; Rosen et al., 1979, 1980;

Westbrook and Gallager, 1975). Overall, the axillary lymph nodes showed metastatic carcinoma in 0% to 4.5% of women with *in situ* (ductal or lobular) carcinomas (Ashikari et al., 1977; Gillis et al., 1960; Kouchoukos et al., 1967; Rosen, 1980a; Silverstein, 1997; Solin et al., 1996; Von Rueden and Wilson, 1984). The frequency of nodal metastases approaches zero in those studies based on mammographically detected DCIS.

Treatment of Ductal Carcinoma *In Situ*

Three treatment options are currently available to the patient: *(1)* mastectomy, *(2)* lumpectomy alone, and *(3)* lumpectomy with radiotherapy. Tamoxifen therapy or some functionally similar compound following lumpectomy may prove to be another option as we learn more about the hormonal manipulations in controlling breast disease. Because axillary lymph node metastases are rare, a watch policy for the axilla has been considered safe (van Dongen et al., 1989). The optimal management of the contralateral breast in patients with DCIS has not been established, but some form of follow-up would be prudent. The follow-up should be life-long and include careful palpation of the breasts by an experienced clinician two to four times a year, along with annual mammography. Treatment for the many variants of DCIS could be more individualized after considering the type and extent of the DIN in the biopsy, the presence or absence of a family history of breast carcinoma, the patient's age, and the patient's level of anxiety.

In selecting the optimal treatment for a given patient's DCIS, a combination of tumor characteristics, host features, expected results for a given approach, and patient preferences should be considered. Even a mastectomy is not an absolute cure, with recurrences of 0 to 4.4% reported. Radiation appears to reduce chances of recurrence after lumpectomy, within the follow-up periods available. Interestingly, tamoxifen appears to have reduced the rate of subsequent breast carcinoma among 13,388 women who participated in the National Surgical Adjuvant Breast Project (NSABP) Breast Cancer Prevention Trial (BCPT) (F.A. Tavassoli, personal communication with Dr. Norman Wolmark). Among 6707 women on placebo, there were 9 cancers/1000 women/year compared to 4.9 cancers/1000 women/year among 6681 women treated with tamoxifen. Both invasive and noninvasive cancers were noted in both groups with relatively similar properties.

Special Studies, Hormone Receptors, and Molecular Markers

The heterogeneity of DCIS is also apparent at the functional level, with variable expression of ER, p53, and c-erbB-2, along with biclonality by DNA ploidy analysis in a given tumor (Leal et al., 1995; Symmans et al., 1995). The expression of various biomarkers in the spectrum of DIN is illustrated in Table 15–9. High-grade DCIS is associated with nuclear pleomorphism, large tumor cell size, presence of intraluminal necrosis, a greater degree of angiogenesis, presence of p53 and c-erbB-2 expression, and absence of ER, PR, and bcl-2 expression, whereas low-grade DCIS is associated with minimal nuclear pleomorphism, smaller tumor cell size, absence of necrosis, less angiogenesis, ER, PR, and bcl-2 expression, and absence of p53 and c-erbB-2 expression. High-grade DCIS also shows an increased frequency of LOH, compared to low-grade DCIS.

Estrogen receptor, progesterone receptor, and Bcl-2. In our experience with over 200 cases of DCIS, ER, PR, and bcl-2 are almost always expressed by low-grade DCIS, unless the lesion displays apocrine differentiation (Tavassoli and Man, 1995; Tavassoli et al., 1996). The expression of bcl-2 generally parallels that of ER. Correlation of bcl-2 expression in well-differentiated DCIS has been confirmed by others (Kapucuoglu et al., 1997). Estrogen receptor has been noted in 60% to 98% of low-grade DCIS, in contrast to 14% to 74% of high-grade DCIS cases (Allred et al., 1994; Bose et al., 1996; Bur et al., 1992; Chaudhuri et al., 1993; Giri et al., 1989; Helin et al., 1989; Hiramatsu et al., 1995; Pallis et al., 1992a; Poller et al., 1993b; Rosen, 1987; Wilbur and Barrows, 1993; Zafrani et al., 1994). Progesterone receptor also generally parallels ER expression (Allred et al., 1994; Bose et al., 1996; Millis et al., 1996; Tavassoli and Man, 1995; Wilbur and Barrows, 1993) and has been identified immunohistochemically in 20% to 95% of low-grade DCIS, whereas 0% to 74% of high-grade DCIS have displayed PRs (Marshall et al., 1997; McDivitt et al., 1968, 1992; Moinfar et al., 1998). These findings provide additional support for the more poorly differentiated nature of the cells in comedocarcinoma.

p53. p53 is expressed predominantly in high-grade DCIS and not in low-grade DCIS (Douglas-Jones et al., 1997). The expression of p53 has ranged from 0% to 21% among low-grade DCIS to 3% to 67% among high-grade DCIS (Allred et al., 1994; Davidoff et al., 1991a,b; Douglas-Jones et al., 1997; Millis et al., 1996; Poller et al., 1993a). Among the 200 cases of DCIS we studied, we did not observe expression of p53 by low grade DCIS (Tavassoli and Man, 1995). p53 expression is associated not only with high-grade DCIS but also with a high mitotic index (Rajan et al., 1997). The variations reported for p53 expression are quite wide, probably reflecting different approaches to grading DCIS, differences in antibodies used, and various approaches to the interpretation of results.

C-erbB-2/HER-2/neu. One of the biomarkers utilized extensively in a number of studies on a variety of breast carcinomas is c-erbB-2 or Neu protein. Neu-protein overexpression was detected immunohistochemically in nearly all specimens showing DCIS with large nuclear size, poor cytonuclear differentiation, and high mitotic rate, and, in contrast, was detected in almost none of the well-differentiated small-cell DCIS lesions tested (Van de Vijver et al., 1988; Wilbur and Barrows, 1993). Neu-protein has membrane receptor characteristics and is homologous with the epidermal growth factor receptor (EGFR). Its presence in large-cell DCIS (comedocarcinoma) has been interpreted as an expression of rapid growth (Van de Vijver et al., 1988). C-erbB-2 immunoexpression has been observed in 0% to 50% of low-grade DCIS, compared to 50% to 100% of high-grade DCIS (Allred et al., 1992, 1994; Barnes, 1993; Bose et al., 1996; De Potter et al., 1993, 1995; Lodato and Maguire, 1990; Millis et al., 1996; Poller et al., 1994; Ramachandra et al., 1990; Van de Vijver et al., 1988). c-erbB-2 gene amplification has been confirmed in 48% of 27 DCIS by a differential polymerase chain reaction (PCR) (Liu et al., 1992). Expression of c-erbB-2 protein appears to be related to cellular proliferation

(Poller et al., 1994; Ramachandra et al., 1990).

Proliferation rate. Another aspect of the different variants of DCIS that has been evaluated and compared is the proliferation rate. The expression of Ki-67 has varied from 23% to 42% in low-grade DCIS to 37% to 40% for high-grade DCIS (Bobrow et al., 1994; Zafrani et al., 1994). The growth rate of comedo carcinoma is more rapid than that of other types of intraductal carcinoma. Comedocarcinomas are composed of a more anaplastic cell population that displays a higher proliferation rate as determined by thymidine labeling-index (TLI), compared to other types of DCIS (Schmitt et al., 1995). The utility of TLI as a prognostic factor and its value in determining the optimal therapeutic regimen for an individual patient with DCIS has not been defined, however.

Epidermal growth factor receptor (EGFR/c-erbB-1/HER-1). The protein epidermal growth factor (EGF) has a role in normal and neoplastic cell proliferation and interacts with a transmembrane receptor, the EGFR. Epidermal growth factor receptor is expressed in normal mammary epithelium, but not to the level observed in some carcinomas. In one study, expression of (EGFR) was noted predominantly in the myoepithelial cells of DCIS, but a few cases of DCIS showed simultaneous expression of ER, PR, and EGFR in the luminal epithelial cells (Agthoven et al., 1994). In general, EGFR expression has been noted in 45% of breast carcinomas (Klijn et al., 1992).

Nm23. Immunohistochemical expression of *nm23*, a putative metastasis suppressor gene, has been detected in 18 non-comedo DCIS, but not in 7 cases of comedo DCIS (Royds et al., 1993).

Ploidy. Ploidy is another feature of malignancies that often correlates with their behavior. An aneuploid DNA content in DCIS seems to be related to high-grade lesions and early recurrence after excisional biopsy (Carpenter et al., 1987; Pallis et al., 1992b; Satallof et al., 1993). About 30% of DCIS and atypical intraductal hyperplasias have displayed aneuploidy. A vast majority of low-grade DCIS lesions are diploid (Allred et al., 1994; Locker et al., 1990; Satallof et al., 1993), whereas aneuploidy has been identified in a high proportion (55% to over 90%) of high-grade DCIS (comedocarcinomas) (Aasmundstad and Haugen, 1990; Allred et al., 1994; Crissman et al., 1990; Locker et al., 1990; Ohtake et al., 1995). Among 26 cases of DCIS associated with invasive carcinoma, 22 (88.4%) displayed aneuploid cells. Of 16 cases of concurrent DCIS and invasive carcinoma, both components of the carcinoma were aneuploid in 11 cases, both were diploid in 1, and in 4 cases the DCIS was aneuploid, whereas the invasive component was diploid. Chromosome aneuploidy was observed in 7 of 10 (70%) DCIS patients (5 of whom had associated invasive carcinoma) (Visscher et al., 1996).

Angiogenesis. In Bose et al.'s (1996) in comedo and non-comedo DCIS immunohistochemical study of angiogenesis using factor VIIIRA and CD34, they rarely found any vessels in the peribasement membrane (BM) region of normal ducts. New vessels were noted in the immediate vicinity of the BM in ducts with DCIS. Evidence of angiogenesis was found in 80% of DCIS, a ring of neovascularity was more complete in cases of comedocarcinoma than in noncomedo DCIS. Guidi et al. (1994) found periductal angiogenesis in around 21 of 55 (38%) cases of pure DCIS. The angiogenesis was unrelated to histologic subtype of the DCIS, the proliferative index, or HER-2/neu expression.

Stromal changes. The stromal changes around ducts with DCIS have also been studied and show stromolysins and lysyl oxidase by immunohistochemistry. Lysyl oxidase expression has also been detected by *in situ* hybridization in myofibroblast and myoepithelial cells around DCIS (Peyrol et al.; 1997). Immunohistochemically detectable (using E9 antibody) metallothionin (MT) has been found more frequently in comedo DCIS (Douglas-Jones et al., 1995, 1997). Myoepithelial cells are also uniformly positive with MT.

Morphometry. Morphometric studies have shown that the mean diameter of ducts containing DCIS with necrosis is 470 μm, compared to a mean diameter of 192 μm for DCIS without necrosis (Mayr et al., 1991). Furthermore, necrosis is found in 94% of ducts larger than 180 μm in radius, compared to 34% of ducts less than 180 μm in size. These findings provide indirect evidence for the existence of a hypoxic compartment in DCIS that could explain the higher local failure rate after conservative surgery and irradiation in cases of comedocarcinoma.

34BetaE12 (high-molecular-weight cytokeratin)—a molecular marker of significant diagnostic value. Recent data in our laboratory have shown that determination of the immunoprofile for the high-molecular-weight cytokeratin antibody cocktail 34BetaE12 is useful in distinguishing between AIDH/DCIS and IDH (Moinfar et al., 1999). Intraductal hyperplasia characteristically stains strongly positive with 34BetaE12 whereas AIDH/DCIS fails to demonstrate immunoreactivity (Moinfar et al., 1999; Figs. 15–26 to 15–28). Together with the morphologic features, use of this immunostain may facilitate the interpretation of difficult lesions as hyperplasia versus AIDH or DCIS.

Molecular analysis for tumor suppressor genes. Both oncogenes and tumor suppressor genes may be altered in mammary carcinogenesis. Genetic alterations in putative and recognized tumor suppressor genes have been measured by assessment of LOH at a number of chromosomal loci. Using the microdissection technique, LOH has been detected on chromosome 17p in 29%–50% of DCIS lesions, as well as on a number of other chromosomes (1p, 3p, 6q, 7q, 11q,16q, 17q, etc.) (Chen and Sahin, 1996; Fujii et al., 1996; Lakhani et al., 1995; Munn et al., 1995, 1996; Noguchi et al., 1994a,b; Radford et al., 1993; Stratton et al., 1995; Teixeira et al., 1996). Identical allelic loss has been found in DCIS and its associated invasive carcinoma (Zhuang et al., 1995); 80% of DCIS and 50% of IDH and AIDH shared LOH patterns with concurrent invasive carcinomas (O'Connell et al., 1994). Interestingly, the incidence of LOH at 17p D17S796 and 16q D16S413 for DCIS is similar to the frequency of LOH at these loci in AIDH (Tham et al., 1989; Tokunaga et al., 1993). Furthermore, both DCIS and AIDH have been shown to

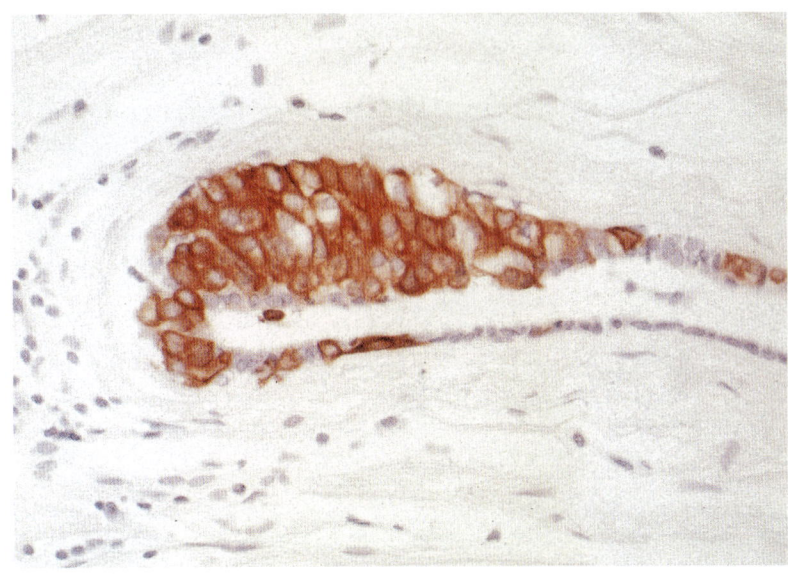

Figure 15–26. Ductal intraepithelial neoplasia, grade 1a (DIN 1a)—intraductal hyperplasia. A focus of intraductal hyperplasia (as well as normal breast epithelium in this case) is strongly immunoreactive for the high-molecular-weight cytokeratin cocktail CK 903 (immunostain for CK 903, high power).

be monoclonal (Lakhani et al., 1995b; Radford et al., 1993). Given the similarity in LOH found in AIDH and DCIS as well as in the monoclonality of both processes, Lakhani et al. (1995b) have suggested that AIDH be grouped with DCIS. Allelic imbalance in the region of the *BRCA1* gene in DCIS of the breast (with or without associated benign or invasive disease) has been noted, and was observed on chromosome 17q12–23 in 74% of cases of DCIS (Stratton et al., 1995). Among nine non-comedo DCIS analyzed for LOH using a series of microsatellite markers, a high level of allele loss at the FHIT and ATM genes was noted (Man et al., 1996).

Results in our lab showed that among a small number of recurrent DCIS cases analyzed for LOH, the recurrent lesions shared identical LOH with the original (primary) tumor, but the recurrent lesions had additional LOH not present in the primary tumors (Lininger et al., 1998). This finding suggests that the recurrent lesion is most likely due to recurrence of residual DCIS, with genetic progression.

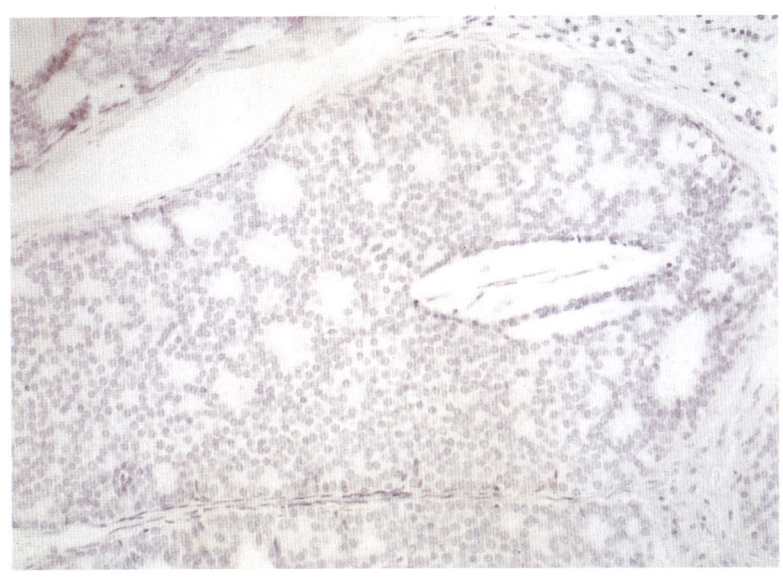

Figure 15–27. Ductal intraepithelial neoplasia, grade 1c (DIN 1c)—ductal carcinoma *in situ* (DCIS), grade 1, cribriform pattern. A large duct contains intraductal carcinoma, grade 1, cribriform pattern, which shows the absence of immunoreactivity with CK 903 (immunostain for CK 903, medium-high power).

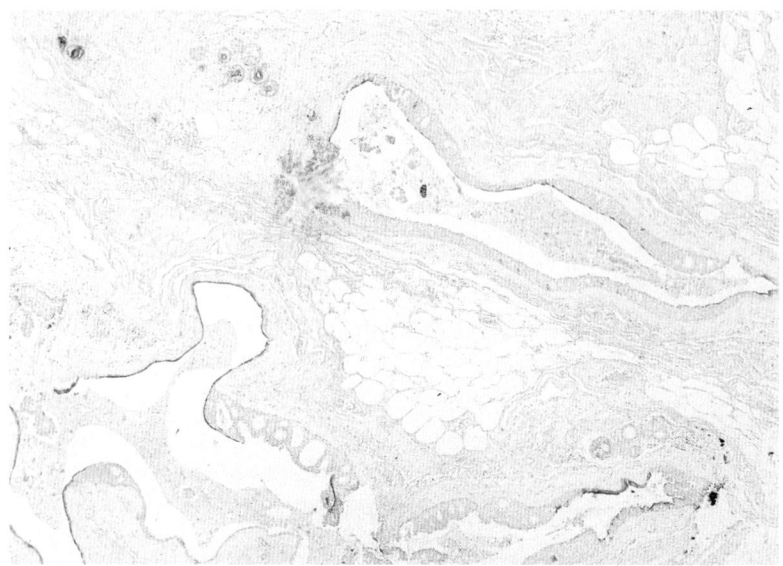

Figure 15–28. Ductal intraepithelial neoplasia, grade 1c (DIN 1c)—ductal carcinoma *in situ* (DCIS), grade 1, cribriform and solid pattern. This low-power view of intraductal carcinoma demonstrates loss of immunoreactivity with CK 903, while the normal, residual overlying breast epithelium remains strongly positive (immunostain for CK 903, low power).

LOBULAR NEOPLASIA

As follow-up information became available on women with LCIS who, for some reason or other, did not have a mastectomy, some investigators—notably Haagensen—began to question whether the lesion warranted a designation of carcinoma and, hence, a mastectomy (Dall'Olmo et al., 1975). The term *lobular neoplasia* (LN) was introduced by Haagensen to cover the entire spectrum of lobular disease ranging from lesions that display only partial lobular involvement to those showing massive distension of acini in numerous lobules. Our personal preference is to use the designation of LN for the entire spectrum of changes within the lobules, rather than splitting the spectrum into atypical lobular hyperplasia (ALH) and lobular carcinoma *in situ* (LCIS) on the basis of features of questionable therapeutic or absolute prognostic value.

Clinical Features and Significance of Lobular Neoplasia

Lobular neoplasia (LN) or lobular carcinoma *in situ* (LCIS) is identified in 0.3% to 3.8% of all breast biopsies (Azzopardi, 1979; Giordano and Klopp, 1973; Haagensen, 1986; Lambird and Shelley, 1969; Wheeler et al., 1974), or about 1.5% of all biopsies performed for benign breast lesions (Andersen, 1974a; Lambird and Shelley, 1969).

Wheeler and Enterline (1976) noted that ALH accounted for 0.4% of all biopsies in their practice, while LCIS accounted for 0.8%, or a total of 1.2% when the two are grouped together. Variations in the reported frequency of the disease are due to differences in criteria, extent of sampling, and the thoroughness of the microscopic evaluation. Patients with LN range in age from 15 years (Ackerman et al., 1993) to over 90 years of age; the median age ranges from 44 to 50 years (Andersen, 1974a; Benfield et al., 1972; Carson et al., 1994; Ciatto et al., 1992; Lewison and Finney, 1968; Newman, 1966; Page et al., 1991; Rosen, 1980c; Rosen et al., 1978; Salvadori et al., 1991; Singletary, 1994). The average age of women with LCIS (45 years) (Rosen, 1980c) is approximately 10 years younger than that of patients with infiltrating duct carcinoma (55 years) and 15 years younger than that of patients with infiltrating lobular carcinoma (60 years). Most of the patients are premenopausal (Lattes, 1980), with 80% (Rosner et al., 1980) to 89% (Haagensen et al., 1983) of the lesions presenting in women less than 54 years of age. Lobular neoplasia is less common in African-American women than in Caucasian women (Ashikari et al., 1974). It is exceptionally uncommon in males, because of the lack of lobular development, and when present, it invariably occurs in males showing lobular development secondary to hormonal therapy, or in the setting of endogenous hormonal perturbations secondary to various disease states.

Additional important characteristics of LN that were noted by Foote and Stewart (1941) and subsequent investigators are summarized below:

1. Lobular neoplasia is predominantly a pathologic diagnosis; it does not produce a palpable mass, rather, it is generally an incidental finding in patients biopsied for other reasons.

2. The lesions are generally multifocal and multicentric, as well as frequently bilateral. The frequency of multicentricity has ranged from 47% (Andersen, 1974d) to 93% (Newman, 1963); the frequency of bilaterality has been as low as 9% in smaller series and up to 59% in larger ones (Benfield et al., 1972; Rosen et al., 1979; Snyder, 1966; Urban, 1967).

3. With prolonged follow-up exceeding 20 years and based on autopsy findings, up to a third of the lesions will progress to an invasive carcinoma (Nielsen et al., 1984) of either the lobular (small cell) or other histologic type.

Microscopic Features

Lobular neoplasia is characterized by a solid, occlusive proliferation of a relatively uniform population of loosely cohesive, and often small, round cells with sparse cytoplasm (Fig. 15–29; see Table 15–8 for a summary of the cytologic and architectural features of LN). In about 30%–40% of cases, there is a pagetoid extension into adjacent terminal ducts (Fig. 15–30). The morphologic appearances of the lesions within this spectrum vary depending upon the degree of acinar distension and the proportion of acini involved within a lobule. The cells of classic LN are often small and uniform, with rather indistinct cell margins and sparse cytoplasm. Occasionally, the cells may display minor variations in size and may even develop abundant granular, eosinophilic cytoplasm with apocrine-like features. Sometimes, the cells show secretory differentiation (Andersen and Vendelboe, 1981; Battifora, 1975; Eusebi et al., 1977; Gad and Azzopardi, 1975). Intracytoplasmic lumens, mucous globules (Andersen and Vendelboe, 1981),

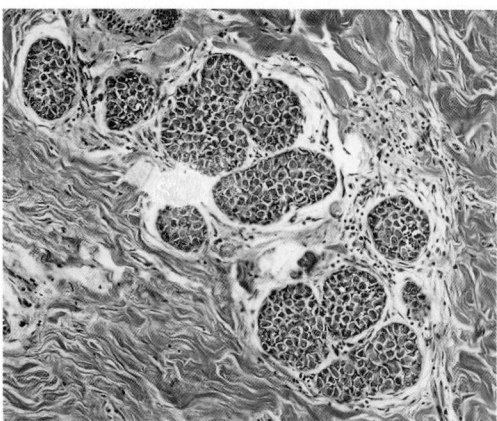

Figure 15–29. Lobular neoplasia (LN 2). The ductules in this terminal duct–lobular unit are all filled and distended by a proliferation of loosely cohesive LN cells, but the individual ductules are still clearly separate with intervening stroma. An occasional intracytoplasmic vacuoles is also present (H&E, ×160).

and a signet-ring cell appearance have also been observed and are not uncommon. The nuclei of LN cells are generally round and uniform, but occasionally display variation in size and shape. When the cells assume an apocrine appearance, the nuclei may display prominent nucleoli. The proliferating cells may appear closely packed and coherent, loosely cohesive, or completely loose and detached. It is extremely rare to observe dis-

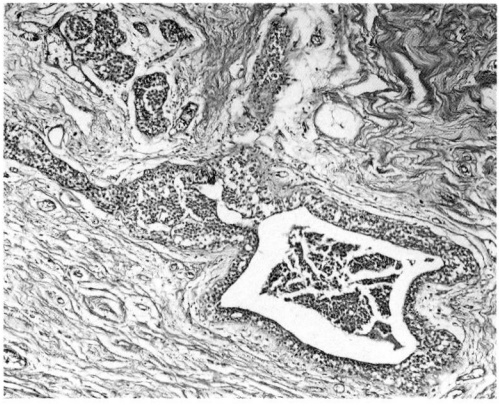

Figure 15–30. Lobular neoplasia (LN 2), with pagetoid extension. Extensive pagetoid spread of LN is present along this elongated duct profile, as well as LN cells filling and minimally extending ductules in an adjacent terminal duct–lobular unit (H&E, low power).

tinct cell margins evident even among LN cells that appear coherent. The native epithelial cells in the TDLUs are either completely replaced or simply displaced and lifted by the proliferating cells (Fig. 15–31). Sometimes this pagetoid ductal involvement may be the only change evident in the biopsy (Fechner, 1972; Page et al., 1988).

Lobular Neoplasia
Classification System

To convey the extent and degree of advancement of these lobular changes, we have graded the alterations as LN 1 to LN 3, based on the extent and degree of proliferation (Table 15–3). To qualify as LN 1, there should be partial or complete replacement or displacement of the normal epithelial cells of acini within one or more lobules by a proliferation of LN cells that may or may not fill the lumens, but without any evidence of distension of the acini (Fig. 15–32) when compared to adjacent uninvolved acini. LN 2 should display more abundant proliferation of LN cells that fill and distend some or all acini, but the acinar outlines should remain distinct and separate from one another with persistence of intervening lobular stroma (Fig. 15–29); residual lumens may persist in some acini. To warrant a designation of LN 3, either an occlusive epithelial

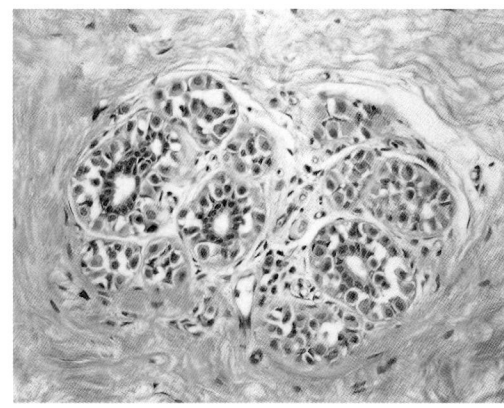

Figure 15–32. Lobular neoplasia (LN 1). Focal pagetoid extension of LN cells beneath residual epithelial-lined lumens of this small terminal duct–lobular unit is seen, in association with ductules that are filled but not distended by the loosely cohesive LN cells (H&E, ×250).

proliferation distending the acini to the point that they appear to be almost confluent—macroacini of Haagensen et al. (1978) (Figs. 15–33 and 15–34)—or acinar distension by a population of signet ring cells proliferating in a solid occlusive manner within the acini should be present (Figs. 15–35 and 15–36); residual lumens are absent and generally there is involvement of multiple acini. In our experience, LN 1 and LN 3 are quite rare, whereas LN 2 is the most common.

Ductal Involvement
by Lobular Neoplasia

Pagetoid involvement of the ducts adjacent to TDLUs involved by LN is very common

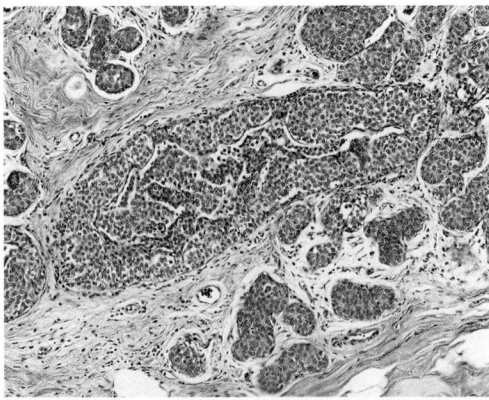

Figure 15–31. Lobular neoplasia (LN 2). A central duct with pagetoid extension and significant proliferation of LN cells displaces centrally the residual overlying epithelium. In addition, multiple adjacent ductules in this terminal duct–lobular unit are filled and distended by LN cells, but the acini remain well defined, separated by intervening stroma (H&E, ×120).

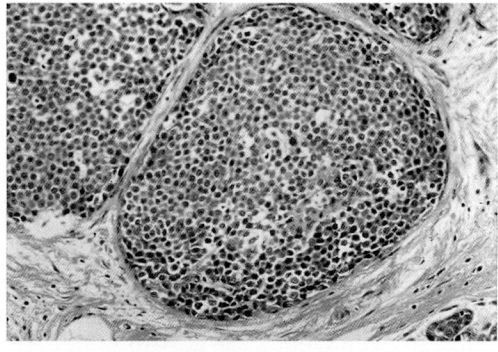

Figure 15–33. Lobular neoplasia (LN 3). Ductules showing massive distension by LN cells indicate LN 3, type 1 (H&E, medium-high power).

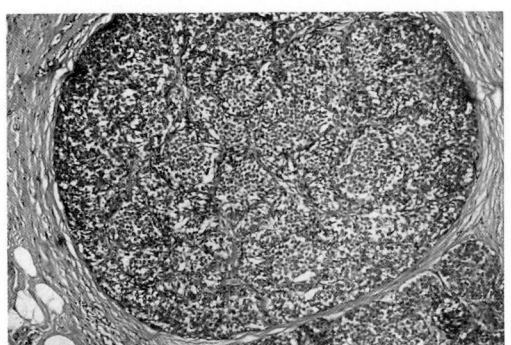

Figure 15–34. Lobular neoplasia (LN 3). This proliferation qualifies as LN 3, type 1, because LN cells massively distend the ductules in this lobule to the point that the acinar stroma appears almost confluent. The interacinar stroma is barely evident (H&E, low power).

(Andersen, 1974b; Fechner, 1972; Fisher and Fisher, 1977; Haagensen, 1986; McDivitt et al., 1967; Rosen et al., 1978; Tulusan et al., 1985; Wheeler and Enterline, 1976). In some cases, the ducts are more extensively involved by LN than the lobules (Haagensen, 1986). One of the characteristic and recognizable patterns of LN, even at low power, is the "clover-leaf" pattern of ductal involvement (Haagensen, 1986; Fig. 15–37).

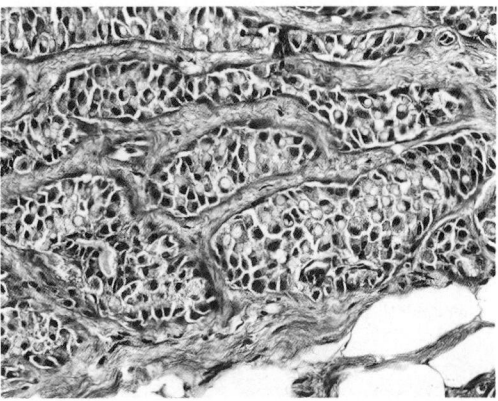

Figure 15–36. Lobular neoplasia, signet-ring cell type (LN 3). In this higher-power view, the signet-ring LN cells demonstrate prominent intracytoplasmic mucin vacuoles that distend the cytoplasm and compress the nucleus, often to a crescent-shaped structure (H&E, ×300).

Necrosis and Microcalcifications

Necrosis and microcalcification rarely occur in lobular neoplasia and do not necessarily or invariably imply a ductal lesion. Although microcalcification may occur in both grades 2 and 3 of LN, necrosis is mainly seen in LN3 lesions that show extensive involvement of numerous lobules and massive acinar distension. The presence of intracytoplasmic lumens in the proliferating cells surround-

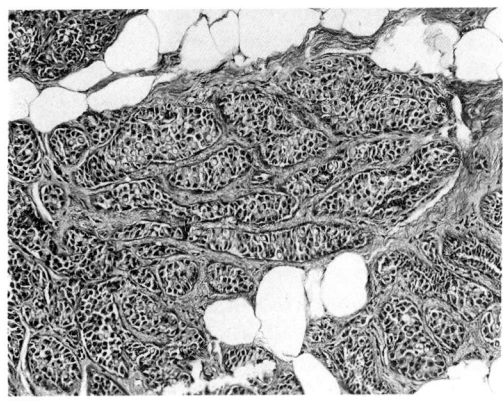

Figure 15–35. Lobular neoplasia, signet-ring cell type (LN 3). Here LN 3, type 2, or signet-ring cell type, is indicated, based on a population of loosely cohesive LN cells showing prominent intracytoplasmic vacuoles (signet ring cells) that fill and distend multiple ductules within this lobule. This variant may not demonstrate significant acinar distension (H&E, ×150).

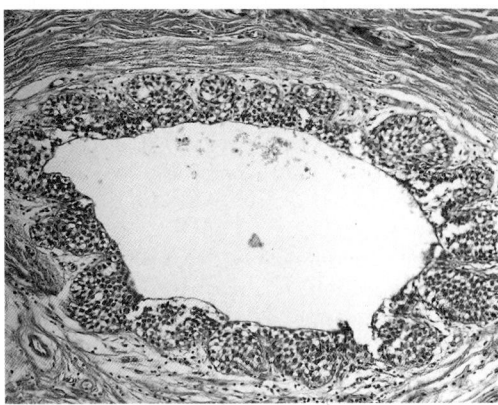

Figure 15–37. Lobular neoplasia (LN 2), clover-leaf pattern. The acini emanating circumferentially from this dilated duct are filled and slightly distended by LN cells, forming a clover-leaf pattern, an appearance characteristic of LN. (H&E, ×160).

ing the areas of necrosis is good evidence of the lobular nature of such proliferations. Since necrosis is apparently a reflection of a far-advanced LN, such lesions should be managed like a grade 2 DCIS. If LN with necrosis or with pleomorphic cells is present at or close to the resection margin, re-excision is suggested.

Myoepithelial Cell Layer and Basement Membrane

The appearance of the myoepithelial (ME) cell layer is quite variable in LN (Broders, 1932; Bussolati, 1980; Eusebi et al., 1977). In some cases, it presents as a distinct layer in its original, normal location, In others, it is displaced and disrupted, with some cells pushed or dislodged into the bolus of cellular proliferation. Finally, in a small number of LN 3 lesions, it is hardly visible on H&E–stained slides; immunostains for actin show widening of the intermyoepithelial cell gaps. The basement membrane around the acini is generally intact.

Lobular Neoplasia Involving Sclerosing Adenosis, Radial Scar, Fibroadenoma, and Collagenous Spherulosis

Lobular neoplasia may extend into or develop within areas of sclerosing adenosis (SA) and radial scar, where it may be confused with an invasive carcinoma (Fechner, 1981). Evaluation of the lesion at low magnification is crucial for its recognition since the nodular or lobulated outline and the presence of streaming, compressed ductules at the periphery of the lesion are best evident at low magnification. If doubts persist regarding the possibility of invasion, immunostains for actin can be used to unmask the ME cell layer around the ductules of SA filled by LN cells.

Lobular neoplasia is the most common lesion described to involve the fibroadenoma, accounting for more than 50% of such atypical epithelial proliferations within fibroadenomas (Yoshida et al., 1985). The predominance of LN involving fibroadenomas is in sharp contrast to the relative rarity of lobules within fibroadenomas and to the relative low (5% to 15%) overall frequency of lobular carcinomas among all breast carcinomas.

Involvement of collagenous spherulosis by lobular neoplasia (Figs. 15–38 and 15–39) may be confused with cribriform DCIS (Sgroi and Koerner, 1995); the distinctive spherules and the orientation of actin-positive myoepithelial cells around them helps resolve the problem.

Differential Diagnosis of Lobular Neoplasia

Distinction from atypical intraductal hyperplasia and ductal carcinoma in situ within the terminal duct–lobular unit. As previously mentioned, both lesions with ductal and lobular patterns may originate in the TDLU (Wellings et al., 1975). Features that help identify the relatively solid variants of ductal growth patterns within the TDLU include formation of multiple, albeit minuscule, secondary lumens, rosette-like arrangement of the nuclei, and distinctive cell margins bestowing a mosaic pattern upon the solid proliferation. The presence of large cells with abundant cytoplasm and pleomorphism associated with any of these features would further support interpretation of the lesion as ductal rather than lobular.

Features that favor lobular neoplasia include loosely cohesive cells and the presence of intracytoplasmic lumens (Battifora, 1975) or secretory globules (Andersen and Vendelboe, 1981) and mucin positivity. The presence of intracellular sialomucin is another feature that may help distinguish LN from ductal carcinomas in the TDLU (Gad and Azzopardi, 1975). Gad and Azzopardi (1975) found that the mucosubstance in LN cells is alcianophilic and periodic acid-Schiff (PAS) positive after diastase digestion.

Despite the variety of helpful features mentioned above, it is sometimes impossible to make such a distinction. Such lesions have been designated as either atypical hyperplasia with mixed ductal and lobular features or *in situ* carcinoma with ductal and lobular features, depending on the degree of cytologic atypia, extent, duct, or lobular expansion, and necrosis present. These lesions would also be designated under the translational classification designation mammary intraepithelial neoplasia (MIN), not further classified, and assigned the appropriate grade (MIN 1–3), akin to the LN classification.

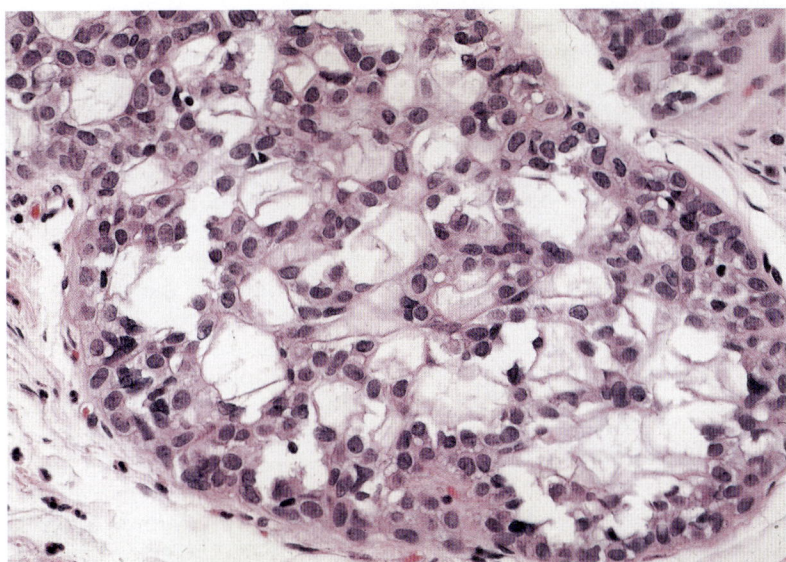

Figure 15–38. Lobular neoplasia, involving collagenous spherulosis (LN 2). In collagenous spherulosis, LN may be confused with ductal carcinoma *in situ* of the cribriform type; the distinctive spherules (collagenous or mucinous) and the orientation of the myoepithelial cell nuclei around the spherules help to eliminate the confusion (H&E, high power).

Coexistence of lobular neoplasia and ductal carcinoma in situ. Various investigators have commented on the simultaneous finding of LN and intraductal or invasive ductal carcinoma within a biopsy as well as within a single TDLU (Haagensen, 1986; Haagensen et al., 1983; Rosen, 1980b). The frequency of this coexistence has been noted to range from 12% to 16% (Haagensen, 1986; Rosen, 1980b). Haagensen (1986) found that pa-

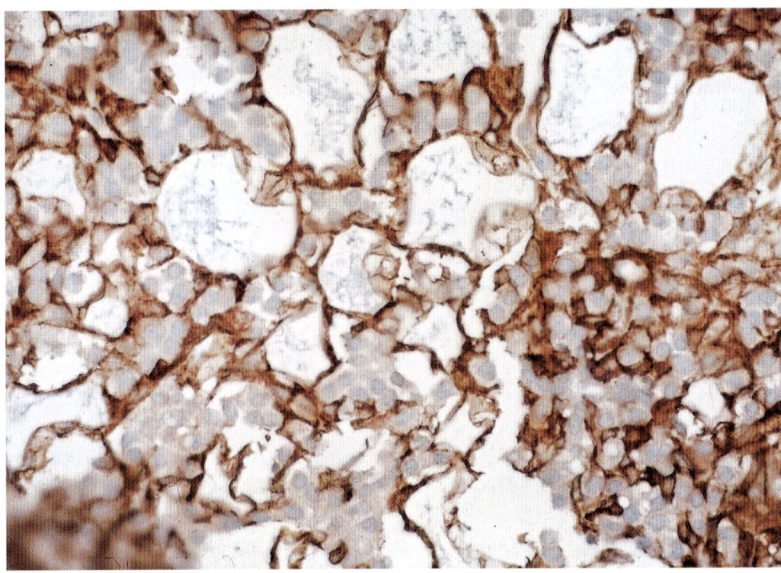

Figure 15–39. Lobular neoplasia, involving collagenous spherulosis (LN 2). The myoepithelial cell layer lining the luminal spaces is highlighted by strong immunoreactivity with smooth muscle actin (immunostain for smooth muscle actin; high power).

tients in whom LN occurred alone were generally younger than the group of patients having LN associated with other forms of breast carcinoma. Biopsies from the latter group displayed LN with loss of cell cohesion, macroacini, and maximal amounts of the lesion more frequently. We have noted a particularly frequent association of LN with the flat type of ductal intraepithelial neoplasia (DIN 1b)—LN is present in almost 30% of cases showing the latter.

Results of Short-Term (5 Years) and Long-Term Follow-up of Patients After Diagnostic Biopsy and No Further Therapy

Five studies have prospectively assessed the frequency of subsequent invasive carcinomas in the ipsilateral and contralateral breast within 5 years after a biopsy diagnosis of lobular carcinoma *in situ.* Using our three-tiered grading system for LN, members of the National Surgical Adjuvant Breast Project (NSABP) (Fisher et al., 1996) graded cases of lobular disease, but they continued to use the designation of LCIS; they found that this grading system can predict lesions that are more likely to recur and progress. Among 63 women with lesions designated as LN 1 (LCIS 1), none developed subsequent invasive carcinoma, one of 81 (1%) women with LN2 (LCIS 2) and three of 38 (8%) women with LN 3 (LCIS 3) developed subsequent invasive carcinoma in the ipsilateral breast, while two patients developed subsequent invasive carcinoma (one mucinous and one invasive lobular) in the contralateral breast within a 5-year period of follow-up (Fisher et al., 1996; Table 15–2). Overall, subsequent ipsilateral invasive carcinoma developed in 2.2% of 182 women with all grades of LN (LCIS), while subsequent contralateral invasive carcinoma developed in 1.1% of women within 5 years.

Among 149 patients with LCIS in two other prospective studies (Ozzello, 1971; Salvadori et al., 1991), 7.7% developed invasive ipsilateral carcinoma, but the margins were not noted. The fourth study (Zurrida et al., 1996) found 4 (2.5%) subsequent invasive carcinomas in the ipsilateral breast and 4 (2.5%) in the contralateral breast among 157 women with LCIS within 5 years of a diagnostic and therapeutic biopsy. Within a

median follow-up period of 5 years, 12% of 69 Danish women with LCIS developed subsequent invasive carcinoma in the ipsilateral breast (Ottesen et al., 1993). No contralateral recurrences occurred. The findings in this Danish study are significantly different from those of practically all other studies.

Comparison of the long-term follow-up results of different studies is difficult because of variations in the criteria used for the diagnosis of LCIS as well as differences in the sampling and evaluation of the specimens. For example, Andersen (1974a,c, 1977) and Wheeler and Enterline (1976) diagnosed LCIS when only a single lobule showed the typical pattern of proliferation, whereas Hutter and Foote (1969) required involvement of at least two to three lobules for a diagnosis of LCIS. Haagensen et al.'s series (Haagensen, 1986; Haagensen et al., 1978) probably includes some lesions that would qualify as atypical lobular hyperplasia (ALH) by the criteria utilized by most other investigators. Rosen et al. (1978, 1981) provided no firm criteria for separating the cases of ALH from LCIS. Nonetheless, these studies have provided a large amount of information regarding the clinical significance of lobular neoplasia. Women with ALH, as defined by Page et al. (1985), have a risk for subsequent development of invasive carcinoma that is 4 to 5.3 times that of the general population (Dupont and Page, 1985; Page, 1986; Page and Dupont, 1990; Page et al., 1985). Of 126 women with ALH in their study, 16 (13%) developed subsequent invasive carcinoma; they did so within an average of 11.9 years (Page et al., 1985). Sixty-nine percent of the invasive carcinomas were in the ipsilateral breast (Page et al., 1985).

Excluding Page et al.'s 1985 study, which specifically addresses ALH, and subtracting the number of patients from various published reports who had previous or current invasive breast carcinoma and who had had a mastectomy within 6 months of the biopsy from 1174, the number of women in 18 separate studies who had lesions diagnosed as either LCIS or LN, 181 (15.4%) women developed invasive carcinoma (Andersen, 1974a, 1977; Benfield et al., 1965; Giordano and Klopp, 1973; Haagensen, 1986; Haagensen et al., 1978; Hutter et al., 1968; Page et al., 1991; Rosen et al., 1978, 1981). Of these 1174 women, 102 (8.7%) developed carcinoma in the ipsilateral breast, while 79 (6.7%) did so in the contralateral breast. Therefore, both breasts are at risk for the subsequent development of invasive carcinoma, with the ipsilateral breast at slightly higher risk.

In a subsequent study of Haagensen's patients over a longer period of follow-up (median:18 years), approximately one-third of 236 women with LN subsequently developed invasive carcinoma, which is 5.4 times (95% CI 4.2–7.0) the rate of the general population (Bodian et al., 1996). The risk for subsequent development of carcinoma remained high for over 20 years. The risk for all women was 13% at 10 years and 23% at 20 years; it continued to increase to 35% for those women who survived 35 years after their initial diagnosis of LN. Furthermore, the relative risk increased substantially if a second biopsy showed LN as well—the relative risk increased from 4.9 (95% CI 3.7–6.4) after one biopsy with LN to 16.1 (95% CI 6.9–31.8) after a second biopsy with LN (Bodian et al., 1996). This is a significant addition to our understanding of LN.

Andersen (1979) calculated the risk for subsequent development of invasive carcinoma in patients with LCIS to be about 12 times that expected in comparable Danish women without LCIS. The calculated ratio of observed to expected carcinomas was 9:1 in two studies (Page et al., 1991; Rosen et al., 1978), and 6.9:1 in another (Haagensen et al., 1978). Haagensen's data are given for the time frame for developing subsequent carcinoma. Rosen et al. (1978) found an increased "hazard rate" in later years.

In most series, only a small proportion of the subsequent carcinomas developed within 10 years of the diagnostic biopsy. Haagensen's data (1986) indicate that the probability of developing carcinoma in both breasts increases uniformly up to 25 years following treatment by biopsy alone. During the first 10 years after a biopsy diagnosis of LCIS, only 17% of all subsequent invasive carcinomas in the ipsilateral breast and about 20% of those predicted to develop in the contralateral breast manifest themselves. In Page et al.'s series (1991), the absolute risk of infiltrating breast carcinoma after LCIS was 17% at 15 years. Ottesen et al. (1993), however, reported significantly different outcomes in a group of 69 women

with LCIS treated by excision only as part of a prospective trial from the Danish Breast Cancer Cooperative Group (DBGG-83) accrued from 1982 to 1987. Eight women (12%) developed subsequent invasive carcinomas, all in the ipsilateral breast, within a 5-year follow-up period.

Judging from two series published in 1978 (Haagensen et al., 1978; Rosen et al., 1978), it appears that dividing this spectrum of lobular changes into ALH and LCIS has no prognostic significance. These studies concluded that a variety of qualitative and quantitative features generally used to subdivide the changes into LCIS and ALH are not of prognostic significance. The features evaluated by these studies as possible prognostic factors included the presence of cysts, perilobular lymphocytic infiltrate, persistence of central lumen, distension of acini, involvement of one or more lobules, macroacini, variation in cell type, loss of cell cohesion, closely packed hyperchromatic cells, and presence of an admixture of small and large cells. The only two features for which the subsequent risk was found to be higher than that for all other patients with LN were the presence of closely packed hyperchromatic cells (Haagensen et al., 1978) and an admixture of small and large cell types (Rosen et al., 1978). However, only 12 patients had the former characteristic and 12 had the latter—too few to be considered significant. The grading system we use for LN effectively separates those lesions with a very limited likelihood of progression (LN 1) from those with greater chance of recurrence or subsequent progression within 5 years after diagnosis (Fisher et al., 1996).

Two subsequent studies (Page et al., 1985, 1991), suggested that the lesions at the lowest end of the proliferative spectrum are associated with a lower risk for subsequent development of carcinoma. Furthermore, in a population of 10,542 women with otherwise benign breast biopsies, Page et al. (1985) discovered 126 cases of atypical lobular hyperplasia with proper follow-up and only 39 cases (0.5%) of lobular carcinoma *in situ* (Page et al., 1991) with long-term follow up. Obviously, Page et al. (1991) are far more conservative in diagnosing LCIS than Rosen et al. (Rosen, 1980, 1980b,c). The latter group interpreted only 13 cases as ALH during the period when they diagnosed 99 cases (only 83 of which had proper follow-up evaluation) of LCIS (1.3%) among their breast biopsies. The fact that both Rosen et al. (1981) and Page et al. (1991) concluded that the relative risk for subsequent development of invasive carcinoma is 9.0 for women with LCIS while using significantly different criteria and analytic approach indicates that the value of splitting this spectrum into two prognostically distinct groups has not been confirmed.

Influence of Family History of Breast Carcinoma

The presence of a family history of breast carcinoma in a sister, mother, or daughter of a patient with ALH doubles the risk from around 5.3 to 11 times that of women who have nonproliferative lesions without a family history of breast carcinoma (Dupont and Page, 1985; Page et al., 1985). In effect, a woman with ALH and a family history of breast carcinoma has the same risk as one with DCIS.

It is not well known if and how the presence of additional risk factors may alter the prognosis of patients with either a diagnosis of LN or LCIS. An increase in risk has been noted by Haagensen et al. (1972, 1978) in patients who have a family history of breast carcinoma and gross cystic disease in addition to lobular neoplasia; the ratio of observed-to-expected subsequent carcinomas rose from 7.2 for all women with LN but without a family history of breast carcinoma or gross cystic disease to 11.8 for those who also had a positive family history and gross cystic disease. In Rosen et al.'s study (1978), 5 of 12 (42%) of women with a family history of breast carcinoma subsequently developed invasive carcinoma, compared to 22 of 62 (36%) of women without a positive family history. The differences between a positive and negative family history was not significant. Page et al. (1991) concluded that family history did not further affect the risk.

Location and Type of Subsequent Invasive Carcinomas

In patients who are treated by biopsy alone, the subsequent invasive carcinoma is of the small-cell infiltrating (lobular) type in 43% of the patients (Haagensen, 1986). Haagensen categorized 90% of the subsequent invasive carcinomas detected through the course of close periodic follow-up in his series as well differentiated. Tulusan et al. (1985) observed that 46% of invasive carcinomas identified prior to, simultaneous with, or after a diagnosis of LCIS are of the invasive lobular, or small cell type.

Rosen et al. (1979) tabulated the findings from 3 studies, including their own, whereby the mastectomy specimens performed for a biopsy diagnosis of LCIS were evaluated for the presence of residual LCIS and infiltrating carcinoma. They found residual LCIS in 60% to 65% of the cases, and identified an invasive carcinoma in 4% to 6% of the mastectomy specimens. The residual LCIS involved quadrants other than the biopsy site in 80% of the cases.

In Page et al.'s series (1991), 10 subsequent invasive carcinomas developed in 9 patients. Seven of these were pure lobular or lobular variants, two were tubular, and one was ductal of no particular type. All eight subsequent invasive carcinomas were in the ipsilateral breast in Ottesen et al.'s (1993) study; four of these were infiltrating duct carcinomas, one was a pure infiltrating lobular carcinoma, one was a tubulolobular carcinoma, one was a combined lobular and ductal carcinoma, and one was a small cell, carcinoid-like carcinoma.

All subsequent invasive carcinoma in the ipsilateral breast and half of those in the contralateral breast were of the lobular type in Fisher et al.'s series (1996). All the ipsilateral carcinomas occurred in the same quadrant as the initial reference biopsy. A vast majority of the initial diagnostic biopsies in these women were described as having margins free of tumor.

As mentioned earlier, in the absence of invasive carcinoma, LN has not been associated with axillary lymph node metastases.

Management of Patients with Lobular Neoplasia

The appropriate management of patients with LN/LCIS has been an enigma, with divergent viewpoints expressed since the recognition of the lesion (Andersen, 1977; Andersen et al., 1980; Benfield et al., 1969; Giordano and Klopp, 1973; Gump, 1990; Haagensen, 1986; Hutter, 1984; Tobon and Price, 1972). Simple mastectomy was recommended by Foote and Stewart (1941).

This recommendation was followed by many as the treatment of choice (Barnes et al., 1959; Godwin, 1952; Lewison and Finney, 1968). Some advised modified radical mastectomy (Hutter and Foote, 1969; Newman, 1966). Because of the high incidence of bilaterality, Newman (1963) suggested an ample biopsy of the contralateral breast, which subsequently became common practice (Benfield et al., 1965; Hutter et al., 1968; Newman, 1966; Urban, 1967), while others went so far as to suggest bilateral mastectomy on prophylactic or therapeutic grounds (Barnes, 1959; Benfield et al., 1969, 1972). For many years, mastectomy with or without contralateral breast biopsy (Donegan and Perez-Mesa, 1972; Rosen, 1980a,b,c; Rosen et al., 1978, 1981) was the only treatment offered to patients with lobular neoplasia (LCIS). Fortunately, a few practitioners persistently questioned mastectomy as too radical and considered a more conservative approach of close observation after the biopsy (Ackerman and Katzenstein, 1977; Andersen, 1977; Dall'Olmo et al., 1975; Haagensen et al., 1972, 1978; Toker and Goldberg, 1971; Wheeler et al., 1974).

Wheeler et al. (1974) and Haagensen et al. (1978) were among the first to argue against mastectomy as the treatment for patients with LCIS (LN) and actually proposed the alternative approach of life-long periodic follow-up for patients whose biopsies showed lobular neoplasia. These recommendations were way ahead of their time.

Currently, however, there is general agreement that when either LCIS, LN, or ALH occurs, the breasts should be regarded as a single organ. Therefore, since both breasts are at almost equal risk for subsequent development of invasive carcinoma, there appear to be two alternative approaches to treatment: bilateral mastectomy or periodic follow-up for the remainder of the patient's life, with or without tamoxifen or other agents for cancer prevention.

Given the relatively young age of many patients with lobular neoplasia, the relatively long interval between detection of lobular disease and the development of most subsequent invasive carcinomas, the low mortality rate from breast carcinoma within a 10-year follow-up (Andersen, 1977), and our inability to predict which breast will manifest the subsequent invasive carcinoma, periodic follow-up seems more justifiable. The follow-up should include examination of both breasts by a physician two to four times a year. The follow-up regimen should also include annual mammography for patients over 40 years of age, if the breast tissue density allows mammographic assessment. Inclusion of tamoxifen or other agents as part of a breast cancer prevention trial could be another consideration in patients who are selected for conservative management. It is important to keep in mind that the benefits and risks of tamoxifen therapy remain speculative at present. It is also possible that utilization of tamoxifen at this stage of disease may lead to development of resistance to its effects. Could this eventually prove a disadvantage to patients who might have benefited from addition of tamoxifen to the treatment of their subsequent invasive carcinoma?

When both LN and DCIS (non-necrotic variants) are present in a mammographically directed biopsy, the issue becomes more complex. Haagensen et al. (1983) found that 92 (31%) of 282 carcinomas present in 237 women who had concurrent LN reflected a variety of intraductal carcinomas. Of these 92 patients, 32% had axillary node metastases; this is a high percentage, considering the rarity of axillary node metastases associated with intraductal carcinoma alone, and the absence of any documented case of axillary node metastases associated with LN alone. There are no good data available to help in the management of these patients, using a more conservative approach to treatment.

It is important that both physician and patient understand the ensuing risks involved in choosing a specific form of therapy and be of the necessity of long-term follow-up over the remainder of the patient's life in the event of conservative management. The ideal approach is to assemble an interdisciplinary team composed of a radiologist, surgeon, pathologist, and oncologist, preferably with an epidemiologist/statistician and social worker/ psychologist to follow all these patients in a systematic manner. The patient's family history and level of anxiety would weigh considerably in the ultimate decision. Genetic studies may prove valuable in the selection of patients for different therapeutic approaches that undoubtedly will become more varied as our knowledge of cancer genetics progresses.

Why some women develop subsequent invasive carcinoma, while others fail to do so, remains an unexplained aspect of this disease and an area that requires continued investigation.

Questions Raised by the Changing Trends in Treatment of Breast Carcinoma

Considering the current recommendation of lumpectomy for invasive carcinomas, particularly those that present as tumors less than 2 cm in size and with no evidence of lymph node metastases, one might question if the presence of concurrent LN in this group would in any way alter the prognosis or management of the patient. There is minimal information available in the literature that might be of any help in this regard. Haagensen et al. (1983) compared the ratio of observed-to-expected carcinomas in the contralateral breast in three groups of women: (1) women with unilateral carcinoma and no prior LN treated by mastectomy; (2) patients with unilateral carcinoma and concurrent LN also treated by mastectomy; (3) women with LN followed after biopsy and who subsequently developed invasive carcinoma. The ratio of observed-to-expected carcinoma for the first group was 3 to 1; for group 2, it was 8.3 to 1, and for the third group, it was 9.4 to 1. Compared to all patients with carcinoma, the risk for a contralateral breast carcinoma was three times as high for postmenopausal woman and twice as high for premenopausal women with concurrent LN and carcinoma. Simultaneous breast carcinoma was five times more frequent in women who had concurrent LN and carcinoma than in those with no prior lobular neoplasia. Ninety-one of the 282 carcinomas with concurrent LN were of the invasive small cell (lobular) type; 45% of these cases had axillary node metastases. This was comparable to the 40.3% frequency of axillary node metastases found in women with cancer in general.

We also need to know how many (and which) lesions (e.g., LN, DCIS, ordinary infiltrating duct carcinoma, tubular carcinoma, colloid carcinoma, lobular carcinoma, etc.) may coexist in a biopsy before changing recommendations for treatment from conservative management to more aggressive therapy.

Hormone Receptors and Tumor Markers

Using immunohistochemical staining, 10 examples of classic LCIS composed of uniform small cells were evaluated for ER expression by Giri et al. (1989). Nine of the 10 cases of LCIS showed variable expression of ER, and 6 of these (60%) displayed significant nuclear staining. Among cases of LN evaluated by a panel of markers including HER-2/neu/c-erbB-2, collagen type IV, B72.3, and BER-EP4 at the AFIP, the only marker that displayed a consistently positive reaction in 14 examples of LN was type IV collagen. The positive reaction to type IV collagen was evident around the acini containing the neoplastic cells, indicating persistence of the basal lamina. All 14 lesions were negative for c-erb-B2, only 1 showed positivity for B72.3, and 1 for BER-EP4. Eleven of 14 intraductal carcinomas, in contrast, showed a positive reaction for BER-EP4. The 14 invasive lobular carcinomas differed from LN mainly in their reaction to collagenase; 11 of the 14 cases displayed absolutely no positivity with collagen type IV. One example of LCIS evaluated by Nesland et al. (1985) displayed a positive reaction for CEA, prekeratin, and casein, but failed to react with lactalbumin.

Casein has been found in the cytoplasm of 5 examples of LCIS and 21 infiltrating lobular carcinomas (Eusebi et al., 1977). In addition, α lactalbumin and lactoferritin were identified in both infiltrating and in situ lobular carcinoma.

Since these earlier studies, many additional cases of LN have been evaluated for a variety of markers and ploidy. In general, LN is ER and PR positive (Bur et al., 1992; Fisher et al., 1996) but negative for c-erbB-2 (Fisher et al., 1996; Porter et al., 1991; Ramachandra et al., 1990). Lobular neoplasia is also predominantly diploid (Fisher et al., 1996; Pallis et al., 1992b); ploidy of the rare pleomorphic variant will probably be different, but these lesions have not been studied in much detail.

Application of recent techniques for assessment of LOH in lobular lesions may unravel some of early events in the development of LN (Lakhani et al., 1995b; Nayar et al., 1997) and its progression to more advanced lesions. In one study, LOH at chromosome 11q13 (INT2, PYGM) was identified in about one-third of informative lobular lesions, including ALH, LCIS, and invasive lobular carcinoma (Nayar et al., 1997). None of the four informative cases of pure ALH displayed LOH. Two of 11 (18%) cases of ALH associated with LCIS and ductal lesions, including one infiltrating ductal carcinoma, showed LOH. The identical nature of the LOH in the one associated with infiltrating duct carcinoma raises the possibility that the so-called LOH may have been an early solid stage of the ductal process. None of the four ALH cases associated with infiltrating lobular carcinoma showed LOH. The frequency of LOH was higher (50%) among LCIS associated with invasive carcinoma (Nayar et al., 1997). In another study (Lakhani et al., 1995a), LOH was detected in 11 of 37 (30%) informative cases at 16q (D16S413), 3 of 41 (7%) at 17p (D17S796), 4 of 9 (44%) at 17q (D17S250) and 3 of 9 (33%) at 13q (D13S267); however, no significant difference was found for samples from pure LCIS versus those from LCIS associated with invasive disease.

The role of the intercellular adhesion molecule and tumor suppressor gene E-cadherin has been studied in both ductal and lobular carcinomas of the breast and has been found to be especially important in lobular disease. Simultaneous loss of E-cadherin and α-, β-, and γ-catenin is reported to be an important step in the formation of LCIS, as a precursor to invasive lobular carcinoma (De Leeuw et al., 1997). In one sutdy, LCIS adjacent to invasive lobular carcinoma showed simultaneous loss of E-cadherin and α- and β-catenins in nine cases (De Leeuw et al., 1997). E-cadherin expression has also been reported to be absent in six cases of LCIS unassociated with invasive carcinoma, in contrast to demonstration of expression in 150 cases of DCIS (also unassociated with an invasive component) (Vos et al., 1997). Furthermore, Vos et al. (1997) reported the presence of identical truncating mutations and LOH of the wild-type E-cadherin gene locus in the LCIS component as well as in the adjacent invasive lobular carcinoma in two cases.

Comparative genomic hybridization analysis has been performed on LCIS and ALH, with interesting results. Lu et al. (1998) found loss of material from chromosomes 16p, 16q, 17p, and 22q and gain of material from 6q, with a similar high frequency in both LCIS and ALH. The results are consistent with LCIS and ALH representing the same genetic stage of development.

REFERENCES

Aasmundstad T, Haugen O. (1990) DNA ploidy in intraductal breast carcinomas. *Eur J Cancer* 26:956–959.

Ackerman BL, Otis C, Steuber K. (1993) Lobular carcinoma *in situ* in a 15-year old girl: a case report and review of the literature. *Plast Reconstr Surg* 94:714–718.

Ackerman LV, Katzenstein AL. (1977) The concept of minimal breast cancer and the pathologists role in the diagnosis of 'early carcinoma.' *Cancer* (Suppl) 39:2755–2763.

Allred D, Clark G, Molina R, Tandon A, Schnitt S, Gilchrist K, Osborne C, Tormey D, McGuire W. (1992) Overexpression of HER-2/neu and its relationship with other prognostic factors change during the progression of *in situ* to invasive breast cancer. *Hum Pathol* 23:974–979.

Allred D, O'Connell P, Fuqua S. (1993) Biomarkers of early breast neoplasia. *J Cell Biochem* 17G:125–131.

Allred DC, O'Connell P, Fuqua SAW, Osborne CK, et al. (1994) Immunohistochemical studies of early breast cancer evolution. *Breast Cancer Res Treat* 32:13–18.

Alpers C, Wellings S. (1985) The prevalence of carcinoma *in situ* in normal and cancer-associated breasts. *Hum Pathol* 16:796–807.

Anastassiades O, Lakovou E, Stavridou N, Gogas J, et al. (1993) Multicentricity in breast cancer: a study of 366 cases. *Am J Clin Pathol* 99:238–243.

Andersen JA. (1974a) Lobular carcinoma *in situ*. A long-term follow-up in 52 cases. *Acta Pathol Microbiol Scand (A)* 82:519–533.

Andersen JA. (1974b) Lobular carcinoma *in situ* of the breast with duct involvement: frequency and possible influence on prognosis. *Acta Pathol Microbiol Scand (A)* 82:655–662.

Andersen JA. (1974c) Lobular carcinoma *in situ*: a histologic study of 52 cases. *Acta Pathol Microbiol Scand (A)* 82:735–741.

Andersen JA. (1974d) Multicentric and bilateral appearance of lobular carcinoma *in situ* of the breast: a retrospective study. *Acta Pathol Microbiol Scand (A)* 82:730–734.

Andersen JA. (1977) Lobular carcinoma *in situ* of the breast. An approach to rational treatment. *Cancer* 39:2597–2602.

Andersen JA, Fechner RE, Lattes R, Rosen PP, Toker C. (1980) Lobular carcinoma *in situ* (lobular neoplasia) of the breast (a symposium). *Pathol Annu* 1492:193–223.

Andersen JA, Vendelboe ML. (1981) Cytoplasmic mucous globules in lobular carcinoma *in situ*. *Am J Surg Pathol* 5:251–255.

Ashikari R, Hajdu SI, Robbins GF. (1971) Intraductal carcinoma of the breast (1960–1969). *Cancer* 28:1182–1187.

Ashikari R, Huvos AG, Snyder RE. (1977) Prospective study of non-infiltrating carcinoma of the breast. *Cancer* 39:435–439.

Ashikari R, Huvos AG, Snyder RE, et al. (1974) A clinicopathologic study of atypical lesions of the breast. *Cancer* 33:310–317.

Agthoven TV, Timmermans M, Foekens JA, et al. (1994) Differential expression of estrogen, progesterone, and epidermal growth factor receptors in normal, benign, and malignant human breast tissues using dual staining immunohistochemistry. *Am J Pathol* 144:1238–1246.

Association of Directors of Anatomic and Surgical Pathology. (1993) Association recommendation: Immediate management of mammographically detected breast lesions. *Am J Surg Pathol* 17(8):850–851.

Azzopardi JG. (1979) *Problems in Breast Pathology*, pp. 128–146; 192–233; 266–273. W.B. Saunders, Philadelphia.

Baker LH. (1982) Breast Cancer Detection Demonstration Project: five-year summary report. *CA Cancer J Clin* 32:194–225.

Barnes JP. (1959) Bilateral lobular carcinoma *in situ* of the breast. *Texas State J Med* 55:581–584.

Barnes D. (1993) c-erbB-2 amplification in mammary carcinoma. *J Cell Biochem* 17G:132–138.

Barnes R, Masood S. (1990) Potential value of hormone receptor assay in carcinoma *in situ* of breast. *Am J Clin Pathol* 94:533–537.

Battifora H. (1975) Intracytoplasmic lumina in breast carcinoma. A helpful histopathologic feature. *Arch Pathol* 99:614–617.

Bellamy COC, McDonald C, Salter DM, Chetty U, et al. (1993) Noninvasive ductal carcinoma of the breast: the relevance of histologic categorization. *Hum Pathol* 24:16–23.

Benfield JR, Fingerhut AG, Warner NE. (1969) Lobular carcinoma of the breast—1969. A therapeutic proposal. *Arch Surg* 99:129–131.

Benfield JR, Fingerhut AG, Warner NE. (1972) A multidisciplinary view of lobular breast carcinoma. *Am Surg* 38:115–116.

Benfield JR, Jacobson M, Warner NE. (1965) *In situ* lobular carcinoma of the breast. *Arch Surg* 91:130–135.

Bhathal PS, Brown RW, Lesueur GC, Russell IS. (1985) Frequency of benign and malignant breast lesions in 207 consecutive autopsies in Australian women. *Br J Cancer* 51:271–278.

Black M, Barclay T, Cutler S, Hankey B, Asire A. (1972) Association of atypical characteristics of benign breast lesions with subsequent risk of breast cancer. *Cancer* 29:338–343.

Blood C, Zetter B. (1990) Tumor interactions with the vasculature: angiogenesis and tumor metastasis. *Biochim Biophys Acta* 1032:89–118.

Bobrow LG, Happerfield LC, Gregory WM, Springall RD, et al. (1994) The classification of ductal carcinoma *in situ* and its association with biological markers. *Semin Diagn Pathol* 11:199–207.

Bocker W. (1997) Preneoplasia of the breast. *Verh Dtsch Ges Pathol* 81:502–513.

Bocker W, Bier B, Freytag G, et al. (1992) An immunohistochemical study of the breast using antibodies to basal and luminal keratins, alpha-smooth muscle actin, vimentin, collagen IV and laminin. Part 1: normal breast and benign proliferative lesions. *Virchows Arch A Pathol Anat* 421:315–322.

Bocker W, Decker T, Ruhnke M, Schneider W. (1997) Ductal hyperplasia and ductal carcinoma *in situ*: Definition—classification—differential diagnosis. *Pathologe* 18:3–18.

Bodian CA, Perzin KH, Lattes R. (1996) Lobular neoplasia. Long-term risk of breast cancer and relation to other factors. *Cancer* 78:1024–1034.

Bodian CA, Perzin KH, Lattes R, Hoffmann P. (1993a) Reproducibility and validity of pathologic classifications of benign breast disease and implications for clinical applications. *Cancer* 71:3908–3913.

Bodian C, Perzin K, Lattes R, Hoffmann P, Abernathy T. (1993b) Prognostic significance of benign proliferative breast disease. *Cancer* 71:3896–907.

Bodis S, Siziopikou KP, Schnitt SJ, Harris JR, et al. (1996) Extensive apoptosis in ductal carcinoma *in situ* of the breast. *Cancer* 77:1831–1835.

Bose S, Lesser ML, Norton L, Rosen PP. (1996) Immunophenotype of intraductal carcinoma. *Arch Pathol Lab Med* 120:81–85.

Broders AC. (1932) Carcinoma *in situ* contrasted with benign penetrating epithelium. *JAMA* 99:1670–1674.

Bur ME, Zimarowski MJ, Schnitt SJ, Baker S, Lew R. (1992) Estrogen receptor immunohistochemistry in carcinoma *in situ* of the breast. *Cancer* 69:1174–1181.

Burbano RR, Neto JB, de Paula Philbert PM, Casartelli C. (1996) Mammary epithelial hyperplasias: alterations related solely to proliferation? *Breast Cancer Res Treatment* 41:95–101.

Bussolati G. (1980) Actin-rich (myoepithelial) cells in lobular carcinoma *in situ* of the breast. *Virchows Arch Cell Pathol* 32:165–176.

Bussolati G, Botta G, Gugliotta P. (1980) Actin-rich (myoepithelial) cells in ductal carcinoma-*in-situ* of the breast. *Virchows Arch B Cell Path* 34:251–259.

Cady B. (1993) Duct carcinoma *in situ*. *Surg Oncol Clin North Am* 2:75–91.

Carpenter R, Gibbst N, Matthews J, Cooke T. (1987) Importance of cellular DNA content in pre-malignant breast disease and pre-invasive carcinoma of the female breast. *Br J Surg* 74:905–906.

Carson W, Sanches-Forgach E, Stompter P, Penetrante R, et al. (1994) Lobular carcinoma *in situ* without surgery as an appropriate therapy. *Ann Surg Oncol* 1:141–146.

Carter C, Corle D, Micozzi M, Schatzkin A, Taylor P. (1988) A prospective study of the development of breast cancer in 16,692 women with benign breast disease. *Am J Epidemiol* 128:467–477.

Carter D, Smith RL. (1977) Carcinoma *in situ* of the breast. *Cancer* 40:1189–1193.

Chaudhuri B, Crist K, Mucci S, Malafa M, Chaudhuri P. (1993) Distribution of estrogen receptor in ductal carcinoma *in situ* of the breast. *Surgery* 113:134–137.

Chen T, Sahin A. (1996) Deletion map of chromosome 16q in ductal carcinoma *in situ* of the breast: refining a putative tumor suppressor gene region 1. *Cancer Res* 55:5605–5609.

Cheng L, Al-Kaisi NK, Liu AY, Gordon NH. (1997) The results of intraoperative consultations in 181 ductal carcinomas *in situ* of the breast. *Cancer* 80:75–79.

Ciatto S, Bonardi R, Cataliotti L, Cardona G. (1990) Intraductal breast carcinoma. Review of a multicenter series of 350 cases. *Tumori* 76:552–554.

Ciatto S, Cattallotti L, Cardona G, et al. (1992): Risk of infiltrating breast cancer subsequent to lobular carcinoma *in situ. Tumori* 78:244–246.

Crissman JD, Visscher DW, Kubus J. (1990) Image cytophotometric DNA analysis of atypical hyperplasias and intraductal carcinomas of the breast. *Arch Pathol Lab Med* 114:1239–1253.

Cutuli B, Dilhuydy JM, De Lafontan B, Berlie J, et al. (1997) Ductal carcinoma *in situ* of the male breast. Analysis of 31 cases [see comments]. *Eur J Cancer* 33:35–38.

Dall'Olmo CA, Ponka JL, Horn RC Jr, Riu R. (1975) Lobular carcinoma of the breast *in situ.* Are we too radical in its treatment? *Arch Surg* 110:537–542.

Davidoff AM, Kerns, B-JM, Iglehart JD, Marks JR. (1991a) Maintenance of p53 alterations throughout breast cancer progression. *Cancer Res* 51:2605–2610.

Davidoff AM, Kerns B-JM, Pence JC, et al. (1991b) p53 alterations in all stages of breast cancer. *J Surg Oncol* 48:260–267.

Dawson PJ, Baekey PA, Clark RA. (1995) Mechanisms of multifocal breast carcinoma: an immunocytochemical study. *Hum Pathol* 26:965–969.

De Leeuw WJ, Berx G, Vos CB, Peterse JL, van de Vijver MJ, Litvinov S, Van Roy F, Cornelisse CJ, Cleton-Jansen AM. (1997) Simultaneous loss of E-cadherin and catenins in invasive lobular breast cancer and lobular carcinoma *in situ. J Pathol* 183:404–411.

De Potter CR, Foschini MP, Schelfhout A-M, et al. (1993) Immunohistochemical study of neu protein overexpression in clinging *in situ* duct carcinoma of the breast. *Virchows Arch A Pathol Anat Histopathol* 422:375–380.

De Potter CR, Schelfhout A-M, Verbeeck P, et al. (1995) neu overexpression correlates with extent of disease in large cell ductal carcinoma *in situ* of the breast. *Hum Pathol* 6: 601–606.

Done SJ, Arneson NCR, Ozcelik H, et al. (1998) p53 mutations in mammary ductal carcinoma *in situ* but not in epithelial hyperplasias. *Cancer Res* 58:785–789.

Done SJ, Kneafsey P, Alexander F, Miller AB. (1996) Nuclear grading and necrosis in DCIS in the National Breast Cancer Screening Study. Use of a histologic scoring system to predict outcome in patients. *Mod Pathol* 9:17A.

Donegan WL, Perez-Mesa CM. (1972) Lobular carcinoma: an indication for elective biopsy of the second breast. *Ann Surg* 176:178–187.

Douglas-Jones AG, Gupta SK, Attanoos RL, et al. (1996) A critical appraisal of six modern classifications of ductal carcinoma *in situ* of the breast (DCIS): correlation with grade of associated invasive carcinoma. *Histopathology* 29:397–409.

Douglas-Jones AG, Navabi H, Morgan JM, Jasani B. (1997) Immunoreactive p53 and metallothionein expression in duct carcinoma *in situ* of the breast. *Virchows Arch* 430:373–379.

Douglas-Jones AG, Schmid KW, Bier B, Horgan K, et al. (1995) Metallothionein expression in duct carcinoma *in situ* of the breast. *Hum Pathol* 26:217–222.

Dupont WD, Page DL. (1985) Risk factors for breast cancer in women with proliferative breast disease. *N Engl J Med* 312:146–151.

Dupont W, Parl F, Hartmann W, Brinton L, Winfield A, Worrell J, Schuyler P, Plummer W. (1993) Breast cancer risk associated with proliferative breast disease and atypical hyperplasia. *Cancer* 71:1258–1265.

Elston C. (1984) The assessment of histological grade in breast cancer. *Aust N Z J Surg* 54:11–15.

Elston C, Ellis I. (1991) Pathological prognostic factors in breast cancer. I. The value of histological grade in breast cancer: experience from a large study with long-term follow-up. *Histopathology* 19:403–410.

Elston C, Gresham G, Rao G, et al. (1982) The cancer research campaign (Kings Cambridge) trial for early breast cancer—pathological aspects. *Br J Cancer* 45: 655–669.

Ernster V, Barclay J, Kerlikowske K, Grady D, Henderson I. (1996) Incidence of and treatment for ductal carcinoma *in situ* of the breast. *JAMA* 275:913–918.

Eusebi V, Feudale E, Foschini M, Micheli A, Conti A, Riva C, Di Palma S, Rilke F. (1994) Long-term follow-up of *in situ* carcinoma of the breast. *Semin Diagn Pathol* 11:223–235.

Eusebi V, Collina G, Bussolati G. (1989a) Carcinoma *in situ* in sclerosing adenosis of the breast: an immunocytochemical study. *Semin Diagn Pathol* 6:146–152.

Eusebi V, Foschini M, Cook M, et al. (1989b) Long-term follow up of *in situ* carcinoma of the breast with special emphasis on clinging carcinoma. *Semin Diagn Pathol* 6:165–173.

Eusebi V, Pich A, Macchiorlatti E, Bussolati G. (1977) Morpho-functional differentiation in lobular carcinoma of the breast. *Histopathology* 1:307–314.

Ewertz M, Holmberg L, Karjalainen S, Tretli S, Adami HO. (1989) Incidence of male breast cancer in Scandinavia, 1943–1982. *Int J Cancer* 43(1):27–31.

Fechner RE. (1971) Ductal carcinoma involving the lobule of the breast. A source of confusion with lobular carcinoma *in situ. Cancer* 28:274–281.

Fechner RE. (1972) Epithelial alterations in the extralobular ducts of breasts with lobular carcinoma. *Arch Pathol* 93:164–171.

Fechner RE. (1981) Lobular carcinoma *in situ* in sclerosing adenosis. A potential source of confusion with invasive carcinoma. *Am J Surg Pathol* 5:233–239.

Fechner RE. (1996) Letters to the Editor: Breast frozen sections. *Am J Surg Pathol* 20(10):1296–1297.

Fisher B. (1979) Breast-cancer management: alternatives to radical mastectomy. *N Engl J Med* 301: 326–328.

Fisher ER, Fisher B. (1977) Lobular carcinoma of the breast: an overview. *Ann Surg* 85:377–385.

Fisher ER, Constantino J, Fisher B, Palekar AS, et al. (1996) Pathologic findings from the National Surgical Adjuvant Breast Project (NSABP) protocol B-17. Five year observations concerning lobular carcinoma *in situ. Cancer* 78:1403–1416.

Fletcher R, Fletcher S, Wagner E, eds. (1982) *Clinical Epidemiology—The Essentials.* Williams & Wilkins, Baltimore.

Foote FW, Stewart FW. (1941) Lobular carcinoma *in situ*: a rare form of mammary cancer. *Am J Pathol* 17:491–495.

Foote FW, Stewart FW. (1945) Comparative studies of cancerous versus non-cancerous breasts. *Ann Surg* 121:6–53

Foschini MP, Fornelli A, Peterse JL, et al. (1996) Microcalcifications in ductal carcinoma *in situ* of the breast: histochemical and immunohistochemical study. *Hum Pathol* 27:178–183.

Fowble B, Hanlon AL, Fein DA, et al. (1997) Results of conservative surgery and radiation for mammographically detected ductal carcinoma *in situ* (DCIS). *Int J Radiat Oncol Biol Phys* 38:949–957.

Fromowitz F, Viola M, Chao S, et al. (1987) ras p21 expression in the progression of breast cancer. *Hum Pathol* 18:1268–1275.

Fujii H, Marsh C, Cairns P, Sidransky D, et al. (1996) Genetic divergence in the clonal evolution of breast cancer. *Cancer Res* 56:1493–1497.

Gad A, Azzopardi JG. (1975) Lobular carcinoma of the breast: a special variant of mucin-secreting carcinoma. *J Clin Pathol* 28:711–716.

Garfinkel L. (1993) Current trends in breast cancer. *CA Cancer J Clin* 43:5–6.

Gillis DA, Dockerty MB, Clagett OT. (1960) Preinvasive intraductal carcinoma of the breast. *Surg Gynecol Obstet* 110:555–562.

Gimbrone M, Cotran R, Leapman S, Folkman J. (1974) Tumor growth and neovascularization: an experimental model using the rabbit cornea. *J Natl Cancer Inst* 52:413–427.

Gimbrone M, Leapman S, Cotran R, Folkman J. (1972) Tumor dormancy *in vivo* by prevention of neovascularization. *J Exp Med* 136:261–276.

Giordano JM, Klopp CT. (1973) Lobular carcinoma *in situ*: incidence and treatment. *Cancer* 31:105–109.

Giri DD, Dundas SAC, Nottingham JF, Underwood JCE. (1989) Oestrogen receptors in benign epithelial lesions and intraduct carcinomas of the breast: an immunohistochemical study. *Histopathology* 15:575–584.

Godwin JT. (1952) Chronology of lobular carcinoma in the breast. Report of a case. *Cancer* 5:259–266.

Goldstein NS, Murphy T. (1996) Intraductal carcinoma associated with invasive carcinoma of the breast: a comparison of the two lesions with implications for intraductal carcinoma classification systems. *Am J Clin Pathol* 106:312–318.

Griffin A, Frazee RC. (1993) Treatment of intraductal breast cancer—noncomedo type. *Am Surg* 59:106–109.

Guerry P, Erlandson RA, Rosen PP. (1988) Cystic hypersecretory hyperplasia and cystic hypersecretory duct carcinoma of the breast: pathology, therapy, and follow-up of 39 patients. *Cancer* 61:1611–1620.

Guidi AJ, Fischer L, Harris JR, Schnitt SJ. (1994) Microvessel density and distribution in ductal carcinoma *in situ* of the breast. *J Natl Cancer Inst* 86:614–619.

Gump FE. (1990) Lobular carcinoma *in situ*. Pathology and treatment. Breast cancer: strategies for 1990's. *Surg Clin North Am* 70:873–883.

Gusterson B, Machin L, Gullick W, Gibbs N, Powles T, Elliott C, Ashley S, Monaghan P, Harrison S. (1988b) c-erbB-2 expression in benign and malignant breast disease. *Br J Cancer* 58:453–457.

Gusterson B, Machin L, Gullick W, Gibbs N, Powles T, Price P, McKinna A, Harrison S. (1988) Immunohistochemical distribution of c-erbB-2 in infiltrating and *in situ* breast cancer. *Int J Cancer* 42:842–845.

Haagensen CD. (1986) *Diseases of the Breast*, 3rd ed, pp. 118–124, 192–249. W.B. Saunders, Philadelphia.

Haagensen CD, Lane N, Bodian C. (1983) Coexisting lobular neoplasia and carcinoma of the breast. *Cancer* 51:1468–1482.

Haagensen CD, Lane N, Lattes R. (1972) Neoplastic proliferation of the epithelium of the mammary lobules: adenosis, lobular neoplasia, and small cell carcinoma. *Surg Clin North Am* 52:497–524.

Haagensen CD, Lane N, Lattes R, Bodian C. (1978) Lobular neoplasia (so-called lobular carcinoma *in situ*) of the breast. *Cancer* 42:737–769.

Harrison M, Coyne JD, Gorey T, Dervan PA. (1996) Comparison of cytomorphological and architectural heterogeneity in mammographically detected ductal carcinoma *in situ*. *Histopathology* 28:445–450.

Helin HJ, Helle MJ, Kallioniemi O-P, Isola JJ. (1989) Immunohistochemical determination of estrogen and progesterone receptors in human breast carcinoma: correlation with histopathology and DNA flow cytometry. *Cancer* 63:1761–1767.

Hiramatsu H, Bornstein VA, Recht A, et al. (1995) Local recurrence after conservative surgery and radiation therapy for ductal carcinoma *in situ*. Possible importance of family history. *Cancer J Sci Am* 1:55–61.

Hittmair AP, Lininger RA, Tavassoli FA. (1998) Ductal carcinoma *in situ* (DCIS) in the male breast: morphologic study of 94 cases of pure DCIS and 30 cases of DCIS associated with invasive carcinoma. *Cancer* 83:2139–2149.

Holland PA, Knox WF, Potten CS, et al. (1997) Assessment of hormone dependence of comedo ductal carcinoma *in situ* of the breast. *J Natl Cancer Inst* 89:1059–1065.

Holland R, Hendriks J, Verbeek A, Mravunac M, Schuurmans Stekhoven J. (1990) Extent, distribution, and mammographic/histological correlations of breast ductal carcinoma *in situ*. *Lancet* 335:519–522.

Holland R, Peterse J, Millis R, et al. (1994) Ductal carcinoma *in situ*: a proposal for a new classification. *Semin Diagn Pathol* 11:167–180.

Holland R, Veling S, Mravunac M, Hendriks J. (1985) Histologic multifocality of Tis, T1–2 breast carcinomas: implications for clinical trials of breast conserving treatment. *Cancer* 56:979–990.

Hutchinson W, Thomas D, Hamlin W, Roth G, Peterson A, Williams B. (1980) Risk of breast cancer in women with benign breast disease. *J Natl Cancer Inst* 65:13–20.

Hutter RVP. (1984) The management of patients with lobular carcinoma *in situ* of the breast. *Cancer* 53:798–802.

Hutter RVP, et al. (1986) Consensus meeting. Is "fibrocystic disease" of the breast precancerous? *Arch Pathol Lab Med* 110:171–173.

Hutter RVP, Foote FW. (1969) Lobular carcinoma *in situ*: long-term follow-up. *Cancer* 24:1081–1085.

Hutter RVP, Foote FW Jr, Farrow JH. (1968) *In situ* lobular carcinoma of the female breast 1939–1968. In: *Breast Cancer—Early and Late*. pp. 201–226. Year Book, Chicago.

Ichihara S, Aomaya H. (1994) Intraductal carcinoma of the breast arising in sclerosing adenosis. *Pathol Int* 44:722–726.

Ichihara S, Koshikawa T, Nakamura S, et al. (1997) Epithelial hyperplasia of usual type expresses both S100-alpha and S100-beta in a heterogeneous pattern but ductal carcinoma *in situ* can express only S100-alpha in a monotonous pattern. *Histopathology* 30:533–541.

Jacquemier J, Hassoun J, Torrente M, Martin P. (1990) Distribution of estrogen and progesterone receptors in healthy tissue adjacent to breast lesions at various stages—immunohistochemical study of 107 cases. *Breast Cancer Res Treat* 15:109–117.

Kapucuoglu N, Losi L, Eusebi V. (1997) Immunohistochemical localization of Bcl-2 and Bax proteins in *in situ* and invasive duct breast carcinomas. *Virchows Arch* 430:17–22.

Karpas C, Leis H, Oppenheim A, Mersheimer W. (1965) Relationship of fibrocystic disease to carcinoma of the breast. *Ann Surg* 162:1–8.

Kasami M, Vnencak-Jones CL, Manning S, et al. (1997) Loss of heterozygosity and microsatellite instability in breast hyperplasia. No obligate correlation of these genetic alterations with subsequent malignancy. *Am J Pathol* 150:1925–1932.

Kerlikowske K, Barclay J, Grady D, et al. (1997) Comparison of risk factors for ductal carcinoma *in situ* and invasive breast cancer. *J Natl Cancer Inst* 89:76–82.

Kern W, Brooks R. (1969) Atypical epithelial hyperplasia associated with breast cancer and fibrocystic disease. *Cancer* 24:668–675.

Killeen J, Namiki H. (1991) DNA analysis of ductal carcinoma *in situ* of the breast. *Cancer* 68:2602–2607.

King JM. (1994) A practical approach to breast ductal carcinoma *in situ* and tumors with an extensive intraductal component. *Pathology* 26:90–93.

Klijn JGM, Berns PMJJ, Schmitz PIM, Foekens JA. (1972) The clinical significance of epidermal growth factor receptor (EGFR) in human breast cancer: a review on 5232 patients. *Endocr Rev* 13:3–17.

Kodlin D, Winger E, Morgenstern R. (1977) Chronic mastopathy and breast cancer: a follow-up study. *Cancer* 39:2603–2607.

Kouchoukos NT, Ackerman LV, Butcher HR Jr. (1967) Prediction of axillary nodal metastases from the morphology of primary mammary carcinomas. *Cancer* 20:948–960.

Kramer WM, Rush BF Jr. (1973) Mammary duct proliferation in the elderly. *Cancer* 31:130–137.

Lagios MD, Margolin FR, Westdahl PR, Rose MR. (1989) Mammographically detected duct carcinoma *in situ*. Frequency of local recurrence following tylectomy and prognostic effect of nuclear grade on local recurrence. *Cancer* 63:618–624.

Lagios MD, Westdahl PR, Margolin FR, Rose MR. (1982) Duct carcinoma *in situ*: relationship of extent of noninvasive disease to the frequency of occult invasion, multicentricity, lymph node metastases, and short term treatment failures. *Cancer* 50:1309–1314.

Lakhani SR, Collins N, Stratton MR. (1995a) Loss of heterozygosity in lobular carcinoma *in situ* of the breast. *J Clin Pathol Mol Pathol* 48:M74–M78.

Lakhani S, Collins N, Stratton M, Sloane J. (1995b) Atypical ductal hyperplasia of the breast: clonal proliferation exhibiting loss of heterozygosity on chromosomes 16q and 17p. *J Clin Pathol* 48:611–615.

Lakhani S, Slack D, Hamoudi R, Collins N, Stratton M, Sloane J. (1996) Detection of allelic imbalance indicates that a proportion of mammary hyperplasia of usual type are clonal, neoplastic proliferations. *Lab Invest* 74:129–135.

Lambird PA, Shelley WM. (1969) The spatial distribution of lobular *in situ* mammary carcinoma. Implications for size and site of breast biopsy. *JAMA* 210:689–693.

Landis SH, Murray T, Bolden S, Wingo PA. (1998) Cancer statistics, 1998. *CA Cancer J Clin* 48:6–29.

Lattes R. (1980) Lobular neoplasia (lobular carcinoma *in situ*) of the breast: a histological entity of controversial clinical significance [review article]. *Pathol Res Pract* 166:415–429.

Leal CB, Schmitt FC, Bento MJ, et al. (1995) Ductal carcinoma *in situ* of the breast: histologic categorization and its relation to ploidy and immunohistochemical expression of hormone receptors, p53, and c-erbB-2 protein. *Cancer* 75:2123–2131.

Lewison EF, Finney GG Jr. (1968) Lobular carcinoma *in situ* of the breast. *Surg Gynecol Obstet* 126:1280–1286.

Lininger RA, Fujii H, Man YG, Gabrielson E, Tavassoli FA. (1998) Comparison of loss of heterozygosity in primary and recurrent intraductal carcinoma of the breast. *Mod Pathol* 11:1151–1159.

Lininger RA, Tavassoli FA. (1997) Atypical intraductal hyperplasia of the breast. In: *Ductal Carcinoma In Situ* (Silverstein MJ, ed.) pp. 195–222. Williams and Wilkins, Baltimore.

Liu E, Thor A, He M, et al. (1992) The *HER2* (c-*erb*B-2) oncogene is frequently amplified in *in situ* carcinomas of the breast. *Oncogene* 7:1027–1032.

Locker AP, Horrock C, Gilmour AS, et al. (1990) Flow cytometric and histological analysis of ductal carcinoma *in situ* of the brest. *Br J Surg* 77:564–567.

Lodato RF, Maguire HC Jr. (1990) Immunohistochemical evaluation of c-*erb*B-2 oncogene expression in ductal carcinoma *in situ* and atypical ductal hyperplasia of the breast. *Mod Pathol* 3:449–453.

London SJ, Connolly JL, Schnitt SJ, Colditz GA. (1992) A prospective study of benign breast disease and the risk of breast cancer. *JAMA* 267:941–944.

Lu YJ, Osin P, Lakhani SR, Di Palma S, Gusterson BA, Shipley JM. (1998) Comparative genomic hybridization analysis of lobular carcinoma *in situ* and atypical lobular hyperplasia and potential roles for gains and losses of genetic material in breast neoplasia. *Cancer Res* 58:4721–4727.

Ma L, Boyd N. (1992) Atypical hyperplasia and breast cancer risk: a critique. *Cancer Causes Control* 3:517–525.

Malmusi M, Ackerman AB. (1998) Apoptosis is a type of necrosis 1. Part I. The importance of historical perspective and definition. *Dermatopathol Pract Concepts* 4:15–27.

Man S, Ellis IO, Sibbering M, et al. (1996) High levels of allele loss at the FHIT and ATM genes in noncomedo ductal carcinoma *in situ* and grade 1 tubular invasive breast cancers. *Cancer Res* 56:5484–5489.

Margolin F, Lagios M. (1986) Mammographic detection of early breast cancer; ten years experience in a community hospital. *West J Med* 144:46–48.

Marshall LM, Hunter DJ, Connolly JL, Schnitt SJ, Byrne C, London SJ, Colditz GA. (1997) Risk of breast cancer associated with atypical hyperplasia of lobular and ductal types. *Cancer Epidemiol Biomarkers Prev* 6:297–301.

Mayr NA, Staples JJ, Robinson RA, Vanmetre JE, Hussey DH. (1991) Morphometric studies in intraductal breast carcinoma using computerized image analysis. *Cancer* 67:2805–2812.

McDivitt RW, Hutter RVP, Foote FW Jr, Stewart FW. (1967) *In Situ* lobular carcinoma: a prospective follow-up study indicating cumulative patient risks. *JAMA* 201:82–86.

McDivitt R, Stevens J, Lee N, Wingo P, Rubin G, Gersell D, and the Cancer and Steroid Hormone Study Group. (1992) Histologic types of benign breast disease and the risk for breast cancer. *Cancer* 69: 1408–1414.

McDivitt RW, Stewart FW, Berg JW. (1968) *Tumors of the Breast. Atlas of Tumor Pathology*, 2nd Series, Fascicle 2. Armed Forces Institute of Pathology, Washington, DC.

Meyer J. (1986) Cell kinetics of histologic variants of *in situ* breast carcinoma. *Breast Cancer Res Treat* 7:171–180.

Merino MJ, LiVolsi VA. (1981) Signet ring carcinoma of the female breast: a clinicopathologic analysis of 24 cases. *Cancer* 48:1830–1837.

Millis RR, Bobrow LG, Barnes DM. (1996) Immunohistochemical evaluation of biological markers in mammary carcinoma *in situ*: correlation with morphological features and recently proposed schemes for histological classification. *The Breast* 5: 113–122.

Millis RR, Thynne GSJ. (1975) *In Situ* intraduct carcinoma of the breast: a long term follow-up study. *Br J Surg* 62:957–962.

Moinfar F, Man YG, Lininger RA, Tavassoli FA. (1999) Use of keratin 34BE12 as an adjunct in the diagnosis of mammary intraepithelial neoplasia—ductal type (benign and malignant intraductal) proliferations of the breast. *Am J Surg Pathol* 23:1048–1058.

Moinfar F, Man YG, Bratthauer G, Tavassoli FA. (1999) Genetic abnormalities in ductal intraepithelial neoplasia—flat type ("clinging carcinoma *in situ*") of the breast. *Mod Pathol* (in press).

Moriya T, Silverberg SG. (1994) Intraductal carcinoma (ductal carcinoma *in situ*) of the breast (A comparison of pure noninvasive tumors with those including differential proportions of infiltrating carcinoma). *Cancer* 74:2972–2978.

Moriya T, Silverberg SG. (1995) Intraductal carcinoma (ductal carcinoma *in situ*) of the breast. (Analysis of pathologic findings of 85 pure intraductal carcinomas). *Int J Surg Pathol* 3:83–92.

Moskowitz M, Gartside P, Wirman J, McLaughlin C. (1980) Proliferative disorders of the breast as risk factors for breast cancer in a self-selected screened population: pathologic markers. *Radiology* 134:289–291.

Munn KE, Walker RA, Menasce L, Varley JM. (1996) Allelic imbalance in the region of the *BRCA1* gene in ductal carcinoma *in situ* of the breast. *Br J Cancer* 73:636–639.

Munn KE, Walker RA, Varley JM. (1995) Frequent alterations of chromosome 1 in ductal carcinoma *in situ* of the breast. *Oncogene* 10:1652–1657.

Mustonen M, Raunio H, Paakko P, Soini Y. (1997) The extent of apoptosis is inversely associated with bcl-2 expression in premalignant and malignant breast lesions. *Histopathology* 31:347–354.

Nayar R, Zhuang Z, Merino MJ, Silverberg SG. (1997) Loss of heterozygosity on chromosome 11q13 in lobular lesions of the breast using tissue microdissection and polymerase chain reaction. *Hum Pathol* 28: 277–282.

Nesland JM, Holm R, Johannessen JV. (1985) Ultrastructural and immunohistochemical features of lobular carcinoma of the breast. *J Pathol* 145:39–52.

Newman P. (1990) Breast cancer incidence is on the rise—but why? *J Natl Cancer Inst* 82:998–1000.

Newman W. (1963) *in situ* lobular carcinoma of the breast. Report of 26 women with 32 cancers. *Ann Surg* 157:591–599.

Newman W. (1966) Lobular carcinoma of the breast. Report of 73 cases. *Ann Surg* 164:305–314.

Nielsen M, Jensen J, Andersen J. (1984) Precancerous and cancerous breast lesions during lifetime and at autopsy. A study of 83 women. *Cancer* 54:612–615.

Nielsen M, Thomsen J, Primdahl S, Dyreborg U, Andersen J. (1987) Breast cancer and atypia among young and middle-aged women: a study of 110 medicolegal autopsies. *Br J Cancer* 56:814–819.

Noguchi S, Aihara T, Koyama H, et al. (1994a) Discrimination between multicentric and multifocal carcinoma of the breast through clonal analysis. *Cancer* 74:872–877.

Noguchi S, Motomura K, Inaji H, et al. (1994b) Clonal analysis of predominantly intraductal carcinoma and precancerous lesions of the breast by means of polymerase chain reaction. *Cancer Res* 54:1849–1853.

O'Connell P, Pekkel V, Fuqua S, et al. (1994) Molecular genetic studies of early breast cancer evolution. *Br Cancer Res Treat* 32:5–12.

Ohtake T, Abe R, Kimijima I, et al. (1995) Intraductal extension of primary invasive breast carcinoma treated by breast conserving surgery: computer graphic three dimensional reconstruction of the mammary duct lobular systems. *Cancer* 76:32–45.

Ohuchi N, Furuta A, Mori S. (1994) Management of ductal carcinoma *in situ* with nipple discharge: Intraductal spreading of carcinoma is an unfavorable pathologic factor for breast-conserving surgery. *Cancer* 74:1294–1302.

Ottesen G, Graversen H, Blichert-Toft M, Zedeler K, Andersen J, on behalf of the Danish Breast Cancer Cooperative Group. (1992) Ductal carcinoma *in situ* of the female breast: short-term results of a prospective nationwide study. *Am J Surg Pathol* 16: 1183–1196.

Ottessen GL, Graversen HP, Blichert-Toft M, Zedeler K, et al. (1993) Lobular carcinoma *in situ* of the female breast: short-term results of a prospective nationwide study. *Am J Surg Pathol* 17:14–21.

Ozaki D, Kondo Y. (1995) Comparative morphometric studies of benign and malignant intraductal proliferative lesions of the breast by computerized image analysis. *Hum Pathol* 26:1109–1113.

Ozzello L. (1971) Ultrastructure of intra-epithelial carcinomas of the breast. *Cancer* 25:1508–1515

Page DL. (1986) Cancer risk assessment in benign breast biopsies. *Hum Pathol* 17:871–874.

Page DL, Anderson TJ, Rogers LW. (1988) Epithelial hyperplasia. In: *Diagnostic Histopathology of the Breast* (Page DL, Anderson TJ, eds.) pp. 145–156; 174–184. Churchill Livingstone, Edinburgh.

Page DL, Dupont WD. (1990) Anatomic markers of human premalignancy and risk of breast cancer. *Cancer* 66:1326–1335.

Page DL, Dupont WD, Rogers LW, Rados MS. (1985) Atypical hyperplastic lesions of the female breast: a long term follow-up study. *Cancer* 55:2698–2708.

Page DL, Kidd TE, Dupont WD, Simpson JF, Rogers LW. (1991) Lobular neoplasia of the breast: higher risk for subsequent invasive cancer predicted by more extensive disease. *Hum Pathol* 22:1232–1239.

Page D, Vander Zwaag R, Rogers L, et al. (1978) Relation between component parts of fibrocystic disease complex and breast cancer. *J Natl Cancer Inst* 61: 1055–1063.

Palazzo J, Hyslop T. (1996) Non-invasive proliferative breast lesions: reproducibility of current diagnostic criteria among community and academic based pathologists. *The Breast Journal* 4:XXX–XXX.

Palli D, Del Turco M, Simoncini R, Bianchi S. (1991) Benign breast disease and breast cancer: a case–control study in a cohort in Italy. *Int J Cancer* 47: 703–706.

Pallis L, Skoog L, Falkmer U, Wilking N, et al. (1992b) The DNA profile of breast cancer *in situ*. *Eur J Surg Oncol* 18:108–111.

Pallis L, Wilking N, Cedermark B, et al. (1992a) Receptors for estrogen and progesterone in breast carcinoma *in situ*. *Anticancer Res* 12:2113–2116.

Peyrol S, Raccurt M, Gerard F, Gleyzal C, et al. (1997) Lysyl oxidase gene expression in the stromal reaction to *in situ* and invasive ductal breast carcinoma. *Am J Pathol* 150:497–506.

Poller D, Roberts J, Bell R, Elston C, Blamey R, Ellis I. (1993a) p53 protein expression in mammary ductal carcinoma *in situ*: relationship to immunohistochemical expression of estrogen receptor and c-erbB-2 protein. *Hum Pathol* 24:463–468.

Poller D, Silverstein M, Galea M, et al. (1994) Ductal carcinoma *in situ* of the breast: a proposal for a new simplified histological classification association between cellular proliferation and c-erbB-2 protein expression. *Mod Pathol* 7:257–262.

Poller D, Snead D, Roberts E, Galea M, Bell J, Gilmour A, Elston C, Blamey R, Ellis I. (1993b) Oestrogen receptor expression in ductal carcinoma *in situ* of the breast: relationship to flow cytometric analysis of DNA and expression of the c-erbB-2 oncoprotein. *Br J Cancer* 68:156–161.

Porter PL, Garcia R, Moe R, Corwin DJ, et al. (1991) C-erbB-2 oncogene protein in *in situ* and invasive lobular neoplasia. *Cancer* 68:331–334.

Powell RW, McSweeney MD, Wilson C. (1983) X-ray calcifications as the only basis for breast biopsy. *Ann Surg* 197:555–559.

Quinn CM, Ostrowski JL, Parkin GJS, et al. (1997) Ductal carcinoma *in situ* of the breast: the clinical significance of histological classification. *Histopathology* 30:113–119.

Radford DM, Fair K, Thompson AM, et al. (1993) Allelic loss on chromosome 17 in ductal carcinoma *in situ* of the breast. *Cancer Res* 53:2947–250.

Rajan PB, Scott DJ, Perry RH, Griffith DM. (1997) p53 protein expression in ductal carcinoma *in situ* (DCIS) of the breast. *Br Cancer Res Treat* 42:283–290.

Ramachandra S, Machin L, Ashley S, et al. (1990) Immunohistochemical distribution of c-erbB-2 in *in situ* breast carcinoma—a detailed morphological analysis. *J Pathol* 161:7–14.

Rasbridge SA, Millis RR. (1995) Carcinoma *in situ* involving sclerosing adenosis: a mimic of invasive breast carcinoma. *Histopathology* 27:269–273.

Ringberg A, Palmer B, Linnell F. (1982) The contralateral breast at reconstructive surgery after breast cancer operation—a histological study. *Breast Cancer Res Treat* 2:151–161.

Rosai J. (1991) Borderline epithelial lesions of the breast. *Am J Surg Pathol* 15:209–221.

Rosen PP. (1980a) Axillary lymph node metastases in patients with occult noninvasive breast carcinoma. *Cancer* 46:1298–1306.

Rosen PP. (1980b) Coexistent lobular carcinoma *in situ* and intraductal carcinoma in a single lobular-duct unit. *Am J Surg Pathol* 4:241–246.

Rosen PP. (1980c) Lobular carcinoma *in situ*: recent clinicopathologic studies at Memorial Hospital. *Pathol Res Pract* 166:430–455.

Rosen PP. (1987) The pathology of breast carcinoma. In: *Breast Diseases* (Harris JR, Hellman S, Henderson IC, eds.) p 149. J.B. Lippincott, Philadelphia.

Rosen P. (1991) Letter to the editor: "borderline" breast lesions. *Am J Surg Pathol* 15:1100–1102.

Rosen PP, Braun DW, Lyngholm B, Urban JA, Kinne DW. (1981) Lobular carcinoma *in situ* of the breast: preliminary results of treatment by ipsilateral mastectomy and contralateral breast biopsy. *Cancer* 47: 813–819.

Rosen PP, Brown DW, Kinne DE. (1980) The clinical significance of preinvasive breast breast carcinoma. *Cancer* 46:919–925.

Rosen PP, Lieberman PH, Braun DW Jr, Kosloff C, Adair F. (1978) Lobular carcinoma *in situ* of the breast: detailed analysis of 99 patients with average follow-up of 24 years. *Am J Surg Pathol* 2:225–251.

Rosen PP, Scott M. (1984) Cystic hypersecretory duct carcinoma of the breast. *Am J Surg Pathol* 8:31–41.

Rosen PP, Senie R, Schottenfeld D, et al. (1979) Non-invasive breast carcinoma. Frequency of unsuspected invasion and implications for treatment. *Ann Surg* 189:377–382.

Rosner D, Bedwani RN, Vana J, Baker HW, Murphy GP. (1980) Non-invasive breast carcinoma. Results of a national survey by the American College of Surgeons. *Ann Surg* 192:139–147.

Royds JA, Stephenson TJ, Rees RC, Shorthouse AJ, et al. (1993) Protein expression in ductal *in situ* and invasive human breast carcinoma. *J Natl Cancer Inst* 85:727–731.

Rubin E, Visscher D, Alexander R, Urist M, Maddox W. (1988) Proliferative disease and atypia in biopsies performed for nonpalpable lesions detected mammographically. *Cancer* 61:2077–2082.

Ryan J, Coady C. (1962) Intraductal epithelial proliferation in the human breast—a comparative study. *Can J Surg* 5:12–19.

Salvadori B, Bartoli C, Zurrida S, et al. (1991) Risk of invasive cancer in women with lobular carcinoma *in situ* of the breast. *Eur J Cancer* 27:35–37.

Satallof DM, Russin VI, Sohn M, Seinige UL. (1993) DNA flow cytometric analysis in ductal carcinoma *in situ* of the breast. *Breast Dis* 6:195–205.

Schmitt FC, Leal C, Lopes C. (1995) p53 protein expression and nuclear DNA content in breast intraductal proliferations. *J Pathol* 176:223–241.

Schnitt S, Connolly J, Tavassoli F, Fechner R, Kempson R, Gelman R, Page D. (1992) Interobserver reproducibility in the diagnosis of ductal proliferative breast lesions using standardized criteria. *Am J Surg Pathol* 16:1133–1143.

Schnitt SJ, Silen W, Sadowsky NL, Connolly JL, Harris JR. (1988) Current concepts: ductal carcinoma *in situ* (intraductal carcinoma of the breast). *N Engl J Med* 318:898–903.

Schuh ME, Nemoto R, Penetrante RB, et al. (1986) Intraductal carcinoma. Analysis of presentation, pathologic findings, and outcome of disease. *Arch Surg* 121:1303–1307.

Schwartz GF, Lagios MD, Carter D, et al. (1997) Consensus conference on the classification of ductal carcinoma *in situ. Cancer* 80:1798–1802.

Schwartz GF, Patchefsky AS, Feig SA, et al. (1980) Clinically occult breast cancer: multicentricity and implications for treatment. *Ann Surg* 91:8112.

Schwartz GF, Patchefsky AS, Finkelstein SD, Sohn SH, et al. (1989) Nonpalpable *in situ* ductal carcinoma of the breast. Predictors of multicentricity and microinvasion and implications for treatment. *Arch Surg* 124:29–32.

Scott MA, Lagios MD, Axelsson K, et al. (1997) Ductal carcinoma *in situ* of the breast: reproducibility of histological subtype analysis. *Hum Pathol* 28:967–973.

Seidman JD, Ashton M, Lefkowitz M. (1996) Atypical apocrine adenosis of the breast: a clinicopathologic study of 37 patients with 8.7–year follow-up. *Cancer* 77:2529–2537.

Sgroi D, Koerner FC. (1995) Involvement of collagenous spherulosis by lobular carcinoma *in situ*. Potential confusion with cribriform ductal carcinoma *in situ. Am J Surg Pathol* 19:1366–1370.

Silver SA, Tavassoli FA. (1998) Mammary ductal carcinoma *in situ* with microinvasion. *Cancer* 82:2382–2390.

Silverberg S, Chitale A. (1973) Assessment of significance of proportions of intraductal and infiltrating tumor growth in ductal carcinoma of the breast. *Cancer* 32:830–837.

Silverstein MJ. (1997) Van Nuys experience by treatment. In: *Ductal Carcinoma In Situ*. (Silverstein MJ, ed.) pp. 443–447. Williams and Wilkins, Baltimore.

Silverstein MJ, Barth A, Poller DN, et al. (1995a) Ten-year results comparing mastectomy to excision and radiation therapy for ductal carcinoma *in situ* of the breast. *Eur J Cancer* 31:1425–1427.

Silverstein MJ, Lagios MD, Craig PH, et al. (1996) A prognostic index for ductal carcinoma *in situ. Cancer* 77:2267–2274.

Silverstein MJ, Poller DN, Waisman JR, et al. (1995b) Prognostic classification of breast ductal carcinoma-*in-situ. Lancet* 345:1154–1157.

Silverstein MJ, Rosser RJ, Gierson ED, et al. (1988) Axillary lymph node dissection for intraductal carcinoma: is it indicated? *Cancer* 59:1819–1824.

Silverstein M, Gierson ED, Colburn Wj, et al. (1994) Can intraductal breast cancer be excised completely by local e-xcision? Clinical and pathologic predictors. *Cancer* 73:2985–2989.

Silverstein JJ, Waisman JR, Gamagami P, et al. (1990) Intraductal carcinoma of the breast (208 cases). Clinical factors influencing treatment choice. *Cancer* 66:102–108.

Singletary SE. (1994) Lobular carcinoma *in situ* of the breast: a 31 year experience at the University of Texas M.D. Anderson Cancer Center. *Breast Dis* 7:157–163.

Siziopikou KP, Prioleau JE, Harris JR, Schnitt SJ. (1996) bcl-2 expression in the spectrum of preinvasive breast lesions. *Cancer* 77:499–506.

Sloane JP, Amendoeira I, Apostolikas N, Bellocq JP, Bianchi S, Boecker W, Bussolati G, Coleman D, Connolly CE, Dervan P, Eusebi V, De Miguel C, Drijkoningen M, Elston CW, Faverley D, Gad A,

Jacquemier J, Lacerda M, Martinez-Penuela J, Munt C, Peterse JL, Rank F, Sylvan M, Tsakraklides V, Zafrani B. (1998) Consistency achieved by 23 European pathologists in categorizing ductal carcinoma *in situ* of the breast using five classifications. European Commission Working Group on Breast Screening Pathology. *Hum Pathol* 29:1056–1062.

Smart CR, Myers MH, Gloeckler LA. (1978) Implications from SEER data on breast cancer management. *Cancer* 41:787–789.

Smith H, Lu W, Beng G, et al. (1993) Molecular aspects of early stages of breast cancer progression. *J Cell Biochem* 176:144–152.

Snyder RE. (1966) Mammography and lobular carcinoma *in situ. Surg Gynecol Obstet* 122:255–260.

Solin LJ, Fowble BL, Yeh I-T, et al. (1992) Microinvasive ductal carcinoma of the breast treated with breast-conserving surgery and definitive irradiation. *Int J Radiat Oncol* 23:961–968.

Solin LJ, Kurtz J, Fourquet A, et al. (1996) Fifteen-year results of breast-conserving surgery and definitive breast irradiation for the treatment of ductal carcinoma *in situ* of the breast. *J Clin Oncol* 14:754–763.

Stratton MR, Collins N, Lakhani SR, Sloane JP. (1995) Loss of heterozygosity in ductal carcinoma *in situ* of the breast. *J Pathol* 175:195–201.

Sunshine JA, Moseley HS, Fletcher WS, Krippaehne WW. (1985) Breast carcinoma *in situ*: a retrospective review of 112 cases with a minimum 10 year follow-up. *Am J Surg* 150:44–51.

Symmans WF, Liu J, Knowles DM, Inghirami G. (1995) Breast cancer heterogeneity: evaluation of clonality in primary and metastatic lesions. *Hum Pathol* 26:210–216.

Tavassoli FA. (1998) Ductal carcinoma *in situ*: introduction of the concept of ductal intraepithelial neoplasia. *Mod Pathol* 11:140–154.

Tavassoli FA. (1999) *Pathology of the Breast*, 2nd ed. Appleton & Lange, Norwalk, CT.

Tavassoli F, Man Y. (1995) Morphofunctional features of intraductal hyperplasia, atypical intraductal hyperplasia, and various grades of intraductal carcinoma. *Breast J* 1:155–162.

Tavassoli FA, Norris HJ. (1990) A comparison of the results of long-term follow-up for atypical intraductal hyperplasia and intraductal hyperplasia of the breast. *Cancer* 65:518–529.

Tavassoli F, Norris H. (1994) Intraductal apocrine carcinoma: a clinicopathologic study of 37 cases. *Mod Pathol* 7:813–818.

Tavassoli FA, Pestaner JP. (1995) Pseudoinvasion in intraductal carcinoma. *Mod Pathol* 8:380–383.

Tavassoli FA, Purcell AP, Bratthauer GL, Man YG. (1996) Androgen receptor expression along with loss of bcl-2, ER, and PR expression in benign and malignant apocrine lesions of the breast: implication for therapy. *Breast J* 2:261–269.

Teixeira MR, Pandis N, Gerdes A-M, et al. (1996) Cytogenetic abnormalities in an *in situ* ductal carcinoma and five prophylactically removed breasts from members of a family with hereditary breast cancer. *Br Cancer Res Treat* 38:177–182.

Tellem M, Prive L, Meranze D. (1962) Four-quadrant study of breasts removed for carcinoma. *Cancer* 15:10–17.

Temple WJ, Lindsay RL, Magi E, Urbanski SJ. (1991) Technical considerations for prophylactic mastectomy in patients at high risk for breast cancer. *Am J Surg* 161(4):413–415.

Tham K-T, Dupont WD, Page DL, Gray GF Jr, Rogers LW. (1989) Micropapillary hyperplasia with atypical features in female breasts, resembling gynecomastia. *Prog Surg Pathol* 10:101–109.

Tobon H, Price HM. (1972) Lobular carcinoma *in situ*. *Cancer* 30:1082–1091.

Toker C, Goldberg JD. (1971) The small cell lesion of mammary ducts and lobules. *Pathol Annu* 12:217–249.

Tokunaga M, Land CE, Aoki Y, et al. (1993) Proliferative and nonproliferative breast disease in atomic bomb survivors. *Cancer* 72:1657–1665.

Tsutsumi Y, Naber S, DeLellis R, et al. (1990) neu oncogene protein and epidermal growth factor receptor are independently expressed in benign and malignant breast tissues. *Hum Pathol* 21:750–758.

Tulusan AH, Egger H, Ober KG. (1985) Lobular carcinoma *in situ* and its relation to invasive breast cancer. In: *Early Breast Cancer. Histopathology, Diagnosis, and Treatment* (Zander J, Baltzer J, eds.) pp. 48–51. Springer-Verlag, New York.

Umekita Y, Takasaki T, Yoshida H. (1994) Expression of p53 protein in benign epithelial hyperplasia, atypical ductal hyperplasia, non-invasive and invasive mammary carcinoma: an immunohistchemical study. *Virchows Archiv* 424:491–494.

Urban JA. (1967) Bilaterality of cancer of the breast—biopsy of the opposite breast. *Cancer* 20:1867–1870.

Urban JA. (1969) Biopsy of the "normal" breast in treating breast cancer. *Surg Clin North Am* 49:291–301.

Van Agthoven TV, Timmermans M, Foekens JA, et al. (1994) Differential expression of estrogen, progesterone, and epidermal growth factor receptors in normal, benign, and malignant human breast tissues using dual staining immunohistochemistry. *Am J Pathol* 144:1238–1246.

Van de Vijver MJ, Peterse JL, Mooi WJ, et al. (1988) neu-protein overexpression in breast cancer. Association with comedo-type ductal carcinoma *in situ* and limited prognostic value in stage II brest cancer. *N Engl J Med* 319:1239–1245.

Van Dongen JA, Fentiman IS, Harris JR, et al. (1989) *In situ* breast cancer: The EORTC consensus meeting. *Lancet* 2:25–27.

Visscher DW, Wallis TL, Crissman JD. (1996) Evaluation of chromosome aneuploidy in tissue sections of preinvasive breast carcinomas using interphase cytogenetics. *Cancer* 77:315–320.

Von Rueden DG, Wilson RE. (1984) Intraductal carcinoma of the breast. *Surg Gynecol Obstet* 158:105–111.

Vos CB, Cleton-Jansen AM, Berx G, de Leeuw WJ, ter Haar NT, van Roy F, Cornelisse CJ, Peterse JL, van de Vijver MJ. (1997) E-cadherin inactivation in lobular carcinoma *in situ* of the breast: an early event in tumorigenesis. *Br J Cancer* 76:1131–1133.

Ward BA, McKhann CF, Ravikumar TS. (1992) Ten-year follow-up of breast carcinoma *in situ* in Connecticut. *Arch Surg* 127:1392–1395.

Watson P, Safneck J, Le K, et al. (1993) Relationship of c-*myc* amplification to progression of breast cancer from *in situ* to invasive tumor and lymph node metastasis. *J Natl Cancer Inst* 85:902–907.

Webber BL, Heise H, Neifeld JP, Costa J. (1981) Risk of subsequent contralateral breast carcinoma in a population of patients with *in situ* carcinoma. *Cancer* 47:2928–2932.

Weidner N. (1995) Intratumor microvessel density as a prognostic factor in cancer. *Am J Pathol* 147:9–19.

Wellings SR, Jensen HM. (1973) On the origin and progression of ductal carcinoma in the human breast. *J Natl Cancer Inst* 50:1111–1118.

Wellings SR, Jensen HM, Marcum RG. (1975) An atlas of subgross pathology of the human breast with special reference to possible precancerous lesions. *J Natl Cancer Inst* 55:231–273.

Westbrook KC, Gallager HS. (1975) Intraductal carcinoma of the breast. A comparative study. *Am J Surg* 130:667–670.

Wheeler JE, Enterline HT. (1976) Lobular carcinoma of the breast, *in situ* and infiltrating. *Pathol Annu* 11:161–188.

Wheeler JE, Enterline HT, Roseman JM, et al. (1974) Lobular carcinoma *in situ*: long-term follow-up. *Cancer* 34:554–563.

Wilbur D, Barrows G. (1993) Estrogen and progesterone receptor and c-erbB-2 oncoprotein analysis in pure *in situ* breast carcinoma: an immunohistochemical study. *Mod Pathol* 6:114–120.

Yoshida Y, Takaoka M, Fukumoto M. (1985) Carcinoma arising in fibroadenoma: case report and review of the world literature. *J Surg Oncol* 29:132–140.

Zafrani B, Leroyer A, Fourquet A, et al. (1994) Mammographically detected ductal *in situ* carcinoma of the breast analyzed with a new classification. A study of 127 cases: correlation with estrogen and progesterone receptors, p53 and c-erbB-2 proteins, and proliferative activity. *Semin Diagn Pathol* 11:208–214.

Zhuang Z, Merino MJ, Chuaqui R, Liotta LA, et al. (1995) Identical allelic loss on chromosome 11q13 in microdissected *in situ* and invasive human breast cancer. *Cancer Res* 55:467–471.

Zurrida S, Bartoli C, Galimberti V, Raselli R, et al. (1996) Interpretation of the risk associated with unexpected finding of lobular carcinoma *in situ*. *Ann Surg Oncol* 3:57–61.

16

UTERINE CERVIX

Jorge Albores-Saavedra, Michael Gilcrease,
and Donald Earl Henson

A spectrum of premalignant lesions is known to occur in the uterine cervix before the development of invasive squamous cell carcinoma. These lesions can be readily detected by cytologic examination, which is responsible for the dramatic reduction in invasive squamous cell carcinoma in the United States over the past 50 years. Although deaths resulting from cervical carcinoma are now relatively low in the United States, carcinoma of the uterine cervix is one of the leading causes of cancer deaths among women in developing countries. There are 340,000 new cases and 160,000 deaths resulting from cervical cancer each year in developing countries (Parkin et al., 1993). In the United States, in contrast, there are 14,500 new cases of invasive cervical cancer each year, and the incidence of squamous carcinoma *in situ* is now 3.5 times that of invasive squamous cell carcinoma of the cervix (Sherman and Kurman, 1998).

The premalignant lesions usually arise from the metaplastic squamous epithelium of the transformation zone. Since the 1960s, epidemiologic studies have linked the development of these premalignant lesions to sexually transmitted diseases. Human papillomavirus (HPV) structural proteins, DNA, or both have been demonstrated in most premalignant and malignant lesions by immunocytochemical, DNA hybridization, and polymerase chain reaction (PCR) studies (Gissmann et al., 1984; Jenson and Lan-

caster, 1990; Kurman et al., 1988; Lancaster et al., 1983; Pfister, 1984; Tase et al., 1989; Wilczynski et al., 1988). In this chapter, we will discuss the current terminology, etiology, microscopic features, and differential diagnosis of these lesions, along with pathologic considerations in their evaluation and treatment. Recent molecular findings will also be addressed, and the pathologic and clinical aspects of microinvasive squamous cell carcinoma and the precursors of a group of uncommon cervical carcinomas will be described.

TERMINOLOGY

Terms currently used to describe precancerous lesions of the cervix include *dysplasia*, *carcinoma* in situ, and *cervical intraepithelial neoplasia* (CIN) (Richart, 1968). The first, adopted by the World Health Organization (Scully et al., 1994) is subdivided into mild, moderate, and severe. The last is further subdivided into three grades of CIN: CIN I is equated with mild dysplasia, CIN II with moderate dysplasia, and CIN III with severe dysplasia and carcinoma *in situ*. Use of the term CIN III obviates the morphologic distinction between severe dysplasia and carcinoma *in situ*. Clinically, there is no difference in the management of these lesions.

The term *flat condyloma* was initially introduced to describe histologic evidence of HPV infection (koilocytosis) and mild dysplasia. The terminology was meant to imply that the mild dysplasia associated with this lesion is a benign viral change distinct from true dysplasia, which is preneoplastic (Meisels and Fortin, 1976; Purola and Savia, 1977). Similarly, the term *atypical condyloma* was applied to moderate and severe dysplasia showing associated HPV changes (Meisels et al., 1981). However, since most cervical lesions are now thought to be associated with HPV infection, regardless of whether koilocytosis is identified, it seems more prudent to retain the term cervical intraepithelial neoplasia (CIN) and include in the report whether or not histologic evidence of HPV infection is present (Editorial, 1983).

A new reporting system designed to replace the Papanicolaou classification for exfoliative cytology of cervical and vaginal lesions was proposed at a meeting in Bethesda, Maryland in 1988 (Workshop, 1989) and subsequently modified in 1991 (Luff, 1992; Table 16–1). In the Bethesda System, cells showing changes associated with HPV (koilocytosis) and mild dysplasia (CIN I) are classified as *low-grade squamous intraepithelial lesions* (LGSIL). Moderate to severe dysplasia (CIN II and CIN III) and carcinoma *in situ* (CIN III) are classified as high-grade squamous intraepithelial lesions (HGSIL). Although the Bethesda System was designed for reporting results of cytologic examinations, some consider extending the Bethesda System to histopathology as well.

ETIOLOGY

The most consistently demonstrated etiologic factors for cervical dysplasia and squamous cell carcinomas of the uterine cervix are early intercourse and multiple sexual partners. The male is clinically silent but serves as a primary reservoir for the etiologic agent. Monogamous women have an increased risk of developing cervical cancer if their sexual partners are sexually active with many women or previously had sexual relations with women with cervical carcinoma. Therefore, most cervical dysplasias and squamous cell carcinomas of the uterine cervix are considered sexually transmitted diseases.

There is a firmly established association between HPV infection and the development of cervical dysplasia and squamous cell carcinoma of the cervix. The association has been demonstrated in both retrospective and prospective epidemiologic studies (Schiffman et al., 1993). Preliminary observations documented HPV genus-specific structural antigens, DNA sequences, or both in 90% of cervical dysplasias and squamous carcinomas *in situ* of the uterine cervix (Lancaster et al., 1983; Okagaki et al., 1983), and studies from many countries have confirmed these findings by PCR amplification (Bosch et al., 1995).

There are more than 60 known genotypes of HPV, and about 20 of these preferentially infect the squamous epithelium of the anogenital tract. Many result in latent infections or show an association with benign condylomas (condylomata acuminata and plana). Most of the benign and low-grade HPV-associated lesions do not appear to progress to higher-grade lesions, so cocarcinogens and host susceptibility factors (such as depressed host immunity) have been considered necessary for malignant transformation to occur. The HPV, then, appears to be necessary but not sufficient for the development of high-grade dysplasia, carcinoma *in situ*, and invasive squamous cell carcinoma of the uterine cervix.

Kurman and colleagues (1983) reported that 95% of women with mild dysplasia, 77% with moderate dysplasia, 64% with severe dysplasia, and 44% with squamous carcinoma *in situ* showed histologic evidence of HPV infection. The histologic features that they considered to correlate best with infection were koilocytosis and/or any two of the following: nuclear wrinkling, binucleation and multinucleation, dyskeratosis, and papillary projections. The HPV antigens were demonstrated in nearly 80% of mild dysplasias, 16% of moderate dysplasias, and 3% of severe dysplasias (when contiguous microscopic sections from the same paraffin block were examined by immunoperoxidase methods). They did not detect HPV antigens in squamous carcinomas *in situ* or metaplastic squamous epithelium.

When present, the HPV antigens were detected in the nucleus and confined to the upper layers of the epithelium, primarily in koilocytic cells. The koilocytic cells contain-

Table 16.1. The 1991 Bethesda System

Adequacy of the specimen
Satisfactory for evaluation
Satisfactory for evaluation but limited by (specify reason)
Unsatisfactory for evaluation (specify reason)

General categorization (optional)
Within normal limits
Benign cellular changes: see Descriptive Diagnosis
Epithelial cell abnormality: see Descriptive Diagnosis

Descriptive diagnosis
Benign cellular changes
  Infection
    Trichomonas vaginalis
    Fungal organisms morphologically consistent with *Candida* sp.
    Predominance of coccobacilli consistent with shift in vaginal flora
    Bacteria morphologically consistent with *Actinomyces* sp.
    Cellular changes associated with herpes simplex virus
    Other
  Reactive changes
  Reactive cellular changes associated with
    Inflammation (includes typical repair)
    Atrophy with inflammation ("atrophic vaginitis")
    Radiation
    Intrauterine contraceptive device (IUD)
    Other

Epithelial cell abnormality
  Squamous cell
    Atypical squamous cells of undetermined significance: qualify[a]
    Low-grade squamous intraepithelial lesion encompassing HPV[b] and mild
      dysplasia (CIN I)
    High-grade squamous intraepithelial lesion encompassing moderate and severe
      dysplasia and CIS (CIN II and CIN III)
    Squamous cell carcinoma
  Glandular cell
    Endometrial cells, cytologically benign, in a postmenopausal woman
    Atypical glandular cells of undetermined significance: qualify[a]
    Endocervical adenocarcinoma
    Endometrial adenocarcinoma
    Extrauterine adenocarcinoma
    Adenocarcinoma, not otherwise specified
    Other malignant neoplasms: specify

Hormonal evaluation (applies to vaginal smear only)
  Hormonal pattern compatible with age and history
  Hormonal pattern incompatible with age and history: specify
  Hormonal evaluation not possible due to (specify)

---

[a]Atypical squamous or glandular cells of undetermined significance should be further qualified as to whether a reactive or a premalignant/malignant process is favored.

[b]Cellular changes of human papillomavirus (HPV) (previously termed "koilocytosis," "koilocytotic atypia" or "condylomatous atypia") are included in the category of low-grade squamous intraepithelial lesion.

---

ing HPV antigen, however, could not be distinguished morphologically from those that were antigen negative. In 85% of cases with demonstrable HPV antigens, the positive cells were located over a zone of proliferating basal or parabasal cells showing varying degrees of nuclear atypia. The capsid antigens were never expressed in the proliferating cells. The presence of HPV antigens reflects the assembly of infectious virions; lesions demonstrating HPV antigens, therefore, are potentially contagious. The frequency of HPV protein expression in epithelium is inversely proportional to the extent of proliferation, which may explain why they were not detected in carcinoma *in situ* lesions and invasive squamous cell carcinomas. In contrast, DNA hybridization studies have shown the presence of the HPV genome in nearly all cases of dysplasia and squamous carcinoma *in situ* (Lancaster et al., 1983; Okagaki et al., 1983).

The HPV infections involving squamous mucosa of the anogenital tract can be divided into three general categories: *(1)* latent infections, which exhibit no clinically or pathologically detectable changes; *(2)* active infections associated with benign flat or exophytic lesions; and *(3)* infections associated with squamous dysplasia, carcinoma *in situ*, or invasive squamous carcinoma. Lesions in the last category appear frequently within or adjacent to benign flat (predominantly) or exophytic lesions. The seven most prevalent and frequently studied mucosotropic viruses can be similarly divided into three groups that impart low, intermediate, and high risk for the development of cervical squamous carcinoma. The HPV types 6 and 11 are associated almost always with lesions of low malignant potential. The HPV types 31, 33, and 35 are associated with lesions of intermediate malignant potential, and HPV types 16 and 18 are associated with most cases of severe dysplasia, carcinoma *in situ*, and invasive squamous carcinoma. In particular, aggressive cervical cancers in young women are often associated with type 18, as well as adenocarcinomas and endocrine tumors of the cervix. The latter include carcinoids, large cell neuroendocrine carcinomas, and small cell carcinomas of the cervix (Mannion et al., 1998; Wistuba et al., 1997). There is a high frequency of HPV infection in both adenocarcinoma *in situ* and invasive adenocarcinoma of the cervix (Okagaki et al., 1989), and the increasing frequency of cervical adenocarcinoma is thought to be causally related to HPV infection (Duggan et al., 1995; Schwartz and Weiss, 1986).

The presence of similar HPV types in mild dysplasia and flat condyloma supports the concept of grouping these together as low-grade lesions. The distribution of HPV types in moderate dysplasia, particularly HPV 16, resembles the distribution seen in severe dysplasia and squamous carcinoma *in situ*, which supports grouping these together as high-grade lesions. The cellular DNA ploidy pattern also appears to correlate with the grade: low-grade lesions are diploid, whereas high-grade lesions are usually polypoid or aneuploid.

MICROSCOPIC FEATURES OF SQUAMOUS DYSPLASIA AND CARCINOMA *IN SITU*

Cervical dysplasia usually begins in the transformation zone, more commonly in the anterior lip of the cervix. The various degrees of dysplasia are characterized by atypical cells that do not involve the full thickness of the epithelium. The proliferating cells in dysplasia are basal and parabasal cells that show evidence of maturation near the surface. Dysplastic lesions are divided into three grades according to the severity and extent of the changes observed. *Mild dysplasia* (CIN I) consists of atypical cells that occupy the deep aspect but do not extend above the lower third of the epithelium. Koilocytotic cells are often present in the superficial layers, and the epithelium maintains evidence of maturation (Fig. 16–1). *Koilocytotic cells* are defined as superficial or intermediate cells showing enlarged hyperchromatic, wrinkled nuclei, perinuclear halos, and distinct cell borders. They are often binucleated or multinucleated. Mitotic figures may be seen in the lower one-third of the epithelium in mild dysplasia but are not seen in the overlying superficial layers with koilocytotic cells.

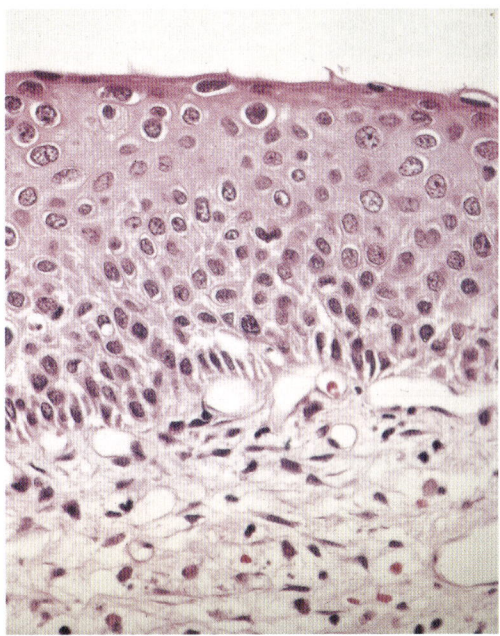

Figure 16–1. Mild squamous dysplasia (CIN I). Some of the koilocytotic cells show meganuclei.

Moderate dysplasia (CIN II) consists of atypical cells that occupy the lower one-third and extend into the middle one-third of the epithelium. There is generally more cytologic atypia and a greater number of mitotic figures than in mild dysplasia. Severe dysplasia (CIN III) involves almost the full thickness of the epithelium. The superficial-most layer still shows evidence of maturation, but the remaining epithelium is replaced by atypical cells showing loss of polarity, nuclear enlargement, and hyperchromasia. Mitotic figures, including atypical ones, are frequently seen (Figs. 16–2 and 16–3). All grades of dysplasia may show hyperkeratosis and parakeratosis (Fig. 16–4). The term carcinoma *in situ* is appropriate when the full thickness of the epithelium is replaced by neoplastic cells (Figs. 16–5 and 16–6).

These criteria cannot be applied to the evaluation of cytologic preparations, however, since the architectural features of cervical dysplasia cannot be evaluated in cervicovaginal smears. On the basis of cytologic criteria alone, premalignant lesions are classified in the Bethesda System into LGSIL and HGSIL categories. Cytologic features of the former, encompassing changes associated with HPV (koilocytosis) and mild dysplasia, include abundant cytoplasm and distinct cell borders. Criteria for LGSIL lesions include nuclear enlargement at least three times the area of normal intermediate cell nuclei, moderate variation in nuclear size and shape, and hyperchromasia. Binucleation and multinucleation are common,

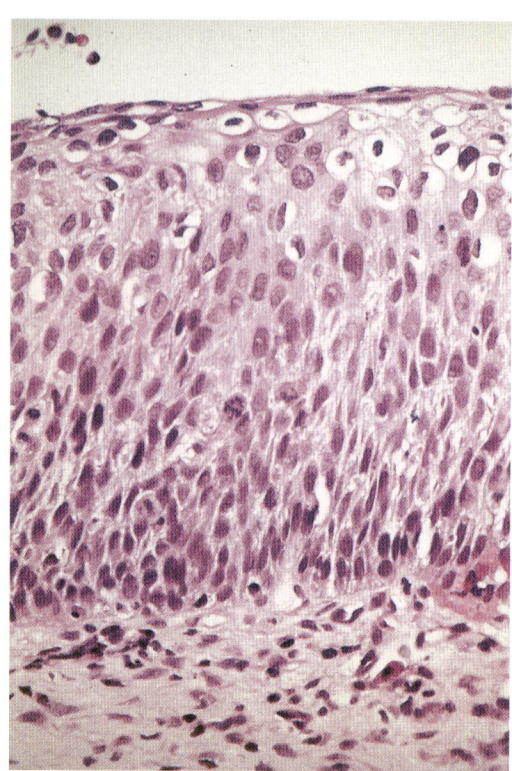

Figure 16–3. Severe squamous dysplasia (CIN III). Higher magnification of dysplastic and koilocytotic cells.

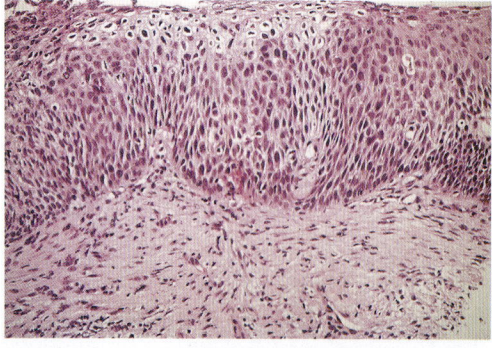

Figure 16–2. Severe squamous dysplasia (CIN III). The atypical squamous cells involve nearly the full thickness of the epithelium. The upper layers of the epithelium show koilocytotic cells.

and nucleoli are only rarely present. Well-defined perinuclear halos with a peripheral rim of dense cytoplasm is characteristic but must be accompanied by the nuclear changes described above (Figs. 16–7 and 16–8).

In contrast, HGSIL lesions are identified in cytologic smears by nuclear abnormalities within predominantly small cells with delicate lacy or metaplastic-appearing cytoplasm. Cells within this category have a very high nuclear-to-cytoplasmic (N/C) ratio, hyperchromasia with either finely or coarsely granular chromatin, and irregular nuclear outlines (Fig. 16–9 and 16–10). These cells usually occur singly but are sometimes in syncytial-like aggregates.

Cytologic abnormalities that fall short of the criteria for LGSIL or HGSIL but appear more atypical than those attributable to reactive changes are regarded as *atypical squamous cells of undetermined significance* (ASCUS).

Both dysplasia and carcinoma *in situ* fre-

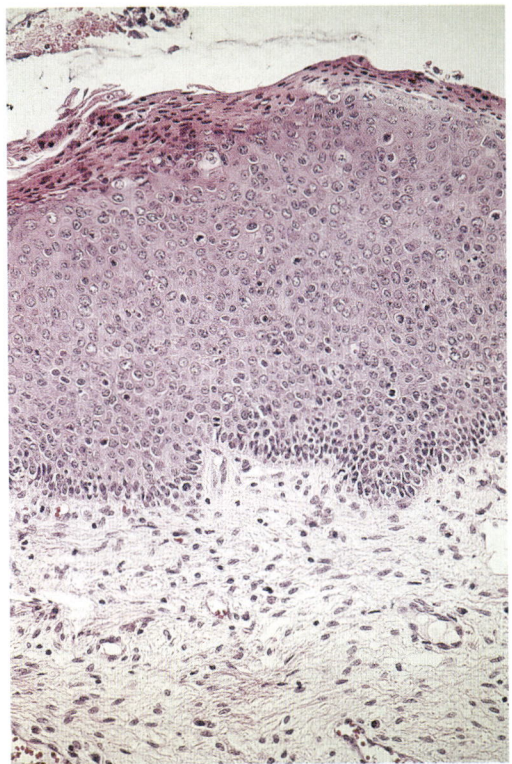

Figure 16–4. Severe squamous dysplasia with parakeratosis (CIN III).

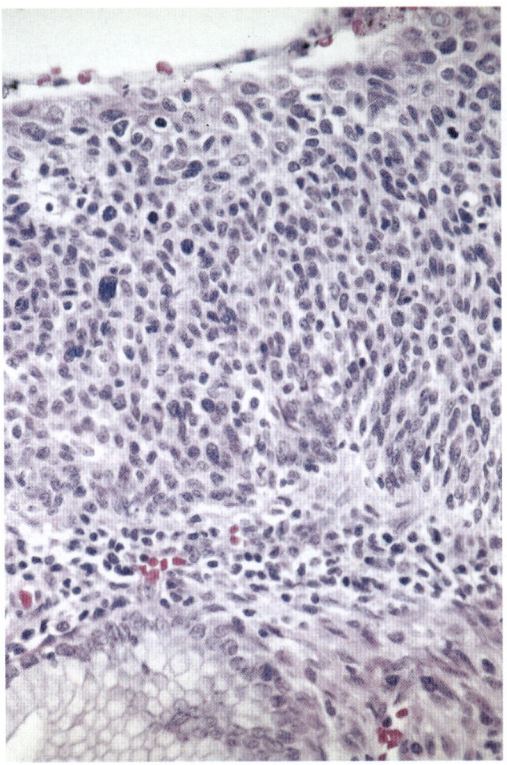

Figure 16–6. Squamous cell carcinoma *in situ* (CIN III). The neoplastic rounded cells have replaced the full thickness of the epithelium.

quently extend into endocervial glands (Fig. 16–11). Involvement of deep and closely packed glands by carcinoma *in situ* can be mistaken for stromal invasion. However, in contrast to invasive squamous carcinoma, glands involved by carcinoma *in situ* appear as solid nests with smooth, round margins (Fig. 16–12). Rarely, carcinoma *in situ* may extend into the endometrium or vaginal mucosa.

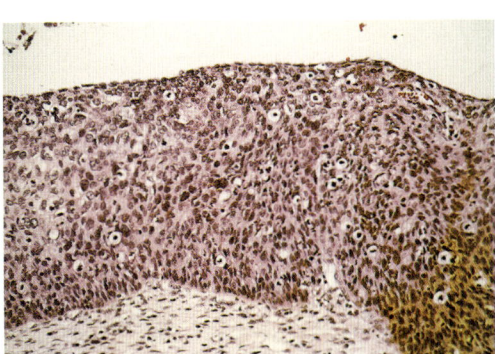

Figure 16–5. Squamous carcinoma *in situ* (CIN III). The full thickness of the epithelium is replaced by undifferentiated neoplastic epithelial cells.

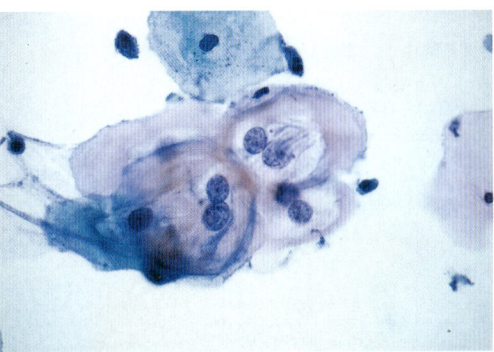

Figure 16–7. Low-grade squamous intraepithelial lesion (LGSIL). Pap smear shows diagnostic koilocytotic cells.

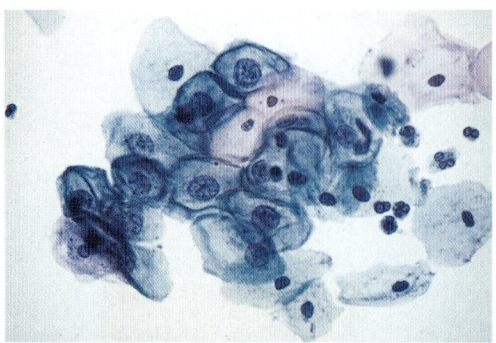

Figure 16–8. Low-grade squamous intraepithelial lesion (LGSIL). Smear shows cells with nuclear enlargement and hyperchromasia.

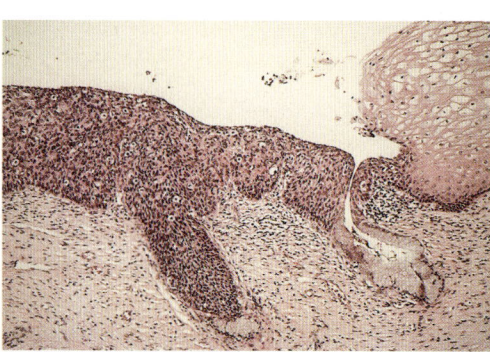

Figure 16–11. Squamous cell carcinoma *in situ* extending into superficial endocervical glands (CIN III).

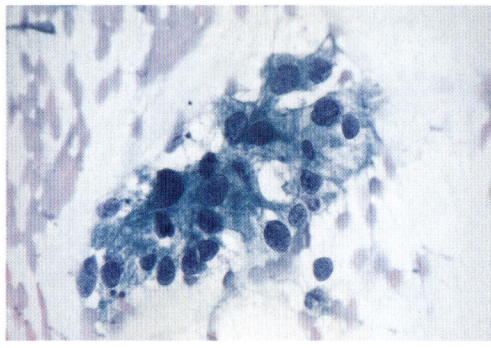

Figure 16–9. High-grade squamous intraepithelial lesion (HGSIL). Cell clusters are composed of cells with a high nuclear-to-cytoplasmic ratio and hyperchromatic nuclei with coarse chromatin.

DIFFERENTIAL DIAGNOSIS

Two lesions must be considered in the differential diagnosis of cervical squamous dysplasia: transitional cell metaplasia and immature squamous metaplasia. *Transitional cell metaplasia* occurs preferentially in postmenopausal women and has no malignant potential. It originates from the transformation zone and exocervix and sometimes extends into endocervical glands. Microscopically, transitional cell metaplasia is characterized by epithelium with crowded nuclei and without obvious maturation. Many cells show oval or spindled nuclei with tapered ends which are oriented vertically and contain small inconspicuous nucleoli and longitudinal grooves. Focally, these nu-

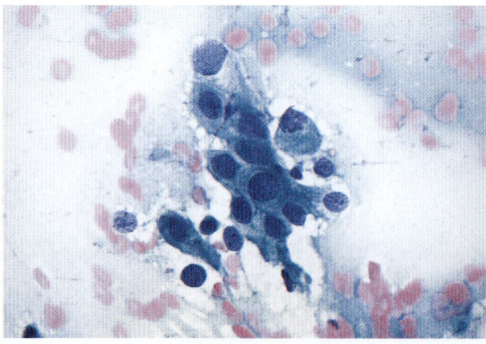

Figure 16–10. High-grade squamous intraepithelial lesion (HGSIL). The small cells in high-grade lesions show scant, delicate cytoplasm reminiscent of endocervical cells.

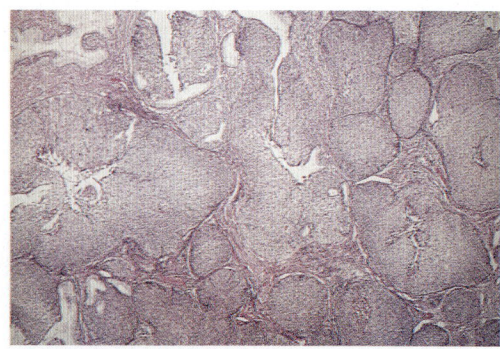

Figure 16–12. Squamous cell carcinoma *in situ* extending to numerous deep endocervical glands mimicking stromal invasion (CIN III).

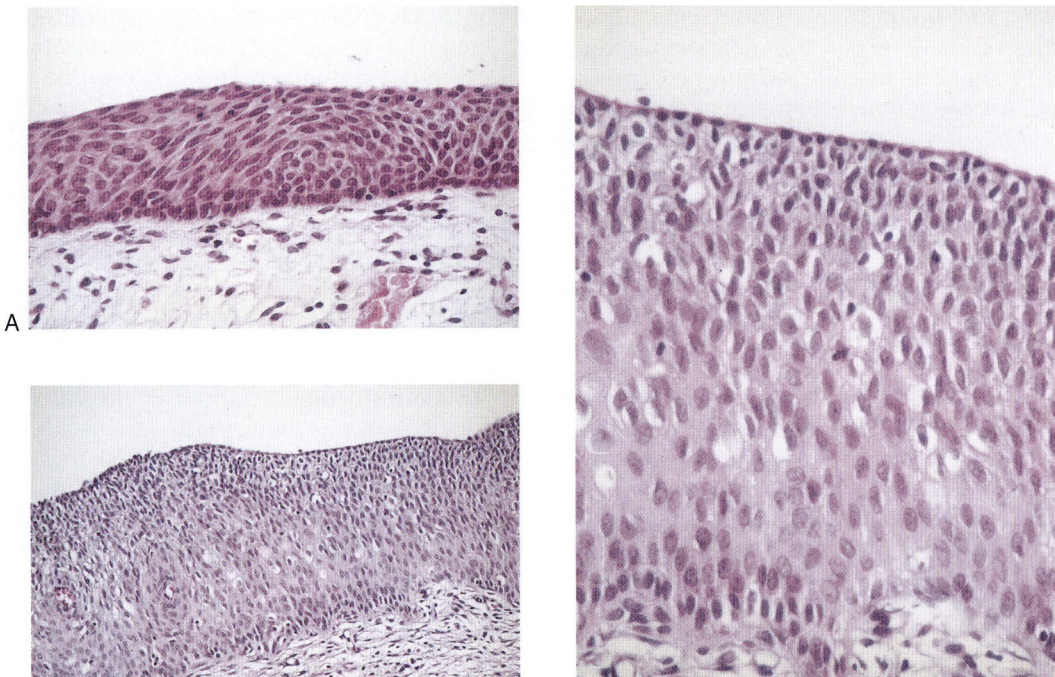

Figure 16–13. *A:* Transitional cell metaplasia. Many of the nuclei are ovoid and show a streaming pattern. No cytologic atypia or mitotic figures are present. *B:* In this example, the epithelium is thickened and the superficial ovoid nuclei are vertically oriented. Umbrella-like cells are seen on the surface. *C:* Higher magnification showing ovoid nuclei, some of which contain grooves.

clei often show characteristic streaming or swirling patterns (Figs. 16–13). Although the cytoplasm may show perinuclear halos, it is not known whether transitional cell metaplasia is an HPV-related lesion or a normal physiologic change (Egan and Russell, 1997; Weir et al., 1997). In contrast to severe dysplasia and carcinoma *in situ*, transitional cell metaplasia lacks cellular disorganization and prominent atypia, and it exhibits little mitotic activity.

Immature squamous metaplasia is composed of parabasal squamous cells often admixed with residual mucinous cells. The immature squamous cells show round to oval hyperchromatic nuclei with smooth nuclear membranes and usually more eosinophilic cytoplasm than high-grade dysplasia. Mitotic figures may be seen in the superficial or deep layers of the epithelium, but they are rarely abnormal. Immature squamous metaplasia lacks the degree of cellular crowding, disorganization, pleomorphism, and mitotic activity seen in severe dysplasia and carci-

noma *in situ*. Nevertheless, immature squamous metaplasia may be difficult to distinguish from severe dysplasia. Immature metaplastic lesions, which resemble but do not fulfill morphologic criteria for CIN III, are sometimes referred to as *atypical immature metaplasia*. At present, atypical immature metaplasia is regarded as a poorly characterized lesion with uncertain biological and clinical significance (Geng et al., 1999).

NATURAL HISTORY

Although there is variation in available data, most studies demonstrate that most lesions with mild dysplasia will either regress or persist, whereas severe dysplasia and carcinoma *in situ* are more likely to progress to invasive carcinoma. A long-term follow-up study by Nasiell and co-workers (1983) of 894 patients with moderate dysplasia showed findings similar to many other studies. Regression occurred in 54%, persistence in

16%, and progression in 30% of patients. Progression occurred after a mean follow-up of 51 months. In contrast, the progression rate for carcinoma *in situ* ranges from 30% to 50%. The latent period from carcinoma *in situ* to microinvasive squamous cell carcinoma is 7 to 10 years, and 10 to 15 years from carcinoma *in situ* to clinically apparent invasive carcinoma (Möbius, 1985).

The rate of progression depends, among other factors, on the type of associated HPV. Moreover, dysplastic lesions with multiple molecular changes may be at increased risk of progressing to invasive carcinoma (Wistuba et al., 1997). It has recently been shown that the frequency of telomerase activity and the degree of RNA telomerase component (hTR) expression are increased in high-grade cervical dysplasia, independent of HPV infection (Yashima et al., 1998). Whether this up-regulation of hTR expression is a marker for the development of invasive carcinoma remains to be determined.

The biologic behavior of dysplastic lesions, especially the low-grade lesions, cannot be predicted with certainty on the basis of histology. However, mild dysplasia with marked koilocytotic atypia in the overlying layers of the epithelium was shown in one study to correlate with infection by high- or intermediate-risk types of HPV (Ziol et al., 1998). Marked koilocytotic atypia was, therefore, considered an early sign of progression.

Another histologic criterion for predicting which dysplastic lesions will progress is the presence of abnormal mitotic figures (Fu et al., 1981). By measuring the chromosomal pattern of different intraepithelial lesions with microspectrophotometry (Dudzinski et al., 1987; Kashyap et al., 1990), it has been demonstrated that cells with abnormal mitotic figures are aneuploid. Therefore, one can make the diagnosis of an aneuploid lesion by identifying abnormal mitotic figures. In a retrospective study, 85% of the dysplastic lesions that regressed were euploid or polyploid, whereas 95% that persisted were aneuploid. All lesions that progressed to invasive carcinoma were aneuploid (Fu et al., 1981).

PATHOLOGIC CONSIDERATIONS IN MANAGEMENT

The cytologic evaluation of cervicovaginal smears is a rapid and relatively inexpensive way of screening for clinically silent, premalignant lesions of the cervix. Mass cytology screening programs have been responsible for a dramatic decrease in cervical cancer. Nevertheless, false-negative rates averaged around 20% prior to the use of modern cytologic screening techniques (Gad and Koch, 1978). Many false-negative cases were the result of inadequate sampling, which is partially overcome by scraping the circumference of the cervix and then aspirating the endocervical canal to increase the number of exfoliated cells in the sample.

In clinical studies, the use of colposcopy with cytology has reduced the false-negative rate to 3% (Vonka et al., 1984). A prospective study at Georgetown University showed that approximately 12% of women had HPV sequences detected in DNA isolated from exfoliated cervical cells. In contrast, only 6% showed abnormal cytology (Lorincz et al., 1986), suggesting that the frequency of HPV infection of the cervix in the general population is higher than anticipated, and that DNA hybridization may be twice as sensitive as conventional cytology screening techniques. New liquid-based collection methods used to prepare thin-layer slides have resulted in decreased false-negative rates compared to conventional techniques, and future developments in computer-assisted slide review may continue to improve cytologic screening procedures.

The appropriate management of cytologic lesions in the ASCUS category is controversial. Approximately 25–60% of ASCUS smears reveal CIN on cervical biopsy (Davey et al., 1996), but it is difficult to predict which of these lesions are at greatest risk for having or subsequently developing CIN based on morphology alone. A number of ancillary studies which can be performed on cytologic specimens may improve the predictive value of an ASCUS or LGSIL pap smear. These include ploidy or cytogenetic analysis (Kurtycz et al., 1996), proliferation antigen Ki-67 labeling (Dunton et al., 1997), detection of nuclear matrix protein expression (Xu et al., 1998), and HPV testing (Wright et al., 1998).

The correlation of cytologic, colposcopic, and histologic findings is essential to the proper evaluation and treatment of precancerous lesions of the cervix. This correlation requires close communication between the pathologist and gynecologist. When evaluating cervical biopsies, the pathologist should pay special attention to several factors that can result in inadequate or inappropriate treatment if not brought to the attention of the clinician. The pathology report should specifically state whether dysplasia or carcinoma *in situ* involves endocervical glands. This is important because the outpatient loop electrical procedure (LEEP), the most common method of treating high-grade dysplasia, has a limited depth of destruction. The LEEP excisions may not completely eradicate deep intraepithelial lesions. Positive margins of cone biopsies are associated with a high recurrence rate, so the status of margins for cone biopsies should also be stated in the pathology report.

Most genital HPV-associated lesions should be regarded as sexually transmitted diseases in which the infectious agent is still present. Even if a lesion is adequately treated, there is the possibility that the male cohort could reinfect the cervix if he has an HPV-associated lesion. Therefore, the male partner should be carefully evaluated for the presence of papillomas on the shaft, corona, or urethra of the penis.

MOLECULAR PATHOLOGY OF SQUAMOUS DYSPLASIA AND CARCINOMA

Integration of HPV DNA into the host genome is probably the earliest event in the development of squamous carcinoma of the cervix. However, since only a small number of HPV-infected women develop cervical carcinoma, other factors probably play a role in tumor progression.

Recent studies have shown that progressive deletions of one or more regions at 3p (especially 3p14.2 and the FHIT gene and 3p21) are frequent and early events in the development of high-grade dysplasia and invasive squamous carcinoma of the cervix (Jones et al., 1994; Mitra et al., 1994; Rader et al., 1997; Wistuba et al., 1997). It is possible that squamous epithelial cells require 3p mutations along with HPV integration for malignant transformation to occur (Wistuba et al., 1997). Microsatellite alterations have been found at chromosome 3p loci and in the RB gene in one-third of dysplastic cervical lesions. Moreover, inactivation of p53 and RB proteins has been demonstrated by

formation of complexes with the E6 and E7 proteins, respectively, of high-risk oncogenic HPV strains. This may be the major mechanism of inactivation of these gene products in the pathogenesis of cervical carcinoma (Dyson et al., 1989; Kurman, 1994; Scheffner, 1990). Mutations of the *p53* gene, in contrast, are not common in cervical dysplasia and carcinoma (Pao et al., 1994; Paquette et al., 1993).

As amplification of particular oncogenes, including Ha-*ras*, c-*myc*, and *erb*-2, has been observed in severe dysplasia and carcinoma *in situ* (CIN III), identification of amplified oncogenes may ultimately prove useful for determining which CIN lesions are likely to recur (Pinion et al., 1991). In invasive squamous carcinoma of the cervix, loss of heterozygosity on all chromosomal arms is relatively common. The most frequent mutations identified in invasive carcinoma, in addition to those at 3p loci, involve 5p (53%), 4q (46%), 6p (43%), and 18q (35%) (Mitra et al., 1994; Mullokandov et al., 1995; Rader et al., 1997). The pathogenetic significance of these additional mutations is unclear.

MICROINVASIVE SQUAMOUS CELL CARCINOMA

Squamous cell carcinomas which invade the cervical stroma in one or more places no more than 3 mm below the epithelial basement membrane are classified as *microinvasive squamous cell carcinomas* if no lymphatic or blood vessel invasion is identified (Creasman et al., 1998). Microinvasive squamous cell carcinomas are not recognized as malignant tumors on gross examination, and they appear to have an extremely low potential for metastasis. In fact, squamous cell carcinomas with up to 5 mm of stromal invasion (microcarcinomas) generally behave as *in situ* carcinomas when no vascular invasion is identified (Östör, 1993). Obviously, thorough evaluation and free margins are critical in making this assessment.

Two patterns of microinvasion are recognized. The first consists of tongues of malignant squamous cells still connected to the carcinoma *in situ* but extending into the superficial stroma. The second pattern is characterized by small nests of malignant squamous cells that lie in the superficial stroma but are detached from the overlying *in situ* carcinomas (Figs. 16–14 and 16–15). Carcinoma *in situ* extending into endocervical glands may similarly show foci of microinvasion (Figs. 16–16 and 16–17). The depth of invasion in this case is measured from the basement membrane of the involved endocervical gland rather than from the surface. A lymphoplasmacytic infiltrate and a desmoplastic reaction are often seen around such microinvasive foci. As small tumor nests may show retraction artifact simulating vascular invasion (Östör, 1993), immunostains for the endothelial markers CD31 and CD34 may be helpful to exclude or confirm vascular invasion.

With the widespread use of LEEP, more cases of microinvasive squamous cell carcinoma are being detected (Killackey et al., 1986; Murdoch et al., 1992). Conization appears to be the treatment of choice. If conization margins are positive, a simple hysterectomy seems appropriate (Roman et al., 1997).

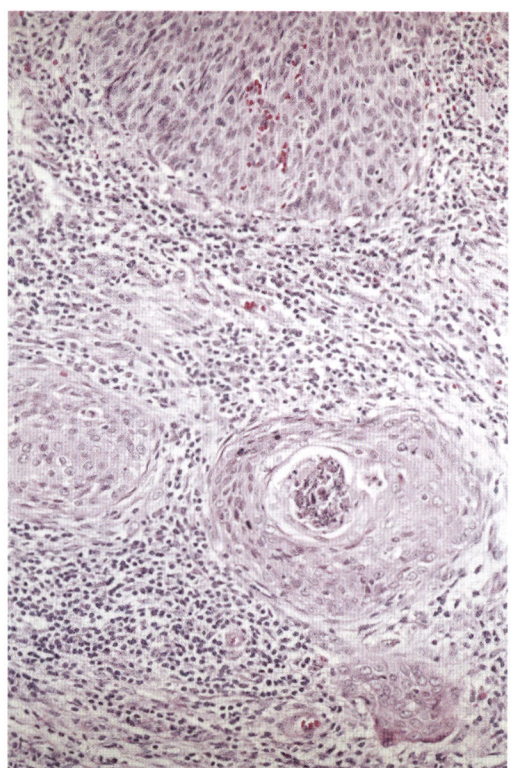

Figure 16–15. Foci of microinvasive squamous cell carcinoma with overlying carcinoma *in situ*. A chronic inflammatory infiltrate is also present.

PAPILLARY SQUAMOUS CARCINOMA

Papillary squamous carcinoma is an uncommon variant of squamous cell carcinoma which, if well differentiated, can be confused with squamous papilloma and condyloma. This variant often shows a noninvasive component. However, it should be kept in mind that small superficial biopsies may reveal only the noninvasive component of the tumor.

Papillary squamous carcinoma should be distinguished from condyloma acuminatum, which shows papillary fronds supported by thin fibrovascular stalks. The squamous epithelium of condyloma acuminatum lacks marked cytologic atypia, and the intermediate and superficial layers contain koilocytes. If koilocytes are not seen in such a lesion, it should be regarded as a squamous papilloma. Most papillary squamous carcinomas, in contrast, show enough cytologic atypia to

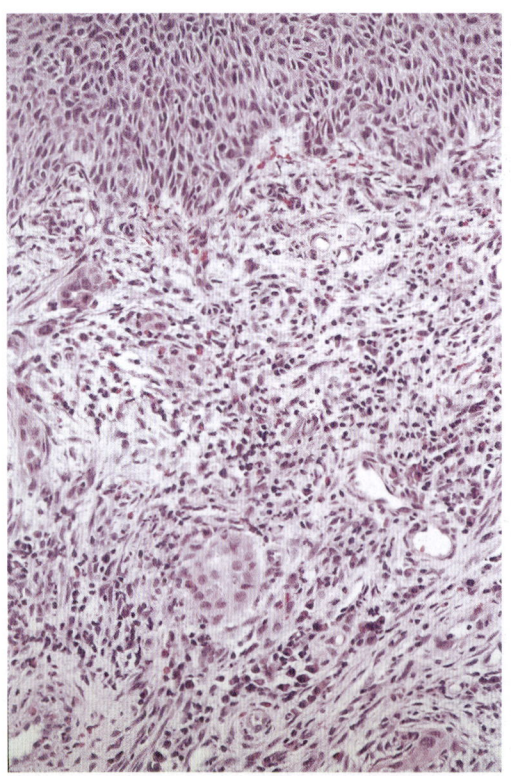

Figure 16–14. Three foci of microinvasion and the overlying carcinoma *in situ* are shown.

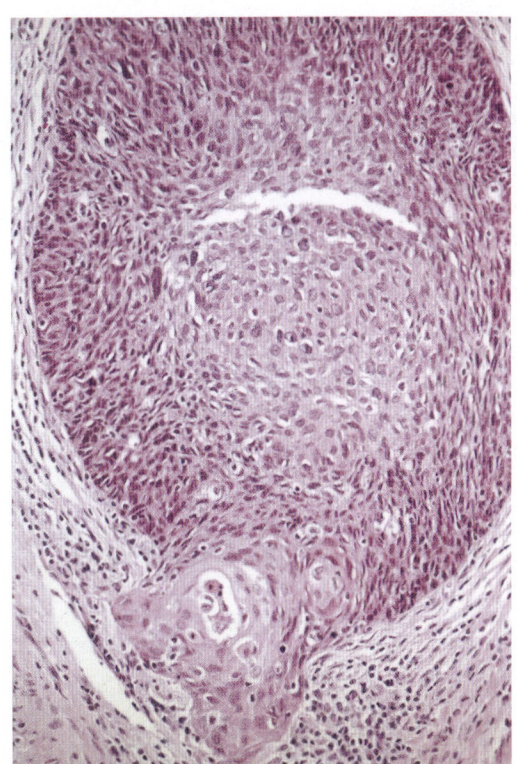

Figure 16–16. Endocervical gland distended by squamous cell carcinoma *in situ* with a single focus of microinvasion which is better differentiated and keratinized.

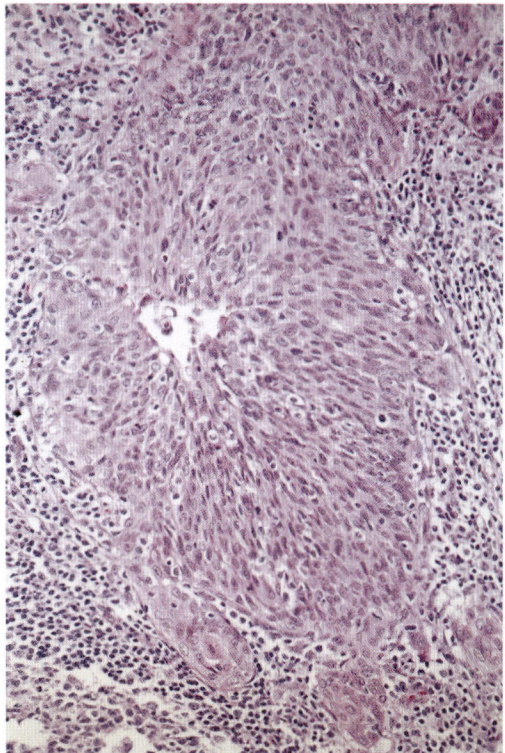

Figure 16–17. Endocervical gland replaced by squamous cell carcinoma *in situ* showing multiple foci of microinvasion, most of which are still attached to the *in situ* carcinoma.

allow recognition as carcinoma (Koenig et al., 1997; Fig. 16–18).

VERRUCOUS CARCINOMA

Verrucous carcinoma is an exceedingly rare but distinctive type of very well–differentiated squamous cell carcinoma (Kraus and Perez-Mesa, 1966). It exhibits round or pointed papillary projections that lack central fibrovascular cores. The deep margin of the tumor consists of bulbous or rounded masses of cells that infiltrate the underlying stroma in a pushing fashion. Because of this feature, proving stromal invasion is often very difficult. There is minimal cytologic atypia and mitotic activity. Despite the large size verrucous carcinomas of the cervix may attain, they seldom metastasize. For this reason, distinguishing verrucous carcinoma from well-differentiated squamous carcinoma can be prognostically useful.

TRANSITIONAL CELL CARCINOMA

Tumors indistinguishable from transitional cell carcinomas of the urinary tract have been described in the uterine cervix (Albores-Saavedra and Young, 1995). The vast majority show a papillary architecture and are invasive. Some exhibit an endophytic growth pattern mimicking inverted transitional cell papillomas (Albores-Saavedra and Molberg, 1997). A few tumors may be entirely papillary and noninvasive (Fig. 16–19). Papillary transitional cell carcinomas are associated with HPV infection (Lininger et al., 1998). Type 16 of HPV, in particular, is present in a significant proportion of these tumors. Papillary cervical carcinomas that show both squamous and transitional cell differentiation are designated *squamotransitional cell carcinomas* (Koenig et al., 1997). These tumors similarly contain a noninvasive papillary component.

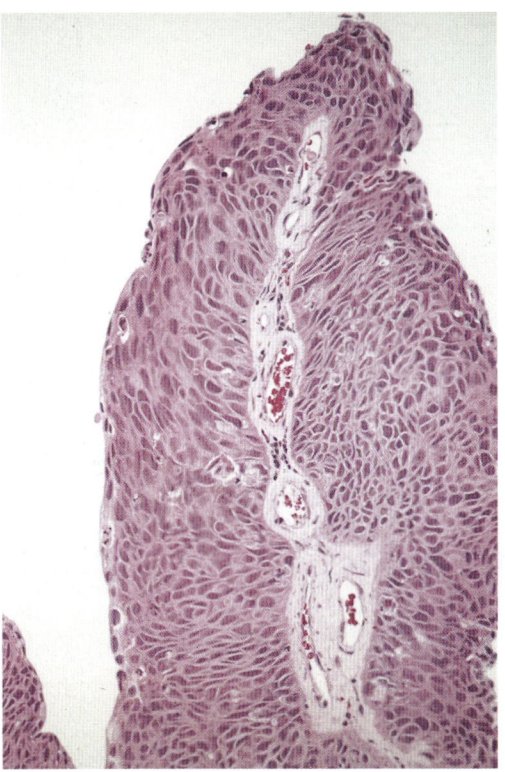

Figure 16–18. Noninvasive moderately differentiated papillary squamous carcinoma in a biopsy sample. The hysterectomy specimen showed foci of invasion.

ADENOCARCINOMA *IN SITU*

Adenocarcinoma *in situ* is an uncommon lesion of the endocervical glands. The average age of occurrence is 40 years, which is about 10 years lower than the mean age at which invasive adenocarcinoma is diagnosed. The lower age of occurrence of the former is consistent with the concept of adenocarcinoma *in situ* as a precursor of invasive adenocarcinoma, which now constitutes 12% to 18.5% of all carcinomas of the uterine cervix (Brand et al., 1988; Tamimi and Figge, 1982). Additional reasons for considering adenocarcinoma *in situ* a "preinvasive lesion" include the following: *(1)* the lesion can be histologically identical to invasive adenocarcinoma, except that it is confined to the endocervical glands; *(2)* the cells comprising adenocarcinoma *in situ* can be identical to those of invasive tumors; and *(3)* adenocarcinoma *in situ* is frequently seen at the periphery of invasive adenocarcinomas (Betsill and Clark, 1986; Christopherson et al., 1979; Gloor and Ruzicka, 1982; Qizilbash, 1975).

In the U.S., there has been an absolute as well as a relative increase in adenocarcinoma of the cervix since the early 1970s (Schwartz and Weiss, 1986). The relative increase is due to the reduction in the incidence of squamous cell carcinoma resulting from widespread cytologic screening. Nevertheless, the actual rate of adenocarcinomas of the cervix increased from 1.7 (per million women per year) in 1973–1975 to 3.8 in 1979–1982 in women under 35 years of age. In contrast to the frequency at which precursors to squamous cell carcinoma are identified in cervicovaginal smears, detection of adenocarcinoma *in situ* by cytologic screening is much less common.

Morphologically, the endocervical glands in adenocarcinoma *in situ* usually maintain their lobular growth pattern. One or several lobules are typically involved. Occasionally, however, a single gland is partially or completely replaced by adenocarcinoma cells (Figs. 16–20 and 16–21). Intraglandular budding, papillary infoldings, and focal cribriform patterns may be seen. The glandular epithelium is pseudostratified, showing atypical cells with nuclear enlargement and hyperchromasia, diminished mucin production, and mitotic activity with occasional atypical mitotic figures (Fig. 16–22). Three types of adenocarcinoma *in situ* have been recognized: endocervical; endometrioid, which is the most common; and intestinal (Figs. 16–23 to 16–25). The last type exhibits goblet cells, endocrine cells, and even Paneth cells (Jaworski, 1990).

Dysplasia and carcinoma *in situ* of the squamous epithelium often coexist with adenocarcinoma *in situ* (Friedell and McKay, 1953; Jaworski et al., 1988; Weisbrot et al., 1972). This association suggests that the same etiologic agent may play a role in malignant transformation of the analogue common to both metaplastic squamous epithelium and endocervical glandular cells, the subcolumnar reserve cell (Christopherson et al., 1979). With *in situ* hybridization techniques, HPV DNA was detected in 70% of cases of adenocarcinoma *in situ* in one study (Tase et al., 1989). Type 18 of HPV was the predominant type found in both adenocar-

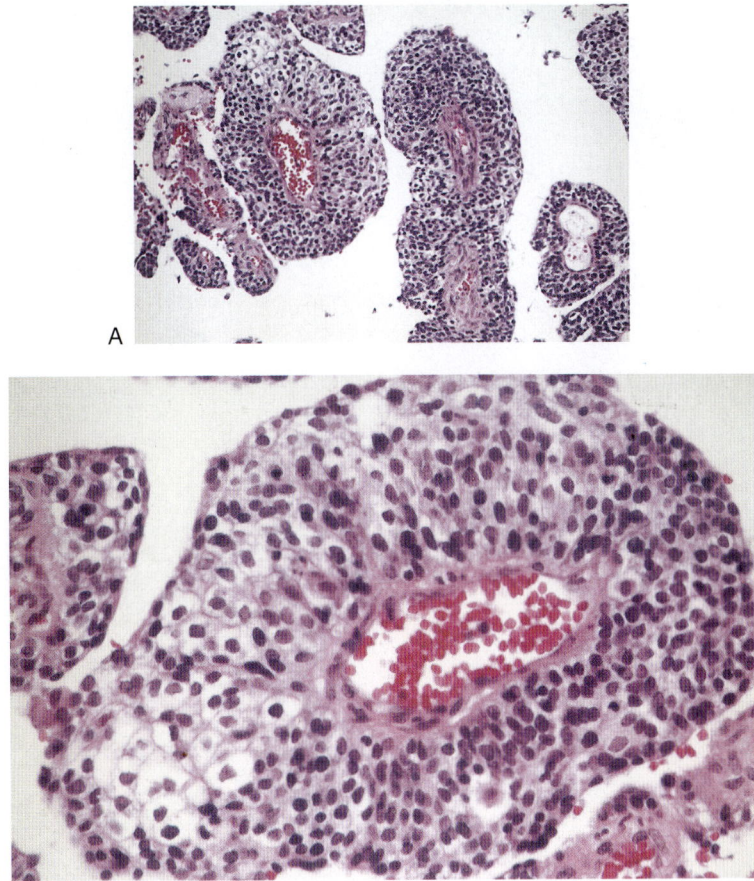

Figure 16–19. *A:* Noninvasive papillary transitional cell carcinoma of the cervix. The hysterectomy specimen showed stromal invasion. *B:* Higher magnification of papillary structure lined by neoplastic cells.

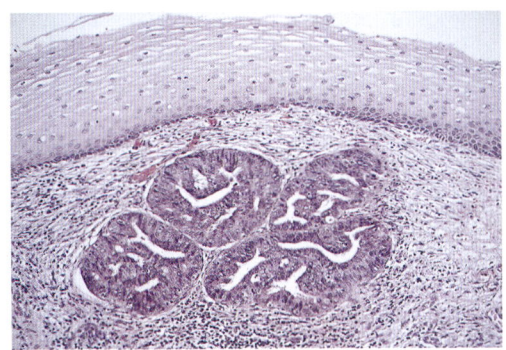

Figure 16–20. Adenocarcinoma *in situ* located beneath the squamous epithelium. Low-power view showing the lobular growth pattern of the neoplastic glands.

cinoma *in situ* and microinvasive adenocarcinoma. Similarly, HPV types 16 and 18 were detected by PCR in 15 of 36 cases (42%) of adenocarcinoma *in situ* in a subsequent study (Lee et al., 1993). It therefore appears that HPV plays a role in the etiology of adenocarcinoma *in situ*, perhaps acting as a direct transforming agent on the columnar epithelium and eventually leading to neoplastic progression.

Increased telomerase activity has recently been detected in adenocarcinoma *in situ*. Both the frequency of telomerase activity and the degree of its RNA component expression are increased in adenocarcinoma *in situ*, and each increase is independent of HPV infection. Whether this up-regulation is a marker for the subsequent development of invasive adenocarcinoma remains to be determined (Yashima et al., 1998).

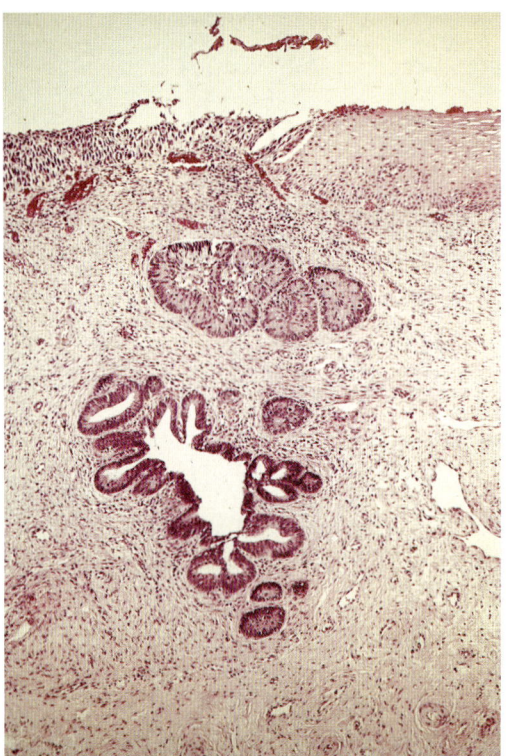

Figure 16–21. Superficial and deep endocervical glands maintain their lobular growth pattern in this adenocarcinoma *in situ.* The overlying squamous mucosa is dysplastic.

Adenocarcinoma *in situ* can be readily diagnosed in histologic material obtained by endocervical curettage, cone biopsy, and hysterectomy (Bousfield et al., 1980; Christopherson et al., 1979; Gloor and Ruzicka, 1982; Krumins et al., 1977; Qizilbash, 1975;

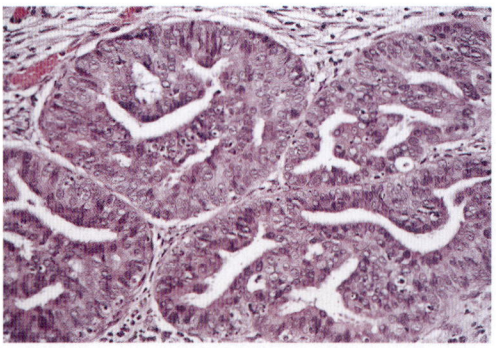

Figure 16–22. Higher magnification of Figure 16–20 showing a lobule composed of glands lined by neoplastic columnar cells.

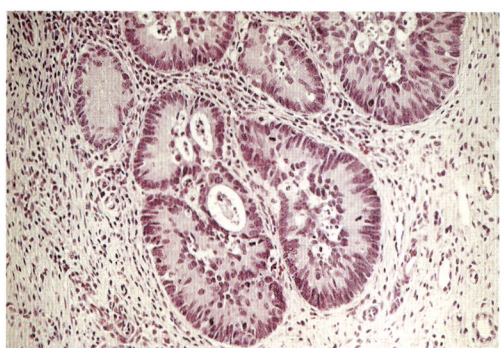

Figure 16–23. Adenocarcinoma *in situ.* Higher magnification of Figure 16–21 shows glands arranged in a lobular pattern.

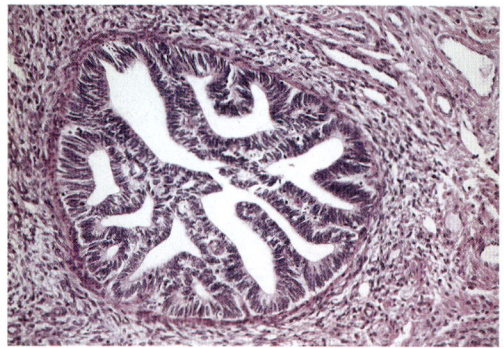

Figure 16–24. Adenocarcinoma *in situ.* This endometrioid neoplastic gland has small papillary structures that fuse, producing a cribriform pattern.

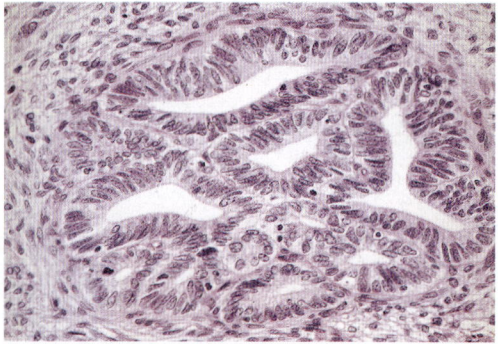

Figure 16–25. Adenocarcinoma *in situ.* This lobule is composed of individual neoplastic glands with an endometrioid appearance.

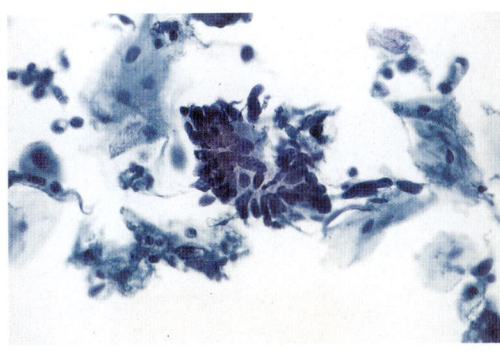

Figure 16–26. Atypical glandular cells of undetermined significance (AGUS), probably adenocarcinoma *in situ.* The columnar cells show nuclear stratification and feathering.

Weisbrot et al., 1972). In cytologic preparations, it is more difficult to distinguish *in situ* from invasive endocervical adenocarcinoma. Often, however, adenocarcinoma *in situ* shows nuclear atypia exceeding that seen in reactive change but falling short of changes typical of invasive adenocarcinoma. Cells showing such changes are classified in the Bethesda System as atypical glandular cells of undetermined significance (AGUS).

They appear as crowded sheets and strips of glandular cells which have lost the honeycombing pattern typical of normal endocervical glandular epithelium. Characteristic features include sheets of cells with feathery edges and palisading nuclei. In addition, there is nuclear enlargement, elongation, and stratification accompanied by hyperchromasia, with small or inconspicuous nucleoli (Figs. 16–26 and 16–27). The presence

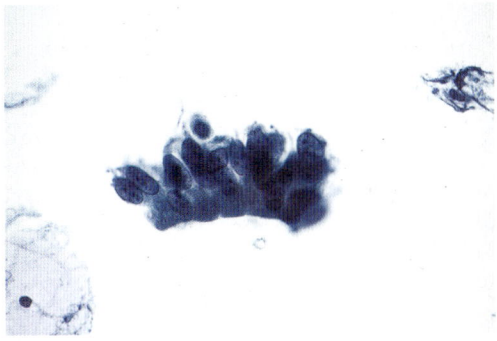

Figure 16–27. Atypical glandular cells of undetermined significance (AGUS), probably adenocarcinoma *in situ.* The nuclei are hyperchromatic with inconspicuous nucleoli.

of irregular chromatin clearing, a markedly uneven chromatin distribution, macronucleoli or a tumor diathesis would increase the likelihood of invasive adenocarcinoma. However, some of these features may be absent in well-differentiated invasive adenocarcinomas.

Because adenocarcinoma *in situ* may be focal and is frequently associated with squamous intraepithelial lesions, it is easily overlooked (Brown and Wells, 1986). Surgical removal of the involved endocervical glands is curative. Östör et al. (1997) followed 77 patients with adenocarcinoma *in situ* and microinvasion that were treated by different surgical modalities. They concluded that conization with free margins is adequate treatment for these patients. If the margins are involved by tumor, a simple hysterectomy is curative. Others emphasize, however, that adenocarcinoma *in situ* may be multicentric. A conization specimen may therefore show negative margins but not remove the entire lesion (Im et al., 1995). They advocate hysterectomy as the procedure of choice. Awareness of the existence of adenocarcinoma *in situ* and careful examination of cytologic smears and biopsies of the cervix should lead to increased diagnosis and improved treatment of this preinvasive lesion.

DIFFERENTIAL DIAGNOSIS

Adenocarcinoma *in situ* must be distinguished from a wide variety of lesions. These include reactive atypia of endocervical glands, microglandular hyperplasia, irradiation effect, endometriosis, Arias-Stella reaction, tubal metaplasia, endocervical tunnel clusters, transitional cell metaplasia, ectopic prostatic tissues, and minimal deviation adenocarcinoma. Reactive atypia of endocervical glands is usually seen in the setting of severe acute and chronic inflammation. The atypical columnar cells exhibit large elongated, hyperchromatic or vesicular nuclei, sometimes with prominent nucleoli. Although mitotic figures may be noted, the atypical cells are usually not stratified. Moreover, they frequently alternate with normal columnar cells, and lymphocytes and neutrophils may be admixed with the columnar cells.

Microglandular hyperplasia is typically a polypoid lesion, seen most frequently in pregnancy or in association with the use of oral contraceptives (Taylor et al., 1967). The same lesion, however, can occur in women without increased exogenous or endogenous hormonal stimulation (Greeley et al., 1995). Histologically, microglandular hyperplasia shows a lobular growth pattern. It consists of small, closely packed glands with little intervening stroma. The glands are lined by cuboidal or columnar mucin-containing cells with uniform basal, hyperchromatic nuclei (Fig. 16–28). The columnar cells often contain subnuclear and supranuclear vacuoles and resemble early secretory endometrium. Focal areas of associated squamous metaplasia are common. Although cytologic atypia and mitotic figures are usually lacking, some examples of microglandular hyperplasia with cytologic atypia have been reported (Young and Scully, 1989a).

Endocervical glands showing irradiation effect may also be confused with endocervical adenocarcinoma *in situ*. Irradiated endocervical cells may appear columnar or flat, and they may exhibit large hyperchromatic or vesicular nuclei with prominent nucleoli. The cytoplasm may be deeply eosinophilic or vacuolated (Lesack et al., 1996). Multinucleated cells may be seen, but nuclear stratification and mitotic figures are usually absent. Moreover, a low N/C ratio is usually maintained (Fig. 16–29). A history of previous radiotherapy is obviously useful in arriving at the correct diagnosis.

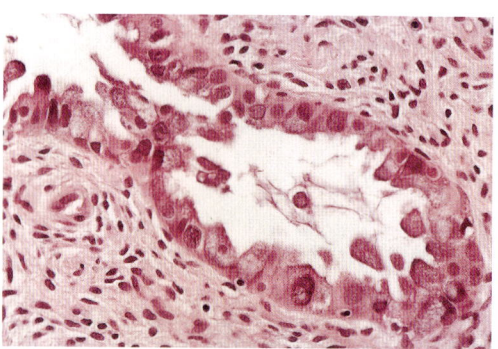

Figure 16–29. Irradiation effect. An endocervical gland shows cells with vesicular nuclei and prominent nucleoli admixed with cells showing hyperchromatic, smudged nuclei. A low nuclear-to-cytoplasmic ratio is maintained.

Endometriosis of the cervix is most often easily distinguished from adenocarcinoma *in situ*, as the former contains both endometrial glands and stroma (Gardner, 1962). However, sometimes only scant stroma is appreciated. The glands may show either proliferative or secretory activity. During pregnancy, Arias-Stella reaction identical to that seen in the endometrium may involve endocervical glands. This feature, if not recognized, could be confused with adenocarcinoma *in situ* of the endocervix (Cove, 1979; Fig. 16–30). In this circumstance, a helpful finding is the simultaneous presence of decidual change involving the endocervical stroma.

Endocervical glands with tubal metaplasia are lined by ciliated and peg cells similar to those of the normal tubal mucosa (Suh and Silverberg, 1990; Fig. 16–31). Foci of tubal metaplasia lack a lobular architecture. Mild cytologic atypia is often seen in tubal metaplasia, and in some cases the atypia is so severe that its appearance approaches that of adenocarcinoma *in situ* (Schlesinger and Silverberg, 1999). Such metaplastic cells are more likely to be confused with adenocarcinoma *in situ* in cytologic preparations than in histologic material, particularly if cilia are not visible or inconspicuous. More troublesome histologically is the occasional presence of metaplastic endometrial glands which may coexist with tubal metaplasia. These endometrial glands lack accompanying stroma and sometimes show mitotic fig-

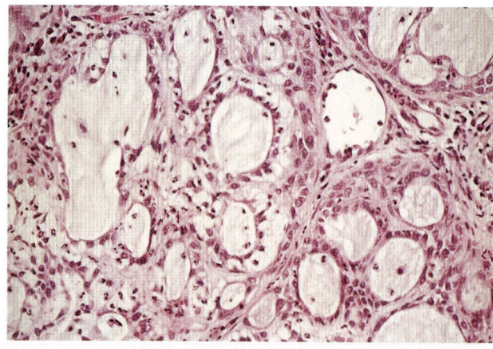

Figure 16–28. Microglandular hyperplasia. The glands are small, closely packed, and separated by scant edematous stroma.

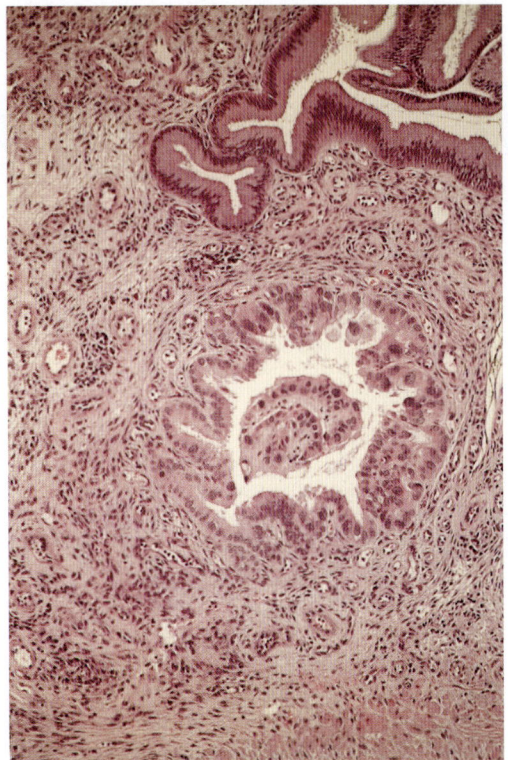

A

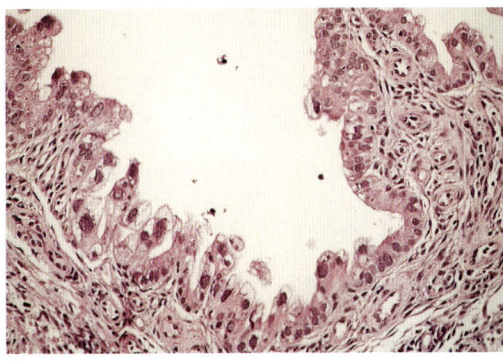

B

Figure 16–30. *A:* Arias-Stella reaction. Endocervical gland is lined by atypical cells with large hyperchromatic nuclei. *B:* In this gland the columnar cells show clear cytoplasm with hobnailing and hyperchromatic nuclei.

ures; they are easily confused with adenocarcinoma *in situ* (Oliva et al., 1995; Fig. 16–32).

Mesonephric remnants are normally scattered within the deep cervical stroma. When they become hyperplastic, they appear as

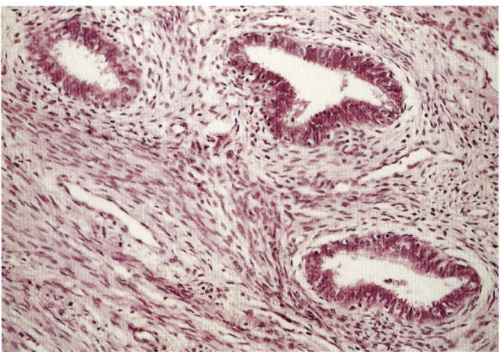

Figure 16–31. Tubal metaplasia. The three metaplastic glands do not show a lobular growth pattern. They are lined by columnar cells, some of which are ciliated.

well-defined lobules of tubular structures that may extend to the cervical epithelium (Fig. 16–33). The tubules are lined by a single layer of cuboidal cells with scant pale or clear cytoplasm and bland nuclei with finely granular chromatin. Although the tubules lack mucin, periodic acid-Schiff (PAS)–positive hyaline material can be seen in the tubular lumina (Ferry and Scully, 1990; Siedman and Tavassoli, 1995). The distinctive appearance of this entity should allow it to be readily distinguished from adenocarcinoma *in situ*. However, tubal metaplasia and mesonephric remnants may coexist with adenocarcinoma *in situ* and thereby cause confusion.

Noncystic endocervical tunnel clusters are usually noted as an incidental finding in

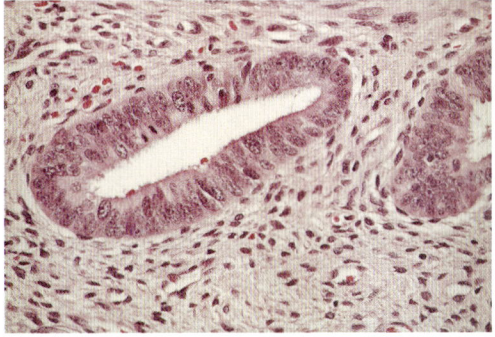

Figure 16–32. Metaplastic endometrial glands. These glands, which are not surrounded by endometrial stroma, were found adjacent to an area of tubal metaplasia.

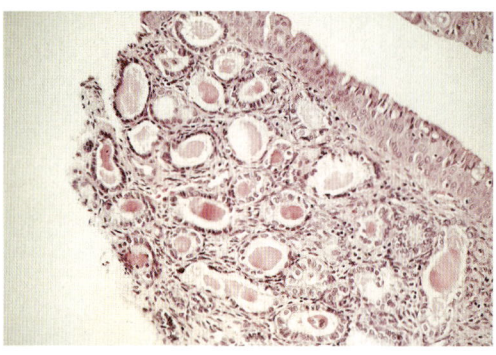

Figure 16–33. Hyperplasia of mesonephric remnants. A lobule composed of tubules containing eosinophilic material is seen immediately beneath the endocervical epithelium.

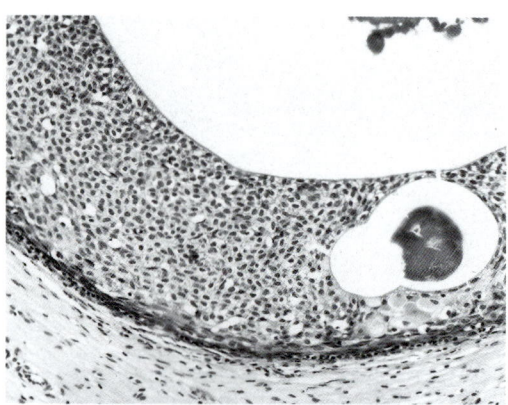

Figure 16–35. Transitional cell metaplasia. An endocervical gland is partially replaced by stratified, transitional type epithelium containing a microcyst.

middle-aged women and are not associated with gross abnormalities. They are composed of closely packed, small, nondilated endocervical glands often showing a well-defined lobular pattern. The glands are often arranged around a central endocervical cleft, and they are lined by cuboidal or columnar cells that occasionally have large hyperchromatic or vesicular nuclei with prominent nucleoli. Such atypical glands may simulate adenocarcinoma *in situ* (Jones and Young, 1996).

Another incidental finding in middle-aged women is *atypical oxyphilic metaplasia.* This lesion consists of endocervical glands lined by cuboidal or columnar cells with abundant oxyphilic cytoplasm and large hyperchromatic nuclei (Fig. 16–34). Occasional multinucleated cells are admixed with the columnar cells, and apical snouts are

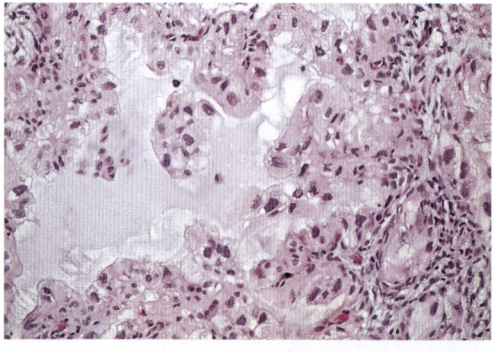

Figure 16–34. Atypical oxyphilic metaplasia. The endocervical glands are lined by large cells with oxyphilic cytoplasm and hyperchromatic nuclei.

rarely observed. Mitotic figures are consistently absent (Jones and Young, 1997).

A common metaplastic lesion occurring preferentially in postmenopausal women is *transitional cell metaplasia.* When it involves the endocervical glands, it may simulate adenocarcinoma *in situ* (Fig. 16–35). Some examples show a close resemblance to Walthard cell nests. Others show small mucin-containing cystic spaces that suggest glandular differentiation (Egan and Russell, 1997; Weir et al., 1997).

Prostatic tissue in the stroma of the uterine cervix is an exceedingly rare abnormality which probably results from either a metaplastic process or a developmental defect. Because of the papillary and cribriform architecture of the prostatic glands, this entity can be mistaken for adenocarcinoma *in situ* (Larraza-Hernandez et al., 1997). Immunostains for prostate specific antigen are very useful in establishing the diagnosis (Fig. 16–36).

The extremely well–differentiated adenocarcinoma of the cervix known as minimal deviation adenocarcinoma or adenoma malignum can be misinterpreted as adenocarcinoma *in situ*, especially when it involves the deep endocervical glands. However, the former consists of glands that are irregular in size and shape, deeply invade the stroma, and lack the lobular pattern of adenocarcinoma *in situ*. Moreover, cytologic atypia is more pronounced in adenocarcinoma *in situ* than in minimal deviation adenocarci-

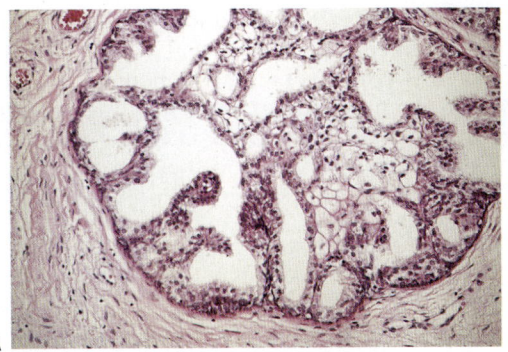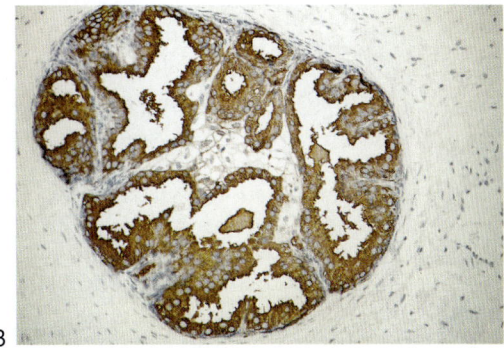

Figure 16–36. *A:* Ectopic prostatic tissue. The prostatic glands show a cribriform and papillary architecture. *B:* Strong diffuse positivity for prostate-specific antigen [courtesy of Dr. Oscar Larraza].

noma, which usually shows a desmoplastic response and, less frequently, vascular or perineural invasion (Kaku and Enjoji, 1983; Gilks et al., 1989).

Invasive adenocarcinomas that secondarily involve the endocervical glands, especially endometrial adenocarcinomas, should also be distinguished from adenocarcinoma *in situ*. This may be facilitated by fractional curettage, examination of the hysterectomy specimen, or observation of a transition from normal endocervical epithelium to malignant epithelium (Maier and Norris, 1980). Immunocytochemistry may also aid in the differential diagnosis (Azumi et al., 1991; Dabbs et al., 1986; Maes et al., 1988). Most endocervical adenocarcinomas are carcinoembryonic antigen (CEA) positive and vimentin negative, whereas the majority of endometrial adenocarcinomas show the opposite staining profile. Since there is some overlap in the expression of these markers,

however, the immunocytochemical findings cannot be considered definitive in any individual case.

Another important consideration is the distinction of adenocarcinoma *in situ* from early invasive carcinoma. Some authors have emphasized the presence of small buds of squamoid cells projecting into the stroma, with subsequent formation of microacini, as diagnostically useful features of early invasion. However, the histologic recognition of stromal invasion is often subjective and sometimes impossible to establish with certainty. Moreover, there can be great difficulty in distinguishing vascular invasion from retraction artifact. Therefore, until more is learned about early stromal invasion and the factors involved in the host reponse to invasive tumor, the diagnostic criteria for microinvasive adenocarcinoma will remain controversial (Jaworski, 1990; Taylor et al., 1967).

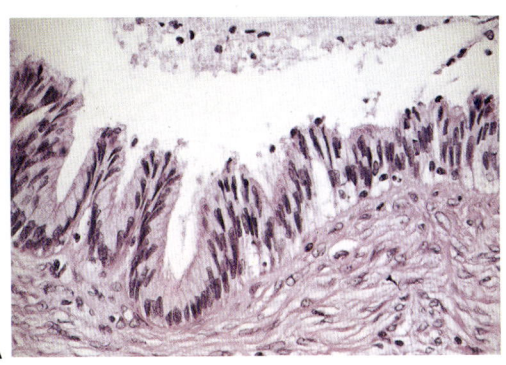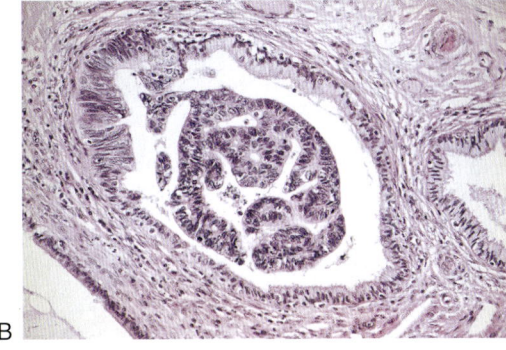

Figure 16–37. *A:* Part of an endocervical gland is replaced by atypical columnar cells interpreted as glandular dysplasia. *B:* Changes of dysplasia and carcinoma *in situ* in a single gland.

DYSPLASIA OF ENDOCERVICAL GLANDS

Cases of endocervical glandular dysplasia have been described with histologic changes less severe than those of well-differentiated adenocarcinoma. The nuclei in such lesions are smaller, the chromatin is not as coarse, there are generally fewer mitotic figures, and the nucleoli are small and round (Bousfield et al., 1980; Casper et al., 1997; Gloor and Hurliman, 1986). When these atypical glandular changes are seen adjacent to adenocarcinoma *in situ* and are not associated with acute and chronic inflammation, we regard them as truly dysplastic and part of the morphologic spectrum of adenocarcinoma *in situ* (Figs. 16–37). However, some investigators do not recognize the existence of endocervical glandular dysplasia (Goldstein et al., 1998), or they believe that a significant proportion of cases resembling glandular dysplasia may represent reactive lesions of

the endocervical columnar epithelium (Jaworski et al., 1988; Tase et al., 1989). Because of this controversy, the noncommital term glandular atypia has been suggested for this lesion. The HPV DNA is less common in glandular atypia not associated with squamous dysplasia than in adenocarcinoma *in situ* (Anciaux et al., 1997).

VILLOGLANDULAR ADENOCARCINOMA

This rare variant of well-differentiated endocervical adenocarcinoma occurs preferentially in young women and is usually associated with a major noninvasive papillary component. Superficial biopsy samples frequently show only this noninvasive component. However, subsequent hysterectomy specimens usually reveal foci of invasive adenocarcinoma. Stromal infiltration is often

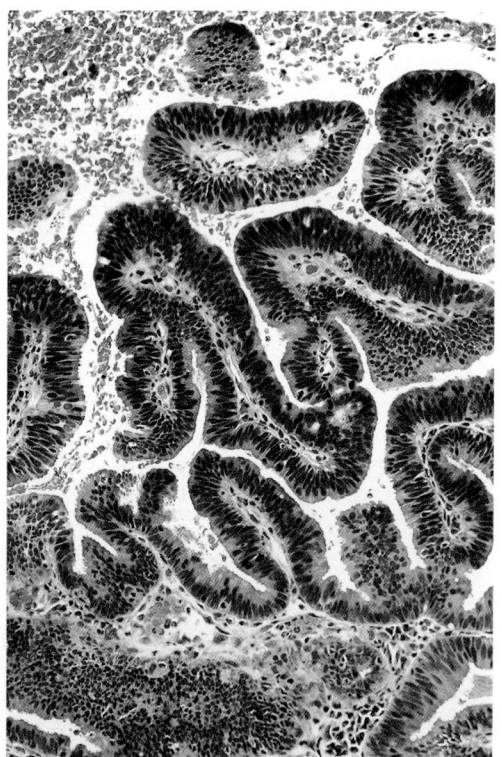
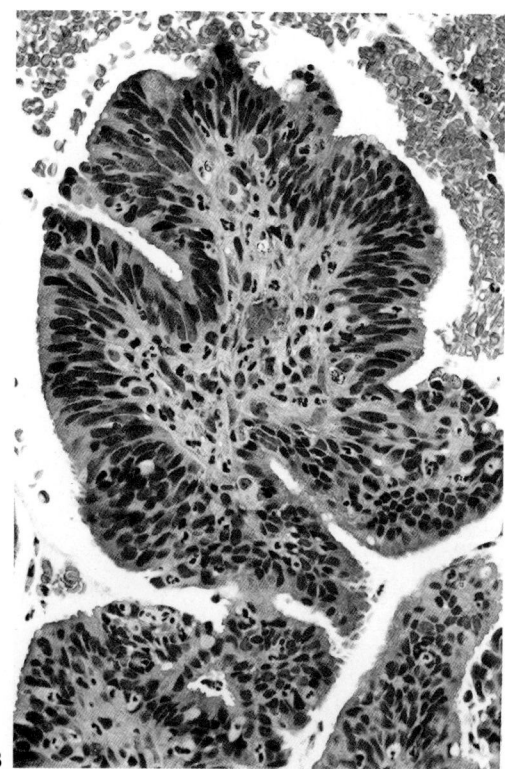

A   B

Figure 16–38. Villoglandular adenocarcinoma. *A:* The papillary structures are lined by pseudostratified columnar cells with an endometrioid appearance. No stromal invasion is seen. *B:* Higher magnification showing the elongated hyperchromatic nuclei.

superficial, which explains the excellent prognosis associated with these tumors (Jones et al., 1993; Stamatakos and Tavassoli, 1997; Young and Scully, 1989).

Villoglandular adenocarcinomas are composed of arborizing papillary structures lined by columnar cells with an endometrioid appearance (Figs. 16–38). The nuclei are elongated, hyperchromatic, and pseudostratified. When neoplastic cells contain abundant cytoplasmic mucin, the tumor may be confused with a villous adenoma. In general, there is only a mild to moderate degree of cytologic atypia and few mitotic figures.

The preinvasive phase of other malignant neoplasms of the cervix, including small cell carcinoma, large cell neuroendocrine carcinoma, carcinoid (Albores-Saavedra et al., 1997), adenoma malignum (Gilks et al., 1989), adenoid cystic carcinoma, clear cell carcinoma (Young and Scully, 1990), and papillary serous carcinoma (Zhou et al., 1998), have not been characterized.

REFERENCES

Albores-Saavedra J, Gersell D, Gilks CB, et al. (1997) Terminology of endocrine tumors of the cervix: results of a workshop Sponsored by the College of American Pathologists and the National Cancer Institute. *Arch Pathol Lab Med* 12:34–39.

Albores-Saavedra J, Molberg KH. (1997) Inverted transitional cell papilloma of the uterine cervix. *Pathol Case Rev* 2:34–37.

Albores-Saavedra J, Young RH. (1995) Transitional cell neoplasms (carcinomas and inverted papillomas) of the uterine cervix. A report of five cases. *Am J Surg Pathol* 19:1138–1145.

Anciaux D, Lawrence WD, Gregoire L. (1997) Glandular lesions of the uterine cervix: Prognostic implications of human papillomavirus status. *Int J Gynecol Pathol* 16:103–110.

Azumi N, Jones M, Joyce J, et al. (1991) Endometrial and endocervical adenocarcinomas: immunohistochemical studies and differentiating markers. *Mod Pathol* 4:54A.

Betsill WL, Jr, Clark AH. (1986) Early endocervical glandular neoplasia. I. Histomorphology, and cytomorphology. *Acta Cytol* (Baltimore) 30:115–126.

Bosch FX, Manos MM, Muñoz et al. (1995) Prevalence of human papillomavirus in cervical cancer: a world perspective. *J Natl Cancer Inst* 87:796–802.

Boshart M, Gissmann L, Ikenberg H, et al. (1984) New type of papillomavirus DNA, its presence in genital cancer biopsies and in cell lines derived from cervical cancer. *EMBO J.* 3:1151–1157.

Bousfield L, Pacey F, Young Q, et al. (1980) Expanded cytologic criteria for the diagnosis of adenocarcinoma *in situ* of the cervix and related lesions. *Acta Cytol* 24:283–296.

Brand L, Berek JS, Hacker NF. (1988) Controversies in the management of cervical adenocarcinoma. *Obstet Gynecol* 71:261–269.

Brown LJ, Wells M. (1986) Cellular glandular atypia associated with squamous intraepithelial neoplasia: a premalignant lesion? *J Clin Pathol* 39:22–28.

Casper GR, Östör AG, Quinn MA. (1997) A clinicopathologic study of glandular dysplasia of the cervix. *Gynecol Oncol* 64:166–70.

Christopherson WM, Nealon N, Gray LA Sr. (1979) Noninvasive precursor lesions of adenocarcinoma and mixed adenosquamous carcinoma of the cervix uteri. *Cancer* 44:975–983.

Clement PB, Young RH, Scully RE. (1990) Stromal endometriosis of the uterine cervix. A variant of endometriosis that may simulate a sarcoma. *Am J Surg Pathol* 14:449–455.

Cove H. (1979) The Arias-Stella reaction occurring in the endocervix in pregnancy. Recognition and comparison with adenocarcinoma of the endocervix. *Am J Surg Pathol* 3:567–568.

Creasman WT, Zaino RJ, Major FJ, DiSaia PJ, et al. (1998) Early invasive carcinoma of the cervix (3 to 5 mm invasion): risk factors and prognosis. *Am J Obstet Gynecol* 178:62–65.

Crum CP, Ikenberg H, Richart RM, Gissmann L. (1984) Human papilloma virus type 16 and early cervical neoplasia. *N Engl J Med* 310:880–883.

Cuzick J, Terry G, Ho L, et al. (1992) Human papillomavirus type 16 DNA in cervical smears as predictor of high grade cervical cancer. *Lancet* 339:959–960.

Dabbs DJ, Geisinger KR, Norris HT. (1986) Intermediate filaments in endometrial and endocervical carcinomas. *Am J Surg Pathol* 10:568–576.

Davey DD, Nielson ML, Naryshkin S, et al. (1996) Atypical squamous cells of undetermined significance: current laboratory practices of participants in the College of American Pathologists Interlaboratory Comparison Program in cervicovaginal cytology. *Arch Pathol Lab Med* 120:440–44.

Dudzinski MR, Haskill SJ, Fowler WC, et al. (1987) DNA content in cervical neoplasia and its relationship to prognosis. *Obstet Gynecol* 69:373–377.

Duggan MA, McGregor SE, Benoit JL, et al. (1995) The human papilllomavirus status of invasive cervical adenocarcinoma: a clinicopathological and outcome analysis. *Hum Pathol* 26:319–325.

Dunton CJ, VanHoeven KH, Kovatich AJ, et al. (1997) Ki-67 antigen staining as an adjunct to identifyng cervical intraepithelial neoplasia. *Gynecol Oncol* 64:451–455.

Dyson N, Howley PM, Munger K, et al. (1989) The human papillomavirus 16 E7 oncoprotein is able to bind to the retinoblastoma gene product. *Science* 243:934–37.

Editorial. (1983) Statement of caution. Interpretation of papillomavirus-associated lesions of the epithelium of uterine cervix. *Am J Obstet Gynecol* 146:125.

Egan AJM, Russell P. (1997) Transitional (urothelial) cell metaplasia of the uterine cervix: morphological assessment of 31 cases. *Int J Gynecol Pathol* 16:89–98.

Ferry JA, Scully RE. (1990) Mesonephric remnants, hyperplasia and neoplasia in the uterine cervix. A study of 49 cases. *Am J Surg Pathol* 14:1100–1111.

Friedell GH, McKay DG. (1953) Adenocarcinoma *in situ* of the endocervix. *Cancer* 6:887.

Fu YS, Berek J, Hillbaine LH. (1987) Diagnostic problems of in situ and invasive adenocarcinomas of the uterine cervix. *Appl Pathol* 5:47–56.

Fu YS, Reagan JW, Richart RM. (1981) Definition of precursors. *Gynecol Oncol* 12 (Suppl.):220–231.

Gad C, Koch F. (1978) The limitation of screening effect. A review of cervical disorders in previously screened women. *Acta Cytol* 21:719–722.

Gardner HL. (1962) Cervical endometriosis, a lesion of increasing importance. *Am J Obstet Gynecol* 84:170–173.

Geng L, Connolly DC, Isaacson C, et al. (1999) Atypical immature metaplasia (AIM) of the cervix. Is it related to high-grade squamous intraepithelial lesion (HSIL)? *Hum Pathol* 30:345–351.

Gilks CB, Young RH, Aguirre P, DeLellis RA, Scully RE. (1989) Adenoma malignum (minimal deviation adenocarcinoma) of the uterine cervix: a clinicopathological and immunohistochemical analysis of 26 cases. *Am J Surg Pathol* 13:717–729.

Gissmann L, Boshart M, Durst M, et al. (1984) Presence of human papillomavirus in genital tumors. *J Invest Dermatol* 83 (Suppl.):26–28.

Gloor E, Hurlimann J. (1986) Cervical intraepithelial glandular neoplasia (adenocarcinoma in situ and glandular dysplasia): a correlative study of 23 cases with histologic grading, histochemical analysis of mucins, and immunohistochemical determination of the affinity for four lectins. *Cancer* 58:1272–1280.

Gloor E, Ruzicka J. (1982) Morphology of adenocarcinoma in situ of the uterine cervix: a study of 14 cases. *Cancer* 49:294–302.

Goldstein NS, Ahmad E, Hussain M, et al. (1998) Endocervical gland atypia. Does a preneoplastic lesion of adenocarcinoma in situ exist? *Am J Clin Pathol* 110:200–209.

Greeley C, Schroeder S, Silverberg S. (1995) Microglandular hyperplasia of the cervix: a true "pill" lesion. *Int J Gynecol Pathol* 14:50–54.

Im DD, Duska LR, Rosenshein NB. (1995) Adequacy of conization margins in adenocarcinoma in situ of the cervix as a predictor of residual disease. *Gynecol Oncol* 59:179–182.

Jablonska S, Dabrowski J, Jakubowicz K. (1972) Epidermodysplasia verruciformis as a model in studies on the role of papovavirus in oncogenesis. *Cancer Res* 32:583–589.

Jaworski RC. (1990) Endocervical glandular dysplasia, adenocarcinoma in situ, and early invasive (microinvasive) adenocarcinoma of the uterine cervix. *Semin Diagn Pathol* 7:190–204.

Jaworski RC, Pacey NF, Greenberg ML, Osborn RA. (1988) The histologic diagnosis of adenocarcinoma in situ and related lesions of the cervix uteri. Adenocarcinoma in situ. *Cancer* 61:1171–1181.

Jenson AB, Lancaster WD. (1990) Association of human papillomavirus with benign, premalignant and malignant anogenital lesions. In: *Papillomavirus and Human Cancer* (Pfister H, ed.) pp. 11–43. CRC Press, Boca Raton, FL.

Jones MH, Koi S, Fujimoto I, Hasumi K, et al. (1994) Allelotype of uterine cancer by analysis of RFLP and microsatellite polymorphisms: frequent loss of heterozygosity on chromosome arms 3p, 9q, 10q, and 17p. *Genes Chromosomes Cancer* 9:119–123.

Jones MR, Silverberg SG, Kurman RJ. (1993) Well-differentiated villoglandular adenocarcinoma of the uterine cervix: a clinicopathological study of 24 cases. *Int J Gynecol Pathol* 12:1–7.

Jones M, Young RH. (1996) Endocervical type A (noncystic) tunnel clusters with cytologic atypia: a report of 14 cases. *Am J Surg Pathol* 20:1312–1318.

Jones M, Young RH. (1997) Atypical oxyphil metaplasia of the endocervical epithelium: a report of six cases. *Int J Gynecol Pathol* 16:99–102.

Kaku T, Enjoji M. (1983) Extremely well differentiated adenocarcinoma ("adenoma malignum") *Int J Gynecol Pathol* 2:28–41.

Kashyap V, Das DK, Luthra UK. (1990) Microphotometric DNA analysis in moderate dysplasia of the uterine cervix. Correlation to the progression and regression of the lesion. *Acta Oncol* 29:755–759.

Killackey MA, Jones WB, Lewis JL. (1986) Diagnostic conization of the cervix. Review of 460 consecutive cases. *Obstet Gynecol* 67:766–770.

Koenig C, Turnicky RP, Kankam CF, Tavassoli FA. (1997) Papillary squamotransitional cell carcinoma of the cervix: a report of 32 cases. *Am J Surg Pathol* 21:915–921.

Kraus FT, Perez-Mesa C. (1966) Verrucous carcinoma. Clinical and pathologic study of 105 cases involving oral cavity, larynx and genitalia. *Cancer* 19:26–38.

Krumins I, Young O, Pacey NF, et al. (1977) The cytologic diagnosis of adenocarcinoma in situ of the cervix uteri. *Acta Cytol* 21:320–329.

Kurman RJ. (1994) *Blaustein's Pathology of the Female Genital Tract*, pp. 229–326. Springer-Verlag, New York.

Kurman RJ, Jenson AB, Lancaster WD. (1983) Papillomavirus infection of the cervix. II. Relationship to intraepithelial neoplasia based on the presence of specific viral structural proteins. *Am J Surg Pathol* 7:39–52.

Kurman RJ, Jenson AB, Sinclair C, Lancasster W-D. (1984) Detection of human papillomaviruses by immunocytochemistry. In: *Advances in Immunocytochemistry* (DeLellis RA, ed.) pp 201. Masson Publishing, New York.

Kurman RJ, Sanz LE, Jenson AB, et al. (1982) Papillomavirus infection of the cervix. I. Correlation of histology with viral structural antigens and DNA sequences. *Int Gynecol Pathol* 1:17–28.

Kurman RJ, Schiffman MH, Lancaster WD, et al. (1988) Analysis of individual human papillomavirus types in cervical neoplasia: a possible role for the type 18 in rapid progression. *Am J Obstet Gynecol* 159:293–296.

Kurman RJ, Shah KH, Lancaster WD, Jenson AB. (1981) Immunoperoxidase localization of papillomavirus antigens in cervical dysplasia and vulvar condylomas. *Am J Obstet Gynecol* 140:931–935.

Kurtycz D, Nuñez M, Arts T, et al. (1996) Use of fluorescent in situ hybridization to detect aneuploidy in cervical dysplasia. *Diagn Cytopathol* 15:46–51.

Lancaster WD, Kurman RJ, Sanz LE, et al. (1983) Human papillomavirus: detection of viral DNA sequences and evidence of molecular heterogeneity in metaplasias and dysplasias of the uterine cervix. *Intervirology* 20:202–212.

Larraza-Hernandez O, Molberg KH, Lindberg G, Albores-Saavedra J. (1997) Ectopic prostatic tissue in the uterine cervix. Case report. *Int J Gynecol Pathol* 16:291–293.

Lee KR, Howard P, Heintz NH, et al. (1993) Low prevalence of human papillomavirus types 16 and 18 in cervical adenocarcinoma *in situ*, invasive adenocarcinoma and glandular dysplasia by polimerase chain reaction. *Mod Pathol* 6:433–437.

Lesack D, Wahab I, Gilks CB. (1996) Radiation-induced atypia of endocervical epithelium: a histological, immunohistochemical and cytometric study. *Int J Gynecol Pathol* 15:242–247.

Lininger RA, Wistuba II, Gazdar A, Koenig C, Tavassoli FA, Albores-Saavedra J. (1998) Human papillomavirus type16 is detected in transitional cell carcinomas and squamotransitional cell carcinomas of the cervix and endometrium. *Cancer* 83:521–527.

Lorincz AT, Lancaster WD, Kurman R, et al. (1986) Characterization of human papillomavirus in cervical neoplasias and their detection in routine clinical screening. In: *Proceedings, Banbury Conference.*

Luff RD. (1992) The Bethesda System for Reporting Cervical/Vaginal Cytologic Diagnoses. Report of the 1991 Bethesda Workshop. *Hum Pathol* 23:719–721.

Maes G, Flemen GJ, Bara J, et al. (1988) The distribution of mucins, carcinoembryonic antigen, and mucus-associated antigens in endocervical and endometrial adenocarcinomas. *Int J Gynecol Pathol* 7:112–122.

Maier RC, Norris HJ. (1980) Coexistence of cervical intraepithelial neoplasia with primary adenocarcinoma of the endocervix. *Obstet Gynecol* 56:361–364.

Mannion C, Park WS, Man YG, et al. (1998) Endocrine tumors of the uterine cervix: morphologic assessment, expression of human papillomavirus, and evaluation for loss of heterozygosity on 1p, 3p, 11q, and 17p. *Cancer* 83:1391–1400.

Meisels A, Fortin R. (1976) Condylomatous lesions of the cervix and vagina. I. Cytologic patterns. *Acta Cytol* 20:505–509.

Meisels A, Roy M, Fortier M, et al. (1981) Human papillomavirus infections of the cervix. The atypical condyloma. *Acta Cytol* 25:7–16.

Mitra AB, Murty VV, Li RG, et al. (1994) Allelotype analysis of cervical carcinoma. *Cancer Res* 54:4481–4487.

Möbius G. (1985) The value of cytodiagnosis in cervix cancer precursors and the latency and progression of carcinoma *in situ. Pathol Res Pract* 180:670–674.

Mullokandov MR, Kholodilov NG, Atkin NB, et al. (1995) Genomic alterations in cervical carcinoma: losses of chromosome heterozygosity and human papilloma virus tumor status. *Cancer Res* 56:197–205.

Murdoch JB, Grimshaw RN, Morgan PR, et al. (1992) The impact of loop diathermy on management of early invasive cervical cancer. *Int J Gynecol Cancer* 2: 129–133.

Nasiell K, Nasiell M, Vaclavinkova V. (1983) Behavior of moderate cervical dysplasia during long-term follow-up. *Obstet Gynecol* 61:609–614.

Okagaki T. (1984) Female genital tumors associated with human papillomavirus infection, and the concept of genital neoplasm-papilloma syndrome (GENPS) *Pathol Annu* (Part 2):31.

Okagaki T, Tase T, Twiggs LB, et al. (1989) Histogenesis of cervical adenocarcinoma with reference to human papillomavirus-18 as a carcinogen. *J Reprod Med* 34:639–644.

Okagaki T, Twiggs LB, Zachow KR, et al. (1983) Identification of human papillomavirus DNA in cervical and vaginal intraepithelial neoplasia with molecularly cloned virus-specific DNA probes. *Int J Gynecol Pathol* 2:152–159.

Oliva E, Clement PB, Young RH. (1995) Tubal and tuboendometrioid metaplasia of the uterine cervix. Unemphasized features that may cause problems in differential diagnosis: a report of 25 cases. *Am J Clin Pathol* 103:618–23.

Orth G, Jablonska S, Breitburd F, et al. (1980) Epidermodysplasia verruciformis: a model for viral oncogenesis in man. *Cold Spring Harbor Conf Cell Prolix* 7:259.

Östör A. (1993) Studies on 200 cases of early squamous cell carcinoma of the cervix. *Int J Gynecol Pathol* 12: 193–207.

Östör A, Rome R, Quin M. (1997) Microinvasive adenocarcinoma of the cervix: a clinicopathologic study of 77 women. *Obstet Gynecol* 89:88–93.

Pao CC, Kao SM, Chen JH, et al. (1994) State of mutational alterations of p53 and retinoblastoma susceptibility genes in papillomavirus-negative small cell cervical carcinomas. *Am J Clin Pathol* 102:665–670.

Paquette RL, Lee YY, Wilczynski SP, et al. (1993) Mutations of p53 and human papillomavirus infection in cervical carcinoma. *Anticancer Res* 13:1107–1111.

Parker SL, Tong T, Bolden S, Wingo PA. (1997) Cancer Statistics, 1997. *CA Cancer J Clin* 47:10–11.

Parkin DM, Pisani P, Ferlay J. (1993) Estimates of the worldwide incidence of eighteen major cancers in 1985. *Int J Cancer* 54:594–606.

Pfister H. (1984) Biology and biochemistry of papillomaviruses. *Rev Physiol Biochem Pharmacol* 99:111–181.

Pinion SB, Kennedy JH, Miller RW, MacLean AB. (1991) Oncogene expression in cervical intraepithelial neoplasia and invasive cancer of cervix. *Lancet* 337:819–820.

Purola E, Savia E. (1977) Cytology of gynecologic condyloma acuminatum. *Acta Cytol* 21:26–31.

Qizilbash AH. (1975) *In situ* and microinvasive adenocarcinoma of the uterine cervix. A clinical, cytologic and histologic study of 14 cases. *Am J Clin Pathol* 64: 155–170.

Rader JS, Kamarasova T, Huettener PC, et al. (1997) Allelotyping of all chromosomal arms in invasive cervical cancer. *Oncogene* 13:2737–2741.

Richart RM. (1968) Natural history of cervical intraepithelial neoplasia. *Clin Obstet Gynecol* 5:748–784.

Richart RM. (1987) Causes and management of cervical intraepithelial neoplasia. *Cancer* 60 (Suppl.): 1951–1959.

Roman LD, Felix JC, Muderspach LI, et al. (1997) Risk of residual invasive disease in women with microinvasive squamous cancer in a conization specimen. *Obstet Gynecol* 90:759–764.

Scheffner M, Wernessw BA, Huibregtse JM, et al. (1990) The E6 oncoprotein encoded by human papillomavirus types 16 and 18 promotes the degradation of p53. *Cell* 63:1129–1136.

Schiffman MH, Bauer HM, Hoover RN, et al. (1993) Epidemiologic evidence showing that human papillomavirus infections causes most cervical intraepithelial neoplasia. *J Natl Cancer Inst* 85:958–964.

Schlesinger C, Silverberg SG. (1999) Endocervical adenocarcinoma *in situ* of tubal type and its relation to atypical tubal metaplasia. *Int J Gynecol Pathol* 18:1–4.

Schwartz SM, Weiss NS. (1986) Increased incidence of adenocarcinoma of the cervix in young women in the United States. *Am J Epidemiol* 124:1045–1047.

Scully RE, Bonfiglio TA, Kurman RJ, et al. (1994) *Histological Typing of Female Genital Tract Tumours.* World Health Organization, 2nd ed., Springer-Verlag, New York.

Sherman ME, Kurman RJ. (1998) Intraepithelial carcinoma of the cervix: reflections on half a century of progress. *Cancer* 83:2243–2246.

Siedman JD, Tavassoli FA. (1995) Mesonephric hyperplasia of the uterine cervix. A clinicopathologic study of 52 cases. *Int J Gynecol Pathol* 14:293–299.

Stamatakos MD, Tavassoli FA. (1997) Villoglandular papillary adenocarcinoma of the cervix. Case report and review of the literature. *Pathol Case Rev* 2:38–42.

Suh KS, Silverberg SG. (1990) Tubal metaplasia of the uterine cervix. *Int J Gynecol Pathol* 9:122–128.

Tamimi HK, Figge DC. (1982) Adenocarcinoma of the uterine cervix. *Gynecol Oncol* 13:335–344.

Tase T, Okagaki T, Clark BA, et al. (1989) Human papillomavirus DNA in adenocarcinoma *in situ,* microinvasive adenocarcinoma of the uterine cervix, and coexisting cervical squamous intraepithelial neoplasia. *Int J Gynecol Pathol* 8:8–17.

Taylor HB, Irey NS, Norris HJ. (1967) Atypical endocervical hyperplasia in women taking oral contraceptives. *JAMA* 202:637–639.

Vonka V, Kanka J, Jelinek J, et al. (1984) Prospective study of the relationship between cervical neoplasia and herpes simplex type-2 virus. I. Epidemiological characteristics. *Int J Cancer* 33:49–60.

Weir MM, Bell DA, Young RH. (1997) Transitional cell metaplasia of the uterine cervix and vagina. An underrecognized lesion that may be confused with high grade dysplasia. A report of 59 cases. *Am J Surg Pathol* 21:507–510.

Weisbrot I, Stabinsky C, Davis AM. (1972) Adenocarcinoma *in situ* of the uterine cervix. *Cancer* 29:1179–1187.

Wilczynski SP, Walker J, Liao SY, et al. (1988) Adenocarcinoma of the cervix associated with human papillomavirus. *Cancer* 62:1331–1336.

Willet GD, Kurman RJ, Reid R, et al. (1989) Correlation of the histologic appearance of intraepithelial neoplasia of the cervix with human papillomavirus types. *Int J Gynecol Pathol* 8:18–25.

Wistuba II, Montellano FD, Milchgrub S, et al. (1997) Deletions of chromosome 3p are frequent and early events in the pathogenesis of uterine cervical carcinoma. *Cancer Res* 57:3154–3158.

Workshop. (1989) The 1988 Bethesda System for Reporting Cervical/Vaginal Cytologic Diagnosis. *JAMA* 262:931–934.

Wright TC, Lorincz A, Ferris DG, et al. (1998) Reflex human papillomavirus deoxyribonucleic acid testing in women with abnormal Papanicolaou smears. *Am J Obstet Gynecol* 178:962–966.

Xu B, Keesee S, Meyer J, et al, (1998) The use of NMP179, a unique nuclear matrix marker, for prediction of behavior of cases designated as ASCUS: a pilot study. *Acta Cytol* 42:1226.

Yashima K, Ashfaq R, Nowak J, et al. (1998) Telomerase activity and expression of its RNA component in cervical lesions. *Cancer* 82:1319–1327.

Young RH, Scully RE. (1989a) Atypical forms of microglandular hyperplasia of the cervix simulating carcinoma. *Am J Surg Pathol* 13:50–56.

Young RH, Scully RE. (1989b) Villoglandular papillary adenocarcinoma of the uterine cervix. A clinicopathologic analysis of 13 cases. *Cancer* 63:1773–1779.

Young RH, Scully RE. (1990) Invasive adenocarcinoma and related tumours of the uterine cervix. *Semin Diagn Pathol* 7:205–227.

Zhou C, Gilks CB, Hayes M, Clement PB. (1998) Papillary serous carcinoma of the uterine cervix. A clinicopathologic study of 17 cases. *Am J Surg Pathol* 22:113–120.

Ziol M, Di Tomaso C, Biaggi A, et al. (1998) Virological and biological characteristics of cervical intraepithelial neoplasia grade I with marked koilocytotic atypia. *Hum Pathol* 29:1068–1073.

17

ENDOMETRIUM

Brigitte M. Ronnett, Mark E. Sherman, and Robert J. Kurman

Endometrial carcinoma is the most common malignant neoplasm of the female genital tract. Factors associated with unopposed estrogenic stimulation, such as obesity, exogenous hormone use, and endometrial hyperplasia, are related to the development of the most common form of endometrial carcinoma—that is, the endometrioid subtype (Bokhman, 1983). More recent studies have confirmed this association by demonstrating elevated serum estrogen levels in patients with endometrioid carcinoma (Brinton et al., 1992; Potischman et al., 1996). It also has been recognized that some forms of endometrial carcinoma appear to be unrelated to hormonal factors and hyperplasia (Sherman et al., 1997). Serous carcinoma is the prototypic endometrial carcinoma that is not related to estrogenic stimulation. In the past two decades, clinicopathologic, immunohistochemical, and molecular genetic studies have provided additional data to allow for the development of a dualistic model of endometrial carcinogenesis. In this model two types of precursor lesions are proposed for the two pathways of endometrial carcinogenesis. *Atypical hyperplasia* (AH) is recognized as the precursor for the endometrioid type of endometrial carcinoma and *endometrial intraepithelial carcinoma* (EIC) as the precursor for serous carcinoma, the most common nonendometrioid subtype of endometrial carcinoma. The following discussion summarizes current knowledge about the relationship of these precursor lesions to the various forms of endometrial carcinoma.

ATYPICAL ENDOMETRIAL HYPERPLASIA AND ITS RELATIONSHIP TO ENDOMETRIOID CARCINOMA OF THE ENDOMETRIUM

CLASSIFICATION AND BEHAVIOR OF ENDOMETRIAL HYPERPLASIAS

In the past, the terms *adenomatous hyperplasia* and *atypical hyperplasia* were used to denote proliferative lesions of the endometrium with varying degrees of architectural complexity and cytologic atypia (Buehl et al., 1964; Campbell and Barter, 1961; Gusberg, 1947; Gusberg and Kaplan, 1963; Gusberg et al., 1954; Hertig and Sommers, 1949; Hertig et al., 1949; Novak and Rutledge, 1948; Vellios, 1974). In addition, the term *carcinoma in situ* was proposed to describe small lesions, with or without glandular crowding, having the cytologic features of carcinoma but lacking invasion (Buehl et al., 1964; Hertig and Sommers, 1949; Hertig et al., 1949; Tavassoli and Kraus, 1978; Vellios, 1974; Welch and Scully, 1977). However, because carcinoma *in situ* was never clearly defined, the term was abandoned and, in retrospect, many of these lesions would be classified today as *hyperplasia with eosinophilic change*. Recently, Spiegel (1995) applied the term to an entirely different set of lesions that are associated with serous carcinoma (see below), adding further ambiguity to the historical confusion surrounding its clinical and biological significance. Pathologists have recognized for decades that endometrial cancer precursors are morphologically and biologically heterogeneous. However, early studies designed to clarify the significance of these lesions were limited by the lack of standardized diagnostic criteria, failure to consider cytologic and architectural features separately, and inclusion of irradiated patients, which may have altered the natural history of the lesions studied (Beutler et al., 1963; Chamlian and Taylor, 1970; Gusberg, 1947; Hertig and Sommers, 1949; Hertig et al., 1949; McBride, 1959; Vellios, 1974; Welch and Scully, 1977). Many of these limitations have been addressed in more recent studies. Kurman et al. (1985) reported a retrospective follow-up study of 170 patients with untreated endometrial hyperplasias that were classified according to architectural and cytologic features identified in endometrial curettings. Women were followed from 1 to 27 years before undergoing hysterectomy in order to delineate the histologic features associated with an increased risk of progression to carcinoma. Lesions were classified as *hyperplasia* or *atypical hyperplasia* according to the absence or presence of nuclear atypia. One-third of the patients with hyperplasia and atypical hyperplasia were asymptomatic after the curettage, presumably because of regression of the lesion, and required no further treatment. Of the patients who required additional hormonal or surgical treatment, 69% with hyperplasia and 39% with atypical hyperplasia regressed. The proliferative process persisted in 28% of women with hyperplasia and in 27% of those with atypical hyperplasia. Two (2%) of 122 patients with hyperplasia progressed to carcinoma whereas 11 (23%) of the 48 women with atypical hyperplasia progressed to carcinoma ($p = 0.001$) (Table 17–1). In a similar study, Gusberg and Kaplan (1963) found that 20% of their group of patients with "severe adenomatous hyperplasia" had uterine carcinoma when hysterectomy was done shortly after curettage, but only 11% of those who were followed developed carcinoma.

In their study, Kurman et al. also assessed the degree of glandular complexity and crowding in an effort to identify a subgroup of lesions with an increased risk of progression to carcinoma. Thus, a proliferative lesion displaying minimal to moderate glandular complexity and crowding but lacking cytologic atypia was termed *simple hyperplasia* (Figs. 17–1 and 17–2), whereas one with marked glandular crowding was termed *complex hyperplasia* (Fig. 17–3). An endometrial proliferation displaying minimal to moderate glandular complexity and crowding accompanied by cytologic atypia was designated *simple atypical hyperplasia* (Figs. 17–4 and 17–5), whereas one demonstrating marked glandular crowding and cytologic atypia was designated *complex atypical hyperplasia* (Figs. 17–6 and 17–7). Progression to carcinoma occurred in 1 (1%) of 93 patients with simple hyperplasia, in 1 (3%) of 29 patients with complex hyperplasia, in 1 (8%) of 13 patients with simple atypical hyperplasia, and in 10 (29%) of 35 patients with complex atypical hyperplasia (Table 17–2). Simple atypical hyperplasia is an uncommon lesion. In most hyperplastic lesions, the degree of glandular crowding and complexity and level of cytologic atypia are concordant. Thus, cytologic atypia was the most useful criterion for identifying a patient with a significantly increased risk of developing carcinoma, with the presence of superimposed glandular complexity and crowding placing the patient at greater risk. This study established the classification of endometrial hyperplasias that was adopted by the World Health Organization (WHO) (Table 17–3; Scully et al., 1994). A more recent study of the behavior of endometrial hyperplasia found that most cases of endometrial hyperplasia without atypia regressed spontaneously, whereas those with complex atypical hyperplasia were much more likely to persist

Table 17–1. Follow-up of Hyperplasia in Comparison with Atypical Hyperplasia (170 Patients)

Finding	Patients n	Regressed n (%)	Persisted n (%)	Progressed to Carcinoma	
				n (%)	P
Hyperplasia	122	97 (80)	23 (19)	2 (2)	0.001
Atypical hyperplasia	48	8 (58)	9 (19)	11 (23)	0.001

Adapted from Kurman et al., 1985, with permission.

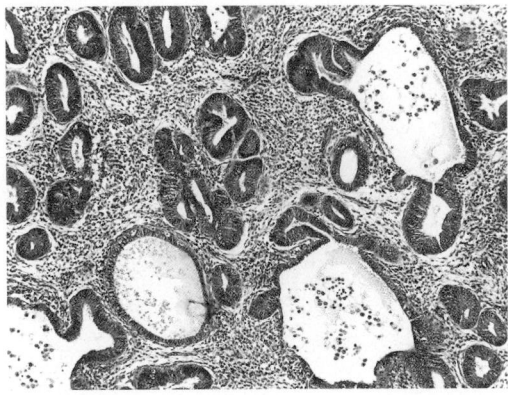

Figure 17–1. Simple hyperplasia without atypia. Glands are slightly crowded, cystically dilated, and have focal glandular outpouchings.

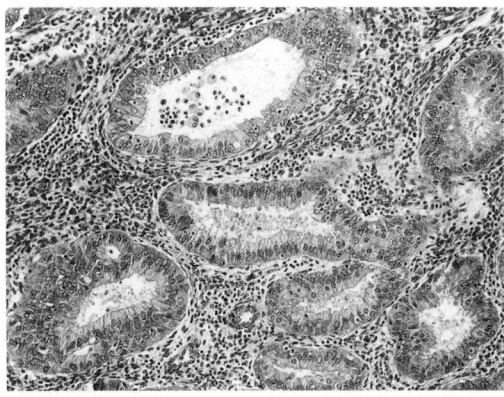

Figure 17–4. Simple atypical hyperplasia. Glands are slightly crowded with a moderate amount of intervening stroma.

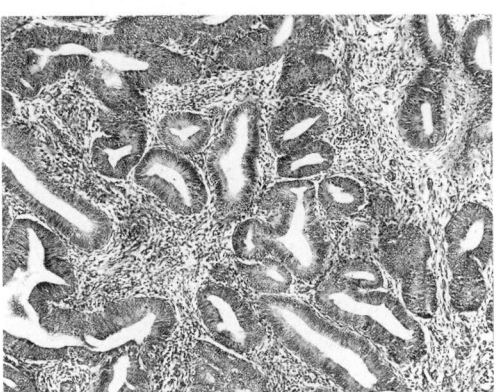

Figure 17–2. Simple hyperplasia without atypia. Glands are slightly more crowded than in Figure 17–1 but they are not arranged in a back-to-back fashion and there is minimal glandular complexity.

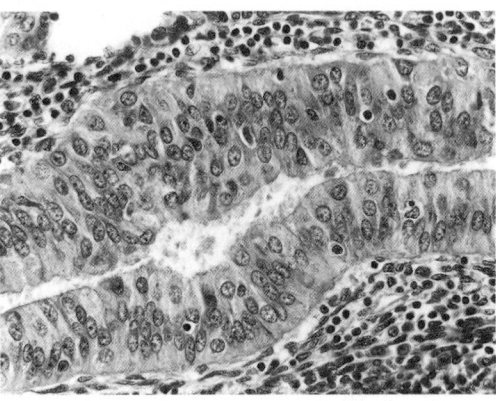

Figure 17–5. Simple atypical hyperplasia. Higher magnification of Figure 17–4 demonstrates cytologic atypia characterized by loss of cellular polarity, nuclear enlargement and rounding, coarse and vesicular chromatin, and occasional prominent nucleoli.

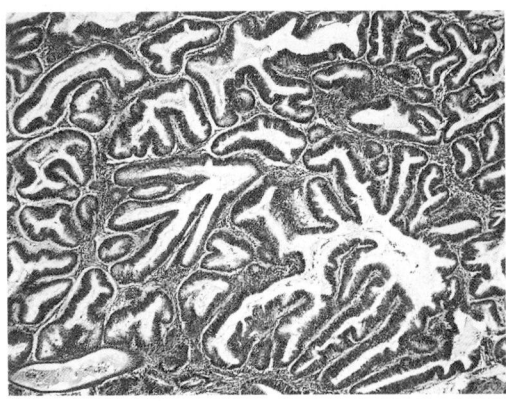

Figure 17–3. Complex hyperplasia without atypia. Glands are crowded in a back-to-back fashion with minimal intervening stroma. Gland outlines are complex rather than simple.

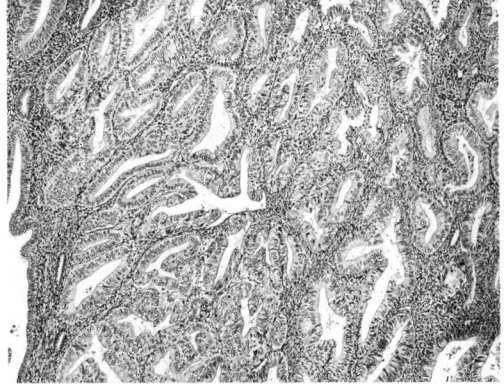

Figure 17–6. Complex atypical hyperplasia. Despite marked glandular crowding, individual glands are completely surrounded by stroma. The glands are not confluent and the stroma shows no evidence of desmoplasia.

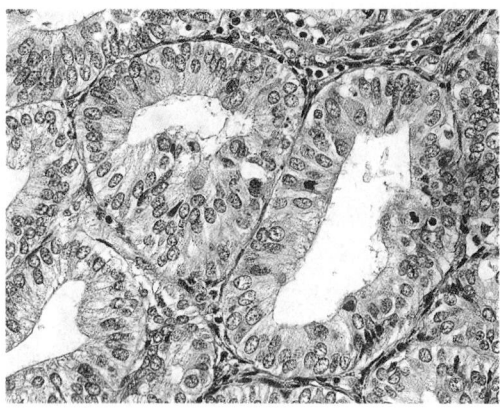

Figure 17–7. Complex atypical hyperplasia. Crowded glands display loss of polarity, nuclear rounding, chromatin irregularities, nucleoli, and occasional mitotic figures.

(Terakawa et al., 1997). Another recent study confirmed the significance of cytologic atypia in predicting an increased risk of associated endometrial carcinoma in hysterectomy specimens (Hunter et al., 1994). Since the vast majority of atypical hyperplasias have complex architecture, complex atypical hyperplasia is associated with a significant risk of persistence and progression to carcinoma. Hence, this lesion is regarded as a direct precursor of well-differentiated endometrioid carcinoma of the endometrium. However, hyperplasia is identified in a prior endometrial specimen or in the hysterectomy specimen in only 35%–75% of women with endometrial carcinoma (Ayhan and Yarali, 1991; Beckner et al., 1985; Bokhman, 1983; Deligdisch and Cohen, 1985; Gucer et al., 1998; Kaku et al., 1996). In those reports that specified the number of hyperplasias that were classified as atypical, 14–36% of women with endometrial carcinoma had associated atypical hyperplasia

Table 17–3. Classification of Noninvasive Endometrial Proliferations

I. Hyperplasia
  A. Simple hyperplasia
  B. Complex hyperplasia
II. Atypical hyperplasia
  A. Simple atypical hyperplasia
  B. Complex atypical hyperplasia

(Gucer et al., 1998; Kaku, 1996). It is unclear whether failure to identify an associated atypical hyperplasia in all cases of endometrioid carcinoma reflects overgrowth of a preexisting hyperplasia by carcinoma or the development of carcinoma through a different pathway.

Some investigators have attempted to use computerized nuclear and architectural morphometric analyses of endometrial hyperplasias to predict coexistent carcinoma in hysterectomy specimens (Ausems et al., 1985; Baak, 1986; Baak et al., 1988, 1992; Dunton et al., 1996). Nuclear morphometry alone has been shown to be insufficiently sensitive and specific to properly distinguish atypical hyperplasias that are associated with carcinoma from those that are not (Ausems et al., 1985; Baak, 1986). The combination of architectural and nuclear morphometric features has been shown to identify 63%–100% of the cases of atypical hyperplasia analyzed that did not have coexistent or subsequent carcinoma. However, not all patients with atypical hyperplasia assessed as high risk for carcinoma based on morphometry had carcinoma detected on follow-up (Baak et al., 1988, 1992; Dunton et al., 1996). Although morphometric analysis is now available in many centers, it is costly and labor intensive and therefore not practical for most laboratories.

Table 17–2. Follow-up of Hyperplasia: Comparison of Cytologic and Architectural Abnormalities (170 Patients)

Finding	Patients n	Regressed n (%)	Persisted n (%)	Progressed to Carcinoma n (%)
Simple hyperplasia	93	74 (80)	18 (19)	1 (1)
Complex hyperplasia	29	23 (80)	5 (17)	1 (3)
Simple atypical hyperplasia	13	9 (70)	3 (23)	1 (8)
Complex atypical hyperplasia	35	20 (57)	5 (14)	10 (29)

Adapted from Kurman et al., 1985, with permission.

PATHOLOGIC DISTINCTION OF ATYPICAL HYPERPLASIA FROM WELL-DIFFERENTIATED ENDOMETRIOID CARCINOMA

To determine specific and reproducible criteria for distinguishing atypical hyperplasia and so-called carcinoma-*in situ* from well-differentiated carcinoma in curettings, Kurman and Norris (1982) reviewed 204 curettings from the Armed Forces Institute of Pathology (AFIP) files. Cases showing the most severe forms of atypical hyperplasia, including examples of what have been regarded as carcinoma *in situ* and well-differentiated carcinoma, were selected and compared with the findings in nonirradiated hysterectomy specimens obtained within 1 month of the curettage. Degrees of cellular atypia, stratification, mitotic activity, and the presence or absence of stromal invasion (see below) were recorded. Of these features, stromal invasion was the most useful criterion for predicting the presence of a clinically significant carcinoma that had invaded the myometrium, including those that had metastasized (King et al., 1984; Kurman and Norris, 1982).

Identification of stromal invasion depended on the presence of one of the following: *(1)* an irregular infiltration of glands associated with cellular, reactive-appearing fibroblastic stroma (desmoplastic response); *(2)* a confluent glandular and/or cribriform pattern in which individual glands, uninterrupted by stroma, merge; and *(3)* an extensive papillary pattern. The processes that manifested the aforementioned features of invasion had to be sufficiently extensive to involve half of a low-power field measuring 4.2 mm in diameter without intervening stroma (Kurman and Norris, 1982; Norris et al., 1983). Originally, replacement of the endometrial stroma by masses of squamous epithelium was considered a rare manifestation of invasion but this criterion has subsequently been modified. Currently, masses of squamous epithelium that replace the endometrium (greater than a 2 mm^2 area) are interpreted as evidence of stromal invasion only if associated with a desmoplastic response or a confluent glandular pattern (Kurman and Norris, 1994). These three features are detailed below.

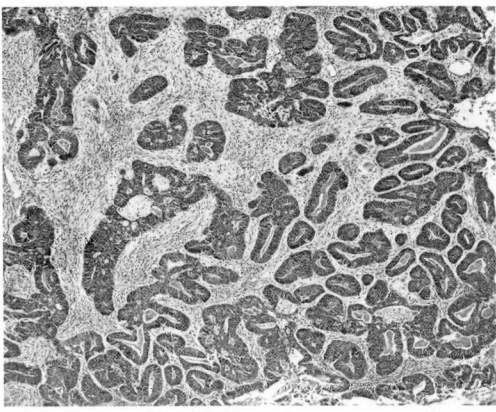

Figure 17–8. Well-differentiated endometrioid carcinoma. Glands are surrounded by a desmoplastic stroma that reflects stromal invasion. [From Kurman, R.J., and Norris, H.J.: Evaluation of criteria for distinguishing atypical endometrial hyperplasia from well-differentiated carcinoma. Cancer 49:2547–2559, 1982; with permission.]

1. A desmoplastic stromal response is characterized by altered stroma containing densely arranged, parallel, reactive fibroblasts that are more spindle shaped than the stromal cells of proliferative or hyperplastic endometrium (Figs. 17–8 to 17–10). Collagen is often prominent, unlike proliferative and hyperplastic endometria, in which it is inconspicuous. The desmoplasia is frequently maintained when neoplastic glands invade the myometrium. Frag-

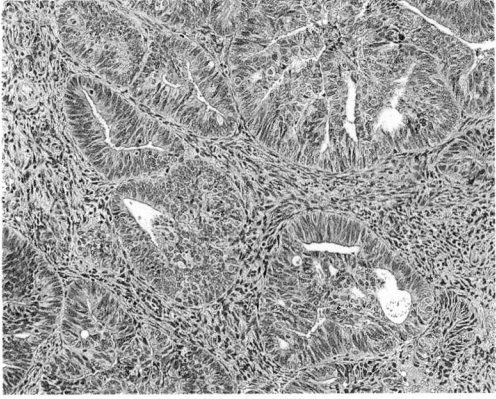

Figure 17–9. Well-differentiated endometrioid carcinoma. Endometrial stroma is altered and replaced by fibroblasts, resulting in a desmoplastic reaction that reflects invasion.

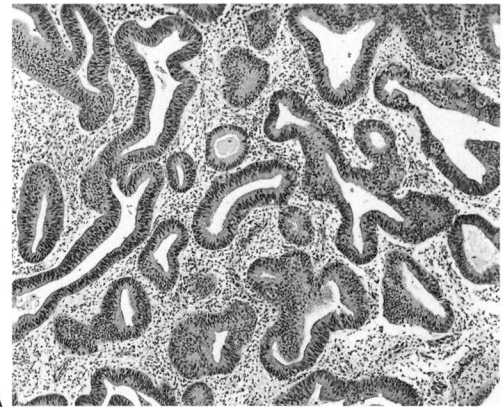
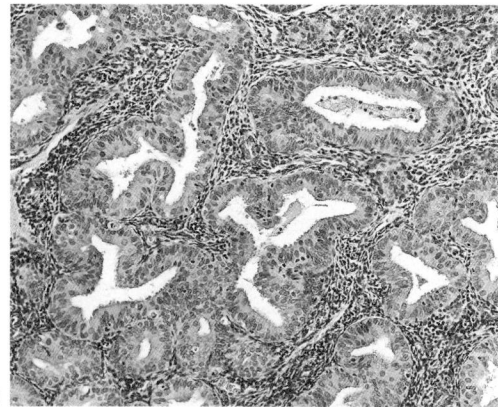

Figure 17–10. Two examples of endometrial hyperplasia that lack stromal desmoplasia *A:* Simple hyperplasia without atypia. *B:* Complex atypical hyperplasia. Glands in both examples are surrounded by stroma that resembles that seen in proliferative endometrium. The stroma surrounding the glands in B is compressed by the closely packed hyperplastic glands. There is no desmoplastic reaction and thus stromal invasion is absent.

ments of polyps, including the atypical adenomyomatous polyp identified by Mazur (1981), or tissue from the lower uterine segment has a fibrous stroma that can be difficult to distinguish from desmoplastic stroma. In such instances, features other than the altered stroma should be used to determine whether stromal invasion is present (see below).

2. Confluent glandular or cribriform growth is characterized by glands that are fused and lack intervening normal stroma (Figs. 17–11 and 17–12).

3. Complex papillary patterns in which multiple branching fibrous processes are lined by atypical columnar epithelium are also considered to represent carcinoma (Fig. 17–13). Hyperplasia may form papillary projections lined by stratified atypical epithelial cells, but these are confined within glandular lumina and lack fibrovascular cores.

When stromal invasion was present in curettings, residual carcinoma was found in the uterus in half the cases; of these, one-third were moderately or poorly differentiated and one-fourth deeply invaded the myometrium (Table 17–4). Seven percent of women with carcinomas (stromal invasion identified in curettings) had extrauterine metastases at hysterectomy, and half of the women died of tumor.

Increasing degrees of nuclear atypia, mi-

totic activity, and stratification of cells in curettings were associated with a higher frequency of carcinoma in the subsequent hysterectomy specimen in the above study (Kurman and Norris, 1982) but were of limited value because even a mild degree of these changes was associated with carcinoma in nearly one-third of the cases. Of the residual carcinomas identified, 20% were moderately or poorly differentiated and 10% invaded the middle or outer third of the myometrium. The presence of nuclear atypia, mitotic activity, and stratification of cells in curettings, therefore, did not permit the

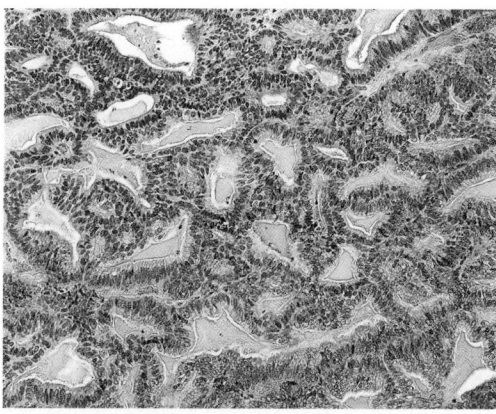

Figure 17–11. Well-differentiated endometrioid carcinoma. Confluent glandular pattern reflects stromal invasion.

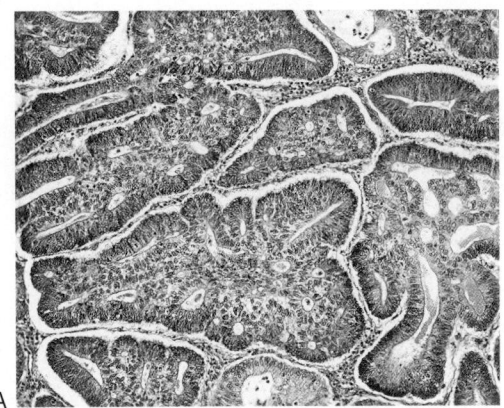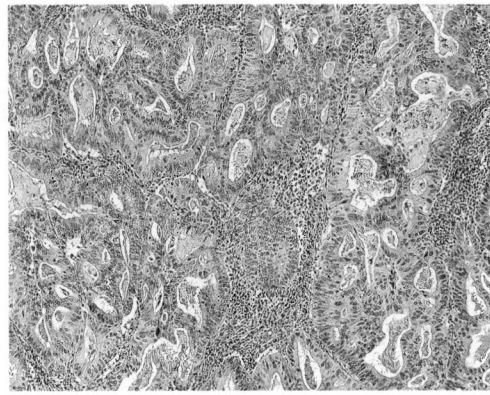

A   B

Figure 17–12. Well-differentiated endometrioid carcinomas. Two examples illustrate the cribriform pattern of stromal invasion. [*A* from Kurman and Norris, 1982, with permission.]

recognition of a biologically significant lesion in the uterus.

When stromal invasion was absent in the curettings, carcinoma was found in the uterus in only 17% of cases, and all the carcinomas were well differentiated and either confined to the endometrium or only superficially invasive (Table 17–5). None of the 89 patients whose lesions in curettings lacked stromal invasion had a recurrence. The finding of carcinoma in the uterus in 17% of patients who demonstrated only atypical hyperplasia in curettings was no higher than anticipated because similar findings had been reported by others (Campbell and

Barter, 1961; Tavassoli and Kraus, 1978). Two more recent studies, however, found higher frequencies of endometrial carcinoma (43% and 50%) in hysterectomy specimens following a diagnosis of atypical hyperplasia (Janicek and Rosenshein, 1994; Widra et al., 1995). Of the carcinomas detected in both studies, 43% were stage 1C or greater. These studies included patients who had been diagnosed by either curettage or biopsy but there were no significant differences in the frequencies with which carcinoma was detected at hysterectomy in those patients who received a curettage compared to those who had been biopsied. However, in one of these studies, the biopsy and curettage specimens were not reviewed to confirm that features of stromal invasion were absent in these specimens (Janicek and Rosenshein, 1994).

Thus, stromal invasion is the most useful feature for distinguishing atypical hyperplasia from well-differentiated carcinoma in curettings. The above findings also indicate

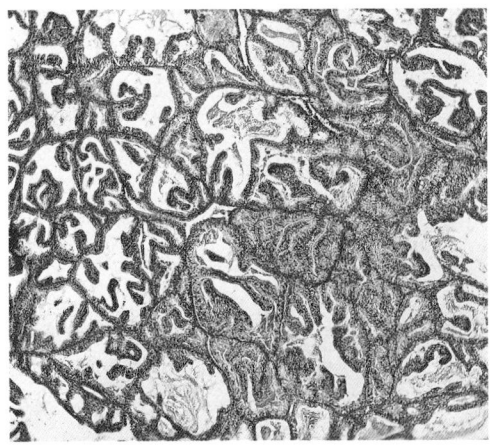

Figure 17–13. Well-differentiated endometrioid carcinoma. A complex papillary pattern is a manifestation of stromal invasion. [From Kurman and Norris, 1982, with permission.]

Table 17–4. Residual Carcinoma in 115 Uteri After Curettage Showing No Stromal Invasion

Finding	Number (%)
Residual carcinoma	58 (50)
Grade 1	38 (66)
Grade 2	14 (24)
Grade 3	6 (10)
Myometrial invasion	42 (72)
Inner third	28 (48)
Middle and outer thirds	14 (24)

Adapted from Kurman et al., 1982, with permission.

Table 17–5. Residual Carcinoma in 89 Uteri After Curettage Showing No Stromal Invasion

Finding	Number (%)
Residual carcinoma	15 (17)
Grade 1	15
Myometrial invasion	7
Depth of invasion	
1 mm or less	5
2 to 4 mm	2

Adapted from Kurman et al., 1982, with permission.

that the presence and absence of stromal invasion in curettings are correlated, respectively, with the finding of more aggressive versus low-grade carcinomas in hysterectomy specimens. More recently, another study has demonstrated that clinically significant endometrial proliferations, i.e., those that have a high likelihood of myometrial invasion, can be recognized when either sufficient architectural complexity or nuclear atypia, including prominence of nucleoli, is present (Longacre et al., 1995). In addition, the strong association of a desmoplastic stromal response with a myoinvasive lesion was confirmed.

REPRODUCIBILITY OF DIAGNOSIS OF ENDOMETRIAL HYPERPLASIA, ATYPICAL HYPERPLASIA, AND WELL-DIFFERENTIATED CARCINOMA

Few studies have addressed the reproducibility of the diagnosis of endometrial hyperplasia and its distinction from well-differentiated carcinoma. One study that compared diagnostic reproducibility using the 1975 and 1994 WHO classifications of endometrial hyperplasia and carcinoma found that interobserver agreement was fair to moderate with both systems (Skov et al., 1997). A subsequent study of 100 endometrial biopsy and curettage specimens ranging from proliferative endometrium to well-differentiated carcinoma found substantial interobserver agreement for diagnoses of hyperplasia and well-differentiated carcinoma but only moderate agreement for the diagnosis of atypical hyperplasia (Table 17–6; Kendall et al., 1998). Of numerous histologic features evaluated, the only feature that was associated with distinction of atypical hyperplasia from hyperplasia without atypia in multivariable logistic regression analysis was the presence of nucleoli. The features that were associated with the distinction of carcinoma from atypical hyper-

Table 17–6. Intra- and Interobserver Reproducibility of Diagnoses of Hyperplasia, Atypical Hyperplasia, and Well-Differentiated Carcinoma of the Endometrium

Intraobserver agreement for Diagnosis of Proliferative Endometrium, Hyperplasia, Atypical Hyperplasia, Well-Differentiated Carcinoma			
Pathologist	Kappa Value	% Agreement	Interpretation
1	0.67	76	Substantial
2	0.69	77	Substantial
3	0.70	77	Substantial
4	0.77	83	Substantial
5	0.85	89	Almost perfect

Interobserver agreement for 4 diagnostic categories[a]				
Diagnosis	Round 1	Interpretation	Round 2	Interpretation
Proliferative endometrium	0.86	Almost perfect	0.86	Almost perfect
Hyperplasia	0.65	Substantial	0.60	Substantial
Atypical hyperplasia	0.42	Moderate	0.47	Moderate
Well-differentiated carcinoma	0.79	Substantial	0.83	Almost perfect

[a]Kappa values.

Data from Kendall et al. (1998).

Table 17–7. Correlation of Histologic Features with Diagnoses of Hyperplasia, Atypical Hyperplasia, and Well-Differentiated Carcinoma of the Endometrium

Hyperplasia versus Atypical Hyperplasia		
Histologic Feature	Univariate Analysis[a]	Multivariate Analysis[a]
Nuclear enlargement	5	1
Vesicular change	5	1
Nuclear pleomorphism	5	—
Chromatin irregularities	4	1
Loss of polarity	4	1
Nuclear rounding	3	—
Nucleoli	3	3
Glandular confluence	1	—
Atypical Hyperplasia versus Well-Differentiated Carcinoma		
Histologic Feature	Univariate Analysis[b]	Multivariate Analysis[b]
Glandular confluence	5	4
Stromal alteration	4	3
Necrosis	4	1
Nuclear enlargement	2	—
Abnormal mitoses	2	—
Fibrosis	1	—
Nuclear pleomorphism	1	—
Nuclear enlargement	1	—
Mitotic activity	1	1

[a]Number of pathologists showing an association by logistic regression analysis with the diagnosis of atypical hyperplasia and the listed feature.

[b]Number of pathologists showing an association by logistic regression analysis with the diagnosis of well-differentiated carcinoma and the listed feature.

Data from Kendall et al. (1998).

plasia included stromal alteration (stromal desmoplasia) and glandular confluence (Table 17–7). Thus, interobserver agreement was lowest for atypical hyperplasia, indicating that further refinement of the histologic criteria used to make the diagnosis of atypical hyperplasia is needed.

MOLECULAR GENETIC CHARACTERIZATION OF ENDOMETRIAL HYPERPLASIA

Numerous studies have begun to characterize the molecular genetic alterations that characterize endometrial hyperplasias. Analyses have focused on monoclonality, certain nuclear proteins, tumor suppressor genes, and oncogenes. Monoclonality has been demonstrated in some atypical endometrial hyperplasias, including some not associated with concomitant carcinoma and some not associated with carcinoma, supporting the concept that this lesion is a cancer precursor (Jovanovic et al., 1996; Mutter et al., 1995). Mutation of *p53*, a tumor suppressor gene involved in cell cycle regulation, has not been found in endometrial hyperplasias and is found in only a small proportion of endometrioid carcinomas. The latter are nearly always high grade (Kohler et al., 1993; Lax et al., 1997). Thus, *p53* mutation appears to be a relatively late event in a small subset of endometrioid carcinomas. This contrasts with the role that *p53* mutations appear to play in the pathogenesis of serous carcinomas (see below). Mutations of the *PTEN* tumor suppressor gene, which have been found in approximately 40%–60% of endometrioid carcinomas, have been detected in approximately 20% of endometrial hyperplasias with and without atypia unassociated with carcinoma. These data suggest that inactivation of this gene is an early event in the development of some endometrioid carcinomas (Levine et al., 1998; Maxwell et al., 1998; Tashiro et al., 1997a). Microsatellite instability, which has been detected in approximately 20% of sporadic endometrioid carcinomas in most studies, has been observed in some complex atypical hyperplasias associated with synchronous endometrioid carcinoma but has not been detected in the small number of pure atypical hyperplasias evaluated (Burks et al., 1994; Caduff et al., 1996; Catasus et al., 1998; Duggan et al., 1994; Kobayashi et al., 1995; Levine et al., 1998; Mutter et al., 1996; Risinger et al., 1993; Sherman and Kurman, 1998). These data suggest that microsatellite instability may occur later in the development of some endometrioid carcinomas, as does mutation of *PTEN*. K-*ras* mutations, which have been detected in 20%–40% of endometrioid carcinomas, have been identified in 12%–16% of atypical hyperplasias evaluated (Enomoto et al., 1991; Sasaki et al., 1993). These findings suggest that ras mutation also may be an early event in the development of a subset of endometrioid carcinomas. Thus, endometrial hyperplasias share some genetic alterations with endometrioid carcinomas, implying that the two lesions are pathogenetically linked. In contrast, serous carcinoma and its putative precursor lesion (EIC) lack these genetic changes, supporting the concept that serous carcinoma develops through a different pathway (see below).

It is important to note that a clear understanding of the significance of various genetic alterations requires analysis of data with respect to careful histological subtyping of the lesions studied. Many earlier studies, including some cited above, reported alterations in endometrial carcinomas without specifying whether they occurred in endometrioid or serous subtypes. Because the pathogeneses of these two types differ, genetic studies should be performed only on carcinomas and precursor lesions that have been meticulously classified.

MANAGEMENT OF ENDOMETRIAL HYPERPLASIA

Management of patients with endometrial hyperplasia should be based on the histologic diagnosis and clinical factors. Women of any age with hyperplasia lacking cytologic atypia (simple or complex) can be treated conservatively because these lesions are associated with an extremely low risk (1% to 3%) of progression to carcinoma. Appropriate management of women with atypical hyperplasia depends on the age of the patient and other factors. Kurman and Norris (1982) reported that the likelihood of finding residual carcinoma in the uterus after a diagnosis of carcinoma in a curettage specimen was considerably lower in women under the age of 35 years and increased sharply with age (Fig. 17–14). Only one of nine patients under the age of 35 years with hyperplasia or atypical hyperplasia had carcinoma in a subsequent hysterectomy specimen and this neoplasm was well differentiated and confined to the endometrium (Table 17–8). Thus, hormonal suppression with exogenous progestins or by induction of ovulation can be considered for women who wish to remain fertile. However, close follow-up is required and data on long-term safety and reproductive success are limited. One recent study found that 62% of women under 40

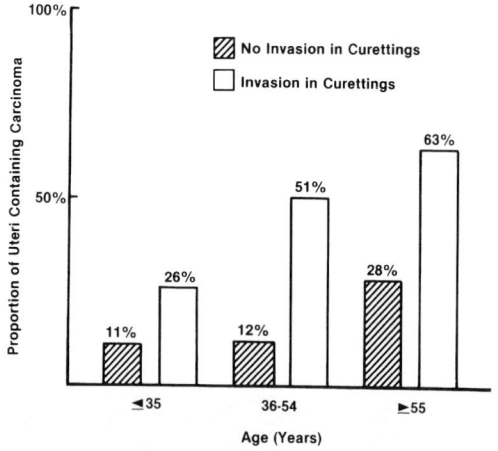

Figure 17–14. The likelihood of finding residual carcinoma in the uterus increases with age even when stromal invasion is not present in curettings.

Table 17–8. Hysterectomy Findings in Women 35 Years and Younger

Finding	Present in Stromal Invasion Curettings (n = 19)	Stromal Invasion Absent in Curettings (n = 9)
Atypical hyperplasia	8 (42)	3 (33)
Residual cancer	5 (26)	1 (11)
Grade 1	5 (100)	1 (100)
Endometrium only	1 (20)	1 (100)
Myometrium (inner third)	4 (80)	0

years of age treated with progestins alone for endometrial carcinoma responded to the hormonal therapy, although 23% of these later developed recurrent disease. Ninety percent of the patients were alive without evidence of disease during the follow-up period (Kim et al., 1997). A more recent study of progestin treatment of atypical hyperplasia and well-differentiated carcinoma in women under age 40 found that 75% of women with carcinoma and 95% with atypical hyperplasia had regression of their lesions. In addition, all patients were alive without evidence of progressive disease during the follow-up period (Randall and Kurman, 1997). Thus, in premenopausal women who wish to preserve fertility, endometrial proliferations encompassing both atypical hyperplasia and well-differentiated carcinoma can be regarded as a single clinicopathologic entity for management purposes. Histologic distinction of atypical hyperplasia from well-differentiated carcinoma is not critical because both lesions are highly responsive to progestin therapy. In perimenopausal and menopausal women who are receiving exogenous estrogens, termination of estrogen therapy, even for atypical hyperplasia, suffices because these proliferations are iatrogenic and regress after the stimulus for their growth has been removed. In perimenopausal and postmenopausal women who are not receiving estrogens, a hysterectomy is indicated, even though one-third of the lesions in women of this age-group also regress.

DUALISTIC MODEL OF ENDOMETRIAL CARCINOGENESIS

Some investigators have proposed that endometrial carcinomas can be divided into two types, type I and type II, based primarily on their clinical presentation (Bokhman, 1983; Kurman and Norris, 1982; Table 17–9). *Type I* carcinomas are associated with unopposed estrogenic stimulation and, as mentioned already, endometrial hyperpla-

Table 17–9. Pathogenetic Types of Endometrial Carcinoma and Precursor Lesions

Feature	Type I	Type II
Histologic type(s)	Endometrioid	Serous, clear cell
Precursor lesion	Atypical hyperplasia	Endometrial intraepithelial carcinoma[a]
Non-neoplastic endometrium	Proliferative or hyperplastic	Atrophic
Hyperestrogenism	Frequently present	Absent
Menopausal status	Pre- and perimenopausal	Postmenopausal
Associated clinical findings	Obesity, diabetes mellitus	None recognized
Myometrial invasion	Often superficial	Often deep
Metastatic spread	Less common	Common
Prognosis	Favorable	Poor

[a]Precursor lesion for serous carcinoma, also designated carcinoma *in situ* and uterine surface carcinoma; no precursor yet recognized for clear cell carcinoma.

sia. These tumors occur most often in perimenopausal white women. Histologically, they are nearly always well- to moderately differentiated endometrioid adenocarcinoma. Myometrial invasion is usually superficial and confined to the inner half of the uterine wall and metastatic spread is unusual. Associated hyperplasia has been reported in 35%–75% of cases (Ayhan and Yarali, 1991; Beckner et al., 1985; Bokhman, 1983; Deligdisch and Cohen, 1985; Gucer et al., 1998; Kaku et al., 1996). Thus, the carcinomas that develop in patients with hyperplasia and atypical hyperplasia are relatively indolent and have a favorable prognosis.

In the dualistic model of endometrial carcinogenesis *type II*, endometrial carcinoma is a high-grade neoplasm that occurs in older postmenopausal women. There is usually no history of unopposed estrogenic stimulation, and associated endometrial hyperplasia is extremely unusual. Typically, the adjacent endometrium is atrophic. Serous carcinoma is the archetypal type II carcinoma (Hendrickson et al., 1982; Sherman et al., 1992); some clear cell carcinomas and high-grade endometrioid carcinomas (often with high-grade squamous components) may also be included (Alberhasky et al., 1982; Christopherson et al., 1982). Type II neoplasms often demonstrate deep myometrial invasion and vascular involvement and have a poor prognosis.

ENDOMETRIAL INTRAEPITHELIAL CARCINOMA AND ITS RELATIONSHIP TO SEROUS CARCINOMA OF THE ENDOMETRIUM

Serous carcinoma is the most common nonendometrioid carcinoma in the type II group of neoplasms. The aggressive nature of serous carcinoma is demonstrated by the reported poor prognosis of tumors that are confined to polyps or stage IA (Carcangiu et al., 1997; Lee and Belinson, 1991; Silva and Jenkins, 1990). Serous carcinoma is composed of complex papillae or glands lined by cells with highly atypical pleomorphic nuclei displaying hyperchromasia, prominent nucleoli, and frequent hobnail-type cells with smudged chromatin. A subset of serous carcinomas is composed purely or predominantly of glands rather than papillae. Architecturally, this variant closely resembles well-differentiated (FIGO grade 1) endometrioid carcinoma. However, the nuclear atypia is marked (grade 3), identical to that seen in the papillary pattern of serous carcinoma. Recognition of the glandular variant of serous carcinoma is critical for both patient management and interpretation of molecular genetic studies of endometrial carcinogenesis. As discussed below, these neoplasms are aggressive even when minimally invasive, and misclassification as a grade 1 endometrioid carcinoma can lead to inappropriate clinical management. Misclassification also obscures the role of various genetic alterations, such as *p53* mutation, in endometrial carcinogenesis by inflating the proportion of endometrioid carcinomas that are reported to harbor *p53* mutations.

Serous carcinoma is frequently associated with a putative precursor lesion, termed *endometrial intraepithelial carcinoma* (EIC), which is characterized by markedly atypical nuclei, identical to those of invasive serous carcinomas, lining the surfaces and glands of the atrophic endometrium adjacent to the serous carcinoma (Figs. 17–15 and 17–16) (Ambros et al., 1995; Sherman et al., 1992). This lesion also has been referred to as *carcinoma in situ* (Spiegel, 1995) and *uterine surface carcinoma* (Zheng et al., 1998). Endometrial intraepithelial carcinoma also can be found in uteri without evidence of an invasive serous carcinoma, frequently in association with a polyp (Figs. 17–17 and 17–18).

Recent studies have demonstrated immunohistochemical overexpression of p53 protein, loss of heterozygosity (LOH) of chromosome 17p, and corresponding *p53* gene mutations in a high proportion of serous carcinomas and EIC (Figs. 17–19 and 17–20; Sherman et al., 1995; Tashiro et al., 1997b). The finding of diffuse, intense staining for p53 is highly correlated with identification of *p53* mutation in these cases. Lack of immunoreactivity for p53, however, does not exclude the presence of a mutation in *p53* because mutations have been detected in a small number of serous carcinomas that were nonreactive for p53 because of the formation of a truncated and/or unstable protein (Tashiro et al., 1997b). Identical *p53* gene mutations have been found in the EIC

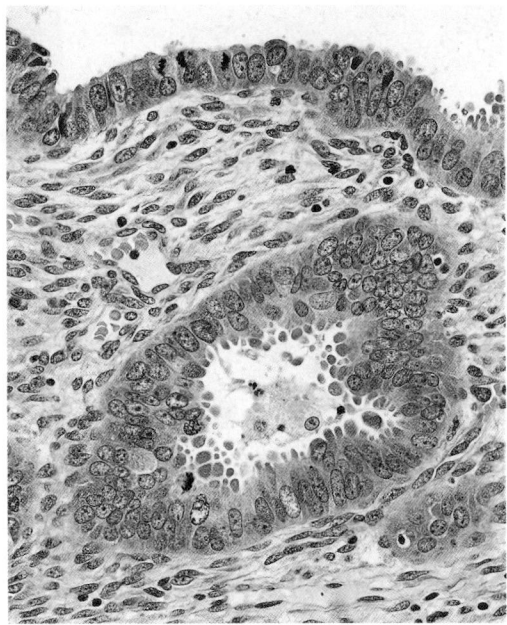

Figure 17–15. Endometrial intraepithelial carcinoma. Cells with markedly atypical nuclei line the surface endometrium and an underlying gland, without evidence of stromal invasion. Nuclei are enlarged and demonstrate prominent nucleoli and chromatin irregularities. Numerous mitotic figures are evident.

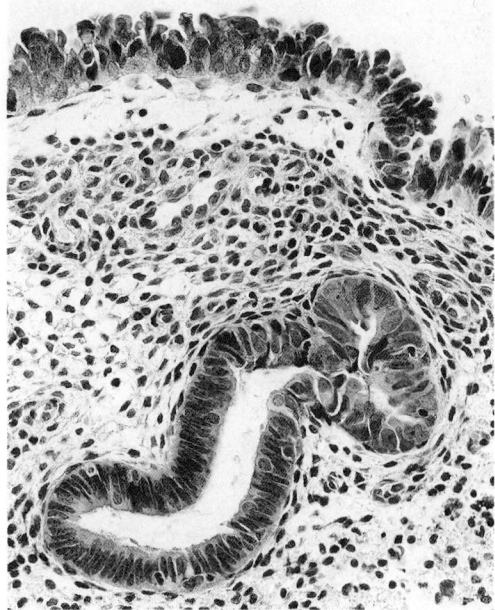

Figure 17–16. Endometrial intraepithelial carcinoma. Cells containing markedly atypical nuclei line the surface endometrium and the right portion of an underlying gland, without evidence of stromal invasion. Many of the cells have a hobnail appearance with smudged, hyperchromatic nuclei.

and adjacent serous carcinoma in several cases. Examples of pure EIC unassociated with serous carcinoma have also been shown to contain *p53* mutations. In addition, a case of pure EIC has been shown to contain *p53* mutation in the absence of LOH chromosome 17p, suggesting that *p53* mutation occurs early in the evolution of serous carcinoma (Tashiro,1997). The finding of EIC unassociated with invasive carcinoma and the presence of identical *p53* mutations in both lesions provide further support for the view that EIC is the precursor lesion of serous carcinoma. Additional observations that support the concept that serous carcinoma is pathogenetically distinct from endometrioid carcinoma include uncommon microsatellite instability and lack of *PTEN* mutations in serous carcinomas (Tashiro et al., 1997a,c). Future analyses that identify genetic alterations in EIC lesions that are commonly found in serous carcinomas will strengthen the pathogenetic link between this putative precursor lesion and serous carcinoma.

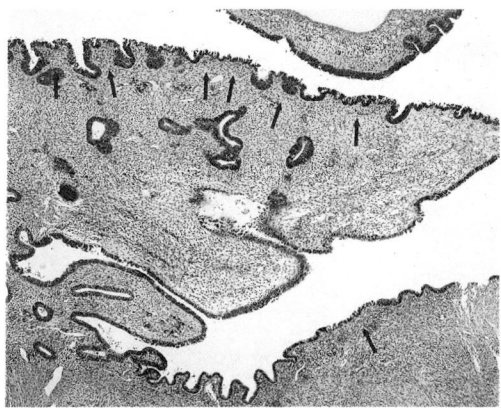

Figure 17–17. Endometrial polyp with foci of endometrial intraepithelial carcinoma (arrows). Foci of endometrial intraepithelial carcinoma line the surface of the polyp and adjacent atrophic endometrium. These foci are recognized at low magnification by a subtle papillary appearance.

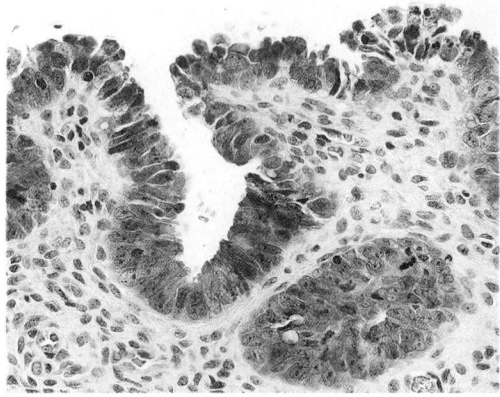

Figure 17–18. Endometrial intraepithelial carcinoma (higher magnification of an area of Figure 17–17). The lesion involves the surface and an underlying gland. Some cells contain markedly atypical nuclei with prominent nucleoli and others have smudged hyperchromatic nuclei.

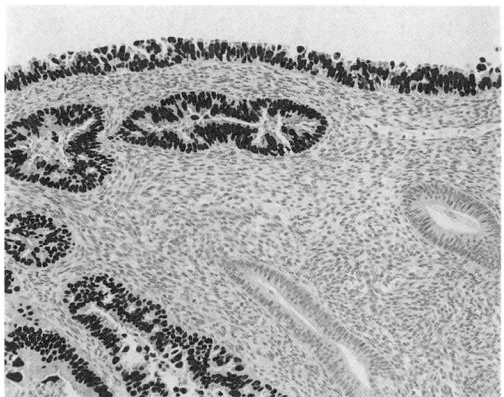

Figure 17–20. Endometrial intraepithelial carcinoma (immunohistochemical stain for p53 on serial section of lesion in Fig. 17–19). Nuclei in the neoplastic epithelium are diffusely and strongly positive for p53, whereas those within the normal glands are negative.

The distinction of extensive EIC from early serous carcinoma has not been defined. We propose that crowded glands involved by EIC within a polyp or within the endometrium be classified as *extensive EIC* when the proliferation lacks a confluent glandular pattern and demonstrates no evidence of stromal desmoplasia (stromal invasion) and is less than 1 cm in greatest dimension. Lesions that demonstrate glandular confluence or stromal desmoplasia

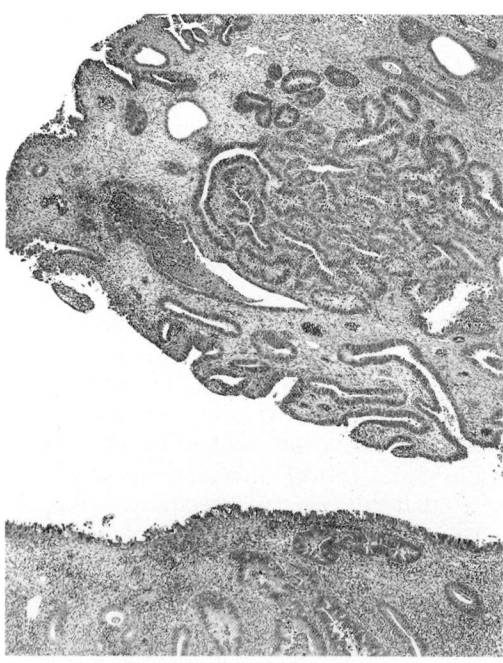

Figure 17–21. Endometrial polyp and adjacent endometrium with extensive endometrial intraepithelial carcinoma versus minimal uterine serous carcinoma. The center of the polyp contains a crowded proliferation of neoplastic glands that is partially confluent, suggesting early stromal invasion, and measures less than 1 cm.

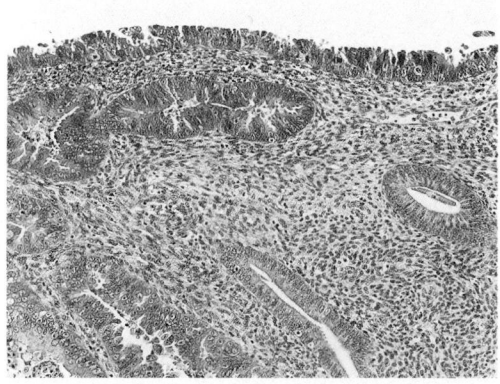

Figure 17–19. Endometrial intraepithelial carcinoma. Cells containing markedly atypical nuclei with prominent nucleoli replace the epithelium of the surface and several glands in the left portion of the field. Two glands in the lower right portion of the field are normal.

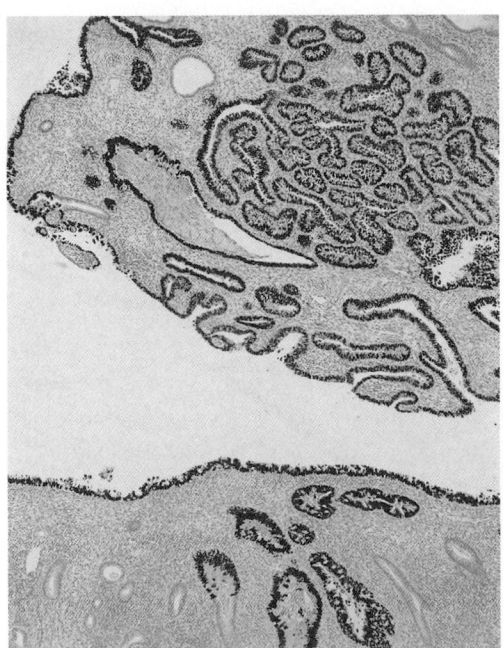

Figure 17–22. Endometrial polyp and adjacent endometrium with endometrial intraepithelial carcinoma minimal uterine serous carcinoma (immunohistochemical stain for p53 on serial section of lesion in Fig. 17–21). Neoplastic epithelium is highlighted by a strong, diffusely positive reaction for p53, whereas benign glands are negative.

and measure less than 1 cm can be designated "minimal uterine serous carcinoma" (Wheeler, 2000) (Figs. 17–21 and 17–22). When either glandular confluence or stromal invasion is present and the proliferation exceeds 1 cm in greatest dimension, we would classify the lesion as *serous carcinoma.* It is important to note, however, that metastatic serous carcinoma can be found in other sites in the genital tract and in the abdomen in the absence of demonstrable invasion in uteri with EIC, indicating that EIC is capable of metastasizing without first invading the stroma of the endometrium (Warren et al., 1998).

A recent study reported strong expression of p53 in surface endometrial lesions that lacked marked nuclear atypia (Zheng et al., 1998). The authors suggested that the definition of EIC be expanded to include surface epithelium containing less atypical cells that are strongly positive for p53 by immunohistochemistry. These investigators proposed the term *uterine surface carcinoma* for this lesion. We have made similar observations but are reluctant to render a diagnosis of carcinoma for lesions that lack the morphologic features of carcinoma on routine hematoxylin and eosin stains despite strong immunohistochemical expression of p53. A variety of metaplastic and reactive processes can display substantial cytologic atypia and closely resemble EIC. Preliminary data based on a small number of cases indicate that these lesions do not overexpress p53 (Zheng et al., 1998). However, a larger number of cases needs to be analyzed by immunohistochemical and molecular genetic methods before these minimally atypical, p53-positive lesions are classified as early manifestations of serous carcinoma. Anecdotally, we have seen cases in which surface endometrial lesions displaying smudgy, presumably degenerative nuclear atypia have demonstrated moderate numbers of p53-positive nuclei but the subsequent hysterectomy specimens failed to reveal carcinoma.

OTHER TYPES OF ENDOMETRIAL CARCINOMAS

Clear cell carcinoma is another type of endometrial carcinoma that is included among the type II neoplasms. It is composed of clear, hobnail, and eosinophilic cells arranged in solid, papillary, or tubulocystic patterns. Some clear cell carcinomas more closely resemble endometrioid carcinomas whereas others are cytologically more similar to serous carcinomas. A recent immunohistochemical analysis of p53, Ki-67 (proliferation marker), and estrogen and progesterone receptor expression that compared clear cell carcinomas to serous and endometrioid carcinomas found that the immunohistochemical profile of clear cell carcinomas differs from that of the other types (Lax et al., 1998). In particular, clear cell carcinomas, like serous carcinomas, tend to lack hormone receptor expression, but they do not display the striking immunoreactivity for p53 that is typical of most serous carcinomas. However, some do express hormone receptors and others are immunoreactive for p53. Proliferation indices of clear cell carcinomas are higher than those of endometrioid carcinomas but not as elevated as those of serous carcinomas. These results suggest that clear cell carcinoma may evolve through a different pathway than serous and endometrioid carcinomas or that clear cell carcinomas represent a heterogeneous group of neoplasms, some of which are related to endometrioid carcinomas and others that are more closely related to serous carcinomas. A unique precursor lesion of clear cell carcinoma has not been identified. Nonetheless, clear cell carcinomas are high-grade neoplasms that are clinicopathologically similar to other type II carcinomas.

Currently, we believe that a dualistic model of endometrial carcinogenesis synthesizes most of the known clinicopathological and molecular genetic features of endometrial carcinomas and their precursor lesions. In this model, endometrioid carcinomas are thought to arise from atypical hyperplasia in the setting of excess estrogenic stimulation. Endometrioid carcinomas tend to occur in pre- and perimenopausal women and are often indolent. In contrast, serous carcinomas are thought to evolve through a precursor lesion termed *endometrial intraepithelial carcinoma* in the setting of an atrophic endometrium. Serous carcinomas typically occur in postmenopausal women and are unrelated to estrogenic stimulation. These carcinomas are aggressive even when minimally invasive. Clear cell carcinomas share some features with serous carcinomas but are less well characterized and do not have a recognized unique precursor lesion. Additional molecular genetic studies will be required to determine whether clear cell carcinoma can be subsumed within the dualistic model and to elucidate other distinctive alterations that support the dualistic model of endometrial carcinogenesis.

REFERENCES

Alberhasky RC, Connelly PJ, Cristopherson WM. (1982) Carcinoma of the endometrium. IV. Mixed adenosquamous carcinoma. *Am J Clin Pathol* 77:655–664.

Ambros RA, Sherman ME, Zahn CM, Bitterman P, Kurman RJ. (1995) Endometrial intraepithelial carcinoma: a distinctive lesion specifically associated with tumors displaying serous differentiation. *Hum Pathol* 26:1260–1267.

Ausems EW, van der Kamp JK, Baak JP. (1985) Nuclear morphometry in the determination of the prognosis of marked atypical endometrial hyperplasia. *Int J Gynecol Pathol* 4:180–185.

Ayhan A, Yarali H. (1991) Endometrial carcinoma: a pathologic evaluation of 142 cases with and without

associated endometrial hyperplasia. *J Surg Oncol* 46: 182–184.

Baak JP. (1986) Further evaluation of the practical applicability of nuclear morphometry for the prediction of the outcome of atypical endometrial hyperplasia. *Anal Quant Cytol Histol* 8:46–48.

Baak JP, Nauta JJ, Wisse-Brekelmans EC, Bezemer PD. (1988) Architectural and nuclear morphometrical features together are more important prognosticators in endometrial hyperplasias than nuclear morphometrical features alone. *J Pathol* 154:335–341.

Baak JP, Wisse-Brekelmans EC, Fleege JC, van der Putten HW, Bezemer PD. (1992) Assessment of the risk on endometrial cancer in hyperplasia, by means of morphological and morphometrical features. *Pathol, Res Pract* 188:856–859.

Beckner ME, Mori T, Silverberg SG. (1985) Endometrial carcinoma: nontumor factors in prognosis. *Int J Gynecol Pathol* 4:131–145.

Beutler HK, Dockerty MB, Randall LM. (1963) Precancerous lesions of the endometrium. *Am J Obstet Gynecol* 86:433–443.

Bokhman JV. (1983) Two pathogenetic types of endometrial carcinoma. *Gynecol Oncol* 15:10–17.

Brinton LA, Berman ML, Mortel R, Twiggs LB, Barrett RJ, Wilbanks GD, Lannom L, Hoover RN. (1992) Reproductive, menstrual, and medical risk factors for endometrial cancer: results from a case–control study. *Am J Obstet Gynecol* 167:1317–1325.

Buehl IA, Vellios F, Carter JE, Huber CP. (1964) Carcinoma *in situ* of the endometrium. *Am J Clin Pathol* 42:594–601.

Burks RT, Kessis TD, Cho KR, Hedrick L. (1994) Microsatellite instability in endometrial carcinoma. *Oncogene* 9:1163–1166.

Caduff RF, Johnston CM, Svoboda-Newman SM, Poy EL, Merajver SD, Frank TS. (1996) Clinical and pathological significance of microsatellite instability in sporadic endometrial carcinoma. *Am J Pathol* 148:1671–1678.

Campbell PE, Barter RA. (1961) The significance of atypical endometrial hyperplasia. *J Obstet Gynecol* 68:668–672.

Carcangiu ML, Tan LK, Chambers JT. (1997) Stage IA uterine serous carcinoma. A study of 13 cases. *Am J Surg Pathol* 21:1507–1514.

Catasus L, Machin P, Matias-Guiu X, Prat J. (1998) Microsatellite instability in endometrial carcinomas: clinicopathologic correlations in a series of 42 cases. *Hum Pathol* 29:1160–1164.

Chamlian DL, Taylor HB. (1970) Endometrial hyperplasia in young women. *Obstet Gynecol* 36:659–666.

Christopherson WM, Alberhasky RC, Connelly PJ. (1982) Carcinoma of the endometrium: I. A clinicopathologic study of clear-cell carcinoma and secretory carcinoma. *Cancer* 49:1511–1523.

Deligdisch L, Cohen CJ. (1985) Histologic correlates and virulence implications of endometrial carcinoma associated with adenomatous hyperplasia. *Cancer* 56:1452–1455.

Duggan BD, Felix JC, Muderspach LI, Tourgeman D, Zheng J, Shibata D. (1994) Microsatellite instability in sporadic endometrial carcinoma. *J Natl Cancer Inst* 86:1216–1221.

Dunton CJ, Baak JP, Palazzo JP, van Diest PJ, McHugh M, Widra EA. (1996) Use of computerized morphometric analyses of endometrial hyperplasias in the prediction of coexistent cancer. *Am J Obstet Gynecol* 174:1518–1521.

Enomoto T, Inoue M, Perantoni AO, Buzard GS, Miki H, Tanizawa O, Rice JM. (1991) K-*ras* activation in premalignant and malignant epithelial lesions of the human uterus. *Cancer Res* 51:5308–5314.

Gucer F, Reich O, Tamussino K, Bader AA, Pieber D, Scholl W, Haas J, Petru E. (1998) Concomitant endometrial hyperplasia in patients with endometrial carcinoma. *Gynecol Oncol* 69:64–68.

Gusberg SB. (1947) Precursors of corpus carcinoma estrogens and adenomatous hyperplasia. *Am J Obstet Gynecol* 54:905–927.

Gusberg SB, Kaplan AL. (1963) Precursors of corpus cancer. IV. Adenomatous hyperplasia as stage 0 carcinoma of the endometrium. *Am J Obstet Gynecol* 87:662–678.

Gusberg SB, Moore DB, Martin F. (1954) Precursors of corpus cancer. II. A clinical and pathological study of adenomatous hyperplasia. *Am J Obstet Gynecol* 68:1472–1481.

Hendrickson M, Ross J, Eifel P, Martinez A, Kempson R. (1982) Uterine papillary serous carcinoma. A highly malignant form of endometrial adenocarcinoma. *Am J Surg Pathol* 6:93–108.

Hertig AT, Sommers SC. (1949) Genesis of endometrial carcinoma. I. Study of prior biopsies. *Cancer* 2:946–956.

Hertig AT, Sommers SC, Bengloff H. (1949) Genesis of endometrial carcinoma. III. Carcinoma *in situ. Cancer* 2:964–971.

Hunter JE, Tritz DE, Howell MG, DePriest PD, Gallion HH, Andrews SJ, Buckley SB, Kryscio RJ, van Nagell JR Jr. (1994) The prognostic and therapeutic implications of cytologic atypia in patients with endometrial hyperplasia. *Gynecol Oncol* 55:66–71.

Janicek MF, Rosenshein NB. (1994) Invasive endometrial cancer in uteri resected for atypical endometrial hyperplasia. *Gynecol Oncol* 52:373–378.

Jovanovic AS, Boynton KA, Mutter GL. (1996) Uteri of women with endometrial carcinoma contain a histopathological spectrum of monoclonal putative precancers, some with microsatellite instability. *Cancer Res* 56:1917–1921.

Kaku T, Tsukamoto N, Hachisuga T, Tsuruchi N, Sakai K, Hirakawa T, Amada S, Saito T, Kamura T, Nakano H. (1996) Endometrial carcinoma associated with hyperplasia. *Gynecol Oncol* 60:22–25.

Kendall BS, Ronnett BM, Isacson C, Cho KR, Hedrick L, Diener-West M, Kurman RJ. (1998) Reproducibility of the diagnosis of endometrial hyperplasia, atypical hyperplasia, and well-differentiated carcinoma. *Am J Surg Pathol* 22:1012–1019.

Kim YB, Holschneider CH, Ghosh K, Nieberg RK, Montz FJ. (1997) Progestin alone as primary treatment of endometrial carcinoma in premenopausal women. Report of seven cases and review of the literature. *Cancer* 79:320–327.

King A, Seraj IM, Wagner RJ. (1984) Stromal invasion in endometrial adenocarcinoma. *Am J Obstet Gynecol* 149:10–14.

Kobayashi K, Sagae S, Kudo R, Saito H, Koi S, Nakamura Y. (1995) Microsatellite instability in endometrial carcinomas: frequent replication errors in tumors of early onset and/or of poorly differentiated type. *Genes Chromosomes Cancer* 14:128–132.

Kohler MF, Nishii H, Humphrey PA, Saski H, Marks J,

Bast RC, Clarke-Pearson DL, Boyd J, Berchuck A. (1993) Mutation of the *p53* tumor-suppressor gene is not a feature of endometrial hyperplasias. *Am J Obstet Gynecol* 169:690–694.

Kurman RJ, Kaminski PF, Norris HJ. (1985) The behavior of endometrial hyperplasia. A long-term study of "untreated" hyperplasia in 170 patients. *Cancer* 56:403–412.

Kurman RJ, Norris HJ. (1982) Evaluation of criteria for distinguishing atypical endometrial hyperplasia from well-differentiated carcinoma. *Cancer* 49:2547–2559.

Kurman RJ, Norris HJ. (1994) Endometrial hyperplasia and related cellular changes. In: *Blaustein's Pathology of the Female Genital Tract*, 4th ed. (Kurman RJ, ed.), pp. 411–437. Springer-Verlag, New York.

Lax SF, Kendall B, Tashiro H, Slebos R, Hedrick L. (1997) Comparison of *p53* and K-*ras* mutations in uterine endometrioid and serous carcinomas suggests different molecular genetic pathways. *Mod Pathol* 10:104A–104A.

Lax SF, Pizer ES, Ronnett BM, Kurman RJ. (1998) Clear cell carcinoma of the endometrium is characterized by a distinctive profile of p53, Ki-67, estrogen, and progesterone receptor expression. *Hum Pathol* 29:551–558.

Lee KR, Belinson JL. (1991) Recurrence in noninvasive endometrial carcinoma. Relationship to uterine papillary serous carcinoma. *Am J Surg Pathol* 15:965–973.

Levine RL, Cargile CB, Blazes MS, van Rees B, Kurman RJ, Ellenson LH. (1998) PTEN mutations and microsatellite instability in complex atypical hyperplasia, a precursor lesion to uterine endometrioid carcinoma. *Cancer Res* 58:3254–3258.

Longacre TA, Chung MH, Jensen DN, Hendrickson MR. (1995) Proposed criteria for the diagnosis of well-differentiated endometrial carcinoma. *Am J Surg Pathol* 19:371–406.

Maxwell GL, Risinger JI, Gumbs C, Shaw H, Bentley RC, Barrett JC, Berchuck A, Futreal PA. (1998) Mutation of the *PTEN* tumor suppressor gene in endometrial hyperplasias. *Cancer Res* 58:2500–2503.

Mazur MT. (1981) Atypical polypoid adenomyomas of the endometrium. *Am J Surg Pathol* 5:473–482.

McBride JM. (1959) Pre-menopausal cystic hyperplasia and endometrial carcinoma. *J Obstet Gynecol Br Emp* 66:288–296.

Mutter GL, Boynton KA, Faquin WC, Ruiz RE, Jovanovic AS. (1996) Allelotype mapping of unstable microsatellites establishes direct lineage continuity between endometrial precancers and cancer. *Cancer Res* 56:4483–4486.

Mutter GL, Chaponot ML, Fletcher JA. (1995) A polymerase chain reaction assay for non-random X chromosome inactivation identifies monoclonal endometrial cancers and precancers. *Am J Pathol* 146:501–508.

Norris HJ, Tavassoli FA, Kurman RJ. (1983) Endometrial hyperplasia and carcinoma. Diagnostic considerations. *Am J Surg Pathol* 7:839–847.

Novak E, Rutledge F. (1948) Atypical endometrial hyperplasia simulating adenocarcinoma. *Am J Obstet Gynecol* 55:46–63.

Potischman N, Hoover RN, Brinton LA, Siiteri P, Dorgan JF, Swanson CA, Berman ML, Mortel R, Twiggs LB, Barrett RJ, Wilbanks GD, Persky V, Lurain JR.

(1996) Case–control study of endogenous steroid hormones and endometrial cancer. *J Natl Cancer Inst* 88:1127–1135.

Randall TC, Kurman RJ. (1997) Progestin treatment of atypical hyperplasia and well-differentiated carcinoma of the endometrium in women under age 40. *Obstet Gynecol* 90:434–440.

Risinger JI, Berchuck A, Kohler MF, Watson P, Lynch HT, Boyd J. (1993) Genetic instability of microsatellites in endometrial carcinoma. *Cancer Res* 53: 5100–5103.

Sasaki H, Nishii H, Takahashi H, Tada A, Furusato M, Terashima Y, Siegal GP, Parker SL, Kohler MF, Berchuck A. (1993) Mutation of the Ki-*ras* protooncogene in human endometrial hyperplasia and carcinoma. *Cancer Res* 53:1906–1910.

Scully RE, Bonfiglio TA, Kurman RJ, Silverberg SG, Wilkinson EJ. (1994) Histologic Typing of Female Genital Tract Tumours (International Histological Classification of Tumours), 2nd ed. pp. 1–189. Springer-Verlag, New York.

Sherman ME, Bitterman P, Rosenshein NB, Dlgado G, Kurman RJ. (1992) Uterine serous carcinoma. A morphologically diverse neoplasm with unifying clinicopathologic features. *Am J Surg Pathol* 16:600–610.

Sherman ME, Bur ME, Kurman RJ. (1995) p53 in endometrial cancer and its putative precursors: evidence for diverse pathways of tumorigenesis. *Hum Pathol* 26:1268–1274.

Sherman ME, Kurman RJ. (1998) Evolving concepts in endometrial carcinogenesis: importance of DNA repair and deregulated growth. *Hum Pathol* 29:1035–1038.

Sherman ME, Sturgeon S, Brinton LA, Potischman N, Kurman RJ, Berman ML, Mortel R, Twiggs LB, Barrett RJ, Wilbanks GD. (1997) Risk factors and hormone levels in patients with serous and endometrioid uterine carcinomas. *Mod Pathol* 10:963–968.

Silva EG, Jenkins R. (1990) Serous carcinoma in endometrial polyps. *Mod Pathol* 3:120–128.

Skov BG, Broholm H, Engel U, Franzmann MB, Nielsen AL, Lauritzen AF, Skov T. (1997) Comparison of the reproducibility of the WHO classifications of 1975 and 1994 of endometrial hyperplasia. *Int J Gynecol Pathol* 16:33–37.

Spiegel GW. (1995) Endometrial carcinoma *in situ* in postmenopausal women. *Am J Surg Pathol* 19:417–432.

Tashiro H, Blazes MS, Wu R, Cho KR, Bose S, Wang SI, Li J, Parsons R, Ellenson LH. (1997a) Mutations in *PTEN* are frequent in endometrial carcinoma but rare in other common gynecological malignancies. *Cancer Res* 57:3935–3940.

Tashiro H, Isacson C, Levine R, Kurman RJ, Cho KR, Hedrick L. (1997b) *p53* gene mutations are common in uterine serous carcinoma and occur early in their pathogenesis. *Am J Surg Pathol* 150:177–185.

Tashiro H, Lax SF, Gaudin PB, Isacson C, Cho KR, Hedrick L. (1997c) Microsatellite instability is uncommon in uterine serous carcinoma. *Am J Pathol* 150:75–79.

Tavassoli FA, Kraus FT. (1978) Endometrial lesions in uteri resected for atypical endometrial hyperplasia. *Am J Clin Pathol* 70:770–779.

Terakawa N, Kigawa J, Taketani Y, Yoshikawa H, Yajima A, Noda K, Okada H, Kato J, Yakushiji M, Tanizawa O, Fujimoto S, Nozawa S, Takahashi T, Hasumi K, Furuhashi N, Aono T, Sakamoto A, Furusato M. (1997) The behavior of endometrial hyperplasia: a prospective study. Endometrial Hyperplasia Study Group. *J Obstet Gynaecol Res* 23:223–230.

Vellios F. (1974) Endometrial hyperplasia and carcinoma *in situ*. *Gynecol Oncol* 2:152–161.

Warren CD, Horak C, Isacson C, Hedrick Ellenson L. (1998) Extrauterine serous tumors in minimally invasive USC are metastatic. *Mod Pathol* 11:116A–116A.

Welch WR, Scully RE. (1977) Precancerous lesions of the endometrium. *Hum Pathol* 8:503–512.

Wheeler DT, Bell KA, Kurman RJ, Sherman ME. (2000) Minimal uterine serous carcinoma: Diagnosis and clinicopathologic correlation. *Am J Surg Pathol* 24:797–806.

Widra EA, Dunton CJ, McHugh M, Palazzo JP. (1995) Endometrial hyperplasia and the risk of carcinoma. *Int J Gynecol Cancer* 5:233–235.

Zheng W, Khurana R, Farahmand S, Wang Y, Zhang ZF, Felix JC. (1998) p53 immunostaining as a significant adjunct diagnostic method for uterine surface carcinoma. *Am J Surg Pathol* 22:1463–1473.

18

OVARY

Debra A. Bell and Robert E. Scully

Cancer of the ovary, the fifth most common form of fatal cancer in women (Landis et al., 1999), is a heterogeneous disease in terms of the diverse origins, different age distributions, and varying biologic characteristics of its subtypes (Scully, 1979; Scully et al., 1998). The three main forms of ovarian cancer are *(1)* the malignant epithelial-stromal tumors, which are thought to be derived ultimately from the surface "epithelium" (modified pelvic mesothelium) and adjacent ovarian stroma; *(2)* tumors composed of steroid hormone–secreting cells, mostly granulosa cell tumors and Sertoli-Leydig cell tumors; and *(3)* malignant germ cell tumors. These three categories account for approximately 90%, 6%, and 3% of ovarian cancers, respectively. Precancerous and early cancerous lesions corresponding to the clinically evident forms of each type of ovarian cancer require separate consideration.

MALIGNANT SURFACE EPITHELIAL-STROMAL TUMORS

Epithelial-stromal tumors are divided into three categories according to their cytologic and architectural features, which correlate with their biologic behavior: *benign, borderline* (proliferating; of low malignant potential), and *malignant* (invasive) (Scully et al., 1998; Serov et al., 1973). Each of these categories is designated further according to its cell type as *serous* (resembling fallopian tube epithelium), *mucinous* (resembling endocer-

vical or gastrointestinal epithelium), *endometrioid* (resembling endometrial epithelium), *clear cell* (resembling certain changes in endometrial glandular cells during pregnancy), and *transitional cell* (resembling uroepithelium). There is evidence that some mucinous tumors and transitional cell tumors may have origins other than the surface epithelium (germ cells for both mucinous and transitional cell tumors and rete ovarii additionally for the latter), but for convenience, all the neoplasms characterized by these two cell types are classified within the epithelial-stromal category. The evidence for the surface epithelial origin of the malignant epithelial forms of these tumors is considerable:

1. The surface epithelium and its derivatives, surface epithelial inclusion glands (Fig. 18–1), may be characterized by any of the types of epithelium encountered in these neoplasms with differing degrees of frequency (common for serous and endometrioid epithelium and rare for mucinous, clear cell, and transitional epithelium) (Blaustein et al., 1981).
2. Tumors containing various admixtures of the five types of epithelium may be encountered.
3. Precancerous changes have been identified rarely in the surface epithelium and its inclusion glands.
4. Tiny macroscopic or microscopic carcinomas have been described that are

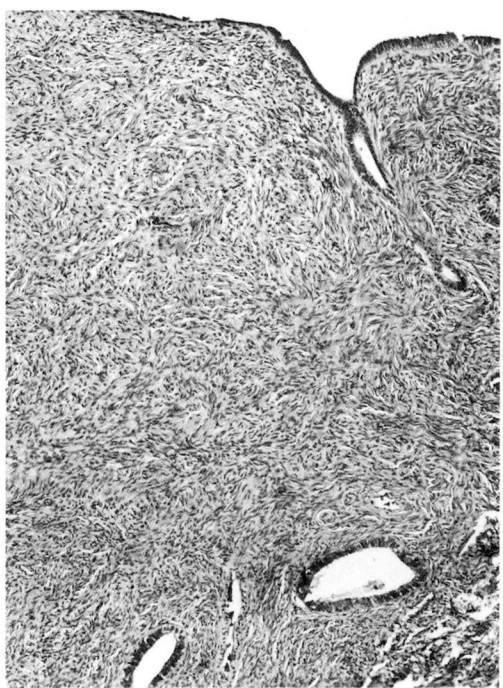

Figure 18–1. Surface epithelium and surface epithelial inclusion glands. One of the glands appears to have been formed by pinching off of the surface epithelium.

usually located on or just beneath the ovarian surface and are often associated with cytologic atypia in nearby surface epithelial inclusion glands (Bell and Scully, 1994; Fig. 18–2).

5. Tumor markers associated with surface epithelial cancers have been demon-

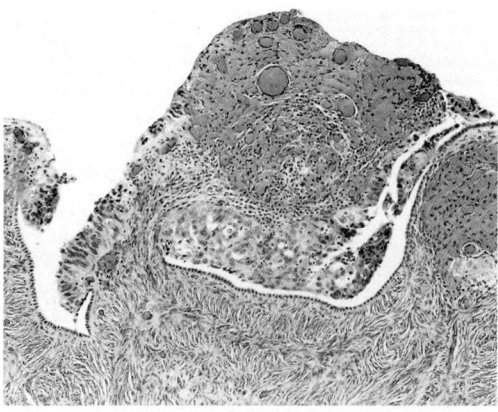

Figure 18–2. Surface growth of malignant epithelium associated with a fibrovascular adhesion.

strated immunohistochemically in surface epithelial inclusion glands (Bell ad Scully, unpublished data; Blaustein et al., 1982; Cordon-Cardo et al., 1985; Kabawat et al., 1983; Nouwen et al., 1987).

6. Occasional carcinomas arise in association with preexisting benign lesions (benign epithelial tumors and endometriosis) containing epithelium closely resembling that of surface epithelium (Puls et al., 1992).

Precancerous lesions of the ovary in the surface epithelial category may be divided into two subtypes for purposes of discussion: lesions that appear *in situ* in surface epithelium or surface epithelial inclusion glands; and benign ovarian epithelial lesions comprising tumors and endometriosis.

PRECANCEROUS LESIONS OF SURFACE EPITHELIUM AND SURFACE EPITHELIAL INCLUSION GLANDS

Despite the widespread acceptance of the origin of surface epithelial cancers from the ovarian surface epithelium and its inclusion glands, only rarely have putative precursor lesions been described at these sites. Two types of lesions have been suggested as possible precursors: proliferative and metaplastic changes; and cytologic atypia. Ovaries have been examined for such lesions in four settings: *(1)* prophylactic oophorectomy specimens from patients with a strong family history of ovarian cancer and breast cancer or both, or with known *BRCA1* or *BRCA2* gene mutations; *(2)* uninvolved ovaries contralateral to ovarian carcinomas or benign or borderline epithelial tumors or a combination of these tumors; *(3)* surface epithelium and epithelial inclusion glands adjacent to invasive ovarian carcinomas; and *(4)* ovaries removed after positive or suspicious *cul de sac* aspirates performed to screen for ovarian cancer.

Unfortunately, most studies of the surface epithelium are limited by its fragility; it is usually denuded by allowing the surface to dry intraoperatively or by touching or rubbing it during removal or gross pathologic examination (Gillett, 1991). As a result, often all that remains for microscopic examination is residual intact epithelium either *in*

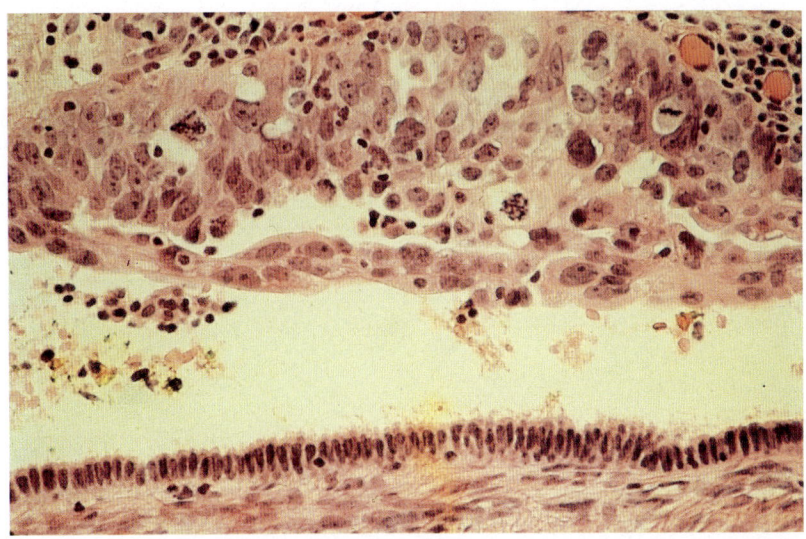

Figure 18–3. Close-up of surface carcinoma and normal surface epithelium with which the carcinoma was continuous.

sulci below a gyriform surface or under the protective umbrella of fibrous adhesions.

Only rare examples of lesions showing significant epithelial atypia (severe dysplasia or carcinoma *in situ*) (Figs. 18–2 to 18–5) have been reported (Bell and Scully, 1994; Graham and Graham, 1967; Graham et al., 1964, 1965; Gusberg and Deligdisch, 1984; Hutson et al., 1995). These lesions are characterized by stratification of cells lining the ovarian surface or epithelial inclusion glands with loss of nuclear polarity and marked nuclear pleomorphism, hyperchromasia, and chromatin clumping (Figs. 18–3 and 18–5). In their study of *cul de sac* aspirates obtained for

ovarian cancer screening, Graham and coworkers identified these changes adjacent to a microscopic serous carcinoma in 1 patient (Graham et al., 1965) and in the surface epithelium of 20 additional patients with malignant cells in their aspirates (Graham et al., 1964; Graham and Graham, 1967). Bell and Scully (1994) noted severe cytologic atypia in 3 of 14 women with incidentally detected microscopic or tiny gross invasive ovarian carcinomas, and Gusberg and Deligdisch (1984) noted such changes in 2 of 3 women whose ovaries had been removed prophylactically because of the finding of ovarian carcinoma in an identical

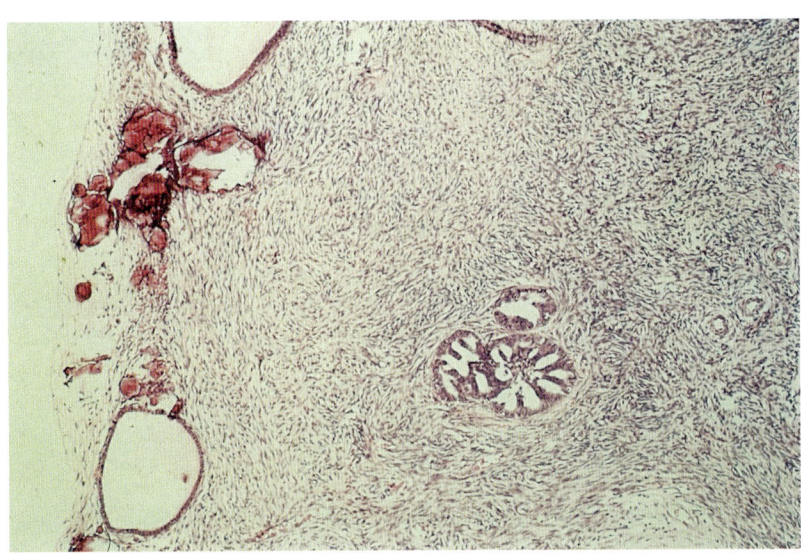

Figure 18–4. Superficial surface epithelial inclusion glands and calcifications (left) and inclusion glands showing severe cytologic atypia (center).

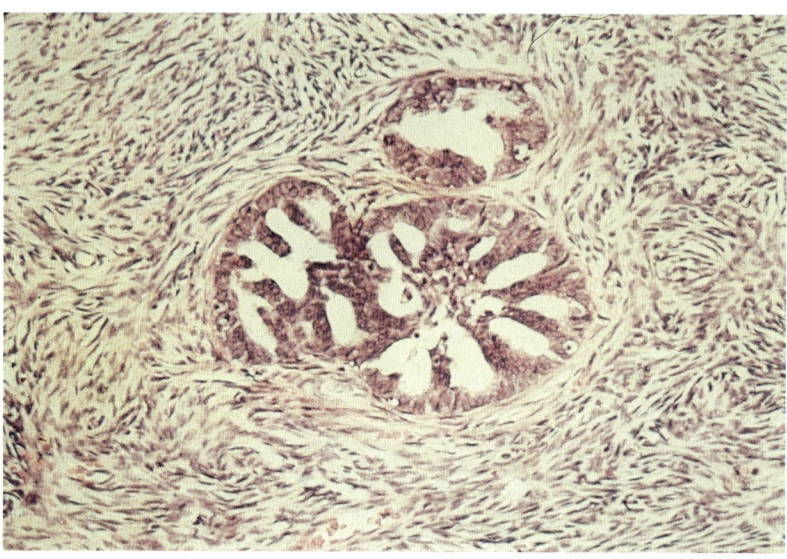

Figure 18–5. Higher power of inclusion glands showing severe cytologic atypia. [From Scully, 1982, with permission.]

twin. Mild to moderate atypia was noted in the third twin, and has also been reported in surface epithelium adjacent to grossly visible or microscopic ovarian carcinomas (Bell and Scully, 1994; Gil and Deligdisch, 1989; Plaxe et al., 1990; Tsukahara et al., 1982). In contrast, severe cytologic atypia has not been noted to date in prophylactic oophorectomy specimens from patients with a strong family history of ovarian cancer or *BRCA* mutations and in uninvolved ovaries contralateral to ovarian carcinoma. Sherman and co-workers (1999) identified mild atypia of the surface epithelium more frequently in the ovaries of women at increased risk for ovarian carcinoma (prophylactically removed ovaries from women with a strong family history of ovarian cancer or known *BRCA* mutations, or ovaries contralateral to ovarian cancer) than controls (Fig. 18–6). Although this difference was statistically significant, the number of cases was small. Werness and colleagues (1999) were unable to identify a difference in the frequency of atypia in prophylactically removed ovaries and controls on light microscopic examination, but demonstrated a statistically significant increase in nuclear enlargement and chromatin heterogeneity in prophylactically removed ovaries morphometrically. Werner et al. (2000) recently reported *in situ* ovarian carcinoma in a single patient with *BRCA1* and loss of

heterozygosity at *BRCA1* and *TP53*. Several other groups have failed to demonstrate epithelial atypia in the prophylactic oophorectomy specimens from women with a strong family history of ovarian cancer (Salazar et al., 1996) or with known *BRCA1* or *BRCA2* mutations (Stratton et al., 1999). Two groups of investigators have noted mild atypia of the surface epithelium in uninvolved ovaries contralateral to ovarian carcinomas or borderline tumors (Sherman et al., 1998; Tresserra et al., 1998); the latter group, however, failed to detect atypia in epithelial inclusion glands. Several other investigators were un-

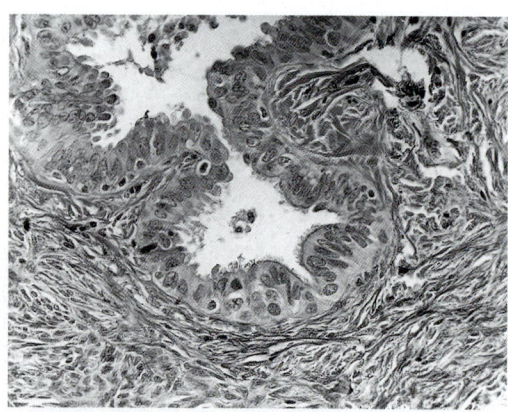

Figure 18–6. Epithelial inclusion gland with tubal metaplasia and mild cytologic atypia.

able to demonstrate a statistically significant increase in atypia in ovaries contralateral to ovarian tumors over control ovaries (Resta et al., 1993; Westoff et al., 1993).

Although early studies had suggested that proliferative or metaplastic changes of the ovarian surface epithelium such as papillae, stratification and tufting, and metaplasia are precursors of ovarian carcinoma (Fraumeni et al., 1975), similar findings have been reported to be increased in frequency in only one more recent large series of prophylactic oophorectomy specimens from women with a strong family history of ovarian cancer (Salazar et al., 1996). In this study an examination of ovaries from 20 women in this category revealed two microscopic or tiny gross carcinomas, one of serous and the other of endometrioid type. Surface papillomatosis, the number of inclusion glands, deep epithelial invaginations, epithelial pseudostratification, and stromal proliferation were statistically more frequent in the prophylactic oophorectomy cases than the 20 controls. The investigators were not blinded, however, to the risk status of the study group and the controls. Two of three groups (Sherman et al., 1998; Stratton et al., 1999) more recently failed to demonstrate any differences in the frequency of these histologic features between cases and controls. The only light microscopic finding of a third group of authors (Werness et al., 1999) was the presence of more surface epithelial inclusion glands in prophylactically removed than control ovaries. In each of the last three studies the pathologic review was performed without knowledge of the risk status of the patients.

Studies of uninvolved ovaries contralateral to unilateral ovarian carcinomas have also yielded variable results regarding proliferative changes. Mittal and co-workers (1993) found an increased number of inclusion glands and a greater frequency of serous metaplasia in uninvolved ovaries contralateral to ovarian carcinoma than in age-matched controls (Fig. 18–6), and Tresserra and colleagues (1998) noted an increase in deep cortical invaginations. Bell and Scully (unpublished data) found that a significantly greater number of surface epithelial inclusion glands in ovaries contralateral to carcinoma had undergone tubal metaplasia than control ovaries, and Resta and co-workers (1993) found that epithelial hyperplasia or squamous, mucinous, endometrioid, or tubal metaplasia were more common in the surface epithelium and surface epithelial inclusion glands in benign ovaries removed because of endometrial carcinoma or polycystic ovarian disease, and in benign ovaries contralateral to ovarian neoplasms than in benign ovaries of women without these diseases. Sherman and co-workers (1999) and Westoff and co-workers (1993), in contrast, reported no differences in proliferative features between uninvolved ovaries contralateral to ovarian carcinomas and controls.

Definitive conclusions based on the above studies are not possible because they were retrospective and varied in design. It is likely that at least in some of the studies the prophylactically removed ovaries had been handled with greater care by the surgeon and pathologist to preserve the surface epithelium than control ovaries removed for predominantly benign gynecologic disease. Also, in all of the studies a greater number of sections were obtained from the prophylactically removed ovaries. With regard to study design, the pathologists were aware of the risk status of the patients in several studies. Also, the gynecologic disorders of women whose ovaries were used for controls varied from study to study, with some having hormone-related lesions, such as endometrial hyperplasia and leiomyomas, and others having non–hormone-related conditions such as cervical lesions and prolapse. Despite these limitations, a few trends in the data are apparent.

Severe atypia of the surface epithelium and surface epithelial inclusion glands is identified only rarely in "high-risk" ovaries in the absence of ipsilateral carcinoma. This finding and the morphologic appearance of the lesions, which is similar to carcinoma *in situ* (CIS) at other sites, suggest that such changes are precursor lesions. The findings by Sherman and coworkers (1999) and Werness and co-workers (1999) of subtle cytologic atypia in women at high risk for ovarian cancer raises the possibility that such changes are also premalignant, but such a conclusion must be confirmed by additional studies. The data evaluating proliferative and metaplastic changes as possible precursor lesions are inconclusive.

Because of limitations of size and cell number, molecular genetic studies such as mutational analysis and investigation of loss of heterozygosity (LOH) have not been per-formed on putative precursor lesions of the surface epithelium and surface epithelial in-clusion glands. Such studies utilizing highly accurate microdissection techniques (Em-mert-Burke et al., 1996) are presently un-derway in several laboratories. A small number of immunohistochemical studies on surface epithelium and surface epithelial inclusion glands have shown that various tu-mor markers found in ovarian carcinoma, in-cluding carcinoembryonic antigen (EA), beta human chorionic gonadotropin, and human placental lactogen, are frequently present in epithelial inclusion glands (Blaustein et al., 1982), particularly those lined by columnar or tubal-type epithelium. Other tumor markers, including CA-125, hu-man milk fat globule, placental-like alkaline phosphatase, and CA19-9, are expressed more often in surface epithelial inclusion glands than in surface epithelium (Kabawat et al., 1983; Nouwen et al., 1987). E-cadherin, an intercellular adhesion molecule (Maines-Bandiera and Auersperg, 1997; Sundfeldt et al., 1997), and c-erbB2 (Wang et al., 1992) are also expressed in surface epithelial inclusion glands and carcinoma, but not in surface ep-ithelium itself. Bell and Scully (unpublished data) have noted an increased frequency of placental-like alkaline phosphatase staining in surface epithelial inclusion glands con-tralateral to carcinoma compared to age-matched controls. Hutson and co-workers (1995) demonstrated a greater frequency of p53 overexpression in epithelial inclusion glands associated with ovarian carcinoma than in those within "normal" ovaries. These studies suggest that the epithelium of surface epithelial inclusion glands is more similar to that of carcinoma than the surface epithe-lium itself. This conclusion is consistent with the intraovarian rather than surface origin of most epithelial cancers.

BENIGN TUMORS AS PRECURSORS OF CARCINOMA

Whether surface epithelial cancers arise in preexistent benign epithelial tumors of the same cell type and, if so, how often they do so, are difficult to determine and warrant further investigation. Benign ovarian neo-plasms are almost always removed as soon as they are detected, and therefore their nat-

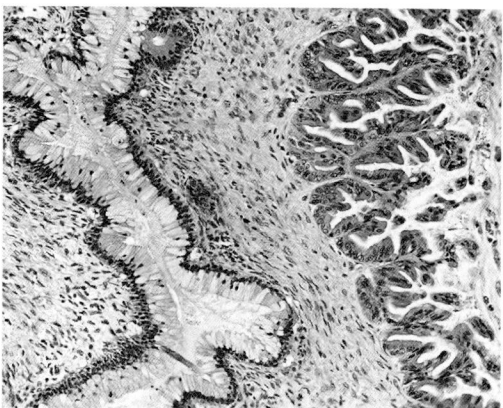

Figure 18–7. Mucinous cystadenoma (left) and a cystic tumor of borderline malignancy (right).

ural history is largely unknown. Evidence of a benign to malignant transformation is largely circumstantial and includes *(1)* a gen-erally observed older-age incidence of carci-nomas than benign tumors of the same cell type; *(2)* the frequent observation of various combinations of benign, borderline, and in-vasive neoplasia within the same specimen (Puls et al., 1992; Figs. 18–7 to 18–9); and *(3)* a reported fivefold increase in the fre-quency of benign epithelial tumors in first- and second-degree relatives of women with ovarian carcinoma (Bourne et al., 1991).

The age distributions of benign, border-line, and invasive surface epithelial-stromal tumors are difficult to establish with cer-tainty, differing from one series to another for several possible reasons:

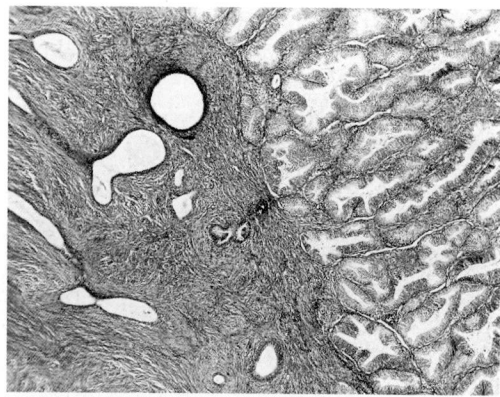

Figure 18–8. Endometrioid adenofibroma (left) and an adenocarcinoma (right).

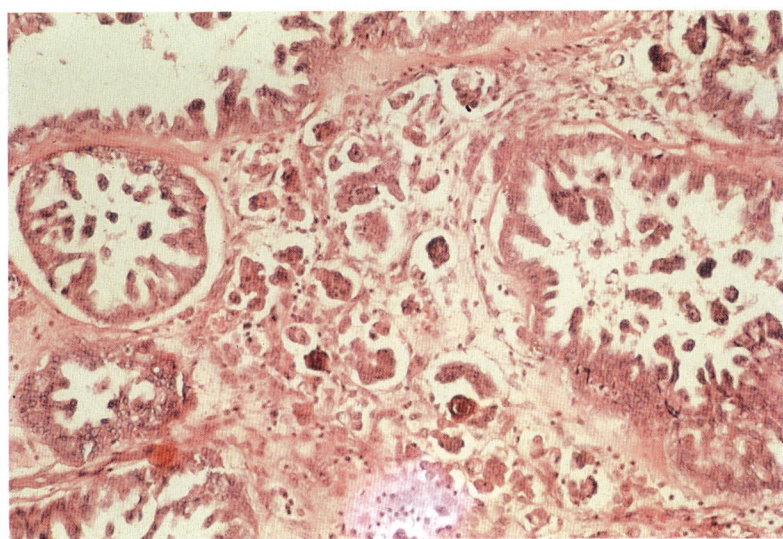

Figure 18–9. Central microscopic focus of serous carcinoma in a tumor that was otherwise of borderline malignancy.

1. Variations exist in the diagnostic criteria for these three categories of neoplasia among individual pathologists.
2. Borderline tumors, which are not specifically designated "carcinomas" by reporting pathologists, are consequently grossly underrepresented in cancer registries (Stalsberg et al., 1983a,c).
3. Conversely, tumors of borderline type, particularly those occurring in young women, are grossly overrepresented in pathology-consultation material because their clinical management differs from that of carcinoma and often requires diagnosis by an expert.

Despite these problems, most investigators have reported progressively higher mean ages for benign, borderline, and invasive tumors in both the serous and mucinous categories, with average ages for the combined categories being 44, 48, and 56 years, respectively (Table 18–1). The differences between benign and invasive tumors are more uniformly agreed upon than those between benign and borderline and those between borderline and invasive tumors. Parallel figures are not available for endometrioid and clear cell neoplasms because of the rarity of their benign and borderline forms. Relatively few borderline and invasive Brenner tumors have been reported, but most of them have been discovered in older women

(average age for borderline, 60 years; for invasive, 63 years) (Hallgrímsson and Scully, 1972; Miles and Norris, 1972; Roth and Sternberg, 1971; Rybak et al., 1981; Woodruff et al., 1981; Yoonessi and Abell, 1979); in contrast, the mean age incidence of benign Brenner tumors is under 50 years (Berge and Borglin, 1967; Ehrlich and Roth, 1971; Fox et al., 1972; Jorgensen et al., 1970; Silverberg, 1971; Waxman, 1979; Yoonessi and Abell, 1979).

Several recent studies have attempted to quantify the association of benign and malignant elements in specimens of ovarian carcinoma. In one investigation (Puls et al., 1992), 28 of 31 (90%) mucinous carcinomas were found to contain benign-appearing epithelium and in 8 of these cases (26% of the total), a transition was observed between the two types of epithelium. Benign epithelium was found in 22 of 39 (56%) serous carcinomas, with a transition observable in 11 of them (28% of the total). In another study of 189 epithelial cancers of the ovary from 156 patients (Scully et al., 1995), benign epithelium was identified in 74% of mucinous carcinomas, 46% of endometrioid carcinomas, and 39% of clear cell carcinomas; in contrast, benign epithelium was encountered in only 15% and 31% of serous carcinomas and mixed serous–transitional cell carcinomas, respectively. In the cases of serous carcinoma and mixed serous–transitional cell carcinoma, the benign epithelium invariably oc-

Table 18–1. Mean Age Incidences Associated with Three types of Serous and Mucinous Tumors[a]

Reference	Type of Cases	Cases (n)	Benign Cases Age (n)	Borderline Cases Age (n)	Invasive Cases Age (n)
Katsube et al. (1982), USA (population)	Serous	110 B,Bo,M		43 (12)	56 (26)
	Muc	60 B,Bo,M		35 (6)	59 (6)
Stalsberg et al. (1983a) UICC (Cancer Registry)	Serous	1143 Bo,M		51 (63)	55 (1080)
	Muc	427 Bo,M		51 (61)	53 (366)
Russell (1979), Australia (hospital)	Serous	460 B,Bo,M	45 (227)	48 (70)	56 (163)
	Muc	362 B,Bo,M	44 (293)	48 (52)	52 (17)
Chenevart and Gloor (1980), Switzerland(hospital)	Serous	381 B,Bo,M	49 (286)	46 (24)	60 (71)
	Muc	241 B,Bo,M	45 (194)	51 (29)	62 (18)
Stalsberg et al. (1983b), Norway (hospital)	Serous	148 B,Bo,M	48 (91)	56 (14)	53 (43)
	Muc	120 B,Bo,M	42 (94)	55 (17)	64 (9)
Salazar (1983), USA (hospital)	Serous	224 B,Bo,M	42 (110)	40 (10)	59 (104)
	Muc	126 B,Bo,M	43 (73)	48 (10)	45 (43)
Isarangkul (1984), Thailand (hospital)	Serous	85 B,Bo,M	42 (58)	42 (9)	58 (18)
	Muc	173 B,Bo,M	37 (141)	38 (18)	50 (14)
Grönroos et al. (1969)	All types	152 Bo,M		49 (61)	55 (91)
Aure et al. (1981), Norway (hospital)	All types	990 Bo,M		46 (161)	52 (829)
Bjorkholm et al. (1982), Sweden (hospital)	Serous	1310 Bo,M		50 (213)	56 (1097)
	Muc	344 Bo,M		53 (127)	55 (217)
Hart and Norris (1973) (consult)	Muc,St1	136 Bo,M		35 (97)	35 (39)

[a]B, benign; Bo, borderline; M, malignant; Muc, mucinous; St, stage. [a]Ages of affected patients are reported in years.

cupied 25% or less of the tumor, and it was difficult in most cases to be certain whether the benign epithelium was residual surface epithelium, the epithelium of a surface epithelial inclusion gland, or the residuum of a serous cystadenoma. In contrast, there was a significant component of benign epithelium (over 25%) in the mucinous carcinomas in 48% of the cases and the benign epithelium was predominant in 22%. Analogous figures for endometrioid and clear cell adenocarcinomas were 33% and 6%, and 32% and 5%, respectively. Transitions between the benign and malignant epithelium appeared to be present in 8% of the serous carcinomas, 18% of the mixed serous–transitional cell carcinomas, 52% of the clear cell carcinomas, 57% of the endometrioid carcinomas, and 80% of the mucinous carcinomas. The above studies suggest that epithelial cancers, particularly those of mucinous type, arise from preexisting benign lesions.

Although the results of these studies suggest that many epithelial cancers, particularly those in the mucinous category, arise from a preexisting benign tumor, the possibility exists that at least in some cases, the benign-appearing epithelium reflects maturation of obviously malignant-appearing epithelium into benign-appearing epithelium. The latter explanation is based on the observation that metastatic adenocarcinomas, particularly from the gastrointestinal tract and pancreas (Young and Scully, 1991), occasionally contain cysts lined by benign-appearing epithelium that under the circumstances obviously reflects maturation of malignant epithelium. In the metastatic tumors, the benign-appearing epithelium typically lines cysts in a diffuse distribution, sometimes with a gradual transition to atypical or malignant epithelium. Since a similar maturation of malignant epithelium is seen only rarely in the extraovarian primary tumor in these cases, it is possible that either pressure of the cyst contents or the presence of some unknown substance within the cyst fluid or the surrounding stroma induces this maturation in the ovary. Maturation of malignant epithelium seems unlikely, however, in cases in which the carcinoma arises more or less abruptly as a minor component of an otherwise uniformly benign-appearing cystic tumor. In other cases, differentiation between transformation from benign to malignant epithelium and cancerous epithelial maturation is not as clear-cut. Clinical follow-up with ultrasonography of benign-appearing ovarian cystic tumors may help to solve the problem of the frequency of their malignant transformation, but because of the average 10–15 years age difference of patients with benign and malignant epithelial tumors, demonstration of this sequence may require prolonged follow-up examination.

An enigmatic tumor that has been estimated to account for up to 10% of tumors initially diagnosed as serous borderline tumors of the ovary is the serous borderline tumor with microinvasion of the stroma (Bell and Scully, 1990; Tavassoli, 1988). In this tumor, single neoplastic cells, small clusters of cells, or larger cribriform groups of cells invade the stroma, forming foci less than 10 sq mm in area; occasionally, vascular space invasion is seen. Although this type of tumor might represent a link between serous borderline tumors and serous carcinomas, so far, limited follow-up data on relatively small series of cases have shown no evidence that otherwise typical serous borderline tumors with microinvasive foci have a worse prognosis than serous borderline tumors without microinvasion; also, curiously, the architecture of the microinvasive tumor differs from that of a typical serous carcinoma, and the infiltrating cells do not elicit the characteristic stromal response seen in the latter.

In the past several years, a number of studies have addressed the issue of development of ovarian epithelial cancers from preexisting tumors by utilization of molecular genetic techniques. These studies have generally been based on the assumptions that precursor lesions should exhibit a subset of the genetic alterations that are present in invasive, preferably "early" invasive, tumors and that adjacent precursor lesions and invasive carcinomas should be monoclonal. To date, the results of these investigations have indicated that genetic alterations differ in serous, endometrioid, and mucinous carcinomas, suggesting that each of these tumor types has a distinct pathogenesis (Jacobs and Lancaster, 1996; McCluskey and Dubeau, 1997; Mok et al., 1999).

Most studies of serous neoplasms have shown different molecular changes in cystadenomas, borderline tumors, and carcinomas, indicating that in most cases each of these tumor types develops via different genetic pathways (Jacobs and Lancaster, 1996; Matias-Guiu, 1998; McCluskey and Dubeau, 1997; Mok et al., 2000). p53 mutations and immunohistochemical overexpression are uncommon in benign and borderline serous tumors, whereas approximately 60% of serous carcinomas have detectable mutations or overexpression of p53. Serous borderline tumors have a higher rate of K-*ras* mutation (28%) than serous carcinomas (6%). Loss of heterozygosity is relatively infrequent in benign and borderline serous tumors but is commonly seen at multiple sites in serous carcinomas.

Exceptions to these findings are those of Zheng and co-workers (1995) and Wolf et al. (1996), which indicate that benign cysts in continuity with serous carcinomas have similar cytogenetic and mutational changes, suggesting that such cysts already have genetic abnormalities that predispose them to malignant transformation. Alternatively, these findings may reflect differentiation of malignant epithelium into a benign-appearing epithelium (Liu and Nuzum, 1995).

Greater similarities in mutation rate and overexpression of oncogenes and tumor suppressor genes have been reported in borderline and malignant mucinous tumors than serous tumors. Most studies have shown similar rates of K-*ras* mutations in mucinous borderline tumors and mucinous carcinomas, ranging from 50% to 86% (Mandai et al., 1998; Matias-Guiu and Prat, 1998; Mok et al., 2000). Mandai and co-workers (1998) have noted similarities in K-*ras* mutation patterns in benign, borderline, and malignant areas in mucinous tumors, which suggest that mucinous tumors may have an adenoma–carcinoma sequence of development. Another finding compatible with this sequence of development is the lower rate of *p53* mutations in mucinous borderline tumors than in mucinous carcinomas (13% vs. 40%) (Matias-Guin and Prat, 1998; Mok et al., 1999).

ENDOMETRIOSIS AS A PRECURSOR OF CARCINOMA

Endometriosis, a common ovarian lesion, is an acknowledged site of origin of surface epithelial cancers, particularly endometrioid and clear cell carcinomas, and rarely, other types of surface epithelial carcinoma, endometrioid stromal sarcoma, and malignant mesodermal mixed tumor (Clement, 1990; Clement and Scully, 1987; Mostoufizadeh and Scully, 1980; Scully et al., 1966, 1998). Endometrioid carcinoma has been reported to originate directly from endometriotic tissue in up to 24% of the cases in various series. Ipsilateral ovarian endometriosis has been detected in 11% to 31%, ovarian endometriosis of unspecified laterality in 9% to 20%, and pelvic endometriosis in 11% to 28% of cases of ovarian endometrioid carcinoma (Aure et al., 1971; Curling and Hudson, 1975; Czernobilsky et al., 1970; De Priest et al., 1992; Fathalla, 1967; Heaps et al., 1990; Kurman and Craig, 1972; McMeekin et al., 1995; Russell, 1979; Scully et al., 1966). Women whose endometrioid carcinoma has arisen in endometriosis have been a decade or more younger and have presented with lower-stage disease than those with ovarian endometrioid carcinoma in general, providing supportive evidence for the precancerous role of this disorder.

Russell (1979) reported a 47% frequency of pelvic endometriosis in 30 cases of clear cell carcinoma of the ovary, and Aure and colleagues (1971) demonstrated a 24% frequency of ovarian endometriosis in 59 cases of the same type of tumor; both of those figures were surprisingly higher than the figures given by the same authors for the association of endometriosis with endometrioid carcinoma (28% and 9%, respectively). Al-though isolated examples of serous and mucinous carcinoma have been reported to originate in endometriosis, the association of these tumors in general with that disorder is not significant. Russell (1979) found only a 2.5% frequency of pelvic endometriosis in 163 cases of serous carcinoma and a 6% frequency in 17 cases of mucinous carcinoma; and Aure and associates (1971) detected no ovarian endometriosis in 283 cases of serous carcinoma and only an 0.8% frequency in 203 cases of mucinous carcinoma. Rutgers and Scully (1988a), however, reported the finding of ovarian endometriosis in 30% of cases of mucinous borderline tumors of endocervical-like (müllerian) type, which accounted for 15% of the mucinous borderline tumors in their series; in contrast, there was no significant association of ovarian endometriosis and the more common mucinous borderline tumor of intestinal type. Borderline tumors of mixed müllerian epithelial cell types also have a frequent association with ovarian endometriosis (Rutgers and Scully, 1988b).

Because carcinoma of the endometrium often arises on a background of hyperplasia with cytologic and architectural atypicality, one might expect that a proportion of carcinomas arising in endometriosis would have similar precursors. Hyperplasia with varying degrees of architectural and cytologic atypia resembling that seen in the endometrium (Figs. 18–10 and 18–11), however, has been

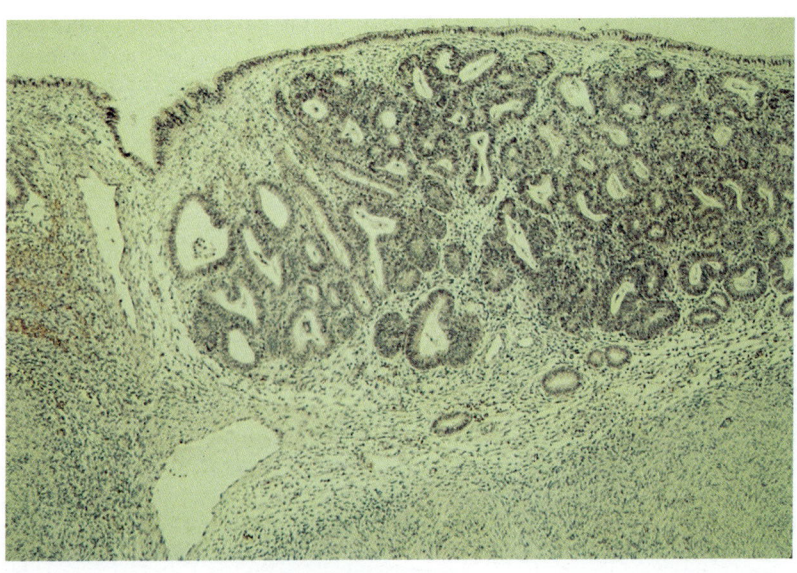

Figure 18–10. Severely atypical complex hyperplasia arising within endometriosis, a pattern encountered more often in the endometrium.

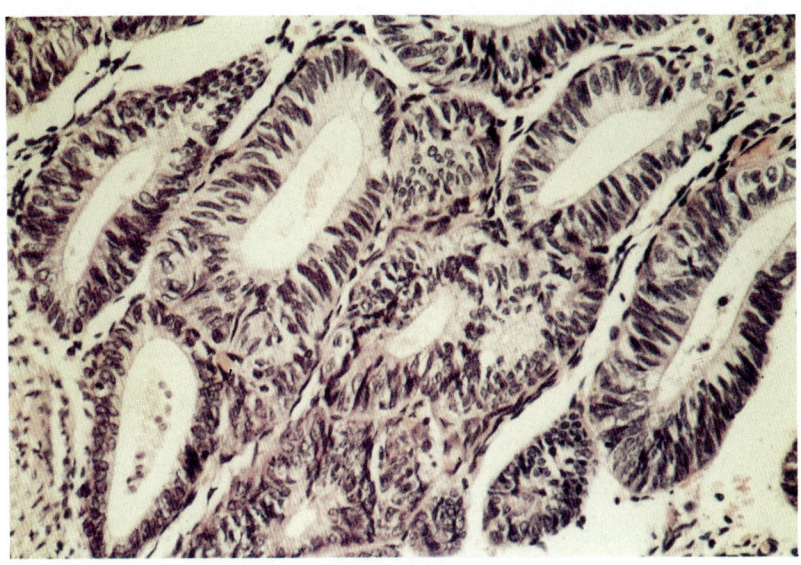

Figure 18–11. Focus of severely atypical complex hyperplasia in the lining of an endometriotic cyst.

recorded in ovarian endometriotic tissue only rarely (Czernobilsky and Morris, 1979; De la Cuesta et al., 1996; LaGrenade and Silverberg, 1988; Mostoufizadeh and Scully, 1980; Scully, 1979; Seidman, 1996). The prognostic significance of such changes is unclear because follow-up data have been limited to only a small number of women. Seidman (1996) reported follow-up information on 13 women with complex atypical hyperplasia and 7 women with "early carcinoma," arising in ovarian endometriosis. All the women with complex atypical hyperplasia were followed for a mean of 8.5 years and survived without the development of carcinoma; however, most of the lesions were completely excised. Similarly, the four women with "adenomatous hyperplasia" in ovarian endometriosis in the report of Czernobilsky and Morris (1979) were followed for 3 to 5 years without recurrence or the development of carcinoma, although 10 of their 11 patients with "adenomatous hyperplasia" or severe atypia of cyst-lining epithelium were treated by oophorectomy, presumably excising completely the atypical lesion. We have observed one case, however, in which the left ovary of a 55-year-old woman, which contained severely atypical endometriotic tissue (Fig. 18–11), was dissected away from the pelvic wall; she received estrogen therapy for 3 years and subsequently returned with an endometrioid adenocarcinoma that had arisen in the

area where ovarian tissue had presumably been left behind (Fig. 18–12). The outcome in this case is interesting in light of epidemiologic studies that have demonstrated a significant increase in the incidence of endometrioid carcinoma of the ovary in women on estrogen therapy (Cramer et al., 1983; Weiss et al., 1982) and in view of the number of reported cases of carcinoma developing in endometriosis in women receiving replacement therapy with estrogens unopposed by progesterone (Clement, 1990).

Two additional atypical lesions encountered in endometriosis—but rarely, if ever,

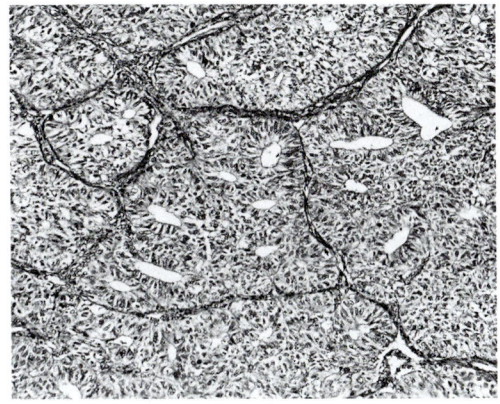

Figure 18–12. Endometrioid adenocarcinoma, grade 3 of 3, attached to pelvic wall at the site of the endometriotic cyst in Figure 18–11 that had been dissected away 3 years previously.

in the endometrium—are characterized by cells showing varying degrees of atypia lining endometriotic cysts without endometrial glandular hyperplasia. In the first type, which comprises most of these cases, the lining epithelium is composed of a single layer of large polygonal cells with abundant eosinophilic cytoplasm and large hyperchromatic, often smudged, nuclei (Fig. 18–13). Acute inflammation is frequently present (Ballouk et al., 1994; Fukunaga et al., 1997; Seidman, 1996). In the second, less common type, large polygonal cells and hobnail cells are present with epithelial stratification and tufting. These cells may have eosinophilic, clear, or vacuolated cytoplasm and may contain intracytoplasmic mucin; their nuclei are usually markedly hyperchromatic and pleomorphic. This type of epithelium may also be associated with acute inflammation (Ballouk et al., 1994; Chalas et al., 1991; Czernobilsky and Morris, 1979; De la Cuesta et al., 1996; Moll et al., 1990; Seidman, 1996). Seidman (1996) obtained follow-up on 20 of 37 women with these two types of cyst-lining atypias and found that the patients were all alive without the development of carcinoma after a mean of 8.6 years; "most" of the lesions, however, were completely excised. Czernobilsky and Morris (1979) reported that seven women with the second type of lining atypia were followed for 3 to 5 years without the development of carcinoma; again, most of the lesions were completely excised. Seidman (1996) concluded from these data that endometriotic cyst lining atypia was probably reactive or degenerative. In contrast, Moll et al. (1990)

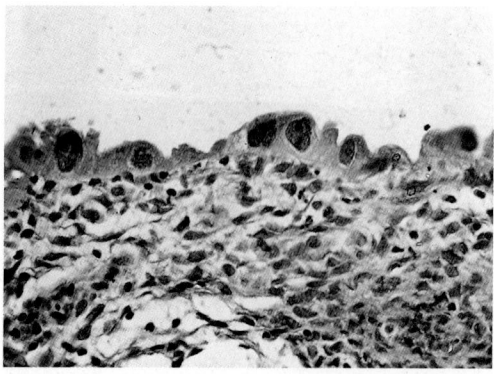

Figure 18–13. Endometriotic cyst lined by large cells with abundant cytoplasm and bizarre nuclei.

described a case in which a resected endometriotic cyst was lined by stratified, severely atypical hobnail cells; 3 years later, the patient had a clear cell carcinoma in the residual ovarian tissue; these authors suggested that such lining changes are preneoplastic. In a study of ploidy of atypical cyst-lining cells, the investigators noted that all of the cases with "mild" atypia and no stratification were diploid, but that three of six cases with "severe" atypia, stratification, and tufting were aneuploid, which suggests a neoplastic potential (Ballouk et al., 1994).

Several groups of investigators have analyzed genetic alterations in endometriosis and endometrioid carcinomas arising in endometriosis. They have shown that most benign-appearing endometriotic cysts are monoclonal (Jiang et al., 1996, Nilbert et al., 1995). Jiang and co-workers (1996, 1998) have shown LOH at several loci in typical endometriosis and have demonstrated that endometriosis and adjacent endometrioid carcinoma share common genetic events such as LOH at the same loci involving the same allele, and have the same pattern of X chromosome inactivation (albeit in only two of two cases examined). These findings support the morphologic conclusion that endometriosis is the precursor of at least some cases of endometrioid carcinoma of the ovary.

Early Carcinoma

Two types of "early" ovarian carcinoma have been described, microscopic or tiny gross *de novo* carcinomas (arising directly from surface epithelium or surface epithelial inclusion glands), which are predominantly of serous type, and small endometrioid carcinomas arising within ovarian endometriosis.

Early *De Novo* Carcinoma

A very small number of microscopic or tiny gross carcinomas have been reported, usually as incidental findings at operations for other gynecologic disorders or, more recently, in prophylactic oophorectomy specimens from patients at high risk for the development of ovarian carcinoma (Bell and Scully, 1994; Chen et al., 1985; Graham et al., 1964, 1965; Salazar et al., 1996; Scully, 1982). The largest study of such cases and the only one to include meaningful follow-up data comprised 14 cases of ovarian carcinomas that had not been recognized preoperatively, intraoperatively, or even on gross examination of the ovaries but were discovered only on microscopic examination (Bell and Scully, 1994). The patients ranged in age from 27 to 65 (mean 50) years. Three women had a family history of ovarian cancer, six did not, and the family history was unknown or unreliable in the remaining cases. All of the tumors were incidental findings in patients operated on because of a gynecologic indication that did not include a suspicion of ovarian cancer.

The tumors ranged in diameter from less than 1 to 7 mm. All of them were unilateral and four appeared to be multifocal. Surface involvement was found in 5 of the 13 cases in which this feature could be evaluated. The tumors had the typical microscopic features of larger clinically apparent tumors of the same cell type and were classified as serous in 10 cases, endometrioid in 1, clear cell in 1, and undifferentiated in two. Twelve of the 14 tumors were grade 2 or 3. Follow-up data of 2 or more years' duration were available for 10 of the 14 patients. Five of the seven patients whose diagnoses had been made prospectively at the time of oophorectomy were alive without recurrence 2 to 12 years postoperatively. At the time of publication of the series, one patient was alive with recurrent tumor and one had died of tumor. Subsequently, at least one patient originally categorized as alive without recurrence had died of tumor. Two of the three women whose ovarian tumors had been diagnosed for the first time on retrospective microscopic examination of previously removed ovaries after the development of peritoneal carcinomatosis 6, 7, and 10 years subsequently died and the third was alive with recurrent tumor.

Clearly, although the data are limited, the prognosis of patients with minute ovarian epithelial cancers is guarded. It is unclear, however, whether the subsequent peritoneal tumor in these women reflected late metastasis from the ovarian carcinoma or the development of a second primary tumor of the peritoneum. Further studies are necessary to answer this question.

Early Carcinoma in Endometriosis

Early carcinoma developing in an endometriotic cyst has also been specifically described in detail in only a few studies. Seidman (1996) reported 11 examples of ovarian endometriosis containing foci that fulfilled the Kurman and Norris (1982) criteria for endometrioid carcinoma of the endometrium. Seven women were followed for a mean of 8.6 years; in "most" of the cases the lesions had been completely excised. Nevertheless, three of them had an adverse outcome. One had a poorly differentiated adenocarcinoma of the anterior vaginal wall 8.1 years later, one had an endocervical-like mucinous borderline tumor in the contralateral ovary 7 years later, and the third patient was found to have "early carcinoma" in foci of endometriosis in the contralateral ovary and the omentum 3 months after the initial diagnosis. Thus, although the prognosis of an individual completely excised example of early carcinoma arising in endometriosis is excellent, carcinoma may arise in residual foci of endometriosis at the same or other sites. For this reason, close follow-up of women with early carcinoma arising in endometriosis is warranted.

SEX-CORD STROMAL TUMORS

GRANULOSA CELL TUMORS

The precursors of granulosa cell tumors and Sertoli-stromal cell tumors are unknown. The discovery of most granulosa cell tumors after the menopause (Stenwig et al., 1979), when the ovary is depleted of its follicles, suggests an origin from ovarian stromal cells. The indolent clinical course of many granulosa cell tumors (with occasional recurrences two or three decades after the initial diagnosis), however, suggests that the presence of these tumors in elderly women may reflect very slow growth of a neoplasm that had arisen from granulosa cells decades earlier. Granulosa cells that persist and proliferate within atretic follicles have also been proposed as a source of granulosa cell tumors (McKay et al., 1953). We have encountered such proliferations in the ovaries of nonpregnant women (Fig. 18–14) and much more often in those of pregnant women (Clement et al., 1988). Except for their size, such proliferations may be indistinguishable from granulosa cell tumors. There is no evidence, however, that these tu-

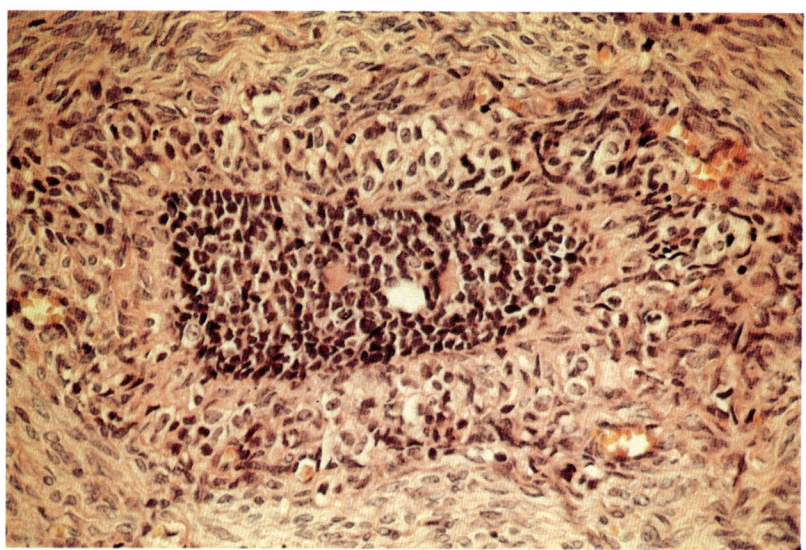

Figure 18–14. Granulosa cells persisting in an atretic follicle.

mor-like lesions are the precursors of clinically evident granulosa cell tumors, and there are no epidemiologic data indicating an association of such tumors with prior pregnancies. Epidemiologic investigations of granulosa cell tumors have not been conducted, to the best of our knowledge. Study of granulosa cell tumors and Sertoli-stromal cell tumors of microscopic size has not yielded histogenetic clues, having shown only tiny tumors lying within otherwise normal-appearing ovarian stroma (Bell and Scully, personal observation).

Thus far, studies of molecular alterations in human granulosa cell tumors have been relatively uninformative with regard to their genesis. p53 is infrequently expressed in these tumors (Costa et al., 1996; Horny et al., 1999; Lui et al., 1996) and mutations of the *p53* tumor suppressor gene (Watson et al., 1997), the Wilms' tumor suppressor gene *WT1* (Coppes et al., 1993), and the *FSH* receptor gene (Fuller et al., 1998) have not been identified. Although α-inhibin is present immunohistochemically in most ovarian sex-cord stromal tumors (Kommoss et al., 1998) and the α-inhibin gene has been shown in knockout mouse models to inhibit granulosa cell tumorigenesis, Watson and co-workers (1997) identified LOH of the α-inhibin gene locus on chromosome 2q in only 1 of 17 human granulosa cell tumors, indicating that this gene is unlikely to be involved in their genesis.

SERTOLI-STROMAL CELL TUMORS

Although testicular "remnants," hilus cells (hilar Leydig cells), and rete ovarii have been identified in the ovarian hilus in most women (Sternberg, 1949), they have not been linked to the development of Sertoli-stromal cell tumors. On the other hand, the existence of transitions between the morphologic patterns of neoplastic and nonneoplastic granulosa cells—such as follicles merging with tubules in gynandroblastomas and the rare finding of typical Leydig cells containing crystals of Reinke within the ovarian stroma and its neoplasms (Sternberg and Roth, 1973)—suggests that at least some Sertoli-stromal cell tumors arise from cells of ovarian type rather than the testicular "remnants" in the ovarian hilus. Also, rarely, Sertoli cell "tumorlets" of obvious granulosa cell origin arise within the basement membrane of atretic follicles during pregnancy (Clement et al., 1988). Finally, tubular transformation of graafian follicles is seen frequently in the canine ovary (Norris et al., 1970; Scully, personal observation). Although acquisition of SRY testis-determining genetic material by granulosa cells and stromal cells would provide an acceptable explanation for the genesis of Sertoli-Leydig cell tumors, polymerase chain reaction (PCR) analysis failed to show the presence of this genetic material in one case (Hittmair et al., 1997).

Sex Cord Tumor with Annular Tubules

An ovarian tumor of great interest from the viewpoint of histogenesis of sex cord–stromal neoplasms is the sex cord tumor with annular tubules (Scully, 1970b; Young et al., 1982). This tumor, which is characterized by a predominance of ring-shaped tubules composed of Sertoli cells (Tavassoli and Norris, 1980), may contain additionally elongated, solid tubules indistinguishable from those of a typical Sertoli cell tumor as well as circumscribed aggregates with small cavities that are indistinguishable from the islands of a microfollicular granulosa cell tumor. The sex cord tumor with annular tubules may occur as a large solitary ovarian mass in an otherwise normal patient or, in approximately one-third of the reported cases, as multiple, bilateral tumorlets in patients with the Peutz-Jeghers syndrome (PJS) (Figs. 18–15 and 18–16), many of whom have a germline mutation in a serine/threonine kinase gene designated *LKB1* or *STK11*. This gene may be a tumor suppressor gene (Hemminki et al., 1998; Jenne et al., 1998). The tumorlets develop multifocally within the ovarian stroma, presumably from follicular granulosa cells, and have not been reported to exceed 3 cm in diameter or pursue a malignant course. In contrast, the large solitary tumors are malignant in 20% to 25% of the cases. Although there is no evidence that the multiple tumorlets give rise to the large tumors, they may be related to and be possible precursors of two types of sex cord–stromal tumors, both of which have been associated with isosexual pseudoprecocity: lipid-rich Sertoli cell tumors (folliculomes lipidiques) (Sohl et al., 1983) and unusual sex cord–stromal tumors with a distinctive microscopic appearance (Young et al., 1983). Small foci resembling the sex cord tumor with annular tubules may be found in the ovaries of children, but appear to have no neoplastic potential (Manivel et al., 1988). Finally, some women with the resistant ovary syndrome have alterations of their follicles that mimic the annular tubules of the sex cord tumor with annular tubules (Case Records of the Massachusetts General Hospital, 1986).

MALIGNANT GERM CELL TUMORS

Lesions that predispose to malignant germ cell tumors in women include dysgenetic gonads associated with a karyotype that almost always contains a Y chromosome or a Y chromosomal fragment (Schellhas, 1974a,b; Scully, 1970a, 1981; Talerman, 1994) and dermoid cysts.

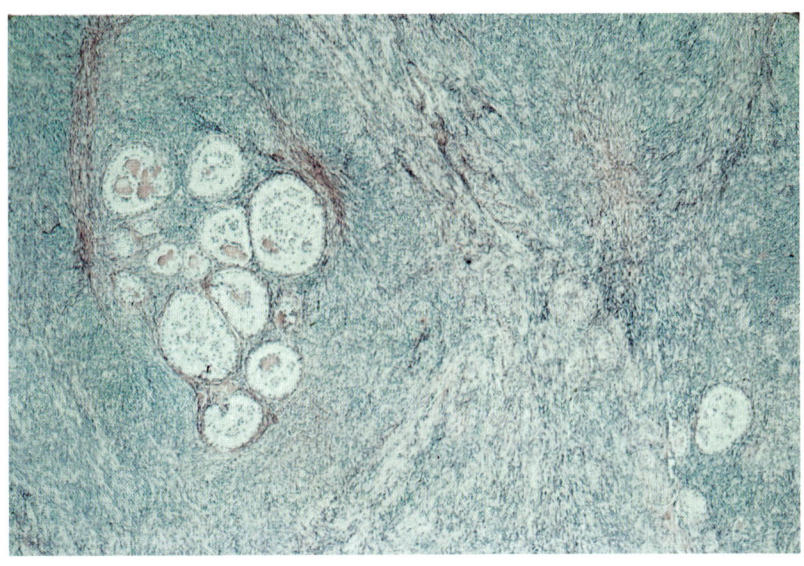

Figure 18–15. Two foci of sex cord tumor with annular tubules in the ovarian cortex of a patient with Peutz-Jeghers syndrome.

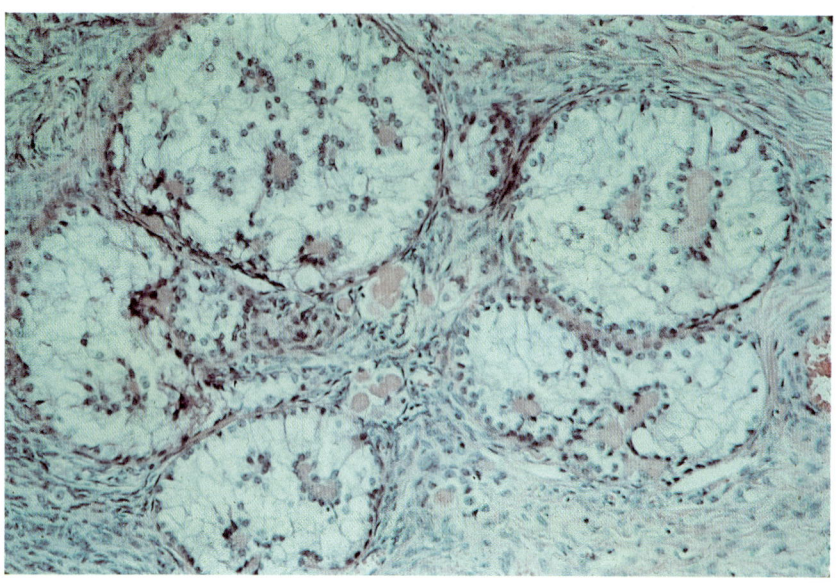

Figure 18–16. Sex cord tumor with annular tubules in a patient with Peutz-Jeghers syndrome.

GONADOBLASTOMA

Approximately 25% of women with a Y chromosome–associated form of gonadal dysgenesis (46 XY pure gonadal dysgenesis; mixed gonadal dysgenesis) have a gonadoblastoma or a malignant pure germ cell tumor by the age of 30 years (Manuel et al., 1976). The most common tumor is the gonadoblastoma (Fig. 18–17) (see also Chapter 22), a mixed germ cell–sex cord–stromal neoplasm that contains germ cells, immature sex cord elements, and, in two-thirds of the cases, stromal derivatives (Leydig or lutein cells) (Fig. 18–18; Scully, 1970a; Scully et al., 1998). An occasional gonadoblastoma arises in the gonad of a fertile woman without evidence of Y chromosome material. Rare patients, most often young children with what appear to be otherwise normal ovaries, have another type of germ cell–sex cord tumor that resembles the gonadoblastoma but differs with respect to several histologic features. This lesion has been designated *germ cell–sex cord tumor, unclassified* (Talerman and van der Harten, 1977; Tavassoli, 1983).

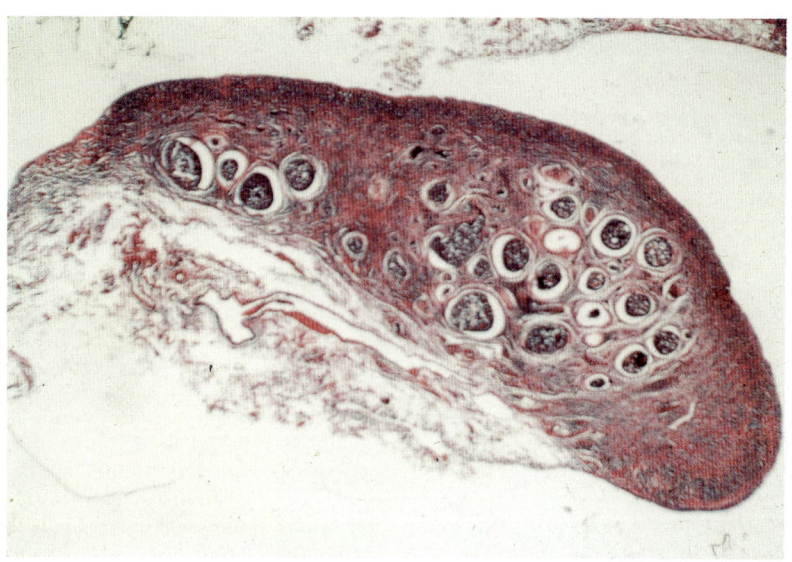

Figure 18–17. Low-power photograph of a gonadoblastoma arising within a streak gonad.

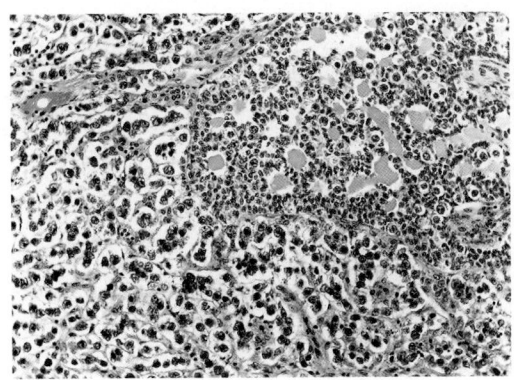

Figure 18–18. Gonadoblastoma (upper right) and dysgerminoma (lower left). The gonadoblastoma contains numerous hyaline bodies composed of basement membrane material. [from Serov et al., 1973, with permission.]

The gonadoblastoma has not shown a capacity to metastasize *per se*, but is generally considered an *in situ* germ cell tumor for two reasons. *(1)* In half the cases, by the time a gonadoblastoma has been detected, its germ cells have escaped from their discrete compartments, shared with the sex cord elements of the tumor, and entered the stromal component to form a germinoma (dysgerminoma, seminoma) (Fig. 18–18), and in an additional 8% of the cases, a nongerminomatous germ cell cancer develops. *(2)* The *in situ* atypical germ cells in gonadoblastomas generally have the same morphologic, immunohistochemical and ploidy features as those of typical testicular intratubular germ cell neoplasia unclassified (carcinoma *in situ*) (Jørgensen et al., 1997).

Several studies have shown in small numbers of cases that dysgerminomas and yolk sac tumors that arise in association with gonadoblastomas are diploid or near diploid, in contrast to most dysgerminomas and yolk sac tumors that arise in otherwise normal ovaries (Baker et al., 1998; Riopel et al., 1998). The authors have suggested that these findings support a different histogenesis for malignant germ cell tumors associated with gonadoblastomas and those in normal ovaries. Malignant germ cell tumors may also arise in dysgenetic gonads, presumably from intratubular germ cell neoplasia, in the absence of evidence of an underlying gonadoblastoma, but it is possible in some cases that the latter was obliter-

ated by the germ cell tumor or was missed as a result of incomplete sampling. Unclassified germ cell–sex cord tumors are rarely malignant *per se* (Talerman and van der Harten, 1977; Tavassoli, 1983), but dysgerminomas and other primitive germ cell tumors have arisen from them (Scully, personal observation).

Since both dysgenetic gonads associated with Y-chromosome material and gonadoblastomas, which can be recognized preoperatively in some cases as calcified pelvic masses, are precancerous, they should be excised as soon as they have been detected.

DERMOID CYST

The *dermoid cyst* is a cystic teratoma composed of mature tissue with a predominance of skin and its appendages (Caruso et al., 1971; Marcial-Rojas and Medina, 1958; Peterson et al., 1955). In contrast to *primitive germ cell* tumors, which are almost always encountered in girls or women of reproductive age, the dermoid cyst is occasionally detected in postmenopausal women, whose ovaries no longer contain recognizable germ cells. This finding is best interpreted as indicative of the leisurely growth rate of a tumor that originated years earlier. Approximately 2% of dermoid cysts contain adult-type malignant tumors, more than 80% of which are squamous cell carcinomas (Fig. 18–19; (Ameigo et al., 1979; Climie and Heath, 1968; Kelley and Scully, 1961; Pins et al., 1996; Waxman and Deppisch, 1983). A few of these carcinomas have been detected *in situ* within cutaneous or respiratory epithelium (Klionsky et al., 1972; Sobel, 1972; Waxman and Deppisch, 1983). The age–incidence data in Table 18–2 provide strong circumstantial evidence that the dermoid cyst is a precancerous lesion. In most cases, it is diagnosed during the third to fifth decades of life (Waxman and Deppisch, 1983). In contrast, squamous cell carcinomas arising in dermoid cysts are detected most often in the fifth to seventh decades; over 90% of these tumors have been found in women 40 years of age or older, and almost half of them in women over 55 years of age. The relatively high frequency of squamous cell carcinomas in the postmenopausal period—during which, as already stated, dermoid cysts are not expected to develop *de*

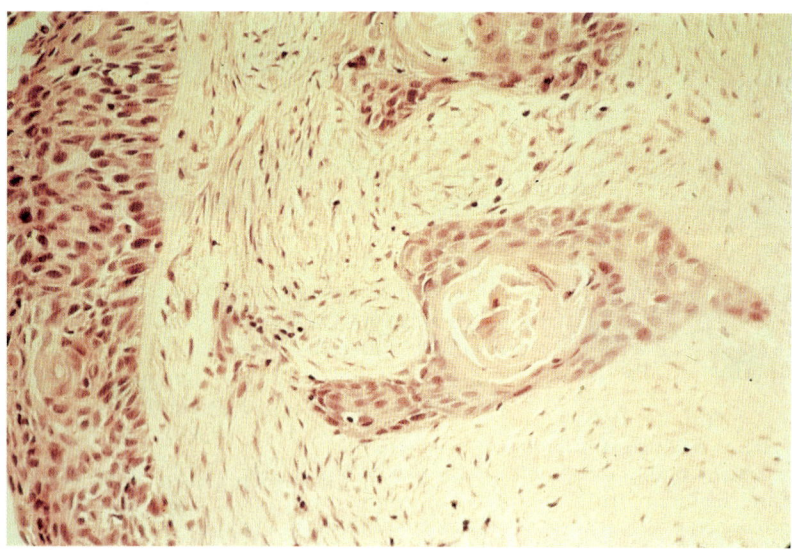

Figure 18–19. Carcinoma *in situ* lining a dermoid cyst with underlying invasive squamous cell carcinoma.

novo—provides convincing evidence that the latter are precancerous in a small proportion of cases. A variety of other malignant tumors arise less frequently within dermoid cysts. These include other cutaneous tumors, such as malignant melanoma and basal cell carcinoma, adenocarcinomas, carcinoids, thyroid carcinomas, and a variety of sarcomas (Stamp and McConnell, 1983). These neoplasms, like squamous cell carcinomas, usually occur in older women, about half of whom are postmenopausal.

An important corollary of the above data, emphasized by Waxman and Deppisch (1983), is that although the frequency of malignant change in a dermoid cyst is less than 1% in patients under the age of 40 years, it is between 4% and 5% in the sixth and seventh decades and 15% in women over 70 years of age. Therefore, dermoid cysts

Table 18–2. Dermoid Cyst[a]

	Benign		Malignant (Squamous Cell Carcinoma)		
Reference	Age Range	Predominant Age (%)	Cases (n)	Age Range	Average Age
Marcial-Rojas and Medina (1958)		11–50 (86)			
Caruso et al. (1971)	10–80	15–45 (80)			
Salazar (1983)		21–40 (61) (average age: 32)			
Peterson et al. (1955, 1956)	2–78	15–50 (92) (most: 20–30)	10	31–78	52
Gloor (1979)		20–59 (80)	6	44–61	52
Climie and Heath (1968) (review)			18	33–68	54
Curling et al. (1979)			10	46–73	60
Amerigo et al. (1979)			5	45–49	51
Stamp and McConnell (1983)			18	36–76	56
Waxman and Deppisch (1983) (review)			162[b]	30 to 10th decade	53

[a]Ages of affected patients are reported in years.

[b]Includes cases other than squamous cell carcinoma.

should be evaluated carefully for the possibility of cancerization, particularly in elderly patients.

NOTE IN PROOF

Since acceptance of this manuscript, Werness and Eltabbakh (Ovarian dysplasia identified by cul-de-sac aspiration: a reexamination of previously reported cases. *Int J Gynecol Pathol* 2000; 19:190–192) reviewed the slides from six of the cases reported by Graham and coworkers as showing significant atypia of ovarian surface epithelium (Graham et al., 1964) and reclassified the changes in these cases as variations in normal ovarian histology.

REFERENCES

Amerigo J, Nogales FFJ, Fernandez-Sanz J, et al. (1979) Squamous cell neoplasms arising from ovarian benign cystic teratoma. *Gynecol Oncol* 8:277–283.

Aure JC, Hoeg K, Kolstad P. (1971) Carcinoma of the ovary and endometriosis. *Acta Obstet Gynecol Scand* 50:63–67.

Aure JC, Hoeg K, Kolstad P. (1981) Clinical and histological studies of ovarian carcinoma. Long-term follow-up of 990 cases. *Obstet Gynecol* 37:1–9.

Baker BA, Frickey L, Yu, I-T, et al. (1998) DNA content of ovarian immature teratomas and malignant germ cell tumors. *Gynecol Oncol* 71:14–18.

Ballouk F, Ross JS, Wolf BC. (1994) Ovarian endometriotic cysts. An analysis of cytologic atypia and DNA ploidy patterns. *Am J Clin Pathol* 102:415–519.

Bell DA, Scully RE. (1990) Ovarian serous borderline tumors with microinvasion. A report of 21 cases. *Hum Pathol* 21:397–403.

Bell DA, Scully RE. (1994) Early *de novo* ovarian carcinoma. A study of fourteen cases. *Cancer* 73:1859–1864.

Berge T, Borglin NE. (1967) Brenner tumors. Histogenetic and clinical studies. *Cancer* 20:308–318.

Bjorkholm E, Pettersson F, Einhorn N. (1982) Long-term follow-up and prognostic factors in ovarian carcinoma. The Radiumhemmet series 1958 to 1973. *Acta Radiol Oncol* 21:413–419.

Blaustein A. (1981) Surface cells and inclusion cysts in fetal ovaries. *Gynecol Oncol* 12:222–233.

Blaustein A, Kaganowicz A, Wells J. (1982) Tumor markers in inclusion cysts of the ovary. *Cancer* 49:722–726.

Bourne TH, Whitehead MJ, Campbell, S, et al. (1991) Ultrasound screening for familial ovarian cancer. *Gynecol Oncol* 43:92–97.

Case Records of the Massachusetts General Hospital. (1986) Case 46-1986. *N Engl J Med* 315:1336–1343.

Caruso PA, Marsh MR, Minkowitz S, et al. (1971) An intense clinicopathologic study of 305 teratomas of the ovary. *Cancer* 27:343–348.

Chalas E, Chumas J, Barbieri R, et al. (1991) Nuclear organizer regions in endometriosis, atypical endometriosis, and clear cell and endometrioid carcinomas. *Gynecol Oncol* 40:260–263.

Chen KT, Schooley JL, Flam MM. (1985) Peritoneal carcinomatosis after prophylactic oophorectomy in familial ovarian cancer syndrome. *Obstet Gynecol* 66:93S-95S.

Chenevart P, Gloor E. (1980) Cystadénomes sereux et muqueux de l'ovaire a la limite de la malignité. *Schweiz Med Wochenschr* 110:531–539.

Clement PB. (1990) Pathology of endometriosis. *Pathol Annu* 25:245–295.

Clement PB, Scully RE. (1987) Extrauterine mesodermal (müllerian) adenosarcoma. A clinicopathologic analysis of five cases. *Am J Clin Pathol* 69:276–283.

Clement PB, Young RH, Scully RE. (1988) Ovarian granulosa cell proliferations of pregnancy: a report of nine cases. *Hum Pathol* 19:657–662.

Climie ARW, Heath LP. (1968) Malignant degeneration of benign cystic teratomas of the ovary. Review of the literature and report of a chondrosarcoma and carcinoid tumor. *Cancer* 22:824–832.

Coppes MJ, Rackley R, Zhao XL, et al. (1993) Analysis of WT1 in granulosa cell and other sex cord–stromal tumors. *Cancer Res* 53:2712–2714.

Cordon-Cardo C, Mattes MJ, Melamed MR. (1985) Immuno-pathologic analysis of a panel of mouse monoclonal antibodies reacting with human ovarian carcinomas and other human tumors. *Int J Gynecol Pathol* 4:121–130.

Costa MJ, Walls J, Ames P, et al. (1996) Transformation in recurrent ovarian granulosa cell tumors: Ki67 (MIB-1) and p53 immunohistochemistry demonstrates a possible molecular basis for the poor histopathologic prediction of clinical behavior. *Hum Pathol* 27:274–281.

Cramer DW, Hutchison GB, Welch WR, et al. (1983) Determinants of ovarian cancer risk. I. Reproductive experiences and family history. *J Natl Cancer Inst* 71:711–716.

Curling OM, Hudson CN. (1975) Endometrioid tumours of the ovary. *Br J Obstet Gynaecol* 82:405–411.

Curling OM, Potsides PN, Hudson CN. (1979) Malignant change in benign cystic teratoma of the ovary. *Br J Obstet Gynaecol* 86:399–402.

Czernobilsky B, Morris WJ. (1979) A histologic study of ovarian endometriosis with emphasis on hyperplastic and atypical changes. *Obstet Gynecol* 53:318–323.

Czernobilsky B, Silverman BB, Mikuta JJ. (1970) Endometrioid carcinoma of the ovary. *Cancer* 26:1141–1152.

De la Cuesta RS, Eichhorn JH, Rice LW, et al. (1996) Histologic transformation of benign endometriosis to early epithelial ovarian cancer. *Gynecol Oncol* 60:238–244.

De Preist PD, Banks ER, Powell DE, et al. (1992) Endometrioid carcinoma of the ovary and endometriosis: the association in postmenopausal women. *Gynecol Oncol* 47:71–75.

Ehrlich CE, Roth LM. (1971) The Brenner tumor. A clinicopathological study of 57 cases. *Cancer* 27:332–342.

Emmert-Buck MR, Bonner RF, Smith PD, et al. (1996) Laser capture microdissection. *Science* 274:998–1001.

Fathalla MF. (1967) Malignant transformation in ovarian endometriosis. *J Obstet Gynaecol Br Commonw* 74:85–92.

Fox H, Agrawal K, Langley FA. (1972) The Brenner tumour of the ovary. A clinicopathological study of 54 cases. *J Obstet Gynaecol Br Commonw* 79:661–665.

Fraumeni JF, Grundy GW, Creagan ET, et al. (1975) Six families prone to ovarian cancer. *Cancer* 36:364–369.

Fukunaga M, Nomura K, Ishikawa E, et al. (1997) Ovarian atypical endometriosis: its close association with malignant epithelial tumours. *Histopathology* 30:249–255.

Fuller PJ, Verity K, Shen Y, et al. (1998) No evidence of a role for mutations or polymorphisms of the follicle-stimulating hormone receptor in ovarian granulosa cell tumors. *J Clin Endocrinol Metab* 83:274–279.

Gil J, Deligdisch L. (1989) Interactive morphometric procedures and statistical analysis in the diagnosis of ovarian dysplasia and carcinoma. *Pathol Res Pract* 185:680–685.

Gillett WR. (1991) Artefactual loss of human ovarian surface epithelium: potential clinical significance. *Reprod Fertil Dev* 3:93–98.

Gloor E. (1979) Tératomes matures benins avec tumeur maligne et tératomes monodermiques malins de l'ovaire. Présentation anatomo-clinique de 10 cas. *Schweiz Med Wochenschr* 109:968–975.

Graham JB, Graham RM. (1967) Cul-de-sac puncture in the diagnosis of early ovarian carcinoma. *J Obstet Gynaecol Br Commonw* 74:371–378.

Graham JB, Graham RM, Schueller EF. (1964) Preclinical detection of ovarian cancer. *Cancer* 17:1414–1432.

Graham RM, Schueller EF, Graham JB. (1965) Detection of ovarian cancer at an early stage. *Obstet Gynecol* 26:151–156.

Grönroos M, Laurén P, Lehto J, et al. (1969) Ovarian cancer and its treatment. *Ann Chir Gynaecol Fenn* 58:83–89.

Gusberg SB, Deligdisch L. (1984) Ovarian dysplasia. A study of identical twins. *Cancer* 54:1–4.

Hallgrímsson J, Scully RE. (1972) Borderline and malignant Brenner tumours of the ovary. *Acta Pathol Microbiol Scand* 80 (suppl. 233):56–66.

Hart WR, Norris HJ. (1973) Borderline and malignant mucinous tumors of the ovary. Histologic criteria and clinical behavior. *Cancer* 31:1031–1045.

Heaps JM, Nieberg RK, Berek JS. (1990) Malignant neoplasms arising in endometriosis. *Obstet Gynecol* 75:1023–1028.

Hemminki A, Markie D, Tomlinson I, et al. (1998) A serine/threonine kinase gene defective in Peutz-Jeghers syndrome. *Nature* 391:184–187.

Hittmair A, Zelger BG, Obrist P, et al. (1997) Ovarian Sertoli-Leydig cell tumor: a SRY gene-independent pathway of pseudomale gonadal differentiation. *Hum Pathol* 28:1206–1210.

Horny HP, Marx L, Krober S, et al. (1999) Granulosa cell tumor of the ovary. Immunohistochemical evidence of low proliferative activity and virtual absence of mutation of the *p53* tumor-suppression gene. *Gynecol Obstet Invest* 47:133–138.

Hutson R, Ramsdale J, Wells M. (1995) p53 protein expression in putative precursor lesions of epithelial ovarian cancer. *Histopathology* 27:367–371.

Isarangkul W. (1984) Ovarian epithelial tumors in Thai women: a histological analysis of 291 cases. *Gynecol Oncol* 17:326–339.

Jacobs I, Lancaster J. (1996) The molecular genetics of sporadic and familial epithelial ovarian cancer. *Int J Gynecol Cancer* 6:337–355.

Jenne DE, Reimann H, Nezu J, et al. (1998) Peutz-Jeghers syndrome is caused by mutations in a novel serine threonine kinase. *Nat Genet* 18:38–43.

Jiang X, Hitchcock A, Bryan EJ, et al. (1996) Microsatellite analysis of endometriosis reveals loss of heterozygosity at candidate ovarian tumor suppressor gene loci. *Cancer Res* 56:3534–3539.

Jiang X, Morland SJ, Hitchcock A, et al. (1998) Allelotyping of endometriosis with adjacent ovarian carcinoma reveals evidence of a common lineage. *Cancer Res* 58:1707–1712.

Jorgensen EO, Dockerty MB, Wilson RB, et al. (1970) Clinicopathologic study of 53 cases of Brenner's tumors of the ovary. *Am J Obstet Gynecol* 108:122–127.

Jørgensen N, Müller J, Jaubert F, et al. (1997) Heterogeneity of gonadoblastoma germ cells: similarities with immature germ cells, spermatogonia and testicular carcinoma in situ cells. *Histopathology* 30:177–186.

Kabawat SE, Bast RCJ, Bhan AK, et al. (1983) Tissue distribution of a coelomic-epithelium-related antigen recognized by the monoclonal antibody OC-125. *Int J Gynecol Pathol* 2:275–285.

Katsube Y, Berg JW, Silverberg SG. (1982) Epidemiologic pathology of ovarian tumors. *Int J Gynecol Pathol* 1:3–16.

Kelley RR, Scully RE. (1961) Cancer developing in dermoid cysts of the ovary. A report of 8 cases, including a carcinoid and a leiomyosarcoma. *Cancer* 14:989–1000.

Klionsky BL, Nickens OJ, Amortegui AJ. (1972) Squamous cell carcinoma in situ arising in adult cystic teratoma of the ovary. *Arch Pathol* 93:161–163.

Kommoss F, Oliva E, Bhan AK, et al. (1998) Inhibin expression in ovarian tumors and tumor-like lesions: an immunohistochemical study. *Mod Pathol* 11:656–664.

Kurman RJ, Craig JM. (1972) Endometrioid and clear cell carcinoma of the ovary. *Cancer* 29:1653–1664.

Kurman RJ, Norris HJ. (1982) Evalution of criteria for distinguishing atypical endometrial hyperplasia from well-differentiated carcinoma. *Cancer* 49:2547–2559.

LaGrenade A, Silverberg SG. (1988) Ovarian tumors associated with atypical endometriosis. *Hum Pathol* 19:1080–1084.

Landis SH, Murray T, Bolden S, et al. (1999) Cancer Statistics, 1999. *CA Cancer J Clin* 49:8–31.

Liu E, Nuzum C. (1995) Molecular sleuthing: tracking ovarian cancer progression [editorial]. *J Natl Cancer Inst* 87:1099–1101.

Liu FS, Ho ES, Lai CR, et al. (1996) Overexpression of p53 is not a feature of ovarian granulosa cell tumors. *Gynecol Oncol* 61:50–53.

Maines-Bandiera SL, Auersperg N. (1997) Increased E-cadherin expression in ovarian surface epithelium: an early step in metaplasia and dysplasia? *Int J Gynecol Pathol* 16:250–255.

Mandai M, Konishi I, Kuroda H, et al. (1998) Heterogeneous distribution of K-ras-mutated epithelia in mucinous ovarian tumors with special reference to histopathology. *Hum Pathol* 29:34–40.

Manivel JC, Dehner LP, Burke B. (1988) Ovarian tumorlike structures, biovular follicles, and binucleated oocytes in children: their frequency and possible pathologic significance. *Pediatr Pathol* 8:283–292.

Manuel M, Katayama KP, Jones HW Jr. (1976) The age of occurrence of gonadal tumors in intersex patients with a Y chromosome. *Am J Obstet Gynecol* 124:293–300.

Marcial-Rojas RA, Medina R. (1958) Cystic teratomas of the ovary. A clinical and pathological analysis of two hundred sixty-eight tumors. *Arch Pathol* 66:577–589.

Matias-Guiu X, Prat J. (1998) Molecular pathology of ovarian carcinomas. *Virchows Arch* 433:103–111.

McCluskey LL, Dubeau L. (1997) Biology of ovarian cancer. *Curr Opin Oncol* 9:645–470.

McKay DG, Hertig AT, Hickey WF. (1953) The histogenesis of granulosa and theca cell tumors of the human ovary. *Obstet Gynecol* 1:125–148.

McMeekin DS, Burger RA, Manetta A, et al. (1995) Endometrioid adenocarcinoma of the ovary and its relationship to endometriosis. *Gynecol Oncol* 59:81–86.

Miles PA, Norris HJ. (1972) Proliferative and malignant Brenner tumors of the ovary. *Cancer* 30:174–186.

Mittal KR, Zeleniuch-Jacquotte A, Cooper JL. (1993) Contralateral ovary in unilateral ovarian carcinoma: a search for preneoplastic lesions. *Int J Gynecol Pathol* 12:59–63.

Mok SC, Lu KH, Ng S, et al. (2000) Molecular pathogenesis of borderline and invasive ovarian tumors. In: *Ovarian Cancer 6,* Jacobs I, Lueslui D, Berchuck A, Blackett T. Oxford Isis Medical Media, in press.

Moll UM, Chumas JC, Chalas E, et al. (1990) Ovarian carcinoma arising in atypical endometriosis. *Obstet Gynecol* 75:537–539.

Mostoufizadeh M, Scully RE. (1980) Malignant tumors arising in endometriosis. *Clin Obstet Gynecol* 23:951–963.

Nilbert M, Pejovic T, Mandahl N, et al. (1995) Monoclonal origin of endometriotic cysts. *Int J Gynecol Cancer* 5:61–63.

Norris HJ, Garner FM, Taylor HB. (1970) Comparative pathology of ovarian neoplasms, IV. Gonadal stromal tumours of canine species. *J Comp Pathol* 80:399–405.

Nouwen EJ, Hendrix PG, Dauwe S, et al. (1987) Tumor markers in the human ovary and its neoplasms. A comparative immunohistochemical study. *Am J Pathol* 126:230–242.

Peterson WF, Prevost EC, Edmunds FT. (1955) Benign cystic teratomas of the ovary. *Am J Obstet Gynecol* 70:368–382.

Peterson WF, Prevost EC, Edmunds FT et al. (1956) Epidermoid carcinoma arising in a benign cystic teratoma. A report of 15 cases. *Am J Obstet Gynecol* 71:173–175.

Pins MR, Young RH, Daly WJ, et al. (1996) Primary squamous cell carcinoma of the ovary. Report of 37 cases. *Am J Surg Pathol* 20:823–833.

Plaxe SC, Deligdisch L, Dottino PR, et al. (1990) Ovarian intraepithelial neoplasia demonstrated in patients with stage I ovarian carcinoma. *Gynecol Oncol* 38:367–372.

Puls LE, Powell DE, DePriest PD, et al. (1992) Transition from benign to malignant epithelium in mucinous and serous ovarian cystadenocarcinoma. *Gynecol Oncol* 47:53–57.

Resta L, Russo S, Colucci GA, et al. (1993) Morphologic precursors of ovarian epithelial tumors. *Obstet Gynecol* 82:181–186.

Riopel MA, Spellerberg A, Griffin CA, et al. (1998) Genetic analysis of ovarian germ cell tumors by comparative genomic hybridization. *Cancer Res* 58:3105–3110.

Roth LM, Sternberg WH. (1971) Proliferating Brenner tumors. *Cancer* 27:687–693.

Russell P. (1979) The pathological assessment of ovarian neoplasms. I. Introduction to the common "epithelial" tumours and analysis of benign "epithelial" tumors. *Pathology* 11:5–26.

Rutgers JL, Scully RE. (1988a) Müllerian mucinous papillary cystadenomas of borderline malignancy: a clinicopathological analysis of 30 cases. *Cancer* 61:340–348.

Rutgers JL, Scully RE. (1988b) Ovarian mixed epithelial papillary cystadenoma of borderline malignancy of müllerian type: a clinicopathological analysis of 36 cases. *Cancer* 61:546–554.

Rybak BJ, Obert WB, Bernacki EG Jr. (1981) Malignant Brenner tumor of the ovary. *Diagn Gynecol Obstet* 3:61–65.

Salazar H. (1983) Epidemiological observations on histologic types of ovarian tumours at Magee-Women's Hospital, a gynecological referral center in Pittsburgh, PA, USA. In: *An International Survey of Distributions of Histologic Types of Tumours of the Testis and Ovary.* (Stalsberg H, ed.) p. 331. UICC. Geneva.

Salazar H, Godwin AK, Daly MB, et al. (1996) Microscopic benign and invasive malignant neoplasms and a cancer-prone phenotype in prophylactic oophorectomies. *J Natl Cancer Inst* 88:1810–1820.

Schellhas HF. (1974a) Malignant potential of the dysgenetic gonad. Part I. *Obstet Gynecol* 44:298–309.

Schellhas HF. (1974b) Malignant potential of the dysgenetic gonad. Part II. *Obstet Gynecol* 44:455–462.

Scully RE. (1970a) Gonadoblastoma. A review of 74 cases. *Cancer* 25:1340–1356.

Scully RE. (1970b) Sex cord tumor with annular tubules. A distinctive ovarian tumor of the Peutz-Jeghers syndrome. *Cancer* 25:1107–1121.

Scully RE. (1979) Tumors of the ovary and maldeveloped gonads. In: *Atlas of Tumor Pathology*, 2nd series; fascicle 16. Armed Forces Institute of Pathology, Washington, DC.

Scully RE. (1981) Neoplasia associated with anomalous sexual development and abnormal sex chromosomes in the intersex child. *Pediatr Adolesc* 8:203–210.

Scully RE. (1982) Minimal cancer of the ovary. *Clin Oncol* 1:379–387.

Scully RE, Bell DA, Abu-Jawdeh GM. (1995) Update on early ovarian cancer and cancer developing in benign ovarian tumors. In: *Ovarian Cancer 3* (Sharp F, Mason P, Blackett T, Berek J, eds.) pp. 139–144. Chapman & Hall Medical, New York.

Scully RE, Young RH, Clement PB. (1998) Tumors of the ovary, maldeveloped gonads, fallopian tube, and broad ligament. In: *Atlas of Tumor Pathology*, 3rd series; fascicle 23. Armed Forces Institute of Pathology, Washington, DC.

Scully RE, Richardson GS, Barlow JF. (1966) The development of malignancy in endometriosis. *Clin Obstet Gynecol* 9:384–411.

Seidman JD. (1996) Prognostic importance of hyperplasia and atypia in endometriosis. *Int J Gynecol Pathol* 15:1–9.

Serov SF, Scully RE, Sobin LH. (1973) Histological typing of ovarian tumours. In: *International Histological Classification of Tumours*, No. 9. World Health Organization, Geneva.

Sherman ME, Lee JS, Burks RT, et al. (1999) Histopathologic features of ovaries at increased risk for carcinoma. A case controlled analysis. *Int J Gynecol Pathol* 18:151–157.

Silverberg S. (1971) Brenner tumors of the ovary. A clinico-pathological study. *Cancer* 28:588–596.

Sobel HJ. (1972) Bowen's disease and senile keratosis arising. *Arch Pathol Lab Med* 94:372–376.

Sohl HM, Azoury RS, Najjar SS. (1983) Peutz-Jeghers syndrome associated with precocious puberty. *J Pediatr* 103:593–595.

Stalsberg H, Bjarnason O, de Carvalho ARL. (1983a) International comparisons of histologic types of ovarian cancer in cancer registry material. In: *An International Survey of Distributions of Histologic Types of Tumours of the Testis and Ovary*, (Stalsberg H, ed.) p. 247. UICC, Geneva.

Stalsberg H, Blom PG, Bostad LH, et al. (1983b) Ovarian tumours and endometriosis in Norway General Hospital material. In: *An International Survey of Distributions of Histologic Types of Tumours of the Testis and Ovary*, (Stalsberg H, ed.) UICC, Geneva.

Stalsberg H, de Carvalho ARL, Correa P. (1983c) International comparisons of histologic types of benign and malignant ovarian tumours in general hospital material. In: *An International Survey of Distributions of Histologic Types of Tumours of the Testis and Ovary* (Stalsberg H, ed.) pp. 313–323. UICC, Geneva.

Stamp GWH, McConnell EM. (1983) Malignancy arising in cystic ovarian teratomas. A report of 24 cases. *Br J Obstet Gynaecol* 90:671–675.

Stenwig J, Hazekamp JT, Beecham JB. (1979) Granulosa cell tumors of the ovary. A clinicopathological study of 118 cases with long-term follow-up. *Gynecol Oncol* 7:136–152.

Sternberg WH. (1949) The morphology, androgenic function, hyperplasia and tumors of the human ovarian hilus cells. *Am J Pathol* 25:493–522.

Sternberg WH, Roth LM. (1973) Ovarian stromal tumors containing Leydig cells. 1. Stromal-Leydig cell tumor and non-neoplastic transformation of ovarian stroma to Leydig cells. *Cancer* 32:940–951.

Stratton JF, Buckley CH, Lowe D, et al. (1999) Comparison of prophylactic oophorectomy specimens from carriers and noncarriers of a *BRCA1* or *BRCA2* gene mutation. *J Natl Cancer Inst* 91:626–628.

Sundfeldt K, Piontkewitz Y, Ivarsson K, et al. (1997) E-cadherin expression in human epithelial ovarian cancer and normal ovary. *Int J Cancer (Pred Oncol)* 74:275–280.

Talerman A. Germ cell tumors of the ovary. (1994) In: *Pathology of the Female Genital Tract*, 4th ed. (Blaustein A, ed.) pp. 849–914. Springer-Verlag, New York.

Talerman A, van der Harten JJ. (1977) A mixed germ cell sex-cord stromal tumor of the ovary associated with isosexual precocious puberty in a normal girl. *Cancer* 40:889–894.

Tavassoli FA. (1983) A combined germ cell-gonadal stromal-epithelial tumor of the ovary. *Am J Surg Pathol* 7:73–84.

Tavassoli FA. (1988) Serous tumor of low malignant potential with early stromal invasion (serous LMP with microinvasion). *Mod Pathol* 1:407–414.

Tavassoli FA, Norris HJ. (1980) Sertoli tumors of the ovary. A clinicopathologic study of 28 cases with ultrastructural observations. *Cancer* 46:2281–2297.

Tresserra F, Grases PJ, Labastida R, et al. (1998) Histological features of the contralateral ovary in patients with unilateral ovarian cancer: a case control study. *Gynecol Oncol* 71:437–441.

Tsukahara Y, Shiozawa I, Sakai Y, et al. (1982) Study on the histogenesis of ovarian tumors—with special reference to five clinical cases with common epithelial tumors detected during the preclinical stage. *Acta Obstet Gynaecol Jpn* 34:959–965.

Wang D, Konishi I, Koshiyama M, et al. (1992) Immunohistochemical localization of c-erbB-2 protein and epidermal growth factor receptor in normal surface epithelium, surface inclusion cysts, and common epithelial tumours of the ovary. *Virchows Arch A Pathol Anat* 421:393–400.

Watson RH, Roy WJJ, Hitchcock DM, et al. (1997) Loss of heterozygosity at the alpha-inhibin locus on chromosome 2q is not a feature of human granulosa cell tumors. *Gynecol Oncol* 65:387–390.

Waxman M. (1979) Pure and mixed Brenner tumors of the ovary. Clinicopathologic and histogenetic observations. *Cancer* 43:1830–1839.

Waxman M, Deppisch LM. (1983) Malignant alteration in benign teratomas. In: *The Human Teratomas. Experimental and Clinical Biology* (Damjanov I, Knowles B, Solter D, eds.) Humana Press, Clifton, NJ.

Weiss NS, Lyon JL, Krishnamurthy S. (1982) Non-contraceptive estrogen use and the occurrence of ovarian cancer. *J Natl Cancer Inst* 68:95–98.

Werness BA, Afify AM, Bielat KL, et al. (1999) Altered surface and cyst epithelium of ovaries removed prophylactically from women with a family history of ovarian cancer. *Hum Pathol* 30:151–157.

Werness BA, Paivatiyan P, Ramus SJ, et al. Ovarian carcinoma *in situ* with gumline *BRCA1* mutation and loss of heterozygosity at *BRCA1* and *TP53*. *J Natl Cancer Inst* 2000; 92:1088–91.

Westhoff C, Murphy P, Heller D, et al. (1993) Is ovarian cancer associated with an increased frequency of germinal inclusion cysts? *Am J Epidemiol* 138:90–93.

Wolf NG, Abdul-Karin FW, Schork NJ, et al. (1996) Origins of heterogeneous ovarian carcinomas. A molecular cytogenetic analysis of histologically benign, low malignant potential malignant potential, and fully malignant components. *Am J Pathol* 149:511–520.

Woodruff JD, Dietrich D, Genadry R, et al. (1981) Proliferative and malignant Brenner tumors. Review of 47 cases. *Am J Obstet Gynecol* 141:118–125.

Yoonessi M, Abell MR. (1979) Brenner tumors of the ovary. *Obstet Gynecol* 54:90–96.

Young RH, Dickersin GR, Scully RE. (1983) A distinctive sex-cord stromal tumor causing sexual precocity in the Peutz-Jeghers syndrome. *Am J Surg Pathol* 7:233–243.

Young RH, Scully RE. (1991) Metastatic tumors in the ovary: a problem-oriented approach and review of the recent literature. *Semin Diagn Pathol* 8:250–276.

Young RH, Welch WR, Dickersin GR, et al. (1982) Ovarian sex-cord stromal tumors with annular tubules. *Cancer* 50:1384–1402.

Zheng J, Benedict WF, Xu H-J, et al. (1995) Genetic disparity between morphologically benign cysts contiguous to ovarian carcinomas and solitary cystadenomas. *J Natl Cancer Inst* 87:1146–1153.

19

LYMPHOID SYSTEM

Michael W. Beaty and Elaine S. Jaffe

The concept of *in situ* lesions has not been generally applied to the lymphoid system. One reason for this is that unlike most cells in the human body, lymphoid cells are normally migratory. Rather than remaining fixed in their tissue environment, they circulate throughout the lymphoid system, following orderly traffic pathways. Benign clonal proliferations of lymphoid cells would therefore not likely remain localized, but would most likely at their inception disseminate throughout the lymphoid system. In fact, benign monoclonal tumors of the lymphoid system have been recognized only recently with the aid of advances in molecular analytical techniques. The relation of premalignant or incipient *in situ* lesions to the development of malignant lymphoma is still under investigation.

Within the lymphoid system, there are areas that are preferentially populated by B or T lymphocytes. For example, the gut-associated lymphoid tissue, including Waldeyer's ring and mesenteric lymph nodes, contains relatively more B cells than T cells. As one would expect, malignant lymphomas arising in these sites are more often of B-cell phenotype. In contrast, T-cell lymphomas more often occur in lymphoid tissues associated with surface epithelium, such as the skin. Compartmentalization of the B and T cells is seen both in the lymph nodes as well as in the spleen and other lymphoid tissues. A lymphoma that remains restricted to its normal environment or compartment may be considered *in situ*. For example, follicular

lymphomas appear to arise morphologically within individual follicles and subsequently "metastasize" to other follicles, giving rise to the characteristic follicular growth pattern. Only late in the course of the disease do the tumor cells lose their homing properties to manifest a diffuse growth pattern.

While polyclonal reactive lymphoid hyperplasias are relatively commonplace, benign monoclonal lymphoid tissues, e.g., solitary plasmacytoma, are relatively unusual. However, certain disease states are associated with an increased risk of developing lymphoproliferative disorders (LPDs), including lymphoma, and these LPDs may be considered incipient neoplastic events (Table 19–1). The basis of the normal immune response is a limited clonal expansion of either T or B cells, or both, usually in response to a particular antigen. Most of these physiological clonal expansions are beyond the limits of routine detection but can be identified using experimental techniques (Callan et al., 1996; Kuppers et al., 1993). However, these benign oligoclonal or monoclonal lymphoid expansions provide the milieu for the emergence of malignant lymphomatous clones, usually with the assistance of additional cytogenetic or oncogenic mutational events.

Immunophenotypic and genetic studies continue to be extremely valuable in the diagnosis of both benign and malignant lymphoid neoplasms. Today we use a wide battery of monoclonal antibodies that are reactive in routinely processed paraffin sec-

Table 19–1. Disease States Associated with Increased Risk of Developing a Lymphoproliferative Disorder

Autoimmune diseases

Helicobacter pylori gastritis
Sjögren's syndrome/rheumatoid arthritis
Hashimoto's thyroiditis
Immunoproliferative small intestinal disease

Lymphotropic viral infections

Epstein-Barr virus
Human herpes virus-8
Human T-cell lymphotropic virus
Hepatitis C virus

Immunodeficiency syndromes

Congenital
Acquired
  Human immunodeficiency virus
  Post-organ transplantation
  Iatrogenic (non-posttransplant)

Other

Celiac Disease

tions, and many of these stains have become essential to malignant hematological diagnoses. Although identification of the cell of origin, whether B, T, or natural killer cell, of a particular neoplasm is important, recognition of additional molecular and cytogenetic abnormalities are equally important in the pathogenesis of lymphoid neoplasms. Molecular biological techniques, namely the polymerase chain reaction (PCR), allow the identification of genetic mutations, chromosomal translocations, antigen receptor gene rearrangements, including both immunoglobulin heavy-chain gene and T-cell receptor gene rearrangements, as well as the monitoring of residual disease. Fluorescence *in situ* hybridization (FISH) techniques are greatly enhancing the ability to detect genetic abnormalities. Moreover, new techniques are emerging, such as the combination of FISH with cell surface markers (FICTION) and comparative genomic hybridization studies, which show promise in their clinical and pathologic utilization (Morgan and Pratt, 1998).

Genotypic studies are being used routinely to detect small clonal populations suggestive of malignancy. Sensitive molecular techniques, e.g., PCR or Southern blot, can detect clonal populations of 1%–5% of cells (Cossman et al., 1988). However, caution

should be exercised in the interpretation of small clones, because clonal expansion, while perhaps a defining characteristic of malignancy, is not necessarily diagnostic of malignancy. As noted above, individual germinal centers may be monoclonal (Kuppers et al., 1993). As these and even more sensitive molecular methods become a daily part of the diagnostic process, more and more examples of nonmalignant or benign clonal lymphoid processes have and will become clinically evident. This is particularly evident in diseases of abnormal immune states, either acquired or congenital, or in cases of persistent antigen stimulation, such as is present in many autoimmune diseases.

One definition of malignancy is autonomous growth. However, there are some lymphoproliferations, e.g., methotrexate-associated LPDs, that are not really autonomous but are still considered neoplastic, either because of chromosomal abnormalities or because if left untreated they will progress. In some clonal disorders, the distinctions between benign and malignant is ambiguous. Certain low-grade lymphomas, such as *Helicobacter pylori*–associated gastric, mucosa-associated lymphoid tissue (MALT) lymphomas, can remain localized for long periods with continued potential curability, raising questions as to whether such tumors truly qualify as lymphoma (Banks and Isaacson, 1999). Yet these neoplasms exhibit monoclonal lymphoid populations, may show genetic abnormalities, are invasive and destructive, and are capable of metastasis and/or progression to a higher grade (Isaacson, 1999a,b). Together, these properties seem to fulfill the requirement for the definition of a malignant process. Also, the conventional therapeutic regimens of surgical excision, localized radiation, and systemic chemotherapy have been expanded to include the use of antimicrobials, withdrawal of specific immunosuppressive drugs, and the use of targeted immunomodulatory agents. The new advances in both our basic understanding of the pathogenesis of incipient lymphoid neoplasia and how they are most appropriately treated are challenging our definitions and boundaries of what it takes to be a malignant neoplasm.

In recent years, the discipline of hematopathology has emphasized the integration of morphologic features and biologic markers for diagnosis. Both the Revised European-American Lymphoma (REAL) (Harris et al., 1994) and the newly proposed World Health Organization (WHO) (Jaffe et al., 1999) lymphoma classification schemes are remarkable for their recognition of distinct disease entities and their use of a multiparameter approach; that is, diseases are defined not just on their respective pathologic findings, rather each entity is defined as a constellation of clinical and laboratory features. As such, the clinical presentation and course of the disease have become as important as the morphologic, immunophenotypic, and genetic features in the diagnosis. Additionally, the site(s) of involvement at presentation are often a signpost for important underlying biologic distinctions (Jaffe, 1999). We have adopted these overriding principles, and the discussions that follow utilize this multiparameter approach in defining the disease states associated with increased risks of developing an incipient LPD.

B-CELL LYMPHOPROLIFERATIVE DISORDERS

PROGRESSIVE TRANSFORMATION OF GERMINAL CENTERS

Progressive transformation of germinal centers (PTGC) is a lesion with distinctive histologic findings, resembling the nodular form of lymphocyte-predominant Hodgkin's disease (NLPHD), and is often seen in association with NLPHD in 20% of cases (Burns et al., 1984). In some instances, both PTGC and NLPHD are seen together in the same lymph node site. In other instances, PTGC precedes the development of NLPHD. In some patients with a documented diagnosis of NLPHD, the diagnosis of PTGC may be made in another anatomic site or in recurrent lymphadenopathy following treatment for NLPHD (Hansmann et al., 1990; Osborne and Butler, 1984). Thus, PTGC may be a preneoplastic lesion that leads to the development of NLPHD. Yet, most lymph nodes with PTGC are benign and not associated with NLPHD (van den Oord et al., 1985) and therefore should not be regarded as a malignant neoplasm; approximately

10% of enlarged lymph nodes showing reactive follicular hyperplasia will contain PTGC (Osborne et al., 1992).

Clinically, PTGC is found in an age population commonly affected by NLPHD; it is more prevalent in males, and most commonly occurs in the fourth to fifth decade of life, further suggesting that the association between PTGC and NLPHD is more than coincidental. Most of the patients present with a solitary asymptomatic enlarged lymph node, usually cervical, and there is often recurrent lymphadenopathy showing reactive follicular hyperplasia with PTGC (Osborne et al., 1992). Interestingly, a syndrome of florid PTGC occurring in adolescent boys and young men (second to third decade) associated with prominent lymphadenopathy without evidence of NLPHD has been described. The NLPHD did not develop in these patients with up to 5 years follow-up (Ferry et al., 1992), therefore recognition of this syndrome is important to avoid overdiagnosis of NLPHD.

Affected lymph nodes may be focally involved, or the PTGC lesions may be extensive and cause architectural obliteration of the node (Fig. 19–1). Histologically, PTGC appears as nodular structures that are at least two to three times the diameter of the surrounding reactive follicles, which often show evidence of hyperplasia. The nodules are composed mainly of immunoglobulin D (IgD)–positive mantle zone B cells, with scattered centroblasts, follicular dendritic cells, and occasional tingible body macrophages. Within the center of the nodules are ill-defined structures that resemble germinal centers, but these are often fragmented, with the germinal center cells dispersed throughout the nodule. Demarcation of the mantle zone is usually difficult to discern. The nodules of PTGC closely resemble those seen in NLPHD. Cells resembling the lymphocyte and histiocyte (L&H) cells, or "popcorn" cells, characteristic of NLPHD may be seen. However, these cells are more infrequent than is typically seen in NLPHD, and are not rosetted by T cells. The distinction between L&H cells and residual germinal center centroblasts is not always straightforward, which can be the cause for some concern in making a diagnosis. Classic Reed-Sternberg cells are not present in either PTGC or NLPHD.

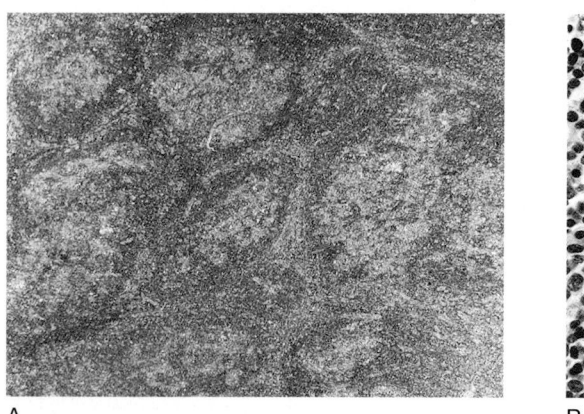
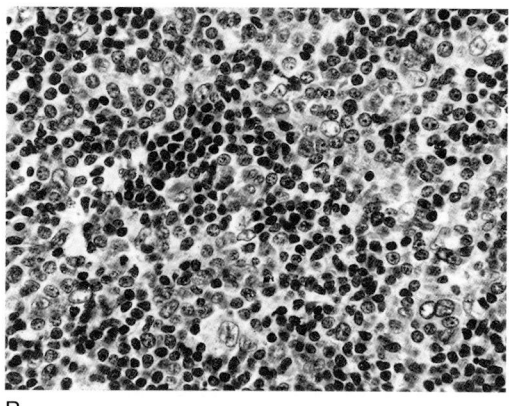

A   B

Figure 19–1. Progressive transformation of germinal centers (PTGC). *A:* Extensive involvement by PTGC causing architectural obliteration of the lymph node. The nodules are large and appear hyperplastic, with vaguely discernable mantle zones. Within the center of the nodules are ill-defined, fragmented germinal centers. *B:* High-power view of one of the altered germinal centers showing follicular center cells admixed with normal lymphocytes. "Popcorn" cells of nodular lymphocyte–predominant Hodgkin's disease (NLPHD) are not seen. Extensive examination should be performed to rule out focal involvement by NLPHD.

Focal involvement of lymph nodes by NLPHD is not uncommon, and immunophenotypic, flow cytometric, and molecular analyses are usually of little help in the differential diagnosis between PTGC and NLPHD. Both L&H cells and residual germinal center cells stain as B cells and are generally negative for both CD15 and CD30. The presence of CD3-positive, CD57-positive T-cell rosettes surrounding L&H cells may be a useful diagnostic feature. In approximately one-third of florid PTGC cases studied, T-cell rosettes were present, but they were notably fewer than those in NLPHD (Nguyen et al., 1999). The formation of T-cell aggregates within the nodules, rather than scattered singly throughout, was also a feature seen more commonly in NLPHD (Nguyen et al., 1999). However, caution should be exercised in the diagnostic use of these immunohistologic features, especially in cases of focal NLPHD or NLPHD containing relatively few to rare L&H cells.

The cells of PTGC are polyconal for immunoglobulin heavy (IgH) chain by conventional molecular methods, e.g., PCR or Southern blot. Polyclonal IgH patterns are also seen with NLPHD, using whole section fresh or frozen tissues. However, recent advances in microdissection techniques for single-cell PCR have shown the L&H cells of NLPHD to represent a monoclonal expansion of B cells (Marafioti et al., 1997; Ohno et al., 1997). Single-cell PCR studies of the occasional atypical cells seen in florid PTGC and recurrent PTGC remain to be done.

The clinical course of PTGC is generally self-limited, although recurrent lymphadenopathy with PTGC is not uncommon (Osborne et al., 1992). Because a node may contain both PTGC and NLPHD, a lymph node showing only the former should be extensively examined for focal involvement by NLPHD. If other significant lymphadenopathy is present in a patient with a previous diagnosis of PTGC, repeat biopsy is indicated to rule out the possibility of NLPHD existing in other nodal sites.

AUTOIMMUNE ASSOCIATED LOW-GRADE MUCOSA-ASSOCIATED LYMPHOID TISSUE LYMPHOMAS

Patients with autoimmune disease have a well-known increased incidence of developing LPDs. The autoimmunity may either precede or complicate an existing LPD, suggesting that autoimmunity is involved in the pathogenesis of the LPD. The vast majority of the known LPDs associated with an underlying autoimmune process are of B-cell origin. With the advent of the new classifi-

Table 19–2. Antigen-Driven Diseases Associated with Mucosa-Associated Lymphoid Tissue Lymphomas

Disease	Tissue Site
Helicobacter pylori gastritis	Stomach
Sjögren's syndrome	Salivary/lacrimal glands
Hashimoto's thyroiditis	Thyroid
Rheumatoid arthritis	Nodal
α heavy chain disease	Duodenum, small bowel

cation schemes (Harris et al., 1994; Jaffe et al., 1999), most of these B-cell LPDs would be classified as low-grade extranodal marginal zone B-cell lymphomas (MZL), arising in mucosa-associated lymphoid tissue (MALT) sites, such as salivary glands, lungs, kidneys, and the gastrointestinal tract (Burke, 1999; Table 19–2). We use the term MALT lymphoma synonymously with extranodal MZL of MALT type.

The development of a LPD from an autoimmune disease stems from persistent local antigenic stimulation, which over time recruits a chronic inflammatory infiltrate in specific tissue sites (Isaacson and Spencer, 1994). The persistent antigenic drive can be of an infectious nature, as in *Helicobacter pylori* gastritis and immunoproliferative small intestinal disease (IPSID), or of autoimmune origin, as seen in Sjögren's syndrome (SS), rheumatoid arthritis (RA), and Hashimoto's thyroiditis (HT) (Isaacson, 1999b). If the antigen stimulus continues unabated, the prelymphomatous chronic inflammatory infiltrate may lead eventually to the emergence of autonomous clones.

The pathophysiological mechanism by which an antigen-driven reactive lymphoid infiltrate transforms into malignant lymphoma is not yet fully understood. The accumulation of antigen-stimulated lymphoid tissue is currently thought to be a T cell–mediated inflammatory process composed of a mixture of B and T cells that show a polyclonal diversity (Jonsson et al., 1999). The exact nature of the T cells associated with the antigen-driven inflammatory processes is still ill defined, although antigen-activated T cells are now thought to be pivotal in sustaining the B-cell lymphoproliferative process (Koulis et al., 1997). This chronic inflammatory infiltrate provides the milieu for the emergence of occult lymphoid clones that can ultimately transform the infiltrate into lymphoma (Jonsson et al., 1999), with the additional assistance of chromosomal abnormalities, oncogene mutations, or both, resulting in escape from T-cell dependency (Guindi, 1999). Preferential usage of particular chains of the T-cell receptor in these lesions, which can be seen with some superantigens expanding T cells with specific V β chains, may be at the heart of the T cell–mediated process (Pivetta et al., 1999). Thus, the interactions between the B and T cells, both of which are activated by local antigens in the reactive infiltrate, may play a critical role in the progression of the prelymphomatous lesions to lymphoma.

The pathologic features of the lymphomas complicating organ-specific autoimmune disease are strikingly homogeneous (Isaacson and Spencer, 1994). The concept of MALT lymphoma comes in large part from our current understanding of gastric lymphomas associated with *H. pylori* infection, which has been the most intensely studied MALT lymphoma since the term was first coined in 1983 (Isaacson and Wright, 1983), and as a result serves as the prototype of the autoimmune-associated LPDs. The concept was later expanded to include extranodal lymphomas involving the salivary gland, thyroid, kidney, and lung (Isaacson and Wright, 1984). Rather than recapitulating features of lymph nodes, the inflammatory infiltrates in the stomach, as well as other organs targeted by autoimmune processes, bear a striking resemblance to the mucosa-associated lymphoid tissues of Peyer's patches. Paradoxically, lymphoid tissue is normally absent in sites where MALT lymphomas occur most often, whereas MALT lymphomas are unusual in normal MALT tissue sites, such as the oral cavity and large bowel (Banks and Isaacson, 1999; Isaacson, 1999a,b).

Although the morphologic, immunophenotypic, and molecular characteristics of MALT lymphoma arising in the setting of chronic antigen stimulation are similar irrespective of the organ involved, the borders between a reactive chronic inflammatory infiltrate or hyperplasia and a low-grade LPD can be quite elusive. To compound the diagnostic difficulty, MALT lymphomas may arise in association with a preexisting or underlying reactive hyperplasia. As previously

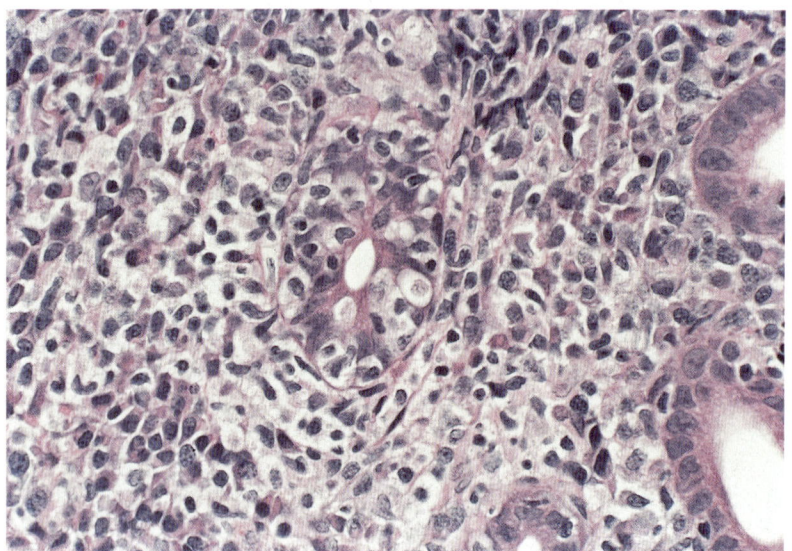

Figure 19–2. Low-grade extranodal marginal zone B-cell lymphoma of mucosa-associated lymphoid tissue (MALT) type (MALT lymphoma) involving the stomach. The atypical lymphoplasmacytic infiltrate is superficial, involving the mucosa and submucosa. A characteristic lymphoepithelial lesion is in the center of the field. *Helicobacter pylori*–like organisms were present in this case in large numbers.

noted, the early lymphoid infiltrates show histologic features that simulate reactive MALT tissues. Reactive germinal centers are surrounded by a polymorphous lymphoid infiltrate showing both plasmacytoid and monocytoid differentiation. As the lesion progresses, aggregates of monocytoid B cells generally invade the glands/acinar structures and the overlying mucosa, forming the hallmark lymphoepithelial lesions (LEL) (Fig. 19–2). The epithelial cells within the LEL show characteristic eosinophilic degenerative changes. Morphologic features helpful in distinguishing MALT lymphoma from benign reactive hyperplasia include increased numbers and destructiveness of the LELs, and anastomosing monocytoid B-cell aggregates seen away from or outside of the LELs. An additional feature that is worrisome for malignant lymphoma is the presence of increased numbers of plasma cells, particularly if they exhibit a sheet-like growth pattern and/or if Dutcher bodies can be identified (Table 19–3). However, these histologic features can be seen to varying de-grees in both antigen-driven reactive hyperplasias and MALT lymphomas.

The polymorphous nature of the lymphoid infiltrates can make the differential diagnosis between an exuberant reactive hyperplasia, or so-called pseudolymphoma, and low-grade MALT lymphoma extremely hazardous even to the most experienced pathologist. Therefore, the use of immunophenotypic studies has become essential in distinguishing prelymphomatous lesions from MALT lymphoma. Immunophenotypically, the lymphomatous infiltrates are composed predominantly of B cells, which express pan B-cell markers CD20, CD22, and express Bcl-2 protein. The B cells lack CD5, CD10, and cyclin D1. Expression of CD23 and CD43 is variable; with upwards of 50% of MALT lymphomas coexpressing CD43. However, in our experience evaluation of CD43 staining can be problematic, due to either the expression of CD43 by normal plasma cells or the presence of numerous CD3-positive T cells, making definitive coexpression by the B cells difficult to interpret. The tumors gener-

Table 19–3. Histologic Criteria for Differentiating Reactive Lymphoid Hyperplasia from Mucosa-Associated Lymphoid Tissue (MALT) Lymphoma

Lymphoid Hyperplasia	*MALT Lymphoma*
Germinal centers common	Germinal centers displaced, or colonized
Occasional lymphoepithelial lesions	Lymphoepithelial lesions common, more destructive
Monocytoid B cells less conspicuous	Aggregates and anastomosing bands of monocytoid B cells
Scattered plasma cells	Sheets of plasma cells, with Dutcher bodies

ally have a low proliferative rate as detected with MIB-1 (Ki-67). In a histologically equivalent lesion, the detection of monoclonal Ig light-chain expression is a prerequisite for a malignant diagnosis (Fig. 19–3). Cytogenetic studies have shown a relatively high percentage of cases (60%) exhibiting trisomy 3 (Wotherspoon et al., 1995). Additional chromosomal abnormalities seen in the MALT lymphomas of autoimmune derivation have been reported, and include both the t(1;14) (Wotherspoon et al., 1992) and t(11;18) (Ott et al., 1997). Oncogene mutations, including *p53* and c-*myc*, have been shown in only a minority of cases, approximately 15% of MALT lymphomas (Du and Isaacson, 1998), and may be related more to progression to higher-grade lymphoma.

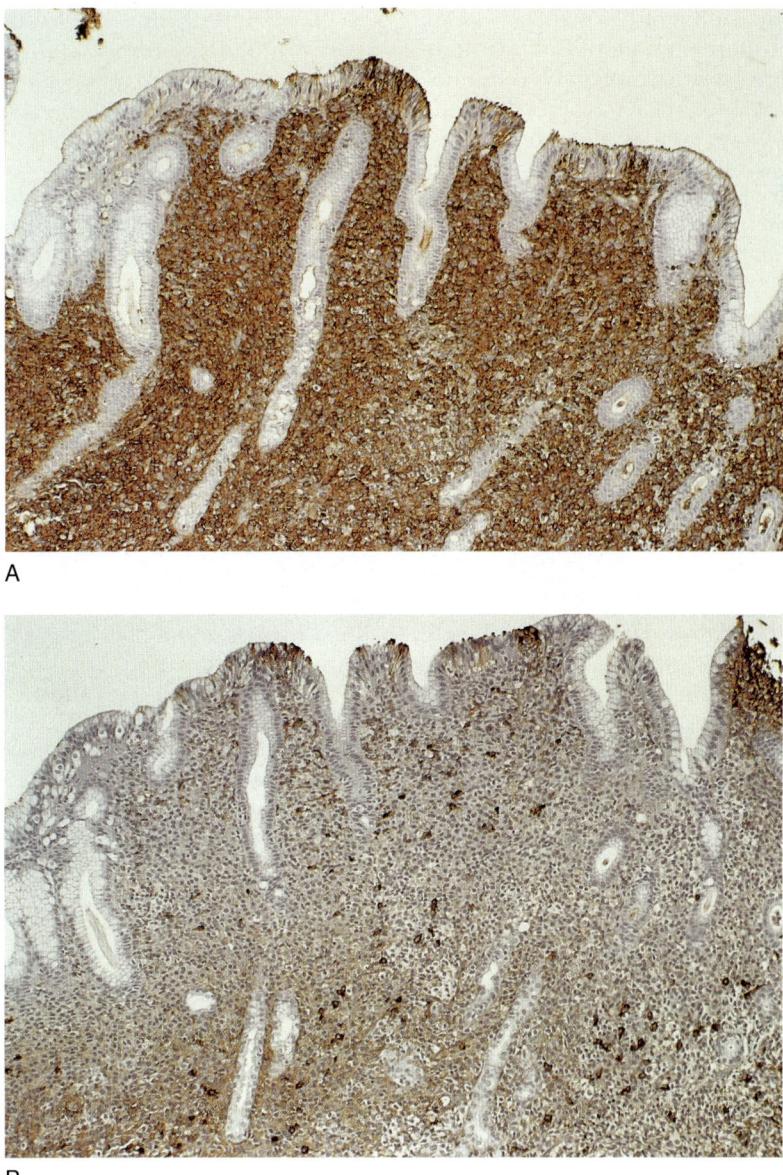

A

B

Figure 19–3. Mucosa-asociated lymphoid tissue lymphoma of the stomach. Immunohistochemical staining for immunoglobulin light chains (*A*, *κ*; *B*, *λ*) shows monoclonal restriction for *κ* light-chain Ig. Detection of monoclonality by either immunohistochemical or molecular methods is extremely helpful in definitively establishing a malignant diagnosis.

Molecular analyses have often been controversial. Most cases of MALT lymphoma have their immunoglobulin (Ig) genes rearranged. Sequencing studies have shown that the most common Ig genes used are for autoantibodies, further evidence suggesting that MALT lymphoma derives from autoreactive B-cell clones and that direct antigen stimulation plays an important role in the clonal expansion of low-grade MALT lymphoma (Du et al., 1996). However, occult oligoclonal and even monoclonal B-cell populations have often been identified through the use of more sensitive molecular methods (e.g., Southern blot, PCR) in morphologically equivalent or even reactive hyperplastic lesions (Nakamura et al., 1998). Identification of monoclones or oligoclones in these lesions has not proven to be a reliable predictor for either morphologic or immunophenotypic evidence of malignancy. Even more interestingly, the finding of clones does not necessarily correlate with clinical evidence of malignancy (Hsi et al., 1996a,b; Quintana et al., 1997). As a result, the concept that monoclonality is the defining characteristic of malignancy has lost validity, particularly with respect to the antigen-driven autoimmune-related MALT lymphomas.

Recent clinicopathological studies have shed light on the clinical behavior of MALT lymphomas. Unlike nodal low-grade B-cell lymphomas, which are usually widely disseminated at the time of diagnosis and are essentially incurable, MALT lymphomas are generally localized at presentation, with two-thirds of cases staged as IE or IIE (The Non-Hodgkin's Lymphoma Classification Project, 1997). The pattern of dissemination of MALT lymphomas is also unusual and distinct from the low-grade nodal lymphoma counterparts. In addition to spread to regional lymph nodes, MALT lymphomas have a propensity to involve other sites of MALT tissues, with sparing of the bone marrow (Burke, 1999; Isaacson, 1999b). Thus, nodal involvement by marginal zone B-cell lymphomas of the MALT type commonly represents spread from a primary extranodal MALT lymphoma (Fig. 19–4). The MALT lymphomas have a long, indolent clinical course; dissemination from the primary site may take decades (Banks and Isaacson, 1999).

Because of the indolent nature of autoimmune-associated MALT lymphomas, localized treatment is generally very effective. Surgical resection of localized disease is effective for superficial lesions. Low-dose radiation therapy has proven effective in localized MALT lymphoma (Schechter et al., 1998) and is particularly suited for sites where surgical excision is unwarranted, such as ocular tissues (Galieni et al., 1997). In cases where a specific antigen is known, such as *H. pylori* infection, eradication of the antigen through the use of appropriate antibiotics is warranted (Wotherspoon, 1998), with a resultant regression of the prelymphomatous infiltrate expected. Unfortunately, for other primary sites of MALT lymphoma disease, such as those associated with Sjögren's syndrome and Hashimoto's thyroiditis, the stimulating antigen can not be so easily eradicated. However, it should be remembered that the potential for very long–term relapse of disease is an important limitation when judging the overall success of managing the MALT lymphomas associated with autoimmunity.

Helicobacter Pylori Gastritis

Helicobacter pylori was first identified as a gastric pathogen in 1984 (Marshall and Warren, 1984). The prevalence of *H. pylori* infection, the foremost cause of peptic ulcer disease in the world, is about 30% in the United States (Covacci et al., 1999), and approaches 80% in developing nations (Fallone, 1999). *H. pylori* infection, particularly the CagA strain, is seen in virtually all cases of low-grade gastric MALT lymphomas (Witherell et al., 1997; Wotherspoon et al., 1991), predating the development of lymphoma by several years, with an odds ratio (OR) of 6.3 for the development of lymphoma (Parsonnet et al., 1994). Gastric lymphomas associated with *H. pylori* infection are the most common and extensively studied of the extranodal MALT lymphomas, thus serving as the model for antigen-associated MALT lymphomas as a whole (Isaacson, 1999a).

Low-grade gastric MALT lymphomas occur in adults in their fifth decade or older, with an equal sex predilection (Burke, 1999). An increasing number of cases are being reported in younger patients. Clinically, patients present with nonspecific symptoms of dyspepsia, showing clinical overlap with

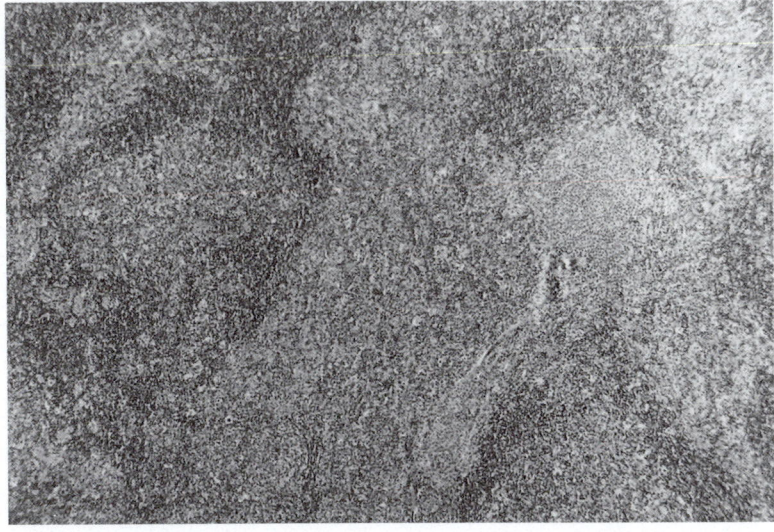

A

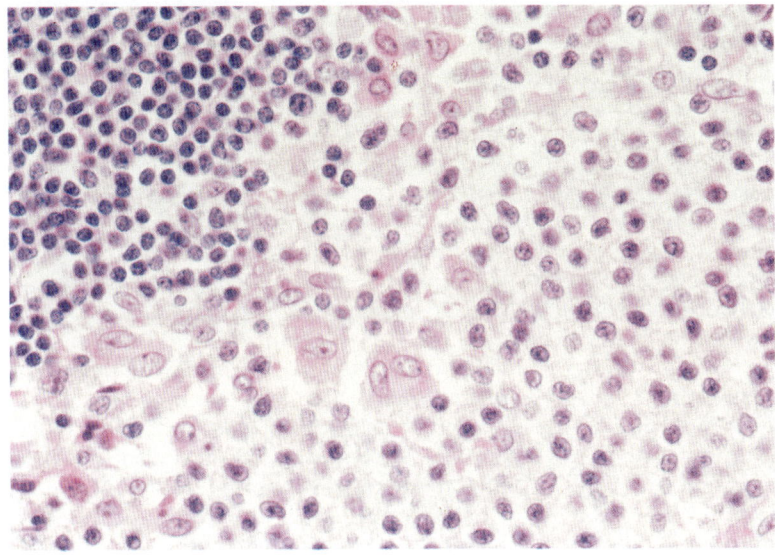

B

Figure 19–4. Nodal marginal zone B-cell lymphoma in a patient with Sjögren's syndrome. *A:* The nodal architecture is disrupted showing expansion of the interfollicular region and marginal zones surrounding lymphoid follicles. *B:* Large aggregates of mono-cytoid cells, with abundant pale cytoplasm, are seen within the sinuses. This lymphoma most likely represents dissemination from a primary extranodal MALT lymphoma of the parotid gland.

gastritis or peptic ulcer disease (Isaacson, 1999). Endoscopic examination usually shows inflamed mucosal gastric folds, with or without ulceration; a mass is usually not seen.

The histologic features, as the name implies, closely resemble those of normal MALT as seen in Peyer's patches. The lymphomatous infiltrate surrounds reactive germinal centers with a marginal zone-like pattern. The cells exhibit both monocytoid and plasmacytoid differentiation, imparting a rather polymorphous appearance to the in-filtrate. An important diagnostic feature is the presence of LEL (Fig. 19–2). Destructive LEL beyond areas of reactive germinal center formation is a helpful morphologic feature in favor of malignancy. However, the differential diagnosis between MALT lymphoma and a florid *H. pylori* gastritis can be extremely difficult, especially in small biopsy specimens. Detection of B-cell monoclonality by either immunohistochemical or molecular means becomes extremely important in definitively establishing a malignant process.

The immunophenotypic features of gastric MALT lymphomas are similar to those seen in MALT lymphomas involving other sites. Most importantly, the B-cell infiltrate of gastric MALT lymphoma shows monoclonal surface immunoglobulin expression, as detected by light-chain restriction (Fig. 19–3). Immunoglobulin heavy-chain (IgH) gene rearrangements are detected in most cases by sensitive molecular techniques, e.g., Southern blot and/or PCR. However, caution is required in interpreting molecular studies, since occult clonal IgH gene rearrangements have been described in *H. pylori*–associated chronic gastritis (Hsi et al., 1996). Continuous antigen stimulation by *H. pylori* of the prelymphomatous gastritis clones leads to progression to MALT lymphoma (Du et al., 1996), with the same clone being involved in extragastric dissemination (Diss et al., 1993).

Clinical behavior of low-grade gastric MALT lymphomas associated with *H. pylori* infection is generally indolent and slow to progress and disseminate; usually it is stage IE or IIE at the time of diagnosis (Isaacson, 1999a). Twenty percent of gastric MALT lymphomas have extragastric spread, usually to regional lymph nodes, spleen, or, less likely, to bone marrow (10%) (Isaacson, 1999b). A striking regression of MALT lymphomas has been shown in 75% of cases through eradication of *H. pylori* infection by appropriate antibiotic therapy (Wotherspoon, 1998). Thus, although gastric MALT lymphomas respond well to conventional therapeutic regimens, including surgery, radiation, and chemotherapy, it is recommended that anti–*H. pylori* therapy be considered first in cases of early low-grade MALT lymphoma. Overall prognosis is excellent; patients with stage IE disease have a 5-year survival rate of >90% (Burke, 1999). Cases that do not respond to antibiotic therapy may have more invasive, higher-grade transformation to large cell lymphoma, and require more aggressive therapeutic approaches.

Sjögren's Syndrome/ Rheumatoid Arthritis

Sjögren's syndrome (SS) and rheumatoid arthritis (RA) are closely related autoimmune diseases characterized by the production of autoantibodies (rheumatoid factor, anti-nuclear antibodies, etc.). Clinically, SS presents with xerostomia and xeropthalmia and may be primary, affecting predominantly middle-aged females, or occur secondarily in association with other autoimmune diseases, most commonly RA, which is a chronic polyarthritis of unknown cause, also affecting middle-aged females (male to female ratio 1:3), usually of insidious onset. Although both of these autoimmune diseases have been associated with an increased risk of B-cell LPD (Kassan et al., 1979; Prior, 1985), the LPDs arising in the setting of RA are further complicated by their close association with immunosuppressive therapy, namely methotrexate, and Epstein-Barr virus (EBV) (Georgescu et al., 1997; Kamel et al., 1995; see section on iatrogenic-induced LPDs for full discussion).

The occurrence of B-cell LPD is one of the major complications of SS, with the risk of developing lymphoma in approximately 6 cases/1000 patients per year (44 times greater than in the normal population) (Kassan et al., 1979). The vast majority of the lymphomas associated with SS are extranodal marginal zone B-cell lymphomas, or MALT lymphomas, which almost invariably arise in the setting of lymphoepithelial sialadenitis (Harris, 1999; Hyjek et al., 1988). The MALT lymphoma may arise in any of the major or minor salivary glands, but the parotid gland is the preferred site.

Clinically, lymphoma should be suspected when patients with SS present with persistent diffuse, bilateral enlargement of the salivary glands. Lymphadenopathy and/or the presence of lung nodules should also raise suspicion of a developing LPD (Mariette, 1999). Lymphoma is more often observed in patients with systemic SS and may appear after several years of an apparently benign, stable course. Predisposing factors to the development of malignant lymphoma in SS include parotidomegaly, splenomegaly, lymphadenopathy, lung nodules, low-dose irradiation, cytotoxic therapy, presence of serum/urinary monoclonal gammopathy, and presence of mixed cryoglobulins (Tzioufas, 1996).

The histopathological lesion occurring in the salivary gland in patients with SS is lymphoepithelial sialadenitis (LESA), known formerly as myoepithelial sialadenitis (MESA) and benign lymphoepithelial lesion (BLEL). Virtually all patients with SS have LESA, and patients with other connective tissue diseases, such as RA, may also develop the lesion (Harris, 1999). The histologic features of LESA, which are remarkably similar to those of MALT lymphomas, are lymphoplasmacytic infiltrates associated with follicular hyperplasia, surrounding and infiltrating salivary acini and ducts, forming lymphoepithelial lesions. The lymphoepithelial lesions may contain prominent aggregates of monocytoid B cells. There is usually both plasmacytoid and monocytoid differentiation of the B cells, giving the infiltrate a polymorphous appearance. Since almost all MALT lymphomas associated with SS arise in a background of LESA, a straightforward diagnosis of malignancy based solely on morphologic criteria may be problematic.

One of the more important morphological features in distinguishing LESA from MALT lymphoma is the number and distribution of the monocytoid B cells (Table 19–3). When monocytoid B cells are seen outside the lymphoepithelial lesions, a diagnosis of MALT lymphoma should be considered (Harris, 1999). Additionally, the presence of increased numbers and/or sheets of plasma cells, particularly if Dutcher bodies can be identified, is also a worrisome feature for indicating MALT lymphoma. In cases of partial involvement of the salivary gland, the distinction between benign LESA and MALT lymphoma based on morphology may be extremely difficult to impossible and requires immunohistochemical analysis, the findings of which are identical to that seen in other MALT lymphomas of different sites. Monoclonality of the lymphoid infiltrate, as detected by immunohistochemical staining for light chains, is an extremely helpful diagnostic feature indicating malignancy.

Molecular criteria for distinguishing benign LESA from low-grade MALT in salivary glands and the significance of genotypically documented clonality in this setting are somewhat controversial. Detection of monoclonal Ig gene rearrangements by molecular analyses have been seen in a high proportion of benign LESA lesions (Hsi et al., 1996b; Quintana et al., 1997), which suggests that most LESA lesions harbor monoclonal or oligoclonal B-cell populations. Interestingly, the occult clonality does not predict progression to clinically overt lymphoma. Thus, acquired salivary gland MALT tissue in the form of LESA may progress to a process that is clonal, but not necessarily malignant. Despite the finding of mono-

clonality, most lymphomas in the salivary gland remain localized for prolonged periods of time and are relatively indolent. When clinically overt lymphoma develops, it usually presents in extrasalivary sites, including regional cervical lymph nodes, lung, stomach, and skin, with the same Ig gene rearrangement and light-chain restriction as the primary salivary lesion (Fig. 19–4).

Treatment and prognosis depend on the type and stage of lymphoma. However, the patient should be completely evaluated for the extent of disease, and if it is localized, surgical resection may be curative for stage I or stage II. If not totally resected, radiation therapy should be considered (Anaya et al., 1996). The 5-year survival rate is >50% for low-grade malignancies. Low-grade MALT lymphomas can progress to a more aggressive grade, and these as well as more clinically aggressive tumors should receive combined modality treatments.

Hashimoto's Thyroiditis

Hashimoto's thyroiditis (HT), or chronic lymphocytic thyroiditis, is an autoimmune disease of adult middle age (fourth–fifth decade), with a striking female predilection. This disease is characterized by the production of autoantibodies against thyroglobulin and/or thyrotropin receptors that alter thyroid function. Malignant lymphoma is the most common malignant complication of HT, with a relative risk of 67 (Holm et al., 1985), and virtually all lymphomas of the thyroid are preceded by HT (Isaacson, 1999b). Most lymphomas of the thyroid gland are of large B-cell type; however; those cases of large cell lymphoma in patients with HT most likely represent histologic progression from a persistent or underlying low-grade MALT lymphoma (Hyjek and Isaacson, 1988).

Clinically, the presentation of lymphoma involving the thyroid is essentially the same as in HT. There is a strong female predominance (male-to-female ratio is 1:4), although the median age at the time of diagnosis of lymphoma is 70, indicating that it may take as long as 20–30 years for lymphoma to develop from HT (Pedersen and Pedersen, 1996). Hypothyroidism and/or goiter is common. Symptoms are related to thyroid enlargement or mass effect, including hoarseness, stridor/dyspnea, and dysphagia (Burke, 1999).

Histologically, the main differential diagnosis includes low-grade MALT lymphoma and chronic lymphocytic thyroiditis. The distinction between the two can be extremely difficult, especially in advanced cases of HT or when the MALT lymphoma arises in a background of HT. Morphologically, MALT lymphomas of the thyroid simulate the features of MALT lymphomas in other sites. There is effacement of the thyroid architecture by dense lymphoplasmacytic infiltrates surrounding residual reactive-appearing germinal centers, which may be prominent. The residual thyroid follicular cells usually show extensive Hürthle cell changes. Lymphoepithelial lesions associated with aggregates of monocytoid B cells are also a common feature, but are not pathognomonic for malignancy. All of these morphologic features can be seen to varying degrees with chronic lymphocytic thyroiditis, as there is a histologic continuum between the HT and MALT lymphoma. Thus, to differentiate between low-grade MALT lymphoma of the thyroid and a marked chronic lymphocytic thyroiditis, immunophenotypic studies are required to demonstrate monoclonality, thereby confirming a diagnosis of malignancy.

Immunophenotypically, light-chain restriction by the infiltrating plasma cells is characteristic of low-grade MALT lymphomas of the thyroid (Hyjek and Isaacson, 1988). Additional immunohistochemical studies for B and T cell marking show similar features as other MALT lymphomas. Immunoglubulin heavy-chain gene rearrangement as detected through molecular methods is a consistent feature. Interestingly, the frequency of occult monoclonal IgH rearrangements found in benign HT is low compared to other autoimmune associated prelymphomatous lesions, such as LESA associated with Sjögren's syndrome or *H. pylori* gastritis. Several studies have failed to demonstrate occult monoclonality in cases of HT, whereas Ig gene rearrangements were detected only in patients with histologic evidence of lymphoma (Hsi et al., 1998; Katzin et al., 1989). This phenomenon may be due in part to the infrequent finding of low-grade MALT lymphomas and/or the long period between the diagnosis of HT and subsequent development of lymphoma.

The development of low-grade MALT lymphoma in the setting of HT is generally slow,

with an indolent clinical course, and clinically low stage at presentation (>75% of patients were stage IE or IIE) (Burke, 1999). Combined modality therapy with or without chemotherapy is the preferred treatment. Patients with low-stage disease treated with surgery and radiation have an 83% survival at 3 years. However, the overall 5-year survival in patients with lymphoma of thyroid is less than 50%, perhaps because of the preponderance of cases showing a more aggressive histologic grade. The following factors have been associated with a poor prognosis: stage III–IV disease, elevated S-urate, hoarseness, and age >66 years (Pedersen and Pedersen, 1996). Close to one-third of patients will have distant relapse, which may take decades to develop.

Immunoproliferative Small Intestinal Disease

The first descriptions of immunoproliferative small intestinal disease (IPSID) come from the mid-1960s, when several reports first described an association between a dietary nutrient malabsorption syndrome and primary intestinal lymphoma (Eidelman et al., 1966; Ramot et al., 1965). The disease, which ultimately came to be known as Mediterranean lymphoma, was clinicopathologically similar to a syndrome characterized by the serum secretion of a partial immunoglobulin heavy chain of the immunoglobulin A (IgA) class, α-heavy-chain disease (Seligmann et al., 1968). However, the processes were considered distinct entities until it was noted that some patients with histologically benign α-heavy-chain disease progressed to small intestinal lymphoma (Rappaport et al., 1972), after which the entities were considered different ends of the spectrum of a single disease process (Meeting of the World Health Organization, 1976), currently classified as IPSID (Martin and Aldoori, 1994).

Immunoproliferative small intestinal disease is a distinct clinicopathological entity that occurs predominantly in younger adults in their second or third decade of life, with equal sex predilection. Most patients are of lower socioeconomic background, live in areas of poor sanitation/hygiene, and are from the Mediterranean basin, including North Africa, Israel, Iran, and Greece (Fine and Stone, 1999). Patients present with a months-to-years duration of a severe malabsorption syndrome, weight loss, and abdominal pain. Clubbing, peripheral edema, and abdominal mass are common findings on physical exam. Endoscopic examination of the small bowel shows diffuse dilation of the duodenum, jejunum, and ileum, with thickened mucosal folds, nodules, and/or ulcers (Halphen et al., 1986). Parasitosis, particularly *Giardia lamblia*, and intestinal bacterial overgrowth are common in these patients.

The pathogenesis of IPSID is thought to be of an origin similar to that of other antigen-derived LPDs, such as *H. pylori*–associated gastric MALT lymphoma. Chronic antigenic stimulation of the intestinal IgA secretory immune system by intestinal microorganisms leads to hyperplasia of lymphoid tissue, with the eventual emergence and expansion of several plasma cell clones. Over time, a structural mutation occurs in a specific clone, resulting in an internal deletion of the V_H and C_H1 regions of the α_1-heavy chain, and an inability to synthesize light chains, resulting in the secretion of α-paraprotein devoid of light chains, rather than intact IgA protein (Seligmann, 1977). The α-heavy-chain protein is secreted by the plasma cells in large amounts into serum, urine, saliva, and intestinal secretions.

The histologic features of IPSID are similar to those of low-grade MALT lymphomas seen in other sites, except that plasma cell differentiation is much more marked, in both the intestinal lamina propria and the draining mesenteric lymph nodes (Isaacson, 1999a). The lymphoplasmacytic infiltrate begins in the lamina propria, and as the disease progresses, extends to full thickness of the bowel wall. Other features of MALT lymphoma, including reactive-appearing germinal centers and aggregates of monocytoid B cells, can be seen. However, lymphoepithelial lesions are not a prominent feature of IPSID. In fact, the epithelium is usually intact, although villous atrophy is a very common finding. Ulceration of the mucosa is a worrisome feature for malignant transformation (Cammoun et al., 1989). Immunohistochemically, the plasma cells are positive for CD79a or MB-1, negative for CD20, and show both surface and cytoplasmic staining for α-heavy chain (Fig. 19–5). As with other autoimmune-related LPDs, occult monoclonal IgH gene rearrangements have been detected in histologically benign-appearing lesions (Smith et al., 1987).

Immunoproliferative small intestinal disease is associated with a relatively poor prognosis because of its advanced stage at the time of diagnosis and its propensity for progression to a higher grade lesion (Fig. 19–6). Because of intestinal bacterial overgrowth, the recommended treatment of early IPSID, low-stage IE or IIE, includes broad-spectrum antimicrobial therapy, which has success in completely eradicating the lesions (Ben-Ayed et al., 1989). This suggests a common pathogenesis with *H. pylori*–associated gastric MALT lymphoma, although no specific organism has yet been implicated in IPSID. In nonresponsive cases or advanced cases with bulky disease, total abdominal radiation combined with non-Hodgkin's lymphoma regimen chemotherapy has a remission rate of 64%, with a 5-year survival rate of about 67% (Fine and Stone, 1999).

FOLLICULAR LYMPHOMA IN SITU

Follicular lymphomas (FL) are common B-cell lymphomas that account for as much as 40% of adult non-Hodgkin's lymphomas in the United States; the incidence is lower elsewhere (Lennert and Feller, 1992). These tumors have distinctive clinicopathologic features, and despite variations in the histologic subtype or grade, they may be regarded as a homogeneous group of lymphomas derived from follicular center cells. Follicular lymphoma is neoplastic and clonal in nature, with a proven cytogenetic abnormality in 70%–95% of cases that involves the translocation of the *bcl*-2 gene on chromosome 18q21 into the IgH joining region on 14q32 (Tsujimoto et al., 1985a; Yunis et al., 1982). The translocation occurs at an early stage of development, during Ig gene rearrangement (Tsujimoto et al., 1985b), and interestingly, occasional cells with rearranged *bcl*-2 genes can be detected in normal lymphoid tissues in normal individuals (Dolken et al., 1996; Limpens et al., 1991). As increasingly more sensitive methods have emerged over the last decade, e.g., PCR for *bcl*-2 gene translocation, the diagnosis of FL is being made earlier in the disease course. Rare cases of *in situ* FL have been diagnosed showing involvement of single or scattered follicles within an otherwise normal lymph node.

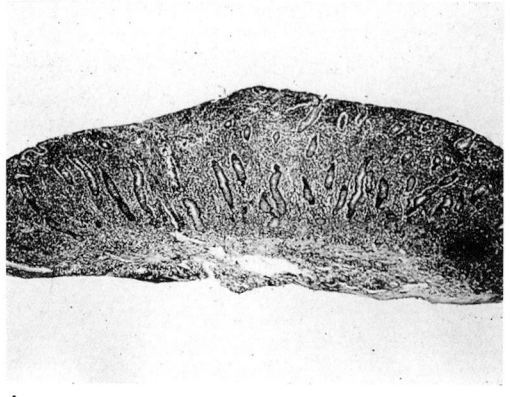

A

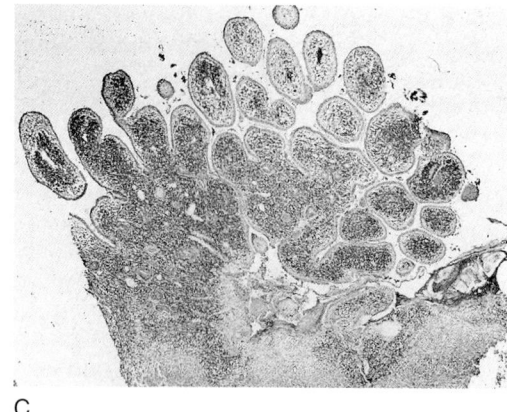

C

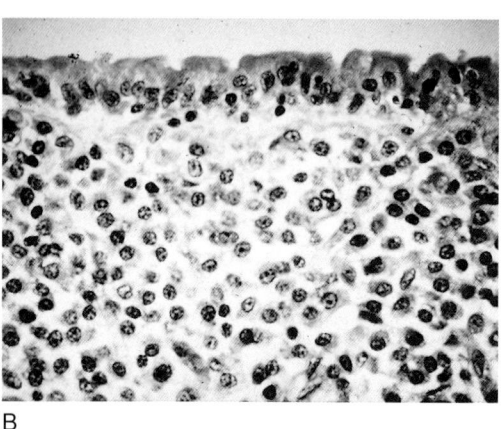

B

Figure 19–5. Immunoproliferative small intestinal disease. *A:* The small bowel shows marked villous atrophy. *B:* The lamina propria shows infiltration by normal-appearing, mature plasma cells. *C:* Virtually all of the plasma cells demonstrate strong reactivity when stained for α heavy chain.

Follicular lymphoma can be considered a form of *in situ* lymphoma in that morphologically, the cells of FL resemble cells of normal lymphoid follicles, and cytologic cri-

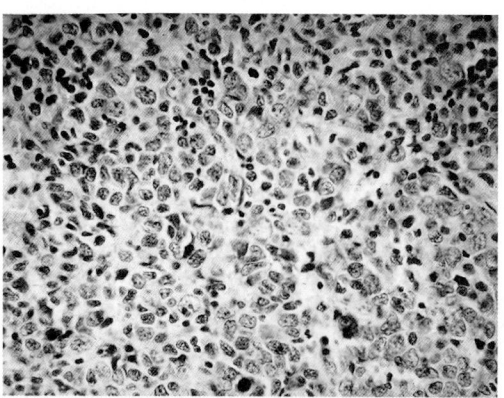

Figure 19–6. Large B-cell lymphoma of a mesenteric lymph node in a patient with immunoproliferative small intestinal disease. The malignant lymphoid cells were shown to contain α heavy chains by immunohistochemical staining.

teria are usually not helpful in distinguishing individual normal lymphocytes from neoplastic follicular B-lymphocytes (Fig. 19–7). Additionally, the FL cells home to B cell–dependent areas throughout the lymphoid system, both in the cortical zone of lymph nodes and in B cell–dependent malpighian corpuscles of the spleen. Thus the disease affects areas normally populated by follicular B cells. The differential diagnosis includes atypical follicular hyperplasias, which are not uncommon and in many cases may be extremely difficult to distinguish from FL. The diagnosis becomes even more problematic in cases of partial nodal involvement of FL, in which only scattered neoplastic follicles may lie hidden among otherwise reactive-appearing hyperplastic germinal centers. Immunophenotypic and/or genotypic studies are thus critical in demonstrating either monoclonality or *bcl*-2 expression or rearrangement, thereby distinguishing FL from atypical follicular proliferations.

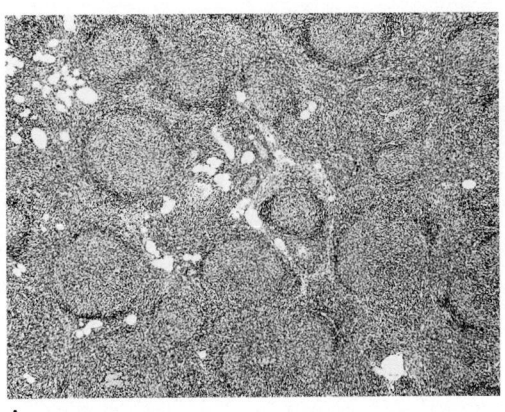
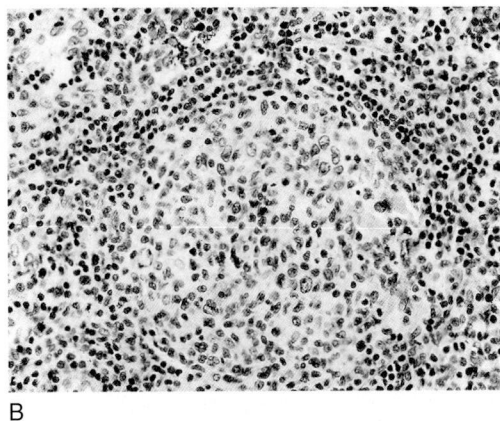

A   B

Figure 19–7. Follicular lymphoma. *A:* Follicular proliferation extends throughout the lymph node effacing the normal nodal architecture. The follicles are generally uniform in size and shape with little intervening normal lymphoid parenchyma. Mantle cuffs may be present but are ill defined. *B:* The cytologic composition of follicular lymphoma mimics the cytologic composition of the normal germinal center. A mixture of cleaved and noncleaved cells is seen.

Immunophenotypically, the malignant cells express B cell–associated antigens CD20, CD19, and CD22; they lack coexpression of CD43 and CD5. The FL cells show monoclonal Ig surface staining and are generally positive for CD10 and Bcl-6. Bcl-2 protein expression is useful in distinguishing reactive from neoplastic follicles and is present in most FL. Staining for IgD is also helpful in that primary follicles, which may have a somewhat monotonous cytologic appearance and show expression of bcl-2 protein, are IgD positive; whereas neoplastic FL follicles are IgD negative.

Circulating t(14;18)-positive cells can persist in a high percentage of FL patients with long-term, complete remission after radiation treatment for stage I and II disease (Finke et al., 1993; Stetler-Stevenson et al., 1988), and over two-thirds of patients tested have had occult clonal lymphoid cells in the bone marrow by PCR, without morphologic evidence of involvement by lymphoma (Berinstein et al., 1993). However, *bcl*-2 gene rearrangements have also been identified in tonsillar and circulating lymphoid cells in normal individuals (Dolken et al., 1996; Limpens et al., 1991).

Despite an indolent clinical course, FL remains largely incurable. Because of the long natural history of FL, a watch-and-wait therapy has apparently not led to reduced survival in asymptomatic patients with advanced-stage disease (stage III or IV). Also, 40%–50% of patients with stage I and II FL show clinical complete remission with local radiation therapy, although relapse occurs in approximately 15% (Mac Manus and Hoppe, 1997). At present it is not known whether detection of occult disease at the time of initial diagnosis or after treatment will be of clinical or prognostic significance.

MONOCLONAL GAMMOPATHY OF UNDETERMINED SIGNIFICANCE/ SOLITARY PLASMACYTOMAS

Benign monoclonal gammopathy, or monoclonal gammopathy of undetermined significance (MGUS), occurs in 1% of the general population. The incidence of small monoclonal serum protein (M protein) spikes increases with age, and 3% of individuals over the age of 70 years will be found to have monoclonal serum protein spikes (Kyle, 1997). A spike of less than 2 g/dl in the absence of lytic bone lesions, anemia, hypercalcemia, more than 10% plasma cells in bone marrow, urinary light chains, or other abnormalities is usually indicative of absence of malignant disease at presentation (Kyle, 1997; Moller-Petersen and Schmidt, 1986). Benign monoclonal gammopathy represents a premyeloma stage that may persist for decades without malignant evolution. Approximately 25% of patients will develop multiple myeloma or another immunoproliferative disorder such as lymphoplasmacytic lymphoma or systemic amyloidosis, usually over a prolonged period of stability (median 10 years) after initial diagnosis (Kyle, 1993). Cytogenetic analyses have shown gains in chromosome 3 and 11 in over 50% of MGUS cases, indicating that MGUS already has the chromosomal characteristics of a plasma cell malignancy (Drach et al., 1995). However, MGUS has a low risk of evolution to malignant LPD when the M-protein value is less than 1.5 g/dl, bone marrow plasma cells are less than 5%, and there are no detectable urinary light chains (Baldini et al., 1996). The development of malignant progression can be abrupt but is usually heralded by clinical symptoms, such as skeletal pain, fever, night sweats, or bruising. Thus, continued clinical follow-up is essential, with reevaluation for possible myeloma or lymphoma if untoward symptoms develop (Kyle, 1997).

Solitary plasmacytomas are rare and may present in bone or soft tissue. The diagnosis is one of exclusion, in that skeletal roentgenograms must show no evidence of lytic lesions, bone marrow biopsy/aspirate must show no evidence of myeloma, and there is no evidence of M protein in the serum or urine (Holland et al., 1992). Like MGUS, plasmacytomas have a propensity to progress into frankly malignant multiple myeloma (MM), generally over a prolonged period of time. Histologically, the tumor consists of sheets of immature or mature plasma cells. Immunophenotypically, the cells express monoclonal immunoglobulin and usually lack pan-B-cell antigens CD19 and CD20. Expression of CD79a and epithelial membrane antigen (EMA) may be positive. Immunoglobulin heavy- and light-chain genes are usually rearranged.

Solitary plasmacytoma of bone is uncommon and occurs in only 3%–5% of patients with plasma cell neoplasms. The disease usually presents with bone pain and is more common in males, with a median age of about 10 years younger than for MM (Kyle, 1997). The axial skeleton is more commonly involved than the appendicular skeleton, with the thoracic vertebrae being the most common site (Frassica et al., 1989). Overt MM develops in 50% of patients with solitary plasmacytoma of bone, usually within 3 years (Holland et al., 1992). Older age, axial lesions, size of lesion, and persistence of M protein following radiation have been shown to be bad prognostic indicators (Bataille and Sany, 1981; Holland et al., 1992). Radiation therapy is effective, and there is no evidence that adjuvant or prophylactic chemotherapy prevents the development of MM. The overall 5-year survival rate is 40%–75% (Kyle, 1997).

Extramedullary solitary plasmacytomas (EMP) are also quite rare, affecting males more than females (ratio 3:1), with a median age of 50–70 years. The EMPs have a predilection for involving head and neck sites, perhaps because of the presence of more abundant lymphoid tissues (Hotz et al., 1999). The tumors are restricted to soft tissues, usually arising in the submucosal tissues of the nasopharynx, sinuses, or oral cavity. Clinically, patient complaints are related to the site of involvement and include hoarseness, epistaxis, and dysphagia (Sulzner et al., 1998). Morphologically, the tumor cells are indistinguishable from those seen in MM or solitary plasmacytomas of bone. Surgical excision may be therapeutic, particularly in easily accessible areas (Meis et al., 1987). While these tumors may present as aggressive locally destructive lesions, their management should be as organ sparing as possible because excellent control can be achieved in most cases (Wax et al., 1993). Radiation is preferred for surgically inaccessible sites. Local recurrences are not uncommon, and although progression to MM is less frequent than in solitary plasmacytoma of bone (20%–50%), it has been reported to develop up to 30 years after the initial diagnosis (Sulzner et al., 1998).

LYMPHOTROPIC VIRUS–ASSOCIATED LYMPHOPROLIFERATIONS

The fraction of human malignancies resulting directly from viral infection are estimated to range from 10%–20% (de The, 1995). While most of these virus-associated cancers are nonhematopoietic, such as hepatitis B/C–associated hepatocellular carcinomas and human papillomavirus (HPV)–associated cervical carcinoma, considerable evidence has accumulated in favor of involvement of viral agents in the pathogenesis of human LPDs (Luppi and Torelli,

1996). Indeed, the pathogenetic importance in the development of specific LPDs of two lymphotropic viruses, Epstein-Barr virus (EBV) and human T-cell lymphotropic virus-I (HTLV-I), has been emphasized by their inclusion in the Revised European-American Lymphoma (REAL) classification scheme (Harris et al., 1994) and the recently proposed World Health Organization (WHO) lymphoma classification (Jaffe et al., 1999). Thus, infection by these viruses may be considered the primary incipient preneoplastic event, only after which malignant transformation can occur.

The association of EBV in the pathogenesis of specific malignancies, particularly Burkitt's lymphoma and undifferentiated nasopharyngeal carcinoma, is well known. Recent evidence based mainly on the detection of EBV DNA/RNA viral sequences has shown pathogenetic associations with a wider spectrum of both pre- and outright malignant LPDs, including lymphomatoid granulomatosis (LG), B-cell LPDs in both acquired and congenital immunocompromised patients, Hodgkin's disease, and various T-cell lymphomas (Niedobitek, 1996; Niedobitek et al., 1997).

The pathogenetic role of EBV in human hematological malignancies is extremely complex and beyond the scope of this discussion, except where it is directly related to the specific entities discussed below. However, there are several areas of practical concern to the surgical pathologist that bear emphasis. The EBV is a ubiquitous virus infecting more than 90% of the human population worldwide (Niedobitek et al., 1997). Primary infection occurs predominantly in early childhood and is commonly asymptomatic; however, if EBV infection is delayed until adulthood, the clinical syndrome of infectious mononucleosis may follow. It is well established that EBV can immortalize B lymphocytes and that following primary infection most individuals carry EBV-infected B cells that can undergo proliferation under appropriate circumstances. Moreover, an intact T-cell surveillance is essential in eradicating EBV-infected B cells (Niedobitek et al., 1997). In an immunocompromised individual, this T-cell response may be lacking, which may result in the uncontrolled proliferation of EBV-infected B cells and subsequent progression to malignant lymphoma.

In addition to EBV, through serological and molecular studies, HTLV-I has been established as the major etiological factor in the development of adult T-cell leukemia/lymphoma (ATLL) (Franchini, 1995). Infection with HTLV-1 is most common in endemic areas, including Japan, Okinawa, the Caribbean basin, and the southeastern United States, where an estimated 10–20 million people are infected (Franchini, 1995). The seroprevalence of HTLV-1 is highest in Japan, with approximately 15% of normal individuals having HTLV-1 antibodies, and the cumulative lifetime risk of developing ATLL in Japan is estimated at 2.5% (Takatsuki, 1997). The pattern of HTLV-1 transmission is predominantly through ingestion of infected breast milk (Hino, 1989), and it is thought that carriers who have acquired their infection early in life are at greatest risk of developing ATLL (Hisada et al., 1998). Sexual intercourse (Murphy et al., 1989) and/or blood transfusions (Osame et al., 1990) are also major routes of infection transmission. For a full discussion of ATLL see the section T-cell Lymphoepithelial Disorders (below).

The last decade of research has identified two additional viral agents with possible pathogenetic relationships to LPDs—human herpesvirus-8 (HHV-8) and hepatitis C virus (HCV). In contrast to the other human herpesviruses, very little is known about the primary infection of HHV-8, although according to seroprevalency studies, the primary mode of transmission appears to be sexual transmission. The seroprevalence of HHV-8 is highest in Africa, with approximately 40% of the general population positive; the United States ranges from 5% to 20%, and the Caribbean basin ranges from 2% to 4% (Chatlynne and Ablashi, 1999). HHV-8 is lymphotropic for B cells and is found in circulating peripheral blood B-lymphocytes of patients with Kaposi's sarcoma (KS) (Mesri et al., 1996). HHV-8 has a well-known and close association with KS, primary effusion lymphoma (PEL), and multicentric Castleman's disease (MCD) (Cesarman and Knowles, 1997), as well as a possible indirect pathogenetic role in MM (Said et al., 1997). The seroprevalency rates of HHV-8 in patients with the acquired immunodeficiency syndrome (AIDS), KS, or MCD are greater than 90% (Chatlynne and Ablashi,

1999). Although the mechanism that leads to malignant transformation of B cells by HHV-8 remains unclear, expression of HHV-8 oncogene and cytokine homologues, including bcl-2 and interleukin-6 (IL-6), respectively, may contribute directly to the pathogenesis of LPDs (Teruya-Feldstein et al., 1998). Monoclonality has been reported in MCD (Hanson et al., 1988; Soulier et al., 1995), and MCD can progress to PEL. Thus, MCD can be considered an incipient neoplasm. Even HHV-8-negative unicentric Castleman's disease can contain monoclonal plasma cells, although progression to lymphoma or multiple myeloma has not been observed (Chilosi et al., 1987; Dworak et al., 1988; Radaszkiewicz et al., 1989).

The HCV, a small, single-stranded, positive-sense RNA virus, is the causative agent of the chronic liver disease non-A, non-B hepatitis (Alter et al., 1989). Infection of the virus is predominantly through parenteral routes, including transfusions and organ transplantation, with approximately 2% of the general population serologically positive for HCV (Bellentani et al., 1999). In addition to its hepatotropic role as a major risk factor for the development of hepatocellular carcinoma in patients with cirrhosis, HCV has been shown to have lymphotropic properties; viral genomic sequences have been found in both T-cell (Shimizu et al., 1992) and B-cell (Ferri et al., 1993) lymphocytes. A striking association between HCV infection and essential mixed cryoglobulinemia (EMC) has been shown, with the vast majority of EMC patients being serologically positive for HCV (Luppi and Torelli, 1996). Similarly, HCV has been associated with certain types of low-grade B-cell lymphomas in patients with EMC, including lymphoplasmacytic lymphoma (LPL), and in noncryoglobulinemic patients with extranodal marginal zone B-cell lymphomas (Lai and Weiss, 1998). Thus, chronic HCV infection seems to play an important pathogenetic role in the clonal B-cell expansion underlying the systemic manifestations of EMC.

Lymphomatoid Granulomatosis

Since its description nearly 30 years ago (Liebow et al., 1972), lymphomatoid granulomatosis (LG), formerly thought to be part of the spectrum of angioimmunoproliferative lesions (AIL) (Jaffe et al., 1989), had been somewhat of an enigma. Lymphomatoid granulomatosis was originally thought to represent a T-cell lymphoproliferative process similar to the nasal-type natural killer (NK)/T–cell lymphoma, or angiocentric lymphoma. Lymphatoid granulomatosis is now known to be a lymphoproliferative B-cell process associated with EBV and an exuberant T-cell reaction, with a wide variation in its clinical course. (Jaffe and Wilson, 1997).

Lymphatoid granulomatosis affects patients of all ages, although most cases occur between the fourth and sixth decades of life. There is a slight male predilection, with a sex ratio of 2.5:1 (Katzenstein et al., 1979). The lung is the most frequently involved organ, and most patients will have pulmonary involvement at some point in the disease. Cough, dyspnea, and chest pain are the most common initial complaints. Multiple organ sites are commonly involved during the course of the disease; skin rashes and neurologic symptoms are seen in up to 20%–50% of cases (Katzenstein et al., 1979; Liebow et al., 1972). Systemic manifestations include fever, malaise, and weight loss. Peripheral blood abnormalities, if present, are generally nonspecific.

Lymphatoid granulomatosis produces nodular mass lesions in most affected organs, namely lung, kidney, liver, and brain (Liebow et al., 1972). Additional sites of involvement include the upper respiratory tract, skin, and gastrointestinal tract, with a striking sparing of lymphoid tissues. Histologically, the lesions have a polymorphous cellular composition, which in addition to the predominant lymphocytes, include plasma cells, immunoblasts, and scattered histiocytes. Neutrophils and eosinophils as well as well-formed granulomas are generally absent. The larger B cells show cytologic atypia, which may be marked with pleomorphic nuclei and prominent nucleoli, resulting in a Reed-Sternberg-like appearance. Occasionally these cells may be multinucleated, further mimicking Hodgkin's disease (Koss et al., 1986). The lymphoid infiltrate, particularly in pulmonary lesions, will show an angiocentric and angiodestructive pattern (Fig. 19–8). Larger lesions and lesions of higher histologic grade usually have prominent parenchymal necrosis (Lipford et al., 1988), which in contrast to Wegener's

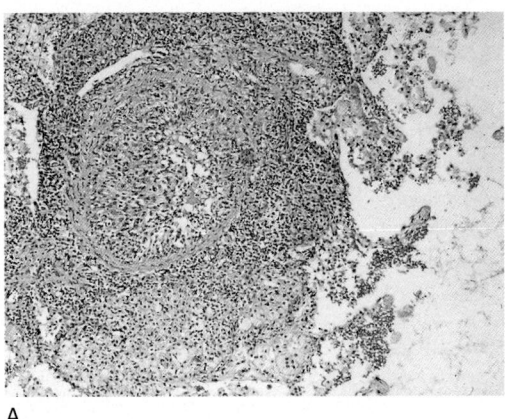
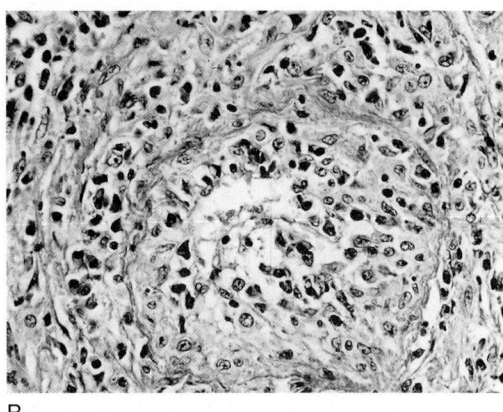

A   B

Figure 19–8. Lymphomatoid granulomatosis of the lung. *A:* The characteristic pulmonary lesion shows a striking angiocentric and angiodestructive lymphoid infiltrate. *B:* The grade I lesions have a polymorphous cellular composition of lymphocytes, plasma cells, immunoblasts, and scattered histiocytes. Lymphocytes may show minimal cytologic atypia.

granulomatosis (WG), is of a coagulative nature and lacks neutrophils and abundant nuclear debris.

Within the lesions, most of the infiltrating lymphocytes are small, reactive CD3-positive T cells, presumably recruited in response to the EBV infection. The B cells represent the minority of the lymphoid cells. The atypical cells are CD20 positive and may be CD30 positive; expression of CD15 is usually negative. Infection with EBV is restricted to the large, atypical B cells and is best seen by *in situ* hybridization, since EBV-latent membrane protein (LMP) expression is variable. The histologic grade of LG is based predominantly on the number of EBV-positive cells in the lesions (Guinee et al., 1994). Low-grade, or grade I, lesions will have infrequent scattered EBV-positive cells with a concentration around vessel walls. In higher-grade II or III lesions, the EBV-positive B cells are more numerous and may sheet out. Grade III lesions may histologically resemble large cell lymphoma (Fig. 19–9). Molecular studies have shown the EBV-infected B cells may be monoclonal, oligoclonal, or even polyclonal for IgH gene rearrangements (Guinee et al., 1994; Wilson et al., 1996).

The clinical presentations of LG and WG can be very similar in that they both frequently present with constitutional symptoms, pulmonary infiltrates, renal and skin lesions. However, pathologically, WG is characterized by a necrotizing vasculitis with

multinucleated giant cells and granuloma formation, which are not histologic features of LG. Histologically, the differential diagnosis of LG also includes nasal/nasal–type NK/T–cell lymphoma. Both lesions are remarkably similar in the angiocentric and angiodestructive lesions associated with coagulative necrosis, and both are associated with EBV. The pattern of EBV-positive cells as identified by *in situ* hybridization is help-

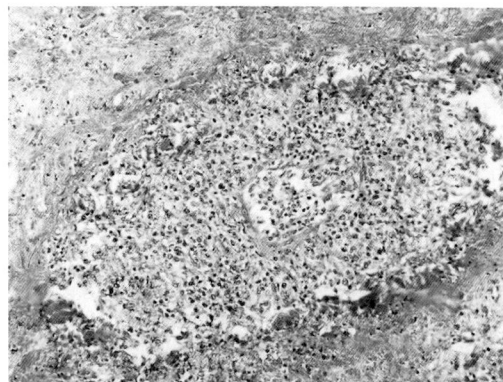

Figure 19–9. Lymphomatoid granulomatosis of the lung. The atypical lymphoid infiltrate extends through the vessel wall, leading to vascular occlusion and extensive pulmonary parenchymal necrosis. The infiltrate in this case is monomorphous, composed predominantly of large lymphoid cells, and would be classified as a grade III lesion, with features of large-cell lymphoma.

ful in distinguishing these two lesions. In LG, the EBV-positive cells are the larger, atypical cells, whereas in nasal/nasal-type NK/T cell lymphoma, the EBV-positive cells are the vastly more numerous T cells. Clinically, these entities have important differences. Nearly all patients with NK/T–cell lymphoma present with histologically aggressive lymphoma involving the nasal cavity and rarely the lung, whereas in LG the opposite distribution is seen, and high-grade lymphoma is only seen in a minority of cases (<30%) (Jaffe and Wilson, 1997).

Most cases of LG occur in otherwise healthy patents, although sporadic cases occur in patients with known underlying immunodeficiencies, either congenital or acquired. These epidemiological associations suggest that patients have some degree of immune compromise resulting in ineffective control of EBV-induced B-cell proliferations (Parkhurst et al., 1994), and most patients with LG, when carefully evaluated, have defects in cytotoxic T-cell function, with reduced levels of CD8-positive T cells (Wilson et al., 1996). In LG, EBV is localized to the B cells, although in some cases, the number of EBV-infected B cells is small and virtually undetectable. Moreover, EBV-positive cells may not be present at all in some sites, e.g., skin, and the vascular effects may actually be mediated by the effects of chemokines, notably IP-10 and Mig, which are up-regulated by EBV expression (Teruya-Feldstein et al., 1996). Thus, EBV is intrinsically linked to all aspects of the pathogenesis of LG.

The clinical behavior varies widely, from an indolent "benign" process to an aggressive large cell lymphoma. In its most indolent form, LG presents with pulmonary or cutaneous lesions, without other symptoms, and resolves spontaneously without therapy, or has a waxing–waning course. More commonly, the clinical course is complicated by constitutional symptoms and involvement of multiple organ sites. Prognosis is poor in these cases, with approximately two-thirds of patients dying within a year of diagnosis (Katzenstein et al., 1979). Cause of death is usually due to extensive pulmonary disease complicated by secondary infection. Several prognostic factors have been identified that predict for a poor clinical outcome, including the presence of neurological disease,

higher histologic grade (II or III), younger age (<25), elevated white blood cell count (WBC), and hepatomegaly (Jaffe and Wilson, 1997). There is no standard therapy for grade I and II lesions, although corticosteroids and/or chemotherapy are the most commonly recommended treatments (Jaffe and Wilson, 1997). However, patients who do not receive complete remission usually develop malignant lymphoma refractory to aggressive therapy (Lipford et al., 1988). Despite more aggressive chemotherapeutic regimens, grade III lesions still have a poor prognosis. Initial clinical trials with interferon-α (IFN-α) have shown remissions in most patients with grade I or II lesions (Wilson et al., 1996). The ability to obtain complete remissions with only immunomodulatory therapy suggests that LG is not an autonomous malignant proliferation.

Angioimmunoblastic T-cell Lymphoma

Angioimmunoblastic lymphadenopathy with dysproteinemia (AILD) is a relatively rare distinct clinicopathologic entity, which initially was thought to be an atypical lymphoproliferative disorder, as a result of an abnormal immune reaction of unknown etiology (Frizzera et al., 1974). It is now considered to be a T-cell lymphoma (Jaffe, 1995b), currently classified as angioimmunoblastic T-cell lymphoma (AILD-T) (Harris et al., 1994; Jaffe et al., 1999). Most lesions show T-cell receptor (TCR) gene rearrangements (Araki et al., 1994; Weiss et al., 1986). A peculiar genotypic feature of AILD-T of particular relevancy to the development of an incipient B-cell LPD is that it is the most common peripheral T-cell lymphoma (TCL) to exhibit occult rearrangements of the IgH genes (10%–30% of cases) (Feller et al., 1988; Griesser et al., 1986). Virtually all cases contain increased numbers of EBV-infected cells, which can be immunohistochemically demonstrated to be B immunoblasts (Anagnostopoulos et al., 1992; Weiss et al., 1992). Rarely, these EBV-infected B cells can evolve into a diffuse large B-cell lymphoma (Abruzzo et al., 1993; Matsue et al., 1998; Nathwani et al., 1978). Therefore, the EBV-positive B immunoblasts represent an incipient clonal process, possibly related to the immunodeficiency associated with the primary disease process.

Angioimmunoblastic T-cell lymphoma is a systemic disease of older adults (median age 62 years), with an equal sex predilection (Pautier et al., 1999). Clinically, the disease is characterized by generalized lymphadenopathy, organomegaly, skin rash, and constitutional symptoms, including fever, night sweats, and weight loss. A variety of serum abnormalities including anemia and polyclonal hypergammaglobulinemia are frequent (Pautier et al., 1999). Patients are usually profoundly immunosuppressed, and recurrent infections are common (Frizzera et al., 1989).

Morphologically, the lymph nodes show effacement of normal architectural features and appear somewhat hypocellular at low power (Fig. 19–10). Although the peripheral subcapsular sinuses are usually patent to dilated, the atypical lymphoid infiltrate can usually be seen extending beyond the nodal capsule. Reactive germinal centers are usually atrophic to absent, but may be hyperplastic in rare cases (Ree et al., 1998; Fig. 19–11). The malignant lymphoid cells form aggregates of "clear" cells, with abundant clear cytoplasm. There is generally a mixed inflammatory background composed of varying elements, including eosinophils, plasma cells, epithelioid histiocytes, and larger immunoblasts, within an anastomosing network of small vessels (Fig. 19–12). One of the distinguishing features of AILD-T is the arborization and proliferation of

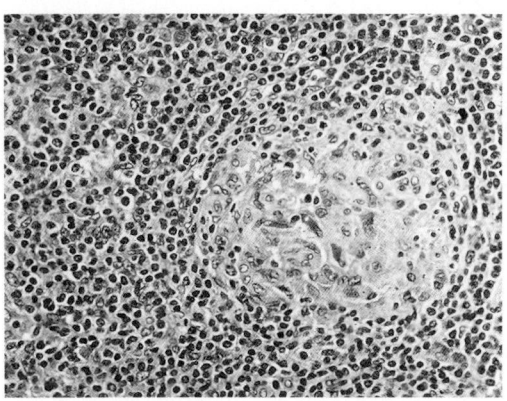

Figure 19–11. Angioimmunoblastic T-cell lymphoma. Germinal centers are either absent or show an atrophic, burned-out appearance. Hyperplastic germinal centers may be present in rare cases.

dendritic or fibroblastic reticular cells associated with the nodal reticular network around the high endothelial venules (Chan, 1999; Jones et al., 1998).

The tumor cells express a T-cell phenotype, CD3, and are usually CD4 positive. CD21 highlights the proliferating reticular cells. As previously noted, most cases will have TCR gene rearrangements, and occasional cases may show IgH gene rearrangements. *In situ* hybridization for EBV highlights scattered immunoblasts in more than 95% of cases, which may be rare to very numerous in number (Weiss et al., 1992). These cells usually show expression of CD20, indicative of a B-cell phenotype. Reports of B-cell lymphomas arising in AILD-T have shown the B-cell lymphomas to be most closely related to the B-cell LPDs arising in other immunodeficiency states, such as posttransplant or congenital immunodeficiencies (Abruzzo et al., 1993; Matsue et al., 1998).

The pathogenesis of incipient B-cell lymphoma arising in AILD-T is not fully understood. The profound immunosuppression associated with the AILD-T itself, as well as treatment with chemotherapeutic agents, may predispose the patient to either a primary or reactivation of EBV infection. With continued immunosuppression, the evolution of polyclonal to oligoclonal and, finally, to monoclonal B-cell expansions may result in B-cell lymphoma (Abruzzo et al., 1993).

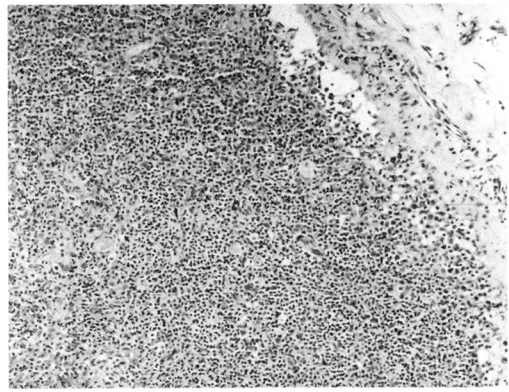

Figure 19–10. Angioimmunoblastic T-cell lymphoma. The lymph node appears somewhat hypocellular with architectural effacement by a diffuse proliferation. However, the cortical sinuses remain patent and are often dilated.

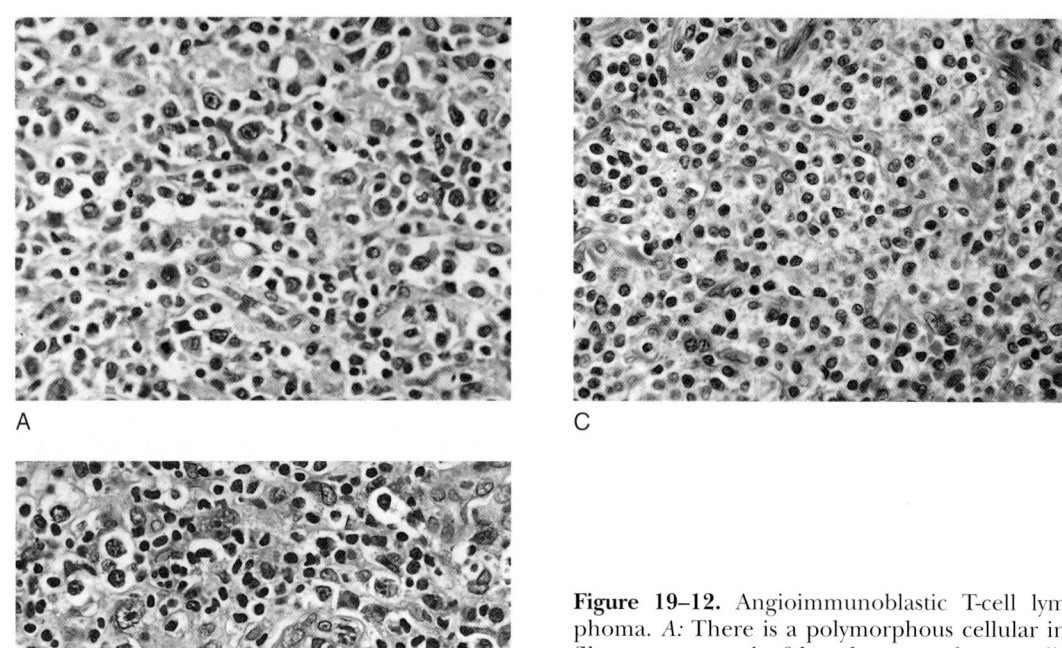

Figure 19–12. Angioimmunoblastic T-cell lymphoma. *A:* There is a polymorphous cellular infiltrate composed of lymphocytes, plasma cells, and large immunoblasts. Many of the large immunoblasts are immunophenotypically B cells. *B:* High endothelial venule within the polymorphous infiltrate, with numerous lymphocytes in transit through the vessel wall. *C:* The malignant lymphoid cells form aggregates of "clear" cells, with abundant pale cytoplasm. Note numerous admixed plasma cells.

Thus, while EBV infection is more a consequence of the AILD-T–associated immunodeficiency than the cause of the disease, it seems to be etiologically linked to the development of a subsequent B-cell lymphoma. Because not all patients with AILD-T develop B-cell lymphoma, additional factors, including defective EBV-cytotoxic T-cell response, down-regulation of latent membrane protein, and/or activation of oncogenes, may contribute to the development of malignant B-cell clones (Knecht et al., 1995; Sallah and Gagnon, 1998).

Most cases of AILD-T present with high-stage (stage III or IV) disease, and the clinical course is moderately aggressive, with occasional spontaneous remissions or protracted responses to steroids. Infectious complications account for most deaths (Frizzera et al., 1989). Age greater than 60 years, anemia, and presence of constitutional symptoms seem to have a negative influence on survival (Pautier et al., 1999).

Prognosis is poor; relapse of disease following conventional chemotherapy is very common (56%), with a median survival of 3 years and an overall 5-year survival of 36% (Pautier et al., 1999).

Multicentric Castleman's Disease

Multicentric Castleman's disease (MCD), or multicentric angiofollicular hyperplasia, is a rare lymphoproliferative disorder first described in the 1970s (Gaba et al., 1978) as distinct from the localized form of the disease (Castleman et al., 1956). Multicentric Castleman's disease is associated with immune abnormalities and an increased risk of malignancy; one third of patients will develop Kaposi's sarcoma and/or malignant B-cell lymphoma (Bowne et al., 1999; Frizzera et al., 1985). HHV-8 sequences have been found in almost all cases of MCD in patients with AIDS and in approximately half of HIV-negative individuals with MCD (Cesarman and Knowles, 1999).

Patients with MCD tend to be older than those diagnosed with localized forms of Castleman's disease, with a median age at diagnosis of 57 years, and a male sex predilection (male-to-female ratio is 2.5:1) (Herrada et al., 1998). Clinically, multiple sites of lymph node enlargement are present, especially peripheral lymphadenopathy. Hepatosplenomegaly is very common, along with a variety of other symptoms, including skin rashes and recurrent infections. Abnormal laboratory findings include anemia, thrombocytopenia, leukopenia, and hypoalbuminemia (Bowne et al., 1999).

Morphologically, at least part of the nodal structure is preserved, while the follicles and interfollicular areas appear abnormal. Lymph nodes showing hyaline-vascular changes, sheets of plasma cells, or both have been described. Most germinal centers have a hyaline-vascular regressed appearance. Immunoblasts may be seen peripheral to the regressed follicles (Fig. 19–13). Scattered hyperplastic follicles may be present. Interfollicular plasmacytosis is usually extreme, forming sheets of mature-appearing plasma cells. Biopsy specimens from different sites may have different histologic appearances.

The plasma cell component of MCD is usually polyclonal by immunohistochemical staining with Ig light chains, and most cases show polyclonal IgH gene patterns by molecular analysis, irrespective of pathologic subtypes, clinical forms, and HIV status. Yet, monoclonal plasma cell populations have been described (Radaszkiewicz and Lennert, 1975), and clonal Ig gene rearrangements have been demonstrated in MCD (Hanson et al., 1988; Soulier et al., 1995). However, no patients with localized Castleman's disease had rearrangements, which suggests that MCD is a disorder distinct from the classical localized variant. Nevertheless, monoclonal plasma cells have been reported in unicentric Castleman's disease (Chilosi et al., 1987). Multicentric Castleman's disease may be an incipient lymphoid malignancy that may progress in some cases to HHV-8–associated lymphoma (Cesarman and Knowles, 1999; Teruya-Feldstein et al., 1998). HHV-8 viral sequences are found in virtually all cases of MCD in patients with AIDS and in human immunodeficiency virus upwards of 50% of (HIV)-negative cases (Soulier et al., 1995).

The role of HHV-8 in the pathogenesis of MCD is poorly understood, and it is not clear whether the HHV-8-positive cases differ clinically from the HHV-8-negative cases in patients without AIDS (Cesarman and Knowles, 1999). Expression of HHV-8 cytokine homologues, namely interleukin-6, may contribute directly to the pathogenesis of MCD (Teruya-Feldstein et al., 1998).

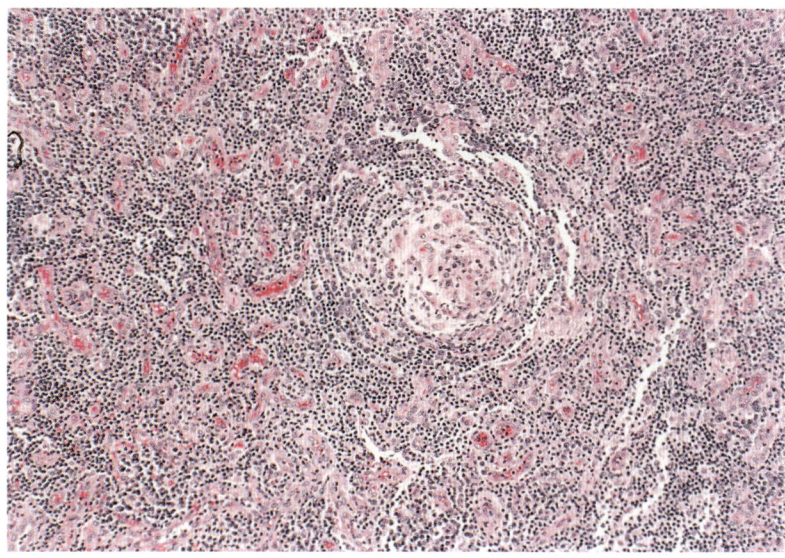

Figure 19–13. Multicentric Castleman's disease. The germinal center shows regressive and atrophic changes. The interfollicular stroma contains numerous vessels with admixed immunoblasts. Plasmacytosis is usually extreme.

The clinical course of MCD is quite aggressive, with a usually fatal outcome; the most common cause of death in patients with MCD is infectious diseases (Herrada et al., 1998). In contrast to unicentric disease, the role of surgery in MCD is limited and should not be considered a realistic option. Systemic therapies in the form of high-dose corticosteroids or multiple-drug chemotherapies have been tried with varied success, and a limited number of cases respond well to low-dose radiotherapy (Bowne et al., 1999). Long-term follow up is recommended because of the high potential of malignant sequelae, KS, and malignant lymphoma.

Essential Mixed Cryoglobulinemia

Essential mixed cryoglobulinemia (EMC) is a benign lymphoproliferative disorder characterized by temperature-sensitive protein complexes formed by polyclonal IgG and monoclonal IgM rheumatoid factors in the absence of clinical evidence of a known underlying disease process, be it neoplastic, infectious, or autoimmune related (Ferri et al., 1998). The prevalence of HCV antibodies in the sera of EMC patients ranges from 30% to 100%, depending on the method of viral detection, with more than 90% of patients having anti-HCV antibodies (Dammacco et al., 1998). A particularly high prevalence of HCV has also been detected in low-grade B-cell lymphomas associated with EMC, namely lymphoplasmacytic lymphoma/immunocytoma (LPL), in up to 30% of patients (Silvestri et al., 1996). In addition, HCV-associated low-grade extranodal marginal zone B-cell lymphomas involving mucosa-associated lymphoid tissues (MALT lymphomas) have been described in noncryoglobulinemic patients, and can appear in the liver, salivary tissues, and ocular tissues (Ascoli et al., 1998).

Essential mixed cryoglobulinemia affects females more than males (3:1), with a mean age of 51 years. Clinically, EMC is characterized by the triad of purpura, weakness, and arthralgias. Patients usually have one or more organ involved; symptoms include chronic hepatitis (in up to two thirds of patients), glomerulonephritis, peripheral neuropathy, skin ulcers, and/or diffuse vasculitis. The diagnosis may be delayed because of either its clinical polymorphism or single-organ manifestations, which may be the only predominant clinical symptom (Ferri et al., 1998).

Histologically, a leukocytoclastic vasculitis is the hallmark lesion, particularly in cutaneous manifestations of EMC. However, the presence of lymphoid aggregates, either in diffuse or nodular growth patterns, in the liver, spleen, kidney, or bone marrow, is highly suggestive of an evolving LPD (Ferri et al., 1998). The lymphocytic infiltrate, as with LPL, is generally rather monotonous, composed of small cells exhibiting plasmacytoid features. Dutcher bodies may be seen. Immunophenotypically, the infiltrates express B-cell antigens CD20, CD22, and CD79a and show surface and cytoplasmic immunoglobulin, usually IgM. The B cells do not coexpress CD5 or CD43 and are CD10 negative.

Molecularly, clonal and polyclonal expansions of B cells can be identified in the peripheral blood. Clonal expansions of the lymphoid aggregates in bone marrow, liver, spleen, and kidneys have all been reported in patients with EMC, thus confirming the lymphoproliferative nature of the process (Ferri et al., 1998; Rasul et al., 1999). Interestingly, a high number of HCV-infected patients without clinical evidence of EMC have been found to have occult clonal Ig gene rearrangements in their peripheral blood B-lymphocytes. The serum levels of rheumatoid factor were increased in all HCV-positive patients with a clonal expansion, suggesting that the expanded B-cell clones belong to the rheumatoid factor producing B-cell subset (Franzin et al., 1995).

Although the exact pathogenetic mechanism of chronic HCV infection leading to the development of EMC is still unknown, persistent antigenic stimulus of the HCV infection may induce complex cellular and humoral autoreactivity, which could greatly expand clones of cryoglobulin-secreting lymphocytes by direct or indirect mechanisms. A subsequent mutational event could lead to the eventual activation of oncogenes, thus resulting in a B-cell lymphoma (Luppi and Torelli, 1996). Thus the clonal B-cell expansion seen in HCV-associated EMC may serve as the incipient neoplastic reservoir for the emergence of an associated low-grade B-cell lymphoma, such as LPL. The antigen-driven properties of HCV may drive the development of the noncryoglobulinemic associated MALT-type lymphomas, which may have originated from lymphoid tissue acquired during long-standing HCV infection, perhaps in much the same way as in *H. pylori*–associated gastric MALT lymphomas (Ascoli et al., 1998). Even so, EMC evolves into frank malignant lymphoma in only a minority of cases, and usually only after a long duration (Miescher et al., 1995).

Treatment with IFN-α is the current therapy of choice for EMC, as IFN-α reduces symptoms of cryoglobulin production and shows antiproliferative and antiviral activity. Just as antibiotic therapy used to eradicate *H. pylori*, aids in the regression of gastric MALT lymphoma, IFN-α appears to be an effective agent for the treatment of mixed cryoglobulinemia and has been shown to decrease disease progression of low-grade lymphomas in HVC-infected patients (Mazzaro et al., 1996).

IMMUNODEFICIENCY-ASSOCIATED LYMPHOPROLIFERATIVE DISORDERS

The incidence of B-cell LPDs, including malignant lymphoma, is significantly higher in individuals who have congenital, acquired, or iatrogenically induced immunodeficiency than in the general population (Knowles, 1999). Although clinically heterogeneous, LPDs occurring in the setting of immunodeficiency, irrespective of the type of immunodeficiency, share several common pathological characteristics: involvement of extranodal sites of disease, diffuse, aggressive histologic grade, B-cell lineage, association with EBV, and generally rapid clinical progression (Elenitoba-Johnson and Jaffe, 1997; Knowles, 1997). The most common, and thus best-studied, immunodeficiency-associated LPDs are those arising in the setting of HIV infection and AIDS, and in the solid-organ post-transplant setting. Less commonly, LPDs arise in association with congenital immunodeficiencies, such as Wiskott-Aldrich syndrome (WAS) and combined variable immunodeficiency disorder (CVID), as well as in the non-post-transplant iatrogenic setting, e.g., LPDs associated with methotrexate therapy.

The EBV plays an important role in the pathogenesis of LPDs arising in immuno-compromised states. The great majority (>90%) of these disorders show evidence of

EBV in the neoplastic cells (Staal et al., 1989), and infection of EBV of the lymphomatous cells generally occurs prior to the development of malignancy (Cleary et al., 1988). The virus is in latency phase and produces latent membrane protein (LMP), a known lymphocyte effector for growth, activation, and transformation (Young et al., 1989). Additional alterations in T-cell mediation, either through impaired production of cytokines IL-1 and IL-2 and/or through reduced proliferation of cytotoxic T cells, ultimately leads to ineffective cytotoxic T-cell control of the EBV-infected B cells (Kamel et al., 1995).

Congenital Immunodeficiency-Associated Lymphoproliferative Disorders

Congenital immunodeficiencies represent a heterogenous group of genetically determined diseases that have specific defects in the cellular/humoral immune systems. These syndromes usually become clinically evident within the first year of life, when they become generally associated with recurrent infections (Rosen et al., 1984a,b). There is a well-known association between congenital immunodeficiency syndromes and the development of LPDs, which make up the majority of related malignancies in this setting (WHO Scientific Study Group, 1995). The clinicopathological heterogeneity of these LPDs reflects the fact that different diseases affect different components of the immune system (Elenitoba-Johnson and Jaffe, 1997). The immunodeficiency syndromes associated with the greatest risk of developing malignant lymphoma include Wiskott-Aldrich syndrome (7.6%) (Perry et al., 1980), ataxia-telangiectasia (10%) (Morrell et al., 1986), and combined variable immunodeficiency disorder (1.4%–7%) (Sander et al., 1992). Other congenital syndromes associated with increased risk of LPDs include severe combined immunodeficiency, X-linked lymphoproliferative disorder, hyper-IgM syndrome, and Job's syndrome (Rosen et al., 1995; Russell et al., 1995; Sullivan and Woda, 1989). Each disease has its own particular risk factors, susceptibility, and specific disease patterns (Table 19–4).

The LPDs occurring in association with congenital immunodeficiency syndromes occur at a younger age than in the general

Table 19–4. Congenital Immunodeficiency-Associated Lymphoproliferative Disorders

Syndrome	Age of Onset	Molecular Defect	Disease Patterns	Risk
Wiskott-Aldrich syndrome	Childhood, boys, median 6 years	WAS gene defects, Xp11.22	CNS: DLBCL, EBV$^{+/-}$	100
Common variable immunodeficiency syndrome	Adulthood	Heterogenous	Nodal: ALH GI: DLBCL, EBV$^+$, PT-LPD-like	30–400
Ataxia-telangiectasia	Childhood, median 9 years	AT gene defects, 11q22-23	ALL, T-PLL, DLBCL, Burkitt's, HD	250
Hyper-IgM syndrome	Early childhood	Xq26 (70%), failure isotope switching	GI/CNS: Burkitt's, DLBCL, EBV$^+$, HD	ND
Severe combined immunodeficiency syndrome	Infancy, early childhood	IL receptor defects, Xq13	Extranodal: DLBCL	80
X-linked lympho-proliferative disorder (Dunce's disease)	Childhood adolescence, boys	Xq25 GI: DLBCL	Fatal IM	ND

ALH, atypical lymphoid hyperplasia; CNS, central nervous system; DLBCL, diffuse large B-cell lymphoma; EBV, Epstein-Barr virus; GI, gastrointestinal; HD, Hodgkin's disease; IL, interleukin; IM, infectious mononucleosis; ND, not determined; PT-LPD, post-transplant lymphoproliferative disorder.

population (WHO Scientific Study Group, 1995). The histopathologic spectrum of lymphoid lesions ranges from mild degrees of nonspecific reactive hyperplasias to atypical lymphoid hyperplasias and malignant lymphoma (Elenitoba-Johnson et al., 1997; Fig. 19–14). Most malignant lymphomas are of a high-grade histologic type and are predominantly of B-cell lineage. They usually occur in extranodal sites, particularly the central

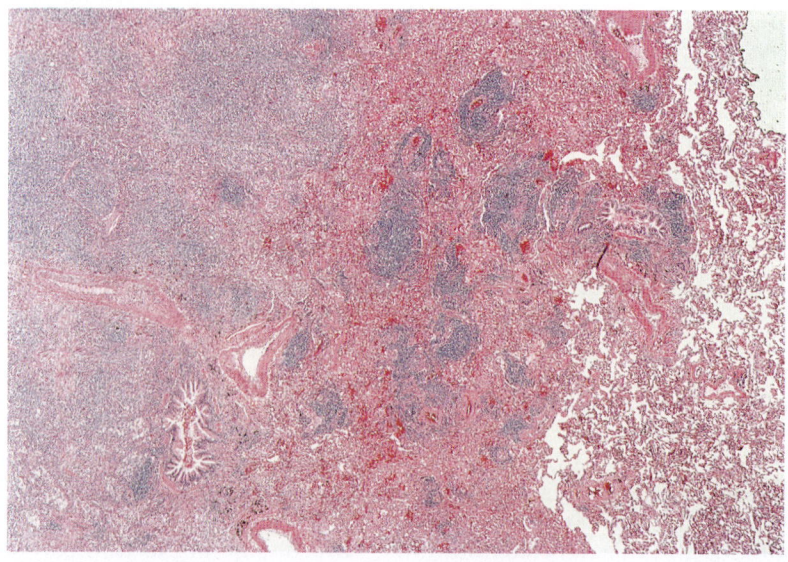

Figure 19–14. Atypical lymphoid hyperplasia of the lung in a patient with common variable immunodeficiency disorder. The nodular peribronchial lesion contains reactive germinal centers within a relatively polymorphous infiltrate composed of small lymphocytes, plasma cells, and larger immunoblasts. Immunohistochemical studies showed a clear predominance of λ light-chain Ig, suggesting the emergence of an occult monoclonal B-cell population. However, Southern blot analysis demonstrated a germline pattern.

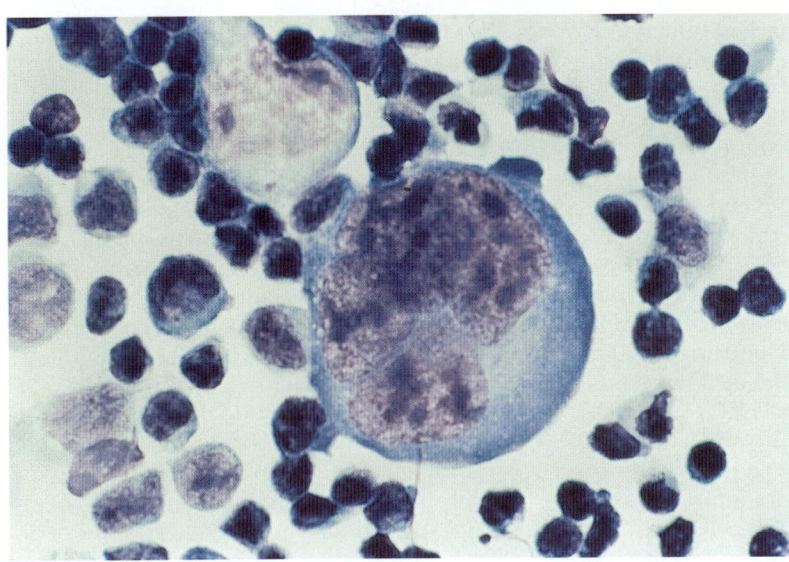

Figure 19–15. A high-grade malignant lymphoma in a patient common variable immunodeficiency disorder who presented with pleural effusions.

nervous system and gastrointestinal tract, and clinically are very aggressive (Fig. 19–15). Immunophenotypic and molecular studies are valuable in the assessment of the clonality of these lymphomas, although Ig gene rearrangements and TCR gene rearrangements in histologically "benign" lymphoid proliferations have been detected (Knowles, 1999). Conversely, morphologically unambiguous malignant lymphoma may not yield monoclonal patterns in rare cases. Furthermore, oligoclonal bands representing separate malignant clones may also be shown (Elenitoba-Johnson et al., 1997).

The exact pathogenesis of the development of congenital immunodeficiency-associated malignant lymphomas generally involves the interplay of polyclonal activation of lymphoid proliferations, abnormal regulation by the dysfunctional immune system, and chromosomal abnormalities (Elenitoba-Johnson et al., 1997). A high percentage of cases (>90%) are associated with EBV (Biemer, 1990; Joncas et al., 1990), which appears to be an important cofactor in the development of LPDs; this suggests that lymphomas arising in the setting of congenital immunodeficiencies have many similarities with lymphomas arising in other clinical settings of immunodeficiency. Additionally, host defects in immunoregulation and/or gene rearrangements probably contribute to lymphomagenesis in patients at risk (Filipovich et al., 1992). Once patients

develop lymphoma their overall survival is poor, with a median survival of 12 months.

AIDS-Related Lymphoproliferative Disorders

Malignant lymphoma is the second most common malignancy associated with HIV infection and is the most common one in intravenous drug abusers and hemopheliacs suffering from AIDS (Beral et al., 1991). The risk of malignant lymphoma in persons with AIDS is 60 times greater than in the normal population, with an incidence of lymphoma in AIDS of between 4% and 10% (Knowles, 1999). Malignant lymphoma occurs in all age-groups and affects all risk groups, regardless of the mode of transmission of the virus.

Patients with HIV who develop malignant lymphoma frequently present with stage III or IV disease (Ioachim et al., 1991), with involvement of extranodal sites, including the gastrointestinal tract, central nervous system, and bone marrow; or the lymphoma may affect unusual sites, such as myocardium, soft tissues, oral cavity, and body cavities (Said, 1997). The tumors generally develop rapidly, forming bulky masses (Knowles et al., 1988). Additionally, there is increased risk for developing Hodgkin's disease in HIV-infected individuals, and these cases usually present with extranodal disease with involvement of bone marrow (Reynolds et al., 1993).

Early in the course of HIV infection, patients have generalized lymphadenopathy.

The lymph nodes show marked follicular hyperplasia and plasmacytosis, while the paracortex may be normal to hyperplastic. Over time, the paracortex becomes depleted and the hyperplastic follicles stand out. A polyclonal hypergammaglobulinemia can be seen in the serum. Clonal B-cell populations have been reported in these hyperplastic nodes (Pelicci et al., 1986). As the disease progresses, progressive lymphoid atrophy occurs, including both the T cell– and B cell–dependent areas. These hyperplastic changes usually precede the development of lymphoma (Ioachim et al., 1991). Almost all lymphomas developing in the setting of AIDS are of intermediate to high-grade histologic types (>90%), the most common types being diffuse, large B-cell lymphoma with or without immunoblastic features, and Burkitt's lymphoma (Said, 1997). Aggressive histologic subtypes of Hodgkin's disease, mixed cellularity and lymphocyte depletion, are the most common.

Immunophenotypically, the AIDS-related lymphomas (95%) express monoclonal surface Ig and/or B-cell associated antigens. The phenotypes are similar to those expressed by the same morphologic type of lymphoma in immunocompetent persons. Most of the remaining AIDS-related lymphomas (5%) are primary effusion lymphomas (PELs) of B-cell lineage derivation that express indeterminant phenotypes (Nador et al., 1996). The vast majority if AIDS-related lymphomas (96%) exhibit clonal Ig heavy- and light-chain gene rearrangements and lack TCR gene rearrangements (Ballerini et al., 1993; Raphael et al., 1994), although rare cases may fail to show monoclonal Ig gene rearrangements by conventional molecular techniques (McGrath et al., 1991). These lesions appear to be analogous to the polyclonal post-transplant lymphoproliferative disorders (discussed below). Alterations in the c-myc gene often occur in these lymphomas (Pelicci et al., 1986), and depending on the detection method, EBV viral sequences can be detected in 35%–65% of cases (Subar et al., 1988). HHV-8 sequences are associated with PELs (Cesarman and Knowles, 1999).

Although HIV genomic sequences are not directly involved in the lymphomagenesis, the production of an array of cytokines and growth factors secondary to the infection serves to induce a state of ongoing B-cell activation, proliferation, and differentiation (Knowles, 1997). Also, the HIV-induced immunosuppression milieu may predispose B cells to genetic mutations that may ultimately lead to progression to lymphoma. Thus, the development of AIDS-related lymphoma is a multistep process, most likely beginning with B-cell hyperplasia and terminating with the acquisition of specific oncogene/tumor suppressor gene alterations, e.g., c-myc and/or p53 (Pelicci et al., 1986).

In general, patients with HIV-associated lymphomas have a poor prognosis. Factors associated with a poor prognosis include central nervous system disease, bone marrow involvement, poor performance status, and other AIDS-defining illnesses (Levine et al., 1991). Interestingly, histologic subtype appears to have little correlation with survival. Aggressive chemotherapy regimens are warranted for the treatment of AIDS-related lymphomas. Patients who fail to respond usually die of their lymphoma within 4 months. However, even those patients with complete response eventually die of other manifestations of AIDS within 2 years (Levine et al., 1991).

Post-Transplantation Lymphoproliferative Disorders

The development of post-transplantation lymphoproliferative disorder (PT-LPD) in patients receiving immunosuppressive therapy secondarily to organ transplantation has been recognized as a major complication since 1969 (Penn et al., 1969). The incidence varies according to the organ transplanted and the type of immunosuppressive therapy received, from 1% in renal transplant to 10% in combined heart/lung transplants and patients receiving cyclosporin A or OKT3 therapy (Knowles, 1999). The vast majority of PT-LPDs (>90%) are associated with EBV infection and are of B-cell lineage (Harris et al., 1997). T-cell LPDs arising in the post-transplant setting are rare, occurring later (median 5 years) after transplantation, and only half are associated with EBV. The PT-LPDs often develop rapidly with multiple sites of involvement, which leads to rapid tumor burden.

Antigen receptor gene rearrangement studies and EBV analyses have shown some lesions to have clonal Ig gene rearrangements, even in cases lacking Ig expression.

Infection by a single clone of EBV has also been shown (Cleary et al., 1984, 1988). Multiple lesions at diverse anatomic sites arising in the same patient may display different Ig gene rearrangements (Chadburn et al., 1995; Cleary et al., 1984). Furthermore, among several clonally distinct PT-LPDs occurring in the same individual, one lesion may have sufficient genetic alterations, e.g., *p53* mutations, indicative of aggressive disease, while another lesion may regress following reduction of immunosuppressive therapy (Chadburn et al., 1997). Thus, PT-LPDs are pathologically heterogeneous with diverse clinical behaviors. The data suggest that each lesion starts from a single B cell driven by EBV and that true dissemination of the clone occurs at a late stage in disease evolution.

Most PT-LPDs can be subclassified into one of three major histologic subtypes: plasmacytic hyperplasia, polymorphic B-cell lymphoproliferative disorder, and malignant lymphoma/multiple myeloma (Knowles et al., 1995). The former is most common in children and young adults, in whom the LPD develops within a few months of transplantation. The lesions generally occur in the tonsils, adenoids, and lymph nodes. Pathological features include preservation of nodal architecture, with an interfollicular expansion of lymphocytes, plasmacytoid lymphocytes, plasma cells, and immunoblasts. Cytologic atypia is minimal. The lesions are composed of a mixture of polyclonal B and T cells lacking clonal Ig heavy- and light-chain and TCR gene rearrangements, as well as oncogene and tumor suppressor gene alterations. Evidence of EBV by *in situ* hybridization is usually present. Most patients with the plasmacytic hyperplasia variant of PT-LPD present with stage I, II, or III disease, and virtually all patients experience regression of the lesions after reduction or discontinuation of immunosuppressive therapy. The prognosis is generally very good, and virtually no one dies as a result of the LPD. Rarely, transformation to a higher histologic grade may occur.

The molecular and clinical behavior of polymorphic B-cell hyperplasia and polymorphic B-cell lymphoma have been shown to be identical and as such have now been categorized as polymorphic lymphoproliferative disorder (PLD) (Knowles et al., 1995). Although PLDs occur at any age, the median age is 43 years, with a median time interval from transplantation to development of approximately 1 year (Knowles, 1999). The lesions occur most frequently in extranodal sites, particularly the lungs and gastrointestinal tract, but may also occur in lymph nodes.

Morphologically, PLDs consist of diffuse polymorphous lymphoid infiltrates that obliterate the underlying tissue architecture. There is considerable variation in the cytologic composition of the lymphoid cells; prominent plasmacytoid differentiation and immunoblasts can occur with or without significant cytologic atypia. Atypical immunoblasts may be highly pleomorphic, sometimes resembling Reed-Sternberg cells (Fig. 19–16). Virtually all PLD contain evidence of necrosis, either with prominent apoptotic debris or diffuse coagulative-type necrosis. Most of the cells are B cells, which may or may not express monoclonal surface Ig by immunohistochemistry. The Ig heavy- and light-chain gene rearrangements are a consistent feature, and they lack TCR gene rearrangements, as well as evidence of *bcl-1*, *bcl-2*, *bcl-6*, *c-myc*, and *p53* gene mutations. Most PLDs contain evidence of infection by a clonal form of EBV and show monoclonal Ig gene rearrangements.

The prognosis for PLD is generally good, although the clinical course is quite variable. In many cases, the lesions regress following reduction or discontinuation of immunosuppressive therapy. However, in some cases the lesions progress despite aggressive chemotherapy (Knowles, 1999).

Some PT-LPDs are histologically identical to diffuse large B-cell lymphoma (DLBCL) or multiple myeloma (MM) occurring in immunocompetent patients. Post-transplant DLBCL and MM frequently occur in older patients, with a median age of 55 years (Knowles, 1999). These lesions tend to involve nodal sites but may also be seen in extranodal sites, including the central nervous system, soft tissue, or bone marrow. Patients usually present with high-stage or disseminated disease (stage III or IV). Those classified as MM may exhibit a monoclonal gammopathy and/or lytic bone lesions.

Morphologically, the post-transplant DLBCL or MM are characterized by their diffuse monomorphic lymphoid infiltrates with obliteration of the nodal architecture. Cytologically, the cells show marked immuno-

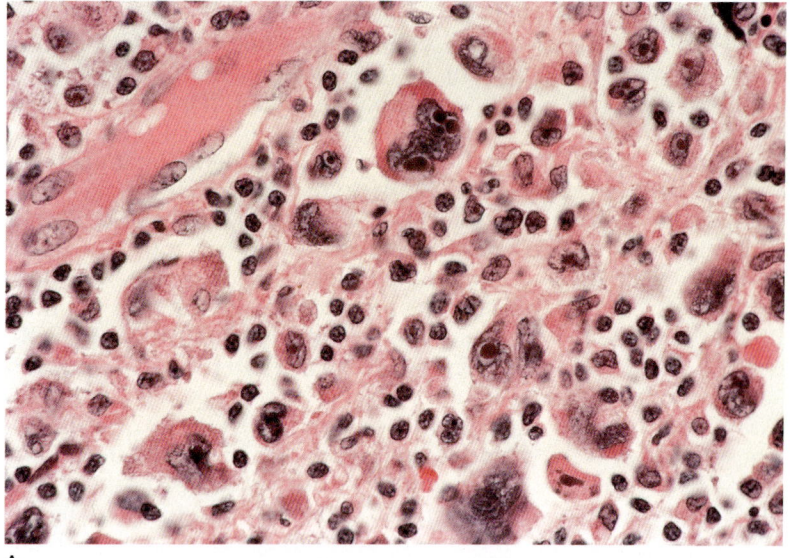

A

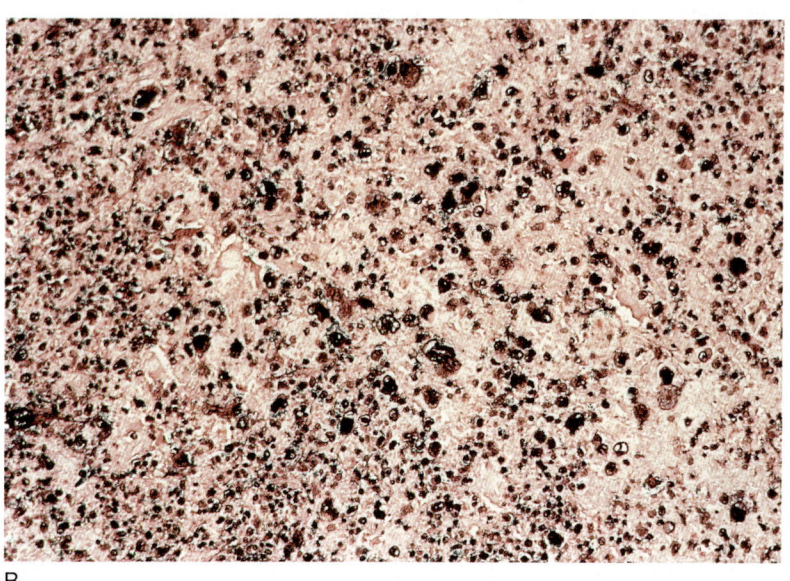

B

Figure 19–16. Polymorphic B-cell lymphoma in a post–heart transplant patient. *A:* Diffuse polymorphic lymphoid infiltrate in a lymph node shows marked cellular pleomorphism, with some of the cells resembling Reed-Sternberg cells. *B: In situ* hybridization for Epstein-Barr virus is positive in virtually every cell.

blastic and/or plasmacytoid features. The cells express B-cell lineage markers and may or may not show monoclonal surface or cytoplasmic Ig expression. However, in all of these lesions their Ig heavy- and usually light-chain genes are rearranged and the lesions show evidence of clonal EBV infection. Importantly, they have oncogene and/or tumor suppressor gene alterations, namely *p53*, *c-myc*, and/or *ras* (Knowles et al., 1995). These patients generally have a poor clinical outcome, as the lesions do not regress after discontinuation therapy. Regression may occur following aggressive chemotherapy, although most patients die within several months of the PT-LPD (Knowles, 1999).

Nontransplantation Iatrogenic-Induced Lymphoproliferative Disorders

Iatrogenic-induced lymphoproliferative disorders (IAT-LPD) have only recently been recognized (Ellman et al., 1991; Kamel et al., 1993). The most common clinical setting in which IAT-LPDs occur is when immunosuppressive therapies, most commonly methotrexate, but also cyclosporin, corticosteroids, and azathioprine, are used for rheumatoid arthritis or related diseases (Kamel, 1997). The clinical situations in which these disorders arise, e.g., rheumatoid arthritis, are not well defined in terms of the degree to which the underlying immune deficits, if any, directly contribute to the development of the LPD (Kamel, 1997). Most lymphomas occurring in rheumatologic patients are likely coincidental and not associated with EBV, and behave as those seen in otherwise healthy individuals. However, several studies have shown an integral role for immunosuppressive therapy in the pathogenesis of IAT-LPDs and have documented the strong association with EBV and regression of such LPDs following discontinuation of the immunosuppressive agent (Salloum et al., 1996; Thomason et al., 1996). This suggests that these LPDs are not autonomous lymphoid neoplasms, but rather EBV-immortalized B-cell proliferations that can be brought under control by the patient if the immunosuppressive therapy is withdrawn.

Patients with rheumatoid arthritis have a 10-fold increase of malignant lymphoma following immunosuppressive therapy and only a 2.5-fold increase in the absence of such treatment (Kamel et al., 1995). Clinically, IAT-LPDs share features similar to those of PT-LPDs, including rapid onset, tendency for involvement of both nodal and extranodal sites, including soft tissues and joint spaces, and a high degree of clinical aggressiveness.

As with post-transplant LPDs, IAT-LPDs show a wide spectrum of morphologies and fall within three main morphologic categories: atypical polymorphous B-cell lymphoproliferative disorder, diffuse high-grade B-cell lymphoma, and lymphoproliferations resembling Hodgkin's disease (Kamel, 1997). The atypical polymorphous LPDs typically consist of a mixture of lymphoid cells at various stages of activation and differentiation, including mature small lymphocytes, immunoblasts, plasmacytoid cells, and plasma cells. Cytologic atypia is not a prominent feature, although focal areas of necrosis may be present. In the diffuse high-grade lymphomas, the most common morphologic pattern resembles diffuse large B-cell lymphoma; the small, noncleaved Burkitt's lymphoma-like pattern is less common. These lymphomas are composed of cytologically malignant cells that sheet out, obliterating any underlying normal architecture. The cells may show immunoblastic, plasmacytoid, pleomorphic, or even Reed-Sternberg-like features (Fig. 19–17).

Immunophenotypically, the malignant cells are B cells, which may be faintly CD20 positive, primarily because of the down-regulation of CD20 by the EBV infection (Garnier et al., 1993). Expression of CD30 is common, as is coexpression of CD43. Since

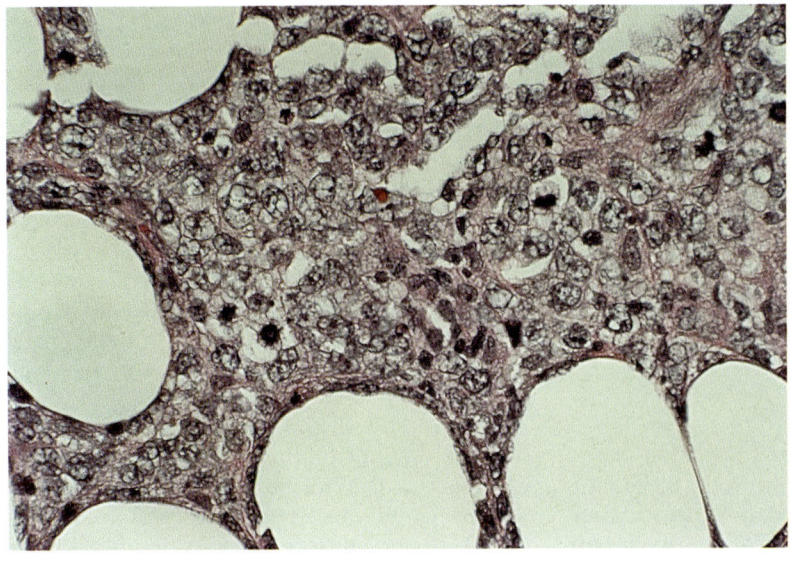

Figure 19–17. Iatrogenic-induced lymphoproliferative disorder in a patient receiving methotrexate for rheumatoid arthritis. The nodal lesion demonstrates the most common morphologic pattern, which resembles diffuse large cell lymphoma. *In situ* hybridization for Epstein-Barr virus was positive in this case.

the vast majority of IAT-LPDs are EBV positive, EBV studies are important in pathologic evaluation of these lesions. The EBV may be detected by expression of LMP, although *in situ* hybridization is far more sensitive in picking up EBV infection. Iatrogenic-induced diffuse large cell lymphomas and some polymorphous B-cell lymphoproliferations will show clonal Ig gene rearrangements, and most will contain clonal EBV strains (Thomason et al., 1996).

Cases of Hodgkin's disease showing unequivocal morphologic and immunophenotypic features have been reported in the IAT setting, including both nodular sclerosis and mixed cellularity subtypes (Kamel et al., 1996). Reed-Sternberg cells are seen in a mixed inflammatory background, with or without the presence of broad fibrous bands. Immunophenotypically, the cells show the classic Hodgkin's phenotype: they express CD30 and CD15 but lack other lymphoid markers; EBV is invariably present.

The clinical behavior of IAT-LPD is variable; some lesions will show spontaneous regression following discontinuation of the immunosuppressive agent, whereas others will progress despite aggressive chemotherapy and result in the patient's death. The morphologic subtype of IAT-LPD does not seem to correlate with clinical outcome or whether the LPD will spontaneously regress on discontinuation of therapy. However, the presence of EBV does have predictive value in that most spontaneously regressing tumors are EBV positive (Kamel et al., 1996; Salloum et al., 1996). The current recommendations include withdrawal of immunosuppressive therapy and observation for a short period of time (4–8 weeks), especially if the lesions are EBV positive (Kamel, 1997). In cases of persistent, relapsing, or progressive disease, more aggressive chemotherapy is warranted.

T-CELL LYMPHOPROLIFERATIVE DISORDERS

ADULT T-CELL LEUKEMIA/LYMPHOMA

Adult T-cell leukemia/lymphoma (ATLL) is a distinctive clinicopathologic entity caused by infection with the human T-cell lymphotropic virus-1 (HTLV-1), generally after many decades following the initial infection. This disease has a worldwide distribution but is most prevalent in the HTLV-1–endemic areas (Franchini, 1995). It affects middle-aged adults, with a median age of 55 years, and shows a slight male predilection (male to female ratio 1.5:1) (Takatsuki, 1997). There are several clinical forms of ATLL, including acute, lymphomatous, chronic, and smoldering variants (Kawano et al., 1985). Although ATLL is generally considered to be an autonomous malignancy, the chronic/smoldering variant forms of the disease may have long, indolent clinical courses, and for the purposes of this discussion, may be thought of as incipient neoplastic processes.

Clinically, the chronic and smoldering variants of ATLL differ significantly from the more common, acute form of the disease (Jaffe, 1995a). The chronic variant presents predominantly with peripheral blood involvement and lacks organomegaly and lymphadenopathy, whereas the smoldering variant is characterized by long-lasting cutaneous lesions and minimal peripheral blood involvement (Fig. 19–18). In contrast, virtually all patients with acute ATLL present with stage IV disease, which is characterized by generalized lymphadenopathy, hepatosplenomegaly, skin lesions, peripheral blood, and central nervous system involvement (Shimoyama, 1991). In the rare lymphomatous form, which is more common in the Caribbean than in Japan, patients present with peripheral lymphadenopathy, but without peripheral blood involvement.

Although not all patients present with peripheral blood involvement, e.g., the smoldering variant, a leukemic phase eventually develops in most cases. Adult T-cell leukemia/lymphoma is characterized by a broad range of morphologic expressions (Jaffe, 1995a) with the most specific pathologic feature being the presence of markedly pleomorphic lymphoid cells in the peripheral blood. The cells have markedly irregular nuclear contours in which the nucleus is divided into multiple lobes, the so-called flower cell. The malignant lymphoid cells are usually distinctive but may resemble Sézary cells when the polylobation of the nucleus is less extreme. Histologic features of lymph node involvement is variable; usually diffuse, polymorphic infiltrates of atypical

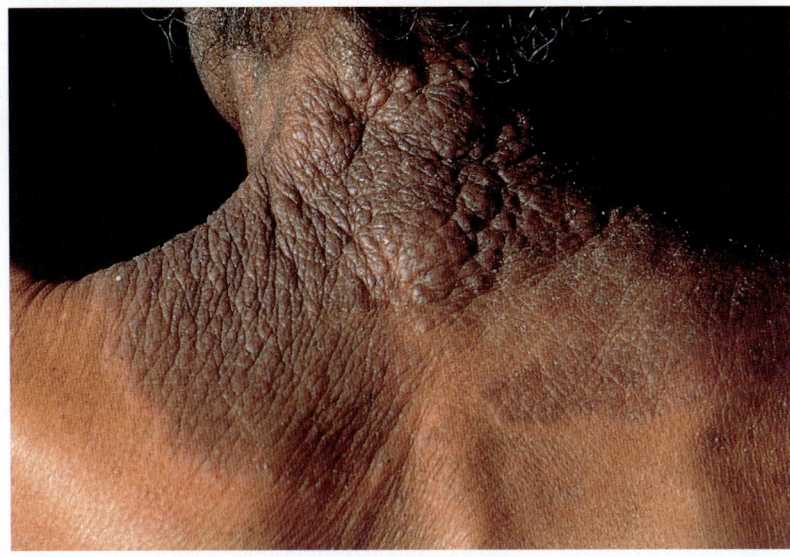

Figure 19–18. Clinical appearance of adult T-cell leukemia/lymphoma, chronic variant, with extensive plaques involving the neck and upper back.

lymphoid cells show the characteristic nuclear pleomorphisms. Reed-Sternberg-like cells may be present, causing a resemblance to Hodgkin's disease, or the infiltrate may be quite monomorphic with large, transformed cells, simulating large B-cell lymphoma. Skin lesions generally show acanthosis and hyperkeratosis of the epidermis. Exocytosis by the atypical cells with or without Pautrier microabscess formation is a consistent feature (Fig. 19–19). Because of the conspicuous epidermotropism by atypical lymphocytes, distinguishing ATLL from mycosis fungoides may be difficult on the basis of morphology alone.

Immunohistochemically, typical ATLL cells have a mature helper T-cell phenotype, expressing CD3, CD4, and CD5; expression of CD7 is usually negative. High expression of CD25 helps differentiate ATLL from other peripheral T-cell lymphomas. Molecular analysis will show the TCR genes rearranged, and clonally integrated HTLV-1 genomes are found in all cases (Chadburn et al., 1991), providing definitive evidence of viral pathogenesis.

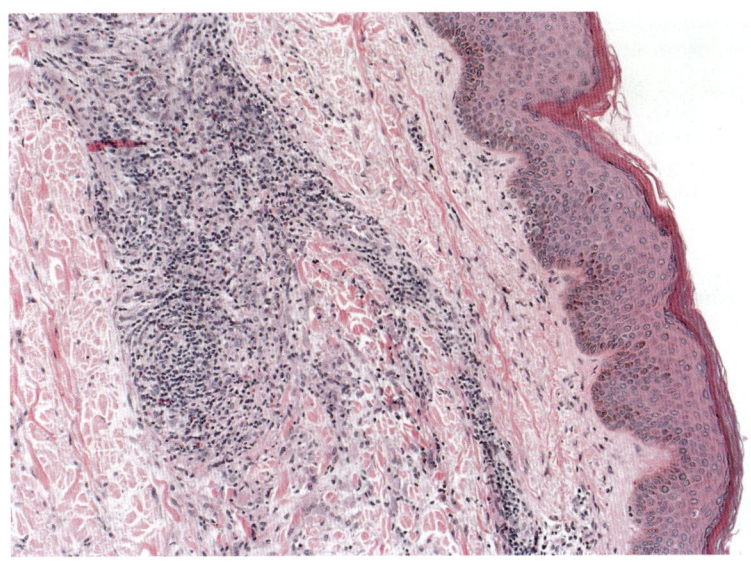

Figure 19–19. Adult T-cell leukemia/lymphoma, chronic variant. A skin biopsy of the same case shown in Figure 19–18 shows acanthosis and hyperkeratosis. The lymphoid infiltrate shows minimal cytologic atypia and is confined primarily to the mid-dermis. Exocytosis with Pautrier microabscess formation is not a prominent feature in this case.

The exact mechanism of HTLV-1 oncogenesis is unknown. The virus infects mature T cells, which go swiftly from a resting state to a proliferative state, similar to EBV in B cells. Thus, HTLV-1 likely affects cell cycling at perhaps different levels, and prevents the infected T cells from reverting to a resting state in the absence of activating antigens or growth factors (Franchini, 1995). As a retrovirus, the genes *gag, pol,* and *env* are present in the usual sequence. However, a unique feature of the HTLV-1 retrovirus is the presence of two genes, *tax* and *rex.* No known homology exists between *tax* and any human oncogene, although *tax* is thought play an interactive role in the transcription of IL-2 and IL-2 receptor α, because *tax*-expressing T cells are hyperresponsive to IL-2 and the CD3 portion of the TCR (Franchini, 1995).

The clinical behavior of ATLL varies widely, from one of an indolent process to a rapidly aggressive fatal disease. The chronic and/or smoldering cases have a more protracted clinical course, with a median survival of usually greater than 2 years. In contrast, the clinical course of acute ATLL is aggressive, with a very poor prognosis and median survival of less than 1 year. High LDH levels (lactate dehydrogenase), hypercalcemia, and elevated WBC in particular are indicators of a bad prognosis. The histologic subtype of ATLL does not appear to influence prognosis (Jaffe et al., 1984). Most ATLL-related deaths are due to opportunistic infections secondary to immunosuppression induced by the HTLV-1 infection. Treatment includes combination chemotherapy, although long-term success is very limited (Pawson et al., 1998). Radioimmunotherapy with 90Y anti-Tac directed toward the IL-2 receptor expressed on ATLL cells may provide a useful approach in treating the more refractory cases (Lehky et al., 1998; Waldmann et al., 1995).

CELIAC DISEASE/GLUTEN-SENSITIVE ENTEROPATHY

Celiac disease (CD), or gluten-sensitive enteropathy, is a chronic malabsorption syndrome of the small intestine caused by exposure to dietary gluten in genetically susceptible individuals. Although considered to be a disease of childhood, adult presentation is becoming increasingly common. Screening with the diagnostic serologic markers for the characteristic anti-gliadin antibodies and anti-endomysial antibodies places the prevalence of CD at around 1:250 (Fasano, 1996). Celiac disease is a human leukocyte antigen (HLA)-associated condition; greater than 90% of cases are associated with HLA DQ2 (Lundin et al., 1994). The overall mortality of CD is twice that of the general population, with most of the excess deaths being directly related to its association with intestinal T-cell LPDs, specifically enteropathy-associated T-cell lymphoma (EATL) and ulcerative jejunitis (Parnell and Ciclitira, 1999). The increase in relative risk of T-cell LPD in CD is approximately 40%, although the exact prevalence of CD-related lymphoma is unknown, because lymphomas can arise in clinically silent or previously undiagnosed CD (Holmes et al., 1989).

The clinical presentation of ulcerative jejunitis and EATL is identical, and many cases of ulcerative jejunitis are complicated by the subsequent development of EATL (Wright, 1997). They both commonly affect adults who have a short history of CD and present with abdominal pain and weight loss. Fewer patients have a history of CD from childhood. Patients usually present with acute emergent abdominal complaints, including perforation, obstruction, and hemorrhage. Both ulcerative jejunitis and EATL occur most commonly in the jejunum as single to multiple ulcerative lesions (Wright, 1997).

Histologically, ulcerative jejunitis and EATL differ somewhat, although the infiltrating lymphoid cells are immunophenotypically identical. In most cases of EATL, cytologic features of malignancy are straightforward. The cells are generally medium to large with abundant pale cytoplasm, but they may appear pleomorphic, immunoblastic, or even small. The malignant infiltrate involves the lamina propria and submucosa and may extend full thickness into the bowel wall (Fig. 19–20). There is usually an accompanying inflammatory infiltrate composed of eosinophils, plasma cells, and other inflammatory cells. Inflammatory mucosal erosions or ulcers are common. The uninvolved areas of the mucosa show characteristic villous atrophy of CD and intense intramucosal lymphocytosis, with distant spread from the dominant tumor mass. However, in some cases, the pathologic features of EATL may be extremely subtle, making it difficult to

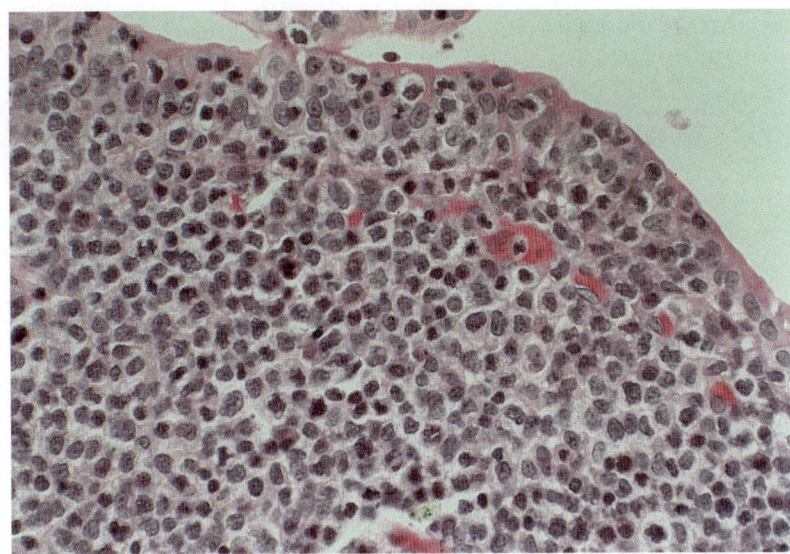

Figure 19–20. Enteropathy-associated T-cell lymphoma. Jejunal biopsy from a patient with celiac disease shows characteristic extensive intramucosal lymphoid infiltrate and intestinal villous atrophy. Cytologically malignant cells are medium to large with abundant cytoplasm.

distinguish EATL from ulcerative jejunitis, in which a tumor mass is absent and only the nonspecific, benign-appearing inflammatory ulcers, villous atrophy, and intraepithelial lymphocytes are present.

The lymphoid cells of both ulcerative jejunitis and EATL show a cytotoxic phenotype that approximates the phenotype of intraepithelial T-cells: they are CD3 positive, but negative for both CD4 and CD8. T-cell intracellular antigen (TIA-1), a cytotoxic granule antigen, is usually positive. The more anaplastic, large-cell variants of EATL may be CD30 positive. Molecular studies of EATL show monoclonal TCR gene rearrangements, and interestingly, monoclonal T cells can be detected in morphologically uninvolved mucosa (Wright, 1997). Monoclonal T-cell populations have been identified in cases of ulcerative jejunitis, in both involved and uninvolved normal mucosa. In cases where ulcerative jejunitis developed or progressed into EATL, the same clone was implicated (Ashton-Key et al., 1997), further suggesting that ulcerative jejunitis represents the benign, prelymphomatous manifestation of EATL.

Both benign and malignant complications of CD occur, although these can often be avoided by early diagnosis and compliance with a gluten-free diet (Murray, 1999). Ulcerative jejunitis shows a limited response to gluten-free diet and careful use of steroid

therapy; surgical resection of the ulcers can also be curative (Green et al., 1993). Nonresponsive CD, or complicated CD, and ulcerative jejunitis are at a higher risk of developing EATL (Carbonnel et al., 1998; Parnell and Ciclitira, 1999). The clinical course of EATL is quite aggressive, and the prognosis is quite poor. Spread to regional mesenteric lymph nodes is not uncommon at the time of diagnosis (Wright, 1997). Therapy for EATL is unsatisfactory; aggressive surgical and chemotherapeutic regimens are most recommended. Survival rates are very low: 1-year survival is 31% and 5-year survival is 11% (Egan et al., 1995).

LOCALIZED PAGETOID RETICULOSIS/WORINGER-KOLOPP DISEASE

Localized pagetoid reticulosis was first described by Woringer and Kolopp in 1939, with the description of a solitary lesion with epidermotropic lymphocytes on the foot of a 13-year-old boy (Woringer and Kolopp, 1939). Since then, the relationship between Woringer-Kolopp disease, or localized pagetoid reticulosis, and mycosis fungoides (MF) has been the subject of much debate as to whether they represent different ends of a spectrum of the same lymphoproliferative process (McNiff et al., 1998). The clinical and pathological features of Woringer-

Kolopp disease, as they are currently understood, suggest either a malignant tumor of low biologic aggressiveness, i.e., unilesional MF, or a benign tumor with a low rate of malignant transformation (pagetoid reticulosis) (Burns et al., 1995).

Woringer-Kolopp disease is rare and presents in younger patients (20% are <15 years) as slowly growing, localized, irregular, somewhat scaly to warty, nonpruritic erythematous plaques that are usually no more than 6 cm in diameter (Jones and Chu, 1981). The lesions typically occur in acral locations, including the palms and soles. The occurrence of histologically similar plaques in a more widespread or disseminated distribution has been called the *Ketron-Goodman variant of pagetoid reticulosis*, and it is unclear whether this variant represents a disseminated form of Woringer-Kolopp disease or a classic, evolving cutaneous T-cell lymphoma/MF (Lacour et al., 1986).

Morphologically, the lesions are indistinguishable from MF. They are characterized by an acanthotic hyperkeratotic epidermis with an infiltrate of enlarged, atypical-appearing mononuclear cells surrounded by a clear zone. The cells invade the epidermis singly or in small clusters. Conspicuous clear spaces around the cells impart a "pagetoid" appearance (Fig. 19–21). Mitotic figures may be present. Within the superficial dermis, a moderate lymphoid infiltrate with cytologic atypia usually accompanies the epidermotropism.

Immunophenotypically, the lymphocytes in Woringer-Kolopp disease show variable expression of T cell–associated antigens, with most cases being positive for CD4 and showing a lack of CD7 expression (Burns et al., 1995). CD8-positive cytotoxic T-cell phenotypes have been described (McNiff et al., 1998; Wood et al., 1988). Some lesions have reported monoclonal TCR gene rearrangements (Wood et al., 1988), particularly in cases manifesting primarily on the palms and soles, giving rise to speculation that these lesions represent a subset of cutaneous T-cell lymphomas of probably low biologic potential (Resnik et al., 1995). Indeed, the differential diagnosis includes early stages of MF, which can be quite problematic, since nearly identical histologic, phenotypic, and genotypic features can be seen in both lesions. Since Woringer-Kolopp disease repre-

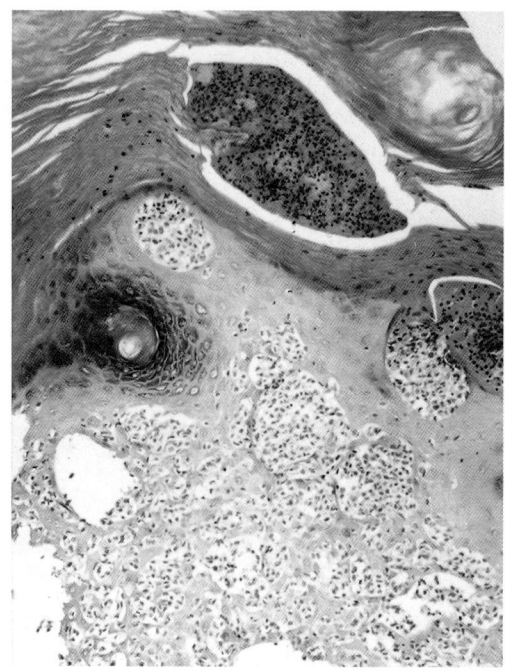

Figure 19–21. Woringer-Kolopp disease of the foot. Atypical lymphoid cells with cerebriform nuclear features extensively infiltrate the epidermis singly and in clusters. Conspicuous clear spaces around the cells impart a "pagetoid" appearance. The patient presented with an isolated lesion on the foot which was resected, but 2 years later the patient developed another, similar lesion on the opposite extremity. Morphologically, the lesion is indistinguishable from mycosis fungoides (MF), and most consider this variant to represent an early, isolated form of MF.

sents phenotypically aberrant T-cell lymphoproliferation in which monoclonality may be demonstrated, we regard these lesions as unilesional MF.

The distinction of Woringer-Kolopp disease from MF is based primarily on clinical grounds. The clinical course of Woringer-Kolopp disease is quite indolent, and the lesions generally remain localized, although this clinical picture is not entirely inconsistent with the course of early stages of MF. Spontaneous regression can occur (McNiff et al., 1998), and prolonged disease-free survival after simple surgical excisions and/or localized radiation is the rule, with rare local recurrences (Burns et al., 1995). Close clinical surveillance and conservative management are recommended.

Table 19–5. Clinicopathological Characteristics of Primary Cutaneous CD30-Positive Lymphoproliferative Disorders

	Lymphomatoid Papulosis	*Cutaneous Anaplastic Large-Cell Lymphoma*
Pathological features		
Depth of involvement	Superficial to deep dermal, sparing subcutis	Superficial to deep, with involvement of subcutis
Epidermotropism	Present	Absent
Inflammatory background	Rich in neutrophils, eosinophils, lymphocytes	Less obvious, neutrophils may be present
CD30$^+$ cells	Scattered	Many, sheeting out
Clinical features		
Lesions	Single, multiple to disseminated	Usually solitary
Spontaneous regression	Always	Usually not
Extracutaneous spread	<5%	Frequent

Adapted from Paulli et al. (1995).

PRIMARY CUTANEOUS CD30-POSITIVE LYMPHOPROLIFERATIVE DISORDERS

Primary cutaneous CD30-positive lymphoproliferative disorders represent a clinical and histologic continuum of a single disease process, ranging from completely benign lymphomatoid papulosis (LyP) to highly malignant primary cutaneous anaplastic large-cell lymphoma (CALCL) (Paulli et al., 1995) (Table 19–5). These disorders account for approximately 20% of all cutaneous T-cell lymphomas. There is a high association with secondary malignant lymphoma with LyP, including mycosis fungoides (Basarab et al., 1998), Hodgkin's disease, and anaplastic large cell lymphoma (LeBoit, 1996; Louvet et al., 1996).

These disorders affect all age-groups, with a peak incidence in the fifth decade of life and a slight male predilection (Paulli et al., 1995). Lymphomatoid papulosis may present as isolated or generalized cutaneous nodules, affecting the extremities, trunk, and/or face. In contrast, CALCL presents generally as a solitary mass (Louvet et al., 1996) and increased clinical evidence of extracutaneous involvement at the time of diagnosis (Fig. 19–22). Constitutional symptoms, or B symptoms, are generally not a feature of either LyP or CALCL, although they are more common in CALCL (Paulli et al., 1995).

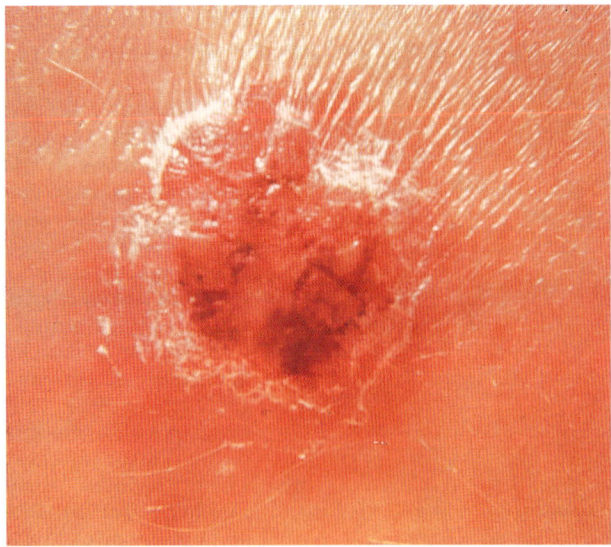

Figure 19–22. Clinical appearance of primary cutaneous anaplastic large cell lymphoma. The lesion appeared as a solitary skin nodule, and the patient subsequently developed regional lymph node involvement.

Morphologically, LyP occurs as perivascular or wedge-shaped dermal atypical lymphoid infiltrates, with sparing of the underlying subcutis. There is considerable variation in the cytologic appearance of the atypical cells, including immunoblasts, Reed-Sternberg cells, or highly pleomorphic cells. The atypical cells usually account for only a minority of the cells in the infiltrate. Ulceration of the overlying epidermis is a common and helpful feature (Fig. 19–23). Lymphomatoid papulosis contains two major histological subtypes, and patients may present with predominantly one type of lesion or a mixture of both types (LeBoit, 1996). Type A, the most common form, resembles morphologically Hodgkin's disease, is generally nonepidermotropic, and contains large immunoblasts that often resemble Reed-Sternberg cells. Mitoses are frequently observed. A rich, mixed inflammatory infiltrate usually accompanies the atypical cells and is composed of neutrophils, eosinophils, and small lymphocytes.

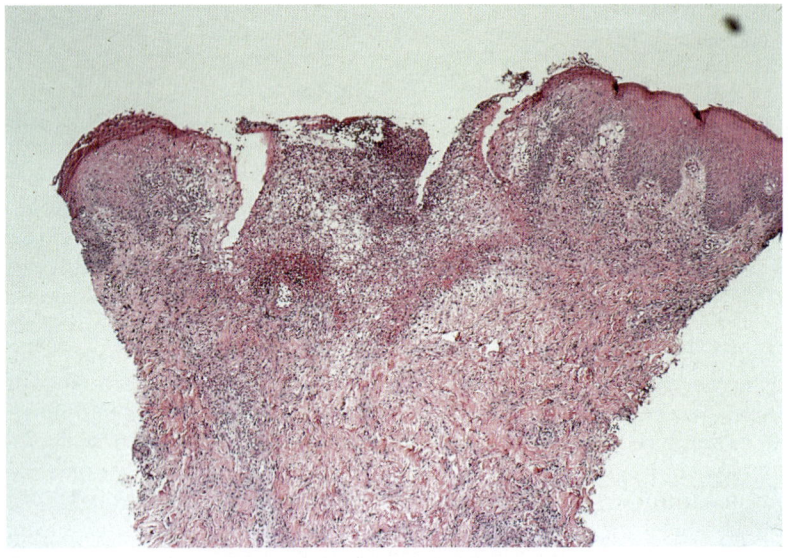

A

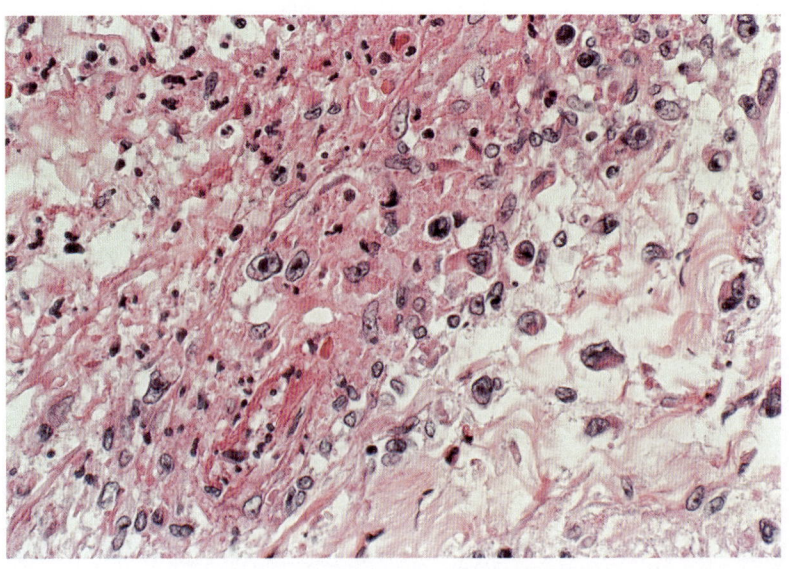

B

Figure 19–23. Lymphomatoid papulosis. *A:* The epidermis shows ulceration, and the superficial dermis contains a superficial to mid-dermal infiltrate with scattered large, pleomorphic, lymphoid cells within a rich inflammatory background. *B:* The atypical cells make up only a minority of the cellular infiltrate, which includes small lymphocytes, neutrophils, and eosinophils.

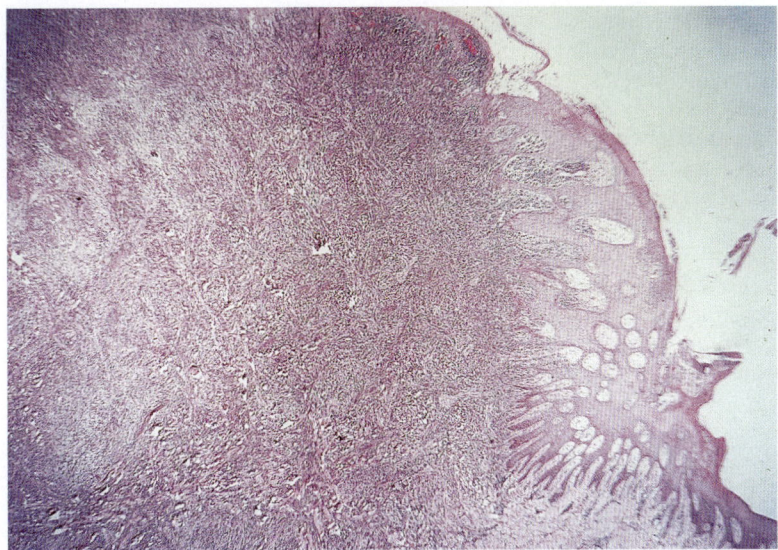

A

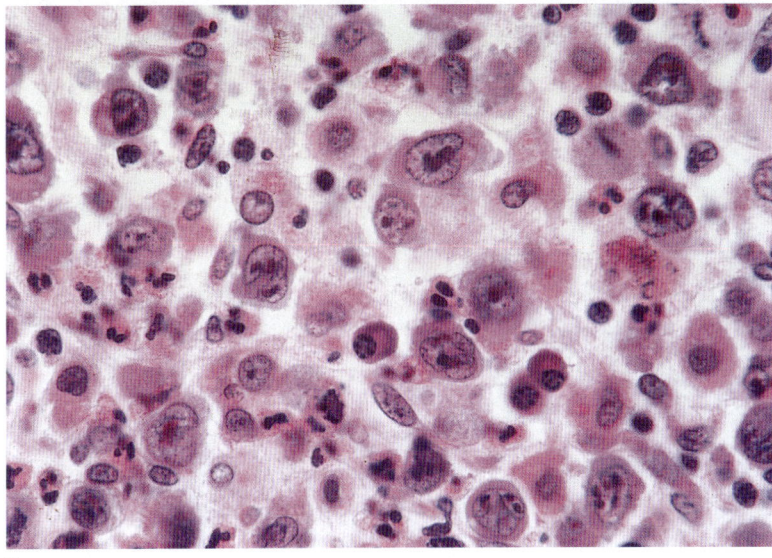

B

Figure 19–24. Primary cutaneous anaplastic large cell lymphoma. *A:* The epidermis shows pseudoepitheliomatous hyperplasia, while the dermis contains a dense cellular infiltrate extending into the deep subcutaneous tissue. *B:* Markedly pleomorphic cells are admixed with lymphocytes, plasma cells, and neutrophils. The atypical cells have abundant amphophilic cytoplasm, and the large vesicular nuclei contain prominent nucleoli. The prominent inflammatory background presents difficulty in the differential diagnosis with lymphomatoid papulosis.

Type B lesions more closely resemble mycosis fungoides and are more epidermotropic with prominent exocytosis of atypical lymphocytes with cerebriform-like nuclei. A mixed inflammatory background is less prominent, and mitoses are less frequent.

In contrast to LyP, CALCL lesions extend deep into the underlying subcutis and usually spare the overlying epidermis. While the malignant cells resemble those seen in LyP lesions, they are more numerous and form sheets, accounting for the majority of cells within the infiltrate (Fig. 19–24). The inflammatory infiltrate is generally confined to the periphery of the lesions. However, considerable borderline overlap exists in the histologic features between LyP and CALCL, making the distinction between LyP and CALCL exceedingly difficult.

The use of ancillary phenotypic and genotypic studies are generally of little value in distinguishing LyP from CALCL. The immunophenotype of the malignant cells seen in both LyP and CALCL is activated helper

T cells with an aberrant phenotype: they express CD4 and lack CD7, although approximately 20% of cases lack T cell–associated antigen expression (LeBoit, 1996). By definition, the malignant cells are CD30 positive; they are usually CD15 and EMA negative. Clonal TCR gene rearrangements can be detected in both LyP and CALCL, and the same clone is generally present in multiple regressing skin lesions. Associated T-cell lymphomas (MF and ALCL) are clonally related in most LyP patients, which suggest that the disease in these patients was initiated by a nonrandom genetic event (Chott et al., 1996; Davis et al., 1992). Various chromosomal abnormalities may be seen, including trisomy 7 and partial deletions of chromosome 10 (Peters et al., 1995). However, the t(2:5) translocation characteristic of nodal anaplastic large-cell lymphomas is absent (DeCoteau et al., 1996). As a result, the NPM:ALK fusion gene product cannot be detected immunohistochemically, thus distinguishing it from systemic ALCL. There is also no indication of EBV (Kadin et al., 1993).

The differential diagnosis of cutaneous CD30-positive LPD includes extranodal involvement of Hodgkin's disease (HD). There may be a striking resemblance to HD when the malignant cells are morphologically and immunophenotypically consistent with Reed-Sternberg cells, especially in the presence of a mixed inflammatory background. However, cutaneous manifestations of HD are extremely rare (Kumar et al., 1996), particularly in the absence of regional nodal disease, and usually represent direct extension from involved lymph nodes (Smith and Butler, 1980). Thus, a diagnosis of cutaneous HD should be made with caution, and only with evidence of nodal disease.

The distinction between LyP and CALCL is extremely important since the two processes may have vastly different clinical outcomes and treatment modalities. Spontaneous regression and self-healing lesions are very helpful characteristic and distinguishing features of LyP, which are less often observed in CALCL. LyP usually pursues a benign, indolent clinical course of recurrent skin nodules over many years, irrespective of the histologic variant. Progression to lymphoma occurs in 10%–20% of patients

(Louvet et al., 1996). Extracutaneous spread is rare in LyP, whereas it occurs in 25%–40% of patients with CALCL (Beljaards et al., 1993; Louvet et al., 1996), in which the development of extracutaneous disease is indicative of a more aggressive clinical course (Paulli et al., 1995). When CALCL is confined to the skin, localized radiation therapy is effective (Kaufmann et al., 1997). However, survival of patients with CALCL having extracutaneous disease following aggressive chemotherapy is still significantly better than for other cutaneous T-cell lymphomas (Beljaards et al., 1993).

REFERENCES

Abruzzo LV, Schmidt K, Weiss LM, Jaffe ES, Medeiros LJ, Sander CA, Raffeld M. (1993) B-cell lymphoma after angioimmunoblastic lymphadenopathy: a case with oligoclonal gene rearrangements associated with Epstein-Barr virus. *Blood* 82:241–246.

Alter HJ, Purcell RH, Shih JW, Melpolder JC, Houghton M, Choo QL, Kuo G. (1989) Detection of antibody to hepatitis C virus in prospectively followed transfusion recipients with acute and chronic non-A, non-B hepatitis. *N Engl J Med* 321:1494–1500.

Anagnostopoulos I, Hummel M, Finn T, Tiemann M, Korbjuhn P, Dimmler C, Gatter K, Dallenbach F, Parwaresch M, Stein H. (1992) Heterogeneous Epstein-Barr virus infection patterns in peripheral T-cell lymphoma of angioimmunoblastic lymphadenopathy type. *Blood* 80;1804–1812.

Anaya JM, McGuff HS, Banks PM, Talal N. (1996) Clinicopathological factors relating malignant lymphoma with Sjogren's syndrome. *Semin Arthritis Rheum* 25:337–346.

Araki A, Taniguchi M, Mikata A. (1994) T cell receptor V beta repertoires of angioimmunoblastic lymphadenopathy-like T cell lymphoma. *Leuk Lymphoma* 16:135–140.

Ascoli V, Lo Coco F, Artini M, Levrero M, Martelli M, Negro F. (1998) Extranodal lymphomas associated with hepatitis C virus infection [see comments]. *Am J Clin Pathol* 109:600–609.

Ashton-Key M, Diss TC, Pan L, Du MQ, Isaacson PG. (1997) Molecular analysis of T-cell clonality in ulcerative jejunitis and enteropathy-associated T-cell lymphoma. *Am J Pathol* 151:493–498.

Baldini L, Guffanti A, Cesana BM, Colombi M, Chiorboli O, Damilano I, Maiolo AT. (1996) Role of different hematologic variables in defining the risk of malignant transformation in monoclonal gammopathy. *Blood* 87:912–918.

Ballerini P, Gaidano G, Gong JZ, Tassi V, Saglio G, Knowles DM, Dalla-Favera R. (1993) Multiple genetic lesions in acquired immunodeficiency syndrome-related non-Hodgkin's lymphoma. *Blood* 81:166–176.

Banks PM, Isaacson PG. (1999) MALT lymphomas in 1997. Where do we stand? *Am J Clin Pathol* 111(1 Suppl. 1):S75–S83.

Basarab T, Fraser-Andrews EA, Orchard G, Whittaker S, Russel-Jones R. (1998) Lymphomatoid papulosis in association with mycosis fungoides: a study of 15 cases. *Br J Dermatol* 139:630–638.

Bataille R, Sany J. (1981) Solitary myeloma: clinical and prognostic features of a review of 114 cases. *Cancer* 48:845–851.

Beljaards RC, Kaudewitz P, Berti E, Gianotti R, Neumann C, Rosso R, Paulli M, Meijer CJ, Willemze R. (1993) Primary cutaneous CD30-positive large cell lymphoma: definition of a new type of cutaneous lymphoma with a favorable prognosis. A European Multicenter Study of 47 patients. *Cancer* 71:2097–2104.

Bellentani S, Pozzato G, Saccoccio G, Crovatto M, Croce LS, Mazzoran L, Masutti F, Cristianini G, Tiribelli C. (1999) Clinical course and risk factors of hepatitis C virus related liver disease in the general population: report from the Dionysos study. *Gut* 44:874–880.

Ben-Ayed F, Halphen M, Najjar T, Boussene H, Jaafoura H, Bouguerra A, Ben Salah N, Mourali N, Ayed K, Ben Khalifa H, et al. (1989) Treatment of alpha chain disease. Results of a prospective study in 21 Tunisian patients by the Tunisian-French intestinal Lymphoma Study Group. *Cancer* 63:1251–1256.

Beral V, Peterman T, Berkelman R, Jaffe H. (1991) AIDS-associated non-Hodgkin lymphoma [see comments]. *Lancet* 337(8745):805–809.

Berinstein NL, Jamal HH, Kuzniar B, Klock RJ, Reis MD. (1993) Sensitive and reproducible detection of occult disease in patients with follicular lymphoma by PCR amplification of t(14;18) both pre- and post-treatment. *Leukemia* 7:113–119.

Biemer JJ. (1990) Malignant lymphomas associated with immunodeficiency states. *Ann Clin Lab Sci* 20:175–191.

Bowne WB, Lewis JJ, Filippa DA, Niesvizky R, Brooks AD, Burt ME, Brennan MF. (1999) The management of unicentric and multicentric Castleman's disease: a report of 16 cases and a review of the literature. *Cancer* 85:706–717.

Burke JS. (1999) Are there site-specific differences among the MALT lymphomas—morphologic, clinical? *Am J Clin Pathol* 111 (1 Suppl 1):S133–S143.

Burns BF, Colby TV, Dorfman RF. (1984) Differential diagnostic features of nodular L & H Hodgkin's disease, including progressive transformation of germinal centers. *Am J Surg Pathol* 8:253–261.

Burns MK, Chan LS, Cooper KD. (1995) Woringer-Kolopp disease (localized pagetoid reticulosis) or unilesional mycosis fungoides? An analysis of eight cases with benign disease. *Arch Dermatol* 131:325–329.

Callan MF, Steven N, Krausa P, Wilson JD, Moss PA, Gillespie GM, Bell JI, Rickinson AB, McMichael AJ. (1996) Large clonal expansions of CD8+ T cells in acute infectious mononucleosis. *Nat Med* 2:906–911.

Cammoun M, Jaafoura H, Tabbane F, Halphen M. (1989) Immunoproliferative small intestinal disease without alpha-chain disease: a pathological study. *Gastroenterology* 96:750–763.

Carbonnel F, Grollet-Bioul L, Brouet JC, Teilhac MF, Cosnes J, Angonin R, Deschaseaux M, Chatelet FP, Gendre JP, Sigaux F. (1998) Are complicated forms of celiac disease cryptic T-cell lymphomas? *Blood* 92:3879–3886.

Castleman B, Iverson L, Menendez V. (1956) Localized mediastinal lymph-node hyperplasia resembling thymoma. *Cancer* 9:822–830.

Cesarman E, Knowles DM. (1997) Kaposi's sarcoma–associated herpesvirus: a lymphotropic human herpesvirus associated with Kaposi's sarcoma, primary effusion lymphoma, and multicentric Castleman's disease [published erratum appears in *Semin Diagn Pathol* (1997) 14:161–162]. *Semin Diagn Pathol* 14:54–66.

Cesarman E, Knowles DM. (1999) The role of Kaposi's sarcoma–associated herpesvirus (KSHV/HHV-8) in lymphoproliferative diseases. *Semin Cancer Biol* 9:165–174.

Chadburn A, Athan E, Wieczorek R, Knowles D. (1991) Detection and characterization of HTLV-I associated T neoplasms in an HTLV-I non-endemic region by polymerase chain reaction. *Blood* 70:1500–1508.

Chadburn A, Cesarman E, Knowles DM. (1997) Molecular pathology of posttransplantation lymphoproliferative disorders. *Semin Diagn Pathol* 14:15–26.

Chadburn A, Cesarman E, Liu YF, Addonizio L, Hsu D, Michler RE, Knowles DM. (1995) Molecular genetic analysis demonstrates that multiple posttransplantation lymphoproliferative disorders occurring in one anatomic site in a single patient represent distinct primary lymphoid neoplasms. *Cancer* 75:2747–2756.

Chan JK. (1999) Peripheral T-cell and NK-cell neoplasms: an integrated approach to diagnosis. *Mod Pathol* 12:177–199.

Chatlynne LG, Ablashi DV. (1999) Seroepidemiology of Kaposi's sarcoma–associated herpesvirus (KSHV). *Semin Cancer Biol* 9:175–185.

Chilosi M, Menestrina F, Lestani M, Bonetti F, Scarpa A, Caligaris-Cappio F, Pizzolo G, Perini A, Fiore-Donati L. (1987) Hyaline-vascular type of Castleman's disease (angiofollicular lymph node hyperplasia) with monotypic plasma cells. An immunohistochemical study with monoclonal antibodies. *Histol Histopathol* 2:49–55.

Chott A, Vonderheid EC, Olbricht S, Miao NN, Balk SP, Kadin ME. (1996) The dominant T cell clone is present in multiple regressing skin lesions and associated T cell lymphomas of patients with lymphomatoid papulosis. *J Invest Dermatol* 106:696–700.

Cleary ML, Nalesnik MA, Shearer WT, Sklar J. (1988) Clonal analysis of transplant-associated lymphoproliferations based on the structure of the genomic termini of the Epstein-Barr virus. *Blood* 72:349–352.

Cleary ML, Warnke R, Sklar J. (1984) Monoclonality of lymphoproliferative lesions in cardiac-transplant recipients. Clonal analysis based on immunoglobulin-gene rearrangements. *N Engl J Med* 310:477–482.

Cossman J, Uppenkamp M, Sundeen J, et al. (1988) Molecular genetics and the diagnosis of lymphoma. *Arch J Pathol* 134:117–127.

Covacci A, Telford JL, Del Giudice G, Parsonnet J, Rappuoli R. (1999) *Helicobacter pylori* virulence and genetic geography. *Science* 284(5418):1328–1333.

Dammacco F, Gatti P, Sansonno D. (1998) Hepatitis C virus infection, mixed cryoglobulinemia, and non-Hodgkin's lymphoma: an emerging picture. *Leuk Lymphoma* 31:463–476.

Davis TH, Morton CC, Miller-Cassman R, Balk SP, Kadin ME. (1992) Hodgkin's disease, lymphomatoid papulosis, and cutaneous T-cell lymphoma derived from a common T-cell clone. *N Engl J Med* 326:1115–1122.

DeCoteau JF, Butmarc JR, Kinney MC, Kadin ME. (1996) The t(2;5) chromosomal translocation is not a common feature of primary cutaneous CD30+ lymphoproliferative disorders: comparison with anaplastic large-cell lymphoma of nodal origin [see comments]. *Blood* 87:3437–3441.

de The G. (1995) Viruses and human cancers: challenges for preventive strategies. *Environ Health Perspect* 103 Suppl 8:269–273.

Diss TC, Peng H, Wotherspoon AC, Pan L, Speight PM, Isaacson PG. (1993) Brief report: a single neoplastic clone in sequential biopsy specimens from a patient with primary gastric-mucosa-associated lymphoid-tissue lymphoma and Sjogren's syndrome [see comments]. *N Engl J Med* 329:172–175.

Dolken G, Illerhaus G, Hirt C, Mertelsmann R. (1996) BCL-2/JH rearrangements in circulating B cells of healthy blood donors and patients with nonmalignant diseases. *J Clin Oncol* 14:1333–1344.

Drach J, Angerler J, Schuster J, Rothermundt C, Thalhammer R, Haas OA, Jager U, Fiegl M, Geissler K, Ludwig H, et al. (1995) Interphase fluorescence in situ hybridization identifies chromosomal abnormalities in plasma cells from patients with monoclonal gammopathy of undetermined significance. *Blood* 86:3915–3921.

Du M, Diss TC, Xu C, Peng H, Isaacson PG, Pan L. (1996) Ongoing mutation in MALT lymphoma immunoglobulin gene suggests that antigen stimulation plays a role in the clonal expansion. *Leukemia* 10:1190–1197.

Du MQ, Isaacson PG. (1998) Recent advances in our understanding of the biology and pathogenesis of gastric mucosa–associated lymphoid tissue (MALT) lymphoma. *Forum (Genova)* 8:162–173.

Dworak O, Tschubel K, Zhou H, Meybehm M. (1988) Angiofollikuläre lymphatische Hyperplasie mit Plasmozytom und Polyneuropathie: Ein Fallbericht mit immunohistochemischer Untersachung. *Klin Wochenschr* 66:591–595.

Egan LJ, Walsh SV, Stevens FM, Connolly CE, Egan EL, McCarthy CF. (1995) Celiac-associated lymphoma. A single institution experience of 30 cases in the combination chemotherapy era. *J Clin Gastroenterol* 21:123–129.

Eidelman S, Parkins R, Rubin CE. (1966) Abdominal lymphoma presenting as malabsorption. A clinicopathologic study of nine cases in Israel and a review of the literature. *Medicine* 45:111–137.

Elenitoba-Johnson KS, Jaffe ES. (1997) Lymphoproliferative disorders associated with congenital immunodeficiencies. *Semin Diagn Pathol* 14:35–47.

Ellman MH, Hurwitz H, Thomas C, Kozloff M. (1991) Lymphoma developing in a patient with rheumatoid arthritis taking low dose weekly methotrexate [see comments]. *J Rheumatol* 18:1741–1743.

Fallone CA. (1999) Determinants of ethnic or geographical differences in infectivity and transmissibility of *Helicobacter pylori*. *Can J Gastroenterol* 13: 251–255.

Fasano A. (1996) Where have all the American celiacs gone? *Acta Paediatr Suppl* 412:20–24.

Feller A, Griesser H, Schilling C, Wacker H, Dallenbach F, Bartels H, Kuse R, Mak T, Lennert K. (1988) Clonal gene rearrangement patterns correlate with immunophenotype and clinical parameters in patients with angioimmunoblastic lymphadenopathy. *Am J Pathol* 133:549–556.

Ferri C, La Civita L, Longombardo G, Zignego AL,

Pasero G. (1998) Mixed cryoglobulinaemia: a crossroad between autoimmune and lymphoproliferative disorders. *Lupus* 7:275–279.

Ferri C, Monti M, La Civita L, Longombardo G, Greco F, Pasero G, Gentilini P, Bombardieri S, Zignego AL. (1993) Infection of peripheral blood mononuclear cells by hepatitis C virus in mixed cryoglobulinemia. *Blood* 82:3701–3704.

Ferry JA, Zukerberg LR, Harris NL. (1992) Florid progressive transformation of germinal centers. A syndrome affecting young men, without early progression to nodular lymphocyte predominance Hodgkin's disease. *Am J Surg Pathol* 16:252–258.

Filipovich AH, Mathur A, Kamat D, Shapiro RS. (1992) Primary immunodeficiencies: genetic risk factors for lymphoma. *Cancer Res* 52 (19 Suppl):5465s–5467s.

Fine KD, Stone MJ. (1999) Alpha-heavy chain disease, Mediterranean lymphoma, and immunoproliferative small intestinal disease: a review of clinicopathological features, pathogenesis, and differential diagnosis. *Am J Gastroenterol* 94:1139–1152.

Finke J, Slanina J, Lange W, Dolken G. (1993) Persistence of circulating t(14;18)-positive cells in long-term remission after radiation therapy for localized-stage follicular lymphoma. *J Clin Oncol* 11:1668–1673.

Franchini G. (1995) Molecular mechanisms of human T-cell leukemia/lymphotropic virus type I infection. *Blood* 86:3619–3639.

Franzin F, Efremov DG, Pozzato G, Tulissi P, Batista F, Burrone OR. (1995) Clonal B-cell expansions in peripheral blood of HCV-infected patients. *Br J Haematol* 90:548–552.

Frassica DA, Frassica FJ, Schray MF, Sim FH, Kyle RA. (1989) Solitary plasmacytoma of bone: Mayo Clinic experience. *Int J Radiat Oncol Biol Phys* 16:43–48.

Frizzera G, Kaneko Y, Sakurai M. (1989) Angioimmunoblastic lymphadenopathy and related disorders: a retrospective look in search of definitions. *Leukemia* 3:1–5.

Frizzera G, Moran EM, Rappaport H. (1974) Angioimmunoblastic lymphadenopathy with dysproteinaemia. *Lancet* 1(7866):1070–1073.

Frizzera G, Peterson BA, Bayrd ED, Goldman A. (1985) A systemic lymphoproliferative disorder with morphologic features of Castleman's disease: clinical findings and clinicopathologic correlations in 15 patients. *J Clin Oncol* 3:1202–1216.

Gaba AR, Stein RS, Sweet DL, Variakojis D. (1978) Multicentric giant lymph node hyperplasia. *Am J Clin Pathol* 69:86–90.

Galieni P, Polito E, Leccisotti A, Marotta G, Lasi S, Bigazzi C, Bucalossi A, Frezza G, Lauria F. (1997) Localized orbital lymphoma. *Haematologica* 82:436–439.

Garnier JL, Cooper NR, Cannon MJ. (1993) Low expression of CD20 and CD23 in Epstein-Barr virus-induced B cell tumors in SCID/hu mice. *Am J Pathol* 142:353–358.

Georgescu L, Quinn GC, Schwartzman S, Paget SA. (1997) Lymphoma in patients with rheumatoid arthritis: association with the disease state or methotrexate treatment [see comments]. *Semin Arthritis Rheum* 26:794–804.

Green JA, Barkin JS, Gregg PA, Kohen K. (1993) Ulcerative jejunitis in refractory celiac disease: enteroscopic visualization. *Gastrointest Endosc* 39:584–585.

Griesser H, Feller A, Lennert K, Minden M, Mak TW. (1986) Rearrangement of the beta chain of the T cell antigen receptor and immunoglobulin genes in lymphoproliferative disorders. *J Clin Invest* 78: 1179–1184.

Guindi M. (1999) Role of *Helicobacter pylori* in the pathogenesis of gastric carcinoma and progression of lymphoid nodules to lymphoma. *Can J Gastroenterol* 13:224–227.

Guinee DJ, Jaffe E, Kingma D, Fishback N, Wallberg K, Krishnan J, Frizzera G, Travis W, Koss M. (1994) Pulmonary lymphomatoid granulomatosis. Evidence for a proliferation of Epstein-Barr virus infected B-lymphocytes with a prominent T-cell component and vasculitis. *Am J Surg Pathol* 18:753–764.

Halphen M, Najjar T, Jaafoura H, Cammoun M, Tufrali G. (1986) Diagnostic value of upper intestinal fiber endoscopy in primary small intestinal lymphoma. A prospective study by the Tunisian-French Intestinal Lymphoma Group. *Cancer* 58:2140–2145.

Hansmann ML, Fellbaum C, Hui PK, Moubayed P. (1990) Progressive transformation of germinal centers with and without association to Hodgkin's disease. *Am J Clin Pathol* 93:219–226.

Hanson CA, Frizzera G, Patton DF, Peterson BA, McClain KL, Gajl-Peczalska KJ, Kersey JH. (1988) Clonal rearrangement for immunoglobulin and T-cell receptor genes in systemic Castleman's disease. Association with Epstein-Barr virus. *Am J Pathol* 131:84–91.

Harris NL. (1999) Lymphoid proliferations of the salivary glands. *Am J Clin Pathol* 111 (1 Suppl 1):S94–S103.

Harris NL, Ferry JA, Swerdlow SH. (1997) Posttransplant lymphoproliferative disorders: summary of Society for Hematopathology Workshop. *Semin Diagn Pathol* 14:8–14.

Harris NL, Jaffe ES, Stein H, Banks PM, Chan JK, Cleary ML, Delsol G, De Wolf Peeters C, Falini B, Gatter KC, et al. (1994) A revised European-American classification of lymphoid neoplasms: a proposal from the International Lymphoma Study Group [see comments]. *Blood* 84:1361–1392.

Herrada J, Cabanillas F, Rice L, Manning J, Pugh W. (1998) The clinical behavior of localized and multicentric Castleman disease. *Ann Intern Med* 128: 657–662.

Hino S. (1989) Milk-borne transmission of HTLV-I as a major route in the endemic cycle. *Acta Paediatr Jpn* 31:428–435.

Hisada M, Okayama A, Shioiri S, Spiegelman DL, Stuver SO, Mueller NE. (1998) Risk factors for adult T-cell leukemia among carriers of human T-lymphotropic virus type I. *Blood* 92:3557–3561.

Holland J, Trenkner DA, Wasserman TH, Fineberg B. (1992) Plasmacytoma. Treatment results and conversion to myeloma. *Cancer* 69:1513–1517.

Holm LE, Blomgren H, Lowhagen T. (1985) Cancer risks in patients with chronic lymphocytic thyroiditis. *N Engl J Med* 312:601–604.

Holmes GK, Prior P, Lane MR, Pope D, Allan RN. (1989) Malignancy in coeliac disease—effect of a gluten free diet. *Gut* 30:333–338.

Hotz MA, Schwaab G, Bosq J, Munck JN. (1999) Extramedullary solitary plasmacytoma of the head and neck. A clinicopathological study. *Ann Otol Rhinol Laryngol* 108:495–500.

Hsi ED, Greenson JK, Singleton TP, Siddiqui J, Schnitzer B, Ross CW. (1996a) Detection of immunoglobulin heavy chain gene rearrangement by polymerase chain reaction in chronic active gastritis associated with *Helicobacter pylori*. *Hum Pathol* 27:290–296.

Hsi ED, Siddiqui J, Schnitzer B, Alkan S, Ross CW. (1996b) Analysis of immunoglobulin heavy chain gene rearrangement in myoepithelial sialadenitis by polymerase chain reaction. *Am J Clin Pathol* 106:498–503.

Hsi ED, Singleton TP, Svoboda SM, Schnitzer B, Ross CW. (1998) Characterization of the lymphoid infiltrate in Hashimoto thyroiditis by immunohistochemistry and polymerase chain reaction for immunoglobulin heavy chain gene rearrangement. *Am J Clin Pathol* 110:327–333.

Hyjek E, Isaacson PG. (1988) Primary B cell lymphoma of the thyroid and its relationship to Hashimoto's thyroiditis. *Hum Pathol* 19:1315–1326.

Hyjek E, Smith WJ, Isaacson PG. (1988) Primary B-cell lymphoma of salivary glands and its relationship to myoepithelial sialadenitis. *Hum Pathol* 19:766–776.

Ioachim HL, Dorsett B, Cronin W, Maya M, Wahl S. (1991) Acquired immunodeficiency syndrome–associated lymphomas: clinical, pathologic, immunologic, and viral characteristics of 111 cases. *Hum Pathol* 22:659–673.

Isaacson P, Spencer J. (1994) Autoimmunity and malignancy. In: *Autoimmune Diseases: Focus on Sjogren's Syndrome* (Isenberg DA, Horsfall AC, eds.) pp. 189–204. Oxford, BIOS Scientific Publishers.

Isaacson P, Wright DH. (1983) Malignant lymphoma of mucosa-associated lymphoid tissue. A distinctive type of B-cell lymphoma. *Cancer* 52:1410–1416.

Isaacson P, Wright DH. (1984) Extranodal malignant lymphoma arising from mucosa-associated lymphoid tissue. *Cancer* 53:2515–2524.

Isaacson PG. (1999a) Gastrointestinal lymphomas of T- and B-cell types. *Mod Pathol* 12:151–158.

Isaacson PG. (1999b) Mucosa-associated lymphoid tissue lymphoma. *Semin Hematol* 36:139–147.

Jaffe ES. (1995a) Adult T-cell leukemia/lymphoma. In: *Surgical Pathology of the Lymph Nodes and Related Organs*, Vol. 16 (Livolsi VA, ed.) pp. 367–374. W.B. Saunders, Philadelphia.

Jaffe ES. (1995b) Angioimmunoblastic T-cell lymphoma: new insights, but the clinical challenge remains [editorial]. *Ann Oncol* 6:631–632.

Jaffe ES. (1999) Hematopathology: integration of morphologic features and biologic markers for diagnosis. *Mod Pathol* 12:109–115.

Jaffe ES, Blattner WA, Blayney DW, Bunn PA, Cossman J, Robert-Guroff M, Gallo RC. (1984) The pathologic spectrum of adult T-cell leukemia/lymphoma in the United States. *Am J Surg Pathol* 8:263–275.

Jaffe ES, Harris NL, Diebold J, Muller-Hermelink HK. (1999) World Health Organization classification of neoplastic diseases of the hematopoietic and lymphoid tissues. A progress report. *Am J Clin Pathol* 111 (1 Suppl 1):S8–12.

Jaffe ES, Lifford EH, Margolick JB, Longo DL, Fauci AS. (1989) Lymphomatoid granulomatosis and angiocentric lymphoma: a spectrum of post-thymic T-cell proliferations. *Semin Respir Med* 10:167–172.

Jaffe ES, Wilson WH. (1997) Lymphomatoid granulomatosis: pathogenesis, pathology and clinical implications. *Cancer Surv* 30:233–248.

Joncas JH, Russo P, Brochu P, Simard P, Brisebois J, Dube J, Marton D, Leclerc JM, Hume H, Rivard GE. (1990) Epstein-Barr virus polymorphic B-cell lymphoma associated with leukemia and with congenital immunodeficiencies [see comments]. *J Clin Oncol* 8:378–384.

Jones D, Jorgensen JL, Shahsafaei A, Dorfman DM. (1998) Characteristic proliferations of reticular and dendritic cells in angioimmunoblastic lymphoma. *Am J Surg Pathol* 22:956–964.

Jones RR, Chu A. (1981) Pagetoid reticulosis and solitary mycosis fungoides. Distinct clinicopathological entities. *J Cutan Pathol* 8:40–51.

Jonsson V, Wiik A, Hou-Jensen K, Christiansen M, Ryder LP, Madsen HO, Geisler C, Hansen MM, Thomsen K, Vorstrup S, Svejgaard A. (1999) Autoimmunity and extranodal lymphocytic infiltrates in lymphoproliferative disorders. *J Intern Med* 245:277–286.

Kadin ME, Vonderheid EC, Weiss LM. (1993) Absence of Epstein-Barr viral RNA in lymphomatoid papulosis. *J Pathol* 170:145–148.

Kamel OW. (1997) Iatrogenic lymphoproliferative disorders in nontransplantation settings. *Semin Diagn Pathol* 14:27–34.

Kamel OW, van de Rijn M, Hanasono MM, Warnke RA. (1995) Immunosuppression-associated lymphoproliferative disorders in rheumatic patients. *Leuk Lymphoma* 16:363–368.

Kamel OW, van, de, Rijn, M, Weiss LM, Del ZG, Hench PK, Robbins BA, Montgomery PG, Warnke RA, Dorfman RF. (1993) Brief report: reversible lymphomas associated with Epstein-Barr virus occurring during methotrexate therapy for rheumatoid arthritis and dermatomyositis [see comments]. *N Engl J Med* 328:1317–1321.

Kamel OW, Weiss LM, van de Rijn M, Colby TV, Kingma DW, Jaffe ES. (1996) Hodgkin's disease and lymphoproliferations resembling Hodgkin's disease in patients receiving long-term low-dose methotrexate therapy. *Am J Surg Pathol* 20:1279–1287.

Kassan S, Thomas T, Moutsopoulos H, Hoover R, Kimberly R, Budman D, Costa J, Decker J, Chused T. (1979) Increased risk of lymphoma in sicca syndrome. *Ann Int Med* 89:888–892.

Katzenstein AL, Carrington CB, Liebow AA. (1979) Lymphomatoid granulomatosis: a clinicopathologic study of 152 cases. *Cancer* 43:360–373.

Katzin WE, Fishleder AJ, Tubbs RR. (1989) Investigation of the clonality of lymphocytes in Hashimoto's thyroiditis using immunoglobulin and T-cell receptor gene probes. *Clin Immunol Immunopathol* 51:264–274.

Kaufmann TP, Coleman M, Nisce LZ. (1997) Ki-1 skin lymphoproliferative disorders: management with radiation therapy. *Cancer Invest* 15:91–97.

Kawano F, Yamaguchi K, Nishimura H, Tsuda H, Takatsuki K. (1985) Variation in the clinical courses of adult T-cell leukemia. *Cancer* 55:851–856.

Knecht H, Martius F, Bachmann E, Hoffman T, Zimmermann DR, Rothenberger S, Sandvej K, Wegmann W, Hurwitz N, Odermatt BF, et al. (1995) A deletion mutant of the LMP1 oncogene of Epstein-Barr virus is associated with evolution of angioimmunoblastic lymphadenopathy into B immunoblastic lymphoma. *Leukemia* 9:458–465.

Knowles DM. (1997) Molecular pathology of acquired immunodeficiency syndrome–related non-Hodgkin's lymphoma. *Semin Diagn Pathol* 14:67–82.

Knowles DM. (1999) Immunodeficiency-associated lymphoproliferative disorders. *Mod Pathol* 12:200–217.

Knowles DM, Cesarman E, Chadburn A, Frizzera G, Chen J, Rose EA, Michler RE. (1995) Correlative morphologic and molecular genetic analysis demonstrates three distinct categories of posttransplantation lymphoproliferative disorders. *Blood* 85:552–565.

Knowles DM, Chamulak GA, Subar M, Burke JS, Dugan M, Wernz J, Slywotzky C, Pelicci G, Dalla-Favera R, Raphael B. (1988) Lymphoid neoplasia associated with the acquired immunodeficiency syndrome (AIDS). The New York University Medical Center experience with 105 patients (1981–1986). *Ann Intern Med* 108:744–753.

Koss MN, Hochholzer L, Langloss JM, Wehunt WD, Lazarus AA, Nichols PW. (1986) Lymphomatoid granulomatosis: a clinicopathologic study of 42 patients. *Pathology* 18:283–288.

Koulis A, Diss T, Isaacson PG, Dogan A. (1997) Characterization of tumor-infiltrating T lymphocytes in B-cell lymphomas of mucosa-associated lymphoid tissue. *Am J Pathol* 151:1353–1360.

Kumar S, Kingma DW, Weiss WB, Raffeld M, Jaffe ES. (1996) Primary cutaneous Hodgkin's disease with evolution to systemic disease. Association with the Epstein-Barr virus. *Am J Surg Pathol* 20:754–759.

Kuppers R, Zhao M, Hansmann ML, Rajewsky K. (1993) Tracing B cell development in human germinal centres by molecular analysis of single cells picked from histological sections. *EMBO J* 12:4955–4967.

Kyle RA. (1993) "Benign" monoclonal gammopathy—after 20 to 35 years of follow-up. *Mayo Clin Proc* 68:26–36.

Kyle RA. (1997) Monoclonal gammopathy of undetermined significance and solitary plasmacytoma. Implications for progression to overt multiple myeloma. *Hematol Oncol Clin North Am* 11:71–87.

Lacour JP, Juhlin L, el Baze P, Barety M, Ortonne JP. (1986) Disseminated pagetoid reticulosis associated with mycosis fungoides: immunomorphologic study. *J Am Acad Dermatol* 14(5 Pt 2):898–901.

Lai R, Weiss LM. (1998) Hepatitis C virus and non-Hodgkin's lymphoma [editorial; comment]. *Am J Clin Pathol* 109:508–510.

LeBoit PE. (1996) Lymphomatoid papulosis and cutaneous CD30+ lymphoma. *Am J Dermatopathol* 18:221–235.

Lehky TJ, Levin MC, Kubota R, Bamford RN, Flerlage AN, Soldan SS, Leist TP, Xavier A, White JD, Brown M, Fleisher TA, Top LE, et al. (1998) Reduction in HTLV-I proviral load and spontaneous lymphoproliferation in HTLV-I-associated myelopathy/tropical spastic paraparesis patients treated with humanized anti-Tac. *Ann Neurol* 44:942–947.

Lennert K, Feller A. (1992) *Histopathology of Non-Hodgkin's Lymphomas.* Springer-Verlag, New York.

Levine AM, Sullivan-Halley J, Pike MC, Rarick MU, Loureiro C, Bernstein-Singer M, Willson E, Brynes R, Parker J, Rasheed S, et al. (1991) Human immunodeficiency virus-related lymphoma. Prognostic factors predictive of survival [see comments]. *Cancer* 68:2466–2472.

Liebow AA, Carrington CR, Friedman PJ. (1972) Lymphomatoid granulomatosis. *Hum Pathol* 3:457–558.

Limpens J, de Jong D, van Krieken J, Price C, Young B, van Ommen G, Kluin P. (1991) Bcl-2 in benign lymphoid tissue with follicular hyperplasia. *Oncogene* 6:2271–2276.

Lipford EH, Margolich JB, Longo DL, Fauci AS, Jaffe ES. (1988) Angiocentric immunoproliferative lesions: a clinicopathologic spectrum of post-thymic T cell proliferations. *Blood* 5:1674–1681.

Louvet S, Dompmartin A, Troussard X, Galateau F, Moreau A, Reman O, Leporrier M, Leroy D. (1996) Spectrum of CD30 lymphoproliferative diseases from lymphomatoid papulosis to anaplastic large cell lymphoma. *Int J Dermatol* 35:842–848.

Lundin KE, Gjertsen HA, Scott H, Sollid LM, Thorsby E. (1994) Function of DQ2 and DQ8 as HLA susceptibility molecules in celiac disease. *Hum Immunol* 41:24–27.

Luppi M, Torelli G. (1996) The new lymphotropic herpesviruses (HHV-6, HHV-7, HHV-8) and hepatitis C virus (HCV) in human lymphoproliferative diseases: an overview. *Haematologica* 81:265–281.

Mac Manus MP, Hoppe RT. (1997) Overview of treatment of localized low-grade lymphomas. *Hematol Oncol Clin North Am* 11:901–918.

Marafioti T, Hummel M, Anagnostopoulos I, Foss HD, Falini B, Delsol G, Isaacson PG, Pileri S, Stein H. (1997) Origin of nodular lymphocyte-predominant Hodgkin's disease from a clonal expansion of highly mutated germinal-center B cells [see comments]. *N Engl J Med* 337:453–458.

Mariette X. (1999) Lymphomas in patients with Sjogren's syndrome: review of the literature and physiopathologic hypothesis. *Leuk Lymphoma* 33:93–99.

Marshall BJ, Warren JR. (1984) Unidentified curved bacilli in the stomach of patients with gastritis and peptic ulceration. *Lancet* 1(8390):1311–1315.

Martin IG, Aldoori MI. (1994) Immunoproliferative small intestinal disease: Mediterranean lymphoma and alpha heavy chain disease. *Br J Surg* 81:20–24.

Matsue K, Itoh M, Tsukuda K, Kokubo T, Hirose Y. (1998) Development of Epstein-Barr virus–associated B cell lymphoma after intensive treatment of patients with angioimmunoblastic lymphadenopathy with dysproteinemia. *Int J Hematol* 67:319–329.

Mazzaro C, Franzin F, Tulissi P, Pussini E, Crovatto M, Carniello GS, Efremov DG, Burrone O, Santini G, Pozzato G. (1996) Regression of monoclonal B-cell expansion in patients affected by mixed cryoglobulinemia responsive to alpha-interferon therapy. *Cancer* 77:2604–2613.

McGrath MS, Shiramizu B, Meeker TC, Kaplan LD, Herndier B. (1991) AIDS-associated polyclonal lymphoma: identification of a new HIV-associated disease process. *J Acquir Immune Defic Syndr* 4:408–415.

McNiff JM, Schechner JS, Crotty PL, Glusac EJ. (1998) Mycosis fungoides palmaris et plantaris or acral pagetoid reticulosis? *Am J Dermatopathol* 20:271–275.

Meeting of the World Health Organization (1976) Alpha-chain disease and related small-intestinal lymphoma: a memorandum. *Bull World Health Organ* 54:615–624.

Meis JM, Butler JJ, Osborne BM, Ordonez NG. (1987) Solitary plasmacytomas of bone and extramedullary plasmacytomas. A clinicopathologic and immunohistochemical study. *Cancer* 59:1475–1485.

Mesri EA, Cesarman E, Arvanitakis L, Rafii S, Moore MA, Posnett DN, Knowles DM, Asch AS. (1996) Human herpesvirus-8/Kaposi's sarcoma–associated herpesvirus is a new transmissible virus that infects B cells. *J Exp Med* 183:2385–2390.

Miescher PA, Huang YP, Izui S. (1995) Type II cryoglobulinemia. *Semin Hematol* 32:80–85.

Moller-Petersen J, Schmidt EB. (1986) Diagnostic value of the concentration of M-component in initial classification of monoclonal gammopathy. *Scand J Haematol* 36:295–301.

Morgan GJ, Pratt G. (1998) Modern molecular diagnostics and the management of haematological malignancies. *Clin Lab Haematol* 20:135–141.

Morrell D, Cromartie E, Swift M. (1986) Mortality and cancer incidence in 263 patients with ataxia-telangiectasia. *J Natl Cancer Inst* 77:89–92.

Murphy EL, Figueroa JP, Gibbs WN, Brathwaite A, Holding-Cobham M, Waters D, Cranston B, Hanchard B, Blattner WA. (1989) Sexual transmission of human T-lymphotropic virus type I (HTLV-I). *Ann Intern Med* 111:555–560.

Murray JA. (1999) The widening spectrum of celiac disease. *Am J Clin Nutr* 69:354–365.

Nador RG, Cesarman E, Chadburn A, Dawson DB, Ansari MQ, Sald J, Knowles DM. (1996) Primary effusion lymphoma: a distinct clinicopathologic entity associated with the Kaposi's sarcoma-associated herpes virus. *Blood* 88:645–656.

Nakamura S, Aoyagi K, Furuse M, Suekane H, Matsumoto T, Yao T, Sakai Y, Fuchigami T, Yamamoto I, Tsuneyoshi M, Fujishima M. (1998) B-cell monoclonality precedes the development of gastric MALT lymphoma in *Helicobacter pylori*–associated chronic gastritis. *Am J Pathol* 152:1271–1279.

Nathwani BN, Rappaport H, Moran EM, Pangalis GA, Kim H. (1978) Malignant lymphoma arising in angioimmunoblastic lymphadenopathy. *Cancer* 41:578–606.

Nguyen PL, Ferry JA, Harris NL. (1999) Progressive transformation of germinal centers and nodular lymphocyte predominance Hodgkin's disease: a comparative immunohistochemical study. *Am J Surg Pathol* 23:27–33.

Niedobitek G. (1996) The role of Epstein-Barr virus in the pathogenesis of Hodgkin's disease. *Ann Oncol* 7 (Suppl 4):11–17.

Niedobitek G, Young LS, Herbst H. (1997) Epstein-Barr virus infection and the pathogenesis of malignant lymphomas. *Cancer Surv* 30:143–162.

The Non-Hodgkins Lymphoma Classification Project (1997) A clinical evaluation of the International Lymphoma Study Group classification of non-Hodgkin's lymphoma. The Non-Hodgkin's Lymphoma Classification Project. *Blood* 89:3909–3918.

Ohno T, Stribley JA, Wu G, Hinrichs SH, Weisenburger DD, Chan WC. (1997) Clonality in nodular lymphocyte-predominant Hodgkin's disease [see comments]. *N Engl J Med* 337:459–465.

Osame M, Janssen R, Kubota H, Nishitani H, Igata A, Nagataki S, Mori M, Goto I, Shimabukuro H, Khabbaz R, et al. (1990) Nationwide survey of HTLV-I-associated myelopathy in Japan: association with blood transfusion. *Ann Neurol* 28:50–56.

Osborne BM, Butler JJ. (1984) Clinical implications of progressive transformation of germinal centers. *Am J Surg Pathol* 8:725–733.

Osborne BM, Butler JJ, Gresik MV. (1992) Progressive transformation of germinal centers: comparison of

23 pediatric patients to the adult population. *Mod Pathol* 5:135–140.

Ott G, Katzenberger T, Greiner A, Kalla J, Rosenwald A, Heinrich U, Ott MM, Muller-Hermelink HK. (1997) The t(11;18)(q21;q21) chromosome translocation is a frequent and specific aberration in low-grade but not high-grade malignant non-Hodgkin's lymphomas of the mucosa-associated lymphoid tissue (MALT-) type. *Cancer Res* 57:3944–3948.

Parkhurst JB, Kuhls TL, Elrod JP, Sexauer CL, Jaffe ES, Peiper SC. (1994) Lymphomatoid granulomatosis in a child with familial chronic active Epstein-Barr virus infection. *Int J Pediatr Hematol Oncol* 1:299–304.

Parnell ND, Ciclitira PJ. (1999) Review article: coeliac disease and its management. *Aliment Pharmacol Ther* 13:1–13.

Parsonnet J, Hansen S, Rodriguez L, Gelb AB, Warnke RA, Jellum E, Orentreich N, Vogelman JH, Friedman GD. (1994) *Helicobacter pylori* infection and gastric lymphoma [see comments]. *N Engl J Med* 330:1267–1271.

Paulli M, Berti E, Rosso R, Boveri E, Kindl S, Klersy C, Lazzarino M, Borroni G, Menestrina F, Santucci M, et al. (1995) CD30/Ki-1-positive lymphoproliferative disorders of the skin—clinicopathologic correlation and statistical analysis of 86 cases: a multicentric study from the European Organization for Research and Treatment of Cancer Cutaneous Lymphoma Project Group. *J Clin Oncol* 13:1343–1354.

Pautier P, Devidas A, Delmer A, Dombret H, Sutton L, Zini JM, Nedelec G, Molina T, Marolleau JP, Brice P. (1999) Angioimmunoblastic-like T-cell non Hodgkin's lymphoma: outcome after chemotherapy in 33 patients and review of the literature. *Leuk Lymphoma* 32:545–552.

Pawson R, Mufti GJ, Pagliuca A. (1998) Management of adult T-cell leukaemia/lymphoma. *Br J Haematol* 100:453–458.

Pedersen RK, Pedersen NT. (1996) Primary non-Hodgkin's lymphoma of the thyroid gland: a population based study. *Histopathology* 28:25–32.

Pelicci PG, Knowles DMd, Arlin ZA, Wieczorek R, Luciw P, Dina D, Basiloco C, Dalla-Favera R. (1986) Multiple monoclonal B cell expansions and c-*myc* oncogene rearrangements in acquired immune deficiency syndrome–related lymphoproliferative disorders. Implications for lymphomagenesis. *J Exp Med* 164:2049–2060.

Penn I, Hammond W, Brettschneider L, Starzl TE. (1969) Malignant lymphomas in transplantation patients. *Transplant Proc* 1:106–112.

Perry GSD, Spector BD, Schuman LM, Mandel JS, Anderson VE, McHugh RB, Hanson MR, Fahlstrom SM, Krivit W, Kersey JH. (1980) The Wiskott-Aldrich syndrome in the United States and Canada (1892–1979). *J Pediatr* 97:72–78.

Peters K, Knoll JH, Kadin ME. (1995) Cytogenetic findings in regressing skin lesions of lymphomatoid papulosis. *Cancer Genet Cytogenet* 80:13–16.

Pivetta B, De Vita S, Ferraccioli G, De Re V, Gloghini A, Marzotto A, Caruso G, Dolcetti R, Bartoli E, Carbone A, Boiocchi M. (1999) T cell receptor repertoire in B cell lymphoproliferative lesions in primary Sjogren's syndrome. *J Rheumatol* 26:1101–1109.

Prior P. (1985) Cancer and rheumatoid arthritis: epidemiologic considerations. *Am J Med* 78(1A):15–21.

Quintana PG, Kapadia SB, Bahler DW, Johnson JT,

Swerdlow SH. (1997) Salivary gland lymphoid infiltrates associated with lymphoepithelial lesions: a clinicopathologic, immunophenotypic, and genotypic study [see comments]. *Hum Pathol* 28:850–861.

Radaszkiewicz T, Hansmann ML, Lennert K. (1989) Monoclonality and polyclonality of plasma cells in Castleman's disease of the plasma cell variant. *Histopathology* 14:11–24.

Radaszkiewicz T, Lennert K. (1975) Lymphogranulomatosis X: klinisches bild, therapie, und prognose. *Dtsch Med Wochenschr* 100:1157–1163.

Ramot B, Shahin N, Bubis J. (1965) Malabsorption syndrome in lymphoma os small intestine. A study of 13 cases. *Israel J Med Sci* 1:221–226.

Raphael MM, Audouin J, Lamine M, Delecluse HJ, Vuillaume M, Lenoir GM, Gisselbrecht C, Lennert K, Diebold J. (1994) Immunophenotypic and genotypic analysis of acquired immunodeficiency syndrome–related non-Hodgkin's lymphomas. Correlation with histologic features in 36 cases. French Study Group of Pathology for HIV-Associated Tumors. *Am J Clin Pathol* 101:773–782.

Rappaport H, Ramot B, Hulu N, Park JK. (1972) The pathology of so-called Mediterranean abdominal lymphoma with malabsorption. *Cancer* 29:1502–1511.

Rasul I, Shepherd FA, Kamel-Reid S, Krajden M, Pantalony D, Heathcote EJ. (1999) Detection of occult low-grade b-cell non-Hodgkin's lymphoma in patients with chronic hepatitis C infection and mixed cryoglobulinemia. *Hepatology* 29:543–547.

Ree HJ, Kadin ME, Kikuchi M, Ko YH, Go JH, Suzumiya J, Kim DS. (1998) Angioimmunoblastic lymphoma (AILD-type T-cell lymphoma) with hyperplastic germinal centers. *Am J Surg Pathol* 22:643–655.

Resnik KS, Kantor GR, Lessin SR, Kadin ME, Chooback L, Cooper HS, Vonderheid EC. (1995) Mycosis fungoides palmaris et plantaris [see comments]. *Arch Dermatol* 131:1052–1056.

Reynolds P, Saunders LD, Layefsky ME, Lemp GF. (1993) The spectrum of acquired immunodeficiency syndrome (AIDS)–associated malignancies in San Francisco, 1980–1987. *Am J Epidemiol* 137:19–30.

Rosen FS, Cooper MD, Wedgwood RJ. (1984a) The primary immunodeficiencies (1). *N Engl J Med* 311:235–242.

Rosen FS, Cooper MD, Wedgwood RJ. (1984b) The primary immunodeficiencies (2). *N Engl J Med* 311:300–310.

Rosen FS, Cooper MD, Wedgwood RJ. (1995) The primary immunodeficiencies. *N Engl J Med* 333:431–440.

Russell SM, Tayebi N, Nakajima H, Riedy MC, Roberts JL, Aman MJ, Migone TS, Noguchi M, Markert ML, Buckley RH, et al. (1995) Mutation of Jak3 in a patient with SCID: essential role of Jak3 in lymphoid development. *Science* 270(5237):797–800.

Said JW. (1997) Human immunodeficiency virus-related lymphoid proliferations. *Semin Diagn Pathol* 14:48–53.

Said JW, Rettig MR, Heppner K, Vescio RA, Schiller G, Ma HJ, Belson D, Savage A, Shintaku IP, Koeffler HP, Asou H, Pinkus G, et al. (1997) Localization of Kaposi's sarcoma-associated herpesvirus in bone marrow biopsy samples from patients with multiple myeloma [see comments]. *Blood* 90:4278–4282.

Sallah S, Gagnon GA. (1998) Angioimmunoblastic lymphadenopathy with dysproteinemia: emphasis on pathogenesis and treatment [see comments]. *Acta Haematol* 99:57–64.

Salloum E, Cooper DL, Howe G, Lacy J, Tallini G, Crouch J, Schultz M, Murren J. (1996) Spontaneous regression of lymphoproliferative disorders in patients treated with methotrexate for rheumatoid arthritis and other rheumatic diseases [see comments]. *J Clin Oncol* 14:1943–1949.

Sander CA, Medeiros LJ, Weiss LM, Yano T, Sneller MC, Jaffe ES. (1992) Lymphoproliferative lesions in patients with common variable immunodeficiency syndrome. *Am J Surg Pathol* 16:1170–1182.

Schechter NR, Portlock CS, Yahalom J. (1998) Treatment of mucosa-associated lymphoid tissue lymphoma of the stomach with radiation alone. *J Clin Oncol* 16:1916–1921.

Seligmann M. (1977) Immunobiology and pathogenesis of alpha chain disease. *Ciba Found Symp* 46: 263–281.

Seligmann M, Danon F, Hurez D, Mihaesco E, Preud'homme JL. (1968) Alpha-chain disease: a new immunoglobulin abnormality. *Science* 162(860): 1396–1397.

Shimizu YK, Iwamoto A, Hijikata M, Purcell RH, Yoshikura H. (1992) Evidence for *in vitro* replication of hepatitis C virus genome in a human T-cell line. *Proc Natl Acad Sci USA* 89:5477–5481.

Shimoyama M. (1991) Diagnostic criteria and classification of clinical subtypes of adult T-cell leukaemia-lymphoma. A report from the Lymphoma Study Group (1984–87). *Br J Haematol* 79:428–437.

Silvestri F, Pipan C, Barillari G, Zaja F, Fanin R, Infanti L, Russo D, Falasca E, Botta GA, Baccarani M. (1996) Prevalence of hepatitis C virus infection in patients with lymphoproliferative disorders. *Blood* 87:4296–4301.

Smith JL Jr, Butler JJ. (1980) Skin involvement in Hodgkin's disease. *Cancer* 45:354–361.

Smith WJ, Price SK, Isaacson PG. (1987) Immunoglobulin gene rearrangement in immunoproliferative small intestinal disease (IPSID). *J Clin Pathol* 40: 1291–1297.

Soulier J, Grollet L, Oksenhendler E, Cacoub P, Cazals-Hatem D, Babinet P, d'Agay MF, Clauvel JP, Raphael M, Degos L, et al. (1995) Kaposi's sarcoma–associated herpesvirus-like DNA sequences in multicentric Castleman's disease. *Blood* 86:1276–1280.

Soulier J, Grollet L, Oksenhendler E, Miclea JM, Cacoub P, Baruchel A, Brice P, Clauvel JP, d'Agay MF, Raphael M, et al. (1995) Molecular analysis of clonality in Castleman's disease. *Blood* 86:1131–1138.

Staal SP, Ambinder R, Beschorner WE, Hayward GS, Mann R. (1989) A survey of Epstein-Barr virus DNA in lymphoid tissue. Frequent detection in Hodgkin's disease [see comments]. *Am J Clin Pathol* 91:1–5.

Stetler-Stevenson M, Raffeld M, Cohen P, et al. (1988) Detection of occult follicular lymphoma by specific DNA amplification. *Blood* 72:1822–1825.

Subar M, Neri A, Inghirami G, Knowles DM, Dalla-Favera R. (1988) Frequent c-*myc* oncogene activation and infrequent presence of Epstein-Barr virus genome in AIDS-associated lymphoma. *Blood* 72: 667–671.

Sullivan JL, Woda BA. (1989) X-linked lymphoproliferative syndrome. *Immunodefic Rev* 1:325–347.

Sulzner SE, Amdur RJ, Weider DJ. (1998) Extramedullary plasmacytoma of the head and neck. *Am J Otolaryngol* 19:203–208.

Takatsuki K. (1997) Kenneth MacGredie Memorial Lectureship. Adult T-cell leukemia/lymphoma. *Leukemia* 11 Suppl 3:54–56.

Teruya-Feldstein J, Jaffe E, Burd P, et al. (1996) Expression of interferon-gamma inducible protein (IP-10) and the macrophage interferon-gamma induced gene (Mig) in lymphomatoid granulomatosis and nasal NK/T cell lymphoma with necrosis and vascular damage. *Blood* 88 (Suppl 1):670a.

Teruya-Feldstein J, Zauber P, Setsuda JE, Berman EL, Sorbara L, Raffeld M, Tosato G, Jaffe ES. (1998) Expression of human herpesvirus-8 oncogene and cytokine homologues in an HIV-seronegative patient with multicentric Castleman's disease and primary effusion lymphoma. *Lab Invest* 78:1637–1642.

Thomason RW, Craig FE, Banks PM, Sears DL, Myerson GE, Gulley ML. (1996) Epstein-Barr virus and lymphoproliferation in methotrexate-treated rheumatoid arthritis. *Mod Pathol* 9:261–266.

Tsujimoto Y, Cossman J, Jaffe E, Croce CM. (1985a) Involvement of the *bcl*-2 gene in human follicular lymphoma. *Science* 228(4706):1440–1443.

Tsujimoto Y, Gorham J, Cossman J, Jaffe E, Croce CM. (1985b) The t(14;18) chromosome translocations involved in B-cell neoplasms result from mistakes in VDJ joining. *Science* 229(4720):1390–1393.

Tzioufas AG. (1996) B-cell lymphoproliferation in primary Sjögren's syndrome. *Clin Exp Rheumatol* 14 Suppl 14:S65–S70.

van den Oord JJ, de Wolf-Peeters C, Desmet VJ. (1985) Immunohistochemical analysis of progressively transformed follicular centers. *Am J Clin Pathol* 83:560–564.

Waldmann TA, White JD, Carrasquillo JA, Reynolds JC, Paik CH, Gansow OA, Brechbiel MW, Jaffe ES, Fleisher TA, Goldman CK, et al. (1995) Radioimmunotherapy of interleukin-2R alpha-expressing adult T-cell leukemia with Yttrium-90-labeled anti-Tac [see comments]. *Blood* 86:4063–4075.

Wax MK, Yun KJ, Omar RA. (1993) Extramedullary plasmacytomas of the head and neck. *Otolaryngol Head Neck Surg* 109:877–885.

Weiss LM, Jaffe ES, Liu XF, Chen YY, Shibata D, Medeiros LJ. (1992) Detection and localization of Epstein-Barr viral genomes in angioimmunoblastic lymphadenopathy and angioimmunoblastic lymphadenopathy-like lymphoma. *Blood* 79:1789–1795.

Weiss LM, Strickler JG, Dorfman RF, Horning SJ, Warnke RA, Sklar J. (1986) Clonal T-cell populations in angioimmunoblastic lymphadenopathy and angioimmunoblastic lymphadenopathy-like lymphoma. *Am J Pathol* 122:392–397.

WHO Scientific Study Group (1995) Primary immunodeficiency diseases. Report of a WHO Scientific Group. *Clin Exp Immunol* 99 Suppl 1:1–24.

Wilson WH, Kingma DW, Raffeld M, Wittes RE, Jaffe ES. (1996) Association of lymphomatoid granulomatosis with Epstein-Barr viral infection of B lymphocytes and response to interferon-alpha 2b. *Blood* 87:4531–4537.

Witherell HL, Hansen S, Jellum E, Orentreich N, Vogelman JH, Parsonnet J. (1997) Risk for gastric lymphoma in persons with CagA+ and CagA− *Helicobacter pylori* infection. *J Infect Dis* 176:1641–1644.

Wood GS, Weiss LM, Hu CH, Abel EA, Hoppe RT, Warnke RA, Sklar J. (1988) T-cell antigen deficiencies and clonal rearrangements of T-cell receptor genes in pagetoid reticulosis (Woringer-Kolopp disease). *N Engl J Med* 318:164–167.

Woringer F, Kolopp P. (1939) Lésion érythématosquameuse polycyclique de l'avant-bras évoluant depuis 6 ans chez un garçonnet de 13 ans: histologiquementinfiltrat intra-épidermique d'appearance tumorale. *Ann Dermatol Venereol* 7:945–948.

Wotherspoon AC. (1998) *Helicobacter pylori* infection and gastric lymphoma. *Br Med Bull* 54:79–85.

Wotherspoon AC, Finn TM, Isaacson PG. (1995) Trisomy 3 in low-grade B-cell lymphomas of mucosa-associated lymphoid tissue. *Blood* 85:2000–2004.

Wotherspoon AC, Ortiz-Hidalgo C, Falzon MR, Isaacson PG. (1991) *Helicobacter pylori*–associated gastritis and primary B-cell gastric lymphoma [see comments]. *Lancet* 338(8776):1175–1176.

Wotherspoon AC, Pan LX, Diss TC, Isaacson PG. (1992) Cytogenetic study of B-cell lymphoma of mucosa-associated lymphoid tissue. *Cancer Genet Cytogenet* 58: 35–38.

Wright DH. (1997) Enteropathy associated T cell lymphoma. *Cancer Surv* 30:249–261.

Young L, Alfieri C, Hennessy K, Evans H, O'Hara C, Anderson KC, Ritz J, Shapiro RS, Rickinson A, Kieff E, et al. (1989) Expression of Epstein-Barr virus transformation–associated genes in tissues of patients with EBV lymphoproliferative disease. *N Engl J Med* 321:1080–1085.

Yunis JJ, Oken MM, Kaplan ME, Ensrud KM, Howe RR, Theologides A. (1982) Distinctive chromosomal abnormalities in histologic subtypes of non-Hodgkin's lymphoma. *N Engl J Med* 307:1231–1236.

20

URINARY BLADDER

Alberto G. Ayala, Jae Y. Ro, Mahul B. Amin, Bogdan Czerniak, and Jorge Albores-Saavedra

Carcinoma of the urinary bladder remains a significant health problem worldwide. The American Cancer Society has estimated that in 2000 there will be 53,200 newly diagnosed cases of urinary bladder carcinoma in the United States and that 12,200 patients will die of this disease (Greenlee et al., 2000). Most malignancies in the urinary bladder are urothelial in origin (Murphy et al., 1994), and clinically three patterns of transitional cell tumors are recognized: carcinoma *in situ,* superficial disease, and invasive disease. *Transitional cell carcinoma in situ* (TCIS) is flat carcinoma involving the urothelial mucosa that, after a variable period of time, may progress to invasive disease. *Superficial disease* refers to papillary tumors of any grade without invasion or with invasion to only the lamina propria (Otto et al., 1995; Pagano et al., 1987; Torti et al., 1987). In general, these lesions are less aggressive and have a lower histologic grade; approximately 10%–15% of them eventually progress to muscle-invasive disease, and they are usually managed conservatively. In contrast, *invasive disease* arises *de novo* in the majority of the cases, and the tumor has already infiltrated the true muscle layer or has gone beyond it at the initial diagnosis. These tumors have a higher histologic grade, and about 50% of patients die of the disease. Hence, these patients require aggressive therapeutic intervention (Johnson and Ayala, 1989).

Urothelial dysplasia is believed to be the most likely precursor of carcinoma *in situ* or invasive carcinoma (Murphy and Soloway, 1982a,b; Nagy et al., 1982). Unfortunately, little is known about dysplasia in the absence of bladder cancer (Murphy and Soloway, 1982a), because urothelial dysplasia is almost always identified in patients subsequent to or coincident with, rather than preceding, urothelial neoplasia. Nevertheless, urothelial dysplasia is considered to be a precursor lesion chiefly because of its association with urothelial carcinoma (Kiemeney et al., 1985; Murphy et al., 1979; Richards et al., 1991). This chapter discusses dysplastic lesions of the bladder, TCIS, and superficial and invasive disease, as well as prognostic factors and molecular aspects of urothelial malignancies.

HISTOLOGIC CONSIDERATIONS

The normal urothelial mucosa averages five to seven cell layers (Leeson et al., 1985; Krause and Cutts, 1986; Petersen, 1986) and has three types of cells: basal, intermediate, and umbrella cells (Fig. 20–1). *Umbrella cells* are large, often multinucleated, and characteristically cover the mucosa (Krause and Cutts, 1986; Leeson et al., 1985; Petersen, 1986). Umbrella cells may be absent from biopsy specimens as they may be dislodged during the biopsy procedure but may be

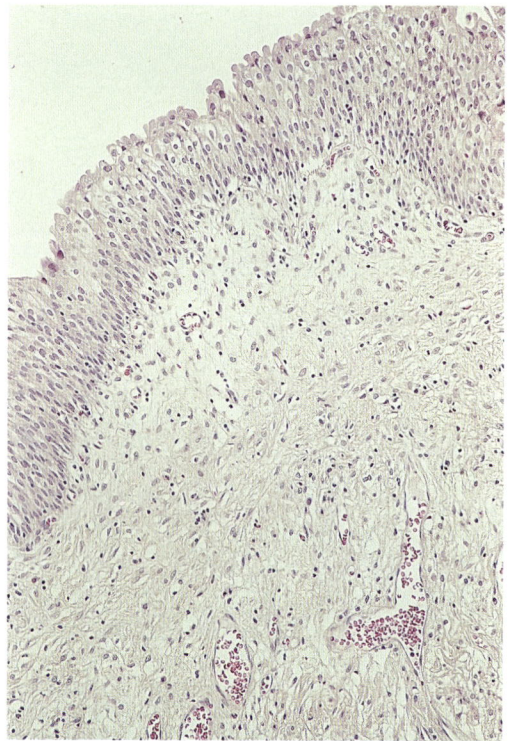

Figure 20–1. Normal bladder mucosa. The normal mucosa contains about 7 to 8 layers of epithelium and is covered by the umbrella cells. Beneath the umbrella cells there are intermediate cells and basal cells. Loose connective tissue and thin-walled vessels constitute the lamina propria.

seen on the surface of low-grade papillary transitional cell carcinomas (Petersen, 1986). The *intermediate cells* are up to six cells thick in the contracted bladder, where they are oriented with the long axis perpendicular to the basement membrane. In the distended state, the intermediate cell layer may be inconspicuous or only one cell thick or flattened. The nuclei are oval with nuclear grooves and have finely granular chromatin. The cytoplasm is relatively abundant and amphophilic and may be vacuolated. The cell membranes are distinct and these cells are attached to each other by desmosomes. The *basal cell layer* is only one cell thick and composed of cuboidal cells that are evident only in the contracted bladder; these cells lie on a thin basement membrane.

The lamina propria consists of a compact layer of fibrovascular connective tissue with a variable number of vessels and smooth muscle fibers, muscularis mucosae (Dixon and Gosling, 1983; Ro et al., 1987a), which are found in 94% to 100% of urinary bladders (Fig. 20–2). In a study of 100 bladder specimens by Ro et al. (1987a), three patterns of distribution of muscle bundles were found: (*1*) smooth muscle fibers forming a continuous layer, a true muscularis mucosae (3 cases among 100 cases examined); (*2*) a discontinuous or interrupted layer of smooth muscle fibers (20 cases); and (*3*) scattered thin bundles of smooth muscle fibers that do not form an obvious layer (71 cases). In six cases, there were no smooth muscle fibers in the lamina propria. These smooth muscle fibers lie parallel to the surface epithelium and are situated approximately midway between the surface epithelium and the proper muscular layer. Large blood vessels are in close association

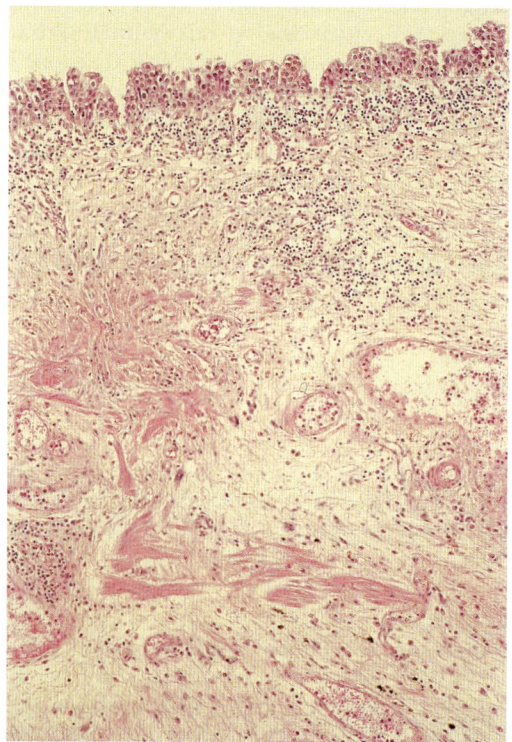

Figure 20–2. Muscularis mucosae. This view exhibits the upper aspect of the urinary bladder, including mucosa, lamina propria, and the muscularis mucosae. The muscularis mucosae is depicted by thin bundles of smooth muscle cells arranged parallel in relation to the mucosa. Notice also the accompanying dilated vessels.

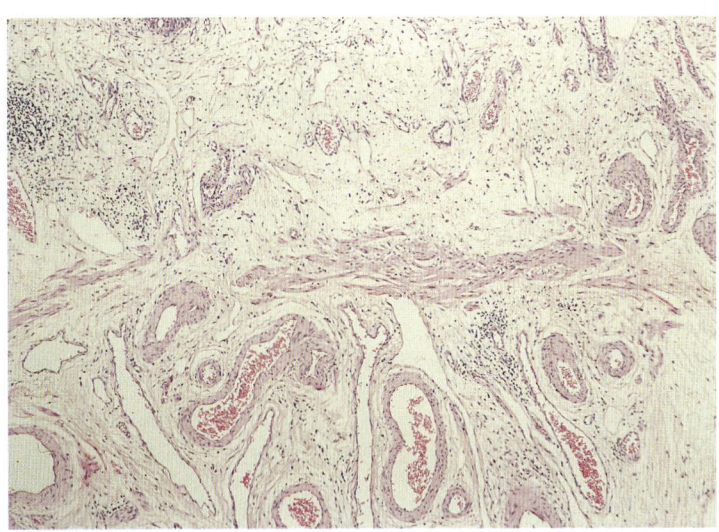

Figure 20–3. Muscularis mucosae. This higher-power view shows the large, thin-walled blood vessels that accompany thin bundles of smooth muscle fibers.

with the fibers of the muscularis mucosae (Fig. 20–3). It is important to be aware of the presence of muscularis mucosae in the lamina propria because the management of tumors invasive to the lamina propria is far different from the management of tumors that invade muscle proper (Ro et al., 1987a).

Another important finding is the presence of adipose tissue in the lamina propria and muscularis propria (Fig. 20–4). In traditional textbooks of histology, there is no information on the presence of fat in these layers. Recently, Philip et al. (1999) reported that adipose tissue is frequently present in the lamina propria and muscularis propria layers of the bladder wall, and is usually scant in the former location and frequently abundant in the latter. Therefore, in transurethral resection of bladder tumor specimens, misinterpretation of tumor infiltrating lamina propria fat as perivesical fat involvement may potentially result in unwarranted aggressive management.

The muscle proper of the bladder (detrussor muscle) consists of haphazardly arranged, thick bundles of smooth muscle that spiral around each ureteral orifice; these fibers increase their thickness around the internal urethral orifice and form the internal sphincter of the bladder. The muscularis is surrounded by a coat of fibroelastic connective tissue, the adventitia, and perivesical fat (Krause and Cutts, 1986; Leeson et al., 1985; Petersen, 1986).

TERMINOLOGY

Although the terminology used to describe bladder lesions is relatively well established, there are areas of controversy regarding the

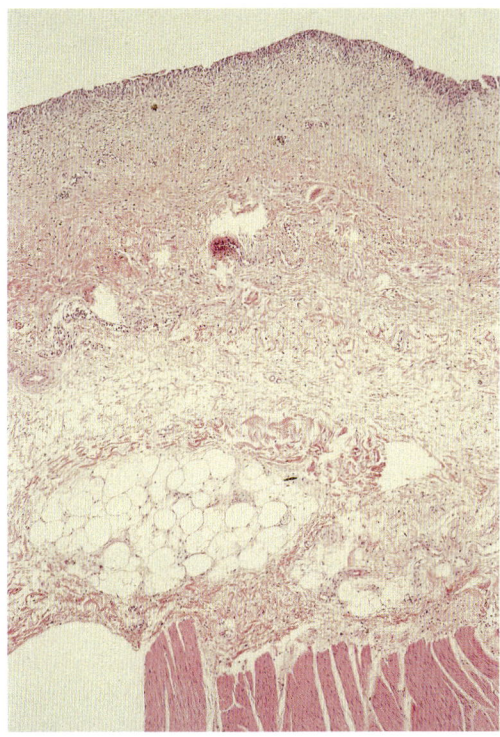

Figure 20–4. The adipose tissue in the lamina propria just above the muscularis propria should not be misinterpreted as adventitial fat.

Table 20–1. The WHO/ISUP Consensus Classification of Urothelial Lesions

Normal

Hyperplasia
　Flat
　Papillary

Flat urothelial
　Reactive (inflammatory) atypia
　Atypia of unknown significance
　Dysplasia
　Carcinoma *in situ*

Papillary urothelial neoplasms
　Urothelial papilloma
　Inverted papilloma
　Papillary urothelial neoplasm of low malignant
　　potential
　Papillary urothelial carcinoma, low grade
　Papillary urothelial carcinoma, high grade

Invasive urothelial carcinoma
　Urothelial carcinoma with lamina propria invasion
　Urothelial carcinoma with muscularis propria
　　(detrussor muscle) invasion

preferred terms as well as their clinical and pathologic relevance.

The terminology included here is based on that proposed by the Consensus Meeting of Urologic Pathologists held in Boston, Massachusetts, at the International Society for Urologic Pathology (ISUP) in 1998 (WHO/ISUP classification; Epstein et al., 1998; Table 20–1). The two systems used prior to this proposed WHO/ISUP Consensus Classification of Urothelial (transitional cell) Neoplasms of the Urinary Bladder were the system by the World Health Organization (WHO) 1973 (Mostofi et al., 1973) and the system espoused in the Armed Forces In-

stitute of Pathology (AFIP) fascicles by Koss (1975) and Murphy et al. (1994).

CONSENSUS CLASSIFICATION OF BLADDER LESIONS

Hyperplasia

Flat urothelial hyperplasia is characterized by a thickened mucosa without cytologic atypia.

Papillary urothelial hyperplasia is characterized by slightly tented, undulating, or papillary growth lined by urothelium of varying thickness without cytologic atypia. Although the lesion may have one or two dilated capillaries at its base, it lacks a well-developed fibrovascular core (Fig. 20–5).

Flat Lesions without Atypia

Reactive atypia has nuclear abnormalities occurring in acutely or chronically inflamed urothelium. Nuclei are enlarged and vesicular and may contain a prominent nucleolus. Mitotic figures may be frequent but are not atypical. Pleomorphism or chromatin alteration is usually absent. There is usually a history of instrumentation, stone, or other inflammatory processes.

Atypia of unknown significance is reserved for those cases in which it is difficult to differentiate reactive from neoplastic atypia (Fig. 20–6).

Flat Lesions with Atypia Believed to Be Neoplastic

Dysplasia (low-grade intra-urothelial neoplasia) (Fig. 20–7), the urothelium has cyto-

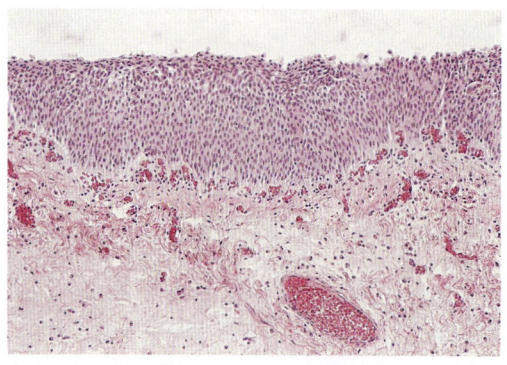

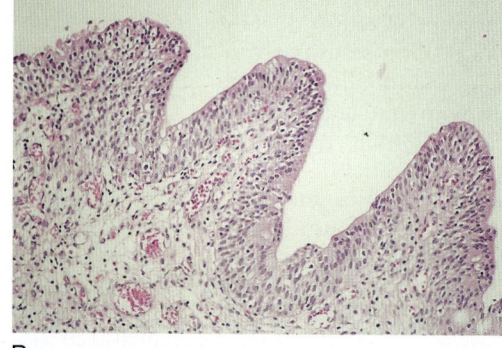

A　　　　　　　　　　　　　　　　B

Figure 20–5. *A*: Flat urothelial hyperplasia with thickened mucosa and no cytologic atypia. *B*: Papillary urothelial hyperplasia shows undulating changes of the mucosa forming pseudopapillae.

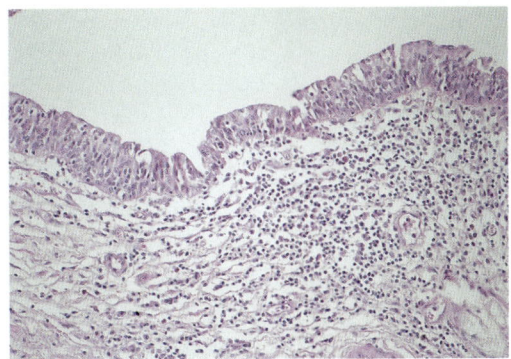

Figure 20–6. Atypia of unknown significance shows a thicker urothelial mucosa than normal and some large nuclei. Some of these large nuclei have a fine nuclear chromatin pattern and small nucleoli and some have hyperchromatic nuclei. Significant variation in size and shape of nuclei is not seen. These changes are associated with inflammation in the lamina propria.

logic and architectural changes believed to be preneoplastic, but these fall short of the diagnostic threshold for urothelial (transitional cell) carcinoma *in situ*. This term encompasses lesions previously diagnosed as mild dysplasia and some cases of moderate dysplasia.

Carcinoma in situ (Fig. 20–8) is characterized by the presence of neoplastic urothelial cells distributed along the entire thickness of the mucosa or only in part of it. In this definition, severe dysplasia and carcinoma *in situ* are considered together as well as lesions that may be represented by a few cells or clusters of pleomorphic cells such as occur in pagetoid spread of carcinoma cells (Fig. 20–9). Some lesions previously diagnosed as moderate dysplasia may also qualify as carcinoma *in situ* according to the slightly expanded definition of carcinoma *in situ* of the WHO/ISUP classification.

Papillary Neoplasms

Papilloma (Fig 20–10) is defined as discrete papillary growth with a central fibrovascular core lined by urothelium of normal thickness and cytology.

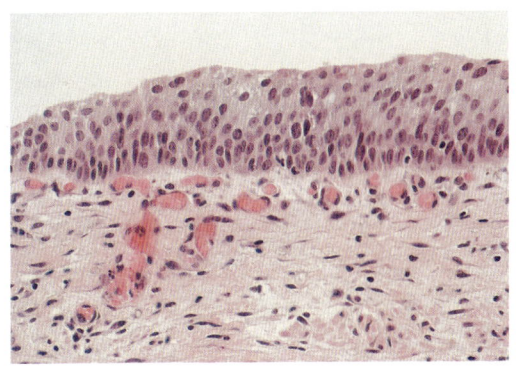

A

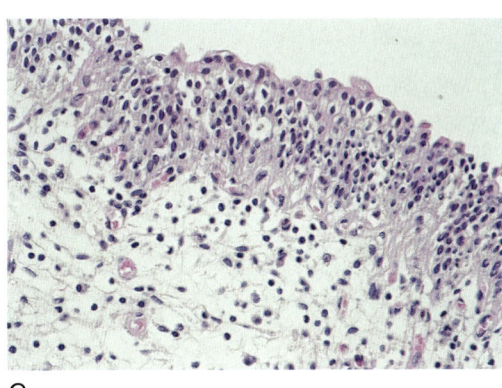

C

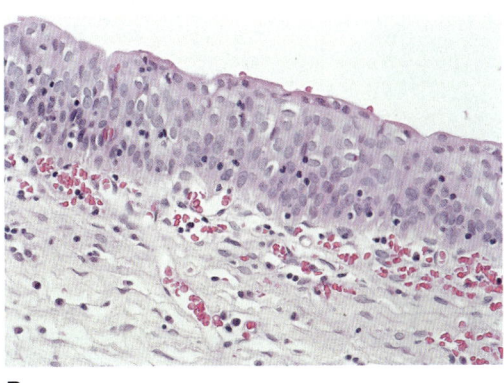

B

Figure 20–7. *A, B:* The thickness of the mucosa in low-grade dysplasia is about normal but there are more nuclei with coarse nuclear chromatin pattern and small nucleoli than expected. Note the engorged vessels in the lamina propria. *C:* The mucosa is slightly thickened and some urothelial cells are hyperchromatic.

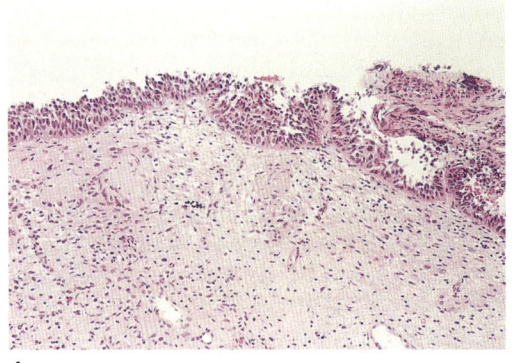

A

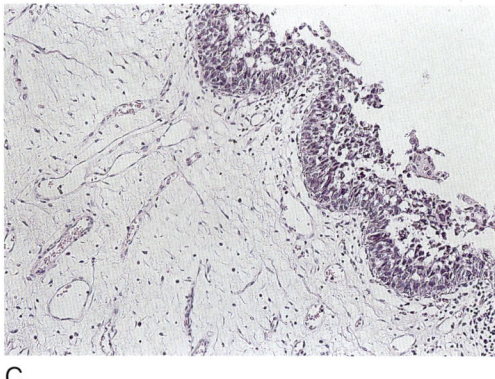

C

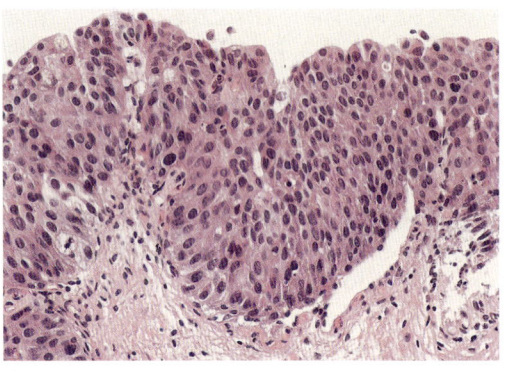

B

Figure 20–8. In transitional cell carcinoma *in situ,* the mucosa is totally replaced by atypical cells that have large irregular nuclei with some mitotic activity (*A*). Some early papillae are also present. *B:* Higher-power view shows distinctive anaplasia and hyperchromatism of the abnormal cells distributed throughout the mucosa. *C:* In this illustration there is sloughing off of the atypical cells.

Inverted urothelial papilloma (Fig. 20–11) consists of numerous invaginations of regular anastomosing cords or trabeculae or columns of urothelial cells extending deep into the underlying lamina propria. The

basal cells are perpendicular to the basal lamina, while the inner cells lie parallel in a horizontal position. The individual cells show no to minimal nuclear atypia, and mitoses are extremely rare or absent.

Papillary urothelial neoplasm of low malignant potential (Fig. 20–12) is characterized by pap-

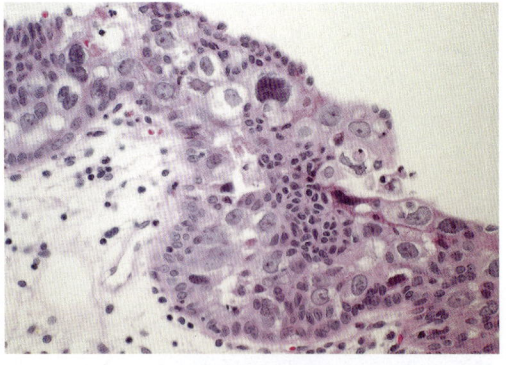

Figure 20–9. In pagetoid spread of transitional cell carcinoma *in situ,* there are large neoplastic urothelial cells with abundant cytoplasm infiltrating the normal mucosa. These neoplastic cells are sharply demarcated from the surrounding normal urothelial cells.

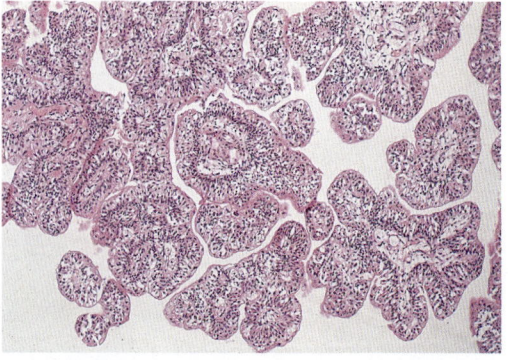

Figure 20–10. Papillary structures in papilloma are lined by normal-looking urothelial cells that have no nuclear atypia. Note the prominent umbrella cell layer.

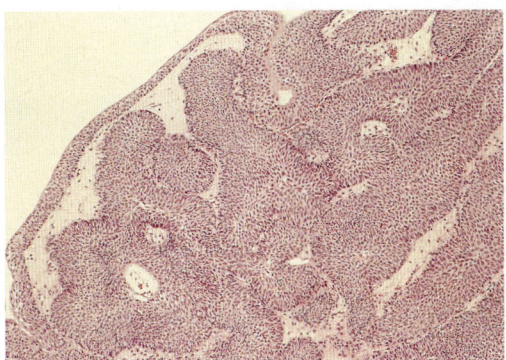

Figure 20–11. An inverted papilloma is a cellular urothelial tumor with bland nuclear features, with some nuclei showing grooves. There is no mitotic activity. Note the prominent in-growth pattern into the lamina propria.

illary growth lined by a proliferation of orderly arranged urothelial cells with minimal nuclear atypia, irrespective of cell thickness. Mitotic activity is rare or absent. This term replaces the term papillary carcinoma, WHO grade 1, and broadens its definition.

Papillary urothelial carcinoma, low grade (Fig. 20–13) is characterized by papillary growth with an orderly arrangement of urothelial cells but with easily recognizable abnormal cytologic features even at scanning magnification. There may be variation in the cell polarity, nuclear enlargement, and variation of nuclear size and shape, but these changes are minimal. This term encompasses lesions

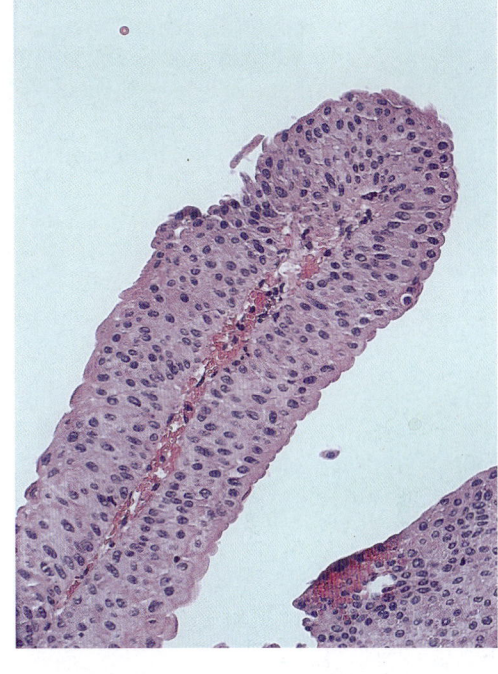

Figure 20–12. A papillary neoplasm of low malignant potential (papillary TCC grade 1) consists of a papillary proliferation lined by slightly abnormal urothelial cells with the absence of mitotic activity.

previously termed WHO grade 2 papillary carcinomas.

Papillary urothelial carcinoma, high grade (Fig. 20–14). A high grade carcinoma shows

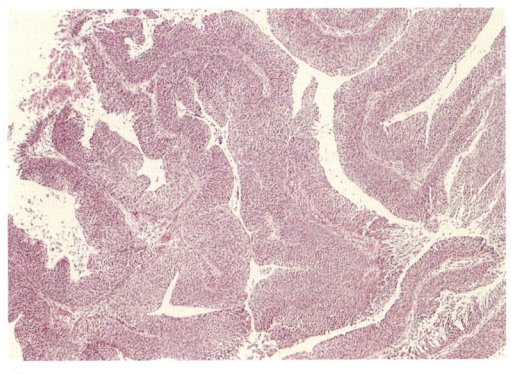

A

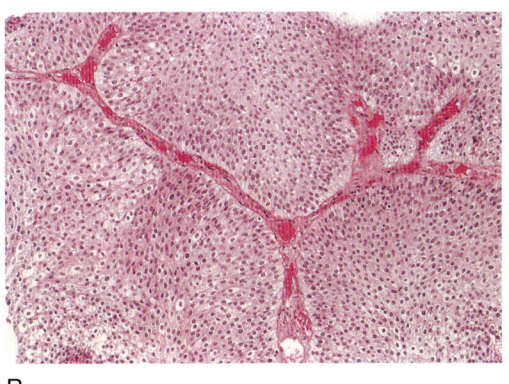

B

Figure 20–13. Papillary transitional cell carcinoma of low-grade malignancy (papillary TCC grade 2). *A:* Numerous, complex and often confluent papillations are lined by a thick layer of urothelium. The nuclei are bland, vary little in size and shape, but they may have some degree of nuclear atypia. Occasional mitoses are seen. *B:* On higher magnification the central fibrovascular core, markedly thickened urothelium, and the retention of uniform, relatively bland nuclear features are evident.

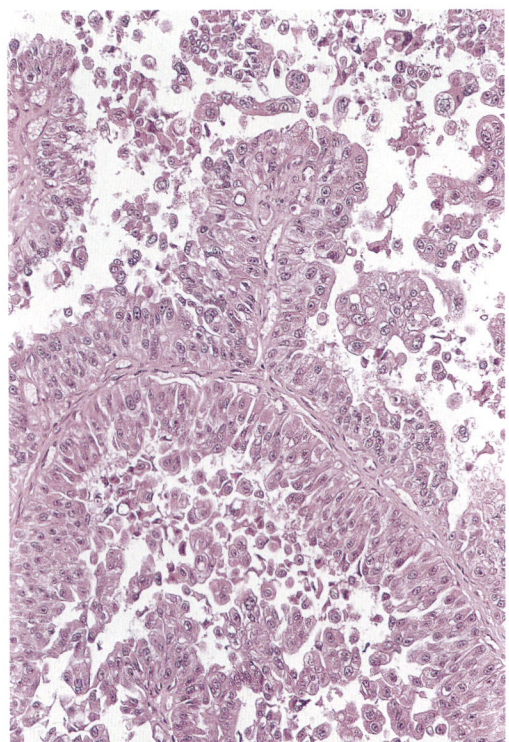

Figure 20–14. Papillary transitional cell carcinoma, high grade (papillary TCC grade 3). Here a papillary neoplasm is lined by cytologically atypical cells. Notice the large nuclei with prominent nucleoli.

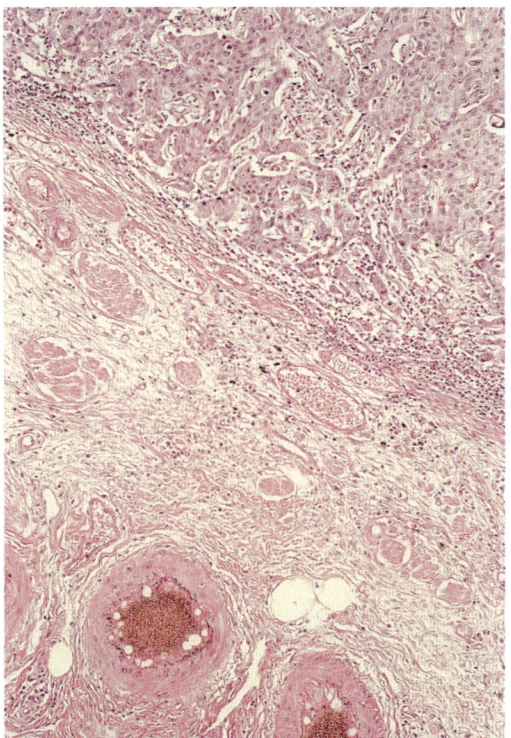

Figure 20–15. Transitional cell carcinoma invading the lamina propria. Interconnecting cords and nests of high-grade carcinoma are seen in the lamina propria. The advancing edge of this tumor is sharply delimited at the level of the muscularis mucosae, where thin bundles of smooth muscle fibers and prominent vessels are present.

a spectrum of pleomorphism ranging from moderate to marked. This term encompasses some WHO grade 2 tumors and all WHO grade 3 tumors.

Invasive Neoplasms

Invasive neoplasms are categorized as tumors invasive into lamina propria (Fig. 20–15) and tumors invading the muscularis propria (Fig. 20–16) and beyond. Invasive tumors are graded in two categories: low grade and high grade.

STAGING

The two most commonly used staging systems in the United States are the Marshall modification of the Jewett and Strong system (Jewett and Strong, 1946; Marshall, 1962) and the American Joint Commission TNM system (American Joint Committee on Can-

cer, 1997). In the former system, stage 0 refers to tumors localized to the urothelium; unfortunately, this system does not separate TCIS from noninvasive papillary carcinoma.

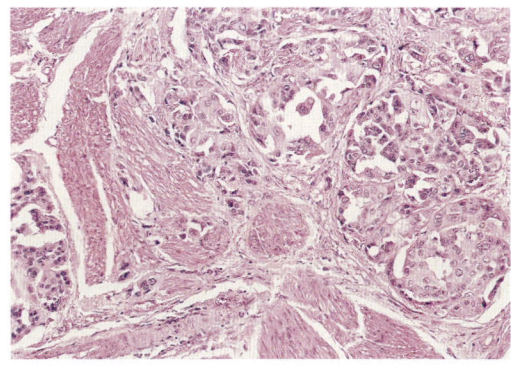

Figure 20–16. Transitional cell carcinoma invading the muscularis propria.

Table 20–2A. Staging Systems for Transitional Cell Carcinoma of the Bladder

JSM	AJCC	Description
	TX	Primary tumor cannot be assessed
	T0	No evidence of primary tumor
0	Tis	Carcinoma *in situ*
0	Ta	Papillary noninvasive carcinoma
A	T1	Tumor invades subepithelial connective tissue
B1	T2a	Tumor invades superficial muscle (inner half)
B2	T2b	Tumor invades deep muscle
C	T3	Tumor invades perivesical fat
	T3a	Microscopically
	T3b	Macroscopically (extravesical mass)
D1	T4	Tumor invades any of the following: prostate, uterus, vagina, pelvic wall, abdominal wall
	T4a	Tumor invades the prostate, uterus, or vagina
	T4b	Tumor invades the pelvic wall or abdominal wall
—	NX	Regional lymph nodes cannot be assessed
—	N0	No regional lymph node metastasis
D1	N1	Metastasis in a single lymph node, ≤ 2 cm
D1	N2	Metastasis in a single lymph node, >2 cm but not more than 5 cm in greatest dimension; or multiple lymph nodes, none more than 5 cm in greatest dimension
D1	N3	Metastasis in a lymph node more than 5 cm in greatest dimension
—	MX	Presence of distant metastasis cannot be assessed
	M0	No distant metastasis
D2	M1	Distant metastasis

AJCC, American Joint Committee on Cancer; JSM, Jewett-Strong (Marshall modification); M, distant metastasis; N, regional lymph nodes; T, primary tumor.

Superficial noninvasive disease in the TNM system, however, recognizes TCIS as stage Tis and noninvasive papillary disease as stage Ta. Thereafter, both systems are relatively similar (Table 20–2A). Tumors that involve the lamina propria are designated stage A or T1 and tumors that invade the muscle proper as B or T2. Stage B or T2 is subdivided into B1 and B2 or T2a and T2b, based on the level of muscularis propria invasion. Stage B1 or T2a is tumor invading superficial detrusor muscle (inner half) and stage B2 or T2b is tumor invading deep detrussor muscle (outer half). In the TNM system, stage T3 tumors invading perivesical tissue are subdivided into T3a for microscopic perivesical invasion and T3b for gross perivesical extension with extravesical mass formation, corresponding to stage C of the Marshall modification of the Jewett and Strong system. Stage D or T4 indicates tumor with spread beyond the bladder wall (fixation, extension into other organs, or metastases). Stage T4 is subdivided into T4a for tumor invading the prostate, uterus, or vagina and T4b for tumor invading the pelvic wall or abdominal wall. See Table 20–2B for additional information concerning the TNM system.

GRADING SYSTEMS

The WHO (Mostofi et al., 1973) grading scheme, a commonly utilized system, divides transitional cell carcinoma (TCC) into three grades. This array of histological variables is reproducible at the extremes (grades 1 and 3) but leaves the grade 2 cancers as a major heterogeneous subgroup. Despite criticism of the grading system, many studies have demonstrated a good correlation of grade with frequency of muscle invasion, metastasis, and survival. Other systems have also

Table 20–2B. TNM Staging System

Primary tumor (T)

TX	Primary tumor cannot be assessed
T0	No evidence of primary tumor
Ta	Noninvasive papillary carcinoma
Tis	Carcinoma *in situ*: "flat tumor"
T1	Tumor invades subepithelial connective tissue
T2	Tumor invades muscle
T2a	Tumor invades superficial muscle (inner half)
T2b	Tumor invades deep muscle (outer half)
T3	Tumor invades perivesical tissue
T3a	Microscopically
T3b	Macroscopically (extravescial massi)
T4	Tumor invades any of the following: prostate, uterus, vagina, pelvic wall, abdominal wall
T4a	Tumor invades prostate, uterus, or vagina
T4b	Tumor invades pelvic wall, or abdominal wall

Regional lymph nodes (N)

(Regional lymph nodes are those within the true pelvis; all others are distant lymph nodes)

NX	Regional lymph nodes cannot be assessed
N0	No regional lymph node metastasis
N1	Metastasis in a single lymph node, 2 cm or less in greatest dimension
N2	Metastasis in a single lymph node, more than 2 cm but not more than 5 cm in greatest dimension; or multiple lymph nodes, none more than 5 cm in greatest dimension
N3	Metastasis in a lymph node more than 5 cm in greatest dimension

Distant metastasis (M)

MX	Distant metastasis cannot be assessed
M0	No distant metastasis
M1	Distant metastasis

Stage grouping

Stage	T	N	M
Stage 0a	Ta	N0	M0
Stage 0is	Tis	N0	M0
Stage I	T1	N0	M0 .
Stage II	T2a	N0	M0
	T2b	N0	M0
Stage III	T3a	N0	M0
	T3b	N0	M0
	T4a	N0	M0
Stage IV	T4b	N0	M0
	Any T	N1	M0
	Any T	N2	M0
	Any T	N3	M0
	Any N		M1

been proposed but have not achieved general use (Bergkvist et al., 1965; Koss, 1975 and 1985; Murphy et al., 1994). The new consensus classification (Epstein et al., 1998) does away with grading of TCC, but its nomenclature can be easily compared with that of the WHO grading system (Mostofi et al, 1973).

INVERTED PAPILLOMA AND INVERTED TRANSITIONAL CELL CARCINOMA

Inverted papilloma, as first described by Paschkis in 1925, accounts for approximately 2.2% tumors of neoplasms of the bladder, renal pelvis, ureter, and urethra (Francis, 1979; Kim and Reiner, 1978; Kunze et al., 1983; Potts and Hirst, 1963; Romanelli, 1986; Theoret et al., 1980). The male-to-female patient ratio is 4:1, and the age range is from 14 to 89 years with a peak in the sixth and seventh decades. Approximately 60% of inverted papillomas occur in people between the ages of 50 and 80 years of age (Francis, 1979; Kim and Reiner, 1978; Kunze et al., 1983; Potts and Hirst, 1963; Romanelli, 1986; Theoret et al., 1980). The symptoms are typically obstructive when the tumor involves the bladder outlet, but hematuria is also quite frequent.

The most common location is in the bladder neck (about 80% of cases), followed by the trigone and the ureteral orifices, but this tumor may occur in any part of the urinary tract (Francis, 1979; Kim and Reiner, 1978; Kunze et al., 1983; Murphy et al., 1994; Potts and Hirst, 1963; Romanelli, 1986; Theoret et al., 1980). Its gross appearance is that of a sessile or pedunculated polyp with a smooth or lobular gray or white surface. Tumors usually measure 1 or 2 cm in diameter but some may be as large as 7.5 cm (Murphy et al., 1994; Trites, 1969). This tumor is typically solitary, although it may rarely be multiple.

The surface of the lesion is smooth, elevated, or pedunculated with an attenuated lining. The lesion consists of numerous invaginations of regular anastomosing cords or trabeculae or columns of urothelial cells extending deep into the underlying lamina propria. The basal cells are perpendicular to the basal lamina, while the inner cells lie parallel in a horizontal position (Cameron and Lupton, 1976; Francis, 1979; Klein, 1974; Kunze et al., 1983; Murphy et al., 1994; Theoret et al., 1980; Trite, 1969). The individual cells show no to minimal nuclear atypia, and mitoses are extremely rare or absent (Fig. 20–11). Often small or large cysts of variable size containing mucin occur in inverted papillomas. Foci of metaplastic "squamoid"

change are not uncommon, but frank squamous differentiation with keratin formation is rare. von Brunn's nests, cystitis cystica, and/or cystitis glandularis are often present near the lesion. Two variants of inverted papilloma, the classical type and the glandular type, have been described (Kunze et al., 1983). The former consists of the typical solid columns or trabeculae as described above, while the second type is characterized by a prominent glandular proliferation morphologically similar to cystitis glandularis. Kunze et al. (1983), reporting on 40 cases, found that 15 were of the trabecular type and 25 were of the glandular type. In our experience, however, the trabecular type is more common.

The histogenesis of inverted papilloma is uncertain, although neoplastic, hamartomatous, hyperplastic, and metaplastic theories have all had their advocates (Kim and Reiner, 1978; Kunze et al., 1983; Potts and Hirst, 1963; Trite, 1969).

The presence of frank pleomorphism, stromal invasion, a florid exophytic papillary component, or necrosis is incompatible with a diagnosis of inverted papilloma. Thus, inverted papilloma has been described in association with TCC either arising in it or associated with it. In addition, inverted TCC may arise *de novo* (Altaffer et al., 1982; Cameron and Lupton, 1976; Khoury et al., 1985; Klein, 1974; Lazarevic and Garret, 1978; Paulsen et al., 1988; Uyama et al, 1980; Whitesel, 1982). Paulsen et al. (1988) reported on seven cases of TCC with inverted features and stressed that an inverted pattern may occur in conventional TCC. Talbert and Young (1989) described an additional case of this type in their report of deceptively benign-appearing bladder cancers and used the designation "inverting transitional cell carcinoma." Amin et al. (1997) reported a series of 18 cases of TCC with inverted growth pattern, 8 of which exclusively or at least focally contained areas resembling inverted papilloma (Fig. 20–17). As stated previously, a striking surface papillary component, significant nuclear atypia, necrosis, irregularity of width of trabeculae with transition into more solid areas, or stromal invasion argues against a diagnosis of inverted papilloma. The chief problem posed by urothelial tumors with an inverted growth

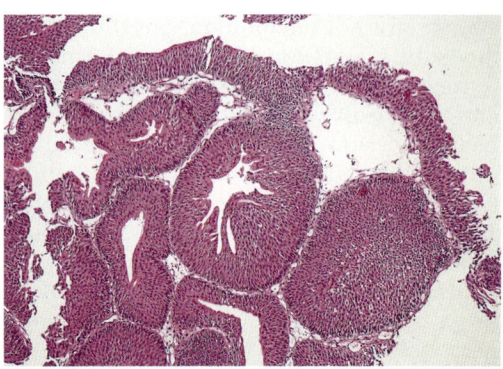

Figure 20–17. Inverted low-grade transitional cell carcinoma is characterized by urothelial growth into the lamina propria. The cells are hyperchromatic but still retain monotony and relatively bland nuclear features.

pattern is the correct assessment of invasion by these tumors; invasion should be recognized only when there is unequivocal destructive stromal invasion by an irregular, jagged infiltrative neoplasm with or without desmoplasia. The biologic potential of inverted papillomas, if strictly and accurately defined, is benign with an extremely low risk of recurrence (Cameron and Lupton, 1976; Francis, 1979; Klein, 1974; Kunze et al., 1983; Theoret et al., 1980; Trites, 1969).

INCIPIENT LESIONS

Unfortunately, little is known about precursor lesions of bladder carcinoma, since the initial event in the overwhelming majority of cases is the discovery of the bladder neoplasm. Unlike cervical or breast precursor lesions, which are relatively easily discovered by the patient or physician, the bladder remains silent until a neoplasm has developed. It is true that dysplastic lesions occur in the bladder urothelium, and a significant amount of knowledge has accumulated regarding these lesions. However, most of what is known relates to the association of carcinoma and dysplasia.

In 1952 Melicow and Hollowell described dysplastic urothelial changes distant from visible tumor. In 1974, Koss et al. mapped 10 urinary bladders removed at surgery for bladder carcinoma and elegantly described the presence of urothelial proliferative changes ranging from hyperplasia to urothelial atypia to carcinoma *in situ* diffusely affecting the bladder mucosa. Koss (1975) stated that urothelial hyperplasia often accompanies bladder tumors and is also undoubtedly the source of papillary neoplasia. Unfortunately, the sequence of events from hyperplasia to dysplasia to carcinoma has not been clearly described in either retrospective or prospective clinical studies.

There are very few studies of dysplasia in the absence of bladder carcinoma (*de novo* dysplasia). Zuk and collaborators (1988) reported on a retrospective study of 15 patients who presented with urothelial dysplasia in the absence of carcinoma; two patients (13%) developed carcinoma *in situ* at a mean follow-up of 4.8 years. In another study on the clinical significance of primary dysplasia utilizing cytologic analysis, it was found that only 1 of 19 patients (5%) developed bladder cancer (Murphy and Miller, 1984). Dysplasia occurs more commonly in patients with urothelial neoplasia. Althausen et al. (1976) and Smith et al. (1983) have shown that patients with dysplasia are more likely to develop muscle-invasive tumors than those without it, and hence dysplasia is a marker for urothelial instability. Cheng et al. (1999) reported 36 patients with isolated urothelial dysplasia in patients with no history of invasive TCC or TCIS. Seven patients (19%) developed progression, three to invasive carcinoma and four to carcinoma *in situ,* with one patient dying of the disease. The authors concluded that urothelial dysplasia is a significant risk for the development of carcinoma *in situ* and invasive carcinoma and those patients with urothelial dysplasia should be followed closely. The biologic potential of dysplasia is summarized in Table 20–3.

These previously mentioned studies suggest that the purported histogenesis of bladder carcinoma is a sequence of events beginning with hyperplasia and proceeding through dysplasia to carcinoma *in situ,* but importantly, they also suggest that not all cases recognizable as dysplasia at the light microscopic level in biopsies or by cytology progress to invasive carcinoma. Screening of patients in the fifth decade of life or above in populations at environmental or occupa-

Table 20–3. Clinical Settings for Dysplasia and Their Biologic Significance

De novo dysplasia

Limited data; 5% to 13% develop bladder tumors

Systemic prospective studies lacking

Dysplasia in patients with noninvasive or superficially invasive transitional cell carcinoma

Increased (but apparently low) risk of recurrence

Increased risk for invasion

Dysplasia in patients with muscle invasive transitional cell carcinoma

Invasive carcinoma overriding prognostic factor

tional risk for bladder cancer may lead to the finding of dysplastic changes.

By microscopy, dysplasia shows a loss of polarity, with more round to polygonal cells showing crowding, nucleomegaly, irregular nuclear contours, altered chromatin distribution, and rare or inconspicuous nucleoli (Figs. 20–7 and 20–8). Prominent nucleoli, brisk mitotic activity, and pleomorphism are usually lacking, and in most instances the thickness of the urothelium is generally unaltered but may be greater. The WHO/ISUP classification (Epstein et al., 1998) defines dysplasia as a lesion containing appreciable cytologic and architectural changes believed to be neoplastic, but falling short of the threshold of TCIS.

TRANSITIONAL CELL CARCINOMA *IN SITU*

Transitional cell carcinoma *in situ* is a proliferation of cytologically malignant urothelial cells confined to the epithelium of the mucosa. It arises *de novo* in patients without a prior or concomitant history of bladder disease in less than 10% of cases but is most commonly seen in patients with a current or prior bladder carcinoma (Lum and Torti, 1985; Smith et al., 1983; Torti and Lum, 1987). Transitional cell carcinoma *in situ* has a great potential for developing subsequent invasive neoplasia, with up to 80% of patients developing invasive carcinoma within 4 years. Patients with multifocal and extensive disease are more likely to have their disease progress than are patients with focal

disease (Lum and Torti, 1985; Smith et al., 1983; Torti and Lum, 1987).

At the University of Texas M.D. Anderson Cancer Center, TCIS has been defined as cytologically malignant cells involving the full thickness of the mucosal epithelium (Ayala and Ro, 1989). In contrast, the definition provided by the consensus WHO/ISUP (Epstein et al., 1998) is wider, as it includes lesions previously interpreted as moderate or severe dysplasia. This consensus definition states that the cells of TCIS, *irrespective of the thickness of involvement of the urothelium*, show loss of polarity, hyperchromasia, nucleomegaly, numerous mitoses, including mitotic activity in the superficial layers, and—most importantly—nuclear pleomorphism. The following features must be recognized: (*1*) the entire thickness of the urothelium does not need to be replaced by atypical cells, but neoplastic cells must be present; patterns of TCIS with less than full-thickness involvement include clinging or denuding TCIS, pagetoid TCIS, and undermining or lepidic growth of TCIS (Fig. 20–18); (*2*) the cells of TCIS do not necessarily have a high nuclear-to-cytoplasmic ratio, but the nuclei must be atypical; and (*3*) an umbrella cell layer may be present. When utilizing the definition of carcinoma *in situ* proposed by the consensus WHO/ISUP classification (Epstein et al., 1998), a comment should be made with regard to the manner in which the diagnosis was made.

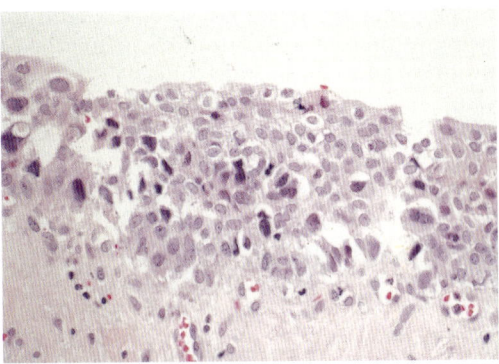

Figure 20–18. Lepidic transitional cell carcinoma *in situ* is characterized by infiltration of neoplastic tumor cells in the mucosa in a burrowing fashion.

The epithelial thickness of TCIS varies, at times being thinner than normal because of shedding resulting from the decreased cohesiveness between tumor cells. Caution should be exercised when the surface epithelium shows fewer than three layers of atypical cells, as the possible sloughing of a maturing surface epithelium may exist. Bladder epithelium may also be involved by TCIS through pagetoid spread. In this mode, malignant cells, either singly or in groups, involve the basal layer or lower third of the otherwise normal mucosa, and the involvement is distant from the major site of the mucosa affected with TCIS (Lum and Torti, 1985; Torti and Lum, 1987). Pagetoid spread may undermine the urothelium, causing it to slough off (Fig. 20–9). The clinical significance of pagetoid TCIS is identical to that of other forms of TCIS. Table 20–4A summarizes the morphologic variations and Table 20–4B the biological significance of TCIS.

Three different clinicopathologic types of TCIS are seen (Lum and Torti, 1985; Torti and Lum, 1987). The most common type (type 1) is the presence of a focus of TCIS immediately adjacent to a papillary tumor. Estimates of the incidence of TCIS in areas adjacent to papillary tumors range from 26% to 40% (Farrow et al, 1977; Schade and Swinney, 1973; Torti and Lum, 1987). In type 2, TCIS is observed distant from the papillary tumor and the intervening mucosa is normal (Soloway et al., 1978). In type 3, TCIS involves totally or near-totally the urothelium, without associated papillary tumors. Radical therapy may be warranted in type 3 (diffuse type), as there is a 50% to 80% incidence of progression to infiltrating cancer in this type (Farrow et al., 1977; Schade and Swinney, 1973; Soloway et al., 1978; Utz et al., 1970).

Involvement of von Brunn's epithelial nests is relatively common and is manifested as a proliferation of atypical cells to a full-blown TCIS replacing the bland urothelium of this proliferative cystitis.

The prostatic urethra and the more centrally occurring prostatic ducts and acini may be involved (Farrow et al., 1976, 1977; Franks and Chesterman, 1956; Johnson et al., 1972; Prout et al., 1987; Schade and Swinney, 1973; Schellhammer and Whitmore, 1976; Soloway et al., 1978; Tomaszewski et al., 1986; Utz et al., 1970; Wishnow and Ro,

Table 20–4A. Morphological Expression of Carcinoma *In Situ*

Small cell carcinoma *in situ*

Large cell carcinoma *in situ*

"Denuding cystitis"

Undermining (lepidic) growth

Pagetoid carcinoma *in situ*

Carcinoma *in situ* involving von Brunn's nests

Carcinoma *in situ* with microinvasion

1988). Since prostatic ductal involvement by TCIS is notoriously silent, a routine biopsy of the prostatic urethra including prostatic tissue is performed in patients with TCIS of the bladder (Franks and Chesterman, 1956; Johnson et al., 1972; Utz et al., 1970). The incidence of TCIS in the prostate has been reported by Farrow et al. (1976) to be as high as 36.8% of patients with TCIS of the bladder and this high incidence probably results because the prostatic urethra and prostatic parenchyma are usually beyond the reach of the topical therapy that is commonly administered in these patients (Farrow et al., 1976; Prout et al., 1987). The main site for involvement is in the verumontanum area, since most prostatic ducts open into this region. Involvement is recognized histologically as an *in situ* change involving ducts, acini, or both. In some cases, there may be a focal breakthrough of the basement membrane and early invasion of the stroma. Wishnow and Ro (1988) found that in 23 patients

Table 20–4B. Carcinoma *In Situ* Clinical Settings With Biological Significance

De novo carcinoma in situ

Potential to progress to invasive carcinoma and death

Biologically appears to be more indolent than previously believed

Carcinoma in situ in patients with noninvasive or superficially invasive transitional cell carcinoma

Increased risk for recurrence

Increased risk for invasion

Increased risk for multifocal disease—renal pelvis, prostatic urethra, etc.

Carcinoma in situ with microinvasion

Low but distinct potential for metastasis and death

with TCIS of the bladder and prostate treated with cystoprostatectomy, only 2 of the 18 patients (11%) with TCIS of the prostate (confined to the prostatic ducts or acini) developed metastases, whereas all 5 patients with prostatic stromal invasion developed metastatic disease.

Transitional cell carcinoma *in situ* can also involve the urethra and periurethral glands (Franks and Chesterman, 1956; Johnson et al., 1972). If the urethra is not removed, tumor can develop at the stump; such a tumor is often difficult to manage.

Nonurothelial mucosa can also be involved by TCIS. Sites described in the literature include the seminal vesicle, ejaculatory duct epithelium, urethral meatus, and collecting ducts of the kidney (Ro et al., 1987; Thomaszewski et al., 1986).

Microinvasive carcinoma has not been accepted as a term or as an entity in bladder carcinoma. Farrow and Utz (1982) defined microinvasive carcinoma as a lesion invading the lamina propria no deeper than 5 mm. In their study, 24 of 70 patients in whom cystectomy was performed for TCIS had foci of microinvasion; the remaining 46 had TCIS alone. A total of six deaths occurred. One death in each group was an operative death. One patient died of metastatic disease in the *in situ* group and three in the microinvasive group. One patient in the microinvasive group also had extensive prostatic duct involvement. The data suggest that microinvasion confers upon the tumor the power to metastasize and cause death in a small but definite proportion of afflicted patients.

SUPERFICIAL DISEASE

Superficial disease includes noninvasive and lamina propria–invasive tumors but does not include TCIS because of its different natural history and behavior (Cutler et al., 1982). At presentation 80% of bladder cancers clinically considered superficial are noninvasive lesions confined to the mucosa, but some superficial tumors are indeed invasive tumors involving the lamina propria. Of the superficial tumors, 60%–65% remain at risk for local recurrences (new occurrences), but never become deeply invasive and pose only a local management problem; the remaining one-third of superficial tumors, however, become invasive with time (Cutler et al., 1982; Heney et al., 1982, 1983). To help identify patients with superficial disease who are at high risk for recurrence or the development of invasive disease, numerous studies on DNA flow cytometry, blood groups, oncogenes, cytogenetic abnormalities, and tumor proliferative activity, as well as conventional prognostic factors, are being evaluated (Heney et al., 1982; Jordan et al., 1987; Lipponen et al., 1991).

HISTOLOGIC GRADING

Histologic assessment of the degree of differentiation of a TCC is very important, since many studies have shown a correlation of grade with frequency of invasion, metastasis, and survival (Abel et al., 1988a, b; Bergkvist et al., 1965; Carbin et al., 1991a,b; Friedell et al., 1976; Ooms et al., 1983; Pauels et al., 1988).

Jordan et al. (1987) reported actuarial 10- and 20-year survival rates for patients with grade 1 TCC of 98% and 93%, respectively. In their study, the cancer did not progress in 84 of 91 patients with grade 1 TCC and the patients had normal life expectancies regardless of the number of recurrences; only 4 of 91 patients (4.4%) died of bladder cancer, and in 3 other patients, grade 1 TCCs progressed to grade 3. In contrast, progressive disease occurred in 62% of 239 patients with grade 3 TCC, with actuarial survival rates of 35% and 28% at 10 and 20 years, respectively. Of the 152 individuals who died of bladder cancers, 142 (93%) had grade 3 TCC, and prognosis was poor even if invasion was not identified in the primary biopsy. Fifty patients with grade 2 TCC fared much better than the patients with grade 3 TCC, with actuarial 10- and 20-year survival rates of 87% and 81%, respectively; six patients died of tumor and five patients developed grade 3 recurrences. Two of the latter five patients later died of tumor. The grade is the primary determinant for risk of muscle invasion, particularly in tumors of the pT1 category.

Carbin et al. (1991a,b) subdivided grade 2 of the WHO grading system into two new subgroups (2a and 2b) on the basis of nuclear pleomorphism and the number of mitoses (modified Bergkvist et al. [1965] system). They found that the behavior of grade 2a bladder tumors was similar to that of grade 1 tumors (5-year survival rate, 92%), whereas the grade 2b cancers were more comparable to grade 3 tumors (5-year survival rate, 43%). They noted that this system had a high reproducibility, with an interobserver agreement of more than 90%. Pauwels et al. (1988) also divided grade 2 tumors into grade 2a (slight cellular variation) and 2b (clear cytologic deviation and a tendency to lose normal polarity) and reported results similar to those of Carbin et al. (1991a,b). The rates of tumor recurrence for tumors of grades 2a and 2b after 1 year were 5% and 31%, respectively; the rates of tumor progression were 4% and 33%, respectively, with progression occurring late in grade 2a carcinomas and fairly early in grade 2b lesions. Pauwels et al. (1988) furthermore proposed that grades 1 and 2a be classified as low grade and that grade 2b tumors be classified as intermediate grade. Blomjous et al. (1990) also subdivided grade 2 TCC on the basis of small nuclei (mean nuclear area $\leq95\ \mu m^2$) and large nuclei ($>95\ \mu m^2$) measured by morphometry, because they found a distinct difference, in terms of recurrence and 5-year survival rate, between patients with grade 2 tumors with small nuclei and those with grade 2 tumors with large nuclei.

The prognostic effect of the recently proposed WHO/ISUP consensus classification (Epstein et al., 1998) needs to be evaluated both retrospectively and prospectively. The papilloma as defined by the 1973 WHO (Mostofi et al., 1973) classification is essentially retained in the new classification; grades 1, 2, and 3 of the 1973 WHO classification are roughly equivalent to papillary urothelial neoplasms of low malignant potential, low-grade carcinoma, and high-grade carcinoma, respectively, in the 1998 WHO/ISUP classification (Epstein et al., 1998).

DEPTH OF INVASION IN SUPERFICIAL DISEASE

In 1946, Jewett and Strong used depth of invasion by tumor as a clinical staging system; this system was later modified by Marshall (1962). The TNM system subsequently incorporated the basic important concepts of this system.

There is a significant difference in behavior between tumors localized to the mucosa and tumors invading the lamina propria (pT1) (Anderstrom et al., 1980; Rubben et al., 1978; Williams et al., 1977). In a study by Abel et al. (1988b), none of the noninvasive mucosal tumors (pTa) progressed to invasion; in contrast, 46% (11 of 24) of the TCC invading the lamina propria (pT1) progressed to invasion of the muscularis propria within 3 years of presentation, and 10 of these 11 patients died of their TCC. Heney et al. (1983) found that only 4% of noninvasive (pTa) tumors progressed. However, there was no significant difference in terms of recurrence between the two groups.

Younes et al. (1990) substaged 31 TCC with lamina propria invasion (pT1) as follows: T1a, invasion of connective tissue superficial to the level of muscularis mucosae (14 patients); T1b, invasion to the level of the muscularis mucosae (3 patients); T1c, invasion through the level of muscularis mucosae but superficial to the muscularis propria (14 patients). They found that 75% of the 17 patients with stage T1a and T1b tumors survived at least 5 years, contrasting with a survival rate of only 11% for the 14 patients with T1c tumors. These results emphasize the importance of the muscularis mucosae as a potential landmark in substaging bladder cancer. Subsequently, two additional studies have shown similar prognostic relevance for the substaging of pT1 TCC (Table 20–5; Angulo et al., 1995; Hasui et al., 1994).

Grade 3 TCCs invading the lamina propria (T1) have a worse prognosis than other superficial tumors, with a recurrence rate of 50% to 74% after transurethral resection alone and a tumor progression rate of 25% to 48% (Cutler et al., 1982; Jake et al., 1987). Jake et al. (1987) further stated that such invasion confers a more malignant nature on the tumor rather than merely increasing the grade of dysplasia shown by the tumor.

Zieger et al. (1998) reported that invasion of the lamina propria was the most significant prognostic factor detected in a multivariate analysis. While 14% of patients with Ta tumors died of disease after 15 years, 63% of the T1 tumors were eventually fatal, reaching the mortality of those of T2 disease. Other independent significant factors were

Table 20–5. Studies of Substage T1 Transitional Cell Carcinoma

Reference	Subclassification	Level of Invasion	Results
Younes et al. (1990)	T1a	Connective tissue superficial to MM	75% 5-year survival
	T1b	To MM	75% 5-year survival
	T1c	Through MM but superficial to MP	11% 5-year survival
Hasui et al. (1994)	T1a	Superficial to MM	6.7% progression
	T1b	Deep to MM	53.5% progression
Angulo et al. (1995)	T1a	Invading lamina propria, but not involving MM	86% 5-year survival
	T1b	Invading submucosa	52% 5-year survival

MM, Muscularis mucosae; MP, muscularis propria.

tumor size and, to a lesser extent, histological grade.

VASCULAR/LYMPHATIC INVASION IN SUPERFICIAL DISEASE

Incidence rates of vascular invasion in superficial tumors range from 2.5% to 7% (Anderstrom et al., 1980; Rubben et al., 1978; Williams et al., 1977). Anderstrom et al. (1980) reported that 10 of 177 patients with superficial bladder tumors showed vascular invasion by tumor cells. Seven of these 10 patients died of widespread bladder carcinoma within 6 years, and the difference in prognosis with and without vascular/lymphatic invasion was statistically significant ($p < 0.01$). Thus, vascular/lymphatic invasion seems to be an important predictor of prognosis in patients with superficial invasion regardless of tumor grade. A major problem with recognition of vascular invasion is that, not infrequently, tumors invasive in the lamina propria exhibit a retraction artifact that potentially may be overdiagnosed as vascular–lymphatic invasion. The results of Ramani et al. (1988) and Larsen et al. (1990), who found that only 40% and 14%, respectively, of instances of morphologically diagnosed vascular invasion could be confirmed by immunohistochemistry, support this conclusion. Hence, strict criteria are required to diagnose vascular invasion, which, if present, suggests that transurethral resection alone may be insufficient to treat the tumors and that more extensive surgery or chemotherapy may need to be considered.

NUMBER AND SIZE OF PAPILLARY TUMORS IN SUPERFICIAL DISEASE

The number of papillary tumors is an important factor for recurrence but not a significant determinant of invasive disease (Grossman, 1996; Jewett and Eversole, 1960; Kaubisch et al., 1991). Lutzeyer et al. (1982) reported recurrence rates in solitary pTa and pT1 tumors of 18% and 33%, respectively; for multiple tumors, the rates were 43% and 46%, respectively. Cutler et al. (1982) showed that patients with a single tumor had a 67% chance of recurrence, in contrast with a 90% chance if they had multiple growths at initial diagnosis. The disease-free interval for patients with multiple tumors was also shorter. Dalesio et al. (1983) found the number of tumors at initial diagnosis to be the single most important factor influencing the new tumor rate. Lerman et al. (1970) also demonstrated significantly different recurrence rates for single lesions (31%) than for multiple lesions (66%). Furthermore, the probability of later-developing invasive carcinoma nearly tripled in patients with multiple lesions on presentation (13.6%) compared with those who presented with a single lesion (4.6%).

Chronology is also an important factor for tumor recurrences. A patient with a first tumor has up to a 45% risk of developing another lesion after transurethral or open resection, but the patient who develops a second tumor has an 84% risk of developing a third lesion (Grossman, 1996).

Heney et al. (1983) reported that progression to muscle invasion occurred in 35%

of patients with superficial tumors larger than 5 cm, compared with 9% of patients with smaller tumors. Pagano et al. (1987), however, reported that tumor size influenced stage but not progression.

STATUS OF NONPAPILLARY UROTHELIUM

An additional prognostic factor of superficial disease is the presence of urothelial dysplasia elsewhere in the bladder mucosa (Pagano et al., 1987). Smith et al. (1983) found that, when dysplasia or TCIS was histologically evident, the recurrence rate was 73% compared with 43% for patients without evidence of concomitant dysplasia. The presence of TCIS with superficial bladder disease increases the risk of invasion to as high as 83%. Althausen et al. (1976) observed that, of the 30% of patients with superficial TCC who developed muscle invasion 5 years after diagnosis, the majority had dysplasia or TCIS in the epithelium adjacent to the primary lesion. Of 78 patients whose tumor biopsy samples contained adjacent mucosa, 12 (15%) had TCIS. Ten (83%) of these developed muscle invasion within 5 years. In contrast, 41 patients (53%) had normal epithelium and in only 3 of these patients (7%) did the tumor progress to muscle invasion. Intermediate between these groups were 25 patients (32%) who had dysplasia elsewhere in the bladder mucosa; of these 25, 9 patients (36%) went on to develop invasive cancer.

MUSCLE-INVASIVE TRANSITIONAL CELL CARCINOMA

Invasive bladder carcinoma differs from noninvasive (superficial) tumors in that the tumors are usually single, almost always nonpapillary, deeply infiltrating, and high grade. The pathologist's role in evaluating biopsies or transurethrally resected specimens from patients with clinical stage B/C (T2/T3) disease is to confirm the diagnosis and evaluate the extent of invasion, namely invasion into the muscularis propria or beyond. The presence of lymphatic and/or vascular invasion should be noted in the report (Fig. 20–19), but the significance of this finding in muscle-invasive tumors is controversial. The prognosis for patients with invasive bladder carcinoma is poor: even with aggressive

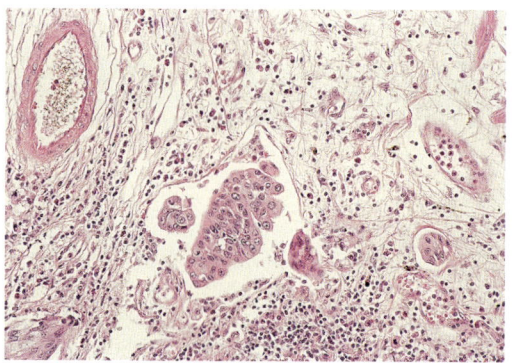

Figure 20–19. Transitional cell carcinoma invading vascular/lymphatic channels.

therapy that includes a combination of surgery, chemotherapy, and/or radiotherapy, the survival rate is no better than 50% at 5 years (Friedell et al., 1976; Johnson and Ayala, 1989; Johnson and Boileau, 1982).

The morphologic appearance of invasive TCC is well known and needs little elaboration. A variety of patterns may be seen. It should be noted, however, that occasionally one does see invasive tumors with relatively bland cytologic features (Talbert and Young, 1989). Invasive TCCs contained areas of either glandular or squamous differentiation in approximately 20% and 7% of the cases, respectively (Friedell et al., 1976; Koss, 1985; Murphy et al., 1994).

OTHER CARCINOMAS OF THE BLADDER AND HISTOLOGIC VARIANTS OF TRANSITIONAL CELL CARCINOMA

An exhaustive list of the histologic diversity of carcinomas of the urinary bladder is provided in Table 20–6.

Squamous carcinoma of the bladder accounts for 3% to 8% of all bladder tumors and has an age and sex distribution similar to that of TCC (Schroder et al., 1986). Risk factors include chronic urinary tract infection, lithiasis, and schistosomiasis. For the diagnosis, a tumor composed almost exclusively of squamous differentiation with intercellular bridges and/or keratinization is required. Many tumors are mixed TCC and squamous carcinoma so that it is not infrequent to have a squamous carcinoma only in a biopsy specimen but a pure TCC or mixed with TCC in the cystectomy specimen

Table 20–6. Classification of Carcinomas of the Urinary Bladder Including Transitional Cell Carcinoma and Its Variants

1. Transitional cell neoplasia	*2. Squamous carcinoma*
Benign	Conventional
Transitional papilloma (WHO grade 0)	Variants:
Inverted papilloma	Verrucous carcinoma
	Sarcomatoid carcinoma
Malignant	
Papillary[a]	*3. Adenocarcinoma*
Typical	Anatomic variants
Variants	Bladder mucosa
With squamous, glandular, or small cell	Urachal
differentiation	With exstrophy
Micropapillary	From endometriosis
Inverted	Histologic variants
Carcinoma *in situ*	Typical intestinal type
Microinvasive carcinoma	Mucinous (including colloid)
Frankly invasive carcinoma	Signet ring cell
Variants containing or exhibiting:	Clear cell
Deceptively benign features	Sarcomatoid carcinoma
Nested pattern (resembling von Brunn's nests)	
Small tubular pattern	*4. Tumors of mixed cell types*
Microcysts	
Inverted pattern	*5. Undifferentiated carcinoma[b]*
Transitional cell carcinoma with clear cell	Small cell carcinoma
features	Lymphoepithelioma-like carcinoma
Transitional cell carcinoma with plasmacytoid	Giant cell carcinoma
features	Not otherwise specified
Squamous differentiation	
Glandular differentiation	*6. Metastatic carcinoma*
Sarcomatoid carcinoma	
Unusual stromal reactions	
Stromal osseous or cartilaginous metaplasia	
Osteoclast-type giant cells	
Prominent lymphoid infiltrate	
Syncytiotrophoblasts	

[a]Papillary tumors may be invasive or noninvasive, and when invasive may be microinvasive or frankly invasive (like nonpapillary tumors).

[b]Refers to tumors that are undifferentiated by light microscopy.

or vice versa. Another rare variant is verrucous carcinoma of bladder (Walther et al., 1986; Fig. 20–20). The prognosis for patients with pure squamous cell carcinomas of the bladder is poor; most patients present with advanced stage. The tumors are refractory to radiation and chemotherapy.

Adenocarcinomas of the bladder constitute about 1% of bladder tumors. Such tumors have a peak incidence in the sixth and seventh decades of life, occurring predominantly in men. Although most cases arise *de novo*, exstrophy of the bladder is a known risk factor. Adenocarcinomas present the usual glandular, papillary, or mucinous appearance and are indistinguishable from enteric (colonic) adenocarcinomas, and some have a signet ring cell appearance. To be classified as signet-ring cell carcinoma, at least 25% of the tumor should have signet ring cells (Grignon et al., 1991a,b; Fig.

20–21). On a stage-by-stage basis, adenocarcinoma has an outcome comparable to that of TCC; however, most adenocarcinomas are diagnosed an advanced stage. A rare variant is clear cell adenocarcinoma that occurs rarely in bladder but is more common in the urethra (Young and Scully, 1985).

Small cell carcinoma (Fig. 20–22) may arise in the bladder either pure or admixed with TCC (Grignon et al., 1992; Mills et al., 1987). Patients with this aggressive form of TCC have a poor prognosis.

Micropapillary TCC (Fig. 20–23), a recently recognized variant of TCC (Amin et al., 1994), is diagnosed at advanced stages and shows frequent vascular invasion. The metastases from patients with this variant tend to retain the micropapillary pattern (Amin et al., 1994a).

Lymphoepithelioma-like carcinoma simulates the nasopharyngeal carcinoma in mor-

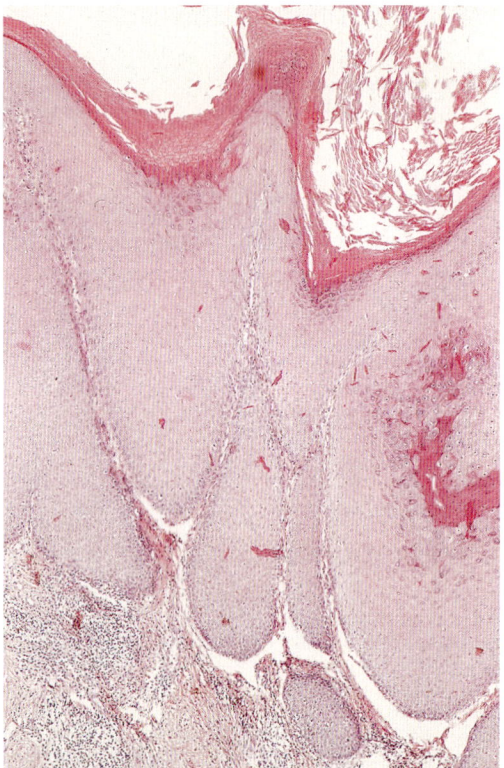

Figure 20–20. Verrucous squamous carcinoma. This is a papillomatous, keratotic, and acanthotic growth with rounded protuberances of cells at the advancing edge. There is neither nuclear atypia nor destructive invasion.

phology (Amin et al., 1994b), and is a high-grade carcinoma with abundant lymphoid infiltrate (Fig. 20–24). This tumor in its pure form responds well to chemotherapy, and patients show a better prognosis than those with the usual type of TCC (Amin et al., 1994b).

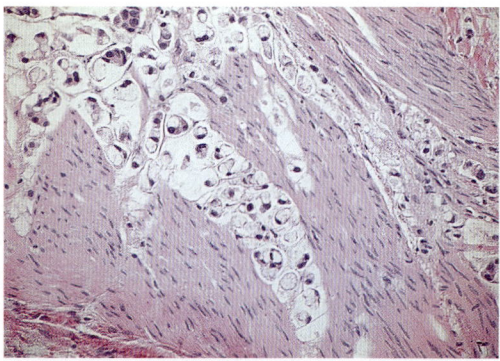

Figure 20–21. Signet-ring cell adenocarcinoma infiltrating muscularis propria.

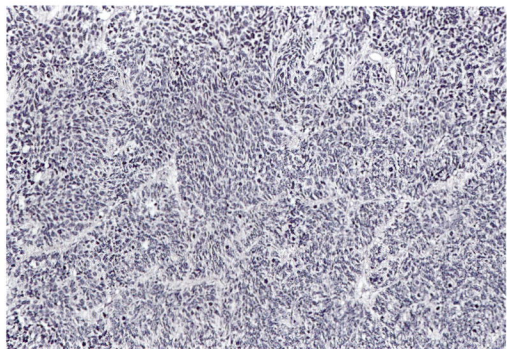

Figure 20–22. Small cell carcinoma. This tumor consists of a cellular proliferation of small cells that have hyperchromatic nuclei with nuclear molding and little cytoplasm.

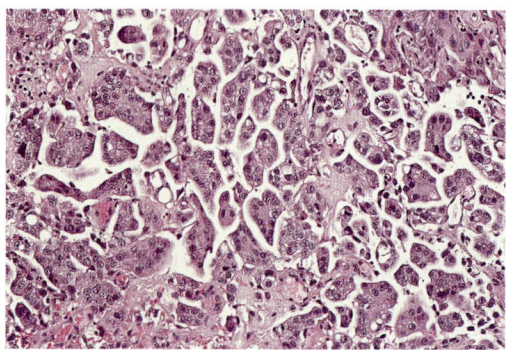

Figure 20–23. Micropapillary transitional cell carcinoma (TCC) characteristically shows small papillary formations that differ from the larger papillary structures of the common TCC. These papillary structures are often contained within spaces that may be retraction artifact or vascular spaces.

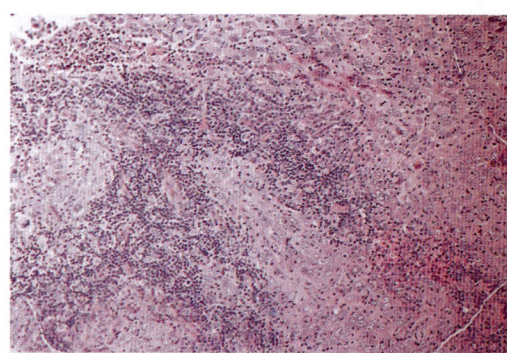

Figure 20–24. Lymphoepithelial like–carcinoma shows a syncytial arrangement of large cells with vesicular nuclei having one or more prominent nucleoli and abundant amphophilic cytoplasm. These cells merge imperceptibly with the lymphocytes and elicit no desmoplastic response of the stroma.

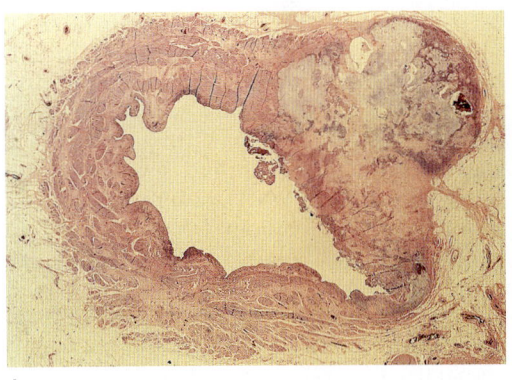

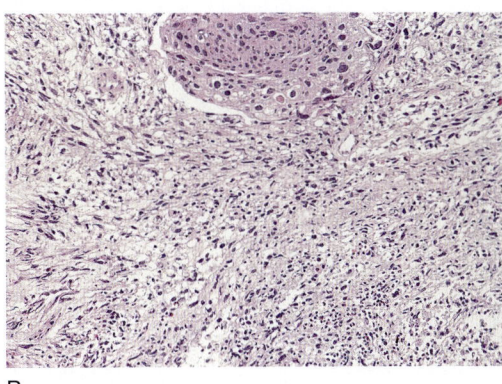

A B

Figure 20–25. *A*: This whole-organ section depicts a large sarcomatoid carcinoma involving the entire thickness of the wall and pushing into the adventitial tissue. The pale gray areas represent a cartilaginous component; the darker areas are epithelial. *B*: High-power view shows the byphasic components of the now obvious carcinoma and sarcoma.

Sarcomatoid carcinoma (carcinosarcoma) is a biphasic malignant tumor with carcinomatous and pleomorphic sarcomatoid components (Fig. 20–25). Patients with this tumor usually present with advanced-stage disease and have a worse prognosis than those with the usual TCC (Ro et al., 1988).

Certain growth patterns of TCC have also been described, including the microcystic TCC (Fig. 20–26; Young and Zuckerberg, 1991), the deceptively benign-looking TCC (Talbert and Young, 1989), and the nested-patterned TCC (Fig. 20–27; Murphy and Deana, 1992); their proper recognition is important to avoid misdiagnosis with von Brunn's nests, cystitis cystica, and nephrogenic adenoma. The nested variant, although histologically banal in its appearance,

is associated with an aggressive outcome: only 3 of 19 patients with adequate follow-up have had no evidence of disease, and no patient with greater than 2 years follow-up has no evidence of disease (Murphy and Deana, 1992). The significance of TCC with choriocarcinoma (Abratt et al., 1988; Young and Eble, 1991) and of TCC with osteoclastic giant cells (Young and Eble, 1991; Zukerberg et al., 1990) is uncertain because only a limited number of cases have been reported; however, those patients had a worse prognosis than patients with the usual TCC. Transitional cell carcinoma exhibiting clear cell features (Kotliar et al., 1995) and plasmacytoid TCC have been described as variants of TCC (Sahin et al., 1991). Two cases of TCC with clear cell changes have been recently

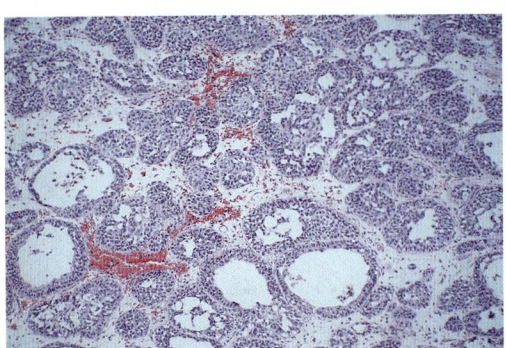

Figure 20–26. Microcystic transitional cell carcinoma is a variant of transitional cell carcinoma that consists of malignant nests of urothelial cells exhibiting cystic structures.

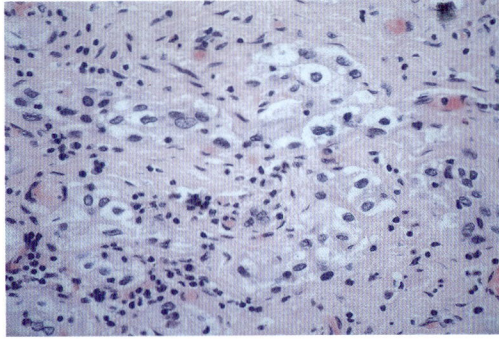

Figure 20–27. Transitional cell carcinoma with a nested pattern has small nests of deceptively bland malignant urothelial cells infiltrating the lamina propria.

described, in which the tumors contained optically clear cells rich in glycogen (Kotliar et al., 1995). Plasmacytoid TCC may be mistaken for plasmacytoma, especially if the patient has evidence of osseous metastasis at presentation (Sahin et al., 1991).

PROGNOSTIC MARKERS

As previously stated, 15%–20% of the cases of superficial disease will progress to muscle invasion (4% or less of the Ta and 30% of the T1 lesions) (Wolf et al., 1983). Furthermore, other studies have shown that progression was greater in grade 3 tumors (28.5%) than in grade 2 tumors (9%) and grade 1 tumors (2.1%) (Chenn et al., 1996; Koontz et al., 1985).

Blood Group Antigen

The disappearance or absence of blood group antigens on the tumor cell surface, demonstrated either by the specific red-cell adherence test or by immunohistochemical analysis, has been associated with progressive disease (Bergman and Javadpour, 1978; Newman et al., 1980; Richie et al., 1980; Sanders et al., 1991; Wick et al., 1989; Yamada et al., 1991). Likewise, the disappearance of the Lewis substance in bladder tumors is associated with an aggressive course (Juhl et al., 1986; Orntoft et al., 1987). The Thomsen-Friedenreich antigen has also been the subject of extensive studies (Blasco et al., 1988; Coon et al., 1982; Langkilde et al., 1991). All of these studies have historical value as they initiated the era of research for accurate prognostic markers in bladder cancer, but they are presently not utilized in clinical practice.

DNA Content and S-phase Fraction

Several studies have related flow cytometric DNA analysis in urothelial neoplasms to tumor recurrence, tumor progression, or survival. In general, nearly all grade 1 TCCs and two-thirds of grade 2 tumors are diploid. Tetraploid tumors are almost exclusively found in grade 2 tumors; most grade 3 tumors and some grade 2 tumors are nontetraploid aneuploid tumors (Blomjous et al., 1988; De Vita et al., 1991; Lipponen et al.,

1991; Masters et al., 1989). Gustafson et al. (1982a,b) examined DNA patterns in relation to tumor recurrence and tumor progression in 229 patients with superficial grade 1 and grade 2 TCC treated by local surgery only. One hundred seventy-five tumors had diploid DNA content, and 54 tumors showed aneuploid DNA content. No progression was found in the 175 patients with diploid tumors, whereas 35% of the 54 aneuploid tumors progressed, with 58% of these patients dying of disease. This was irrespective of tumor grade. The difference in frequency of recurrence between aneuploid and diploid tumors was statistically significant in this study. Multiple grade 2 aneuploid tumors had 1.64 recurrences per year, while multiple grade 2 diploid lesions exhibited 1.19 annual recurrences. From the results of this study, it appears that DNA analysis can help identify those grade 2 TCCs with a propensity for recurrence. In a study by Blomjous et al. (1988), all 16 grade 1 TCCs, 13 of 34 grade 2 TCCs, and none of 11 grade 3 TCCs were diploid tumors. Of the 37 superficial tumors, 25 (68%) were diploid. The data suggest that the initial presence of aneuploidy in superficial bladder cancers is a strong argument for more aggressive treatment. Masters et al. (1989) also reported that patients with aneuploid tumors, with a high proportion of cells in S phase, and with poorly differentiated tumors more frequently developed progressive disease than did patients with diploid tumors, a low proportion of cells in S phase, and well-differentiated tumors. In contrast, Murphy et al. (1986) reported that, although there was a correlation between ploidy and outcome in superficial bladder tumors, this correlation was not independent of tumor grade.

Although differences in S-phase fraction appear to have a significant association with survival, this may not be independent of ploidy, since there is a strong correlation between aneuploidy and high S-phase fraction. Tribukait (1984) reported that only one diploid TCC displayed an S-phase fraction of more than 10% but that most of the aneuploid TCCs (77%) displayed an S-phase fraction of 10% or greater. Sixty-two percent of patients with aneuploid tumors and an S-phase fraction of 10% or greater were dead of disease at 4 years, compared with 5% of those with an S-phase fraction of less than 10%.

Tumor Proliferative Activity

Tumor proliferative activity (TPA) has been shown to be significantly higher in TCC than in normal epithelium (Helpap et al., 1985; Mellon et al., 1990; Pfister et al., 1999). Furthermore, TPA is higher in TCC with muscle invasion than in superficial TCC. Tumor labeling index or S-phase fraction has been correlated with prognosis in bladder tumors. The S-phase fraction can be measured directly by DNA flow cytometry, by incorporation of [³H]thymidine or BrdUrd into tumor DNA, or by immunohistochemical staining of cell-specific antigens such as Ki-67 or proliferating cell nuclear antigen (PCNA), which is expressed only in proliferating cells. Measurement of nucleolar organizer regions, another method for analyzing TPA, has been reported to correlate with tumor grade, stage, and clinical behavior (Lipponen and Eskelinen, 1991).

In general, TPA is higher in muscle-invasive TCC and poorly differentiated tumors than in superficial and well-differentiated tumors. Evidence suggests that this approach to assessing TPA produces simple and reproducible results. The TPA measurements may be helpful in determining which tumors will recur and progress into muscle-invasive tumors within the superficial tumor group (Fradet, 1990). To date, no method of estimating tumor proliferation has consistently yielded prognostic information superior to, or independent of, the more conventional prognostic methods.

Others

Immunostaining for basement-membrane components, such as laminin and type IV collagen, may provide valuable information on early invasion in cases in which the evaluation of invasion is difficult by conventional microscopic examination alone. Loss or lack of basement-membrane materials underlying noninvasive TCC or nests of invasive TCC in the lamina propria may be correlated with subsequent progression to higher clinical stages or vascular invasion. The type 1 pattern (intact basement membrane) has been frequently associated with pTa and low-grade tumors, whereas type 2 pattern (fragmented or lack of basement membrane) is associated with pT1 and high-grade tumors (Schapers et al., 1990).

Human milk fat globulin-2 (HMFG-2) staining occurs in the lumina in well-differentiated superficial tumors, whereas diffuse staining of all cells occurs in invasive TCCs. There is a significant association between the HMFG-2 staining score and T category, as well as between staining score and histologic grade. pTa and grade 1 tumors have low HMFG-2 staining scores, whereas pT1 and grade 3 tumors have high scores. Although there is a poor correlation between staining and recurrence, there is a significant relationship between staining pattern and subsequent progression to muscle invasion and metastatic disease (Conn et al., 1988).

Monoclonal antibody 32-2B to desmosomal glycoprotein may be of value in detecting stromal invasion (Conn et al., 1990). In addition, transferrin receptor positivity has been reported to correlate with increased grade and subsequent recurrence. The role of angiogenesis in bladder tumor development and its putative role in determining tumor progression and recurrence have also been studied (Crew et al., 1996).

Chromosomal Abnormalities

Several studies have demonstrated that the presence of marker (abnormal) chromosomes in superficial papillary tumors predicts invasive potential and an adverse prognosis (Hopman et al., 1991; Pauwels et al., 1987; Sandberg, 1977, 1986; Sekine, 1976; Summers et al., 1981). In a study with 6 to 10 years of follow-up (Hopman et al., 1991; Sekine, 1976) 10% (2/20) of noninvasive papillary TCCs without marker chromosomes recurred during the follow-up period, and only one patient died of tumor. In contrast, 90% (18/20) of noninvasive papillary TCCs with marker chromosomes subsequently recurred, with only one patient death. In a third group, 80% (20/25) of pT1 TCCs with marker chromosomes recurred, and about half (12/25) of the patients died of tumor (Hopman et al., 1991). These findings strongly suggest that the detection of marker chromosomes in superficial TCC may help to predict recurrence and progression.

It is less clear how important the identification of specific chromosomal abnormalities in TCC is in predicting prognosis in superficial bladder cancers. Several reports have found chromosomal abnormalities in chromosomes 1, 5, 7, 9, and 11 in TCC (Hopman et al., 1991; Sekine, 1976; Summers et al., 1981; Waldman et al., 1991). The potential significance of these chromosomal abnormalities is unknown. However, the presence of extra copies of chromosome 7 in TCC is potentially significant because the c-*erb*-B oncogene, which codes for a portion of the epidermal growth factor receptor, is located on chromosome 7. Overexpression of this gene, by increased copy number, may thus be important in the growth of the tumor (Waldman et al., 1991).

Karyotyping of solid tumors is a more precise approach and detects numerical and/or structural abnormalities in chromosomes. However, this method is laborious and tedious. In addition, it is difficult to get enough cells in metaphase from solid tumors. Therefore, tumor cells are cultured to obtain an increased number of cells in metaphase, which creates a potential danger for loss of genetic material and selection of fast-growing subpopulations. Fluorescent *in situ* hybridization (FISH) using specific probes and nonisotopic detection procedures can detect numerical and structural chromosomal aberrations in nonmitotic interphase cells (Van Dekken et al., 1991; Neuhaus et al., 1999). In addition, this technique is a fast and powerful tool to apply to routine paraffin-embedded tissue sections. One study has shown that 88% of diploid tumors have chromosomal aberrations of chromosomes 7 (trisomy), 9 (monosomy), and 10 (trisomy) (Matsuyan et al., 1994).

ONCOGENES

ras Genes

The human *ras* genes (H-, Ki-, and N-*ras*) constitute a prototypic family of cellular transforming genes in which mutations or overexpression can lead to malignant transformation (Czerniak et al., 1990; Reddy et al., 1982). These genes encode a group of closely related 21 kD proteins that bind guanine nucleotides and have guanisine triphosphase (GTPase) activity. The protein is bound to the cytoplasmic surface and serves as a signal transduction molecule that mediates cell proliferation and differentiation. Two mechanisms have been proposed to explain how *ras* genes transform cells (Fig. 20–28). The first possible mechanism involves mutations at codon 12, 13, 59, or 61 (Chakraborty et al., 1991; Reddy et al., 1982). Such mutations are the most frequent alterations identified in human tu-

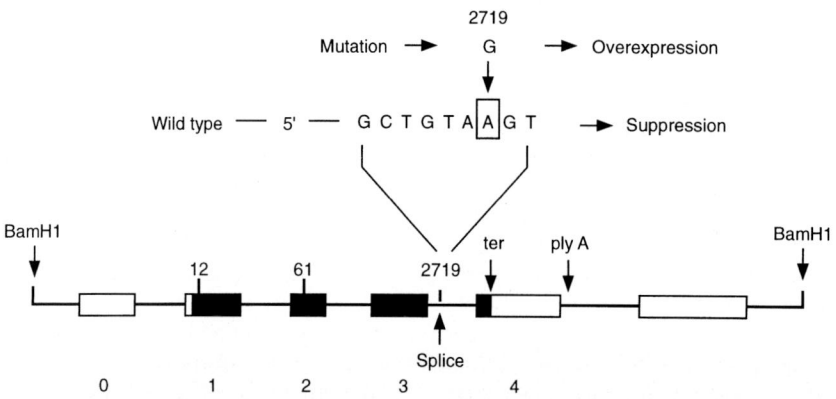

Figure 20–28. Exon–intron organization of K-*ras* gene. Mutations, predominantly of codons 12 and 61, are responsible for transforming activity of the p21 product. Splicing recognition site within the last intron suppresses expression of gene product and protects the cell from its transforming activity. A mutation at position 2719 within splicing recognition site abolishes this mechanism. If it is associated with mutation of coding sequence, it causes overexpression of transforming gene product.

mors, including urothelial malignancies. The mutations in these codons result in amino acid substitutions that affect the GTP binding domain and reduce the enzymatic activity of the protein. The second possible mechanism involves the regulation of *ras* gene expression. It has been shown that an internal splicing mechanism within the last intron (intron D) of the H-*ras* gene plays an important regulatory role mediating the gene expression (Chakraborty et al., 1991; Cohen and Levinson, 1988; Cohen et al., 1989). The sequence around nucleotide 2719 within intron D regulates an alternative splicing mechanism; it suppresses the gene expression by destabilizing transcription and channeling it to a nonproductive pathway. This results in the production of a truncated protein with tumor suppressor gene activity. Hence, the H-*ras* gene seems to be a model gene capable of encoding two antagonistic products: one with transforming activity and the other with tumor suppressor activity. It has been documented that a mutation at position 2710 of intron D abolishes the alternative splicing pathway, causing the overexpression of the gene product. If this mutation is associated with a mutation in the coding sequence, it results in an overexpression of the gene product with strong transforming ability. Mutations of the coding sequence of H-*ras*, especially at codon 12, are relatively frequent in urothelial tumors and can be seen in approximately 30%–40% of the urothelial lesions, but they cannot be related to any particular clinicopathological features and especially not to the aggressive behavior of urothelial carcinoma (Cohen et al., 1988; Czerniak et al., 1992; Czerniak and Herz, 1995). On the contrary, concurrent mutations within the splicing mechanism and the coding sequence, resulting in the overexpression of the transforming gene product, were documented exclusively in high-grade and high-stage tumors, but these are relatively infrequent and can be identified in less than 10% of TCCs. The pathogenetic significance of *ras* genes in urothelial malignancies is still a controversial issue, and there is no strong evidence that they can be used as diagnostic or prognostic markers for TCC (Agnantis et al., 1990; Chesa et al., 1987).

c-*Myc* Gene

The c-*Myc* gene encodes a sequence-specific DNA binding protein (Veyrune et al., 1997). It acts as a ubiquitous transcriptional factor and plays a role in proliferation and cell differentiation. Recently, c-*Myc* has been identified as one of the major regulatory elements of programmed cell death (Veyrune et al., 1997). The c-*Myc* gene contributes to tumorigenesis by the increased levels of the gene product as a result of amplification (Evan et al., 1994; Lemaitre et al., 1996; Vamvakas et al., 1993). Overexpression of c-*Myc* is a frequent finding in many common malignancies and has been associated with much more aggressive behavior, hormonal independence, and, in general, poor outcome. c-*Myc* overexpression in bladder tumors is typically seen in high-grade and high-stage lesions, but c-*Myc* is overexpressed in low-grade superficial papillary tumors (Evan et al., 1994; Lemaitre et al., 1996; Vamvakas et al., 1993).

p53 Gene

The *p53* gene, located on the short arm of chromosome 17, is a tumor-transforming gene that plays a major role in the development of many human malignancies (Levine et al., 1991; McBride et al., 1986; Velculesco and El-Diery, 1996). The gene product was originally identified as a 53 kD phosphoprotein in cells transformed by the SV40 virus (Levine et al., 1991; McBride et al., 1986; Velculesco and El-Diery, 1996). It was later shown that the transforming activity of *p53* is related to point mutations and that the mutated protein has a much longer half-life than the wild-type product (Livingstone et al., 1992). In tumors, *p53* acts predominantly in the homozygotic state, and the loss of its physiologic function is a major contributor to tumorigenesis (Finlay et al., 1989). Occasionally, a gain of new function after mutation may be of biological significance, and the gene can have a contributory effect to neoplastic transformation while it is still in the heterozygotic state. Mutations of *p53*, especially in common epithelial malignancies, are typically amino acid substitutions (Fig. 20–29). The missense mutations terminating the production of the gene product are more frequently observed in soft tissue and bone tumors. In urinary bladder

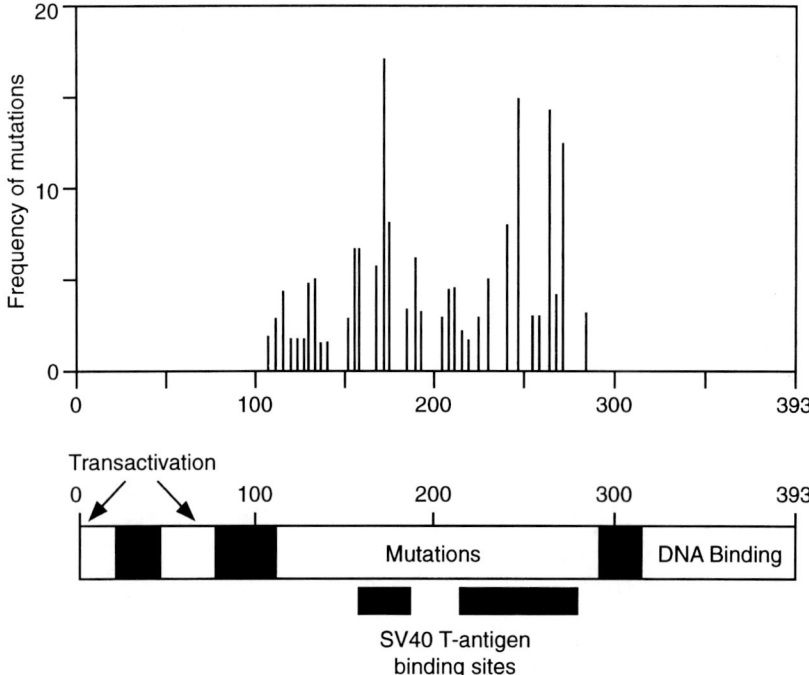

Figure 20–29. Functional organization of p53 protein. The *top panel* shows the distribution of mutations in various human tumors. The mutations cluster in the region coding for SV40 T antigen-binding domain *(bottom panel)*. Distribution of the mutations is according to the human genome database.

tumors, the alterations of *p53* typically develop in the urothelial dysplasia, which progress to carcinoma *in situ* and invasive nonpapillary carcinoma. These alterations can be documented in approximately 50% of high-grade invasive urinary bladder tumors. The presence of altered *p53* in an invasive bladder tumor signifies aggressive behavior of the lesion and is associated with a high propensity for distant metastasis and resistance to chemotherapy and radiation therapy (Czerniak and Herz, 1995).

Rb Gene

The *Rb* gene was originally identified as the gene of retinoblastoma, a rare intraocular malignant neoplasm. It was the first tumor suppressor gene identified, i.e., a gene whose loss of function leads to the development of malignant neoplasms (Lee, 1989), and was originally identified as a germline mutation that predisposes children to the development of retinoblastoma. The gene encodes for a 105 kD protein that is a transcription regulator in all adult cells and which has a strong affinity to react with D-cyclin (Lee, 1989). Loss of *Rb* gene function can be an important contributory mechanism of tumorigenesis, not only in retinoblastoma but also in many other epithelial or nonepithelial malignancies (Dowdy et al., 1993; Friend et al., 1987). The wild-type product of the *Rb* gene has properties of a cell cycle regulatory element (Horowitz et al., 1990). Alterations of the *Rb* gene in human neoplasms are of two main types: deletions and mutations (Fig. 20–30). The first mechanism consists of deletion of large gene segments, leading to the production of a truncated nonfunctioning gene product. The second mechanism involves substitutions of individual nucleotides that alter the gene function by creating improperly positioned initiation and splicing signals or stop codons, as well as causing amino acid substitutions that alter the protein function. In urinary bladder tumors, loss of the *Rb* gene function is a frequent event in the evolution of urothelial dysplasia, car-

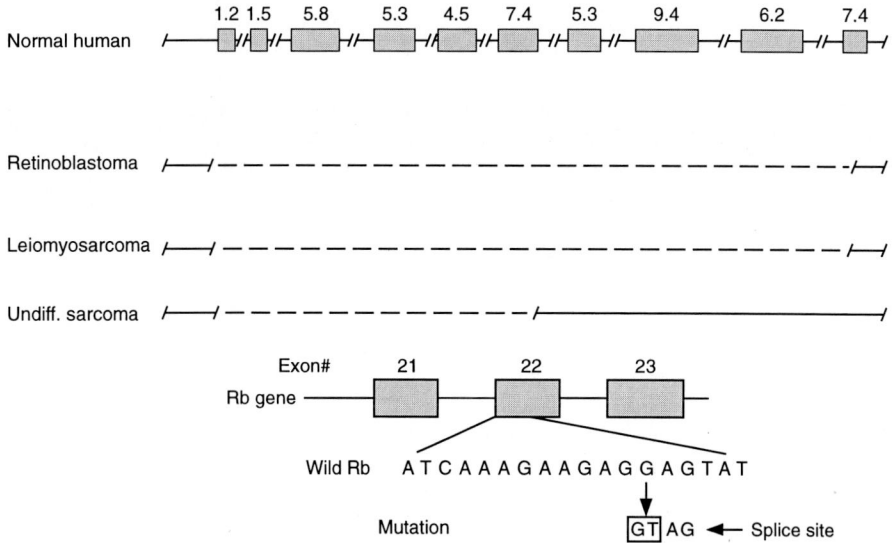

Figure 20–30. Two types of alterations of the *Rb* gene result in functional inactivation of its product, i.e., large deletions and point mutations prematurely terminating mRNA transcription.

cinoma *in situ*, and invasive high-grade non-papillary carcinoma. This loss can be documented in approximately 50% of high-grade invasive tumors and is very infrequently identified in low-grade superficially growing papillary lesions (Xu et al., 1993). Loss of *Rb* gene function is associated with high-stage and high-grade tumors and with tumors that show aggressive clinical behavior. A synergistic effect of alterations involving the *p53* and *Rb* genes has been documented in a study by Xu et al. (1996). The tumors with synchronous alterations of the *p53* and *Rb* genes are significantly more aggressive and exhibit a particularly high propensity for distant metastasis.

ADHESION MOLECULES AND PROTEASES

It is generally accepted that invasive growth and distant metastases are related to the abnormal interaction between tumor cells and normal host stromal elements. The loss of certain adhesion molecules, especially e-cadherin, has been correlated in urinary bladder tumors with progression to invasive disease (Imao et al., 1999). The deregulation of the tumor cell protease network has been postulated to play a major role in the development of invasive growth and metastases in experimental systems, and such deregula-

tion has been related to the aggressive behavior of several common malignancies (Imao et al., 1999). The proteases are produced by tumor cells as inactive proenzymes and are autoactivated by their active forms or other reaction partners in a complex cascade. Typically, several proteases are produced by an individual tumor cell, and each tumor type can have distinct patterns of protease expression responsible for its invasive growth and metastasis. In urinary bladder tumors, two metalloproteinases, MMP-2 and MMP-9, are particularly important for the development of invasive growth and metastasis and may be used as markers of clinically aggressive urothelial carcinoma (Kanayma et al., 1998; Ozdemir et al., 1999).

PATHOGENETIC CONCEPTS OF UROTHELIAL NEOPLASIA

The current so-called dual-track concept of urothelial neoplasia implies that common urothelial tumors of the bladder arise via two distinct but sometimes overlapping pathways: one that leads to papillary TCC and the other that leads to nonpapillary (solid) TCC (Czerniak and Herz, 1995). This concept was developed on the basis of clinicopathologic observations and whole-organ histologic mapping studies of cystectomy specimens conducted more then two decades ago (Koss et al., 1974). These early studies found a progression of urothelial neoplasia from precursor lesions such as dysplasia and carcinoma *in situ* to invasive bladder cancer. Furthermore, virtually every clinically evident lesion was associated with wide, microscopically recognizable changes of the urinary bladder mucosa representing either hyperplasia and/or dysplasia of various degrees. Conversely, invasive bladder cancer represents a progression of the dysplasia–carcinoma *in situ* sequence and typically affects patients without a history of papillary lesions. The precancerous *in situ* lesions progress to invasive cancer via complex stepwise molecular events (Reznikoff et al., 1996; Sarankk et al., 1996).

The picture emerging from individual studies permits several generalizations. (*1*) Low-grade, superficially growing papillary lesions of the bladder, in general, have fewer chromosomal changes than high-grade invasive carcinomas. (*2*) This group of low-grade urothelial lesions is characterized by frequent trisomies of chromosomes 1 and 7 and deletions of chromosome 9. (*3*) High-grade invasive bladder carcinomas develop multiple cumulative rearrangements and deletions of chromosomes with formation of markers that frequently involve chromosomes 3, 11, 17, and 18. Deletions of chromosome 17 in the p11-13 region, which contains putative tumor suppressor genes such as *p53*, are frequently observed in TCCs of high histologic grade and advanced stage. More recently, deletions of chromosomes 8p21, q11.12, 4p16.3, 9p21, and 14q have been postulated to play a role in the progression of urothelial neoplasia to invasive bladder cancer. Numerous studies indicate that several major tumor suppressor and transforming genes, such as *Rb* and *p53*, are more likely to be altered in a nonpapillary pathway than in superficially growing papillary lesions (Czerniak and Herz, 1995).

Experimental data based on cultured urinary bladder tumor cell lines indicate that human urothelial cells can be transformed by alterations of one of at least two main cell cycle regulatory pathways that involve the *p53* and *Rb* genes with tandemly linked CDKN2a (p16[INK4a]) MTS and ARF (p14[INK4b]) at 9p21 (Markl and Jones, 1998; Fig. 20–31A). The locus of closely related CDKN2a/ARF genes encodes two proteins.

The first pathway involves the *CDKN2a* gene, which inhibits the activities of CDK3 cyclin complexes, predominantly CDK4.6/cyclin D and CDK cyclin E, and in turn inhibits the phosphorylation of the Rb protein. An unphosphorylated Rb protein interacts with E2F1 transcription factor, arresting the progression of the cell cycle by preventing the transcription of S-phase gene and inhibiting the G_0-G_1 checkpoint transit (Czerniak et al., 1999).

The second pathway includes the p53 protein as a central regulatory molecule and involves ARF, which induces p53 expression and up-regulates CDKN1a, in turn inhibiting the CDK/cyclin complexes and arresting the cell cycle at any given point. Three major molecular mechanisms for urothelial carcinogenesis have been recently postulated (Chatuverdi et al., 1997; Czerniak et al., 1999; Mark and Jones, 1998). The first and most frequent mechanism involves alterations of *p53* in exons 5–11, followed by the loss of *Rb* gene expression for immortalization of urothelial cells. This mechanism can be identified in approximately 60% of human urinary bladder cell lines. The second, less frequent mechanism, observed in approximately 20% of the cell lines, is an independent synchronous loss of CDKN2a and ARF in a single step, activating the 9p21 locus and resulting in transformation and immortalization of urothelial cells. The third mechanism, also observed in approximately 20% of cell lines, involves a unique alteration of *p53* in exons 1–4 followed by a loss of CDKN2a and ARF functions. This model postulates that the specific alterations of *p53* involving exons 5–11 versus exons 1–4 are followed by distinct, secondary molecular events. Thus, the pattern of *p53* mutations is a prerequisite for subsequent distinctive molecular event in other genes such as *Rb* and the CDKN2a/ARF locus. On the other hand, observations on human tumors indicate that approximately 30% of urinary bladder tumors, especially low-grade superficially growing papillary lesions, do not show any evidence of *p53* or *Rb* altered pathways (Chatuverdi et al., 1997; Czerniak et al., 1999). The presence of concurrent alterations involving these two pathways can be documented in aproximately 25% of bladder tumors and is associated with their high propensity for distant metas-

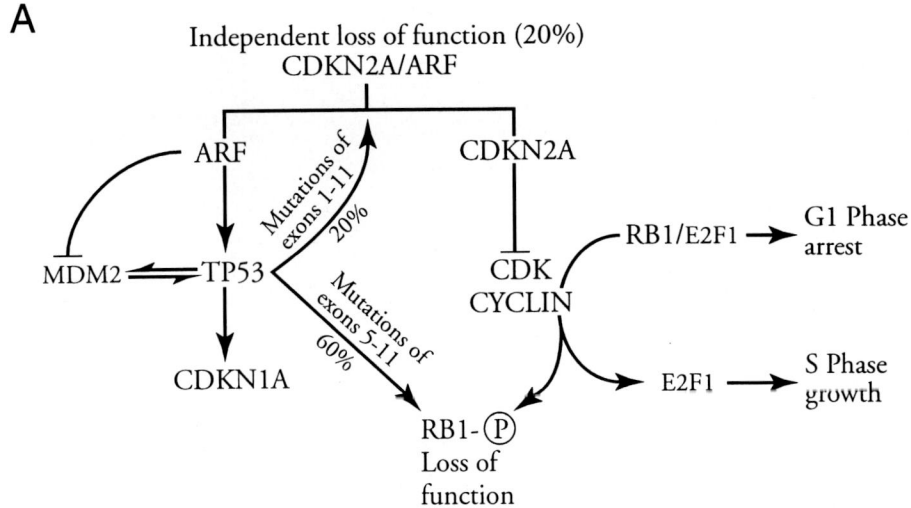

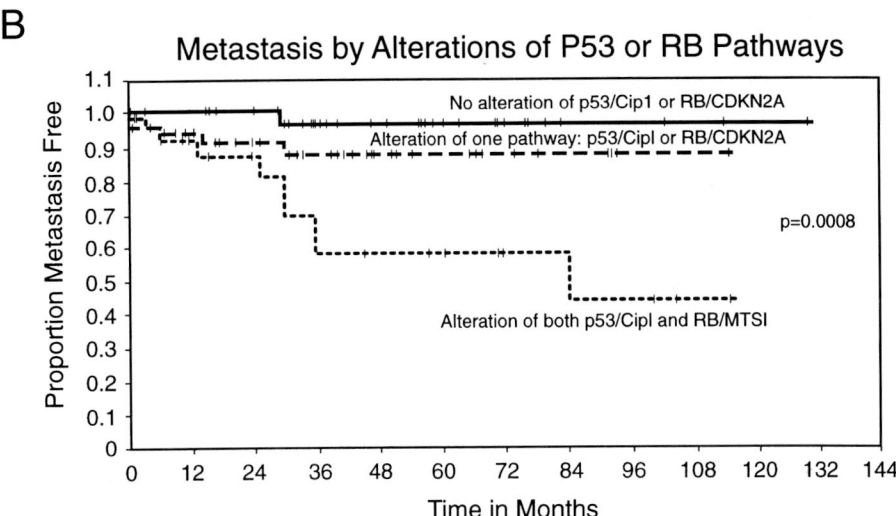

Figure 20–31. Alterations of the critical molecular pathways implicated in playing a role in the development of bladder cancer. *A*: Alterations of p53/Rb and tandemly linked molecules CDKN2a/ARF at the 9p21 locus result in immortalization/transformation of human urothelial cells [Modified from Mark L and Jones (1998) *Cancer Res* 58:5348–5353, with permission.] *B*: Aggressiveness of bladder cancer in relation to synchronous alterations of p53 and Rb pathways. Note that tumors with synchronous alterations of p53/Rb have a particularly high propensity for metastases (Czerniak et al., unpublished data).

tases (Fig. 20–31B). These observations suggest that there are still unknown molecular pathways that operate predominantly in the proliferation and immortalization of urothelial cells and which contribute to the development of urinary bladder tumors. Typical reciprocal staining patterns for Rb and p16 proteins in bladder tumors are shown in Figure 20–32.

Recent studies of urinary bladder cancer progression from precursor conditions to invasive disease have shown that the involvement of several loci on some chromosomes may represent common early events for both pathways of urinary bladder neoplasia preceding the development of clinically and even microscopically recognizable disease (Chatuverdi et al., 1997; Czerniak et al.,

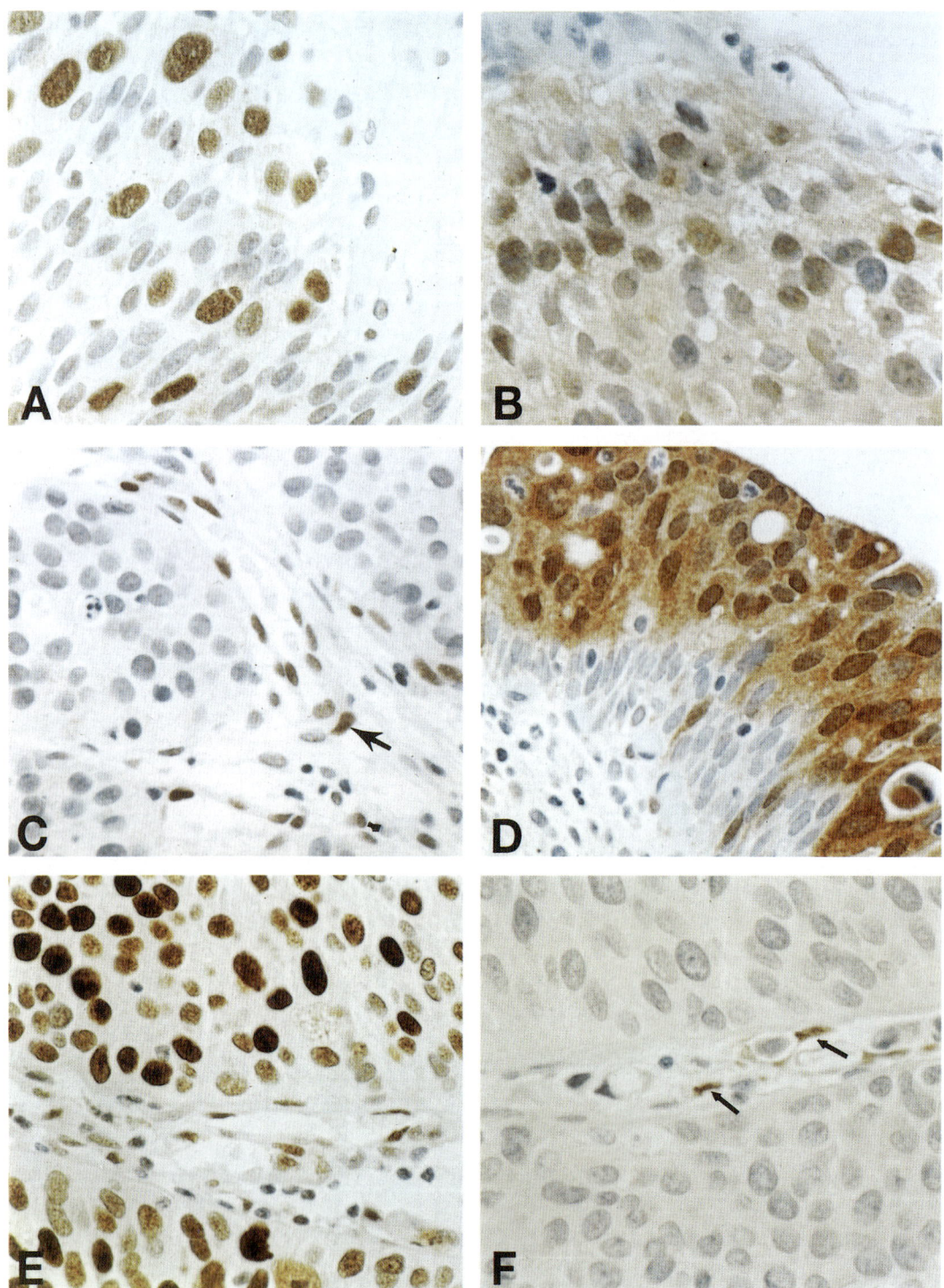

Figure 20–32. Typical case of Rb and p16 staining in bladder tumors. *A, B:* Heterogenous staining of Rb and p16, respectively, is considered normal. A tumor that is Rb negative (*C*) and shows homogenously strong p16 staining (*D*) is shown next. The arrow in C indicates an example of a normal Rb-positive cell used as an internal positive control for Rb-negative cases. Finally, a tumor with homogenously strong Rb (*E*) and negative p16 (*F*) staining is shown. The arrows in F illustrate the presence of normal p16-positive cells [From Benedict et al., (1999) *Oncogene* 18:1197–1203, with permission.]

1999, 2000). Several such loci were recently mapped on chromosomes 9 and 3 (Fig. 20–33). These studies have also documented that alterations in the *p53* and *Rb* gene loci in fact represent early events in the evolution of dysplasia, carcinoma *in situ*, and invasive TCC sequence. It also appears from these studies that virtually every case of urothelial tumor, either papillary or nonpapillary, is preceded by the establishment of a molecularly abnormal clone occupying large portions of the urinary bladder mucosa (Fig. 20–34). The identification of this phenomenon provides a unique opportunity to design molecular markers that can be tested in a noninvasive fashion on voided urine samples of patients with various forms of urothelial neoplasia. Testing of several hy-

pervariable DNA markers that map to such loci on voided urine samples of patients with TCC identified loss of heterozygosity in virtually every case (Chatuverdi et al., 1997; Czerniak et al., 1999). Moreover, the presence of a genetically abnormal clone can also be documented for patients with a history of TCC and no clinically or microscopically detectable lesion at the time of testing. This approach can be used for monitoring recurrence as well as the therapeutic response during the preclinical and even premicroscopic phases. The generation of genetic maps documenting the evolution of chromosomal allelic losses from precursor conditions to invasive disease is now well underway, and such genetic maps will provide a landmark for subsequent, more spe-

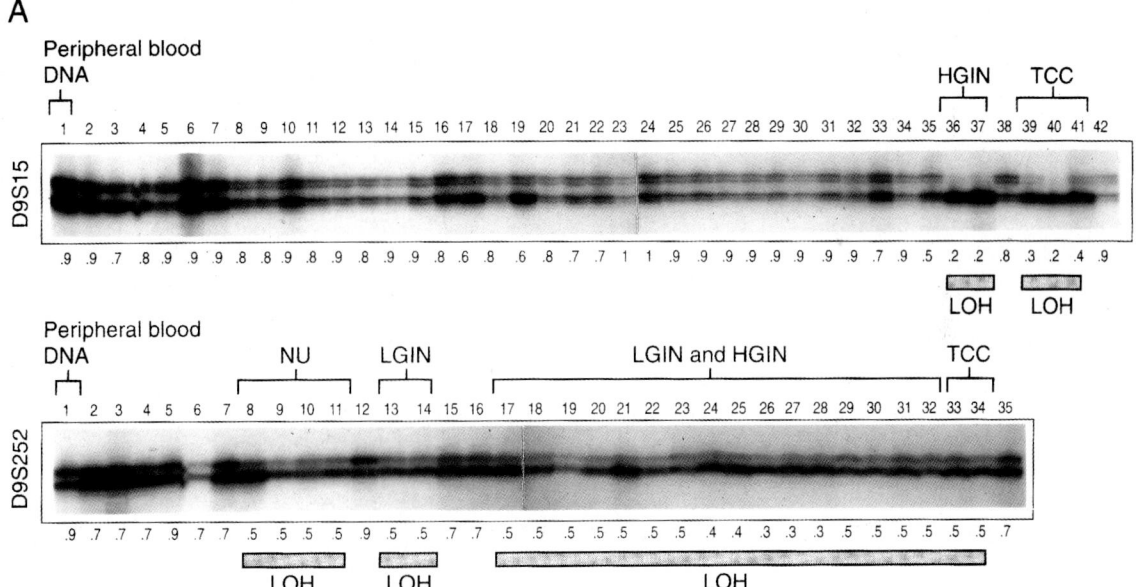

Figure 20–33. Assembly of superimposed histologic and genetic maps. *A*: Examples of two markers tested on multiple mucosal samples from the same cystectomy specimen. Marker D9S15 shows loss of heterozygosity (LOH) in five samples. Samples 36 and 37 correspond to high grade intraurothelial neoplasia (HGIN). Samples 39–41 represent invasive transitional cell carcinoma (TCC). Marker D9S252 shows LOH in multiple samples corresponding to TCC (samples 33 and 34) as well as involving large areas of urinary bladder mucosa that exhibit changes consistent with low grade intraurothelial neoplasia (LGIN) and HGIN (samples 13–14 and 17–32). Samples 8–11 correspond to microscopically normal urothelium with evidence of LOH. Samples 1 in both panels represent allelic patterns of the same marker from peripheral blood of the same patient and serve as control. In summary, marker D9S15 shows LOH restricted to invasive TCC and a small area of mucosa corresponding to advanced precursor intraurothelial conditions, i.e. severe urothelial dysplasia/flat transitional cell carcinoma *in situ* (HGIN). In contrast, marker D9S253 shows LOH involving a large area of urinary bladder mucosa with invasive carcinoma and virtually all stages of intraurothelial precursor conditions as well as adjacent microscopically normal urothelium. The presence of LOH in all samples was confirmed by densitometry and is expressed as optical density (OD) ratio below each sample in both panels; an OD ≤0.5 is indicative of LOH. (*Continued*)

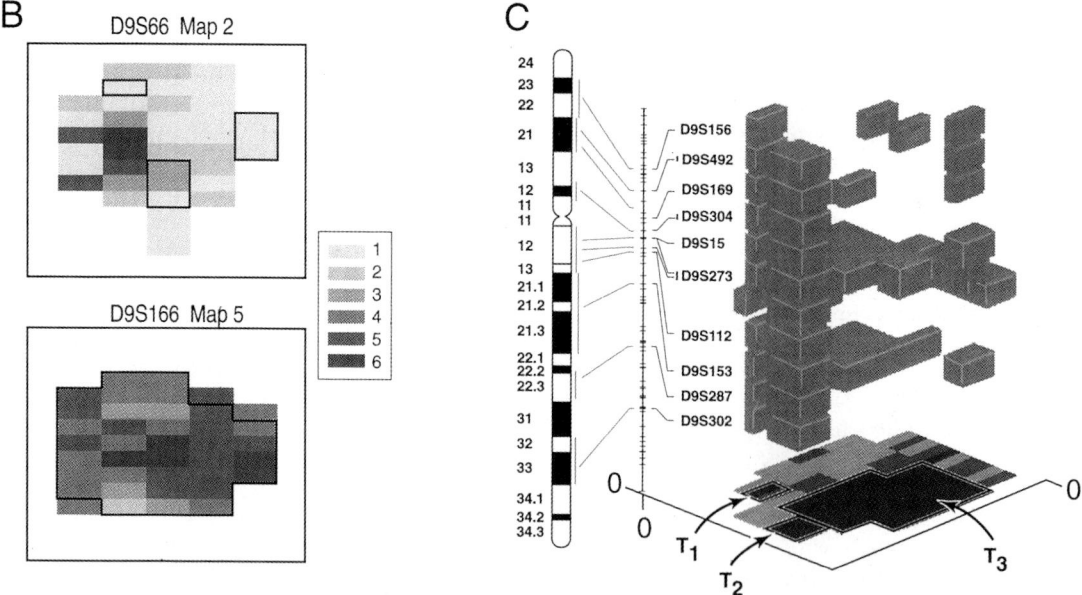

Figure 20–33. (*Continued*) *B*: Examples of superimposed histologic and genetic maps of two cystectomy specimens. Marker D9S66 (*top panel*) shows scattered foci of LOH. Marker D9S166 (*lower panel*) shows a plaque-like LOH involving almost the entire urinary bladder mucosa. Open boxes delineated by black lines indicate areas of urinary bladder mucosa with alterations in a given locus. The background shadowed area represents a histologic map of cystectomy specimen depicting distribution of various intraurothelial precursor conditions and TCC. Histologic map code: 1, normal urothelium; 2, mild dysplasia; 3, moderate dysplasia; 4, severe dysplasia; 5, carcinoma *in situ*; 6, transitional cell carcinoma. *C*: Example of chromosome 9 allelic losses in a single cystectomy specimen with multifocal TCC and assembled by nearest neighbor analysis. The vertical axis represents a chromosome 9 vector with positions of markers and their chromosomal locations. Only altered markers are shown. The shaded blocks represent areas of urinary bladder mucosa with LOH as they relate to progression of neoplasia presented by a histologic map of cystectomy in the background. An area designated T_1 represents a focus of invasive nonpapillary TCC. Areas of T_2 and T_3 represent foci of noninvasive papillary TCC. The histologic map code is the same as in *B*. Note that allelic losses of chromosome 9 show wide involvement of urinary bladder mucosa in loci D9S153 and D9S15. There is accumulation of allelic losses involving multiple loci in areas of mucosa corresponding to the foci of noninvasive papillary TCC (T_1 and T_2) but not in the area of invasive TCC (T3). Scattered, apparently separate loci of allelic losses occur within areas of urinary bladder mucosa with wide field-type allelic losses in other chromosomal regions. [From Czerniak et al. (1999) *Oncogene* 18:1185–1196, with permission.]

Figure 20–34. Genethon vector of chromosome 9 with a list of tested markers and their distances. Chromosomal locations are provided for altered markers only. Markers with solid bars on the left were added to the vector. All the markers are positioned on the vector and on chromosmal bands according to the human genome database (version Oct. 16, 1995). Asterisks on the right side of the markers indicate the statiscally significant association between an altered marker and urothelial neoplasia as established by log odds (LOD) scores. Bars on the left side of the chromosomal vector identify the lost regions associated with the devlopment and progression of urothelial neoplasia. These regions are defined by flanking markers and a size of deleted segment in centimorgans (cM). In general, the diagram shows scattered regions of loss of heterozygosity (LOH) on both arms of chromosome 9 that may contain putative tumor suppressor genes involved in urinary bladder carcinogenesis. The regions defined by the nearest markers flanking the microsatellites exhibiting LOH with signifcant LOD scores are as follows: D9S268-D9S285, (p22-23); D9S52-D9S165, (p11-13); D9S200-D9S175, (q12-13); D9S152-D9S318, (q21); D9S151-D9S277, (q22); ABL-1-D9S158, (q34). These regions show alternating involvement in the development and evolution of urothelial neoplasia as established by superimposed histologic and genetic mapping and the LOD score analysis. The markers and deleted regions implicated to play a role in the development and progression of neoplasia are shown without designation of particular phases of urothelial neoplasia. SHGM, superimposed histologic and genetic mapping of individual cystectomy specimens consecutively numbered 1 through 5; ○, nonaltered marker; ●, altered marker; ⊘ noninformative marker. [From Czerniak et al. (1999), *Oncogene* 18:1185–1196, with permission.]

Sex-averaged map

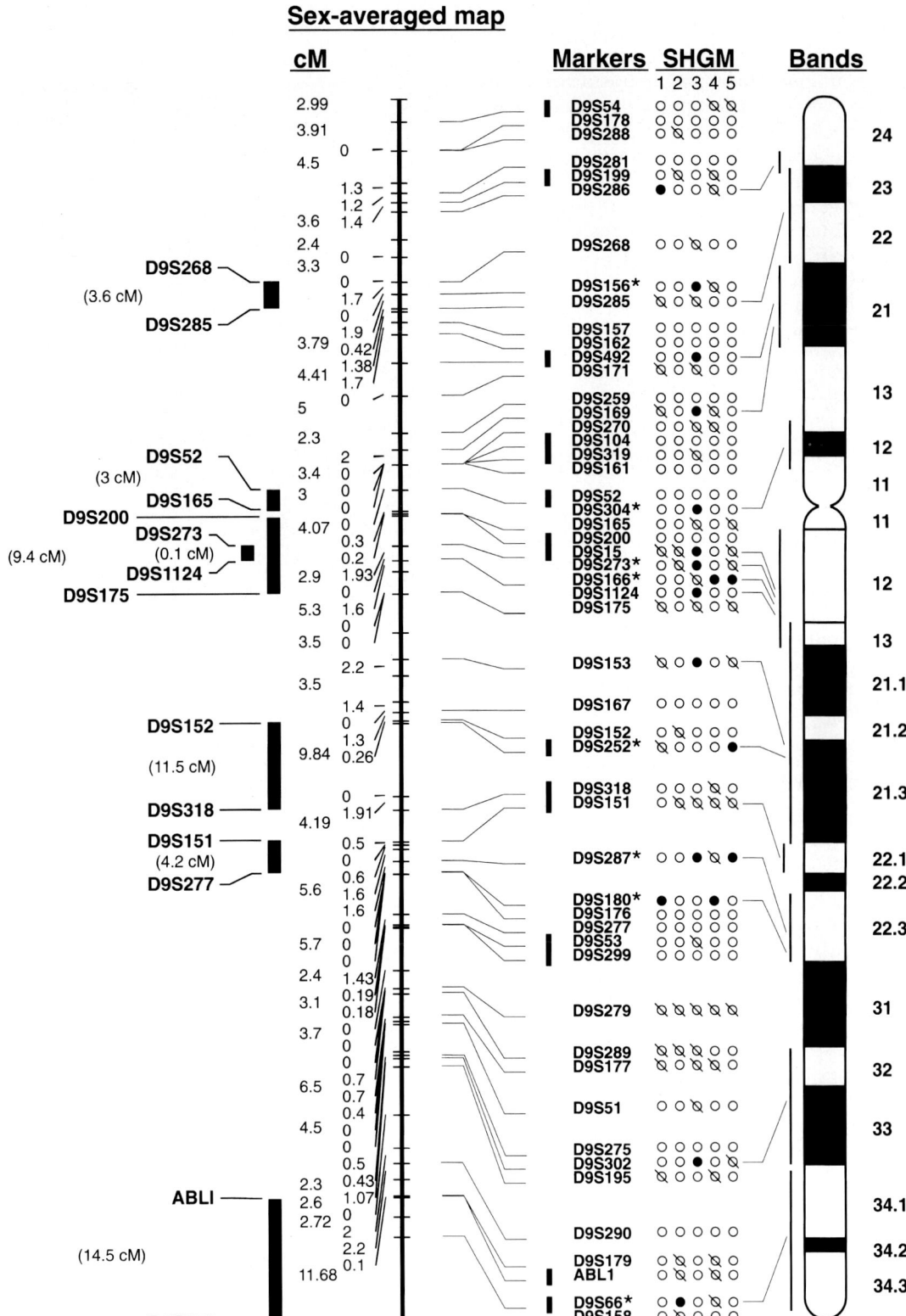

cific studies of urothelial carcinogenesis on a whole genomic scale. An example of deletional map of chromosome 9 is provided in Figure 20–34. Such maps, referred to as *genetic models of cancer progression,* parallel the human genome data and provide important information for the identification of individual genes involved in cancer progression on a total genomic scale (Czerniak et al., 2000). In a practical sense, urinary bladder neoplasia can serve as a unique model for the use of molecular probes, moving our concepts of cancer treatment and prevention not only to the preclinical phase but even to the premicroscopic phase.

DIFFERENTIAL DIAGNOSIS

Tumor-like lesions that mimic incipient neoplasia of the urinary bladder should be considered in the differential diagnosis of urothelial malignancies, as these include von Brunn's nests, cystitis cystica, cystitis glandularis, nephrogenic metaplasia, endocervicosis, endometriosis, inverted papilloma, and pseudosarcomatous myofibroblastic proliferations.

Von Brunn's Nests, Cystitis Cystica, and Cystitis Glandularis

One of the most frequently encountered lesions in bladder biopsy material is so-called proliferative cystitis, which encompasses the morphologic entities von Brunn's nests, cystitis cystica, and cystitis glandularis. Because there is substantial overlap between these changes, particularly between von Brunn's nests and cystitis cystica, we believe these lesions represent different morphological expressions of the same hyperplastic and metaplastic process. *Von Brunn's nests* are found in the subepithelial connective tissue and are composed of well-demarcated, rounded buds of urothelial cells that may or may not retain their connections to the surface urothelium (Fig. 20–35). The number of von Brunn's nests increases with advancing age, and therefore, the frequent association between these nests and bladder tumors, also a disease of older age-groups, is not surprising.

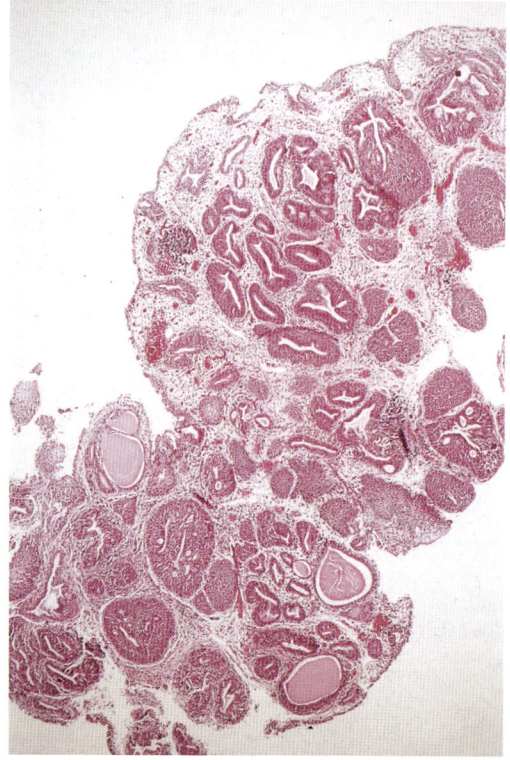

Figure 20–35. Bladder biopsy showing von Brunn's nests and cystitis cystica changes in different stages of evolution.

Cystitis cystica appears to be a variant of von Brunn's nests, with the urothelial cell groups replaced by one or more slit-like spaces or cysts lined by columnar or cuboidal epithelium. The columnar cells that are first seen in the central portion of the nests eventually replace the transitional cells, leading to the formation of cystically dilated glands (Figs. 20–36 and 20–37).

Although von Brunn's nests and cystitis cystica are not premalignant lesions, dysplastic changes, including carcinoma *in situ* of the surface epithelium, may extend into von Brunn's nests and simulate invasive carcinoma. Moreover, carcinoma *in situ* may rarely arise from von Brunn's nests. It is important to recognize this phenomenon and to distinguish it from invasive urothelial carcinoma extending into the subepithelial connective tissue.

Usually an incidental microscopic finding, *cystitis glandularis* may form a polypoid mass in the neck or trigone that can give rise to

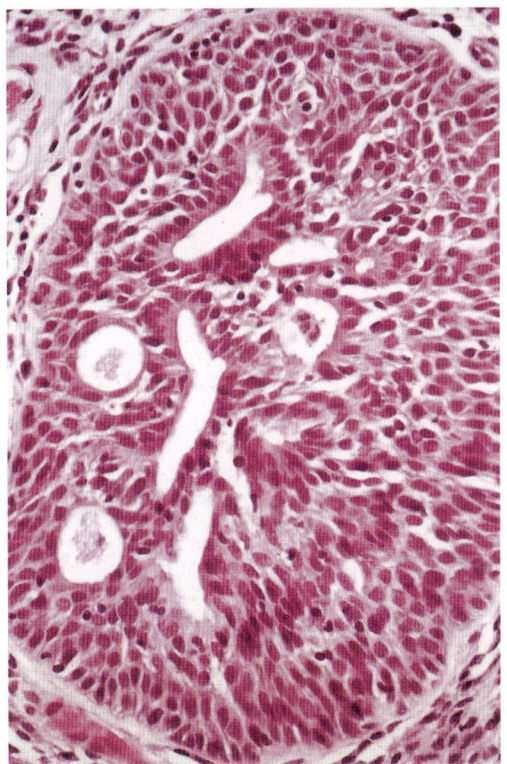

Figure 20–36. Higher magnification of von Brunn's nest with early changes of cystitis cystica.

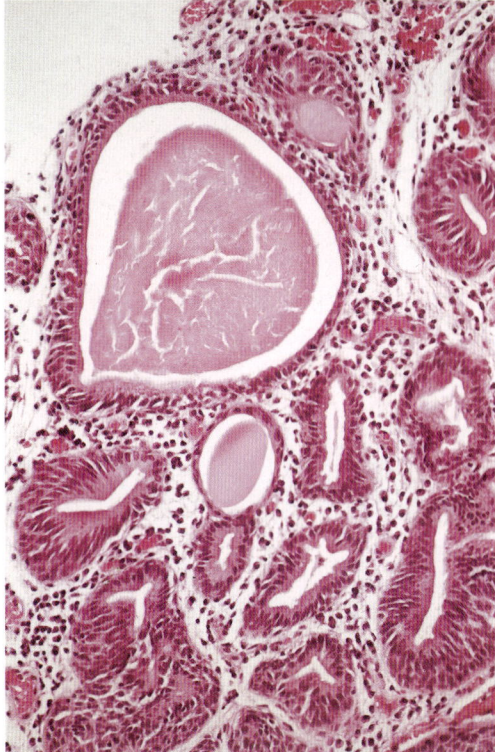

Figure 20–37. Well-developed cystitis cystica.

passage of mucus and hematuria and simulate a malignant neoplasm (Young, 1997). Cystitis glandularis can be focal or diffuse and consists of gland-like structures lined by intestinal-type columnar epithelium, goblet cells, endocrine cells, and, rarely, Paneth cells. Because of these cytologic features it should be regarded as a form of intestinal metaplasia (Maung et al., 1988) which can also occur in the urethra, ureter, and renal pelvis (Navarro and Huggins, 1984). Transition from the normal urothelium to the intestinal epithelium is seen in some cases (Fig. 20–38). In the lamina propria, cystitis glandularis usually has a lobular growth pattern and lacks cytologic atypia, mitotic figures, and invasive properties (Figs. 20–39 and 20–40). Florid cystitis glandularis can be confused with adenocarcinoma, especially when mucin extravasation occurs (Young and Boswick, 1996; Fig. 20–41). The mucin pools, however, do not contain malignant cells. The diffuse form of cystitis glandularis is associated with increased risk for devel-

opment of adenocarcinoma (Young, 1997). Well-differentiated adenocarcinomas of the urinary bladder show randomly distributed glands lined by columnar cells having basally located large hyperchromatic nuclei (Fig. 20–42).

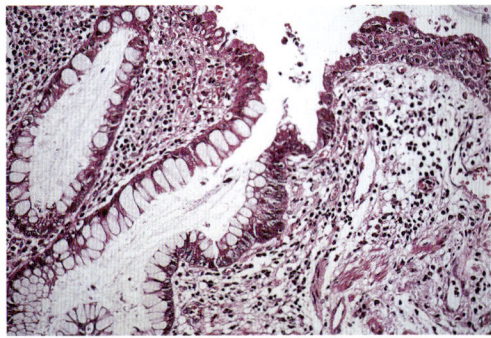

Figure 20–38. Intestinal metaplasia (cystitis glandularis). The transitional epithelium is replaced by mature goblet cells. Two epithelial invaginations give rise to gland-like structures.

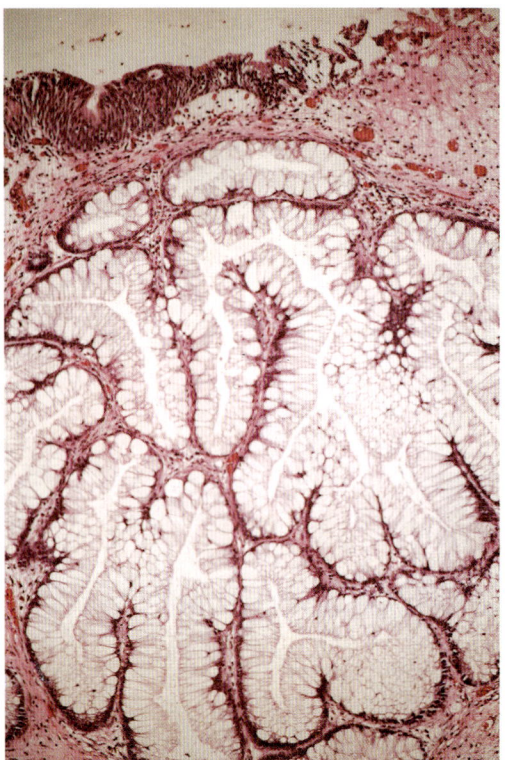

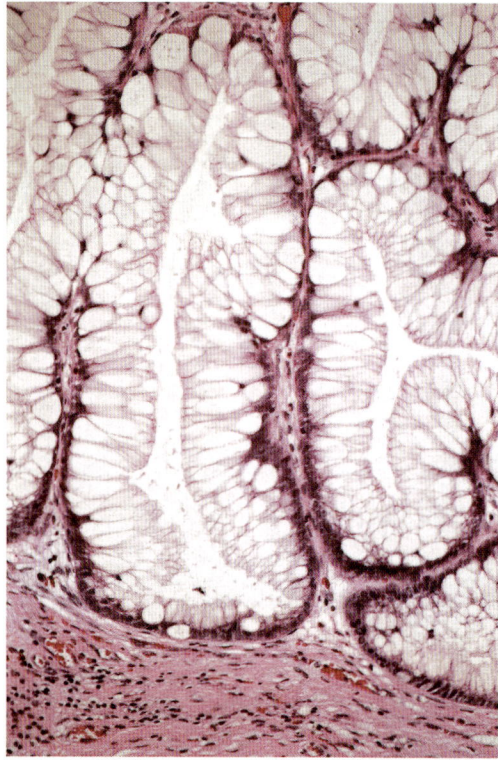

Figure 20–39. Intestinal metaplasia (cystitis glandularis). A well-defined lobule composed of glands lined by mature goblet cells and columnar cells with mucin-containing cytoplasm is present in the lamina propria of the urinary bladder.

Figure 20–40. Intestinal metaplasia (cystitis glandularis). The nuclei of the columnar and goblet cells are basally located and show no nuclear atypia and mitotic activity.

NEPHROGENIC METAPLASIA (ADENOMA)

The resemblance of the tubular structures of this metaplastic lesion to renal tubules is indeed superficial, and its "nephrogenic" origin, in spite of some similarities, has not been proved. The metaplastic nature of this lesion is supported by its occasional coexistence with intestinal metaplasia and endocervicosis. Therefore, the term *nephrogenic metaplasia* is preferable over nephrogenic adenoma for this non-neoplastic lesion.

Nephrogenic metaplasia occurs mostly in the bladder or prostatic urethra exposed to chronic irritation or trauma. The metaplastic process originates in the urothelium and extends to the lamina propria, leading to a pseudoinfiltrative appearance that complicates histologic interpretation (Ford et al., 1985; Malpica et al., 1994; Odze and Begin, 1989). When nephrogenic metaplasia arises

in the urethra it may extend into the prostate, where it can be confused with adenocarcinoma of this organ (Malpica et al., 1994). Nephrogenic metaplasia consists of

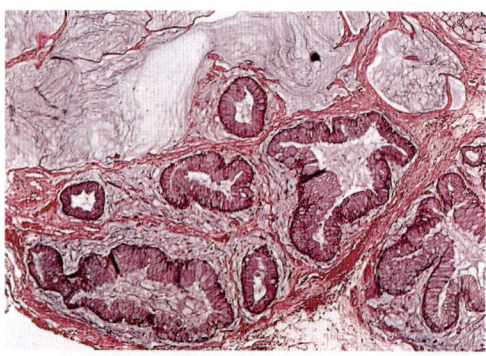

Figure 20–41. Intestinal metaplasia (cystitis glandularis). Abundant extracellular mucin has escaped from the metaplastic glands and simulates adenocarcinoma.

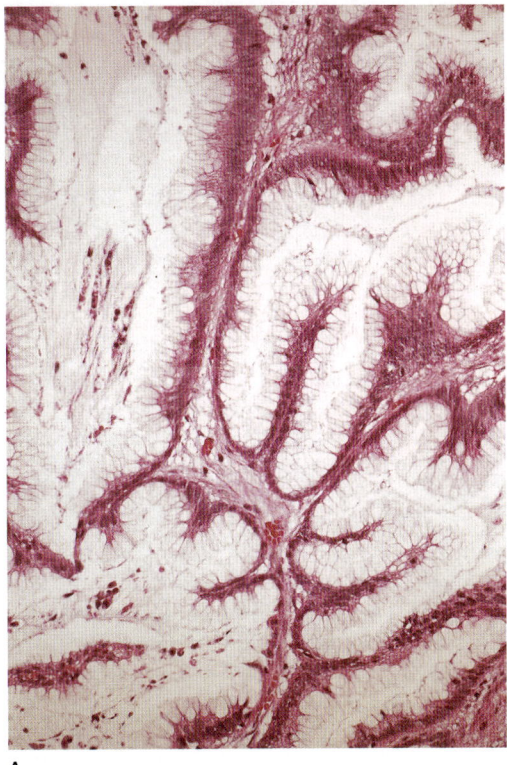

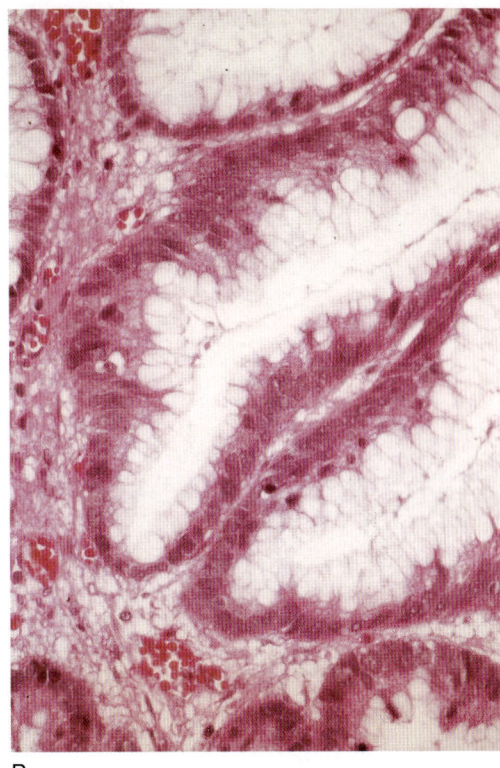

A   B

Figure 20–42. *A*: Well-differentiated mucinous adenocarcinoma confined to the lamina propria. The glands are not arranged in a lobular pattern. *B*: Higher magnification shows nuclear atypia of the mucin-containing columnar cells.

tubular and glandular structures of different sizes mixed with small papillary fronds. Small, medium-sized and cystically dilated tubules may coexist in the same lesion (Fig. 20–43). The small tubular structures often contain mucin and may mimic signet-ring cell adenocarcinoma (Oliva and Young, 1995; Fig. 20–44). Larger tubules are lined by cuboidal or columnar cells, sometimes with apical hyperchromatic or vesicular nuclei and prominent nucleoli (hobnail cells). In some cases a papillary pattern predominates. Nephrogenic metaplasia has no malignant potential but may mimic clear cell carcinoma, especially when the former lesion is composed predominantly of clear cells or the latter shows only mild cytologic atypia (Alsanjari et al., 1995; Cheng et al., 2000; Oliva and Young, 1996; Figs. 20–45 to 20–47). In contrast to nephrogenic metaplasia, clear cell carcinoma overexpresses p53 protein and shows high MIB-1 positivity. Moreover, clear cell carcinoma shows

greater cytologic atypia and mitotic figures than nephrogenic metaplasia (Gilcrease et al., 1998). This lesion can also be confused with the adenomatoid tumor, a benign neoplasm of mesothelial origin, which occurs on

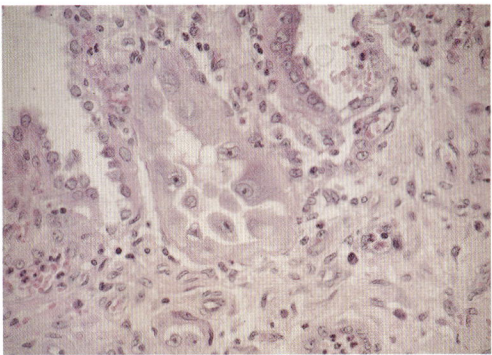

Figure 20–43. Nephrogenic metaplasia. These tubules are lined by cuboidal cells. The central tubule shows hobnail cells with vesicular nuclei and prominent nucleoli.

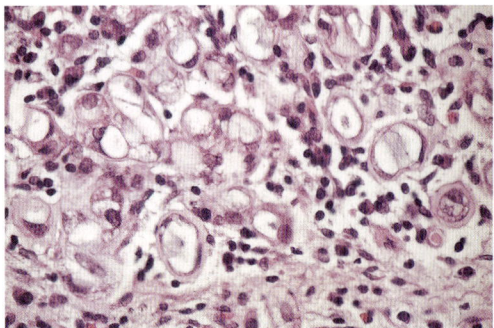

Figure 20–44. Nephrogenic metaplasia. Microcystic structures contain mucin and are lined by flat or cuboidal hyperchromatic cells. This form of nephrogenic metaplasia has been confused with signet-ring cell carcinoma.

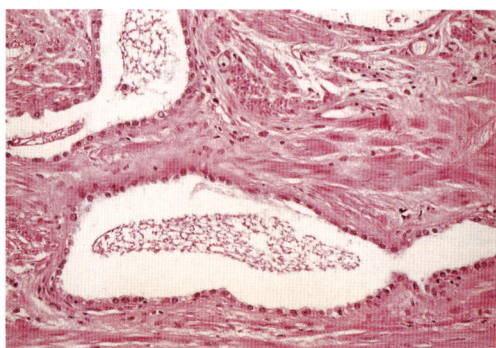

Figure 20–46. Clear cell carcinoma of urinary bladder mimicking nephrogenic metaplasia. The tubules are lined by cuboidal cells with minimal nuclear atypia that invade the muscularis propria.

the external surface of the bladder, most often related to other organs like the uterus or ductus deferens. Nephrogenic metaplasia may coexist with cystitis glandularis and endocervical epithelial metaplasia.

ENDOCERVICOSIS AND ENDOMETRIOSIS

The urothelium of the urinary bladder is rarely replaced by endocervical-type epithelium which may extend to the connective tissue of the lamina propria and muscularis propria (Fig. 20–48). With some frequency, intramural endocervical glands are seen with-

out an overlying mucosal lesion. Occasionally the endocervical glands are surrounded by fibrosis or edema. Extravasation of mucin occurs in a few cases. Endocervicosis may form masses measuring 2 to 3 cm, most often located in the posterior wall or posterior dome of the bladder of young women (Clement and Young, 1992; Nazeer et al., 1996). This lesion should not be confused with adenocarcinoma. We have seen a case of endocervicosis that coexisted with nephrogenic metaplasia. In endometriosis, in addition to endometrial glands, endometrial stroma is also identified (Fig. 20–49). Endosalpingiosis has rarely been observed in the wall of the urinary bladder (Young and Clement, 1996).

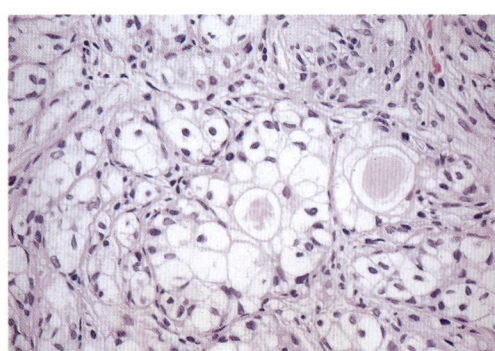

Figure 20–45. Nephrogenic metaplasia, clear cell type. Tubules contain eosinophilic material and are lined by cells with abundant clear cytoplasm. Small nests of clear cells are also present.

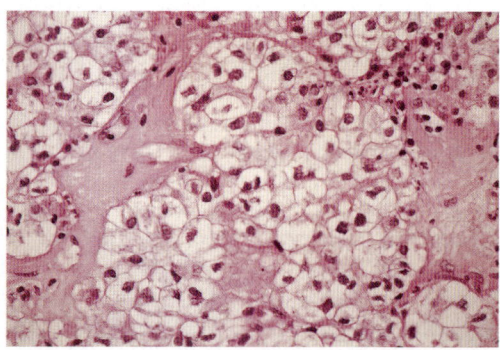

Figure 20–47. Clear cell carcinoma. This tumor shows more cytologic atypia than that seen in nephrogenic metaplasia, clear cell type.

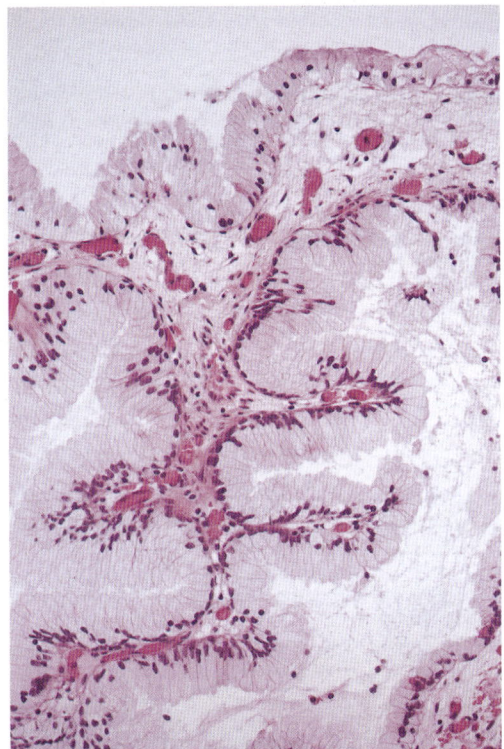

Figure 20–48. Endocervicosis. The transitional epithelium is replaced by columnar epithelium resembling endocervical epithelium. Part of two glands present in the lamina propria are lined by the same type of epithelium.

INVERTED TRANSITIONAL CELL PAPILLOMA

This rare lesion is believed to be the endophytic counterpart of the benign, exophytic transitional cell papilloma. It was first described in the urinary bladder, but it has recently been reported in the renal pelvis, urethra, and uterine cervix (Albores-Saavedra and Molberg, 1997; Kunze et al., 1983). The lesion is characterized by densely cellular anastomosing cords and trabeculae of urothelium in the subepithelial connective tissue covered by thin, normal bladder mucosa. Another rather consistent feature is the presence of cystic structures in the urothelial masses, a finding not seen in exophytic papillomas.

The practicing pathologist should keep in mind that inverted papilloma of bladder has to be differentiated from TCC with an inverted growth pattern. The latter neoplasms show cytologic atypia, mitotic figures, and invasive properties. More detailed description can be seen on page 499.

PSEUDOSARCOMATOUS MYOFIBROBLASTIC PROLIFERATIONS

We have chosen the term *pseudosarcomatous myofibroblastic proliferations* (PMPs) for a group of histologically disturbing lesions of the urinary bladder that we believe are re-

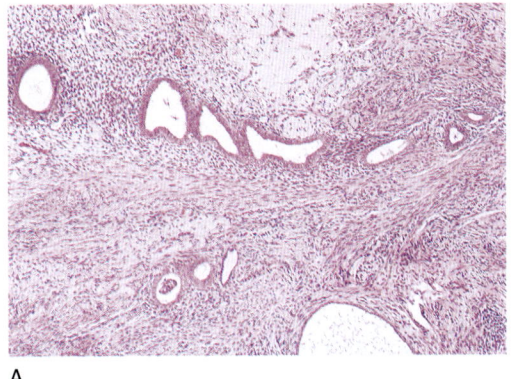

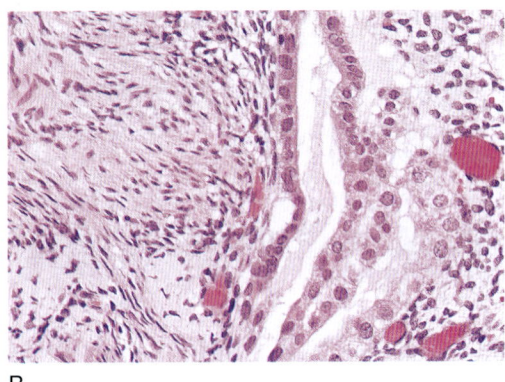

A   B

Figure 20–49. Endometriosis. *A:* Endometrial glands and stroma are seen in the muscularis propria. *B:* Some endometrial glands are lined by columnar cells with mild nuclear atypia.

active and non-neoplastic in nature (Albores-Saavedra et al., 1990). These lesions have been described in both children and adults (Hojo et al., 1995; Lundgren et al., 1994). Inflammatory pseudotumor, pseudosarcomatous fibromyxoid tumor, postoperative spindle cell nodule, and myofibroblastic inflammatory tumor (Coffin et al., 1995; Ro et al., 1986), are some of the terms applied to this lesion, which can occur in many sites. Some of these PMPs may be caused by bacterial infections, while others appear following surgical trauma. Because of their gross appearance, cellularity, mitotic rate, and the "strap" appearance of myofibroblasts, these urinary bladder lesions are often confused with sarcomas, especially leiomyosarcomas and rhabdomyosarcomas. Since some of the PMPs are positive for muscle-specific actin, smooth muscle actin, and desmin, immunohistochemistry does not allow separation from leiomyosarcomas and rhabdomyosarcomas.

Follow-up of PMPs in children and adults indicates that these lesions are benign. Although inflammatory pseudotumor of lymph nodes, spleen, and liver has some histologic similarities to PMPs of the urinary bladder, we believe that the natural history, morphologic features, and probably the etiology of these two lesions differ and therefore should not be included in the same group.

Supported in part by NIH grant CA66723 to B. Czerniak.

REFERENCES

Abel PD, Hall RR, Williams G. (1988a) Should pT1 transitional cell cancers of the bladder still be classified as superficial? *Br J Urol* 62:235–239.

Abel PD, Henderson D, Bennett MK, Hall RR, Williams G. (1988b) Differing interpretations by pathologists of the pT category and grade of transitional cell cancer of the bladder. *Br J Urol* 62:339–342.

Abratt RP, Temple-Comp CRE, Pontin AR. (1988) Choriocarcinoma and transitional cell carcinoma of the bladder—a case report and review of the clinical evolution of disease in reported cases. *Eur J Surg Oncol* 15:149–153.

Agnantis NJ, Constantinidou A, Poulios C, Pintzas A, Kakkanas A, Spandidos DA. (1990) Immunohistochemical study of the *ras* oncogene expression in human bladder endoscopy specimens. *Eur J Surg Oncol* 16:153–160.

Albores-Saavedra J, Manivel JC, Essenfeld H, et al. (1990) Pseudosarcomatous myofibroblastic proliferations in the urinary bladder. *Cancer* 66:1234–1241.

Albores-Saavedra J, Molberg K. (1997) Inverted transitional cell papilloma of the uterine cervix. *Pathol Case Rev* 2:34–37.

Alsanjari N, Lynch MJ, Fisher C, et al. (1995) Vesical clear cell adenocarcinoma. V. nephrogenic adenoma: a diagnostic problem. *Histopathology* 27:43–49.

Altaffer LF III, Wilkerson SY, Jordan GH, Lynch DF. (1982) Malignant inverted papilloma and carcinoma in situ of the bladder. *J Urol* 128:816–818.

Althausen AF, Prout GR, Daly JJ. (1976) Non-invasive papillary carcinoma of the bladder associated with carcinoma *in situ*. *J Urol* 116:575–580.

American Joint Committee on Cancer. (1997) Bladder: TNM classification. In: *Manual for Staging of Cancer*, 5th ed. pp. 241–246. Lippincott-Raven, Philadelphia.

Amin MB, Gomez JA, Young RH. (1997) Urothelial transitional cell carcinoma with endophytic growth patterns: a discussion of patterns of invasion and problems associated with assessment of invasion in 18 cases. *Am J Surg Pathol* 21:1057–1068.

Amin MB, Ro JY, Ayala AG, et al. (1994a) Micropapillary variant of transitional cell carcinoma of the urinary bladder. *Am J Surg Pathol* 18:1224–1232.

Amin MB, Ro JY, Lee KM, et al. (1994b) Lymphoepithelioma-like carcinoma of urinary bladder. *Am J Surg Pathol* 19:466–473.

Anderstrom C, Johansson S, Nilsson S. (1980) The significance of lamina propria invasion on the prognosis of patients with bladder tumors. *J Urol* 124:23–26.

Angulo JC, Lopez JI, Grignon DJ, Sanchez-Chapado M. (1995) Muscularis mucosa differentiates two populations with different prognosis in stage T1 bladder cancer. *Urology* 45:47–53.

Ayala AG, Ro JY. (1989) Premalignant lesions of the urothelium and transitional cell tumors. In: *Pathology of the Urinary Bladder* (Young RH, ed.) pp. 65–101. Churchill Livingstone, New York.

Benedict W, Lerner S, Zhou J, Shen X, Tokunaga H, Czerniak B. (1999) Level of retinoblastoma protein expression correlates with p16 (MTS-1/INK4A/CDKN2) status in bladder cancer. *Oncogene* 18:1197–1203.

Bergkvist A, Ljungquist A, Moberger G. (1965) Classification of bladder tumours based on the cellular pattern. Preliminary report of a clinical-pathological study of 300 cases with a minimum follow-up of eight years. *Acta Chir Scand* 130:371–378.

Bergman S, Javadpour N. (1978) The cell surface antigen A, B or O (H) as an indicator of malignant potential in stage A bladder carcinoma: preliminary report. *J Urol* 119:49–51.

Blasco E, Torrado J, Belloso L, Arocena F, Gutierrez-Hoyos A, Cuadrado E. (1988) T-antigen: a prognostic indicator of high recurrence index in transitional carcinoma of the bladder. *Cancer* 61:1091–1095.

Blomjous CEM, Schipper NW, Baak JPA, van Galen EM, de Voogt HJ, Meyer CJLM. (1988) Retrospective study of prognostic importance of DNA flow cytometry of urinary bladder carcinoma. *J Clin Pathol* 41:21–25.

Blomjous CEM, Vos W, Schipper NW, Uyterlinde AM, Baak JPA, de Voogt HJ, Meijer CJLM. (1990) The prognostic significance of selective nuclear morphometry in urinary bladder carcinoma. *Hum Pathol* 21:409–413.

Brogdon BG, Silbiger ML, Colston JAC. (1965) Cystitis glandularis. *Radiology* 85:470–473.

Cameron KM, Lupton CH. (1976) Inverted papilloma of the lower urinary bladder. *Br J Urol* 48:567–577.

Carbin B-E, Ekman P, Gustafson H, Christensen NJ, Sandstedt B, Silfversward C. (1991a) Grading of human urothelial carcinoma based on nuclear atypia and mitotic frequency. I. Histological description. *J Urol* 145:968–971.

Carbin B-E, Ekman P, Gustafson H, Christensen NJ, Silfversward C, Sandstedt B. (1991b) Grading of human urothelial carcinoma based on nuclear atypia and mitotic frequency. II. Prognostic importance. *J Urol* 145:972–976.

Chakraborty AK, Cichutek K, Duesberg PH. (1991) Transforming function of proto-ras genes depends on heterologous promoters and is enhanced by specific point mutations. *Proc Natl Acad Sci USA* 88:2217–2221.

Chatuverdi V, Li L, Hodges S, et al. (1997) Superimposed histologic and genetic mapping of chromosome 17 alterations in human urinary bladder neoplasia. *Oncogene* 14:2059–2070.

Cheng L, Cheville JC, Neumann RM, Bostwick DG. (1999) Natural history of urothelial dysplasia of the bladder. *Am J Surg Pathol* 23:443–447.

Chenn SS, Chen KK, Lin AT, et al. (1996) The significance of tumour grade in predicting disease progression in stage Ta transitional cell carcinoma of the urinary bladder. *Br J Urol* 78:209–212.

Chesa PG, Rettig WJ, Melamed MR, Old LJ, Niman HL. (1987) Expression of p21^{ras} in normal and malignant human tissues: lack of association with proliferation and malignancy. *Proc Natl Acad Sci USA* 84:3234–3238.

Clement PB, Young RH. (1992) Endocervicosis of the urinary bladder: a report of six cases of a benign müllerian lesion that may mimic adenocarcinoma. *Am J Surg Pathol* 16:533–542.

Coffin CM, Watterson J, Priest JR, et al. (1995) Extrapulmonary inflammatory myofibroblastic tumor (inflammatory pseudotumor): a clinicopathologic and immunohistochemical study of 84 cases. *Am J Surg Pathol* 19:859–872.

Cohen JB, Broz SD, Levinson AD. (1989) Expression of the Ha-ras protooncogene is controlled by alternative splicing. *Cell* 58:461–472.

Cohen JB, Levinson AD. (1988) A point mutation in the last intron responsible for increased expression and transforming activity for the c-Ha-ras oncogene. *Nature* 334:119–124.

Coon JS, Weinstein RS, Summers JL. (1982) Blood group precursor T-antigen expression in human urinary bladder carcinoma. *Am J Clin Pathol* 77:692–699.

Conn IG, Crocker J, Emtage LA, Wallace DMA. (1988) HMFG-2 as a prognostic indicator in superficial bladder cancer. *J Clin Pathol* 41:1191–1195.

Conn IG, Vilela MJ, Garrod DR, Crocker J, Wallace DMA. (1990) Immunohistochemical staining with monoclonal antibody 32-2B to desmosomal glycoprotein 1: its role in the histological assessment of urothelial carcinomas. *Br J Urol* 65:176–180.

Crew JP, O'Brien TS, Harris AL. (1996) Bladder cancer angiogenesis, its role in recurrence, stage progression and as a therapeutic target. *Cancer Metastasis Rev* 15:221–230.

Cutler SJ, Heney NM, Friedell GH. (1982) Longitudinal study of patients with bladder cancer: factors associated with disease recurrence and progression. In: *Bladder Cancer.* A.U.A. Monographs, Vol. 1 (Bonney WW, Prout GR, eds.) pp. 35–46. Williams and Wilkins, Baltimore.

Czerniak B, Chatuverdi V, Li L, Hodges S, Johnston D, Ro JY, Luthra R, Logothetis C, von Eschenback AC, Grossman B, Benedict WF, Bataskis JG. (1999) Superimposed histologic and genetic mapping of chromosome 9 in progression of human urinary ladder neoplasia. Implications for a genetic model of multistep urothelial carcinogenesis and early detection of urinary bladder cancer. *Oncogene* 18:1185–1196.

Czerniak B, Cohen GL, Etkind P, Deitch D, Simmons H, Herz F, Koss LG. (1992) Concurrent mutations of coding and regulatory sequences of the Ha-ras gene in urinary bladder carcinomas. *Hum Pathol* 23:1199–1204.

Czerniak B, Deitch D, Simmons H, Etkind P, Herz LG, Koss LG. (1990) Ha-ras gene codon 12 mutation and DNA ploidy in urinary bladder carcinoma. *Br J Cancer* 62:762–763.

Czerniak B, Herz F. (1995) Molecular biology of common genito-urinary tumors. (Koss LG, ed.). pp. 345–465. In Diagnostic Cytology of the urinary tract. Lippincott-Raven, Philadelphia.

Czerniak B, Li L, Chaturvedi V, Ro J, Johnston D, Hodges S, Benedict W (2000). Genetic modeling of human urinary bladder carcinogenesis. *Genes, Chromosomes Cancer* 27:392–402.

Dalesio O, Schulman CC, Sylvester R, et al. (1983) Prognostic factors in superficial bladder tumors. A study of the European Organization for Research on Treatment of Cancer: Genitourinary Tract Cancer Cooperative Group. *J Urol* 129:730–733.

De Vita R, Forte D, Maggi F, Eleuteri P, Di Silverio F. (1991) Cellular DNA content and proliferative activity evaluated by flow cytometry versus histopathological and staging classifications in human bladder tumors. *Eur Urol* 19:65–73.

Dixon JS, Gosling JA. (1983) Histology and fine structure of the muscularis mucosae of the human urinary bladder. *J Anat* 136:265–271.

Dowdy SF, Hinds PW, Louie K, Ree SI, Arnold A, Weinberg RA. (1993) Physical interaction of the retinoblastoma protein with human D cyclins. *Cell* 73:449–511.

Epstein JI, Amin MB, Reuter VE, Mostofi FK, and the Bladder Consensus Committee. (1998) The World Health Organization/International Society of Urological Pathology consensus classification of urothelial (transitional cell) neoplasms of the urinary bladder. *Am J Surg Pathol* D 22:1435–1448.

Evan G, Harrington E, Fanidi A, Land H, Amati B, Bennett M. (1994) Integrated control of cell proliferation and cell death by the c-myc oncogene. *Philos Trans R Soc Lond* 345:269–275.

Farrow GM, Utz DC. (1982) Observations on microinvasive transitional cell carcinoma of the urinary bladder. *Clin Oncol* 1:609–619.

Farrow GM, Utz DC, Rife CC. (1976) Morphological and clinical observations of patients with early bladder cancer treated with total cystectomy. *Cancer Res* 36:2495–2501.

Farrow GM, Utz DC, Rife CC, Greene LF. (1977) Clinical observations on sixty-nine cases of *in situ* carcinoma of the urinary bladder. *Cancer Res* 37:2794–2798.

Finlay C, Hinds PW, Levine AJ. (1989) The *p53* proto-oncogene can act as a suppressor of transformation. *Cell* 57:1083–1093.

Ford TF, Watson GM, Cameron KM. (1985) Adenomatous metaplasia (nephrogenic adenoma) of urothelium: an analysis of 70 cases. *Br J Urol* 57:427–433.

Fradet Y. (1979) Biological markers of prognosis in invasive bladder cancer. *Semin Oncol* 17:533–543.

Francis RR. (1979) Inverted papilloma in a 14-year-old male. *Br J Urol* 51:327.

Franks LM, Chesterman FC. (1956) Intra-epithelial carcinoma of prostatic urethra, periurethral glands and prostatic ducts ("Bowen's disease of urinary epithelium"). *Br J Cancer* 10:223–225.

Friedell GH, Bell JR, Burney SW, Soto EA, Tiltman AJ. (1976) Histopathology and classification of urinary bladder carcinoma. *Urol Clin North Am* 3:53–70.

Friend SH, Horowita JM, Gerber MR, Wang XF, Bogenmann E, Li FP, Weinberg RA. (1987) Deletions of a DNA sequence in retinoblastomas and mesenchymal tumors: organization of the sequence and its encoded protein. *Proc Natl Acad Sci USA* 84: 9059–9063.

Gilcrease MZ, Delgado R, Vuitch F, Albores-Saavedra J. (1998) Clear cell adenocarcinoma and nephrogenic adenoma of the urethra and urinary bladder: a histopathologic and immunohistochemical comparison. *Hum Pathol* 29:1451–1456.

Greenlee RT, Murray T, Bolden S, Wingo PA. (2000) Cancer Statistics, 2000. *CA Cancer J Clin* 50:7–33.

Grignon DJ, Ro JY, Ayala AG, Johnson DE. (1991a) Primary signet-ring cell carcinoma of the urinary bladder. *Am J Clin Pathol* 95:13–30.

Grignon DJ, Ro JY, Ayala AG, Johnson DE, Ordóñez NG. (1991b) Primary adenocarcinoma of the urinary bladder: a clinicopathologic analysis of 72 cases. *Cancer* 67:2165–2172.

Grignon DJ, Ro JY, Ayala AG, Shum DT, Ordóñez NG, Logothetis CJ, Johnson DE, Mackay B. (1992) Small cell carcinoma of the urinary bladder: a clinicopathologic analysis of 22 cases. *Cancer* 69:527–l536.

Grossman HB. (1996) Superficial bladder cancer: decreasing the risk of recurrence. *Oncology* 10:1617–1624.

Gustafson H, Tribukait B, Esposti PL. (1982a) DNA pattern, histological grade and multiplicity related to recurrence rate in superficial bladder tumours. *Scand J Urol Nephrol* 16:135–139.

Gustafson H, Tribukait B, Esposti PL. (1982b) DNA profile and tumour progression in patients with superficial bladder tumours. *Urol Res* 10:13–18.

Hasui Y, Osada Y, Kitada S, Nishi S. (1994) Significance of invasion to the muscularis mucosae on the progression of superficial bladder cancer. *Urology* 43:782–786.

Helpap B, Schwabe HW, Adolphs HD. (1985) Proliferative pattern of urothelial bladder cancer and urothelial atypias. *J Cancer Res Clin Oncol* 109:46–54.

Heney NM, Ahmed S, Flanagan MJ, et al. (1983) Superficial bladder cancer: progression and recurrence. *J Urol* 130:1083–1086.

Heney NM, Nocks BN, Daly JJ, et al. (1982) Ta and T1

bladder cancer: location, recurrence and progression. *Br J Urol* 54:152–157.

Hojo H, Newton WA, Hamoudi AB, et al. (1995) Pseudosarcomatous myofibroblastic tumor of the urinary bladder in children: a study of 11 cases with review of the literature: an Intergroup Rhabdomyosarcoma Study. *Am J Surg Pathol* 19:1224–1236.

Hopman AHN, Moesker O, Smeets AWGB, Pauwels RPE, Vooijs GP, Ramaekers FCS. (1991) Numerical chromosome 1, 7, 9, and 11 aberrations in bladder cancer detected by *in situ* hybridization. *Cancer Res* 51:644–651.

Horowitz JM, Park SH, Bogenmann E, Cheng JC, Yandell DW, Kaye FJ, Minna JD, Dryja TP, Weinberg RA. (1990) Frequent inactivation of the retinoblastoma anti-oncogene is restricted to a subset of human tumor cells. *Proc Natl Acad Sci USA* 87:2775–2779.

Imao T, Koshida K, Endo Y, et al. (1999) Dominant role of e-cadherin in the progression of bladder cancer. *J Urol* 161:692–698.

Jake G, Loidl W, Seeber G, et al. (1987) Stage T1, grade 3 transitional cell carcinoma of the bladder: unfavorable tumor? *J Urol* 137:39–43.

Jewett HJ, Eversole SL Jr. (1960) Carcinoma of the bladder: characteristic modes of local invasion. *J Urol* 83:383–389.

Jewett HJ, Strong GH. (1946) Infiltrating carcinoma of bladder: relation of depth of penetration of bladder wall to incidence of local extension and metastases. *J Urol* 55:366–372.

Johnson DE, Ayala AG. (1989) Bladder cancer: clinically relevant advances. In: *Systemic Therapy for Genitourinary Cancers* (Johnson DG, Logothetis CJ, von Eschenbach AC, eds.) pp. 3–12. Year Book Medical Publishers, Inc, Chicago, pp 3–12.

Johnson DE, Boileau MA. (1982) Bladder cancer: overview. In: *Genitourinary Tumors: Fundamental Principles and Surgical Techniques* (Johnson DE, Boileau MA, eds.) pp. 399. Grune & Stratton, New York.

Johnson DE, Hogan JM, Ayala AG. (1972) Transitional cell carcinoma of the prostate: a clinical morphological study. *Cancer* 29:287–293.

Jordan AM, Weingarten J, Murphy WM. (1987) Transitional cell neoplasms of the urinary bladder. Can biologic potential be predicted from histologic grading? *Cancer* 60:2766–2774.

Juhl BR, Hartzen SH, Hainau B. (1986) Lewis A antigen in transitional cell tumors of the urinary bladder. *Cancer* 58:222–228.

Kanayama H, Yokota K, Kurokawa Y, et al. (1998) Prognostic values of matrix metalloproteinase-2 and tissue inhibitor of metalloproteinase-2 expression in bladder cancer. *Cancer* 82:1359–1366.

Kaubisch S, Lum BL, Reese J, Freiha F, Torti FM. (1991) Stage T1 bladder cancer: grade is the primary determinant for risk of muscle invasion. *J Urol* 146: 28–31.

Khoury JM, Stutzman RE, Sepulveda RA. (1985) Inverted papilloma of the bladder with focal transitional cell carcinoma: a case report. *Mil Med* 150:562–563.

Kiemeney LAMA, Witjes JA, Heijbroek RP, Debruyne FMJ, Verbeck ALM. (1985) Dysplasia in normal-looking urothelium increases the risk of tumor progression in primary superficial cancer. *J Urol* 133: 395–398.

Kim YH, Reiner L. (1978) Brunnian adenoma (inverted papilloma) of the urinary bladder: report of a case. *Hum Pathol* 9:229–231.

Klein HL. (1974) Inverted papilloma and transitional cell carcinoma of the bladder. *Kimbrough Urol Semin* 8:45–46.

Koontz WW, Heney NM, Soloway MS, et al. (1985) Mitomycin for patients who failed on Tiotepa. The National Bladder Group. *Urology* 26 (Suppl 4):30–31.

Koss LG. (1975) *Tumors of the Urinary Bladder.* Fascicle 11, 2nd series, pp. 9–79, Suppl pp. 514–541 (1985). Armed Forces Institute of Pathology, Washington, DC.

Koss LG, Tiamson EM, Robbins MA. (1974) Mapping of cancerous and precancerous bladder changes. A study of the urothelium in ten surgically removed bladders. *JAMA* 227:281–286.

Kotliar SN, Wood CA, Schaeffer AJ, Oyasu R. (1995) Transitional cell carcinoma exhibiting clear cell features: a differential diagnosis for clear cell adenocarcinoma of the urinary tract. *Arch Pathol Lab Med* 119:79–81.

Krause WJ, Cutts JH. (1986) Urinary system. In: *Concise Text of Histology.* 2nd ed. (Krause WJ, Cutts JH, eds.) pp. 387–389. Williams and Wilkins, Baltimore.

Kunze E, Schauer A, Schmitt M. (1983) Histology and histogenesis of two different types of inverted urothelial papillomas. *Cancer* 51:348–358.

Langkilde NC, Wolf H, Meldgard P, Orntoft TF. (1991) Frequency and mechanism of Lewis antigen expression in human urinary bladder and colon carcinoma patients. *Br J Cancer* 63:583–586.

Larsen MP, Steinberg GD, Brendler CB, et al. (1990) Use of *Ulex europaeus* agglutinin I (UEAI) to distinguish vascular and "pseudovascular" invasion in transitional cell carcinoma of bladder with lamina propria invasion. *Mod Pathol* 3:83–88.

Lazarevic B, Garret R. (1978) Inverted papilloma and papillary transitional cell carcinoma of urinary bladder: report of four cases of inverted papilloma, one showing papillary malignant transformation and review of the literature. *Cancer* 42:1904–1911.

Lee WH. (1989) The molecular basis of cancer suppression by the retinoblastoma gene. *Princess Takamastsu Symp* 20:159–170.

Leeson CR, Leeson TS, Paparo AA. (1985) The urinary system. In: *Textbook of Histology* 5th ed. (Leeson CR, Leeson TS, Paparo AA, eds.) pp. 432–434. W.B. Saunders, Philadelphia.

Lemaitre JM, Buckle RS, Mechali M. (1996) C-myc in the control of cell proliferation and embryonic development. *Adv Cancer Res* 70:95–144.

Lerman RI, Hutter RVP, Whitmore WF. (1970) Papilloma of the urinary bladder. *Cancer* 25:333–342.

Levine AJ, Momand J, Finlay CA. (1991) The *p53* tumor suppressor gene. *Nature* 351:435–456.

Lipponen PK, Eskelinen MJ. (1991) Nucleolar organiser regions (NORs) in bladder cancer: relation to histological grade, clinical stage and prognosis. *Anticancer Res* 11:75–80.

Lipponen PK, Eskelinen MJ, Kiviranta J, Nordling S. (1991) Classic prognostic factors, flow cytometric data, nuclear morphometric variables and mitotic indexes as predictors in transitional cell bladder cancer. *Anticancer Res* 11:911–916.

Livingstone LR, White A, Sprouse J, Livanos E, Jacks T,

Tlsty TD. (1992) Altered cell cycle arrest and gene amplification potential accompanying loss of wild-type p53. *Cell* 70:923–935.

Lum BL, Torti FM. (1985) Therapeutic approaches including interferon to carcinoma *in situ* of the bladder. *Cancer Treat Rev* 12 (Suppl):45–59.

Lundgren L, Aldenborg F, Angervall L, et al. (1994) Pseudomalignant spindle cell proliferations of the urinary bladder. *Hum Pathol* 25:181–191.

Lutzeyer W, Rubben H, Dahm H. (1982) Prognostic parameters in superficial bladder cancer: an analysis of 315 cases. *J Urol* 127:250–252.

Malpica A, Ro JY, Troncoso P, et al. (1994) Nephrogenic adenoma of the prostatic urethra involving the prostate gland: a clinicopathologic and immunohistochemical study of eight cases. *Hum Pathol* 25: 390–395.

Markl IDC, Jones PA. (1998) Presence and location of TP53 mutation determines pattern of CDKN2A/ ARF pathway inactivation in bladder cancer. *Cancer Res* 58:5348–5353.

Marshall VF. (1962) The relation of the preoperative estimate to the pathologic demonstration of the extent of vesical neoplasm. *J Urol* 68:714–723.

Masters JRW, Camplejohn RS, Parkinson MC, Woodhouse CRJ. (1989) DNA ploidy and the prognosis of stage pT1 bladder cancer. *Br J Urol* 64:403–408.

Matsuyam H, Bergre US, Nilsson I, et al. (1994) Nonrandom numerical aberrations of chromosomes 7, 9, and 10 in DNA-diploid bladder cancer. *Cancer Genet Cytogenet* 77:118–124.

Maung R, Kelly JK, Grace DA. (1988) Intestinal metaplasia and dysplasia of prostatic urethra secondary to stricture. *Urology* 32:361–363.

McBride OW, Merry D, Givol D. (1986) The gene for human p53 cellular tumor antigen is located on chromosome 17 short arm. *Proc Nat Acad Sci USA* 83:130–134.

Melicow MM, Hollowell JW. (1952) Intra-urothelial cancer: carcinoma in situ, Bowen's disease of the urinary system. Discussion of 30 cases. *J Urol* 68: 763–772.

Mellon K, Neal DE, Robinson MC, Marsh C, Wright C. (1990) Cell cycling in bladder carcinoma determined by monoclonal antibody Ki67. *Br J Urol* 66: 281–285.

Mills SE, Wolfe JT III, Weiss MA, et al. (1987) Small cell undifferentiated carcinoma of the urinary bladder: a light-microscopic, immunohistochemical, and ultrastructural study of 12 cases. *Am J Surg Pathol* 11:606.

Mostofi FK, Sobin LH, Torlini H. (1973) *Histological Typing of Urinary Bladder Tumours. International Histological Classification of Tumours,* No. 10. World Health Organization, Geneva.

Murphy WM, Beckwith JB, Farrow GM. (1994) *Atlas of Tumor Pathology.* Third Series, Fascicle 11. *Tumors of the Kidney, Bladder, and Related Urinary Structures.* Armed Forces Institute of Pathology, Washington, DC.

Murphy WM, Chandler RW, Trafford RM. (1986) Flow cytometry of deparaffinized nuclei compared to histological grading for the pathological evaluation of transitional cell carcinomas. *J Urol* 135:694–697.

Murphy WM, Deana DG. (1992) The nested variant of transitional cell carcinoma: a neoplasm resembling proliferation of Brunn's nests. *Mod Pathol* 5:240–243.

Murphy WM, Miller AW. (1984) Bladder cancer. In: (Javadpour NE, ed.) pp. 100–102. Williams & Wilkins, Baltimore.

Murphy WM, Nagy GK, Rao MK, Soloway WS, Parija GC, Cox CE, Friedell GH. (1979) Normal urothelium in patients with bladder cancer. *Cancer* 44:1050–1058.

Murphy WM, Soloway MS. (1982a) Developing carcinoma (dysplasia) of the urinary bladder. *Pathol Annu* 17:197–217.

Murphy WM, Soloway MS. (1982b) Urothelial dysplasia. *J Urol* 127:849–854.

Nagy GK, Frable WJ, Murphy WM. (1982) Classification of premalignant urothelial abnormalities: a Delphi study of the National Bladder Cancer Collaborative Group A. *Pathol Annu* 17:219–233.

Navarro JE, Huggins TJ. (1984) Cystitis glandularis: an unusual cause of ureteral obstruction. *Urol Radiol* 6:27–29.

Nazeer T, Ro JY, Tornos C, et al. (1996) Endocervical type glands in urinary bladder: A clinicopathologic study of six cases. *Hum Pathol* 27:816–820.

Newman AJ Jr, Carlton CE Jr, Johnson S. (1980) Cell surface A, B or O (H) blood group antigens as an indicator of malignant potential in stage A bladder carcinoma. *J Urol* 124:27–29.

Odze R, Begin LR. (1989) Tubular adenomatous metaplasia (nephrogenic adenoma) of the female urethra. *Int J Gynecol Pathol* 8:374.

Oliva E, Young RH. (1996) Clear cell adenocarcinoma of the female urethra: a clinicopathologic study of 19 cases. Mod Pathol 9:513–520.

Oliva E, Young RH. (1995) Nephrogenic adenoma of the urinary tract: a review of the microscopic appearances of 80 cases with emphasis on unusual features. *Mod Pathol* 8:722–730.

Ooms ECM, Anderson WAD, Alons CL, Boon ME, Veldhuizen RW. (1983) Analysis of performance of pathologists in the grading of bladder tumors. *Hum Pathol* 14:140–143.

Orntoft TF, Nielsen MJS, Wolf H, et al. (1987) Blood group ABO and Lewis antigen expression during neoplastic progression of human urothelium: immunohistochemical study of type 1 chain structures. *Cancer* 60:2641–2648.

Otto T, Goepel M, Heider KH, Rubben H. (1995): Prognostic factors for bladder cancer. *Urol Res* 23:137–141.

Ozdemir E, Kakehi Y, Okuno H, Yoshida O. (1999) Role of matrix metalloproteinase-9 in the basement membrane destruction of superficial urothelial carcinomas. *J Urol* 161:1359–1363.

Pagano F, Garbeglio A, Milani C, Bassi P, Pegoraro V. (1987) Prognosis of bladder cancer. I. Risk factors in superficial transitional cell carcinoma. *Eur Urol* 13:145–149.

Paschkis R. (1925) Uber Adenoma der Harnblase. *Z Urol Chir* 21:315–325.

Paulsen J, Metwalli N, Wu B, Nochsmovitz L. (1988) Transitional cell carcinoma of bladder with features of inverted papilloma. *Mod Pathol* 1:71A.

Pauwels RP, Smeets WW, Geraedts JP, Debruyne FM. (1987) Cytogenetic analysis in urothelial cell carcinoma. *J Urol* 137:210–215.

Pauwels RPE, Schapers RFM, Smeets AWGB, Debruyne FMJ, Geraedts JPM. (1988) Grading in superficial bladder cancer. (1) Morphological criteria. *Br J Urol* 61:129–134.

Petersen RO. (1986) Urinary bladder. In: *Urologic Pathology*. (Petersen RO, ed.) pp. 279–416. Lippincott, Philadelphia.

Philip AT, Amin MB, Tamboli P, Lee TJ, Ro JY. (1999) Intravesical adipose tissue: a quantitative study of its presence and location with diagnostic implications. *Mod Pathol* 12:104A.

Potts IF, Hirst E. (1963) Inverted papilloma of the bladder. *J Urol* 90:175–179.

Prout GR Jr, Griffin PP, Daly JJ. (1987) The outcome of conservative treatment of carcinoma *in situ* of the bladder. *J Urol* 138:766–770.

Ramani P, Birch BRP, Harlund SJ, et al. (1988) Evaluation of endothelial markers in detecting blood and lymphatic channel invasion in pT1 transitional carcinoma of the bladder. *Histopathology* 19:551–554.

Reddy EP, Reynolds RK, Santos E, Barbacid M. (1982) A point mutation is responsible for the acquisition of transforming properties by the T24 human bladder carcinoma oncogene. *Nature* 300:149–152.

Reznikoff CA, Belair CD, Yeager TR, et al. (1996) A molecular genetic model of human bladder cancer pathogenesis. *Semin Oncol* 23:571–584.

Richards B, Parmar MKB, Anderson CK, et al. (1991) Interpretation of biopsies of normal urothelium in patients with supeficial bladder cancer. *Br J Urol* 67:369–375.

Richie JP, Blute RD Jr, Waisman J. (1980) Immunologic indicators of prognosis in bladder cancer: the importance of cell surface antigens. *J Urol* 123:22–24.

Ro JY, Ayala AG, El-Naggar A. (1987a) Muscularis mucosae of urinary bladder: importance for staging and treatment. *Am J Surg Pathol* 11:668–673.

Ro JY, Ayala AG, El-Naggar A, Wishnow KI. (1987b) Seminal vesicle involvement by in situ and invasive transitional cell carcinoma of the bladder. *Am J Surg Pathol* 11:951–958.

Ro JY, Ayala AG, Ordonez NG, et al. (1986) Pseudosarcomatous fibromyxoid tumor of the urinary bladder. *Am J Clin Pathol* 86:583–590.

Ro JY, Ayala AG, Wishnow K. et al. (1988) Sarcomatoid bladder carcinoma: clinicopathological and immunohistochemical study of 44 cases. *Surg Pathol* 1:359.

Romanelli R. (1986) Inverted urothelial papilloma: report of five cases and review of the literature. *Pathologica* 78:89–97.

Rubben H, Dahm HH, Bubenzer J, et al. (1978) TNM classification of urinary bladder tumours: value of Ta category for non-infiltrating exophytic tumours. In: *Bladder Tumours and Other Topics in Urological Oncology* (Pavone-Macaluso M, Smith PH, Edsmyr F, eds.) pp. 9–12. Plenum Press, London.

Sahin AS, Myhre M, Ro JY, et al. (1991) Plasmacytoid transitional cell carcinoma. Report of a case with initial presentation mimicking multiple myeloma. *Acta Cytol* 35:277–280.

Sandberg AA. (1986) Chromosome changes in bladder cancer: clinical and other correlations. *Cancer Genet Cytogenet* 19:163–175.

Sandberg AA. (1977) Chromosome markers and progression in bladder cancer. *Cancer Res* 37:2950–2956.

Sanders H, McCue P, Graham SD Jr. (1991) ABO (H) antigens and beta-2 microglobulin in transitional cell carcinoma: predictors of response to intravesical Bacillus Calmette-Guerin. *Cancer* 67:3024–3028.

Saran KK, Gould D, Godec CJ, Verman RS. (1996) Genetics of bladder cancer. *J Mol Med* 74:441–445.

Schade RO, Swinney J. (1973) The association of urothelial atypism with neoplasia: its importance in treatment and prognosis. *J Urol* 109:619–622.

Schapers RFM, Pauwels RPE, Havenith MG, Smeets AWGB, van den Brandt PA, Bosman FT. (1990) Prognostic significance of type IV collagen and laminin immunoreactivity in urothelial carcinomas of the bladder. *Cancer* 66:2583–2588.

Schellhammer PF, Whitmore WF Jr. (1976) Transitional cell carcinoma of the urethra in men having cystectomy for bladder cancer. *J Urol* 115:56–60.

Schroder LE, Weiss MA, Hughes C. (1986) Squamous cell carcinoma of bladder: an increased incidence in Blacks. *Urology* 28:288.

Sekine S. (1976) Cytogenetic observations in tumours of the urinary tract and male genitals. *Jpn J Urol* 67:452–464.

Smith G, Elton RA, Beynon LL. (1983) Prognostic significance of biopsy results of normal-looking mucosa in cases of superficial bladder cancer. *Br J Urol* 55:665–669.

Soloway MS, Murphy WM, Rao MK, Cox C. (1978) Serial multiple-site biopsies in patients with bladder cancer. *J Urol* 120:57–59.

Summers JL, Falor WH, Ward R. (1981) A 10-year analysis of chromosomes in non-invasive papillary carcinoma of the bladder. *J Urol* 125:177–178.

Talbert ML, Young RH. (1989) Carcinomas of the urinary bladder with deceptively benign-appearing foci: a report of three cases. *Am J Surg Pathol* 13:374.

Theoret G, Paquin F, Schick E, Martel A. (1980) Inverted papilloma of urinary tract. *Urology* 16:149–151.

Tomaszewski JE, Korat OC, LiVolsi VA, Connor M, Wein A. (1986) Paget's disease of the urethral meatus following transitional cell carcinoma of the bladder. *J Urol* 135:368–370.

Torti FM, Lum BL. (1987) Superficial bladder cancer: risk of recurrence and potential role for interferon therapy. *Cancer* 59:613–616.

Torti FM, Lum BL, Aston D, et al. (1987) Superficial bladder cancer: the primacy of grade in the development of invasive disease. *J Clin Oncol* 5:125–130.

Tribukait B. (1984) Clinical DNA flow cytometry. *Med Oncol Tumor Pharmacother* 1:211–218.

Trites AEW. (1969) Inverted urothelial papilloma: report of two cases. *J Urol* 101:216–219.

Utz DC, Farrow GM. (1984) Carcinoma *in situ* of the urinary tract. *Urol Clin North Am* 11:735–749.

Utz DC, Hanash KA, Farrow GM. (1970) The plight of the patient with carcinoma *in situ* of the bladder. *J Urol* 103:160–164.

Uyama T, Nakamura S, Moriwaki S. (1980) Inverted papilloma of bladder: two cases with questionable malignancy and squamous metaplasia. *Urology* 16:152–154.

Vamvakas S, Bittner D, Koster U. (1993) Enhanced expression of the protooncogenes c-*myc* and c-*fos* in normal and malignant renal growth. *Toxicol Lett* 67:161–172.

Van Dekken H, Schervish EW, Pizzolo JG, Fair WR, Melamed MR. (1991) Simultaneous detection of fluorescent *in situ* hybridization and *in vivo* incorporated BrdU in human bladder tumour. *J Pathol* 164:17–22.

Velculescu VE, El-Diery WS. (1996) Biological and clinical importance of the *p53* tumor suppressor gene. *Clin Chem* 42:858–868.

Veyrune JL, Hesketh J, Blanchard JM. (1997) 3′ untranslated regions of c-*myc* and c-*fos* mRNAs: multifunctional elements regulating mRNA translation, degradation and subcellular localization. *Prog Mol Subcell Biol* 18:35–63.

Waldman FM, Carroll PR, Kerschmann R, Cohen MB, Field FG, Mayall BH. (1991) Centromeric copy number of chromosome 7 is strongly correlated with tumor grade and labeling index in human bladder cancer. *Cancer Res* 51:3807–3813.

Walther M, O'Brien DP, Birch HW. (1986) Condylomata acuminata and verrucous carcinoma of the bladder: case report and literature review. *J Urol* 135:362.

Whitesel JA. (1982) Inverted papilloma of the urinary tract: malignant potential. *J Urol* 127:539–540.

Wick MR, Zarbo RJ, Hitchcock CL. (1989) Special techniques for the pathologic analysis of lesions of the urinary bladder. In: *Pathology of the Urinary Bladder* (Young RH, ed.) pp. 285–349. Churchill Livingstone, New York.

Williams JL, Hammonds JC, Saunders N. (1977) T1 bladder tumours. *Br J Urol* 49:663–668.

Wishnow KI, Ro JY. (1988) Importance of early treatment of transitional cell carcinoma of the prostatic ducts. *Urology* 32:11–12.

Wolf H, Hojgaard K. (1983) Urothelial dysplasia concomitant with bladder tumours as a determinant factor for future new occurrences. *Lancet* 2:134–136.

Wolf H, Olsen PR, Hojhaard K. (1985) Urothelial dysplasia concomitant with bladder tumors: a determinant for future new occurrence in patients treated by full-course radiotherapy. *Lancet* 1:1005–1008.

Xu H-J, Cagle PT, Hu S-X, Benendict WF. (1996) Altered retinoblastoma and p53 protein status in nonsmall cell carcinoma of the lung: potential synergistic effects on prognosis. *Clin Cancer Res* 2:1169–1176.

Xu H-J, Cairns P, Hu S-X, Knowles MA, Benendict WF. (1993) Loss of RB protein expression in primary bladder cancer correlates with loss of heterozygosity at the RB locus and tumor progression. *Int J Cancer* 53:781–784.

Yamada T, Fukui I, Kobayashi T, et al. (1991) The relationship of ABH (O) blood group antigen expression in intraepithelial dysplastic lesions to clinicopathologic properties of associated transitional cell carcinoma of the bladder. *Cancer* 67:1661–1666.

Younes M, Sussman J, True LD. (1990) The usefulness of the level of the muscularis mucosae in the staging of invasive transitional cell carcinoma of the urinary bladder. *Cancer* 66:543–548.

Young RH. (1997) Pseudoneoplastic lesions of the urinary bladder and urethra: a selective review with emphasis on recent information. *Semin Diagn Pathol* 14:133–146.

Young RH, Bostwick DG. (1996) Florid cystitis glandularis with mucin extravasation: a mimic of adenocarcinoma. *Am J Surg Pathol* 20:1462–1468.

Young RH, Clement PB. (1996) Müllerianosis of the urinary bladder. *Mod Pathol* 9:731–737.

Young RH, Eble JN. (1991) Unusual forms of carcinoma of the urinary bladder. *Hum Pathol* 22:948–965.

Young RH, Scully RE. (1985) Clear cell adenocarcinoma of the bladder and urethra: a report of three cases and review of the literature. *Am J Surg Pathol* 9:816–826.

Young RH, Zuckerberg LR. (1991) Microcystic transitional cell carcinomas of the urinary bladder: report of 4 cases. *Am J Clin Pathol* 96:635.

Zieger K, Wolf H, Olsen PR, Hojgaard K. (1998) Long-term survival of patients with bladder tumors: the significance of risk factors. *Br J Urol* 82:667–672.

Zuk RJ, Rogers HS, Matin JE, Baithum SI. (1988) Clinicopathological importance of primary dysplasia of bladder. *J Clin Pathol* 41:1277–1280.

Zukerberg LR, Armin AR, Pisharodi L, et al. (1990) Transitional cell carcinoma of the urinary bladder with osteoclast-type giant-cells: a report of two cases and review of the literature. *Histopathology* 17:407–411.

21

PROSTATE

ALBERTO G. AYALA, BOGDAN CZERNIAK, AND JAE Y. RO

Within the past two decades, there have been significant advances in our understanding of the pathogenesis of prostatic carcinoma and its early detection. The early detection of localized prostatic carcinoma, enhanced by the utilization of sonography (Cooner et al., 1988; Lee et al., 1991), digital rectal examination, measurements of prostate-specific antigen (PSA) and prostatic acid phosphatase (PAP) levels in serum, and the biopsy gun technique for prostatic biopsies, has literally resulted in an explosion of radical prostatectomies for treating localized disease. Clarification of the anatomy of the prostate (McNeal, 1968), which permits correlative sonographic studies (Lee et al., 1989), has also contributed to our understanding of prostatic neoplasia, and cytogenetic and molecular diagnostic techniques have opened the field for future investigation.

BACKGROUND

In 1965 and 1969, McNeal described two potentially premalignant lesions of the prostate as intraductal dysplasia (McNeal, 1965, 1969; McNeal and Bostwick, 1986), which was subsequently designated "ductal acinar dysplasia and atypical adenomatous hyperplasia (AAH) " (McNeal et al., 1991). He challenged the prevailing theory that prostate cancer develops from atrophic epithelium (Franks, 1954a,b) by postulating that it arises from active proliferative epithelium. McNeal

emphasized the multifocality of premalignant lesions and prostatic adenocarcinoma and introduced the concept of zonal anatomy of the prostate (McNeal, 1968). However, it was not until the 1980s that his work gained widespread recognition.

ZONAL ANATOMY

McNeal's concept of zonal anatomy (McNeal, 1968, 1969, 1981, 1988) has been widely accepted among urologists and radiologists because it can be correlated with sonographic findings (Lee et al., 1989).

The prostate gland is a small, pear-shaped organ ($4 \times 3 \times 2$ cm; 20 g) that is almost vertically oriented behind the pubis in the pelvis. The base of the prostate is located toward the bladder, and its apex is toward the inferior aspect of the pelvis. The prostate is traversed by the urethral tube, which manifests a $35°$ anterior angulation at about its longitudinal midpoints. Beginning at the point of angulation, at the lower half of the urethra, the verumontanum protrudes from the posterior urethral wall and extends down for about one-half the length of the distal urethral segment, tapering distally. The ejaculatory ducts open on the convexity of the verumontanum (McNeal, 1968, 1988).

The prostate consists of three distinct zones: a peripheral zone, transition zone and central zone. The *peripheral zone* makes up approximately 70% of the glandular mass, and its ducts, aligned in double rows, open in the lower half of the urethra extending from the base of the verumontanum to the prostatic apex. Most of the distal half of the prostate, including the apex, is constituted by this zone, which ascends posteriorly, covering the central and transition zones (Fig. 21–1). In addition, the peripheral zone partially envelops the lateral aspect of the transition zone, reaching its anterior aspect focally. Because these extensions are seen bilaterally, they are known as the anterior "horns" on sonograms. The peripheral zone is the origin of most prostatic adenocarcinomas (McNeal, 1988). Because of the anatomic location of this zone, lesions are easily accessible for palpation and biopsy via a rectal approach. However, the peripheral zone is relatively inaccessible for transurethral surgical procedures.

The *central zone* is a cone of tissue that represents approximately 25% of the prostate. The base of the central zone is at the seminal vesicles, and its vertex is at the verumontanum. Ducts within the central zone open in the verumontanum in the immediate vicinity of the orifices of the ejaculatory ducts. The central zone surrounds and follows the path of the ejaculatory ducts and shows no clear-cut boundaries with the peripheral zone (Fig. 21–1). However, the configuration of the glandular and ductal structures within this zone is different from that of the glands and ducts of the peripheral and transition zones. Thus, in the central zone, the branching of the duct system is more elaborate than in the peripheral zone, and most of the terminal sacculations are concentrated peripherally. In the peripheral and transition zones, the pattern of duct branching is simplified, showing smaller, rounded sacculations and less prominent intraluminal partitions (McNeal, 1988). In addition, the epithelial lining of the glands in the central zone tends to show nuclear stratification, a feature that may be confused with the proliferative change of prostatic intraepithelial neoplasia (PIN). The central zone rarely gives rise to prostatic carcinoma, but because it surrounds and accompanies the ejaculatory ducts from the seminal vesicles to the urethra, it is a pathway for the spread of carcinoma to the seminal vesicles.

The *transition zone* consists of two independent small lobes situated on the lateral and anterior aspects of the proximal half of the urethra. It represents about 5% of a normal prostate (McNeal, 1988). A band of fibromuscular tissue, previously known as the surgical capsule, surrounds the transition zone and separates it from the peripheral and central zones. Ducts in the transition

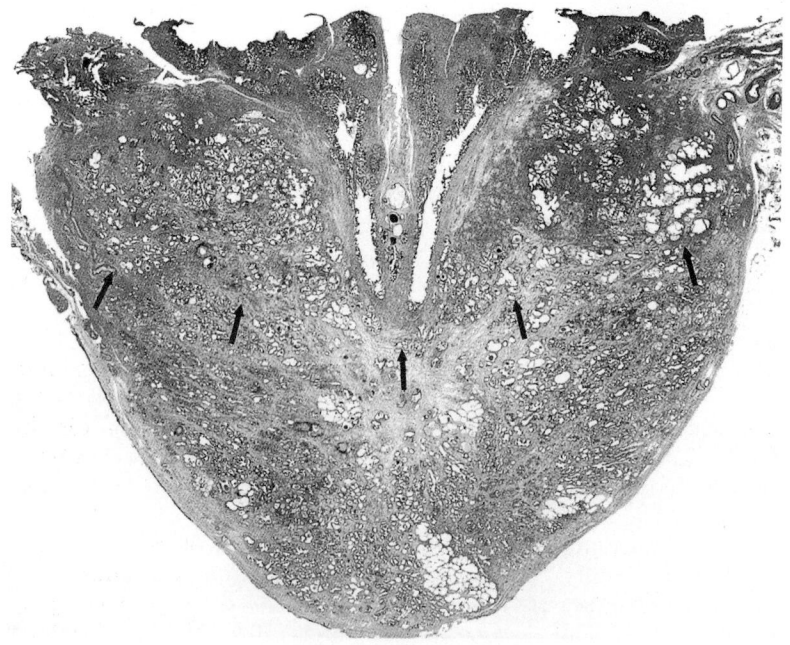

Figure 21–1. Coronal section of the prostate (from apex to base, including seminal vesicles) parallel and posterior to the distal half of the urethra. The central zone (arrows) surrounds the ejaculatory ducts and forms the base of the prostate. The rest of the prostatic parenchyma constitutes the peripheral zone. The transition zone and the urethra are not seen at this level.

zone empty into the posterolateral recesses of the urethral wall at a single point, near the site of urethral angulation. The transition zone is the seat of nodular hyperplasia and its variants, basal cell hyerplasia (BCH), clear cell cribriform hyperplasia (CCCH) and sclerosing adenosis (SA). A distinct adenocarcinoma called "clear cell carcinoma" also arises in this zone (McNeal, 1988).

The *proximal periurethral region*, which represents less than 1% of the glandular volume, may give rise to prostatic hyperplasia. When this occurs, this region becomes the so-called *middle lobe*. This region consists of small periurethral glands and ducts that are contained within the preprostatic sphincter, which surrounds the proximal urethral segment posteriorly and laterally (McNeal, 1988).

The prostate is well circumscribed but does not contain a true complete capsule (Ayala et al., 1989). Most of its posterior area is covered by 1 to 2 mm–thick band of smooth muscle fibers and fibroblasts, which in turn is covered by a thin Denonvillier's fascia, giving the impression that it is a "true" capsule. The remainder of the outer fibromuscular coat, however, is very irregular. In the posterolateral aspect of the prostate, the fibromuscular band loses its tightness bilaterally. Some of the fibers of ill-defined fibromuscular band spring toward the fibroadipose tissue, which contains smooth muscle fibers, nerves, vessels, and lymphatics. The nerves are generally small, consisting of single fibers or small bundles that never achieve a significant diameter. This area is of extreme importance in nerve-sparing surgery (Eggleston and Walsh, 1985; Walsh et al., 1983).

There is no anatomic separation at the junction where the prostate, seminal vesicles, and bladder merge, nor is there anatomic separation between the apex of the prostate and the surrounding soft tissues. The pelvic floor, with its numerous skeletal muscle fibers, covers and penetrates the apex of the prostate and extends upward anteriorly and laterally. This anatomic configuration explains the presence of skeletal muscle fibers anchored within the prostatic stroma. These fibers are numerous in the apex and lower aspect of the anterior and lateral surfaces of the prostate but decrease and eventually disappear toward the supe-

rior aspect. The prominent smooth muscle fibers, skeletal muscle fibers, and fibroblastic stroma cause the anterior aspect of the prostate to appear aglandular. The skeletal muscle fibers are normally present in the prostate glands; thus, the admixture of glandular structures and skeletal muscle do not indicate either malignancy or extraprostatic extension of prostate cancer.

PREMALIGNANT LESIONS

Atypical adenomatous hyperplasia (AAH) and PIN have been thought to represent premalignant processes in the pathogenesis of prostate cancer. Current information, however, indicates that AAH is not a premalignant lesion but a lesion that simulates, and thus must be distinguished from, well-differentiated adenocarcinoma of the prostate. Atypical adenomatous hyperplasia does not show nuclear atypia, which is a feature of PIN, and its premalignant status has not been proved (Amin et al., 1994; Bostwick, 1996). In contrast, PIN demonstrates a close association with prostatic carcinoma in biopsy and prostatectomy specimens (Amin et al., 1994; Bostwick, 1996; Haggman et al., 1997a; Langer et al., 1996; Murphy, 1998; Raviv et al., 1996; Shepherd et al., 1996).

PROSTATIC INTRAEPITHELIAL NEOPLASIA

The nomenclature for atypical lesions of the prostate was inconsistent among reports in the European literature (Helpap, 1980; Kastendieck, 1980) and among these reports and those in the American literature. In 1986, McNeal and Bostwick refined and expanded this histologic criteria for intraductal dysplasia, and in 1987, Bostwick and Brawer proposed that PIN be used to describe these atypical prostatic lesions. The PIN nomenclature was officially adopted in 1989 at the Workshop on Preneoplastic Lesions of the Prostate and included the designations of PIN 1 for low-grade neoplasisa and PIN 2 and PIN 3 for high-grade neoplasia (Table 21–1; Drago et al., 1989).

Prostatic intraepithelial neoplasia is an epithelial proliferation of the ducts and acini that predominantly involves the peripheral

Table 21–1. Grading Criteria for Prostatic Intraepithelial Neoplasia[a]

Criterion	Grade 1	Grade 2	Grade 3
Nuclear size	Markedly increased[b]	Markedly increased	Markedly increased
Variability of nuclear size	Markedly increased[b]	Increased (inconsistent)	Less than grade 2
Cell spacing	Irregular, with focal crowding and multilayering	As in grade 1	As in grade 1; occasional luminal bridging
Chromatin	Normal	Increased[b]	Markedly increased
Nucleoli	Infrequent small, prominent nucleoli	Occasional small, prominent nucleoli	Numerous large, prominent nucleoli[b]

[a]Prostatic intraepithelial neoplasia was referred to as intraductal dysplasia in the McNeal and Bostwick article (1986).

[b]Indicates most characteristics feature or features.

Modified from McNeal JE, Bostwick DG. (1986) Intraductal dysplasia. A premalignant lesion of the prostate. *Hum Pathol* 17:64–71, with permission.

zone of the prostate and rarely involves the transition or central zone. The spectrum of this proliferation ranges from hyperplastic change with minimal atypia to frankly atypical change characteristic of high-grade PIN. Low-grade PIN, or PIN 1, is similar to simple hyperplasia and is characterized by an epithelial proliferation that exhibits nuclear enlargement, anisokaryosis, and irregular nuclear stratification. Although small nucleoli may be seen, they are not prominent or numerous (Fig. 21–2). The category PIN 2 is a step up from PIN 1. Some nuclei exhibit hyperchromatism, whereas others demonstrate a fine chromatin pattern. Large, prominent nucleoli begin to appear, but they are not numerous (Fig. 21–3). Cyto-

plasmic eosinophilia may be observed. The next grade, PIN 3, is characterized by features similar to those of PIN 2 but often demonstrates hyperchromatism and many large, prominent nucleoli like those seen in invasive carcinoma (Fig. 21–4). While occasionally present, mitoses are not characteristic of PIN 2 or PIN 3. On pathology reports, PIN 1 should be described in the "Comment" section and not as a diagnosis because it cannot reproducibly be distinguished from benign prostatic hyperplasia or metaplasias (Epstein et al., 1995). Furthermore, patients shown to have PIN 1 by needle

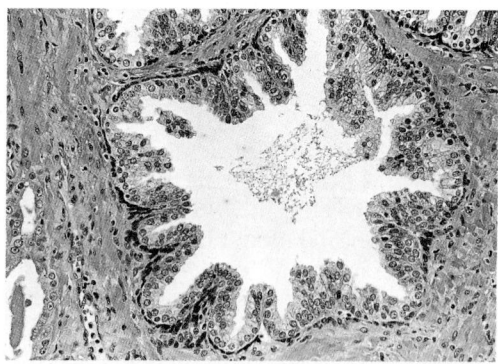

Figure 21–2. Low-grade prostatic intraepithelial neoplasia (PIN-1). A star–like shaped glandular structure shows proliferation of the epithelium with nuclear stratification and some anisonucleosis but no nucleoli. Note a very prominent basal cell layer.

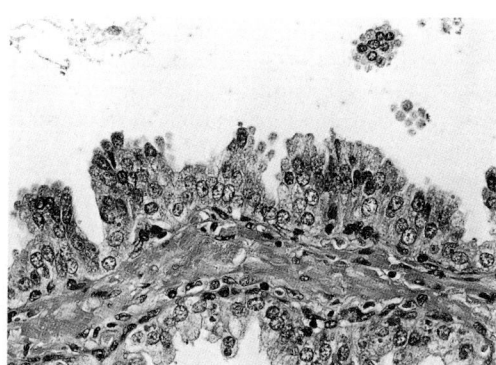

Figure 21–3. This illustration shows the lining of two adjacent glands. The gland that is superiorly located exhibits thickening of the ductal/acinar epithelium with some enlargement of nuclei and the presence of small nucleoli representing PIN-2. In contrast, the gland in the bottom shows some nuclear enlargement but no appreciable nucleoli representing PIN-1 of the former three-tiered grading system.

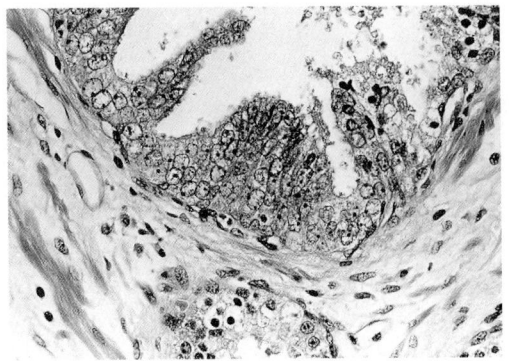

Figure 21–4. High-grade prostatic intraepithelial neoplasia. This duct shows increased cellularity manifested by nuclear stratification. Clearing of nuclei is present as well as numerous prominent nucleoli.

biopsy are at no greater risk of having carcinoma on repeat biopsy (Brawer et al., 1991), and the frequency with which PIN 1 occurs in patients with and without prostate cancers is not different (Troncoso et al., 1989).

High-grade PIN was initially divided into two grades. However, there is no good interobserver agreement on the distinction between them; furthermore, the finding of either PIN 2 or PIN 3 on a needle biopsy specimen is associated with the same risk of finding carcinoma on a subsequent biopsy specimen (Weinstein and Epstein, 1993), and both precede the development of

prostate cancer more frequently than not (Langer et al., 1996; Shepherd et al., 1996; Troncoso et al., 1989; Weinstein and Epstein, 1993).

PROGRESSION OF PROSTATIC INTRAEPITHELIAL NEOPLASIA

Prostatic intraepithelial neoplasia is readily identified under low-power magnification. The glandular structures involved by PIN stand out because they are darker than the surrounding normal or atrophic glandular units (Fig. 21–5). This condition may be a focal process that partially or completely involves a single ductal-acinar unit, but more frequently it is a multifocal process (McNeal and Bostwick, 1986; Troncoso et al., 1989). At inception, the process may consist of an increased number of atypical cells in the lining of the duct or acinus, giving the appearance of a thickened hypercellular wall, but as this proliferation progresses, intraluminal papillae of atypical epithelium are formed that eventually bridge the glandular lumen and produce a papillary arrangement. Later, as the cell mass increases, this arrangement becomes papillary or cribriform (Fig. 21–6). In some ducts, the atypical cellular proliferative process may show a maturation effect toward the center of the lumen, where the cells are smaller and devoid of nuclear atypia (Fig. 21–6A). The basal cell layer remains at least partially intact (Fig. 21–6B) and is easily demonstrated

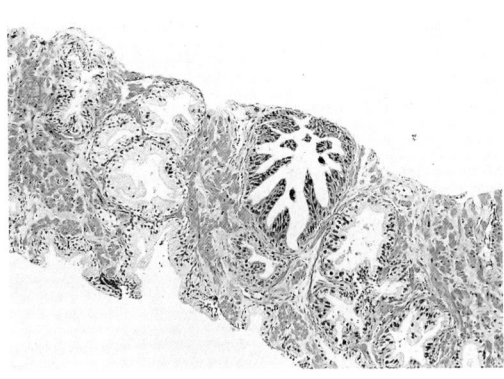

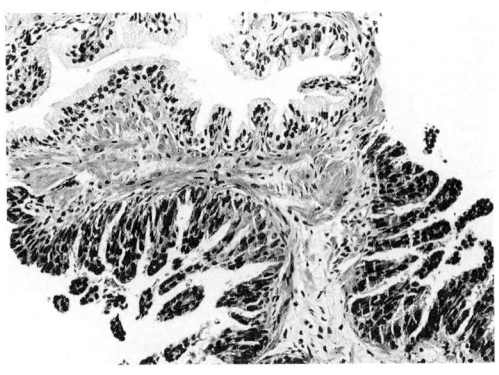

A   B

Figure 21–5. Low-power view of prostatic intraepithelial neoplasia (PIN). *A:* In this needle biopsy the affected ductal structures show increased cellularity contrasting with the surrounding normal glands. *B:* This closer view (different biopsy) of high-grade PIN specimen shows thickened hyperchromatic epithelium that contrasts with an adjacent normal gland.

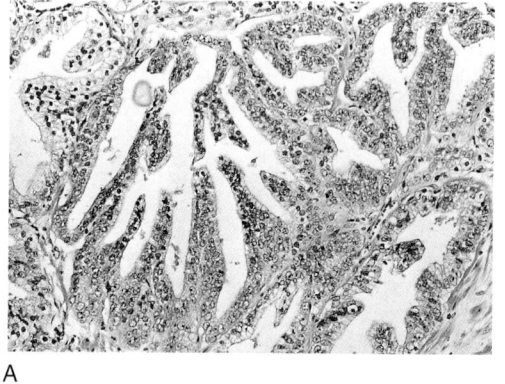

A

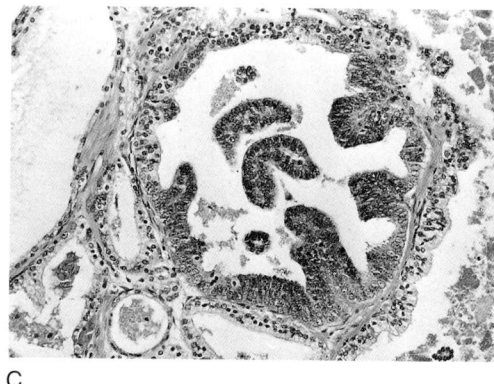

C

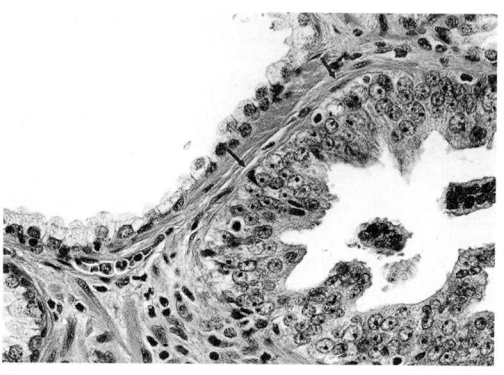

B

Figure 21–6. *A*: Low-power view of papillary high-grade prostatic intraepithelial neoplasia (PIN). As the cells reach the central portion of the duct, their nuclei become smaller and darker, a common occurrence in papillary PIN. *B*: Partial preservation of basal cell layer is present in this illustration of PIN (arrows). *C*: Partial involvement of high-grade PIN is present in this duct.

with a high-molecular-weight antikeratin antibody (basal cell–specific cytokeratin) (Bostwick and Brawer, 1987). When the ducts or acini are filled with a cribriform–papillary proliferation, the process of high-grade PIN reaches the level of intraductal carcinoma *in situ* (Fig. 21–7). At this point,

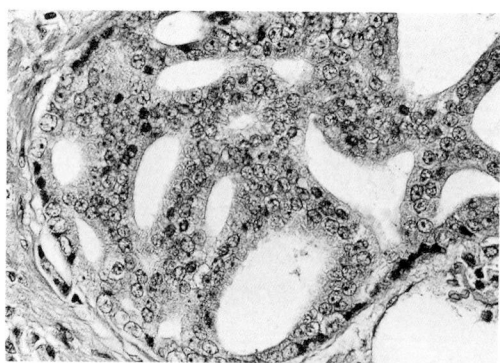

Figure 21–7. This illustration shows the cribriform pattern of prostatic intraepithelial neoplasia. A few dark-staining cells at the periphery of the duct represent an attenuated basal cell layer.

the basal cell layer may be partially interrupted.

As PIN increases in grade, it may progress to invasive carcinoma (Figs. 21–8 and 21–9). Immunohistochemical proof was given by Bostwick and Brawer (1987), who, employing a monoclonal antibody directed against the basal cell layer, demonstrated that it remained intact in the areas of high-grade PIN but disappeared as invasive carcinoma developed. They speculated that high-grade PIN progresses to carcinoma *in situ*, which, after losing its basal cell layer, enables stromal invasion. They cautioned, however, that despite the attractiveness of their hypothesis, there was no definite evidence that PIN progresses to invasive carcinoma (Bostwick and Brawer, 1987).

In several studies (Helpap, 1980; Kastendieck, 1980; Kovi et al., 1988; McNeal and Bostwick, 1986; Oyasu et al., 1986; Troncosco et al., 1989), the authors have evaluated PIN in serially sectioned excised prostates with and without carcinoma and have found that there is a significant increase in the prevalence, extent, and severity of PIN in prostates

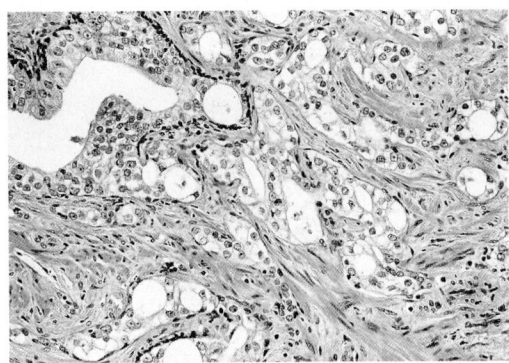

Figure 21–8. Prostatic intraepithelial neoplasia (PIN) and adenocarcinoma. In the upper left corner there is a large glandular structure showing atypical epithelium of high-grade PIN. The nuclear features of the associated carcinoma present in the remainder of the picture are similar to those of the high-grade PIN. Note the prominence of a compressed, dark-staining basal cell layer in the gland with PIN and its absence in the invasive carcinoma.

with carcinoma, which supports the concept that PIN is a precursor of carcinoma.

Troncoso et al. (1989) demonstrated the multifocality of PIN by studying whole-organ sections of the prostates from 100 patients who underwent radical cystoprostatectomies for bladder carcinoma. Prostatic intraepithelial neoplasia was present in 89 prostates and prostatic carcinoma was in 61 cases. All 61 prostates with carcinoma demonstrated PIN, but PIN was present in only 72% of the

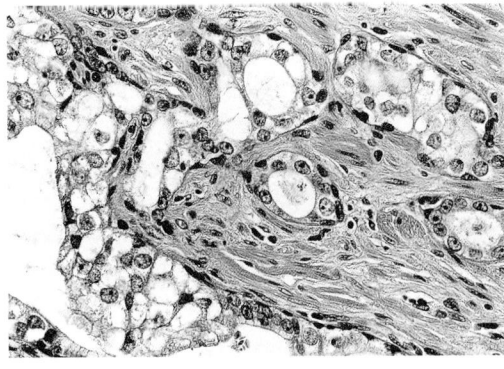

Figure 21–9. Prostatic intraepithelial neoplasia (PIN) and adenocarcinoma. A high-power view illustrates invasive carcinoma manifested by small glands lined by a single cell layer with prominent nucleoli. Note high-grade PIN in the lower left corner.

specimens without carcinoma. The extent of PIN in prostates with carcinoma, as demonstrated by the number and size of the foci, was significantly increased. Of the prostates with carcinoma, 71% had more than 10 foci, with a substantial proportion (28%) displaying more than 20 foci. In contrast, only 15% of the prostates without carcinoma contained more than 10 foci. Large foci of PIN (greater than 4.5 mm) were also found more frequently in prostates with carcinoma (33%) than in those without carcinoma (7%). Prostates with carcinoma also tended to have higher grades of PIN than prostates without carcinoma, and PIN was predominantly localized in the peripheral zone (86%), followed by the central zone (13%) and the transition zone (1%). Furthermore, PIN was found to be immediately adjacent to or within the same low-power field (4.5 mm) of the carcinoma in 62% of cases (Troncoso et al., 1989). Other studies (Epstein, 1994b; McNeal and Bostwick, 1986; Qian et al., 1997b; Skjorten et al., 1997; Wiley et al., 1997) had observations similar to those of Troncoso et al. (1989).

Arguments against use of the PIN nomenclature stem from the facts that low-grade PIN is an accentuation of a hyperplastic change with little nuclear atypia and has been observed equally with or without carcinoma. Because low-grade PIN is not clinically significant (McNeal and Bostwick, 1986; Troncoso et al., 1989), it does not need to be included in the surgical pathology report when found in a biopsy specimen, as mentioned above. However, because high-grade PIN has a high predictive value for the presence of carcinoma (Kovi et al., 1988; McNeal and Bostwick, 1986; Oyasu et al., 1986), it should be included in the surgical pathology report. Patients with high-grade PIN need to be assessed or reassessed with measurements of PSA and PAP serum levels, digital rectal examination, and sonography. Sonographically guided biopsies should also be done regardless of whether suspicious lesions are detected or not. Several studies detected an average of 73% carcinoma on repeat biopsy specimens from patients whose initial biopsy specimens revealed only high-grade PIN, proving PIN to be a highly predictive marker for carcinoma (Brawer et al., 1991; Davidson et al., 1995; Keetch et al., 1995; Weinstein and Epstein, 1993). Finding high-grade PIN on transurethral resection of prostate (TURP) specimens is relatively uncommon and is found primarily in an elderly population. Patients with high-grade PIN on (TURP) appear to be at increased risk of developing prostatic carcinoma, although not to the same degree as patients with high-grade PIN on needle biopsy (Gaudin et al., 1997; Pacelli and Bostwick, 1997).

DIFFERENTIAL DIAGNOSIS OF PROSTATIC INTRAEPITHELIAL NEOPLASIA

Low-grade PIN is subtle and may often be intially misinterpreted as another epithelial proliferation, such as epithelial hyperplasia of the usual type or transitional metaplasia (Amin et al., 1994; Epstein et al., 1995). The usual hyperplasia does not show marked nuclear enlargement, and the uniform nuclei are evenly spaced without nuclear overlap. Transitional metaplasia can be recognized by the presence of a residual luminal layer, longitudinal nuclear grooves, or both. If nucleoli develop in transitional metaplasia, low-grade PIN may be difficult to rule out.

Benign epithelial proliferations included in the differential diagnosis of high-grade PIN are basal cell hyperplasia and clear cell cribriform hyperplasia, which are discussed later in this chapter. Transitional cell carcinoma (TCC) involving prostatic ducts may occasionally resemble high-grade PIN. The cells of the usually high-grade TCC show significant anaplastic features manifested by large nuclei, marked variation in nuclear size, and a coarse chromatin pattern. The cytoplasm is granular and mitoses are usually present (Amin et al., 1994; Cheville et al., 1998; Johnson et al., 1972). The presence of mitotes is a feature not included in the grading scheme of PIN. Mitoses are extremely rare in PIN, and when they are seen in radical prostatectomy or cystoprostatectomy specimens, one should consider the possibility of other diagnoses. We have noticed, however, mitoses in needle biopsy specimens (A.G. Ayala, B. Czerniak, J.Y. Ro, unpublished data). The difference in fixation time, which is very rapid for needle biopsy cores and prolonged for the other specimens, probably plays a role in the mitotic count variance. Cribriform carcinoma is more difficult to differentiate from high-grade PIN. Large expanding ductal-acinar proliferation

of atypical cells with a cribriform pattern, especially when the periphery is irregular, favors a diagnosis of cribriform carcinoma over high-grade PIN. Unfortunately, some cases of cribriform carcinoma may spread in a retrograde fashion, and when this occurs, the basal cell layer may be retained (McNeal and Yemoto, 1996; Rubin et al., 1998).

IMMUNOPHENOTYPIC AND PROLIFERATIVE FEATURES OF PROSTATIC INTRAEPITHELIAL NEOPLASIA

Basal Cell Disruption

The basal and luminal cells of the prostate display different immunoreactivities for keratin. A high-molecular-weight antikeratin monoclonal antibody (34βE12) that recognizes keratin proteins of 49, 51, 57, and 66 Kd specifically labels the basal cells but not the luminal (secretory) cells of the prostatic glandular elements. The basal cell layer present in normal glands and benign epithelial proliferations is absent in carcinoma and may be disrupted in PIN (Brawer et al., 1985). Bostwick and Brawer (1987) have shown that the frequency and extent of basal cell disruption in PIN are related to the PIN grade and that this disruption occurs most frequently and is extensive in high-grade PIN adjacent to foci of carcinoma. In their study, Bostwick and Brawer (1987) identified areas of basal cell disruption in high-grade PIN associated with foci of small glandular outpouchings that lacked basal cells, which they interpreted as immunohistochemical evidence of early invasion. However, one must be cautious in the interpretation of this specific antikeratin. Hedrick and Epstein (1989) found that a small number of foci of high-grade dysplasia showed a disrupted basal cell pattern. Because they had observed a discontinuous pattern of staining with this antibody in normal glands in paraffin-embedded tissue but not in frozen sections, they concluded that the lack of focal immunoreactivity in the basal cell layer could be related to antigen damage during fixation and processing.

DNA Content and Proliferative Activity

Using autoradiography, Helpap showed in 1980 that the thymidine-labeling index of atypical hyperplasia (presumably PIN) was similar to that of poorly differentiated carcinoma and cribriform carcinoma and three times greater than that of simple hyperplasia.

Studies evaluating the number of argyrophilic nucleolar organizer regions (AgNOR) have shown that AgNOR counts increase from benign prostatic hyperplasia (BPH) to PIN to invasive carcinoma and that the AgNOR counts for PIN are significantly higher than those of BPH but are similar to those of invasive carcinoma. These results suggest that PIN and carcinoma share similar proliferative activity, ploidy values, or both (Deschenes and Weidner, 1990; Sesterhenn et al., 1991).

Static DNA cytometry of Feulgen-stained sections has revealed that the DNA content of PIN is intermediate between the DNA content of benign glands and that of carcinoma and that the number of aneuploid nuclei increases as the degree of PIN increases (Amin et al., 1993; Montironi et al., 1990). It is interesting that the ploidy pattern of PIN and that of the concomitant invasive carcinoma are not always similar (Amin et al., 1993; Weinberg and Weidner, 1993). We (unpublished data) and others (Amin et al., 1993) have observed aneuploid nuclei in high-grade PIN adjacent to carcinoma with a diploid DNA content.

Tamboli et al. (1996) studied nuclear proliferative activity using MIB-1 (Ki-67 antigen) antibody on benign glands, areas of high-grade PIN, and adenocarcinoma and demonstrated that the mean Ki-67 antigen expression significantly differed among histologic categories ($P < 0.01$, all three comparisons). They also found that the proliferative index consistently increased along the continuum from benign to malignant and concluded that the MIB-1 proliferative index of high-grade PIN lies between that of a benign and a carcinomatous prostate, supporting the assertion that high-grade PIN is a biologic intermediate in the multistep process of transformation to cancer. Weinstein (1998) reported similar data. Apoptosis with the use of routine hematoxylin-eosin stains and *in situ* end-labeling of fragmented DNA method demonstrated a progressive increase in the rates of apoptosis from benign glands (0.34%–0.38%) to high-grade PIN (1.44%–1.39%) to carcinoma (2.69%–2.75%). The increase in the apoptosis rate in PIN

and carcinoma is, again, indicative of the continuum in the pathogenetic process leading to invasive prostatic carcinoma (Drachenberg et al., 1997).

Immunophenotypic Profile

Multiple studies (Brawer et al., 1985; Nagle et al., 1991; Perlman and Epstein, 1990) have shown not only that high-grade PIN is cytologically similar to invasive carcinoma but also that it shares many immunophenotypic characteristics with invasive prostatic adenocarcinoma. Using frozen sections, Nagle and co-workers (1991) showed that high-grade PIN and invasive carcinoma have significantly increased reactivity to a monoclonal antikeratin antibody, KA4, which is specific for keratins 14, 15, 16, and 19. Although only 4% of cases of BPH showed reactivity, more than 90% of cases of PIN and invasive carcinoma were immunoreactive to this antibody. Furthermore, the luminal cells of PIN showed a significant loss of vimentin expression. Vimentin reactivity was present in the luminal cells in more than 90% of cases of BPH but in only 15% of cases of PIN and was absent in all cases of invasive carcinoma. Finally, PIN and carcinoma showed a similar pattern of binding of the lectin from *Ulex europaeus* (UEA-1). UEA-1 staining was absent in all cases of BPH and present in more than 90% of cases of PIN and invasive carcinoma. The lectin-binding pattern observed in this study (Nagle et al., 1991) is similar to one reported previously (Perlman and Epstein, 1990) and different from those reported in an earlier study by McNeal et al. (1988b), who noted decreased lectin binding in foci of dysplasia. Janssen et al. (1966) reported that carcinoma and high-grade PIN exhibited a significantly higher number of the peanut (*Arachis hypogaea*) lectin acceptors than BPH and low-grade PIN. A-80 is a mucin-like glycoprotein associated with exocrine differentiation that shows little or no expression in normal exocrine cells and typical adenomas, but it is up-regulated in dysplasia and adenocarcinoma of certain organs. Gould et al., (1996) reported that, in the prostate, A-80 showed strong reactivity in PIN and prostatic carcinoma but no reactivity in benign and hyperplastic epithelium, a finding that reflected that of other organs.

Blood group antigen expression [A, B, Le(a), and Le(b)] is also absent in PIN and invasive carcinoma but is present in 5% to 15% of normal cells (Perlman and Epstein, 1990).

A reduction or absence of cytoplasmic staining for PSA, PAP, and Leu-7 in foci of PIN on formalin-fixed, paraffin-embedded tissue was interpreted as representing impaired cellular differentiation (McNeal et al., 1988a). Bostwick et al. (1998a) reported that unlike PSA, the expression of prostate-specific membrane antigen was stronger in carcinoma and high-grade PIN than in benign epithelium. Conversely, PSA showed the greatest reactivity in benign epithelium, with incrementally decreased expression from benign epithelium to high-grade PIN or adenocarcinoma (Bostwick et al., 1998a). Human glandular kallikrein 2 is a potential new tumor marker (Darson et al., 1997) that may be useful as an adjunct to PSA in the diagnosis and monitoring of prostate cancer (Darson et al., 1997). Darson et al. (1997) reported that the intensity and extent of expression for this marker were greater in cancer than in high-grade PIN and greater in high-grade PIN than in benign epithelium.

In summary, evidence for the association between PIN and prostate carcinoma includes the following: (1) cytological features are similar; (2) localization is in the peripheral zone; (3) there is more than three times the proliferative activity of benign glands as well as similar immunophenotypic profiles; (4) the highest grade of PIN may exhibit partial loss of the basal cell layer, as in adenocarcinoma; (5) with high-grade PIN, there is a statistically significant increase in carcinoma; and (6) there are similarities in the cytogenetics and molecular pathology between PIN and prostate carcinoma.

ATYPICAL ADENOMATOUS HYPERPLASIA (ADENOSIS)

In the previous edition of this book, AAH was referred to as *small gland hyperplasia*. The preferred term accorded by a consensus opinion of genitourinary pathologists is AAH (Bostwick et al., 1994). Another popular term, *adenosis*, was initially utilized by Brawn in 1982 and later by Epstein et al. (Epstein, 1994a, 1995; Gaudin and Epstein, 1994). Other names given to this lesion include atypical glandular proliferation, atypi-

cal hyperplasia of small acinar type, and adenocarcinoma *in situ* (Brawn, 1982; Kovi, 1985; McNeal, 1965). The term "atypical" does not refer to cellular atypia but rather to an abnormal small-gland type of arrangement. Thus, this lesion is a proliferation of small glands situated back to back and lined by a single row of epithelial cells, which, unlike those in well-differentiated adenocarcinoma, contain no nucleoli larger than 1 μm (Fig. 21–10). The basal cell layer is seemingly absent, but it can be highlighted with the use of a high-molecular-weight keratin (34βE12). Partial staining of the basal cell layer is the usual pattern seen in this process (Fig. 21–10D). The importance of AAH derives from its similarity to well-differentiated adenocarcinoma of the prostate. Although it has been considered a premalignant lesion in the origin of prostatic adenocarcinoma, this has yet to be proved (Amin et al., 1994; Bostwick, 1996). Srigley (1988) noted that AAH is usually seen in TURP specimens, which indicate its origin in the transition zone, where the origin of prostatic carcinoma is less common. Furthermore, AAH often has an intimate association with nodular hyperplasia. It is reported in 1.6% of TURP specimens and in 0.8% of all needle biopsy specimens (Epstein, 1994a, 1995). It is characteristically found in the transition zone of the prostate, is frequently multifocal, and most often presents as an incidental finding on TURP specimens performed for urinary obstruction. Although AAH mimics well-differentiated adenocarcinoma of the prostate, there is no conclusive evidence suggesting that patients with AAH have an increased risk of harboring or developing adenocarcinoma of the prostate.

WELL-DEFFERENTIATED ADENOCARCINOMA

Most prostatic carcinomas associated with PIN are well-differentiated adenocarcinomas with a Gleason score of up to 6 with a small percentage displaying the cribriform pattern. The cribriform pattern seen in some forms of high-grade PIN has been compared with Gleason's grade 3 cribriform pattern by McNeal et al. (1986), who presented evidence that most examples of the latter are in fact intraductal rather than invasive car-

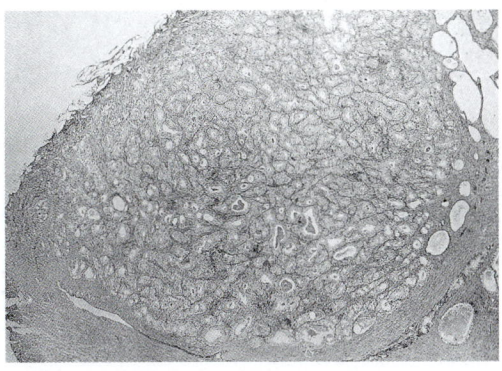

A

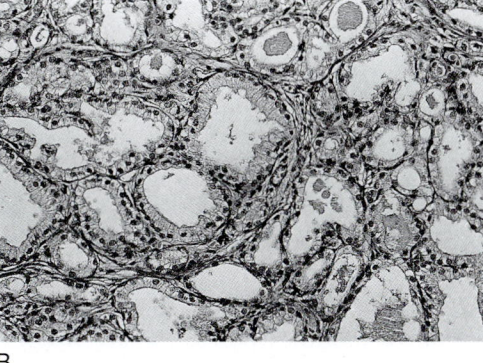

B

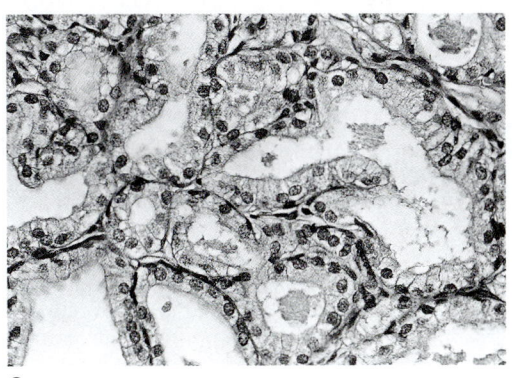

C

Figure 21–10. Atypical adenomatous hyperplasia (adenosis). *A*: This low-power view exhibits a nodule containing numerous, back-to-back small glands. At the periphery of the nodule there are compressed and elongated atrophic ductules. *B*: Medium-power view demonstrates small- to medium-sized glands seemingly lined by a single cell layer of epithelium. *C*: High-power magnification discloses small glands with round monotonous nuclei that are relatively hyperchromatic without prominent nucleoli. The basal cell layer is not visible. *D*: High-molecular cytokeratin demonstrates partial preservation of basal cell layer (color picture).

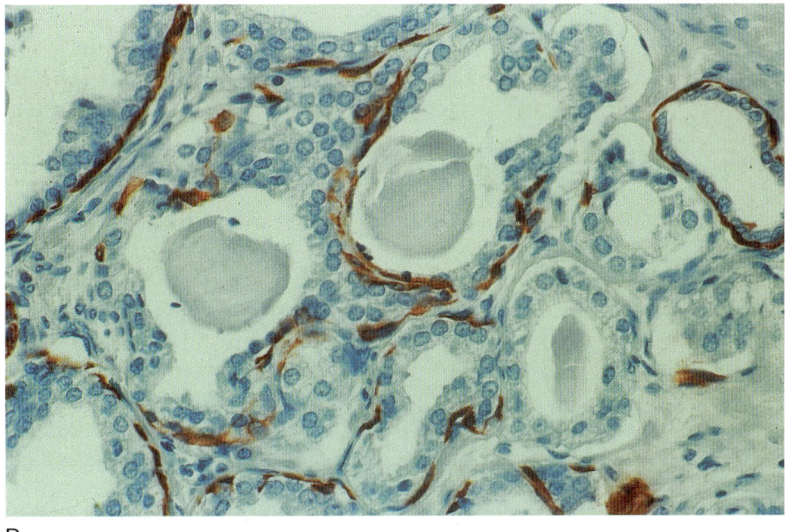

D

cinomas, thus representing in situ evolution from ductal or acinar dysplasia to invasive carcinoma.

Prostatic carcinoma may show various patterns, including acinar, fused acinar, cribriform, papillary, trabecular, and solid (Mostofi and Price, 1973). A well-differentiated ade-nocarcinoma usually exhibits an acinar (small glandular) pattern, which is frequently a concurrent component of other, less-differentiated patterns.

In its most differentiated form, acinar adenocarcinoma may be difficult to distinguish from AAH (adenosis) (Kovi, 1985; Srigley,

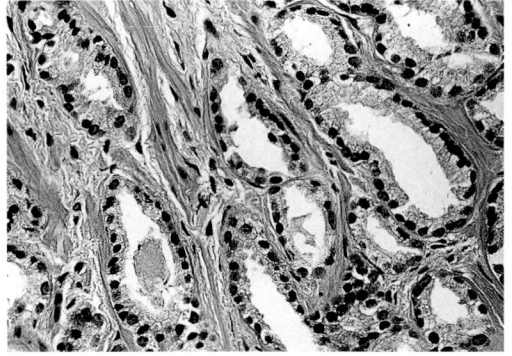

A

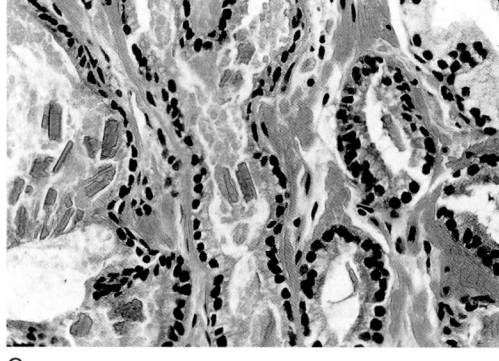

C

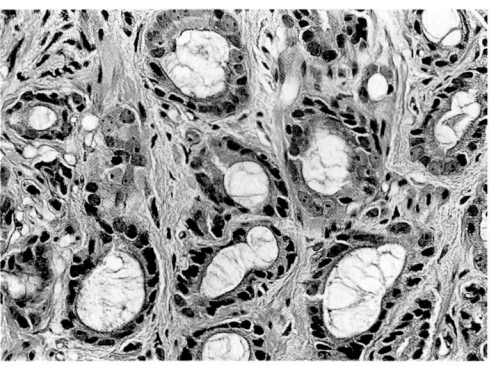

B

Figure 21–11. Well-differentiated adenocarcinoma. *A*: This view shows small glands lined by a single cell layer of cuboidal epithelium. A few prominent nucleoli are also present. *B*: Within the lumina of the glands of the carcinoma there are ill-defined threads of gray–dark material representative of the mucin. *C*: This illustration shows numerous intraluminal crystalloids.

1988). Like AAH, it is made up of a proliferation of small glands whose acini are usually back to back (Fig. 21–11). The advancing border of carcinoma may be infiltrative or at best irregular, and the acini are lined by a single row of epithelial cells whose nuclei generally show a fine chromatin pattern or sometimes exhibit a clear emptiness. The nuclear membrane may be thick, and large nucleoli should be present; their number per nucleus may vary, but more importantly, some of the nucleoli should be large (at least 1 μm in diameter) and prominent (Gleason, 1985). These large nucleoli are often eosinophilic and round. It should be stressed that they may not be present in all of the cells and that in a poor preparation they may not be visible; hence, a good preparation of the specimen is essential. Gleason (1985) stated that perhaps his patterns 1 and 2 might indeed be forms of AAH. One must remember that immunohistochemistry was not available when Gleason designed the grading system. The utilization of a high-molecular-weight cytokeratin antibody is of utmost impor-

tance when a small acinar lesion is being evaluated. Negative staining favors a carcinoma. In contrast, the presence of partial staining of the basal cells favors a diagnosis of AAH. In evaluating high-molecular-weight cytokeratin staining, one must see positive staining in benign glands (internal control). If benign glands are negative, negative staining in a small acinar lesion is meaningless.

In addition to the above-described features, other findings often associated with adenocarcinoma of the prostate include intraluminal mucin and crystalloids. Mucin in prostatic lesions was described in 1967 by Hukill and Vidone and later by Ro and collaborators (1986, 1988a, 1998b). These investigators found neutral mucin in the normal or hyperplastic prostatic epithelium and acid sialomucins (blue with Alcian blue stain or red with mucicarmine stain) in prostatic adenocarcinoma; however, the stainable secretion was present only in the lumina of the neoplastic glands and not in the cytoplasm of the malignant epithelium (Fig. 21–11B). The presence of intraluminal mucin is not diagnostic for carcinoma because it can be seen in AAH, sclerosing adenosis (SA) and nephrogenic adenoma. However, its presence should alert the pathologist to the possibility of a well-differentiated acinar carcinoma (Ro et al., 1997).

Crystalloids were initially described in 1977 by Elizabeth Holmes, who thought that they may aid in the diagnosis of prostatic carcinoma. Ro and collaborators (1986, 1988a) described crystalloids further. Crystalloids are rectangular, sometimes octagonal, nonpolarizing, nonbirefringent formations found within the lumina of the neoplastic glands (Fig. 21–11C). They do not stain with PSA, PAP, mucicarmine, Alcian blue, periodic acid-Schiff (PAS), or kappa and lambda light chains, but intraluminal mucin usually accompanies them. Ultrastructurally, they contain nonspecific amorphous electron-dense material different from Bence Jones protein or corpora amylacea. They are usually seen in well-differentiated prostatic adenocarcinomas but have also been described in poorly differentiated carcinomas, including tumors with papillary or cribriform patterns. Their presence in a small acinar proliferation should raise the suspicion of a well-differentiated adenocarcinoma; however, they are not pathognomonic of carcinoma, because they have also been described in the hyperplastic glands adjacent to carcinoma, AAH, and SA (Anton et al., 1998; Del Rosario et al., 1993; Grignon et al., 1992; Henneberry et al., 1997; Young and Clement, 1987).

Although most adenocarcinomas of the prostate arise from the peripheral zone, there is a type of prostatic carcinoma that arises predominantly in the transition zone; this has been called "clear cell carcinoma" (McNeal et al., 1988c). It is a well-differentiated tumor with an acinar pattern that characteristically presents tall columnar cells with clear cytoplasm and basally located nuclei (Fig. 21–12). The nuclei are large, may be hyperchromatic, and contain prominent nucleoli. Intraluminal crystalloids may be present. The size of the glands varies, and although most are small, some are large, resembling prostatic hyperplasia. These glands often form nodules resembling nodular hyperplasia but may also show infiltrative borders. The clear cell pattern of this carcinomatous variant may occupy 60% to 100% of a given carcinoma. This tumor is usually well differentiated, and most are Gleason's grades 1 to 3. This variant of prostatic carcinoma may arise from precursors other than PIN.

CRIBRIFORM ADENOCARCINOMA

The pattern of cribriform adenocarcinoma of the prostate was recognized by early investigators as having a poor prognosis, but detailed clinicopathologic studies of this

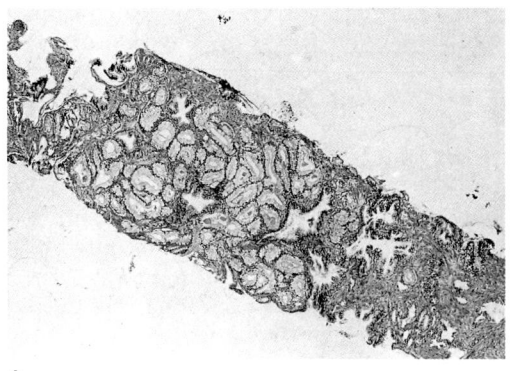
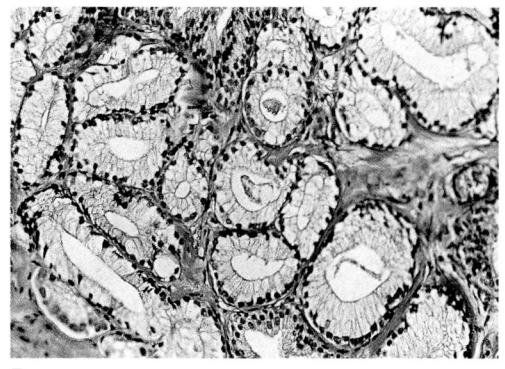

A   B

Figure 21–12. Clear cell adenocarcinoma of transition zone type. *A*: This is a well-differentiated adenocarcinoma composed of small- to medium-sized glands with clear cytoplasm, which simulates benign prostatic hyperplasia. Compare the abnormal glandular proliferation seen in the center of the core with the normal glands. *B*: Characteristically, a single layer of tall, columnar clear cells with basally located nuclei lines the glands of this tumor.

variant have appeared only recently (McNeal et al., 1986). In his grading system, Gleason recognized it as a grade 3 pattern if no necrosis was present and a grade 5 pattern if necrosis was present (Gleason, 1977; Gleason and Mellinger, 1974). Cribriform carcinomas are usually large; in a study of 21 cases of cribriform carcinoma, all tumors were larger than 1.7 cm^3, and 86% showed not only a Gleason's grade 3 pattern but also patterns of Gleason's grades 4 and 5. In that study, 7 of 21 cases of cribriform carcinoma showed a morphologic transition from normal ductal epithelium to cribriform arrangement, passing through the stages of ductal dysplasia with tufting, papillation, and bridging of the lumen. The authors believe that these findings strongly support the concept that cribriform carcinoma arises from an intraductal precursor (McNeal et al., 1986).

On needle biopsy specimens, cribriform carcinoma may be represented by its intraductal component only, but erroneous interpretation of such a finding as invasive carcinoma has not been a clinical problem. As stated above, cribriform carcinomas, albeit predominantly intraductal, are invasive and generally high-volume lesions (McNeal et al., 1986).

LESIONS MIMICKING PROSTATIC CARCINOMA

Several benign prostate lesions may show a small acinar growth pattern similar to that seen in prostatic carcinoma. Such lesions are usually found in older individuals, do not produce specific symptoms, and are detected on TURP resection specimens. These lesions include BCH (Cleary et al., 1983; Grignon et al., 1988), CCCH (Ayala et al., 1986; Frauenhoffer et al., 1991), SA (Grignon, et al., 1992; Young and Clement, 1987), and various forms of atrophy (McNeal, 1988; Moore, 1936; Srigley, 1988).

Nephrogenic adenoma of the prostatic urethra (Bhagavan, et al., 1981; Malpica et al., 1994; Young and Scully, 1986) and ejaculatory duct or seminal vesicle (Arias-Stella and Takano-Moron, 1958; Kuo and Gomez, 1981) can be confused with adenocarcinoma or PIN. They are discussed in Chapter 20 on incipient lesions of the urinary bladder.

BASAL CELL HYPERPLASIA

Although BCH is relatively uncommon, it has distinct histologic characteristics that permit its identification (Cleary, et al., 1983; Grignon, et al., 1988). Its major importance is the possible confusion with adenocarcinoma of the prostate. Basal cell hyperplasia occurs predominantly in patients in the sixth to eighth decades of life who present with obstructive symptoms and whose condition is clinically diagnosed as BPH.

Histologically, BCH shows features similar to those of nodular hyperplasia. There is a nodular growth pattern involving acinar units (Fig. 21–13A), which are characteristically replaced and expanded by a proliferation of small, dark-staining cells, the basal cells. A nodule of BCH evident on low-power examination contains multiple expanded acini that may be well circumscribed but not encapsulated, and thus, may merge into nodules of conventional hyperplasia of the prostate (Cleary et al., 1983; Grignon et al., 1988).

The acini are generally filled with basal cells, but most of the acini show a central lumen (Fig. 21–13). Although lumina are inconspicuous in most cases, sometimes larger lumina are seen to the extreme of reducing the number of basal cells to one or two rows. This pattern, *incomplete BCH*, is likely to be confused with prostate adenocarcinoma (Srigley, 1988). The lumina may contain neutral and acid mucins, which can be stained with PAS, mucicarmine, and Alcian blue. Corpora amylacea and calcifications may be seen in approximately 50% of cases. The individual cells have uniform, oval and hyperchromatic nuclei with a heavy and finely dispersed chromatin and scanty cytoplasm. Nucleoli are generally absent, but inconspicuous small nucleoli may be seen. Mitoses are rare. A striking feature is the peripheral palisading of basal cells, much like those seen in basal cell carcinoma of the skin. Epstein and Armas (1992) reported 12 cases of BCH having prominent nucleolus, nuclear enlargement, hyperchromatism, and moderate pleomorphism. They designated these lesions *atypical BCH,* which must be differentiated from adenocarcinoma and PIN (Devaraj and Bostwick, 1993; Epstein and Armas, 1992).

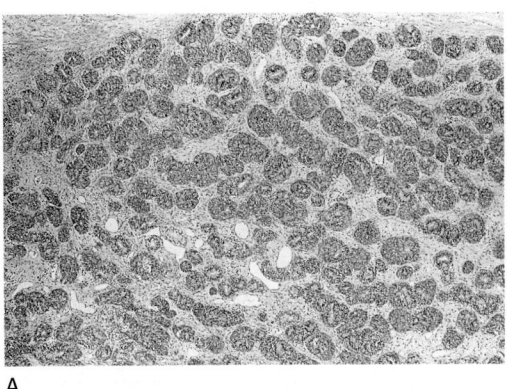 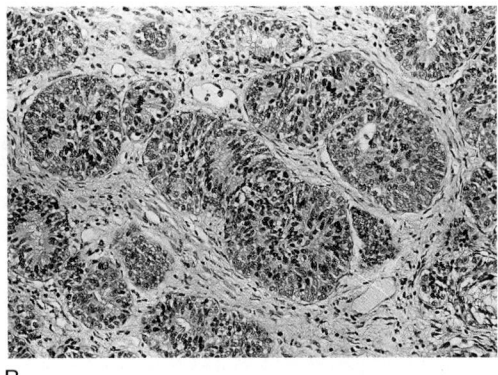

A   B

Figure 21–13. Basal cell hyperplasia. *A*: In this low-power view there is a nodule made up of multiple, small, round aggregates of hyperchromatic cells. Some of these small clusters of cells show a distinctive glandular lumen. *B*: High-power illustration demonstrates that the glandular/ductal structures are completely filled with a proliferation of dark-staining cells. Some luminal differentiation is also noted. The stroma shows increased cellularity.

The cells of BCH, like normal basal cells of the prostate, react to a monoclonal high-molecular-weight antikeratin antibody ($34\beta E12$) but are unreactive to PSA or PAP (Brawer et al., 1985; Grignon et al., 1988). However, the cells lining the lumina within the nests of basal cells demonstrate their secretory activity by their reaction to PSA and PAP immunostaining. A feature that has not been emphasized is the participation of the stroma. There is a subtle but definite proliferation of the stroma, both fibroblastic and myofibroblastic, that can be seen on routine hematoxylin-eosin–stained specimens and that can be easily demonstrated by immunostaining with smooth-muscle actin.

ADENOID BASAL CELL TUMOR

A closely related neoplastic proliferation is the so-called adenoid basal cell tumor (ABT), which histologically is an accentuation of the pattern seen in BCH (Grignon et al., 1988; Reed, 1984). It also arises from the transition zone in elderly persons with prostatic obstruction. Histologically, it consists of large nodules (up to 1 cm in diameter) composed of a proliferation of dark hyperchromatic cells growing in a solid fashion, but many contain single or multiple small lumina (Fig. 21–14). Unlike BCH, in which the

basal cells fill and slightly expand the acini, the nodules of ABT are larger and confluent; the cells are larger than those of BCH, but the nuclear features are similar. The lumina lined by tall columnar secretory epithelial cells contain variable dense eosinophilic and intensely PAS-positive concretions or Alcian blue–positive-acid mucin.

Immunostaining of ABT demonstrates reactivity of the basaloid cells with a monoclonal antikeratin antibody ($34\beta E12$) and positivity of the luminal cells with PSA and PAP. Keratin reactivity is focal and, for the most part, weak. In contrast, S-100 protein

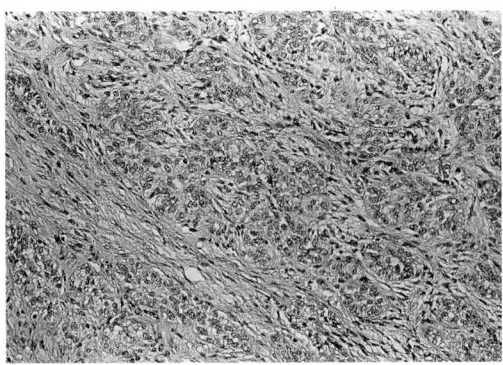

Figure 21–14. Adenoid basal cell tumor. In contrast to basal cell hyperplasia, adenoid basal cell tumor shows a diffuse proliferation of basaloid cells. The stroma is also reactive.

is diffusely positive with variable intensity, staining both the basaloid and the luminal secretory-lining cells (Grignon et al., 1988).

Adenoid cystic carcinoma involving the prostate, whose primary prostatic origin is debated, is rare and believed to represent the malignant counterpart of the spectrum of the BCH and ABT neoplastic complex (Grignon et al., 1988; Young et al. 1988).

CLEAR CELL CRIBRIFORM HYPERPLASIA

This is a rare variant of hyperplasia, which by virtue of its cribriform pattern is likely to be confused with cribriform carcinoma of the prostate (Ayala et al., 1986; Frauenhoffer et al., 1991). It occurs in patients above the sixth decade of life who present with symptoms of urinary obstruction.

Like BCH, CCCH has a growth pattern similar to that of benign nodular hyperplasia. It is characterized by a complex papillary-cribriform proliferation of clear cells involving acini, and is always associated with benign nodular hyperplasia (BPH); in fact in most cases, a gradual transition from BPH to CCCH can be seen.

Microscopically, CCCH almost always involves several acinar units; thus, on low-power examination (Fig. 21–15A), one sees enlarged acinar structures occupying usually more than one-half of a low-power field separated by a scant but reactive fibromuscular stroma. The acinar units are expanded by a proliferation of bland-looking cells that demonstrate a papillary–cribriform pattern. A distinct basal cell layer is present in these acinar units. The cells of CCCH are cuboidal to tall columnar with abundant clear cytoplasm, and their nuclei are uniformly round to oval, with rare small nucleoli (Fig. 21–15A–C). Mitotic activity is not apparent. Although scant glycogen may be present in the cytoplasm of the clear cells, mucin is not found. The cribriform spaces are devoid of acid mucin or crystalloids.

Immunoperoxidase studies reveal the presence of PSA and PAP in the clear cells, denoting their origin from secretory cells. The basal cell layer does not react with these markers, but it is immunoreactive to antik-eratin antibody 34βE12 (Fig. 21–15C; Frauenhoffer, et al., 1991).

The differential diagnosis of CCCH is prin-cipally with cribriform adenocarcinoma of the prostate. Most cribriform carcinomas of the prostate are intraductal and consequently may completely or partially retain the basal cell layer as in high-grade PIN. However, the individual cells of cribriform carcinomas, unlike those of CCCH, demonstrate nuclear atypia, as previously described. In contrast, CCCH shows a proliferation of clear cells with a bland nuclear morphology. Furthermore, cribriform adenocarcinoma, when present, is usually a high-volume disease and frequently shows an aneuploid DNA content. In contrast, all cases of CCCH have shown a diploid DNA content (Frauenhoffer et al., 1991).

SCLEROSING ADENOSIS

Although relatively few cases of SA have been reported in the literature, the lesion is not uncommon (Grignon et al., 1992). From the clinical standpoint, SA does not have symptoms different from those of BPH, with which it is closely associated. Sclerosing adenosis is a lesion of the transition zone and therefore is encountered in specimens obtained through the urethra. In the past, this lesion was called "adenomatoid tumor of the prostate" (Chen and Schiff, 1983) because of its histologic resemblance to that lesion; since the demonstration of its epithelial nature by immunostaining, that name has become obsolete. Young and Clement (1987), noticing its resemblance to SA of the breast, proposed the current term. This lesion does not have malignant potential, but because it resembles small acinar adenocarcinoma, pathologists should be familiar with its histology.

Histologically, SA consists of a proliferation of small glandular structures immersed in a reactive fibromuscular stroma (Fig. 21–16). The lesion may be unicentral or multicentric, and on low-power examination, may consist of a nodule or nodules generally larger than 2 mm in diameter. These nodules may be well circumscribed or may have an irregularly infiltrative border. The acini are compressed by the reactive stroma, and the cell lining may show flattened or cuboidal cells. The cells have round or oval nuclei, which may contain prominent nucleoli; mitoses are not usually seen. The glandular lumina may contain acid mucin and, rarely, crystalloids. On routine histologic examina-

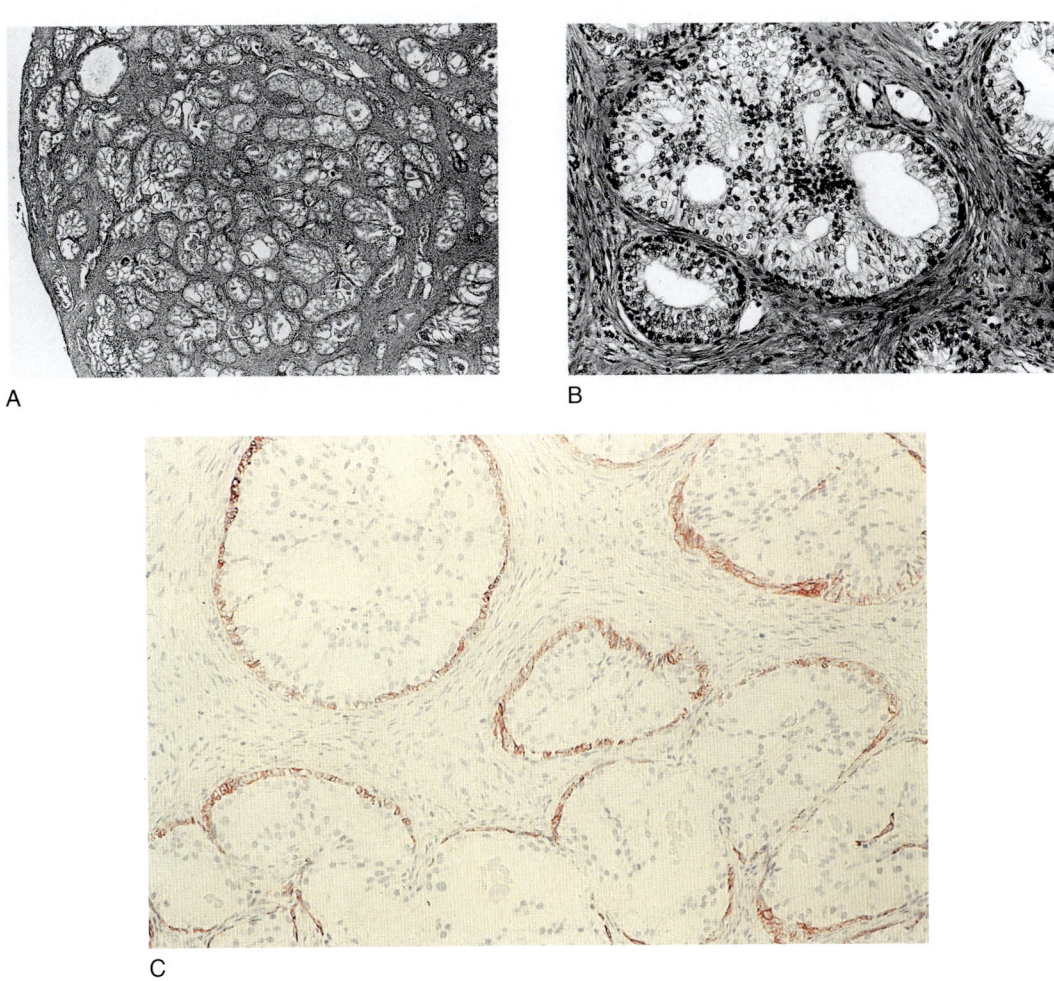

Figure 21–15. Clear cell cribriform hyperplasia. *A:* Low-power view demonstrates enlarged acinar structures containing a proliferation of clear cells with a distintive cribriform arrangement. The stroma is also quite cellular. *B:* High-power magnification shows the cribriform pattern, clear cells, and the presence of a basal cell layer at the periphery of the acinar structure involved. The clear cells contain abundant cytoplasm and the cytoplasmic membranes, separating each cell, are well demarcated. Note also the reactive spindle cell stroma. *C:* The basal cell layer is highlighted by intense immunoreactivity with high-molecular-weight keratin (34βE12).

tion, one observes two cell types lining the acini, but in many cases, the basal cell layer becomes so attenuated that it is difficult to see. In such situations, use of the high-molecular weight antikeratin antibody (34βE12) may clearly demonstrate the basal cell layer. However, it should be stressed that in certain cases the basal cell layer may stain incompletely. In the luminal lining of SA cells, immunostaining with PSA and PAP is positive.

The stroma of SA consists of a proliferation of fibroblasts and myofibroblasts that can be demonstrated by immunostaining with smooth-muscle actin. The differential diagnosis is with well-differentiated adenocarcinoma. Both share the same small glandular pattern, prominent nucleoli, and intraluminal mucin (Grignon et al., 1992; Young and Clement, 1987). However, SA has a basal cell layer, which can be enhanced with the specific antikeratin antibody for basal cells. Partial staining of the basal cell layer is an acceptable indication of SA, in contrast to well-differentiated adenocarci-

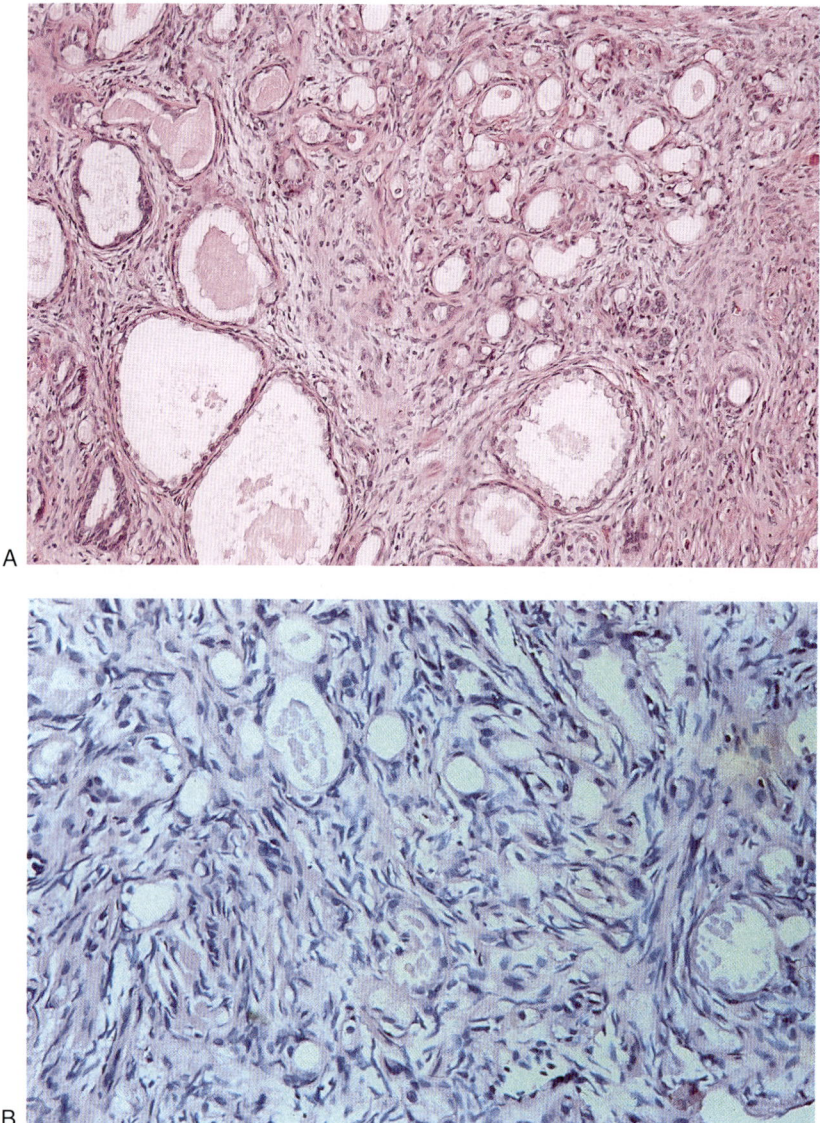

Figure 21–16. Sclerosing adenosis. *A*: In this low-power view, a small gland proliferation with reactive stromal background contrasts with the larger normal glands. *B*: On high-power examination, the glands show variation in size and shape; the shape of the lining cells varies from flat to cuboidal. The basal cell layer is obscured by the stromal proliferation. (*Continued*)

noma. When desmoplasia occurs in prostatic carcinoma, it is generally more fibrocollagenous than cellular. Therefore, the presence of a cellular spindled stroma around the glandular structures should always raise suspicion for SA. In addition to differential diagnostic importance from well-differentiated adenocarcinoma, SA has

an anatomical interest. Apparently SA is the only lesion in which basal cells show myoepithelial cell differentiation. Myoepithelial cell differentiation has been confirmed by positive immunostaining with smooth muscle actin and S-100 protein of basal cells and by electron microscopic analysis (Grignon et al., 1992).

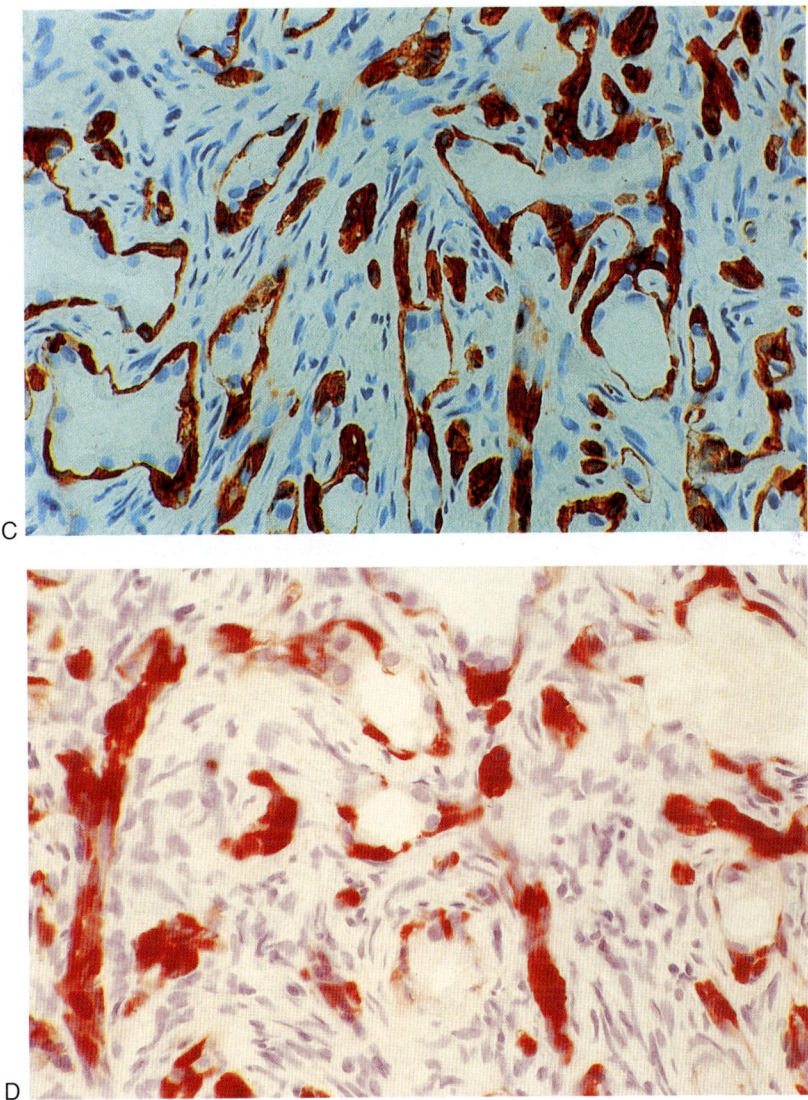

Figure 21–16. (*Continued*) Sclerosing adenosis. *C:* The basal cell layer is highlighted by intense immunoreactivity with high-molecular-weight keratin (34βE12). *D:* SMA and S-100 protein are also positive in the basal cell layer, indicating myoepithelial differentiation.

PROSTATIC ATROPHY

Atrophic changes of the prostate occur in both the peripheral and the transition zones, and their morphologic changes may raise the question of a small acinar carcinoma. Two types of atrophy have been described—simple lobular atrophy and sclerotic atrophy (McNeal, 1988; Moore, 1936; Srigley, 1988). *Simple lobular atrophy* is easily recognized because the structure of the lobule is retained. Thus, generally one sees a large feeding duct surrounded by atrophic acini. The epithelium of the atrophic acini is flat as a result of having lost most of its cytoplasm, but the double cell layer remains and can be enhanced by immunostaining of the basal cell layer with the specific antikeratin antibody. The nuclei are hyperchromatic, and various degrees of luminal dilatation may occur. Although some of the acini remain small, some may become relatively large and cystic. In TURP specimens, this pattern is not difficult to recognize, but

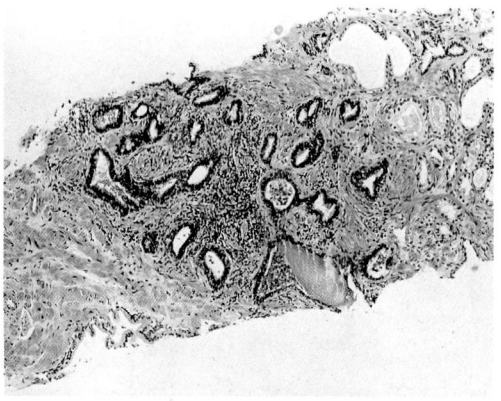

Figure 21–17. Atrophy. This view shows small- to medium-sized glands lined by a hyperchromatic epithelium. Chronic inflammatory cell are present in the center of the illustration.

in a needle biopsy specimen, the question of a small acinar adenocarcinoma may arise (Fig. 21–17).

Generally, sclerotic atrophy is characterized by elongated, compressed, glandular structures that most likely represent distorted ducts. Acinar units are not prevalent, either because they disappear during the atrophic process or because the sclerosing process is limited to the ducts (Fig. 21–18A,B). Whatever the pathogenetic mechanism of this process, the histologic picture may be confused with that of an infiltrating carcinoma. However, no matter how compressed the epithelial layer may be, the ductal/acinar structures retain the basal cell layer (Fig. 21–18C).

Postatrophic hyperplasia may occur in the setting of either simple lobular or sclerotic atrophy (Cheville and Bostwick, 1995; Ruska et al., 1998; Amin et al., 1999; Anton et al., 1999). When this occurs, new acinar budding develops from hyperplastic acini. The glands thus formed are small and lined by cells with clear or granular cytoplasm. They are distinguished from carcinoma in that the cells of atrophy are usually flat, the nuclei are small, and the nucleoli are absent or inconspicuous (Fig. 21–19). The basal cell layer is generally not visible but may be

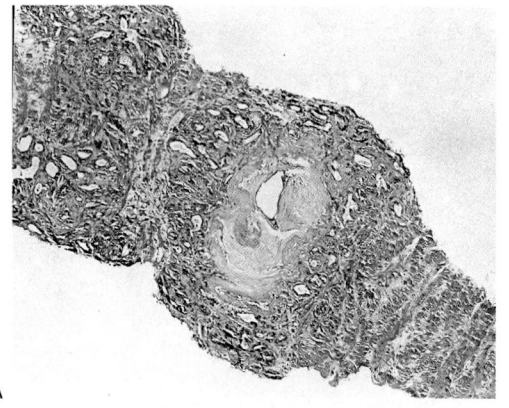

A

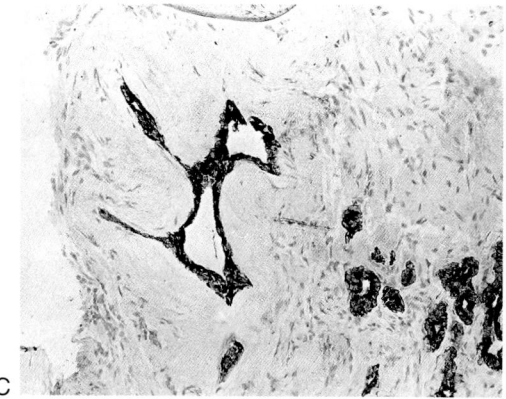

C

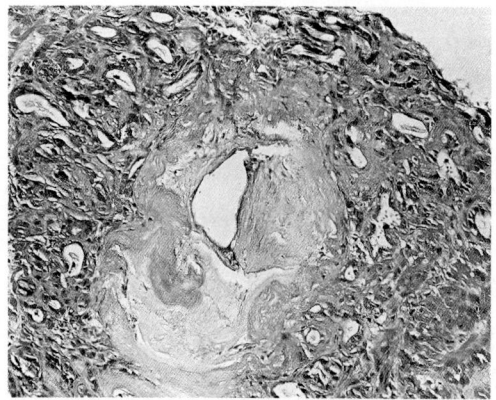

B

Figure 21–18. Sclerotic atrophy. *A:* This low-power view shows a needle biopsy exhibiting a central area of sclerosis surrounded by a small gland proliferation. *B:* Higher power view discloses the central duct surrounded by fibrosis and the small glands lined by hyperchromatic epithelium. *C:* This illustration of the same case shows strong immunoreactivity for high-molecular-weight keratin (34βE12) in all of the cells, indicating their basal cell origin.

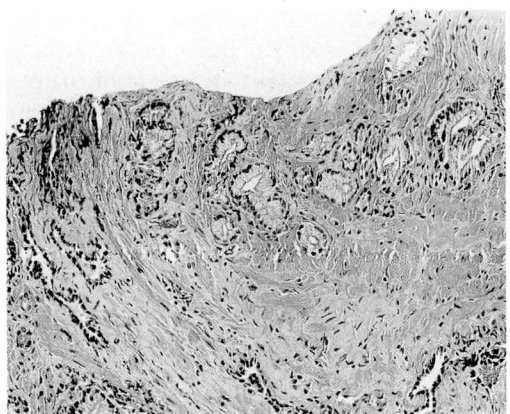

Figure 21–19. Atrophy and adenocarcinoma. In this illustration the small gland proliferation typical of carcinoma is in contrast with the dark, compressed glands of atrophy.

demonstrated with the use of a high-molecular-weight cytokeratin. As a general rule, larger dilated ducts are usually seen in nearby areas.

Prostatic adenocarcinoma with atrophic features has also been reported recently. This rare variant of adenocarcinoma is easily confused with benign acinar atrophy. It can be recognized by a combination of architectural and cytologic changes and usually coexists with a typical microacinar carcinoma. It is important to recognize this pattern to avoid the underdiagnosis of malignancy (Cina and Epstein, 1997; Egan et al., 1997; Kaleem et al., 1998).

In summary, there are many different types of small glandular proliferations of the prostate, and each has a distinctive histologic pattern. The diagnosis of these lesions is usually not complicated. However, the lesions may be confused with well-differentiated adenocarcinoma, so pathologists should be familiar with their morphology.

MOLECULAR BIOLOGY OF PROSTATIC NEOPLASIA

Epidemiological observations suggest that several different factors could be of etiologic importance in prostate tumorigenesis. These include genetic, hormonal, and chemical/environmental factors. However, no overall unifying concept has emerged with respect to the contribution of each of these factors to prostate cancer. Recent data indicate that genetic predisposition plays a role in a subset of familial prostatic cancer. Within the last two decades, there have been numerous technologic developments that contributed to the understanding of many molecular aspects of cell biology and shed light on some of the molecular events that may be responsible for the malignant behavior of human and animal cells. Although at the time of this writing in 2000, no definitive statement can be made as to which of these events are truly responsible for the development and progression of prostatic carcinoma, significant progress has been made toward the understanding of malignant transformation as a biologic phenomenon. In this section, some of the most promising avenues of molecular research on prostate cancer, with emphasis on those events that play a role in the early phases of prostatic neoplasia and its progression to clinically aggressive disease, will be discussed.

The current research on prostatic carcinoma is focused on several phenomena: metastatic phenotype, hormonal dependence, and molecular events of incipient preneoplastic lesions. The progress in clinical management of prostatic carcinoma, combining ultrasound and serum PSA measurement, allowed the identification of an ever-increasing number of small intraprostatic carcinomas or intraepithelial preneoplastic conditions. Retrospective studies indicate that only a small fraction of these lesions will progress to a clinically significant disease and to metastases. Therefore, the identification of molecular markers that may enable the identification of a subset of these early lesions that may progress to clinically aggressive versus indolent lesions is of prime importance. The androgen-dependent growth of prostatic carcinoma offers the opportunity to control their growth by hormonal manipulation. The development of androgen-independent growth is responsible for the ultimate failure of this approach; hence, the elucidation of the underlying molecular mechanism is of great clinical importance.

CHROMOSOMAL ALTERATIONS AND DNA PLOIDY

As is the case with other organs, neoplastic lesions of the prostate often contain cells with chromosomal aberrations. On the chromosomal level, some of the prostatic adenocarcinomas show a normal chromosomal complement (Arps et al., 1993). A subset of prostatic cancer is aneuploid with multiple chromosomal rearrangements (Lundgren et al., 1988, 1992). Clonal chromosomal alterations range from trisomy 7 and loss of chromosome Y to deletions of smaller chromosomes regiones such as 10q24 and 16q (Arps et al., 1993; Babu et al., 1990; Carter et al., 1990b; Micale et al., 1993). Deletion of 10q and possibly of 7q seems to be a recurring theme in prostatic carcinomas. The use of chromosomal transfer techniques has shown that the metastatic phenotype of prostatic cancer cells can be suppressed by chromosome 11 insertion. Specific mapping studies suggest that the loss of a gene located on 11p11.2-13 can play a role in metastatic behavior of these cells (Ichikawa et al., 1992). Chromosome 8 mapping studies have defined a 14 cM minimal deleted fragment mapped to 8p21.2-21.3 region (Bowa et al., 1993). Deletions on other chromosomes have also been documented, most frequently involving chromosomes 8, 10, 16, and 18. The long arm of chromosome 16 shows deletions in 56% of informative cases (Bergerheim et al., 1991).

Fluorescence *in situ* hybridization (FISH) studies of chromosomes 7, 8, 10, 12, and Y revealed similar chromosomal numeric anomalies in PIN and prostate cancer; however, carcinomatous foci contained more anomalies than paired PIN foci. The most common alteration was a gain of chromosome 8, which was associated with advanced stage and high grade of the prostatic carcinoma. This suggests that dominantly activated genes on chromosome 8 may play a role in the progression of prostatic carcinoma (Qian et al., 1995).

Recent studies with the use of hypervariable DNA markers and FISH have revealed allelic losses involving chromosomes 8, 10, and 16 in a large proportion of prostatic cancers (Bergheim et al., 1991; Brothman et al., 1990; Carter et al., 1990b). These studies also provided evidence that losses of 8p, 10q, and 16q frequently occur in early lesions (Bergerheim et al., 1991; Bova et al., 1993), whereas the losses of 10q appeared to be a later event (Trybus et al., 1996). Chromosome 8p deletions are also common in colorectal, hepatocellular, and non-small cell lung cancers (Emi et al., 1992). More specifically, sequences that map within 8p22 appear to be affected in PIN as well as in localized and metastatic prostate cancer (Bova et al., 1993; Macoska et al., 1994; Sakr et al., 1994). The finding of frequent 8p allelic loss in localized low- and high-grade primary tumors and in PIN suggests that 8p deletions are early events in prostatic tumorigenesis (Macoska et al., 1995). Allelic losses involving 8p did not involve all the foci of PIN, which suggests that only a subset of PIN progresses to invasive prostatic carcinoma (Emmert-Buck et al., 1995; Haggman et al., 1996, 1997a,b). Qian et al. (1997a) studied the cribriform pattern of prostate cancer and PIN and demonstrated a gain of chromosomes 7, 12, and Y copies and loss of chromosome 8 in both cancer and PIN. However, the number of chromosomes involved was much higher in carcinoma than in PIN, which implicates that, cumulative genetic alterations are involved in progression of PIN to invasive disease. Bostwick et al. (1998b) studied the distribution of allelic losses at six polymorphic loci on chromosomes 7q, 8p, 8q, and 18q in multiple foci of PIN and carcinoma from completely embedded, mapped whole prostates. Their findings indicated that individual foci of PIN and carcinoma arise independently within the same prostate. However, there were strong genetic similarities between foci of PIN and adjacent carcinoma. This suggests that multiclonal expansion and progression of independent PIN foci may account for the multifocal nature of prostatic carcinomas.

HORMONAL REGULATIONS OF CELL PROLIFERATION

The most important issue of prostate cancer biology is the hormonal growth dependence of these tumors on which androgen ablation therapy is based. Unfortunately, virtually all prostatic carcinomas eventually relapse to an androgen-independent state and some are *de novo* hormone independent. The molecular events responsible for hormonal independence are still poorly understood. It is thought that changes that affect the androgen-signaling pathway, as well as other growth regulatory elements, may be responsible for the androgen-independent status of prostate tumor cells. The androgen-independent cells seem to have a structurally normal androgen receptor gene but with an altered level of expression. Since the antihormonal or hormone ablation demise of prostatic cancer cells is associated with apoptotic tumor cell death, the genes involved in programmed cell death may have a role in the development of hormone independent status (Martikainen et al., 1991). The up-regulation of bcl-2 in prostatic adenocarcinoma has been shown to be associated with the emergence of androgen independence (McDonnell, 1993). This supports the concept that an altered genetic cell death program may, at least in part, be responsible for androgen independence of prostatic cancer.

Transforming and Tumor Suppressor Genes

Among the more than 100 transforming and tumor suppressor genes identified so far, only a few have been documented to play a significant role in the biology of prostatic carcinoma. Thus, the ras family of genes, the p53 and Rb genes as well as the functionally related genes of the p53 and Rb regulatory pathways seem to play a significant role in the biology of these neoplasms.

It has been reported that mutations of ras genes occur in approximately 25% of prostate cancer, but other studies have not confirmed such a high frequency. They occur predominantly in the Ha-ras gene and less frequently in N- or Ki-ras (Carter et al., 1990a; Gumerlock et al., 1991; Moul et al., 1992; Pergolizzi et al., 1993).

The myc oncogene product is an ubiquitous DNA binding protein that regulates cell growth and mediates apoptosis. Overexpression of myc was associated with the development of prostatic dysplasia (PIN) in neonatally estrogenized mice (Pylkkänen et al., 1993). A transfection of mouse urogenital sinus with retrovirus carrying activated myc resulted in acquisition of the hyperplastic phenotype (Thompson et al., 1989).

In human tumors enhanced expression of the c-myc is seen predominantly in high-grade and advanced stage tumors (Buttyan et al., 1987; Fleming et al., 1986).

Studies on the expression of the c-erbB-2 oncogene in PIN and prostate cancer have shown its increased expression in PIN and prostate cancer. In non-neoplastic prostatic glands, increased expression of c-erbB-2 was confined to the basal cells (Myers et al., 1994b). Increased expression of c-erbB-2 in foci of PIN and adjacent cancer further confirms the relationship between these lesions.

p53 mutations occur in 30%–40% of prostatic carcinomas. They seem to correlate with advanced-stage and metastatic phenotypes of prostatic cancers (Bookstein et al., 1993; Effert et al., 1992, 1993; Visakorpi et al., 1992). Loss of heterozygosity at a locus telemetric to p53 correlates with metastatic potential of tumor and suggests the presence of another important tumor suppressor gene in the same locus (Effert et al., 1992, 1993). In general, loss of the 17p and mutations of p53 seem to correlate with a metastatic phenotype of prostatic carcinoma and are considered late events in prostatic tumorgenesis (Macoska et al., 1992). Sporadically, mutations of p53 can be found in BPH (Meyers et al., 1993). They can also occur in PIN and the reported range of p53 mutations in preneoplastic in situ conditions of prostate varies from 6% to 17.5% (Hughes et al., 1995; Myers et al., 1994a). In summary, there is a clear pattern of p53 alterations that shows increasing frequency paralleling progression of prostatic neoplasia from in situ precursor conditions to invasive disease.

Tamboli et al. (1998) have shown that Rb gene expression is typically retained in foci of PIN and adjacent carcinoma. They also found the overexpressed p53 gene in areas corresponding to high-grade PIN and adjacent invasive cancer. The role of telomerase has not yet been well investigated in early phases of prostatic neoplasia. Increased frequency of telomerase upregulation was seen in parallel to progression from PIN to invasive cancer (Koeneman et al., 1998). Down-regulation of some adhesion molecules, such as beta4 integrin, was found in PIN but not in benign prostatic glands (Allen et al., 1998). The up-regulated nm23-H1 gene product was documented in PIN as well as in invasive, localized, and metastatic prostate cancer (Allen et al., 1998). The product of nm23-H1 was shown to be responsible for metastatic phenotype of prostatic cancer and appears to be involved in early events in prostatic neoplasia (Myers et al., 1996).

METASTATIC PHENOTYPE

Clinical observations indicate that prostatic carcinomas can be divided into two major subsets: indolent, local invasive growth and aggressive with a high propensity for metastases. In addition, a small fraction of patients (probably less than 5%) initially present with an indolent form of prostatic carcinoma that (2–5 years after the initials diagnosis) eventually progresses to a highly aggressive small cell or sarcomatoid carcinoma. Therefore, the identification of molecular events governing this phenomenon is of prime clinical significance. As a general rule, multiple transforming and tumor suppressor genes are more frequently altered in aggressive tumors than in clinically indolent lesions, but the correlation is not perfect and significant overlap between these two groups can be found. The putative metastasis suppressor gene was mapped in 1992 to chromosome 11p11.2-12 by microcell-mediated chromosome transfer (Ichikawa et al., 1996; Kovacs et al., 1992). The positional cloning revealed a metastasis suppressor sequence that has mapped to the same region of chromosome 11 and is designated KA/1 (a metastasis suppressor gene for prostate cancer) (Maraj et al., 1998; Yu et al., 1997). KA/1 codes for a 267 amino acid product, which represents a cell membrane protein with transmembrane domains and several N-glycosylation sites. This product represents a member of leukocyte surface glycoproteins of the CD cluster (Yang et al., 1997). In an experimental animal model, this protein suppresses the metastatic phenotype of several cancer cell lines (Yoshida et al., 1998).

APOPTOSIS

Approximately 20 years ago, Kerr et al. (1974, 1980) defined a distinct mode of programmed cell death, which they called *apoptosis*. Since then, the concept of genetically regulated cell death has become increasingly popular among biologists and cancer researchers. The four general major implications of apoptosis are that (1) it is an important mechanism for tissue and organ development and homeostasis, (2) it is regulated by genes with documented transforming and tumor suppressor activities, (3) it is a major response in immunologic and hormonal cell stimulation, and (4) it mediates radiotherapy- and chemotherapy-induced cell death.

Morphologically, apoptosis is characterized by cell shrinkage that leaves a hole or open space around the apoptotic cell. The chromatin becomes highly condensed, and in later stages, fragmentation of cytoplasm and nuclei takes place. Ultrastructurally, apoptosis is characterized by condensation and subsequent segmentation of a cell with intact organelles. On the molecular level, the most distinguishing features of apoptosis are cleavage of DNA and the absence of activated proteolytic enzymes (Chang et al., 1989; Oren, 1992).

The first protein noted to protect cells from apoptosis was bcl-2 (Chang et al., 1989; Cohen, 1991; Stein et al., 1996). Subsequently, the contributions of *myc, abl,* and *p53* have been documented as influential in the regulation of apoptosis. The significance of apoptosis in the biology of neoplasia is defined by the fact that radiotherapy, to some extent chemotherapy, and the response to antihormone therapy result in apoptotic cell death of responsive tumor cells (Soldatenkov et al., 1995; Stephens et al., 1993; Walton et al., 1993; Wang et al., 1995; Williams, 1991; Wyllie et al., 1980). Moreover, spontaneous, sometimes massive, apoptosis is a common feature of some tumors (e.g., Ewing's sarcoma) and is also occasionally seen in some prostatic cancers, typically of high histologic grade (Dorfman and Czerniak, 1998). Hence, it can be anticipated that the genes playing a role in the regulation of apoptosis may have a significant effect on the biology of human cancer, including those that affect the prostate gland. In fact, it has been shown that the overexpression of bcl-2 can help prostatic cancer cells to overcome hormone depletion–related apoptosis and gain hormone-independent growth (Wyllie, 1980). The use of several chemotherapeutic agents, however, may circumvent bcl-2-associated resistance for programmed cell death (Williams and Smith, 1993). Experimental evidence supports the idea that *p53* and bcl-2 have an antagonistic effect on apoptosis. However, the coexistence of mutant *p53* and overexpressed bcl-2 may exert a synergistic effect on a cell's escape from apoptosis. Many other genes may act in a synergistic way or an antagonistic fashion to regulate apoptosis and proliferative cellular activities (Sentman et al., 1991; Vaux et al., 1992). Both of these mechanisms play an important role, first in the immortalization of abnormal preneoplastic clones during early stages in prostatic tumorigenesis, and later in the development of hormone-independent growth and antihormone therapy resistance.

CELL CYCLE ALTERATIONS

It is generally agreed that during cell growth and especially in its exponential phase, cells double their constituents prior to mitosis. Most home-keeping proteins double their content before the onset of DNA replication (Czerniak et al., 1989). It is also of interest that minimal threshold levels of total RNA and proteins are essential for S-phase entry (Fig. 21–20A). Given these parameters, it is possible to separate G cells into early (G1A) and late (G1B) subpopulations. A similar relationship exists on the individual protein (expressed gene) level. It is surprising that many individual cell proteins follow the same overall pattern of cell cycle–related expression (Czerniak et al., 1984, 1987a,b). Moreover, it is very difficult to identify the major differences in their pattern of expression between benign and malignant cells. Through numerous measurements of various cell markers, a similar cell cycle–related pattern of expression has been found in benign and malignant prostatic epithelial cells growing in short-term culture (Czerniak et al., 1989). The levels of some tumor-associated antigens, such as carcinoembryonic antigen (CEA) or epithectin, may be higher in malignant cells than in benign cells but it is not a consistent finding (Herz et al., 1991). The most frequent differences in gene expression patterns between benign and malignant cells are in the increased variability of post-mitotic G1 malignant cells that have resulted from increased asymmetric distribution of gene products after mitosis (Fig.

21–20b) (Czerniak et al., 1992). This is particularly important for explaining the ability of cancer cells to adverse growth conditions through involvement of cell cycle regulatory proteins. This phenomenon was documented in reference to several transforming and tumor suppressor genes in human prostatic cancer cells growing *in vitro*. The increased postmitotic asymmetricity of cancer cells and uneven distribution of their regulatory proteins accounted for the asynchrony of the cycle transverse by placing the cells with higher levels of regulatory protein close to the G1–S transition. This explains why the cells with lower levels of these proteins stay in G1 phase longer (Czerniak et al., 1992).

The traverse of an individual cell across the cell cycle can be envisioned as a pathway of multiple checkpoints that are encountered sequentially (Fig. 21–21A). Multiple, alternative pathways are available in higher cellular organisms with interacting complex regulatory mechanisms. The phenomenon of cancer results in profound deregulation of the system on a genomic scale and, almost certainly, each individual case of cancer has some distinctive alterations. This explains why it is so difficult and perhaps even impossible to link the development and progression of human cancers, including those that originate in the prostate, to a single molecular alteration (Czerniak et al., 1992).

Overall, the factors that mediate cell proliferation can be separated into those that mediate the initiation of proliferation of G0 $\rightarrow$ G1 phase transit and those that are important to maintaining progression through the cell cycle. It appears that G1B $\rightarrow$ S phase transit is an important checkpoint where competency for the S phase is monitored. The second important checkpoint is in the G2 phase, when cell ability to initiate and traverse the mitotic cycle is monitored. The cells can traverse the cell cycle quickly (exponential phase) or slowly. At these checkpoints, the mechanisms for continued proliferative growth, arrest, prolonged residency in a given cell cycle compartment, or apoptotic death are operative and are executed accordingly.

In G0 $\rightarrow$ G1 phase transit and progression throught the G_1 phase, the genes involved in the synthesis of basic DNA units (deoxynucleotides) are activated and provide the foundation for further DNA synthesis

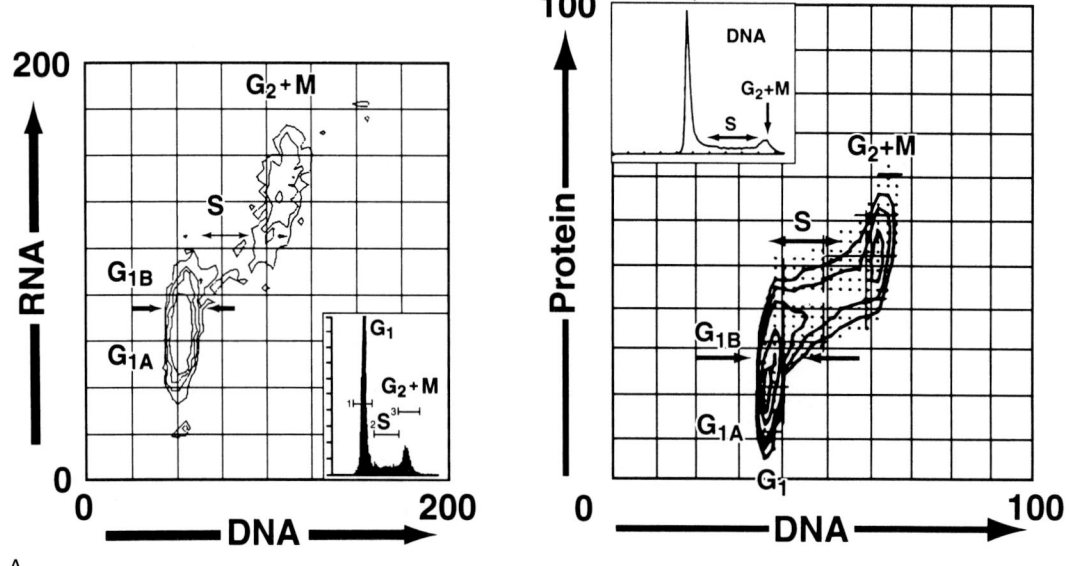

A

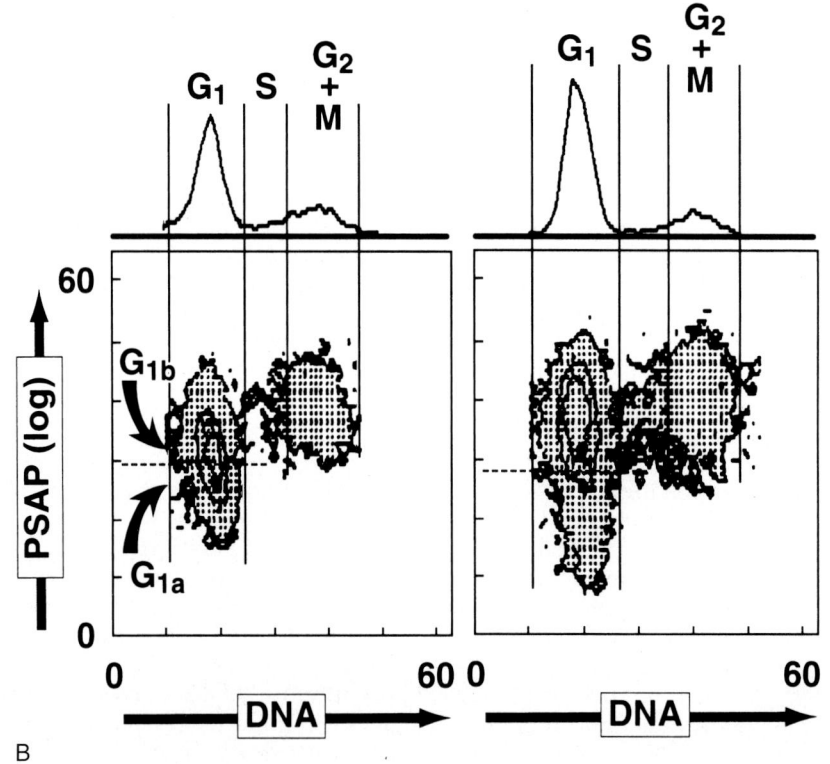

B

(King et al., 1994; Koff et al., 1993; Sherr, 1994). During the G1 phase progression, factors needed for DNA replication are expressed and activated. The S phase is characterized by DNA replication in parallel to histone gene up-regulation. The G2 phase is preparation for the mitotic cycle and is characterized by the synthesis of mitotic regulatory factors and the reorganization of the chromatin structure. Several ubiquitous proteins play an important role in mediating the competency of cells to initiate and traverse the cell cycle (King et al., 1994; Sherr, 1994).

Cyclin-related proteins and their dependent kinases (cdks) have been documented repeatedly as principal regulators of cell cycle progression and signal transduction (Darzynkiewicz et al., 1996; Macoska et al., 1992; Nigg, 1993). In response to extracellular signals, cyclins mediate the phosphorylation of their dependent transcription factors and other proteins that maintain the proliferative state (Fig. 21–21B).

The activities of cdks are controlled in a sequential manner by their cyclin proteins and inhibitors. Activation of cdk4 and cdk6 by D-type cyclins is implicated as a principal regulator of the early G_1 phase (Macoska et al., 1992; Nigg, 1993; Pan et al., 1994; Serrano et al., 1993; Xiong et al., 1993). The discovery of genes that code for cdk inhibitors, such as *p21*(*CIP*-1/*WAF*-1) and *MTS*, indicates that regulation of the cell cycle is extremely complex and involves both positive and negative elements (El-Deiry et al., 1993; Hussussian et al., 1994; Liu et al., 1995; MacLachlan et al., 1995). Activated

cdk4 and cdk6 phosphorylate the Rb protein, which in turn activates the E2F transcription factor (Chellappan et al., 1991; Dowdy et al., 1993). After phosphorylation, E2F acts as a principal activator of multiple genes involved in DNA replication.

The G1-S phase transition checkpoint is one of the most important periods of cell proliferative activities in which the cell ability for DNA synthesis is verified and all elements required for DNA replication must be present in sufficient amounts. It appears that the cdk2–cyclin complex is an important initiator of DNA synthesis in which complexes with p107, Rb, and E2F proteins are formed (Chellappan et al., 1991; Girard et al., 1991). In addition, activated cdk4 participates in the phosphorylation of RPA class proteins that bind single-stranded DNA (Pan et al., 1994). Minimum threshold levels of cyclin E are required for entry into the S phase (Gong et al., 1995). It appears that entry into the S phase is negatively regulated and requires inhibition of some cdks by transforming growth factor β (TGF-β) (Kovacs et al., 1992).

Complex regulatory mechanisms that operate on the promoter level of cell cycle–mediating genes influence the proliferative activities of cells. The regulation of histone gene expression is used as a paradigm of ubiquitous regulatory mechanisms in proliferating cells (Fig. 21–21C; Pauli et al., 1987). In general, the transcription of histone genes is up-regulated at the beginning of the S phase and is suppressed in differentiated or quiescent cells (Baumbach et al., 1984;

Figure 21–20. Cell cycle progression in relation to total RNA and protein content. *A, left*: Dual-parameter flow cytometric measurement of exponentially growing human tumor cells stained with acridine orange for simultaneous measurement of total DNA and RNA content. Cell cycle phases G1, S, and G2+M are identified on the basis of RNA content. Note that minimum threshold content of total RNA is required for entry into S phase [Courtesy Dr. Z. Darzynkiewicz, New York]. *Right*: Dual-parameter flow cytometric measurement of exponentially growing human tumor cells stained with propidium iodide (DNA) and fluorescein (protein). Cell cycle populations in G1, S, and G2+M phases are identified on the basis of DNA content. Note that by using total protein threshold level, the G1 cell population can be separated into G1A and G1B populations. This separation is similar to that seen when studying total RNA content. Minimum threshold level of total protein is required for entry into S-phase [Courtesy Dr. Z. Darzynkiewicz, New York]. *B*: PASP content in cell cycle progression. Two-parameter scattergrams, obtained from simultaneous flow cytometric measurements of green FITC immunoflourescence with anti-PSAP antibody and red PI fluorescence of (*left*) benign and (*right*) malignant primary prostatic epithelial cell cultures, show the distribution of PSAP in relation to the cell cycle. The distinction between cell cycle compartments was done graphically and was based on differences in DNA content, indicated by the continuous vertical lines. The horizontal lines indicate the S-phase threshold of PSAP and separate the G1A and G1B subcompartments. [From Herz F, et al. (1991) *Cell Prolif* 24:321–330, with permission.]

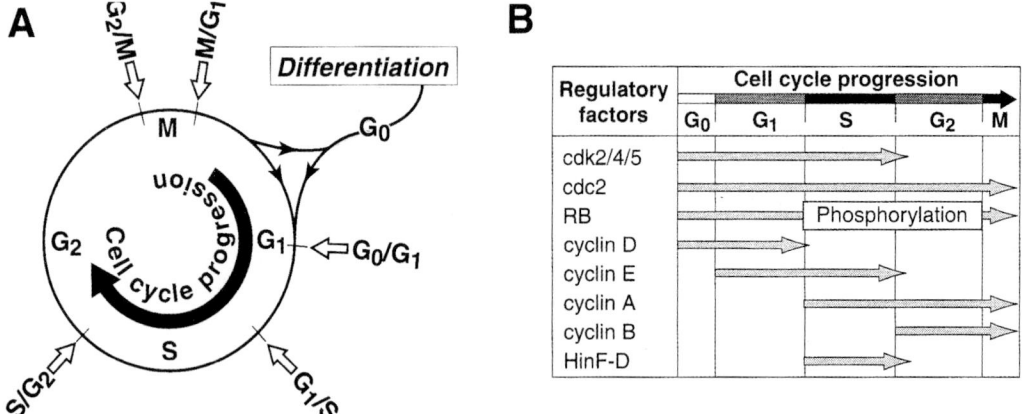

Histone Gene

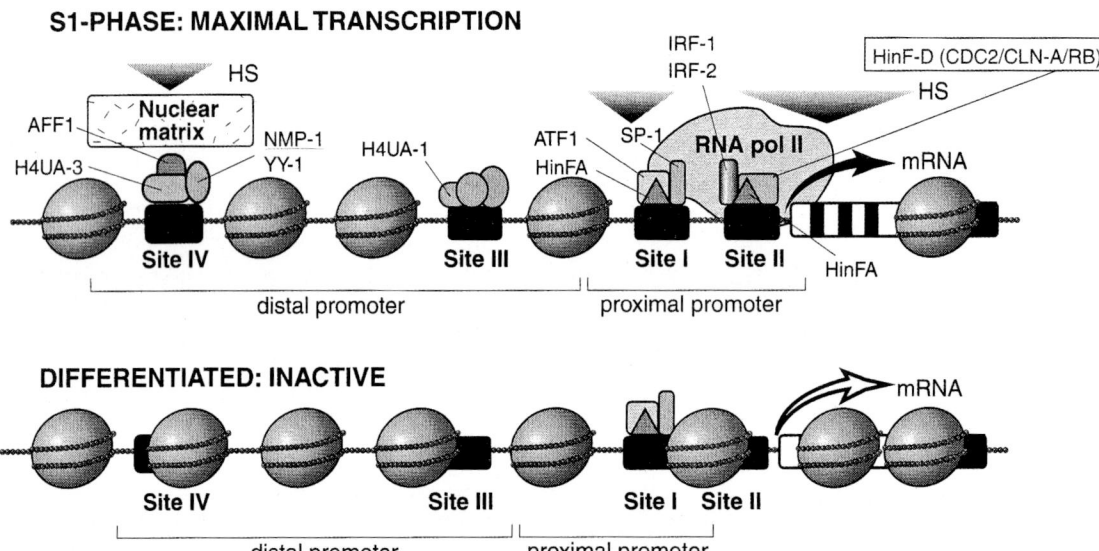

Figure 21–21. Basic regulation of cell cycle. *A*: Cell-cycle progression is depicted as circular sequential events of G0, G1, S, and G2+M phases. Arrows depict checkpoints at the boundaries of G0/S, G1/S, S/G2, and G2/M. Exit from cell cycle with onset of quiescence (G0) or differentiation is also shown. *B*: Cell cycle–dependent patterns of up-regulation of cyclins, their kinases, and Rb protein (with its phosphorylation that occurs at onset of S phase) are shown. *C*: Organization of regulatory elements (promoters) of a histone gene and their interaction with DNA binding factors in proliferated and differentiated (inactive) states. Maximal transcription in S-phase is associated with binding of multiple transcription factors in sites I and II of proximal promoter and sites III and IV of distal promoter. The differentiated (inactive) state is associated with complete inhibition of transcription and dissociation of multiple growth factors from sites I, II, and IV. Occupation at site I is retained in the differentiated (inactive) state. [Adapted from Stein GS, et al. (1996) Mechanisms regulating osteoblast proliferation and differentiation. In: *Principles of Bone Biology* (Bilezikian JP, Raisz LG, Rodan GA, eds.). Academic Press, San Diego.

Pauli et al., 1987). Accordingly, the promoter of the histone gene responds to various regulatory proliferation signals such as those from CDC2, cyclin A, the Rb-related protein, and 1RF-2, among many others (Shakoori et al., 1995; Van Wijnen et al., 1989, 1994; Vaughan et al., 1995). Suppression of histone gene expression at transition to the differentiation or quiescent state is associated with dissocation of the histone gene from the nucelar matrix and from transcription factors at several binding sites within the promoter.

From a conceptual point of view, these ubiquitous molecular regulators of the cell cycle are ultimate targets of tumorigenesis in virtually every human cancer. Their interaction with specific tissue differentiation programs may add additional complicating factors, resulting in the plethora of organ-specific neoplasms, including those that originate in the prostate.

REFERENCES

Allen MV, Smith GJ, Juliano R, Maygarden SJ, Mohler JL. (1998) Down-regulation of the beta4 integrin subunit in prostatic carcinoma and prostatic intraepithelial neoplasia. *Hum Pathol* 29:311–318.

Amin MB, Ro JY, Ayala AG. (1994) Prostatic intraepithelial neoplasia: relationship to adenocarcinoma of prostate. *Pathol Annu* 29:1–30.

Amin MB, Schultz DS, Zarbo RJ, Kubus J, Shaheen C. (1993) Computerized static DNA ploidy analysis of prostatic intraepithelial neoplasia. *Arch Pathol Lab Med* 117:794–798.

Amin MB, Tamboli P, Varma M, Srigley JR. (1999) Postatrophic hyperplasia of the prostate gland: a detailed analysis of its morphology in needle biopsy specimens. *Am J Surg Pathol* 23:918–924.

Anton PC, Chakraborty S, Wheeler TM. (1998) The significance of intraluminal prostatic crystalloids in benign needle biopsies. *Am J Surg Pathol* 22:446–449.

Anton RC, Kattan MW, Chakraborty S, Wheeler TM. (1999) Postatrophic hyperplasia of the prostate: lack of association with prostate cancer. *Am J Surg Pathol* 23:932–936.

Arias-Stella J, Takano-Moron J. (1958) Atypical epithelial changes in the seminal vesicle. *Arch Pathol* 66:761–766.

Arps S, Rodewald A, Schmalenberger B, Carl P, Bressel M, Kastendieck H. (1993) Cytogenetic survey of 32 cancers of the prostate. *Cancer Genet Cytogenet* 66:93–99.

Ayala AG, Ro JY, Babaian R, Troncoso P, Grignon DJ. (1989) The prostate capsule: does it exit? Its importance in the staging and treatment of prostatic carcinoma. *Am J Surg Pathol* 13:21–27.

Ayala AG, Srigley JR, Ro JY, Abdul-Karim FW, Johnson DE. (1986) Clear cell cribriform hyperplasia of the prostate: report of 10 cases. *Am J Surg Pathol* 10:665–671.

Babu VR, Miles BJ, Cerny J, Weiss L, Van Dyke DL. (1990) Cytogenetic study of four cancers of the prostate. *Cancer Genet Cytogenet* 48:83–87.

Baumbach LL, Marashi F, Plumb M, Stein G, Stein J. (1984) Inhibition of DNA replication coordinately reduces cellular levels of core and H1 histone mRNAs: requirement for protein synthesis. *Biochemistry* 23:1618–1625.

Bergerheim US, Kunimi K, Colins VP, Ekman P. (1991) Deletion mapping of chromosomes 8, 10 and 16 in human prostatic carcinoma. *Genes Chromosomes Cancer* 3:215–20.

Bhagavan BS, Tiamson EM, Wenk RE, Berger BW, Hamamoto G, Eggleton JC. (1981) Nephrogenic adenoma of the urinary bladder and urethra. *Hum Pathol* 12:907–916.

Bookstein R, MacGrogan D, Hilsenbeck SG, Sharkey F, Allred DC. (1993) *p53* is mutated in a subset of advanced-stage prostate cancers. *Cancer Res* 53:3369–3373.

Bostwick DG. (1996) Prospective origins of prostate carcinoma. Prostatic intraepithelial neoplasia and atypical adenomatous hyperplasia. *Cancer* 78:330–336.

Bostwick DG, Algaba F, Amin MM, et al. (1994) Consensus statement on terminology: recommendation to use atypical adenomatous hyperplasia in place of adenosis of the prostate. *Am J Surg Pathol* 18:1069–1070.

Bostwick DG, Brawer MK. (1987) Prostatic intraepithelial neoplasia and early invasion in prostate cancer. *Cancer* 59:788–794.

Bostwick DG, Pacelli A, Blute M, Roche P, Murphy GP. (1998a) Prostate specific membrane antigen expression in prostatic intraepithelial neoplasia and adenocarcinoma: a study of 184 cases. *Cancer* 82:2256–2261.

Bostwick DG, Shan A, Qian J, Darson M, Maihle NJ, Jenkins R, Cheng L. (1998b) Independent origin of multiple foci of prostatic intraepithelial neoplasia: comparison with matched foci of prostate carcinoma. *Cancer* 83:1995–2002.

Bova GS, Carter BS, Bussemakers MJ, Emi M, Fujiwara Y, Kyprianou N, Jacobs SC, Robinson JC, Epstein JI, Walsh PC, et al. (1993)Homozygous deletion and frequent allelic loss of chromosome 8p22 loci in human prostate cancer. *Cancer Res* 53:3869–3873.

Brawer MK, Bigler SA, Sohlberg OE, Nagle RB, Lange PH. (1991) Significance of prostatic intraepithelial neoplasia on prostate needle biopsy. *Urology* 38:103–107.

Brawer MK, Peehl DM, Stamey TA, Bostwick DG. (1985) Keratin immunoreactivity in the benign and neoplastic human prostate. *Cancer Res* 45:3663–3667.

Brawn PN. (1982) Adenosis of the prostate: a dysplastic lesion that can be confused with prostate adenocarcinoma. *Cancer* 49:826–833.

Brothman AR, Peehl DM, Patel AM, McNeal JE. (1990) Frequency and pattern of karyotypic abnormalities in human prostate cancer. *Cancer Res* 50:3795–3803.

Buttyan R, Sawczuk IS, Benson MC, Siegal JD, Olsson CA. (1987) Enhanced expression of the c-*myc* protooncogene in high-grade human prostate cancers. *Prostate* 11:327–337.

Carter BS, Epstein JI, Isaacs WB. (1990a) *ras* gene mutations in human prostate cancer. *Cancer Res* 50:6830–6832.

Carter BS, Ewing CM, Ward WS, Treiger BF, Aalders TW, Schalken JA, Epstein JI, Isaacs WB. (1990b) Allelic loss of chromosomes 16q and 10q in human prostate cancer. *Proc Natl Acad Sci USA* 87:8751–8755.

Chang MP, Bramhall J, Graves S, Bonavida B, Wisnieski BJ. (1989) Internucleosomal DNA cleavage precedes diphtheria toxin-induced cytolysis: evidence that cell lysis is not a simple consequence of translation inhibition. *J Biol Chem* 264:15261–15267.

Chellappan SP, Hiebert S, Mudryj M, Horowtiz JM, Nevins JR. (1991) The E2F transcription factor is a cellular target for the RB protein. *Cell* 65:1053–1061.

Chen KT, Schiff, JJ. (1983) Adenomatoid prostatic tumor. *Urology* 21:88–89.

Cheville JC, Bostwick DG. (1995) Postatrophic hyperplasia of the prostate. A histologic mimic of prostatic adenocarcinoma. *Am J Surg Pathol* 19:1068–1076.

Cheville JC, Dundore PA, Bostwick DG, Lieber MM, Batts KP, Farrow GM. (1998) Transitional cell carcinoma of the prostate: a clinicopathologic study of 50 cases. *Cancer* 82:703–707.

Cina SJ, Epstein JI. (1997) Adenocarcinoma of the prostate with atrophic features. *Am J Surg Pathol* 21:289–295.

Cleary KR, Choi HY, Ayala AG. (1983) Basal cell hyperplasia of the prostate. *Am J Clin Pathol* 80:850–854.

Cohen JJ. (1991) Programmed cell death in the immune system. *Adv Immunol* 50:55–85.

Cooner WH, Mosley BR, Ruthford CL Jr, Beard JH, Bass RB, Pond HS, Terry WJ. (1988) Clinical application of transrectal ultrasonography and prostate specific antigen in the search for prostatic cancer. *J Urol* 139:758–761.

Czerniak B, Darzynkiewicz Z, Herz F, Wersto RP, Koss LG. (1989) Flow cytometry in clinical oncology: cell cycle and DNA ploidy in assessing tumor behavior. *Mater Med Pol* 21:3–9.

Czerniak B, Darzynkiewicz Z, Staiano-Coico L, Herz F, Koss LG. (1984) Expression of Ca antigen in relation to cell cycle in cultured human tumor cells. *Cancer Res* 44:4342–4346.

Czerniak B, Herz F, Wersto R, Koss LG. (1987a) Expression of H-*ras* oncogene p21 protein in relation to the cell cycle of cultured human tumor cells. *Am J Pathol* 126:411–416.

Czerniak B, Herz F, Wersto RP, Koss LG. (1992) Asymmetric distribution of oncogene products at mitosis. *Proc Natl Acad Sci USA* 89:4860–4863.

Czerniak B, Herz, Wersto R, Koss LG. (1987b) Modification of Ha-*ras* oncogene expression and cell cycle progression in the human colonic cancer cell line HT-29. *Cancer Res* 47:2826–2830.

Darson MF, Pacelli A, Roche P, Rittenhouse HG, Wolfert RL, Young CY, Klee GG, Tindall DJ, Bostwick DG. (1997) Human glandular kallikrein 2 (hK2) expression in prostatic intraepithelial neoplasia and adenocarcinoma: a novel prostate cancer marker. *Urology* 49:857–862.

Darzynkiewicz Z, Gong J, Juan G, Ardelt B, Traganos F. (1996) Cytometry of cyclin proteins. *Cytometry* 25:1–13.

Davidson D, Bostwick DG, Qian J, Wollan P, Oesterling JE, Rudders RA, Siroky M, Stilmant M. (1995) prostatic intraepithelial neoplasia is a risk factor for adenocarcinoma. Predictive accuracy in needle biopsies. *J Urol* 154:1295–1299.

Del Rosario AD, Bui HX, Abdulla M, Ross JS. (1993) Sulfur-rich prostatic intraluminal crystalloids: a surgical pathologic and electron probe x-ray microanalytic study. *Hum Pathol* 24:1159–1167.

Deschenes J, Weidner N. (1990) Nucleolar organizer regions (NOR) in hyperplastic and neoplastic disease. *Am J Surg Pathol* 14:1148–1155.

Devaraj LT, Bostwick DG. (1993) Atypical basal cell hyperplasia of the prostate: immunophenotypic profile and proposed classification of basal cell proliferations. *Am J Surg Pathol* 17:645–659.

Dorfman HD, Czerniak B. (1998) Bone Tumors. Mosby-Year Book, St. Louis.

Dowdy SF, Hinds PW, Louie K, Reed SI, Arnold A, Weinberg RA. (1993) Physical interaction of the retinoblastoma protein with human D cyclins. *Cell* 73:499–511.

Drachenberg DB, Ioffe OB, Papademetriou JC. (1997) Progressive increase of apoptosis in prostatic intraepithelial neoplasia and carcinoma: comparison between *in situ* end-labeling of fragmented DNA and detection by routine hematoxylin-eosin staining. *Arch Pathol Lab Med* 121:54–58.

Drago JR, Mostofi FK, Lee F. (1989) Introductory remarks and workshop summary. *Urology* 34 (Suppl):2–3.

Effert PJ, McCoy RH, Walther PJ, Liu ET. (1993) *p53* gene alterations in human prostate carcinoma. *J Urol* 150:257–261.

Effert PJ, Neubauer A, Walther PJ, Liu ET. (1992) Alterations of the *p53* gene are associated with the progression of a human prostate carcinoma. *J Urol* 147:789–793.

Egan AJ, Lopez-Beltran A, Bostwick DG. (1997) Prostatic adenocaracinoma with atrophic features: malignancy mimicking a benign process. *Am J Surg Pathol* 21:931–935.

Eggleston JC, Walsh PC. (1985) Radical prostatectomy with preservation of sexual function: Pathological findings in the first 100 cases. *J Urol* 134:1146–1148.

El-Deiry WS, Tokino T, Velculescu VE, Levy DB, Parson R, Trent JM, Lin D, Mercer WE, Kinzler KW, Vogelstein B. (1993) WAF-1, a potential mediator of *p53* tumor suppression. *Cell* 75:817–825.

Emi M, Fujiwara Y, Nakajima T, Tshuchiya E, Tsuda H, Hirohashi, S, Maeda Y, Tsuruta K, Miyaki M, Nakamura Y. (1992) Frequent loss of hetorozygosity for loci on chromosome 8p in hepatocellular carcinoma, colorectal cancer, and lung cancer. *Cancer Res* 52:5368–5372.

Emmert-Buck MR, Vocke CD, Pozzatti RO, Duray PH, Jennings SB, Florence CD, Zhuang Z, Bostwick DG, Liotta LA, Linehan WM. (1995) Allelic loss on chromosome 8p12–21 in microdissected prostatic intraepithelial neoplasia. *Cancer Res* 55:2959–2962.

Epstein JI. (1995) Adenosis (atypical adenomatous hyperplasia): histopathology and relationship to carcinoma: *Pathol Res Pract* 191:888–898.

Epstein JI. (1994a) Adenosis vs. atypical adenomatous hyperplasia of the prostate. *Am J Surg Pathol* 18:1070–1071.

Epstein JI. (1994b) Prostatic intraepithelial neoplasia. *Adv Anat Pathol* 1:123–134.

Epstein JI, Armas OA. (1992) Atypical basal cell hyperplasia of the prostate. *Am J Surg Pathol* 16:1205–1214.

Epstein JL, Grignon DJ, Humphrey PA, et al. (1995) Interobserver reproducibility in the diagnosis of prostatic intraepithelial neoplasia. *Am J Surg Pathol* 19: 873–886.

Fleming WH, Hamel A, MacDonald R, Ramsey E, Pettigrew NM, Johnston B, Dodd JG, Matusik RJ. (1986) Expression of the c-*myc* protooncogene in human prostatic carcinoma and benign prostatic hyperplasia. *Cancer Res* 46:1535–1538.

Franks LM. (1954a) Atrophy and hyperplasia in the prostate proper. *J Pathol Bact* 68:617–621.

Franks LM. (1954b) Latent carcinoma of the prostate. *J Pathol Bacter* 68:603–616.

Frauenhoffer EE, Ro JY, El-Naggar AK, Ordóñez NG, Ayala AG. (1991) Clear cell cribriform hyperplasia of the prostate. Immunohistochemical and DNA flow cytometric study. *Am J Clin Pathol* 95:446–453.

Gaudin PB, Epstein JI. (1994) Adenosis of the prostate: histologic features on transurethral resection specimens. *Am J Surg Pathol* 18:863–870.

Gaudin PB, Sesterhenn IA, Wojno KJ, Mostofi FK, Epstein JI. (1979) Incidence and clinical significance of high-grade prostatic intraepithelial neoplasia in TURP specimens. *Urology* 49:558–563.

Girard F, Strausfeld U, Fernandez A, Lamb NJ. (1991) Cyclin A is required for the onset of DNA replication in mammalian fibroblasts. *Cell* 67:1169–1179.

Gleason DF. (1985) Atypical hyperplasia, benign hyperplasia and well-differentiated adenocarcinoma of the prostate. *Am J Surg Pathol* 9 (Suppl.):53–67.

Gleason DF. (1977) The Veterans Administration Cooperative Urological Research Group. Histological grading and clinical staging of prostatic adenocarcinoma. In: *Urologic Pathology: The Prostate* (Tannenbaum M, ed.): pp. 171–198. Lea & Febiger, Philadelphia.

Gleason DF, Mellinger GT. (1974) The Veterans Administration Cooperative Urological Research Group. The prediction of prognosis for prostatic adenocarcinoma by combined histological grading and clinical staging. *J Urol* 111:58–64.

Gong J, Traganos F, Darzynkiewicz Z. (1995) Threshold expression of cyclin E but not D type cyclins characterizes normal and tumor cells entering S phase. *Cell Prolif* 28:337–346.

Gould VE, Doljanskaia V, Gooch G, Bostwick DG. (1996) Immunolocalization of glycoprotein A–80 in prostatic carcinoma and prostatic intraepithelial neoplasia. *Hum Pathol* 27:547–552.

Grignon DJ, Ro JY, Ordóñez NG, Ayala AG, Cleary KR. (1998) Basal cell hyperplasia, adenoid basal cell tumor, and adenoid cystic carcinoma of the prostate gland: an immunohistochemical study. *Hum Pathol* 19:1425–1433.

Grignon DJ, Ro JY, Srigley JR, Troncoso P, Raymond AK, Ayala AG. (1992) Sclerosing adenosis of the prostate gland: a lesion showing myoepithelial differentiation. *Am J Surg Pathol* 16:383–391.

Gumerlock P, Poonamallee UR, Meyers FJ, deVere White RW. (1991) Activated *ras* alleles in human carcinoma of the prostate are rare. *Cancer Res* 51:1632–1637.

Haggman M, Wojno K, Macoska JA. (1996) Allelic loss of chromosome 8p-sequences in prostatic intraepithelial neoplasia (PIN) and invasive prostate cancer. *J Urol* (part 2) 155:324A.

Haggman MJ, Macoska JA, Wojno KJ, Oesterling JE. (1997a) The relationship between prostatic intraepithelial neoplasia and prostate cancer: critical issues. *J Urol* 158:12–22.

Haggman MJ, Wojno KJ, Pearsall CP, Macoska JA. (1997b) Allelic loss of 8p sequences in prostatic intraepithelial neoplasia and carcinoma. *Urology* 50: 643–647.

Hedrick L, Epstein JI. (1989) Use of keratin 903 as an adjunct in the diagnosis of prostate carcinoma. *Am J Surg Pathol* 13:389–396.

Helpap B. (1980) The biological significance of atypical hyperplasia of the prostate. *Virchows Arch A Pathol Anat* 387:307–317.

Henneberry JM, Kahane H, Humphrey PA, Keetch DW, Epstein JI. (1997) The significance of intraluminal crystalloids in benign prostatic glands on needle biopsy. *Am J Surg Pathol* 21:725–728.

Herz F, Czerniak B, Deitch D, Wersto RP, Simmons DA, Koss LG. (1991) Protein expression in relation to the cell cycle of exponentially growing human prostatic epithelial cells. *Cell Prolif* 24:321–330.

Holmes EJ. (1977) Crystalloids in prostatic carcinoma: relationship to Bence Jones crystal. *Cancer* 39:2073–2080.

Hughes JH, Cohen MB, Robinson RA. (1995) *p53* immunoreactivity in primary and metastatic prostatic adenocarcinoma. *Mod Pathol* 8:462–466.

Hukill PB, Vidone RA. (1967) Histochemistry of mucus and other polysaccharides in tumors. II. Carcinoma of the prostate. *Lab Invest* 16:395–406.

Hussussian CJ, Struewing JP, Goldstein AM, Higgins PA, Ally DS, Sheahan MD, Clark WH Jr, Tucjer AM, Dracopoli NC. (1994) Germline p16 mutations in familial melanoma. *Nat Genet* 8:15–21.

Ichikawa T, Ichikawa Y, Dong J, Hawkins AL, Griffin CA, Isaacs WB, Oshimura M, Barrett JC, Isaacs JT. (1992) Localization of metastasis suppressor gene(s) for prostatic cancer to the short arm of human chromosome 11. *Cancer Res* 52:3486–3490.

Ichikawa T, Nihei N, Kuramochi H, Kawana Y, Killary AM, Rinker-Schaeffer CW, Barrett JC, Isaacs JT, Kugoh H, Oshimura M, Shimazaki J. (1996) Metastasis suppressor genes for prostate cancer. *Prostate* 6:31–35.

Janssen T, Petein M, Van Velthoven R, Van Leer P, Fourmarier M, Vanegas JP, Danguy A, Schulman C, Pasteels JL, Kiss R. (1996) Differential histochemical peanut agglutinin stain in benign and malignant human prostate tumors: relationship with prostatic specific antigen immunostain and nuclear DNA content. *Hum Pathol* 27:1341–1347.

Johnson DE, Hogan JH, Ayala AG. (1972) Transitional cell carcinoma of the prostate. A clinical morphologic study. *Cancer* 29:287–293.

Kaleem Z, Swanson PE, Vollmer RT, Humphrey PA. (1998) Prostatic adenocarcinoma with atrophic features: a study of 202 consecutive completely embedded radical prostatectomy specimens. *Am J Clin Pathol* 109:695–703.

Kastendieck H. (1980) Correlations between atypical primary hyperplasia and carcinoma of the prostate: histological study of 180 total prostatectomies. *Pathol Res Pract* 169:366–387.

Keetch DW, Humphrey P, Stahl D, Smith DS, Catalona WJ. (1995) Morphometric analysis and clinical follow-up of isolated prostatic intraepithelial neoplasia in needle biopsy of the prostate. *J Urol* 154:347–351.

Kerr JF, Harmon B, Searle J. (1974) An electron-microscope study of cell deletion in the anuran tadpole tail during spontaneous metamorphosis with special reference to apoptosis of striated muscle fibers. *J Cell Sci* 14:571–585.

Kerr JF, Searle J. (1980) Apoptosis: its nature and kinetic role. In: *Radiation Biology in Cancer Research*, (Meyn RE, Withers HR, eds.) Raven Press, New York.

King RW, Jackson PK, Kirschner MW. (1994) Mitosis in transition. *Cell* 79:563–571.

Koeneman KS, Pan CX, Jin JK, Pyle JM, Flanigan RC, Shankey TV, Diaz MO. (1998) Telomerase activity, telomere length, and DNA ploidy in prostatic intraepithelial neoplasia (PIN). *J Urol* 160:1533–1539.

Koff A, Ohtsuki M, Polyack K, Roberts JM, Massague J. (1993) Negative regulation of G1 in mammalian cells: inhibition of cyclin E-dependent kinase by TGFβ. *Science* 260:536–539.

Kovacs G, Kiechle-Schwarz M, Schere G, Kung HF. (1992) Molecular analysis of the chromosome 11p region in renal cell carcinomas. *Cell Mol Biol* 38:59–62.

Kovi J. (1985) Miscroscopic differential diagnosis of small acinar adenocarcinoma of prostate. *Pathol Annu* 20:157–196.

Kovi J, Mostofi FK, Heshmat MY, Enterline JP. (1988) Large acinar atypical hyperplasia and carcinoma of the prostate. *Cancer* 61:555–561.

Kuo T, Gomez LG. (1981) Monstrous epithelial cells in human epididymis and seminal vesicles. A pseudomalignant change. *Am J Surg Pathol* 5:483–490.

Langer JE, Rovner ES, Coleman BG, Yin D, Arger PH, Malkowicz SB, Nisenbaum HL, Rowling SE, Tomaszewski JE, Wein AJ, Jacobs JE. (1996) Strategy for repeat biopsy of patients with prostatic intraepithelial neoplasia detected by prostate needle biopsy. *J Urol* 155:228–231.

Lee F, Siders DB, Torp-Pedersen ST, Kirscht JL, McHugh TA, Mitchell AE. (1991) Prostate cancer: transrectal ultrasound and pathology comparison. A preliminary study of outer gland (peripheral and central zones) and inner gland (transition zone) cancer. *Cancer* (Suppl.) 67:1132–1142.

Lee F, Torp-Pedersen ST, Siders DB, Littrup PJ, McLeary RD. (1989) Transrectal ultrasound in the diagnosis and staging of prostatic carcinoma. *Radiology* 170:609–615.

Liu Q, Neuhausen S, McClure M, Frye C, Weaver-Feldhaus J, Gruid NA, Eddington K, Allalunis-Turner MJ, Skolnick MH, Fujimura FK, Kamb A. (1995) CDKN2 (MTS1) tumor suppresor gene mutations in human tumor cell lines. *Oncogene* 10:1061–1067.

Lundgren R, Kristoffersson U, Heim S, Mandahl N, Mitelman F. (1988) Multiple structural chromosome rearrangements, including del(7q) and del(10q), in an adenocarcinoma of the prostate. *Cancer Genet Cytogenet* 35:103–108.

Lundgren R, Mandahl N, Heim S, Limon J, Henrikson H, Mitelman F. (1992) Cytogenetic analysis of 57 primary prostatic adenocarcinomas. *Genes Chromosomes Cancer* 4:16–24.

MacLachlan TK, Sang N, Giordano A. (1995) Cyclins, cyclin-dependent kinases and Cdk inhibitors: implications in cell cycle control and cancer. *Crit Rev Eukaryot Gene Expr* 5:127–156.

Macoska JA, Powell IJ, Sakr W, Lane MA. (1992) Loss of the 17p chromosomal region in a metastatic carcinoma of the prostate. *J Urol* 147:1142–1146.

Macoska JA, Trybus, TM, Benson PD, Sakr WA, Grignon DJ, Wonjo KD, Pietruk T, Powell IJ. (1995) Evidence for three tumor suppressor gene loci on chromosome 8p in human prostate cancer. *Cancer Res* 55: 5390–5395.

Macoska JA, Trybus, TM, Sakr WA, Wolf MC, Benson PD, Powell IJ, Pontes JE. (1994) Fluorescence *in situ* hybridization analysis of 8p allelic loss and chromosome 8 instability in human prostate cancer. *Cancer Res* 54:3824–3830.

Malpica A, Ro JY, Troncoso P, Ordonez NG, Amin MB, Ayala AG. (1994) Nephrogenic adenoma of the prostatic urethra involving the prostate gland: a clinicopathologic and immunohistochemical study of eight cases. *Hum Pathol* 25:390–395.

Maraj BH, Leek JP, Karayi M, Ali M, Lench NJ, Markham AF. (1998) Detailed genetic mapping around a putative prostate-specific membrane antigne locus on human chromosome 11p11.2. *Cytogenet Cell Genet* 81:3–9.

Martikainen P, Kyprinamou N, Tucker RW, Isaacs JT. (1991) Programmed death of non-proliferating androgen-independent prostatic cancer cells. *Cancer Res* 51:4693–4700.

McDonnell TJ. (1993) Cell division versus cell death: a functional model of multistep neoplasia. *Mol Carcinog* 8:209–213.

McNeal JE. (1965) Morphogenesis of prostatic carcinoma. *Cancer* 18:1659–1666.

McNeal JE. (1968) Regional morphology and pathology of the prostate. *Am J Clin Pathol* 49:347–357.

McNeal JE. (1969) Origin and development of carcinoma in the prostate. *Cancer* 23:24–34.

McNeal JE. (1981) Normal and pathologic anatomy of the prostate. *Urology* 17 (Suppl.):11–16.

McNeal JE. (1988) Normal histology of the prostate. *Am J Surg Pathol* 12:619–633.

McNeal JE, Alroy J, Leav I, Redwine EA, Freiha FS, Stamey TA. (1988a) Immunohistochemical evidence for impaired cell differentiation in the premalignant phase of prostate carcinogenesis. *Am J Clin Pathol* 90:23–32.

McNeal JE, Bostwick DG. (1986) Intraductal dysplasia: a premalignant lesion of the prostate. *Hum Pathol* 17:64–71.

McNeal JE, Leav I, Alroy J, Skutelsky E. (1988b) Differential lectin staining of central and peripheral zones of the prostate and alterations in dysplasia. *Am J Clin Pathol* 89:41.

McNeal JE, Redwine EA, Freiha FS, Stamey TA. (1988c) Zonal distribution of prostatic adenocarcinoma. Correlation with histologic pattern and direction of spread. *Am J Surg Pathol* 12:897–906.

McNeal JE, Reese JH, Redwine EA, Freiha FS, Stamey TA. (1986) Cribriform adenocarcinoma of the prostate. *Cancer* 58:1714–1719.

McNeal JE, Villers A, Redwine EA, Freiha FS, Stamey TA. (1991) Microcarcinoma in the prostate: its association with duct-acinar dysplasia. *Hum Pathol* 22: 644–652.

McNeal JE, Yemoto CE. (1996) Spread of adenocarcinoma within prostatic ducts and acini. Morphologic and clinical correlations. *Am J Surg Pathol* 20:802–814.

Meyers FJ, Chi SG, Fishman JR, DeVere White RW, Gumerlock PH. (1993) *p53* mutations in benign prostatic hyperplasia. *J Natl Cancer Inst* 685:1856–1858.

Micale MA, Sandford JS, Powell IJ, Sakr WA, Wolman SR. (1993) Defining the extent and nature of cytogenetic events in prostatic adenocarcinoma: paraffin FISH vs. metaphase analysis. *Cancer Genet Cytogenet* 69:7–12.

Montironi R, Scarpelli M, Sisti S, Braccischi A, Gusella P, Pisani E, Alberti R, Mariuzzi GM. (1990) Quantitative anaylsis of prostatic intraepithelial neoplasia on tissue sections. *Anal Quant Cytol Histol* 12:366–372.

Moore RA. (1936) The evolution and involution of the prostate gland. *Am J Pathol* 12:599–624.

Mostofi FK, Price EB. (1973) Tumors of the male genital system. In: *Atlas of Tumor Pathology*, 2nd series, Fascicle 8, pp. 177–252. Armed Forces Institute of Pathology, Washington, DC.

Moul JW, Friedrichs PA, Lance RS, Theune SM, Chang EH. (1992) Infrequent *ras* oncogene mutations in human prostate cancer. *Prostate* 20:327–338.

Murphy WM. (1998) The relationship between prostatic intraepithelial neoplasia and prostate cancer: critical issues. *J Urol* 159:995–996.

Myers RB, Oelschlager D, Srivastava S, Grizzle WE. (1994a) Accumulation of the *p53* protein occurs more frequently in metastatic than in localized prostatic adenocarcinomas. *Prostate* 25:243–248.

Myers RB, Srivastava S, Oelschlager DK, Brown D, Grizzle WE. (1996) Expression of nm23-H1 in prostatic intraepithelial neoplasia and adenocarcinoma. *Hum Pathol* 27:1021–1024.

Myers RB, Srivastava S, Oelschlager DK, Grizzle WE. (1994b) Expression of p160erbB-3 and p185erbB-2 in prostatic intraepithelial neoplasia and prostatic adenocarcinoma. *J Natl Cancer Inst* 86:1140–1145.

Nagle RB, Brawer MK, Kittelson J, Clark V. (1991) Phenotypic relationships of prostatic intraepithelial neoplasia to invasive prostatic carcinoma. *Am J Pathol* 138:119–128.

Nigg EA. (1993) Targets of cyclin-dependent protein kinases. *Curr Opin Cell Biol* 5:187–193.

Oren M. (1992) The involvement of oncogenes and tumor suppressor genes in control of apoptosis. *Cancer Metastasis Rev* 11:141–148.

Oyasu R, Bahnson RR, Nowels K, Garnett JE. (1986) Cytological atypia in the prostate gland: frequency, distribution and possible relevance to carcinoma. *J Urol* 135:959–962.

Pacelli A, Bostwick DG. (1997) Clinical significance of high-grade prostatic intraepithelial neoplasia in transurethral resection specimens. *Urology* 50:355–359.

Pan ZQ, Amin AA, Gibbs E, Niu H, Huwitz J. (1994) Phosphorylation of the *p34* subunit of human single-stranded, DNA-binding protein in cyclin A–activated G1 extracts is catalyzed by cdk-cyclin A complex and DNA-dependent protein kinase. *Proc Natl Acad Sci USA* 91:8343–8347.

Pauli U, Chrysogelos S, Stein G, Stein J, Nick H. (1987) Protein-DNA interactions in vivo upstream of cell cycle regulated human H4 histone gene. *Science* 236:1308–1311.

Pergolizzi RG, Kreis W, Rottach C, Susin M, Broome JD. (1993) Mutational status of codons 12 and 13 of the N- and K-*ras* genes in tissue and cell lines derived from primary and metastatic prostate carcinomas. *Cancer Invest* 11:25–32.

Perlman EJ, Epstein JI. (1990) Blood group antigen expression in dysplasia and adenocarcinoma of the prostate. *Am J Surg Pathol* 14:810–818.

Pylkkänen L, Mäkelä S, Valve E, Harkonen P, Toïkkanen S, Santti R. (1993) Prostatic dyplasia associated with increased expression of c-myc in neonatally estrogenized mice. *J Urol* 149:1593–1601.

Qian J, Bostwick DG, Takahashai S, Borrell TJ, Herath JF, Lieber MM, Jenkins RB. (1995) Chromosomal anomalies in prostatic intraepithelial neoplasia and carcinoma detected by fluorescence *in situ* hybridization. *Cancer Res* 55:5408–5414.

Qian J, Jenkins RB, Bostwick DG. (1997a) Detection of chromosomal anomalies and c-*myc* gene amplication in the cribriform pattern of prostatic intraepithelial neoplasia and carcinoma by fluorescence *in-situ* hybridization. *Mod Pathol* 10:1113–1119.

Qian J, Wollan P, Bostwick DG. (1997b) The extent and multicentricity of high-grade prostatic intraepithelial neoplasia in clinically localized prostatic adenocarcinoma. *Hum Pathol* 28:143–148.

Raviv G, Janssen T, Zlotta AR, Descamps F, Verhest A, Schulman CC. (1996) Prostatic intraepithelial neoplasia: influence of clinical and pathological data on the detection of prostate cancer. *J Urol* 156:1050–1055.

Reed RJ. (1984) Consultation case. Adenoid basal-cell tumor. *Am J Surg Pathol* 8:699–704.

Ro JY, Ayala AG, Ordóñez NG, Cartwright J, Mackay B. (1986) Intraluminal crystalloids in prostatic adenocarcinoma. Immunohistochemical, electron microscopic, and X-ray microanalytic studies. *Cancer* 57:2397–2407.

Ro JY, Grignon DJ, Amin MB, Ayala AG. (1997) *Atlas of Male Genital Pathology*. W.B. Saunders, Philadelphia.

Ro JY, Grignon DJ, Troncoso P, Ayala AG. (1988a) Intraluminal crystalloids in whole-organ sections of the prostate. *Prostate* 13:233–239.

Ro JY, Grignon DJ, Troncoso P, Ayala AG. (1988b) Mucin in prostatic adenocarcinoma. *Semin Diagn Pathol* 5:273–283.

Rubin MA, De La Taille A, Bagiella E, Olsson CA, O'Toole KM. (1998) Cribriform carcinoma of the prostate and cribriform prostatic intraepithelial neoplasia: incidence and clinical implications. *Am J Surg Pathol* 22:840–848.

Ruska KM, Sauvageot J, Epstein JI. (1998) Histology and cellular kinetics of prostatic atrophy. *Am J Surg Pathol* 22:1073–1077.

Sakr WA, Macoska JA, Benson P, Girgnon DJ, Wolman SR, Pontes JE, Crissman JD. (1994) Allelic loss in locally metastatic, multisampled prostate cancer. *Cancer Res* 54:3273–3277.

Sentman CL, Shutter JR, Hockenbery D, Kanagawa O, Korsemcyer SJ. (1991) bcl-2 inhibits multiple forms of apoptosis but not negative selection in thymocytes. *Cell* 67:879–888.

Serrano M, Hannon GJ, Beach D. (1993) A new regulatory motif in cell-cycle control causing specific inhibition of cyclin D/CDK4. *Nature* 366:704–707.

Sesterhenn IA, Becker RL, Avallone FA, et al. (1991) Image analysis of nucleoli and nucleolar organizer regions in prostatic hyperplasia, intraepithelial neoplasia, and prostatic carcinoma. *J Urogenital Pathol* 1:61–74.

Shakoori AR, van Wijnen AJ, Cooper C, Aziz F, Birnbaum M, Reddy GP, Grana X, DeLuca A, Giordano A, Lian JB, Stein JL, Quesenbery P, Stein GS. (1995) Cytokine-induction of proliferation and expression cdc3 and cyclin A in FDC-P1 myeloid hematopoietic progenitor cells: regulation of ubiquitous and cell cycle dependent histone gene transcription factors. *J Cell Biochem* 59:291–302.

Shepherd D, Keetch DW, Humphrey PA, Smith DS, Stahl D. (1996) Repeat biopsy strategy in men with isolated prostatic intraepithelial neoplasia on prostate needle biopsy. *J Urol* 156:460–462 and 462–463.

Sherr CJ. (1994) G1 phase progression: cycling on cue. *Cell* 79:551–555.

Skjorten FJ, Berner A, Harvei S, Robsahm TE, Tretli S. (1997) Prostatic intraepithelial neoplasia in surgical resections: relationship to coexistent adenocarcinoma and atypical adenomatous hyperplasia of the prostate. *Cancer* 79:1172–1179.

Soldatenkov VA, Prasad S, Notario V, Dritschilo A. (1995) Radiation-induced apoptosis of Ewing's sarcoma cells: DNA fragmentation and proteolysis of poly (ADP-ribose) polymerase. *Cancer Res* 55:4240–4242.

Srigley JR. (1988) Small-acinar patterns in the prostate gland with emphasis on atypical ademimatoms hyperplasia and smaller acinar carcinoma. *Semin Diagn Pathol* 5:254–272.

Stein GS, Lian JB, Stein JL, van Winjnen AJ, Frenkel B, Montecino M. (1996) Mechanisms regulating osteoblast proliferation and differentiation. In: *Principles of Bone Biology* (Bilezikian JP, Raisz LG, Rodan GA, eds.) Academic Press, San Diego.

Stephens LC, Hunter NR, Ang KK, Milas L, Meyn RE. (1993) Development of apoptosis in irradiated murine tumors as a function of time and dose. *Radiat Res* 135:75–80.

Tamboli P, Amin MB, Schultz DS, Linden MD, Jubus J. (1996) Comparative analysis of the nuclear proliferative index (Ki-67) in benign prostate, prostatic intraepithelial neoplasia, and prostatic carcinoma. *Mod Pathol* 9:1015–1019.

Tamboli P, Amin MB, Xu HJ, Linden MD. (1998) Immunohistochemical expression of retinoblastoma and *p53* tumor suppressor genes in prostatic intraepithelial neoplasia: comparison with prostatic adenocarcinoma and benign prostate. *Mod Pathol* 11:247–252.

Thompson TC, Southgate J, Kitchener G, Land H. (1989) Multistage carcinogenesis induced by *ras* and *myc* oncogenes in a reconstituted organ. *Cell* 56:917–930.

Troncoso P, Babaian RJ, Ro JY, Grignon DJ, von Eschenbach AC, Ayala AG. (1989) Prostatic intraepithelial neoplasia and invasive prostatic adencarcinoma in cystoprostatectomy specimens. *Urology* 34 (Suppl.): 52–56.

Trybus TM, Burgess AC, Wojno KJ, Glover TW, Macoska JA. (1996) Distinct areas of allelic loss on chromosomal regions 10p and 10q in human prostate cancer. *Cancer Res* 56:2263–2267.

Van Wijnen AJ, Aziz F, Grana X, DeLuca A, Desai RK, Jaarsveld K, Last TJ, Soprano K, Giordano A, Lian JB, Stein JL, Stein GS. (1994) Transcription of histone H4, H3 and H1 cell cycle genes: promoter factor HiNF-D contains CDC-2, cyclin A and an Rb-related protein. *Proc Natl Acad Sci USA* 91:12882–12886.

Van Wijnen AJ, Wright Kl, Lian JB, Stein JL, Stein GS. (1989) Human H4 histone gene transcription requires the proliferation-specific nuclear factor HiNF-D: auxiliary roles for HiNF-C (Sp1-like) and HiNF-A (high mobility group-like). *J Biol Chem* 264:15034–15042.

Vaughan PS, Aziz F, van Wijnen AJ, Wu S, Harada H, Taniguch T, Soprano K, Stein JL, Stein GS. (1995) Activation of a cell cycle regulated histone gene by the oncogenic transcription factor IRF2. *Nature* 377:362–365.

Vaux DL, Weissman IL, Kim SK. (1992) Prevention of programmed cell death in *Caenorhabditis elegans* by human blc-2. *Science* 258:1955–1957.

Visakorpi T, Kallioniemi OP, Heikkinen A, Koivula T, Isola J. (1992) Small subgroup of aggressive, highly proliferative prostatic carcinomas defined by *p53* accumulation. *J Natl Cancer Inst* 84:883–887.

Walsh PC, Lepor H, Eggleston JC. (1983) Radical prostatectomy with preservation of sexual function: anatomical and pathological considerations. *Prostate* 4:473–485.

Walton MI, Whysong D, O'Conner PM, Hockenbery D, Korsmeyer SJ, Kohn KW. (1993) Constitutive expression of human bcl-2 modulates nitrogen mustard and camptothecin induced apoptosis. *Cancer Res* 53:1853–1861.

Wang J, Bucana CD, Roth JA, Zhang WW. (1995) Apoptosis induced in human osteosarcoma cells is one of the mechanisms for the cytocidal effect of Ad5CMV-*p53*. *Cancer Gene Ther* 2:9–17.

Weinberg DS, Weidner N. (1993) Concordance of DNA content between PIN and concomitant invasive carcinoma. Evidence that PIN is a precursor of invasive prostatic carcinoma. *Arch Pathol Lab Med* 117: 1132–1137.

Weinstein MD. (1998) Digital image analysis of proliferative index: two distinct populations of high-grade prostatic intraepithelial neoplasia in close proximity to adenocarcinoma of the prostate. *Hum Pathol* 29:620–626.

Weinstein MH, Epstein JI. (1993) Significance of high-grade prostatic intraepithelial neoplasia (PIN) on needle biopsy. *Hum Pathol* 24:624–629.

Wiley EL, Davidson P, McIntire DD, Sagalowsky AI. (1997) Risk of concurrent prostate cancer in cystoprostatectomy specimens is related to volume of high-grade prostatic intraepithelial neoplasia. *Urology* 49:692–696.

Williams GT. (1991) Programmed cell death: apoptosis and oncogenes. *Cell* 65:1097–1098.

Williams GT, Smith CA. (1993) Molecular regulation of apoptosis: genetic controls on cell death. *Cell* 74: 777–779.

Wyllie AH. (1985) The biology of cell death in tumors. *Anticancer Res* 5:131–136.

Wyllie AH, Kerr JF, Currie AR. (1980) Cell death: the significance of apoptosis. *Int Rev Cytol* 68:251–306.

Xiong Y, Hannon GJ, Zhang H, Casso D, Kobayashi R, Beach D. (1993) *p21* is a universal inhibitor of cyclin kinases. *Nature* 366:701–704.

Yang X, Welch DR, Phillips KK, Weissman BE, Wei LL. (1997) KAI1, a putative marker for metastatic potential in human breast cancer. *Cancer Lett* 119:149–55.

Yoshida BA, Chekmareva MA, Wharam JF, Kadkhodaian M, Stadler WM, Boyer A, Watabe K, Nelson JB, Rinker-Schaeffer CW. (1998) Prostate cancer metastasis-suppressor genes: a current perspective. *In Vivo* 12:49–58.

Young RH, Clement PB. (1987) Sclerosing adenosis of the prostate. Report of a case. *Arch Pathol Lab Med* 111:363–366.

Young RH, Frierson HF, Mills SE, Kaiser JS, Talbot WH, Bhan AK. (1988) Adenoid cystic-like tumor of the prostate gland. A report of two cases and review of the literature on "adenoid cystic carcinoma" of the prostate. *Am J Clin Pathol* 89:49–56.

Young RH, Scully RE. (1986) Nephrogenic adenoma. A report of 15 cases, review of the literature, and comparison with clear cell adenocarcinoma of the urinary tract. *Am J Surg Pathol* 10:268–275.

Yu Y, Yang JL, Markovic B, Jackson P, Yardley G, Barrett J, Russell PJ. (1997) Loss of KAI1 messenger RNA expression in both high-grade and invasive human bladder cancers. *Clin Cancer Res* 3:1045–1049.

22

TESTIS

Thomas M. Ulbright and Robert E. Scully

Precancerous lesions of the testis comprise three recognized categories: intratubular germ cell neoplasia, the apparent precursor of invasive germ cell tumors in adults; gonadoblastoma, a lesion seen almost exclusively in patients with dysgenetic gonads and abnormal sexual development; and intratubular Sertoli cell tumor, the precursor of certain types of Sertoli cell tumor that only rarely are malignant.

INTRATUBULAR GERM CELL NEOPLASIA

This term was recommended at a consensus conference of pathologists convened in Minneapolis to discuss the classification and nomenclature of testicular tumors (Scully, 1982) and refers to all forms of atypical and malignant lesions of germ cells confined to the lumens of testicular tubules, including those types also having a minimally invasive component (Table 22–1).

The most common form of intratubular germ cell neoplasia is termed the "unclassified" type in the Minneapolis nomenclature. It was first recognized as a precancerous lesion by Skakkebaek (1972b), who subsequently designated it "carcinoma *in situ*" (Skakkebaek, 1972a; Skakkebaek et al., 1982). Other investigators preferred the designations "intratubular malignant germ cells" (Burke and Mostofi, 1988b) and "intratubular atypical germ cells" (Mark and Hedinger, 1965) for the identical lesion. The

term "intratubular germ cell neoplasia, unclassified" (IGCNU) was chosen by the Minneapolis committee instead of "carcinoma *in situ*" because follow-up studies have revealed that both seminomas and nonseminomatous germ cell tumors may develop from it if an orchiectomy is not performed (Andres et al., 1980; Berthelsen et al., 1982; Pryor et al., 1983; Sigg and Hedinger, 1981; Skakkebaek, 1978; Skakkebaek et al., 1981), and most of these tumors are not carcinomas. The terms "atypical germ cells" and "malignant germ cells" describe the cells involved in the process, but not the process itself.

Intratubular germ cell neoplasia, unclassified, is encountered most often by pathologists within the tubules of testes that have been removed from adults with invasive germ cell tumors. The lesion is seen relatively rarely in pure form. In an unselected population of 399 Danish men 18–50 years old who died suddenly, Giwercman and co-workers (1991b) found no case of IGCNU, although three patients (0.8%) had had a history of IGCNU or testicular cancer. Isolated IGCNU is most often identified in patients in the third and fourth decades who have had a biopsy because of cryptorchidism or infertility associated with severe oligospermia or azoospermia. The lesion has been encountered, however, in older patients, and may be the precursor of the rare testicular germ cell tumors found in elderly men (Abell and Holtz, 1968). It is seen only exceptionally in prepubertal patients (see below).

In the earliest stage of IGCNU, which is

Table 22–1. Classification of Intratubular Germ
Cell Tumors

Intratubular germ cell neoplasia, unclassified

Intratubular germ cell neoplasia, unclassified
 With extratubular infiltration ("early" seminoma)

Intratubular seminoma
 Classic
 Spermatocytic

Intratubular embryonal carcinoma

Intratubular germ cell neoplasia, other forms
 Seminoma with syncytiotrophoblast cells
 Syncytiotrophoblast cells
 Yolk sac tumor

only occasionally observed, microscopic examination reveals focal proliferation of cells
closely resembling those of seminoma in
the seminiferous tubules (Fig. 22–1). These
cells, which are large and rounded with
abundant clear cytoplasm and central nuclei
containing one or a few prominent nucleoli,
are widely scattered along the periphery of
tubules in which spermatogenic activity remains (Fig. 22–1; Schulze and Holstein,
1977; Skakkebaek et al., 1982). In the
more commonly encountered late phase of
IGCNU spermatogenic cells have disappeared, larger numbers of atypical cells are
found at the periphery of tubules, and Sertoli cells have been displaced toward the lumen (Fig. 22–2). Mitotic figures are frequent
in the atypical germ cells. The basement

membranes of the affected tubules are often
thickened (Fig. 22–2), and the adjacent lamina propria may be hyalinized. At this stage
the involved tubules are often distributed in
a patchy fashion, with intervening normal-
appearing tubules that lack atypical germ
cells (Fig. 22–3). The atypical germ cells
commonly extend into the rete testis, where
they are scattered in a pagetoid fashion
within the epithelial lining (Lee and
Theaker, 1994; Perry et al., 1994). Prominent involvement of the rete occasionally
produces a complex expansion of the rete
tubular network, which contains an admixture of atypical germ cells and rete epithelial cells (Fig. 22–4). We have seen rare cases
of extensive IGCNU in the rete testis that
produced a palpable mass. In occasional
cases the microscopic features of this process
are confused with those of embryonal carcinoma because of the atypical cells in a glandular pattern; close examination, however,
demonstrates the characteristic morphology
of IGCNU cells and compressed, benign rete
epithelium within the tubular framework of
the rete testis.

The cells of IGCNU have been shown to
have an aneuploid DNA content (de Graaff
et al., 1992; Mosunjac et al., 1998; Müller et
al., 1981, 1985) and an isochromosome 12p
(Vos et al., 1990), which is characteristic of
invasive germ cell tumors. The atypical cells,
like those of seminoma, usually contain
glycogen in their cytoplasm (Fig. 22–5) and

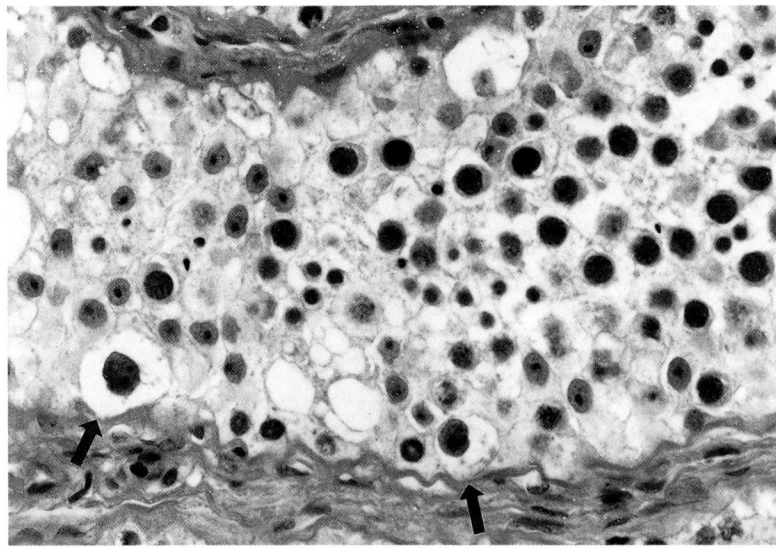

Figure 22–1. Shown here
are two cells (arrows)
with the characteristic
clear cytoplasm, enlarged
nuclei, and prominent
nucleoli of intratubular
germ cell neoplasia, un-
classified type, in a seminiferous tubule with
active spermatogenesis.

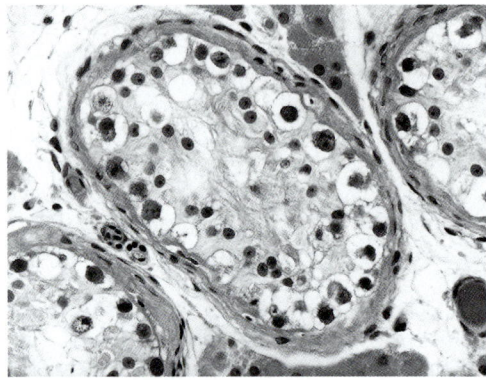

Figure 22–2. The seminiferous tubules show a peripheral arrangement of IGCNU cells, with Sertoli cells displaced toward the lumen. The tubular basement membranes are thickened.

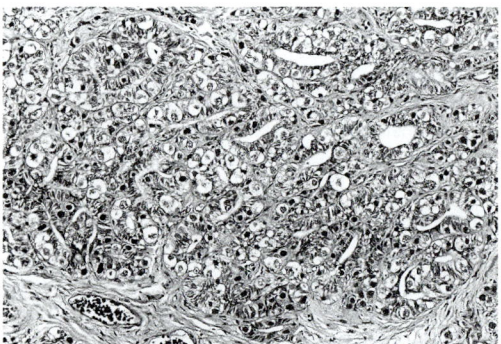

Figure 22–4. The IGCNU cells have extended into the epithelium of the rete testis, so-called pagetoid spread.

are positive immunohistochemically for placental-like alkaline phosphatase (Fig. 22–6) (Bailey et al., 1991; Burke and Mostofi, 1988a,b; Jacobsen and Norgaard-Pedersen, 1984; Koide et al., 1987; Loftus et al., 1990; Niehans et al., 1988), neuron-specific enolase (Niehans et al., 1988), the protein product of the *c-kit* proto-oncogene (Hawkins et al., 1997), and glutathione-*S*-transferase π (Klys et al., 1992), with monoclonal antibodies M2A (Bailey et al., 1991; Giwercman et al., 1988a), 43-9F (Giwercman et al., 1990), TRA-1-60 (Giwercman et al., 1993a; Jørgensen et al., 1993), HB5, HF2, and HE11

(Hiraoka et al., 1997), and, sometimes, for ferritin (Jacobsen et al., 1980; Niehans et al., 1988; Sigg and Hedinger, 1984). In contrast, spermatogonia and Sertoli cells in postpubertal testes are negative for placental-like alkaline phosphatase except that, rarely, focal staining of spermatocytes is seen (Burke and Mostofi, 1988a). Several of the immunohistochemical markers (placental-like alkaline phosphatase and the epitopes recognized by M2A, TRA-1-60, HB5, HF2, and HE11) are normally expressed in the nonneoplastic germ cells of fetuses and neonates (Hiraoka et al., 1997; Jørgensen et al., 1993). Stains for α-fetoprotein and human chori-

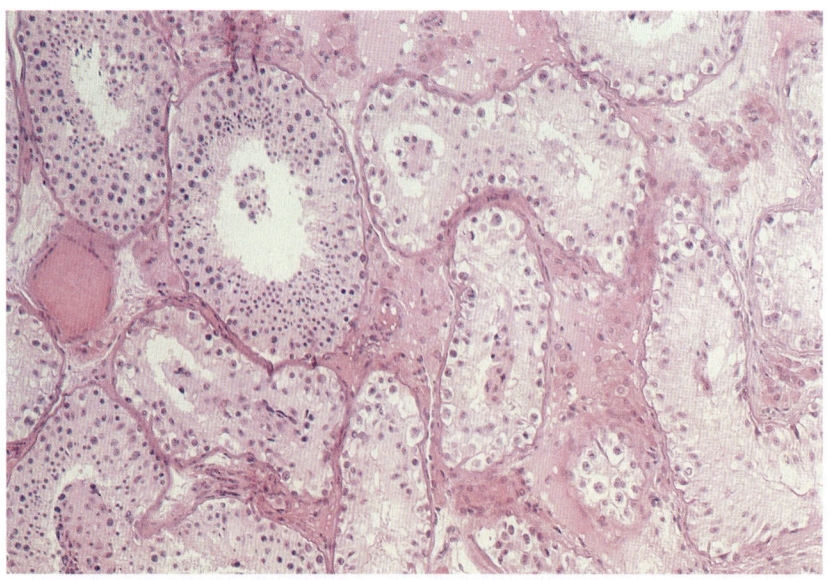

Figure 22–3. This case illustrates the frequently patchy distribution of IGCNU cells which are present in several tubules adjacent to normal tubules with spermatogenesis (left).

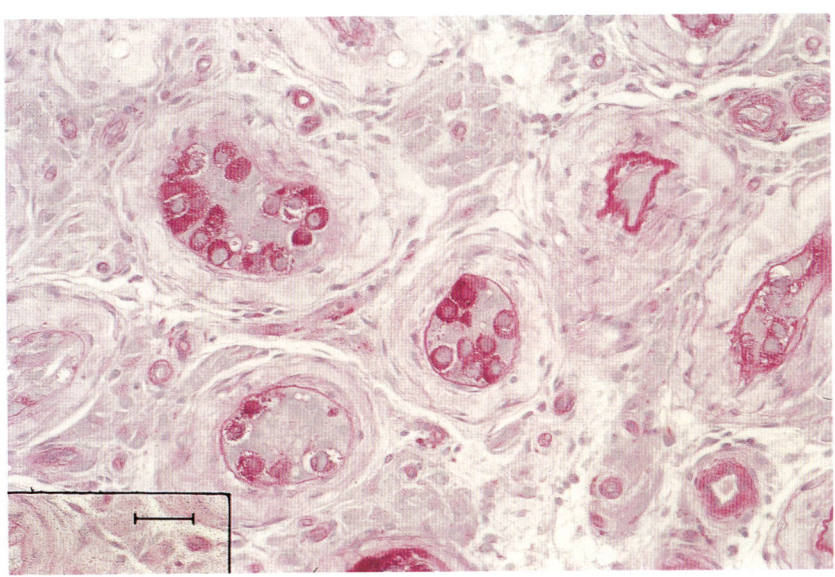

Figure 22–5. A periodic acid-Schiff stain highlights the cells of IGCNU in several shrunken tubules.

onic gonadotropin are negative (Sigg and Hedinger, 1984). On ultrastructural examination, the atypical cells have features similar to those of prespermatogenic cells and seminoma cells (Table 22–2; Albrechtsen et al., 1982; Gondos, 1993; Gondos et al., 1983; Nielsen et al., 1974; Schulze and Holstein, 1977; Sigg and Hedinger, 1984). The cells of IGCNU also have more argyrophilic nucleolar organizer regions (AgNORs) than spermatogonia and Sertoli cells (Loftus et al., 1990; Müller et al., 1994), and synthesize a unique mRNA transcript for platelet-derived

growth factor α-receptor (Mosselman et al., 1996).

The cells of IGCNU may penetrate the wall of the involved tubules and extend into the interstitium (Fig. 22–7). The resultant lesion has been termed "IGCNU with extratubular infiltration" or "microinvasive germ cell tumor" (von Eyben et al., 1981), but it is generally more informative to clinicians to designate it "IGCNU with microinvasive seminoma." The conclusion that the cells of IGCNU and seminoma are equivalent is based on their similar light micro-

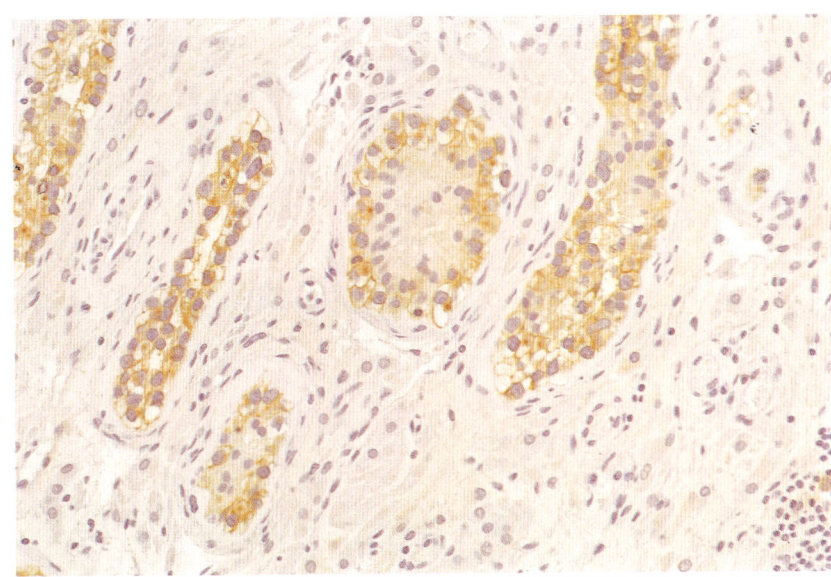

Figure 22–6. The IGCNU cells are highlighted by an immunostain directed against placental alkaline phosphatase, whereas the Sertoli cells and interstitium are negative.

Table 22–2. Ultrastructural Features of Intratubular Germ Cell Neoplasia, Unclassified

Nuclei

Large

Prominent nucleoli

Cytoplasm
  Glycogen
  Polarization of organelles
  Peripheral microfilaments
  Microtubules
  Nuages[a]
  Dense core vesicles[b]
  Annulate lamellae

No intercellular bridges

[a]Accumulations of finely granular, moderately electron-dense material lying free in the cytoplasm (literally, "clouds").

[b]Homogeneous electron-dense material in the centers of otherwise empty-appearing vesicle.

scopic appearance, ultrastructural features, immunohistochemical reactions, cytogenetic findings, number of nucleolar organizer regions, lectin binding patterns, DNA content, and proliferative fractions (Bailey et al., 1986, 1991; de Graaff et al., 1992; de Jong et al., 1990; Delahunt et al., 1990; Ferreiro, 1994; Giwercman et al., 1988a; Malmi and Söderström, 1991; Mosunjac et al., 1998; Müller et al., 1985; Schulze and Holstein, 1977; Vos et al., 1990).

Karyotypic analyses of IGCNU and its associated invasive germ cell tumor are consistent with the concept that the cytogenetic changes in the former, which are similar to those identified in the latter, occur prior to extratubular invasion (Gillis et al., 1994; Looijenga et al., 1993; Oosterhuis et al., 1993) and clonal similarities between the two processes support the conclusion that the latter is derived from the former (van Echten et al., 1995). In other words, IGCNU, although morphologically homogeneous, appears to be genetically diverse with the capability of giving rise to both seminomas and nonseminomatous tumors.

When the cells of IGCNU proliferate to the extent that the Sertoli cells are obliterated and the tubules are distended (Fig. 22–8), the term "intratubular seminoma" (of the classic type) is used (Mostofi and Price, 1973; Schulze and Holstein, 1977). Although we and others (Sigg and Hedinger, 1980) have seen this lesion accompanying seminomas more commonly than nonseminomatous germ cell tumors, its occasional association with the latter tumors suggests that, like IGCNU, intratubular seminoma may give rise to them as well. Nonetheless, because of the striking resemblance to seminoma, even to the extent that it may be infiltrated by lymphocytes and epithelioid histiocytes, the designation "intratubular seminoma" is used.

Intratubular seminoma and IGCNU must be differentiated from several other lesions that may superficially resemble them. Intratubular spermatocytic seminoma is very

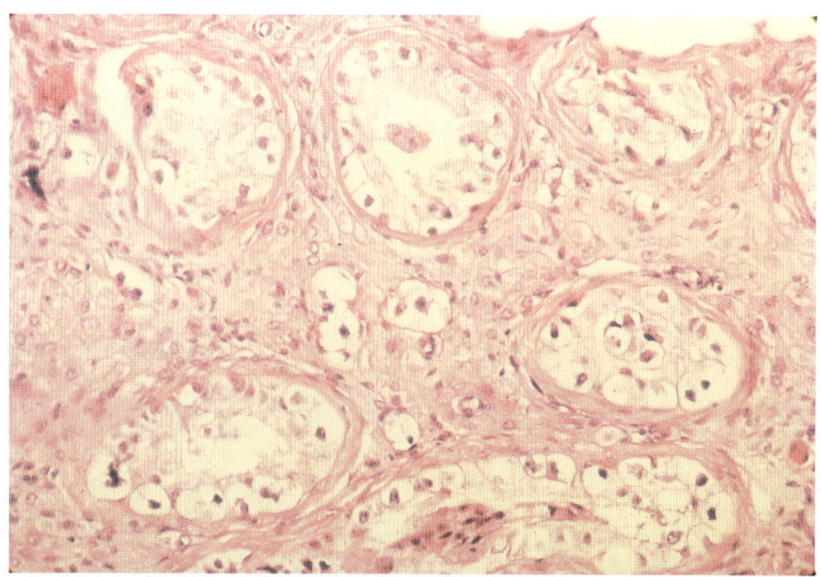

Figure 22–7. Several IGCNU-type cells are present in the interstitium, adjacent to tubules with IGCNU.

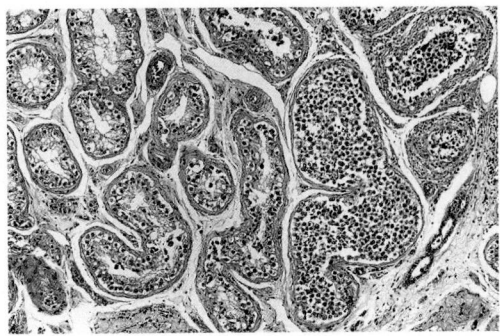

Figure 22–8. Many tubules show the typical pattern of IGCNU, but one is distended by similar cells, a finding classified as intratubular seminoma.

rarely encountered in the absence of an invasive spermatocytic seminoma; its cells, which vary in size, as discussed below, contrast with the homogeneous cell population of IGCNU and intratubular seminoma. Viral orchitis and other forms of orchitis may produce intratubular accumulations of mononuclear inflammatory cells (Morgan, 1976) that can cause confusion with IGCNU or intratubular seminoma, particularly in small biopsy specimens (Fig. 22–9). The usual presence of simultaneous interstitial inflammation, nuclear features that differ from those of seminoma, and immunohistochemical staining are helpful in this differential diagnosis in difficult cases. In granulomatous orchitis, epithelioid histiocytes distend the seminiferous tubules (Aitchison et al., 1990; Lynch et al., 1968) and in one-quarter of cases, Langhans-type giant cells are also present. It is important to recognize, however, that similar-appearing granulomatous reactions may occur within intratubular seminoma (Fig. 22–10), sometimes obscuring the tumor cells and necessitating careful search to confirm their presence. Lymphoma involving the testis grows within the tubules in about one-third of cases (Gowing, 1976), almost always within the confines of the neoplasm. The tumor cells differ from those of intratubular seminoma in that they usually have more irregularly shaped nuclei and scanty cytoplasm lacking glycogen. Also, lymphoma cells are not restricted to the tubules but diffusely involve the interstitium in most cases. We have seen one case of anaplastic large

cell lymphoma of the testis with a prominent intratubular component and comedo-like necrosis that mimicked intratubular embryonal carcinoma (Fig. 22–11; Ferry et al., 1997), as discussed below.

Intratubular germ cell neoplasia, unclassified has been reported in the seminiferous tubules adjacent to seminomas in 64%–89% of cases and adjacent to nonseminomatous germ cell tumors in 75%–100% of cases (Coffin et al., 1985; Jacobsen et al., 1981; Klein et al., 1985; Sigg and Hedinger, 1980; Skakkebaek, 1975). In contrast, intratubular seminoma has been identified in only 44% of testes containing seminomas and 27% of those containing nonseminomatous germ cell tumors (Sigg and Hedinger, 1980). Both IGCNU and intratubular seminoma have also been found within or adjacent to scars in the testes of patients with metastatic seminomas and nonseminomatous germ cell tumors (Azzopardi and Hoffbrand, 1965; Azzopardi et al., 1961). Identification of these lesions in this context provides evidence for regression of an invasive germ cell tumor that has metastasized. The occurrence of IGCNU in testicular biopsy specimens from 8 of 12 patients with retroperitoneal germ cell tumors who lacked palpable testicular tumors supports the conclusion that such retroperitoneal tumors are metastatic from regressed testicular primary tumors in most cases (Chen and Cheng, 1989; Daugaard et al., 1987). In contrast, the absence of IGCNU in testicular biopsy specimens from three patients with mediastinal germ cell tumors without retroperitoneal involvement is consistent with the primary nature of these tumors (Daugaard et al., 1987); a rare case of simultaneous, but apparently independent involvement at both sites has also been reported (Hailemariam et al., 1997).

The precancerous nature of IGCNU is strongly supported by a number of clinical observations, which include its increased frequency on biopsy examination of testes of patients known to be at increased risk for invasive germ cell tumors. For example, biopsies of cryptorchid testes, most of which had been treated by orchidopexy, have shown either IGCNU or, less often, intratubular seminoma in 2% to 3% of cases (Giwercman et al., 1988b, 1989; Nistal et al., 1989); biopsies of testes from infertile men, most of whom

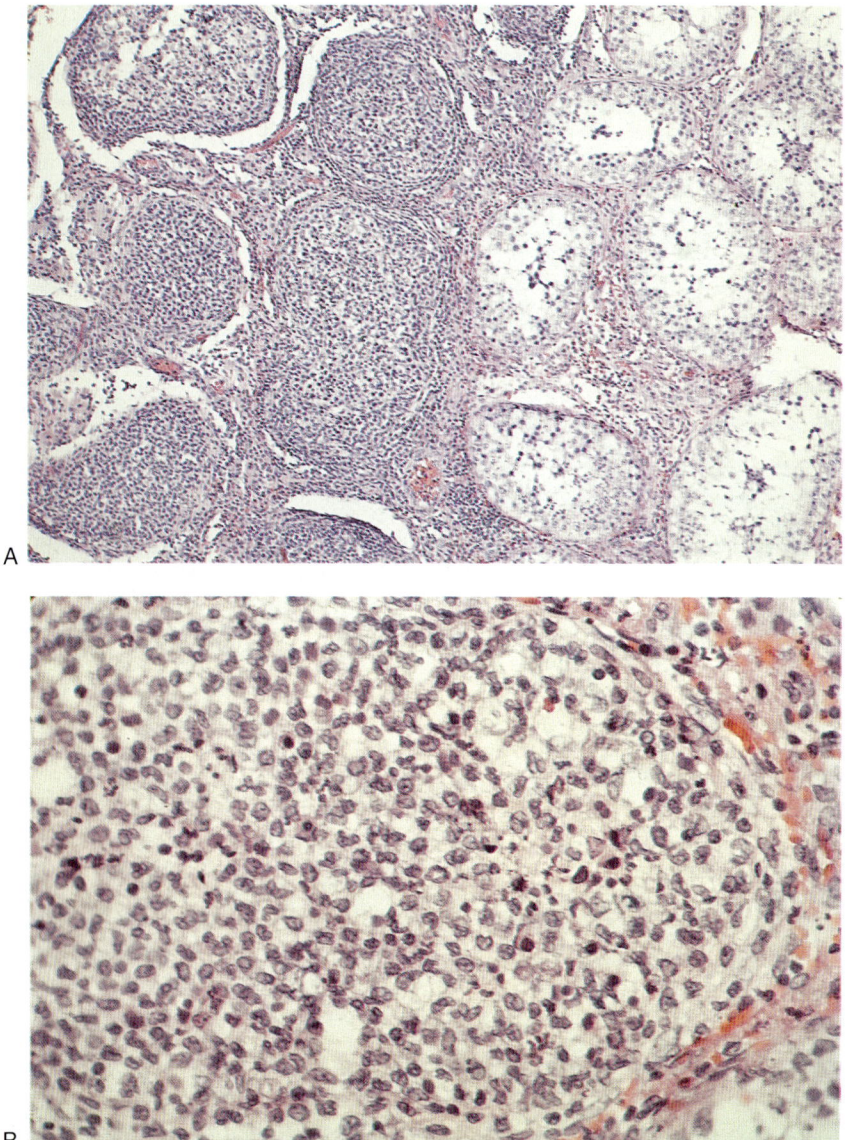

Figure 22–9. *A*: Many tubules are distended by mononuclear inflammatory cells in a case of viral orchitis, potentially causing confusion with intratubular seminoma. Note the accompanying interstitial inflammation. *B*: The lymphoid cells in the tubules have irregular nuclear contours and lack the cytologic features of seminoma or IGCNU cells.

had severe oligospermia or azoospermia, have shown IGCNU in 0% to 1% of cases (Giwercman et al., 1997; Nistal et al., 1989; Skakkebaek, 1978), and biopsies of testes contralateral to invasive testicular germ cell tumors have yielded IGCNU in 4% to 7% of cases (Berthelsen et al., 1982; Dieckmann and Loy, 1998; Dieckmann et al., 1993; Loy and Dieckmann, 1993; Mumperow et al.,

1992; von der Maase et al., 1986), correlating with a similar frequency of bilateral, usually asynchronous occurrence of testicular germ cell tumors (Dieckmann et al., 1993; Scheiber et al., 1987). In patients with a history of either cryptorchidism or a prior invasive germ cell tumor, there was a significantly higher frequency of IGCNU if the testis was atrophic (Berthelsen et al., 1982;

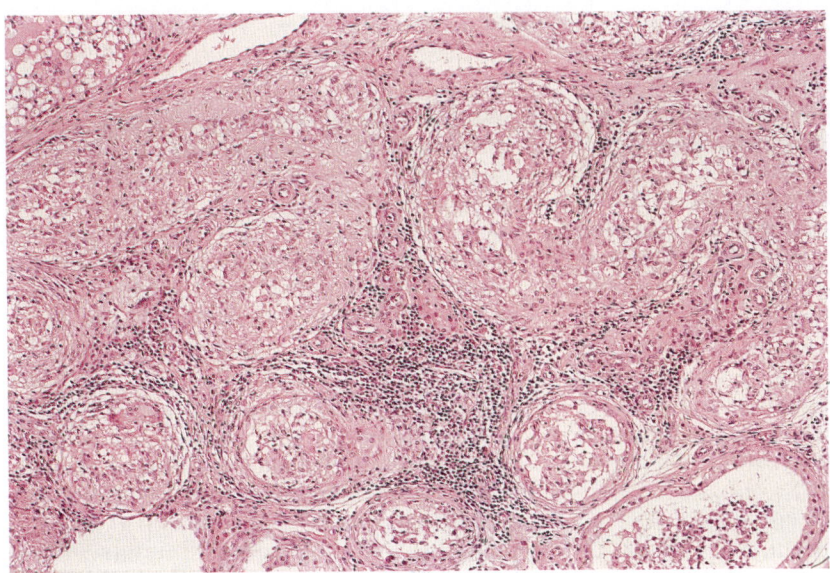

Figure 22–10. This prominent intratubular granulomatous reaction occurred in association with an invasive seminoma.

Dieckmann and Loy, 1998; Harland et al., 1993; Loy and Dieckmann, 1993). For example, in Dieckmann and Loy's (1998) study, which was based on 1954 simultaneous biopsies of the testis contralateral to an invasive germ cell tumor, the presence of testicular atrophy elevated the risk of IGCNU 4.3-fold, although 64% of the cases of IGCNU occurred in nonatrophic testes (Dieckmann and Loy, 1998). The relatively high frequency of IGCNU in the above clinical situations correlates with the increased frequency of germ cell tumors in patients with cryptorchidism, infertility, and a contralateral testicular germ cell tumor. It is also

not surprising that IGCNU is common in the testes (which are almost always undescended) of patients with the androgen insensitivity syndrome (Müller and Skakkebaek, 1984; Nogales et al., 1981; Rutgers and Scully, 1991; Skakkebaek, 1979), since an invasive germ cell tumor develops in about one-third of these patients by the age of 50 years (Manuel et al., 1976). Infants and children with 45,XO/46,XY mixed gonadal dysgenesis have also developed IGCNU (MacMahon and Cussen, 1991; Müller et al., 1985; Wallace and Levin, 1990). Additional support for the precancerous nature of IGCNU is its aforementioned common oc-

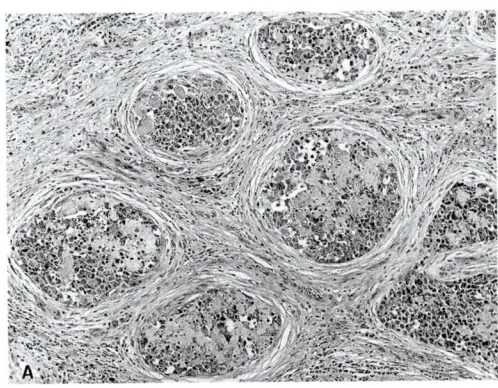
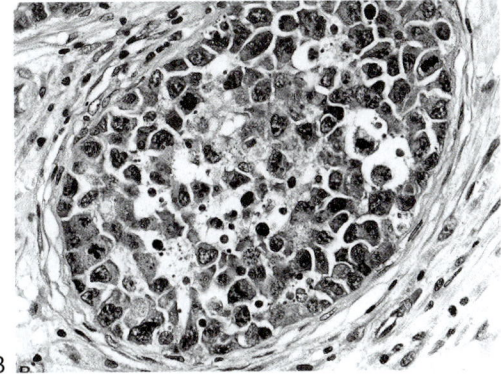

Figure 22–11. *A*: This rare case of anaplastic large cell lymphoma of the testis has a prominent intratubular growth pattern with necrosis that mimics intratubular embryonal carcinoma (see Figure 22–15). *B*: The markedly "twisted" nuclei are a clue to the possibility of lymphoma, but immunostains were required for definitive diagnosis.

currence adjacent to invasive seminomas and nonseminomatous germ cell tumors in postpubertal patients (Coffin et al., 1985; Jacobsen et al., 1981; Klein et al., 1985; Sigg and Hedinger, 1980; Skakkebaek, 1975).

The precancerous nature of IGCNU is confirmed most convincingly by follow-up studies of patients in whom it has been identified on biopsy. In one study, 7 of 19 patients with untreated IGCNU developed invasive tumors on follow-up, with an estimated frequency of invasive tumors of 50% at 5 years (von der Maase et al., 1986). In a compilation of five series of patients with IGCNU (Berthelsen et al., 1982; Burke and Mostofi, 1988b; Pryor et al., 1983; Sigg and Hedinger, 1981; Skakkebaek, 1978), invasive tumors developed in 7 of 16 patients followed for less than 1 year, 9 of 19 patients followed for 1 to 5 years, and 4 of 9 patients followed for longer than 5 years (Fig. 22–12). Thus, invasive tumors developed in 20 of 44 patients on follow-up, which was limited in many cases. The tumors that developed were seminomas in 15 of the cases and nonseminomatous germ cell tumors of various types in the remainder. Although five patients were free of invasive tumor at 6 to 8 years of follow-up, invasive tumors not included in the above series have been documented at 7 years (Andres et al., 1980), 10.5 years (Müller et al., 1984) and 16 years (C.E. Hedinger, personal communication) after a biopsy showing IGCNU.

In contrast to the abundant evidence for the role of IGCNU as the precursor of invasive germ cell tumors in adults, the intratubular precursor of germ cell tumors in prepubertal children has not been identified in the great majority of cases. Several groups of investigators have reported an absence of IGCNU in the adjacent testis in well over 100 cases of prepubertal yolk sac tumors and teratomas (Guinand and Hedinger, 1981; Hawkins et al., 1997; Jøorgensen et al., 1995; Koide et al., 1987; Manivel et al., 1988, 1989; Soosay et al., 1991). Conversely, intratubular lesions identical to IGCNU have been reported in testicular specimens without invasive germ cell tumors, particularly in fetuses and infants under 2 years of age, and rarely in older children. In one study of testicular biopsy specimens obtained at the time of orchidopexy (Hailemariam et al., 1998), 22 of 440 prepubertal patients had intratubular germ cells that resembled those of IGCNU both morphologically and immunohistochemically, but none of the 15 patients with available follow-up information had a germ cell tumor during follow-up intervals of 19.5 to 33.5 (mean 25) years. From another perspective, Parkinson and co-workers (1994) reported the development of invasive germ cell tumors at 11 and 22 years of follow-up in 2 patients among a group of 57 who had negative biopsies at the time of childhood orchidopexy. Cortes et al. (1994) reported a similar sequence of microscopic findings in 2 patients among 828 who were followed after negative biopsies at orchidopexy, but many of their patients were probably not prepubertal.

Despite the above findings, evidence has been presented that atypical germ cells with at least some microscopic features of IGCNU might have led to the development of occasional prepubertal invasive germ cell tumors. Renedo and Trainer (1994) reported the case of a 3-year-old boy with a testicular teratoma in which the adjacent testicular

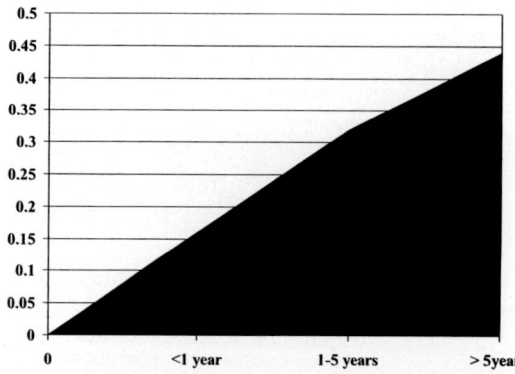

Figure 22–12. The shaded part of the graph represents the proportion of patients with IGCNU in testicular biopsies who developed invasive tumors on follow-up. The proportion beyond 5 years is not well established, but there is little change in the slope, consistent with a progressive process.

tubules contained glycogen-positive atypical germ cells that were negative immunohistochemically for placental-like alkaline phosphatase. On the basis of staining for proliferating cell nuclear antigen (PCNA) and p53, those authors concluded that the atypical intratubular cells were the precursor of the adjacent tumor. Hawkins et al. (1997), however, interpreted the findings in that case as reactive rather than precancerous, having observed similar cells adjacent to a testicular Sertoli cell tumor. We have also seen atypical germ cells that lacked the cytologic and immunohistochemical features of IGCNU in the tubules adjacent to prepubertal germ cell tumors (Fig. 22–13). Stamp et al. (1993) reported the presence of glycogen-positive, placental-like alkaline phosphatase-positive intratubular germ cells adjacent to an immature testicular teratoma in an 8-month-old patient; these cells could have been an incidental finding, however, in view of their more frequent identification in testes from patients in this age group in the absence of an invasive tumor.

Two cases are much more convincing in respect to the precancerous potential of prepubertal atypical germ cells that resemble those of IGCNU. Hu et al. (1992) reported a case of yolk sac tumor in a 15-month-old infant in which adjacent tubules contained cells that were glycogen-rich and focally positive for placental-like alkaline phosphatase. The intratubular lesion was triploid by *in situ* hybridization, whereas the invasive yolk sac tumor cells were tetraploid, leading the authors to exclude that the atypical intratubu-

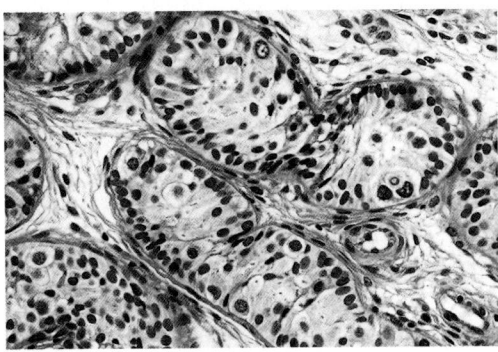

Figure 22–13. "Atypical" germ cells in the tubules of a prepubertal boy with a testicular teratoma. These cells are different from those of IGCNU and are not established to be neoplastic.

lar germ cells reflected tubular invasion by the adjacent tumor. Dorman et al. (1979) reported the case of a 13-year-old boy with bilateral cryptorchidism and an immature testis in which typical IGCNU was found on bilateral biopsy, accompanied by extratubular infiltration of the atypical, seminoma-like cells.

Ancillary evidence that prepubertal atypical germ cells resembling those of IGCNU may be precancerous is their apparently increased frequency in prepubertal patients without invasive germ cell tumors who have had mixed gonadal dysgenesis (MacMahon and Cussen, 1991; Müller et al., 1985; Ramani et al., 1993; Wallace and Levin 1990) or the androgen insensitivity syndrome (Müller and Skakkebaek, 1984a); both syndromes are associated with an increased risk of germ cell tumors. Finally, a lesion resembling IGCNU has also been seen on biopsy of undescended testes of three infants with the prune-belly syndrome in contrast to absence of the lesion in five age-matched control testes (Massod et al., 1991). The authors who reported these findings concluded that patients with this syndrome should be followed carefully for the development of invasive testicular germ cell tumors later in life. An editorial comment mentioned the additional finding of typical IGCNU in a 19-year-old man with the prune-belly syndrome.

Intratubular spermatocytic seminoma was originally described by Masson (1946) in one of his cases of invasive spermatocytic seminoma. He concluded that its occurrence could not be ascribed to intratubular spread of the invasive tumor because of its distance from the latter. Other investigators have also noted the concurrence of intratubular and invasive spermatocytic seminoma (Rosai et al., 1969; Scully, 1961; Talerman, 1980a), and we have seen a single example of exclusively intratubular spermatocytic seminoma, occurring within a 1.5 mm cluster of tubules in the atrophic testis of a 49-year-old-man. This lesion, and examples of intratubular spermatocytic seminoma associated with invasive tumors, have appeared as tubules filled with cells of varying sizes with round, hyperchromatic nuclei and cytoplasm devoid of glycogen (Fig. 22–14), features that contrast with those of IGCNU. Among all of the invasive testicular germ cell tumors in adults, spermatocytic

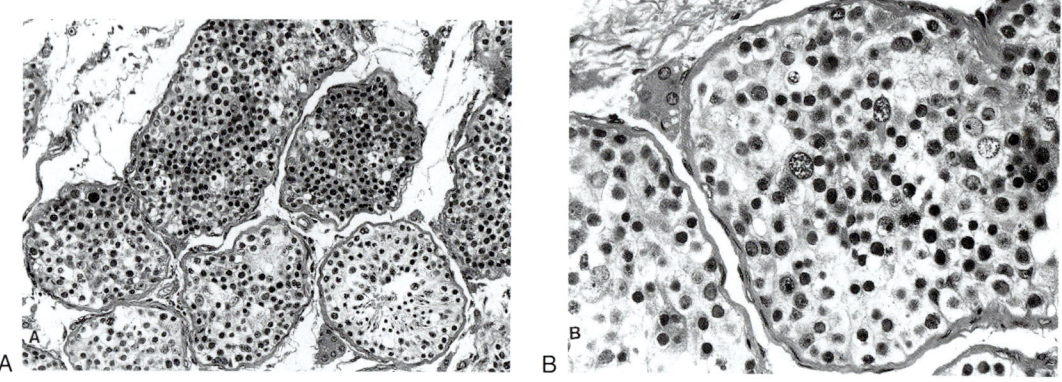

Figure 22–14. *A*: Intratubular spermatocytic seminoma fills several tubules. A tubule at the lower right is not involved. *B*: High magnification shows the polymorphous population of cells in intratubular spermatocytic seminoma, with small, darkly staining, lymphocyte-like cells, cells of intermediate size, and larger cells, some with a "spireme" chromatin.

seminoma is the one type that is not associated with IGCNU (Müller et al., 1987; Skakkebaek et al., 1987).

Intratubular embryonal carcinoma (Akhtar and Sidiki, 1979; Azzopardi et al., 1961; Mostofi, 1980; Mostofi and Price, 1973), to our knowledge, has not been described as an isolated finding in biopsy specimens. It has been seen in seminiferous tubules adjacent to invasive nonseminomatous germ cell tumors and in relation to scars of regressed testicular tumors that have metastasized. Intratubular embryonal carcinoma, like its in-

vasive component, is characterized by cells with nuclei that are larger, darker, and more irregularly shaped than those of seminoma (Fig. 22–15). The lesion frequently undergoes central necrosis, similar to the comedo necrosis often seen in intraductal carcinoma of the breast, and the necrotic material is typically eosinophilic with admixed, basophilic nuclear debris (Fig. 22–15) (Azzopardi et al., 1961). Rare examples of intratubular yolk sac tumor associated with invasive yolk sac tumor in children have been described (Teilum, 1976), and in-

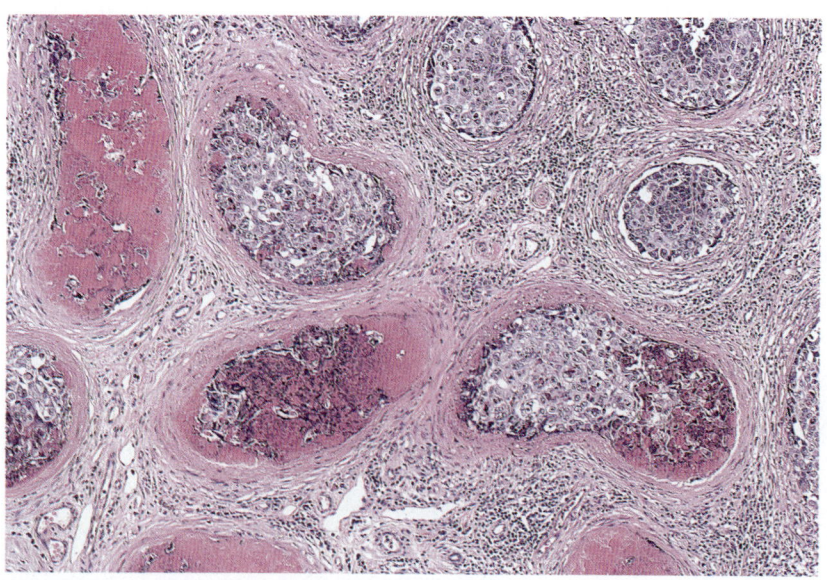

Figure 22–15. This intratubular embryonal carcinoma shows the typical eosinophilic necrotic debris admixed with degenerated nuclear fragments.

tratubular syncytiotrophoblast cells have been found with IGCNU in very infrequent cases of seminoma (Mostofi, 1980; Mostofi and Price, 1973). We are not aware of any reports of intratubular teratoma or chorio-carcinoma.

The selection of patients who should be subjected to biopsy to detect IGCNU before the development of an invasive tumor remains controversial (Herr and Sheinfeld, 1997). The three main categories of candidates are (*1*) those with current or corrected cryptorchidism; (*2*) those with a current or prior contralateral testicular germ cell tumor; and (*3*) infertile patients with azoospermia or severe oligospermia in association with testicular atrophy. Some overlap among these groups may occur. The approximate frequencies of detection of IGCNU in these groups have been presented above. Since testicular atrophy, whether in the context of cryptorchidism, infertility, or a prior testicular cancer, appears to be a significant risk factor for IGCNU (Loy and Dieckmann, 1993), restriction of biopsies to patients who have atrophy in addition to another risk factor results in a higher yield of positive biopsies (Harland et al., 1993), but there remains a significant proportion of patients at risk who do not have testicular atrophy (Loy and Dieckmann, 1993). It does not appear worthwhile to perform a biopsy on at-risk patients before the onset of puberty, since IGCNU is rarely and not always reliably recognized in such patients (Oliver, 1995), as discussed above. In that regard, one patient (Parkinson et al., 1994) had a negative biopsy at 9 years of age, but rebiopsy at the age of 16 years showed IGCNU.

The currently recommended biopsy procedure to detect IGCNU is the securement of one or two specimens 3 mm in diameter (Berthelsen and Skakkebaek, 1981), which permits detection of the great majority of lesions since they are typically multifocal (Berthelsen and Skakkebaek, 1981). In support of the effectiveness of this recommendation is the finding of a testicular germ cell tumor on follow-up examination of up to 8 years in only 1 of more than 1500 patients with infertility, cryptorchidism, or both after negative testicular biopsies (Giwercman and Skakkebaek, 1989). Also, Dieckmann and Loy (1998) reported that invasive germ cell tumors later developed in only 2 of 1858 pa-

tients with negative biopsies of testes contralateral to a germ cell tumor. In occasional cases a lesion that is less extensive than usual may be missed, however, with the recommended procedure (Mumperow et al., 1992). Intratubular germ cell neoplasia, unclassified may not be detected in sclerotic seminiferous tubules of atrophic testes but may persist near the rete testis. Nistal and co-workers (1989) therefore recommended that biopsies be directed posteriorly in such cases to avoid a false negative result.

Some authorities recommend the use of special fixatives for testicular biopsy specimens. Skakkebaek and his group, who have had the most experience with the detection of IGCNU, have used Cleland's fluid and, most recently, Stieve's fluid (formol sublimate). Preservation of immunoreactivity for the usual markers of IGCNU with the use of Cleland's fluid, however, is not consistent; 12 of 23 specimens with IGCNU that had been fixed in Cleland's fluid were negative immunohistochemically for placental-like alkaline phosphatase, whereas fixation in Stieve's fluid, Bouin's solution, and formalin gave uniformly positive results (Giwercman et al., 1991a). The use of Stieve's fluid and Bouin's solution also enabled consistent detection of IGCNU with monoclonal antibodies M2A and 43-9F, although occasional specimens were only weakly reactive (Giwercman et al., 1991a). Almost all formalin-fixed specimens were negative with these two antibodies. In our experience, usage of Bouin's solution has resulted in difficulty with placental-like alkaline phosphatase immunostaining in some cases, and thinly cut, formalin-fixed sections have been a suitable alternative. It is important to test the immunohistochemical methods on similarly processed controls before a particular fixative is selected in clinical practice.

Because of its tendency to progress to invasive germ cell tumors in a high proportion of cases, unilateral IGCNU is usually treated by orchidectomy (Giwercman et al., 1993b). There is evidence that chemotherapy for an invasive tumor can eliminate IGCNU, based on a decreased frequency of a subsequent germ cell tumor in the contralateral testis (van Basten et al., 1997). The testicular tubules provide a partial "sanctuary" for malignant germ cells because of the blood-testis barrier, however, and chemotherapy is therefore not consistently effective in the eradication of IGCNU (Bottomley et al., 1990; Christensen et al., 1998; von der Maase et al., 1988). Bilateral IGCNU is usually managed by bilateral low-dose testicular radiation, which permits preservation of Leydig cell function but causes permanent sterility (Giwercman et al., 1993b).

GONADOBLASTOMA

Gonadoblastoma is a tumor composed of germ cells, which are usually similar to those of IGCNU, seminoma, and dysgerminoma; sex cord elements consistent with immature Sertoli cells or granulosa cells; and, in approximately two-thirds of cases, cells of Leydig or lutein type that lack Reinke crystals (Scully, 1970, 1981).

These tumors are exceptionally rare in otherwise normal testes but occur typically in patients with gonadal dysgenesis. Eighty percent of the patients are phenotypic females, who usually have some degree of virilization, and the remainder are phenotypic males, who almost always have hypospadias, cryptorchidism, and some development of müllerian duct derivatives; gynecomastia is often present as well. On cytogenetic study, patients with gonadoblastoma almost always have either a 46,XY, 45,XO/46,XY, or another form of mosaic karyotype containing a Y chromosome. The phenotypic males in whom gonadoblastoma develops are considered to have dysgenetic male pseudohermaphroditism or mixed gonadal dysgenesis, both of which are now classified as the same disorder by most investigators (Rajfer and Walsh, 1981; Robboy et al., 1982). The confinement of gonadoblastomas to patients with a Y chromosome in almost all cases has led to a search for a gonadoblastoma gene or genes on this chromosome. Iezzoni et al. (1997), using fluorescence *in situ* hybridization in studying three gonadoblastomas from patients with 45,X/46,XY mosaicism, found that a high proportion of tumor nuclei were positive for a Y chromosome compared to the nuclei of non-neoplastic stromal cells. Genetic mapping investigations have defined a "susceptibility" locus containing a putative gonadoblastoma gene or genes near the centromere of the Y chro-

mosome (Salo et al., 1995; Tsuchiya et al., 1995).

Gross examination of a gonadoblastoma reveals a discrete, soft to firm nodule with the consistency depending on the presence or absence of calcification, and its extent, if present. In cases with marked calcification, radiographs may permit visualization of the tumor clinically. In about 20% of cases a streak gonad with ovarian-type stroma can be identified microscopically adjacent to the tumor, and, in a similar proportion of cases, a remnant of dysgenetic testis is encountered. If an invasive germ cell tumor has developed (see below) the gross appearance may reflect its presence; the tumor is usually soft, fleshy, and gray–white if it is a germinoma.

On microscopic examination the germ cells and sex cord cells are generally enclosed within discrete nests surrounded by basement membranes (Fig. 22–16) and are arranged in one or more of three distinctive patterns. The germ cells may form the center of a nest with a peripheral, single-file arrangement of sex cord cells, or the sex cord cells may form a mantle around the germ cells, similar to the corona of immature granulosa cells that surround primordial ova. In addition, the sex cord cells may envelop rounded, hyaline masses composed of basement membrane material that is focally continuous with the basement membrane at the periphery of the nests (Fig. 22–17). Sometimes these hyaline masses coalesce, and laminated calcific deposits within them may merge to form complex, mulberry-shaped calcifications (Fig. 22–18). In about half the cases, the germ cells penetrate the peripheral basement membranes of the nests and invade the adjacent stroma to form a germinoma (Fig. 22–18). In less than 10% of cases, the germ cells differentiate into an invasive non-germinomatous tumor, usually of a higher degree of malignancy than germinoma. A very rare gonadoblastoma contains, in addition to the typical patterns, areas with a more diffuse arrangement of intermixed germ cells and sex cord elements more characteristic of the unclassified form of mixed germ cell–sex cord–stromal tumor (see below; Colafranceschi and Massi, 1995).

Some gonadoblastomas may be clearly intratubular without distortion of testicular architecture, but even when they grow to form

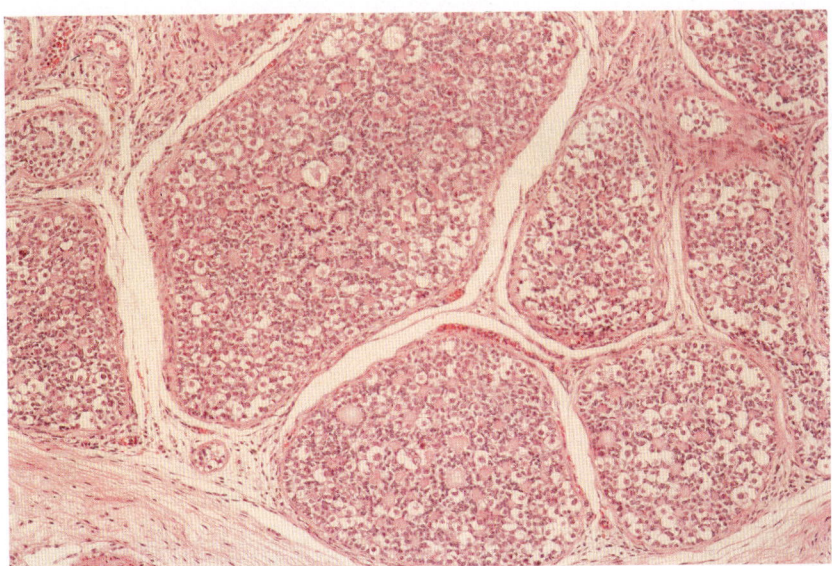

Figure 22–16. Multiple nests of germ cells and sex cord cells comprise this typical gonadoblastoma. Note the hyaline cylinders of basement membrane material.

confluent masses of germ cells and sex cord elements, they appear to retain the characteristics of an *in situ* or premalignant lesion. They do not metastasize in the form of gonadoblastoma, although we have seen an "implant" of gonadoblastoma in the *cul de sac* several months after a biopsy of the primary tumor had been performed, and a sub-serosal uterine implant was described in a case having features of both gonadoblastoma and unclassified mixed germ cell–sex cord–stromal tumor (Colafranceschi and Massi, 1995). The precancerous nature of gonadoblastoma is evidenced by its strong association with invasive germ cell tumors, which are usually discovered synchronously,

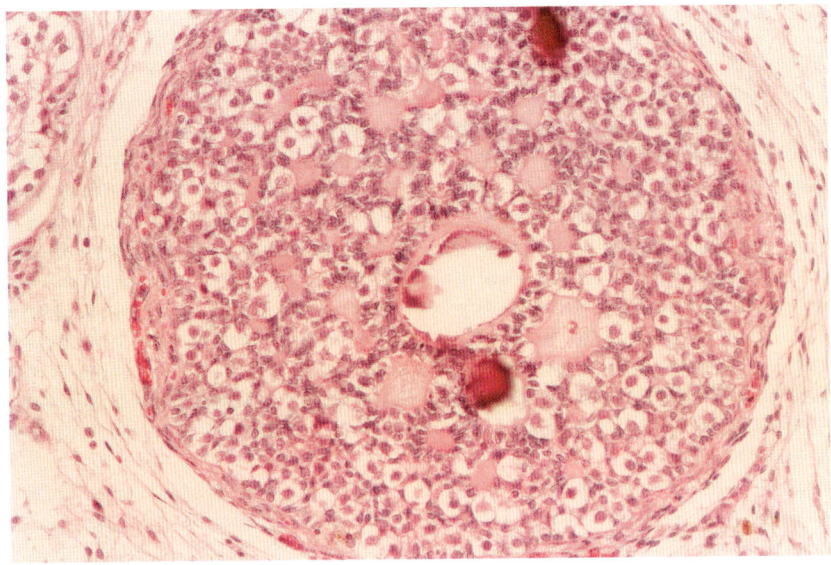

Figure 22–17. This nest of gonadoblastoma shows the germ cells surrounded by sex cord cells, hyaline basement membrane deposits, and focal calcifications.

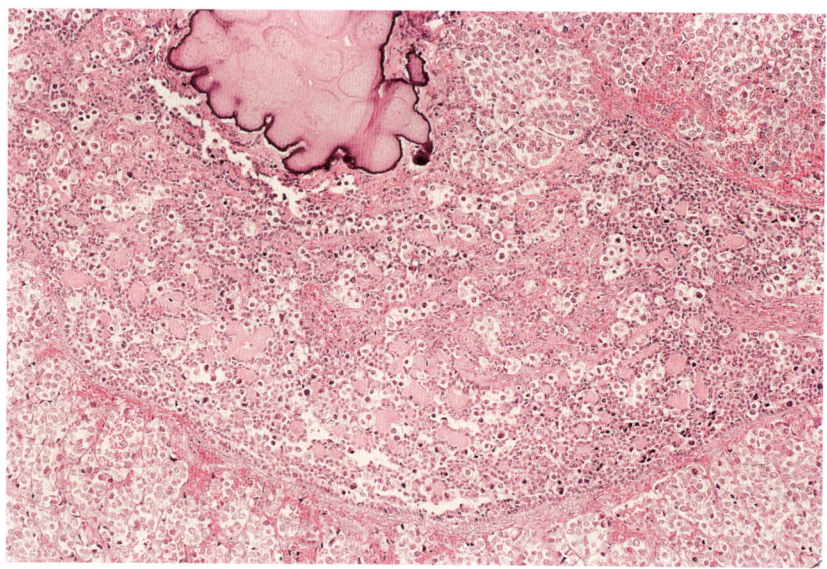

Figure 22–18. An area of gonadoblastoma with a mulberry-shaped calcification is seen in the upper portion of this illustration, with an associated germinoma at the bottom.

although in an occasional case an invasive germ cell tumor occurs in a conserved contralateral gonad after the excision of an apparently unilateral gonadoblastoma. The atypical germ cell component of gonadoblastomas typically exhibits all of the morphological and immunohistochemical characteristics of IGCNU and, like IGCNU, has an aneuploid DNA content (Jørgensen et al., 1997). The absence of immunohistochemical staining for the typical markers of IGCNU in a portion of the germ cells of some gonadoblastomas, however, provides evidence for a non-neoplastic germ cell population in at least some cases and a heterogeneous germ cell component in gonadoblastomas (Jørgensen et al., 1997). Inhibin marks the sex cord cells of gonadoblastoma (Hussong et al., 1997; Kommoss et al., 1998), and the product of the Wilms' tumor gene (WT1) has also been identified in the sex cord cells in one study (Hussong et al., 1997).

Three lesions may be confused with gonadoblastoma. One is the extremely rare mixed germ cell–sex cord–stromal tumor, unclassified (Bolen, 1981; Matoska and Talerman, 1989; Talerman, 1980b). It is composed of a mixture of germ cells that are usually more mature in appearance than those of gonadoblastoma and sex cord elements that are generally admixed within a diffuse

pattern of growth but occasionally in a cord-like or solid tubular pattern. Hyaline bodies and calcification are rarely present, and the patients do not exhibit abnormal sexual development. Some of these cases may be sex cord–stromal tumors that have entrapped spermatogonia, and may not be true mixed tumors of germ cell–sex cord type (Ulbright et al., 1999). One must also be careful not to confuse scattered nonspecific large cells with clear or pale cytoplasm with the germ cells of a mixed germ cell–sex cord stromal tumor or gonadoblastoma; such cells are not uniformly or regularly distributed throughout the tumor as in many cases of the latter two tumors. A second neoplasm that may mimic gonadoblastoma is the sex cord tumor with annular tubules, but this tumor is exceptionally rare in the testis and contains no germ cells. Clusters of small tubules lined by immature Sertoli cells (Sertoli cell nodules) (Hedinger et al., 1967; Stalker and Hendry, 1952) are relatively frequent in cryptorchid testes and may be encountered in descended testes as well. These lesions may contain hyaline bodies and resemble gonadoblastoma, but they generally lack germ cells. Rarely, they contain occasional spermatogonia or, in cases with a coexistent germ cell tumor, may become populated by IGCNU (Fig. 22–19). Unlike gonadoblastoma, however, Sertoli cell nodules are almost invariably incidental mi-

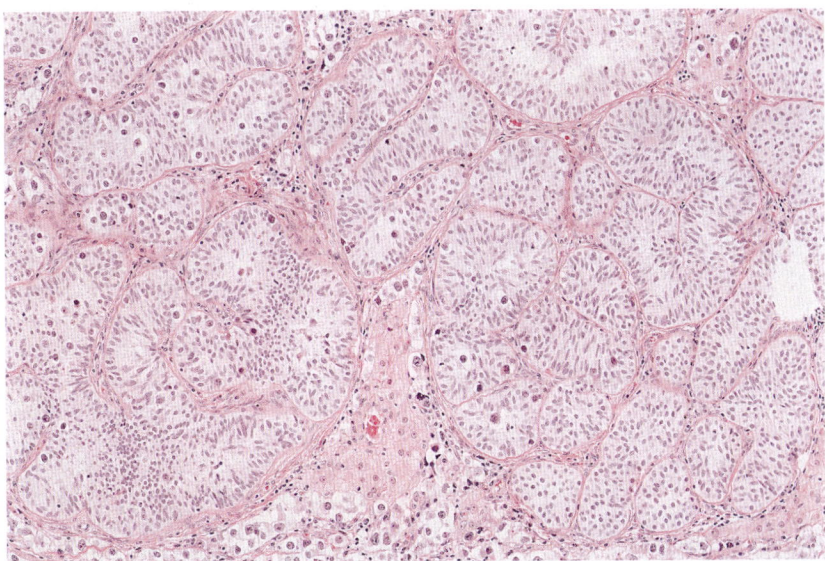

Figure 22–19. A Sertoli cell nodule in a patient with a seminoma has been colonized by IGCNU cells. This may mimic a gonadoblastoma, but the germ cells have a patchy distribution.

croscopic findings and have not been reported in dysgenetic gonads; when they are populated by IGCNU, the atypical germ cells may have a more patchy distribution than in gonadoblastoma (Fig. 22–19).

INTRATUBULAR SERTOLI CELL AND GRANULOSA CELL NEOPLASIA

It is logical to assume that an intratubular growth phase must precede the develop-

ment of invasive Sertoli cell tumors, but no studies are available concerning exclusively intratubular neoplasia of Sertoli cells. We have seen one case of an apparently intratubular Sertoli cell tumor that was an incidental finding in an orchiectomy specimen. It consisted of a circumscribed area of expanded seminiferous tubules that were filled with Sertoli cells (Fig. 22–20). An intratubular component is also a relatively common finding within the large cell calcifying variant of Sertoli cell tumor (Proppe and Scully, 1980) which, although usually be-

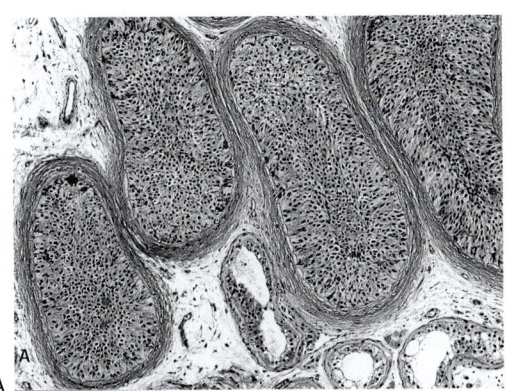
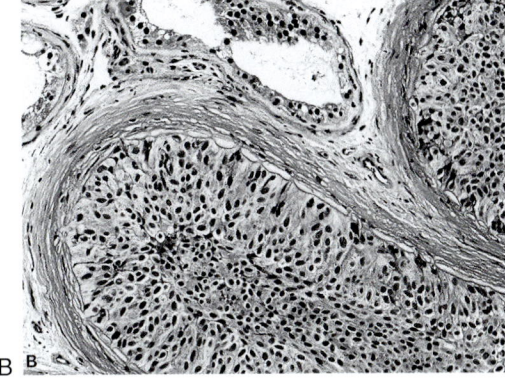

Figure 22–20. *A*: An intratubular Sertoli cell tumor, not otherwise specified, distends several seminiferous tubules. This case lacked an invasive Sertoli cell tumor component. *B*: Higher magnification shows the uniform proliferation of Sertoli cells in the expanded tubules.

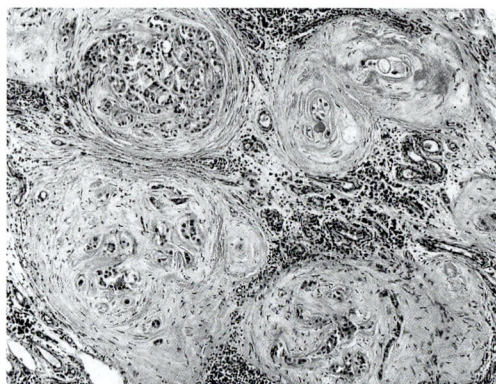

Figure 22–21. Intratubular Sertoli cell tumor of the large cell calcifying type. Note the prominent peritubular sclerosis. This area occurred at the periphery of an invasive tumor.

tratubular component in these cases has shown the characteristic large cells with abundant, eosinophilic cytoplasm, often with laminated calcifications, in expanded seminiferous tubules that frequently show peripheral sclerosis (Fig. 22–21). Patients with the Peutz-Jeghers syndrome may have intratubular as well as infiltrative nodules of Sertoli cell neoplasia, which may be associated with estrogenic manifestations (Ros et al., 1999). These tumors are composed of large cells resembling those of the large cell calcifying Sertoli cell tumor but tend to be associated with less prominent calcification (Fig. 22–22); they also resemble to some extent the sex cord tumor with annular tubules that occurs in the ovary of patients with the Peutz-Jeghers syndrome. In addition, an intratubular component was identified in all 10 examples of sclerosing Sertoli cell tumor reported by Zukerberg et al. (1991). They closely resembled the "foci of immature tubules" or "Sertoli cell nodules" that are commonly identified in cryptorchid testes. One of these 10 tumors was histologically malignant, although it did not metastasize during a limited period of follow-up.

nign, may exhibit malignant pathologic features and metastasize in a minority of cases (Kratzer et al., 1997). One of the originally reported cases was an exclusively intratubular tumor that occurred in the testis of a patient with the androgen insensitivity syndrome (Proppe and Scully, 1980). The in-

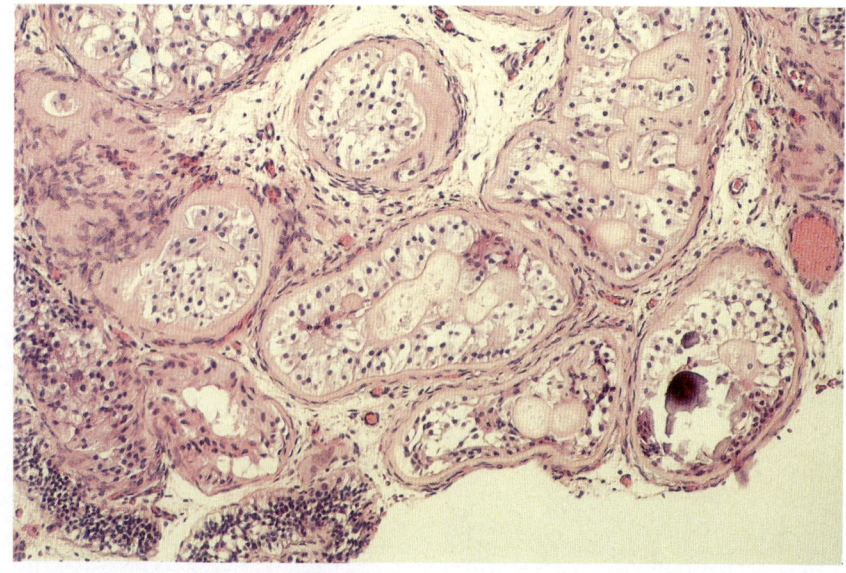

Figure 22–22. Intratubular Sertoli cell neoplasia in a patient with the Peutz-Jeghers syndrome. There are overlapping features with the large cell calcifying Sertoli cell tumor and the sex cord tumor with annular tubules, as seen in the ovary.

REFERENCES

Abell MR, Holtz F. (1968) Testicular and paratesticular neoplasms in patients 60 years of age and older. *Cancer* 21: 852–870.

Aitchison M, Mufti GR, Farrell J, Paterson PJ, et al. (1990) Granulomatous orchitis: review of 15 cases. *Br J Urol* 66:312–314.

Akhtar M, Sidiki Y. (1979) Undifferentiated intratubular germ cell tumor of the testis: light and electron microscopic study of a unique case. *Cancer* 43:2332–2339.

Albrechtsen R, Nielsen MH, Skakkebaek NE, Wewer U. (1982) Carcinoma *in situ* of the testis. Some ultrastructural characteristics of germ cells. *Acta Pathol Microbiol Immunol Scand* [A] 90:301–303.

Andres TL, Trainer TD, Leadbetter GW. (1980) Atypical germ cells preceding metachronous bilateral testicular tumors. *Urology* 15:307–309.

Aneiros J, Zuluaga A, Lopez M, Caracuel M, Gomez M. (1987) Atypical germ cells in prepubertal cryptorchid testes. *Br J Urol* 60:258–260.

Azzopardi JG, Hoffbrand AV. (1965) Retrogression in testicular seminoma with viable metastases. *J Clin Pathol* 18:135–141.

Azzopardi JG, Mostofi FK, Theiss EA. (1961) Lesions of testes observed in certain patients with widespread choriocarcinoma and related tumors. *Am J Pathol* 38:207–225.

Bailey D, Baumal R, Law J, et al. (1986) Production of monoclonal antibody specific for seminomas and dysgerminomas. *Proc Natl Acad Sci USA* 83:5291–5295.

Bailey D, Marks A, Stratis M, Baumal R. (1991) Immunohistochemical staining of germ cell tumors and intratubular malignant germ cells of the testis using antibody to placental alkaline phosphatase and a monoclonal anti-seminoma antibody. *Mod Pathol* 4:167–171.

Berthelsen JG, Skakkebaek NE. (1981) Value of testicular biopsy in diagnosing carcinoma *in situ* testis. *Scand J Urol Nephrol* 15:165–168.

Berthelsen JG, Skakkebaek NE, von der Maase H, Sorensen BL, et al. (1982) Screening for carcinoma *in situ* of the contralateral testis in patients with germinal testicular cancer. *BMJ* 285:1683–1686.

Bolen JW. (1981) Mixed germ cell–sex cord stromal tumor. A gonadal tumor distinct from gonadoblastoma. *Am J Clin Pathol* 75:565–573.

Bottomley D, Fisher C, Hendry WF, Horwich A. (1990) Persistent carcinoma *in situ* of the testis after chemotherapy for advanced testicular germ cell tumours. *Br J Urol* 66:420–424.

Burke AP, Mostofi FK. (1988a) Placental alkaline phosphatase immunohistochemistry of intratubular malignant germ cells and associated testicular germ cell tumors. *Hum Pathol* 19:663–670.

Burke AP, Mostofi FK. (1988b) Intratubular malignant germ cells in testicular biopsies: clinical course and identification by staining for placental alkaline phosphatase. *Mod Pathol* 1:475–479.

Chen KT, Cheng AC. (1989) Retroperitoneal seminoma and intratubular germ cell neoplasia. *Hum Pathol* 20:493–495.

Christensen TB, Daugaard G, Geertsen PF, von der Maase H. (1998) Effect of chemotherapy on carcinoma *in situ* of the testis. *Ann Oncol* 9:657–660.

Coffin CM, Ewing S, Dehner LP. (1985) Frequency of intratubular germ cell neoplasia with invasive testicular germ cell tumors. Histologic and immunocytochemical features. *Arch Pathol Lab Med* 109:555–559.

Colafranceschi M, Massi D. (1995) Gonadoblastoma with coexistent features of mixed germ cell–sex cord stroma tumor: a case report. *Tumori* 81:215–218.

Cortes D, Thorup J, Frisch M, Moller H, et al. (1994) Examination for intratubular germ cell neoplasia at operation for undescended testis in boys. *J Urol* 151:722–725.

Daugaard G, von der Maase H, Olsen J, Rorth M, et al. (1987) Carcinoma-*in-situ* testis in patients with assumed extragonadal germ-cell tumours. *Lancet* 2:528–530.

de Graaff WE, Oosterhuis JW, de Jong B, Dam A, et al. (1992) Ploidy of testicular carcinoma *in situ*. *Lab Invest* 66:166–168.

de Jong B, Oosterhuis JW, Castedo SM, Vos A, et al. (1990) Pathogenesis of adult testicular germ cell tumors. A cytogenetic model. *Cancer Genet Cytogenet* 48:143–167.

Delahunt B, Mostofi FK, Sesterhenn IA, Ribas JL, et al. (1990) Nucleolar organizer regions in seminoma and intratubular malignant germ cells. *Mod Pathol* 3:141–145.

Dieckmann KP, Loy V, Buttner P. (1993) Prevalence of bilateral testicular germ cell tumours and early detection based on contralateral testicular intraepithelial neoplasia. *Br J Urol* 71:340–345.

Dieckmann K-P, Loy V. (1998) The value of the biopsy of the contralateral testis in patients with testicular germ cell cancer: the recent German experience. *APMIS* 106:13–23.

Dorman S, Trainer TD, Lefke D, Leadbetter G. (1979) Incipient germ cell neoplasia in a cryptorchid testis. *Cancer* 44:1357–1362.

Ferreiro JA. (1994) Ber-H2 expression in testicular germ cell tumors. *Hum Pathol* 25:522–524.

Ferry JA, Ulbright TM, Young RH. (1997) Anaplastic large cell lymphoma presenting in the testis. *J Urol Pathol* 5:139–147.

Gillis AJ, Looijenga LH, de Jong B, Oosterhuis JW. (1994) Clonality of combined testicular germ cell tumors of adults. *Lab Invest* 71:874–878.

Giwercman A, Andrews PW, Jørgensen N, Müller J, et al. (1993a) Immunohistochemical expression of embryonal marker TRA-1-60 in carcinoma *in situ* and germ cell tumors of the testis. *Cancer* 72:1308–1314.

Giwercman A, Bruun E, Frimodt-Moller C, Skakkebaek NE. (1989) Prevalence of carcinoma-*in-situ* and other histopathologic abnormalities in testes of men with a history of cryptorchidism. *J Urol* 142:998–1002.

Giwercman A, Cantell L, Marks A. (1991a) Placental-like alkaline phosphatase as a marker of carcinoma-*in-situ* of the testis: comparison with monoclonal antibodies M2A and 43-9F. *APMIS* 99:586–594.

Giwercman A, Lindenberg S, Kimber SJ, Andersson T, et al. (1990) Monoclonal antibody 43-9F as a sensitive immunohistochemical marker of carcinoma *in situ* of human testis. *Cancer* 65:1135–1142.

Giwercman A, Marks A, Bailey D, Baumal R, et al. (1988a) M2A—a monoclonal antibody as a marker for carcinoma-*in-situ* germ cells of the human adult testis. *Acta Pathol Microbiol Immunol Scand* [A] 96:667–670.

Giwercman A, Müller J, Skakkebaek NE. (1988b) Carcinoma *in situ* of the undescended testis. *Semin Urol* 6:110–119.

Giwercman A, Müller J, Skakkebaek NE. (1991b) Prevalence of carcinoma *in situ* and other histopathological abnormalities in testes from 399 men who died suddenly and unexpectedly. *J Urol* 145:77–80.

Giwercman A, Skakkebaek NE. (1989) Carcinoma-*in-situ* (gonocytoma-*in-situ*) of the testis. In: *The Testis* (Burger H, de Kretser, D, eds.) pp. 475–491. Raven Press, New York.

Giwercman A, Thomsen JK, Hertz J, Berthelsen JG, et al. (1997) Prevalence of carcinoma *in situ* of the testis in 207 oligozoospermic men from infertile couples: prospective study of testicular biopsies. *BMJ* 315:989–991.

Giwercman A, von der Maase H, Skakkebaek NE. (1993b) Epidemiological and clinical aspects of carcinoma *in situ* of the testis. *Eur Urol* 23:104–10.

Gondos B. (1993) Ultrastructure of developing and malignant germ cells. *Eur Urol* 23:68–74.

Gondos B, Berthelsen JG, Skakkebaek NE. (1983) Intratubular germ cell neoplasia (carcinoma *in situ*): a preinvasive lesion of the testis. *Ann Clin Lab Sci* 13:185–192.

Gowing NFC. (1976) Malignant lymphoma of the testis. In: *Pathology of the testis* (Pugh, RCB, ed.) pp. 334–355. Blackwell Scientific, Oxford.

Guinand S, Hedinger C. (1981) Cellules germinales atypiques intratubulaires et tumeurs germinales testiculaires de l'enfant. *Ann Pathol* 1:251–257.

Hailemariam S, Engeler DS, Bannwart F, Amin MB. (1997) Primary mediastinal germ cell tumor with intratubular germ cell neoplasia of the testis—further support for germ cell origin of these tumors: a case report. *Cancer* 79:1031–1036.

Hailemariam S, Engeler DS, Bannwart F, et al. (1998) Significance of intratubular germ cell neoplasia (ITGCN) in prepubertal testes of patients with cryptorchidism (CO): correlation with clinical reappraisal after two decades. *Mod Pathol* 11:84A.

Harland SJ, Cook PA, Fossa SD, et al. (1993) Risk factors for carcinoma *in situ* of the contralateral testis in patients with testicular cancer. An interim report. *Eur Urol* 23:115–8.

Hawkins E, Heifetz SA, Giller R, Cushing B. (1997) The prepubertal testis (prenatal and postnatal): its relationship to intratubular germ cell neoplasia: a combined Pediatric Oncology Group and Children's Cancer Study Group. *Hum Pathol* 28:404–410.

Hedinger CE, Huber R, Weber E. (1967) Frequency of so-called hypoplastic or dysgenetic zones in scrotal and otherwise normal human testes. *Virchows Arch A Pathol Anat Histopathol* 342:165–168.

Herr HW, Sheinfeld J. (1997) Is biopsy of the contralateral testis necessary in patients with germ cell tumors? *J Urol* 158:1331–1334.

Hiraoka N, Yamada T, Abe H, Hata J. (1997) Establishment of three monoclonal antibodies specific for prespermatogonia and intratubular malignant germ cells in humans. *Lab Invest* 76:427–438.

Hu LM, Phillipson J, Barsky SH. (1992) Intratubular germ cell neoplasia in infantile yolk sac tumor. Verification by tandem repeat sequence *in situ* hybridization. *Diagn Mol Pathol* 1:118–128.

Hussong J, Crussi FG, Chou PM. (1997) Gonadoblastoma: an immunohistochemical localization of mul-lerian-inhibiting substance, inhibin, WT-1 and p53. *Mod Pathol* 10:1101–1105.

Iezzoni JC, von Kap-Herr C, Golden WL, Gaffey MJ. (1997) Gonadoblastomas in 45,X/46,XY mosaicism: analysis of chromosome distribution by fluorescence *in situ* hybridization. *Am J Clin Pathol* 108:197–201.

Jacobsen GK, Henriksen OB, von der Maase H. (1981) Carcinoma *in situ* of testicular tissue adjacent to malignant germ-cell tumors: a study of 105 cases. *Cancer* 47:2660–2662.

Jacobsen GK, Jacobsen M, Praetorius C. (1980) Ferritin as a possible marker protein of carcinoma-*in-situ* of the testis. *Lancet* 2:533–534.

Jacobsen GK, Norgaard-Pedersen B. (1984) Placental alkaline phosphatase in testicular germ cell tumours and carcinoma-*in-situ* of the testis: an immunohistochemical study. *Acta Pathol Microbiol Immunol Scand [A]* 92:323–329.

Jørgensen N, Giwercman A, Müller J, Skakkebaek NE. (1993) Immunohistochemical markers of carcinoma *in situ* of the testis also expressed in normal infantile germ cells. *Histopathology* 22:373–378.

Jørgensen N, Müller J, Giwercman A, Visfeldt J, et al. (1995) DNA content and expression of tumour markers in germ cells adjacent to germ cell tumours in childhood: probably a different origin for infantile and adolescent germ cell tumours. *J Pathol* 176:269–278.

Jørgensen N, Müller J, Jaubert F, Clausen OP, et al. (1997) Heterogeneity of gonadoblastoma germ cells: similarities with immature germ cells, spermatogonia and testicular carcinoma *in situ* cells. *Histopathology* 30:177–186.

Klein FA, Melamed MR, Whitmore WF Jr. (1985) Intratubular malignant germ cells (carcinoma *in situ*) accompanying invasive testicular germ cell tumors. *J Urol* 133:413–415.

Klys HS, Whillis D, Howard G, Harrison DJ. (1992) Glutathione S-transferase expression in the human testis and testicular germ cell neoplasia. *Br J Cancer* 66:589–593.

Koide O, Iwai S, Baba K, Iri H. (1987) Identification of testicular atypical germ cells by an immunohistochemical technique for placental alkaline phosphatase. *Cancer* 60:1325–1330.

Kommoss F, Oliva E, Bhan A, Young RH, et al. (1998) Inhibin expression in ovarian tumors and tumor-like lesions: an immunohistochemical study. *Mod Pathol* 11:656–664.

Kratzer SS, Ulbright TM, Talerman A, Srigley JR, et al. (1997) Large cell calcifying Sertoli cell tumor of the testis: contrasting features of six malignant and six benign tumors and a review of the literature. *Am J Surg Pathol* 21:1271–1280.

Lee AH, Theaker JM. (1994) Pagetoid spread into the rete testis by testicular tumours. *Histopathology* 24:385–389.

Loftus BM, Gilmartin LG, O'Brien MJ, et al. (1990) Intratubular germ cell neoplasia of the testis: identification by placental alkaline phosphatase immunostaining and argyrophilic nucleolar organizer region quantification. *Hum Pathol* 21:941–948.

Looijenga LH, Gillis AJ, Van Putten WL, Oosterhuis JW. (1993) *In situ* numeric analysis of centromeric regions of chromosomes 1, 12, and 15 of seminomas, nonseminomatous germ cell tumors, and carcinoma *in situ* of human testis. *Lab Invest* 68:211–219.

Loy V, Dieckmann KP. (1993) Prevalence of contralateral testicular intraepithelial neoplasia (carcinoma in situ) in patients with testicular germ cell tumour. Results of the German multicentre study. Eur Urol 23:120–122.

Lynch VP, Eakins D, Morrison E. (1968) Granulomatous orchitis. Br J Urol 40:451–458.

MacMahon RA, Cussen LJ. (1991) Detection of gonadal carcinoma in situ in childhood and implications for management. Aust N Z J Surg 61:667–669.

Malmi R, Söderström KO. (1991) Lectin histochemistry of embryonal carcinoma. APMIS 99:233–243.

Manivel JC, Reinberg Y, Niehans GA, Fraley EE. (1989) Intratubular germ cell neoplasia in testicular teratomas and epidermoid cysts. Correlation with prognosis and possible biologic significance. Cancer 64:715–720.

Manivel JC, Simonton S, Wold SE, Dehner LP. (1988) Absence of intratubular germ cell neoplasia in testicular yolk sac tumors in children. Arch Pathol Lab Med 112:641–645.

Manuel M, Katayama KP, Jones HW. (1976) The age of occurrence of gonadal tumors in intersex patients. Am J Obstet Gynecol 124:293–306.

Mark GJ, Hedinger C. (1965) Changes in remaining tumor-free testicular tissue in cases of seminoma and teratoma. Virchows Arch A Pathol Anat Histopathol 340:84–92.

Massod CA, Cohen MB, Kogan BA, Beckstead JH. (1991) Morphology and histochemistry of infant testes in the prune belly syndrome. J Urol 146:1598–1600.

Masson P. (1946) Étude sur le sèminome. Rev Can Biol 5:361–387.

Matoska J, Talerman A. (1989) Mixed germ cell–sex cord stroma tumor of the testis. A report with ultrastructural findings. Cancer 64:2146–2153.

Morgan AD. (1976) Inflammation and infestation of the testis and paratesticular structures. In: Pathology of the Testis (Pugh RCB, ed.) pp. 79–138. Blackwell Scientific, Oxford.

Mosselman S, Looijenga LH, Gillis AJ, van Rooijen MA, et al. (1996) Aberrant platelet-derived growth factor alpha-receptor transcript as a diagnostic marker for early human germ cell tumors of the adult testis. Proc Natl Acad Sci USA 93:2884–2888.

Mostofi FK. (1980) Pathology of germ cell tumors of testis: a progress report. Cancer 45:1735–1754.

Mostofi FK, Price EB Jr. (1973) Tumors of the Male Genital System. Atlas of Tumor Pathology, 2nd Series, Fascicle 8. Armed Forces Institute of Pathology, Washington D.C.

Mosunjac MB, Mosunjac MI, DeRose PB, Lawson D, Cohen C. (1998) Image cytometric analysis of DNA ploidy and proliferation marker MIB-1 in intratubular germ cell neoplasia and adjacent testicular germ cell tumor. J Urol Pathol 9:197–210.

Müller J, Skakkebaek NE. (1984) Testicular carcinoma in situ in children with the androgen insensitivity (testicular feminisation) syndrome. BMJ 288:1419–1420.

Müller J, Skakkebaek NE, Lundsteen C. (1981) Aneuploidy as a marker for carcinoma-in-situ of the testis. Acta Pathol Microbiol Scand [A] 89:67–68.

Müller J, Skakkebaek NE, Nielsen OH, Graem N. (1984) Cryptorchidism and testis cancer. Atypical infantile germ cells followed by carcinoma in situ

and invasive carcinoma in adulthood. Cancer 54:629–634.

Müller J, Skakkebaek NE, Parkinson MC. (1987) The spermatocytic seminoma: views on pathogenesis. Int J Androl 10:147–156.

Müller J, Skakkebaek NE, Ritzén M, Plöen L, et al. (1985) Carcinoma in situ of the testis in children with 45,X/46,XY gonadal dysgenesis. J Pediatr 106:431–436.

Müller M, Lauke H, Hartmann M. (1994) The value of the AgNOR staining method in identifying carcinoma in situ testis. Pathol Res Pract 190:429–435.

Mumperow E, Lauke H, Holstein AF, Hartmann M. (1992) Further practical experiences in the recognition and management of carcinoma in situ of the testis. Urol Int 48:162–166.

Niehans GA, Manivel JC, Copland GT, Scheithauer BW, et al. (1988) Immunohistochemistry of germ cell and trophoblastic neoplasms. Cancer 62:1113–1123.

Nielsen H, Nielsen M, Skakkebaek NE. (1974) The fine structure of possible carcinoma-in-situ in the seminiferous tubules in the testis of four infertile men. Acta Pathol Microbiol Scand [A] 82:235–248.

Nistal M, Codesal J, Paniagua R. (1989) Carcinoma in situ of the testis in infertile men. A histological, immunocytochemical, and cytophotometric study of DNA content. J Pathol 159:205–210.

Nogales FF Jr, Toro M, Ortega I, Fulwood HR. (1981) Bilateral incipient germ cell tumours of the testis in the incomplete testicular feminization syndrome. Histopathology 5:511–515.

Oliver RT. (1995) Germ cell cancer of the testes. Curr Opin Oncol 7:292–296.

Oosterhuis JW, Gillis AJ, van Putten WJ, de Jong B, et al. (1993) Interphase cytogenetics of carcinoma in situ of the testis. Numeric analysis of the chromosomes 1, 12 and 15. Eur Urol 23:16–21.

Parkinson MC, Swerdlow AJ, Pike MC. (1994) Carcinoma in situ in boys with cryptorchidism: when can it be detected? Br J Urol 73:431–435.

Perry A, Wiley EL, Albores-Saavedra J. (1994) Pagetoid spread of intratubular germ cell neoplasia into rete testis: a morphologic and immunohistochemical study of 100 orchiectomy specimens with invasive germ cell tumors. Hum Pathol 25:235–239.

Proppe KH, Scully RE. (1980) Large-cell calcifying Sertoli cell tumor of the testis. Am J Clin Pathol 74:607–619.

Pryor JP, Cameron KM, Chilton CP, et al. (1983) Carcinoma in situ in testicular biopsies in men presenting with infertility. Br J Urol 55:780–784.

Rajfer J, Walsh PC. (1981) Mixed gonadal dysgenesis—dysgenetic male pseudohermaphroditism. In: Pediatric Adolescent Endocrinology, Vol. 8: The Intersex Child, pp. 105–115. S. Krager, Basel.

Ramani P, Yeung CK, Habeebu SSM. (1993) Testicular intratubular germ cell neoplasia in children and adolescents with intersex. Am J Surg Pathol 17:1124–1133.

Renedo DE, Trainer TD. (1994) Intratubular germ cell neoplasia (ITGCN) with p53 and PCNA expression and adjacent mature teratoma in an infant testis. An immunohistochemical and morphologic study with a review of the literature. Am J Surg Pathol 18:947–952.

Robboy SJ, Miller T, Donahoe PK, Jahre C, et al. (1982) Dysgenesis of testicular and streak gonads in the syndrome of mixed gonadal dysgenesis. Perspective derived from a clinicopathologic analysis of twenty-one cases. *Hum Pathol* 13:700–716.

Ros P, Nistal M, Alonso M, Calvo de Mora J, et al. (1999) Sertoli cell tumour in a boy with Peutz-Jeghers syndrome. *Histopathology* 34:84–86.

Rosai J, Silber I, Khodadoust K. (1969) Spermatocytic seminoma. I. Clinicopathologic study of six cases and review of the literature. *Cancer* 24:92–102.

Rutgers JL, Scully RE. (1991) The androgen insensitivity syndrome (testicular feminization): a clinicopathologic study of 43 cases. *Int J Gynecol Pathol* 10: 126–145.

Salo P, Kaariainen H, Petrovic V, Peltomaki P, et al. (1995) Molecular mapping of the putative gonadoblastoma locus on the Y chromosome. *Genes Chromosome Cancer* 14:210–214.

Scheiber K, Ackermann D, Studer UE. (1987) Bilateral testicular germ cell tumors: a report of 20 cases. *J Urol* 138:73–76.

Schulze C, Holstein AF. (1977) On the histology of human seminoma: development of the solid tumor from intratubular seminoma cells. *Cancer* 39:1090–1100.

Scully RE. (1961) Spermatocytic seminoma of the testis: a report of 3 cases and review of the literature. *Cancer* 14:788–794.

Scully RE. (1970) Gonadoblastoma. A review of 74 cases. *Cancer* 25:1340–1356.

Scully RE. (1981). Neoplasia associated with anomalous sexual development and abnormal sex chromosomes. In: *Pediatric Adolescent Endocrinology: Vol. 8: The Intersex Child,* pp. 203–217. S. Karger, Basel.

Scully RE. (1982) Intratubular germ cell neoplasia (carcinoma *in situ*): what it is and what should be done about it. Lesson 17. In: *World Urology Update Series,* Vol. I (Fraley EE, ed.) pp. 1–8. Continuing Professional Education Center, Princeton.

Sigg C, Hedinger C. (1980) Keimzelltumoren des Hodens und atypische Keimzellen. *Schweiz Med Wochenschr* 110:801–806.

Sigg C, Hedinger C. (1981) Atypical germ cells in testicular biopsy in male sterility. *Int J Androl* 4 (Suppl): 163–171.

Sigg C, Hedinger C. (1984) Atypical germ cells of the testis. Comparative ultrastructural and immunohistochemical investigations. *Virchows Arch A Pathol. Anat Histopathol* 402:439–450.

Skakkebaek NE. (1972a) Possible carcinoma-*in-situ* of the undescended testis. *Lancet* 2:516–517.

Skakkebaek NE. (1972b) Abnormal morphology of germ cells in two infertile men. *Acta Pathol Microbiol Scand [A]* 80:374–378.

Skakkebaek NE. (1975) Atypical germ cells in the adjacent "normal" tissue of testicular tumours. *Acta Pathol Microbiol Scand [A]* 83:127–130.

Skakkebaek NE. (1978) Carcinoma *in situ* of the testis: frequency and relationship to invasive germ cell tumours in infertile men. *Histopathology* 2:157–170.

Skakkebaek NE. (1979) Carcinoma *in situ* of the testis in testicular feminization syndrome. *Acta Pathol Microbiol Scand [A]* 87:87–89.

Skakkebaek NE, Berthelsen JG, Giwercman A, Müller J. (1987) Carcinoma-*in-situ* of the testis: possible origin from gonocytes and precursor of all types of germ cell tumours except spermatocytoma. *Int J Androl* 10:19–28.

Skakkebaek NE, Berthelsen JG, Müller J. (1982) Carcinoma-*in-situ* of the undescended testis. *Urol Clin North Am* 9:377–385.

Skakkebaek NE, Berthelsen JG, Visfeldt J. (1981) Clinical aspects of testicular carcinoma-*in-situ. Int J Androl* 4(Suppl):153–162.

Soosay GN, Bobrow L, Happerfield L, Parkinson MC. (1991) Morphology and immunohistochemistry of carcinoma *in situ* adjacent to testicular germ cell tumors in adults and children: implications for histogenesis. *Histopathology* 19:537–544.

Stalker AL, Hendry WT. (1952) Hyperplasia and neoplasia of the Sertoli cell. *J Pathol Bacteriol* 64:161–168.

Stamp IM, Barlebo H, Rix M, Jacobsen GK. (1993) Intratubular germ cell neoplasia in an infantile testis with immature teratoma. *Histopathology* 22:69–72.

Talerman A. (1980a) Spermatocytic seminoma: clinicopathological study of 22 cases. *Cancer* 45:2169–2176.

Talerman A. (1980b) The pathology of gonadal neoplasms composed of germ cells and sex cord stroma derivatives. *Pathol Res Pract* 170:24–38.

Teilum G. (1976) *Special Tumors of Ovary and Testis and Related Extragonadal Lesions.* J.B. Lippincott, Philadelphia.

Tsuchiya K, Reijo R, Page DC, Disteche CM. (1995) Gonadoblastoma: molecular definition of the susceptibility region on the Y chromosome. *Am J Hum Genet* 57:1400–1407.

Ulbright TM, Srigley JR, Reuter VE, Wojno K, et al. (2000) Sex cord–stromal tumors of the testis with entrapped germ cells: a lesion mimicking unclassified mixed germ cell sex cord–stromal tumors. *Am J Surg Pathol* 24:535–542.

van Basten JP, Hoekstra HJ, van Driel MF, Sleijfer DT, et al. (1997) Cisplatin-based chemotherapy changes the incidence of bilateral testicular cancer. *Ann Surg Oncol* 4:342–348.

van Echten J, van Gurp RJ, Stoepker M, Looijenga LH, et al. (1995) Cytogenetic evidence that carcinoma *in situ* is the precursor lesion for invasive testicular germ cell tumors. *Cancer Genet Cytogenet* 85:133–137.

von der Maase H, Meinecke B, Skakkebaek NE. (1988) Residual carcinoma-*in-situ* of contralateral testis after chemotherapy. *Lancet* 1:477–478.

von der Maase H, Rorth M, Walbom-Jørgensen S, et al. (1986) Carcinoma *in situ* of contralateral testis in patients with testicular germ cell cancer: study of 27 cases in 500 patients. *BMJ* 293:1398–1401.

von Eyben FE, Mikulowski P, Busch C. (1981) Microinvasive germ cell tumors of the testis. *J Urol* 126:842–844.

Vos A, Oosterhuis JW, de Jong B, Buist J, et al. (1990) Cytogenetics of carcinoma *in situ* of the testis. *Cancer Genet Cytogenet* 46:75–81.

Wallace TM, Levin HS. (1990) Mixed gonadal dysgenesis. A review of 15 patients reporting single cases of malignant intratubular germ cell neoplasia of the testis, endometrial adenocarcinoma, and a complex vascular anomaly. *Arch Pathol Lab Med* 114:679–688.

Zukerberg LR, Young RH, Scully RE. (1991) Sclerosing Sertoli cell tumor of the testis: a report of 10 cases. *Am J Surg Pathol* 15:829–834.

23

KIDNEY

John N. Eble

In many neoplastic systems, the sequence of changes leading to cancer is well understood and entities such as dysplasia and carcinoma *in situ* have been defined as milestones along the pathway. This is not the case for most epithelial neoplasms of the renal cortex. The nature of the precursors of renal cell carcinomas has been controversial for more than a century and remains so. The tissue of origin of these carcinomas was itself debated for many years; this is reflected in the misnomer *hypernephroma*, which only lately has largely been eradicated from the literature, although the discovery of brush borders on the lumenal surfaces of some clear cell renal cell carcinomas four decades ago (Oberling et al., 1960) laid to rest the idea that renal cell neoplasms arise from heterotopic adrenal tissue. Evidence that some renal cell neoplasms arise elsewhere in the nephron than the proximal tubule (Eble and Hull, 1984; Störkel et al., 1989) has made the concept of histogenesis more complex. Beyond the question of histogenesis, the existence of benign epithelial neoplasms of the renal cortex, so-called *renal adenoma*, has also been highly controversial. Until recently, these controversies have been heightened by the general acceptance that, despite the morphological diversity of the epithelial neoplasms of the renal cortex, they all could be subsumed under the single rubric *renal cell carcinoma*. This chapter will examine these issues in light of recent morphological, clinical, cytogenetic, and molecular biologic studies which have made great advances in

the knowledge of the beginnings of neoplasia of the epithelium of the renal cortex and have led to the modern classification of renal cell neoplasms shown in Table 23–1 (Störkel et al., 1997).

BENIGN RENAL CELL NEOPLASMS

Papillary Adenoma

Over the years, most pathologic classification schemes of renal epithelial tumors have included adenoma as an entity (Kovacs, 1993; Mostofi et al., 1981; Murphy et al., 1994; Thoenes et al., 1986). However, criteria for distinguishing adenoma from adenocarcinoma in the kidney have been difficult to establish. In the second series Armed Forces Institute of Pathology (AFIP) fascicle, Bennington and Beckwith (1975) said, "The so-called adenoma is a small renal adenocarcinoma which has not yet produced metastasis." More recently, Murphy and co-workers (1994) avowed, "With the exception of oncocytoma, it has not been possible to define an unequivocally benign renal cortical neoplasm using histologic, immunohistochemical, and ultrastructural studies." The details of the history of the controversies concerning the definition of renal adenoma have recently been reviewed (Delahunt and Eble, 1997b).

The increasing numbers of small renal tumors detected with imaging technology give

591

Table 23–1. Classification of Neoplasms of Renal Tubular Epithelium

Benign Neoplasms
Papillary adenoma
Renal oncocytoma
Metanephric adenoma

Malignant neoplasms
Clear cell renal cell carcinoma
Papillary renal cell carcinoma
   Type 1
   Type 2
Chromophobe renal cell carcinoma
   Typical
   Eosinophil
Collecting duct carcinoma
Renal cell carcinoma, unclassified

the issue of renal adenoma clinical importance (Aso and Homma, 1992; Levine et al., 1989; Thompson and Peek, 1988). Jamis-Dow et al. (1996) demonstrated that computed tomography, which, under the best conditions has resolution on the order of 1 mm, is capable of detecting 47% of renal tumors less than 5 mm in diameter and 60% of tumors in the range of 5 mm to 10 mm. For those larger than 15 mm the detection rate is essentially 100%.

The study of renal adenoma has been impeded by the problem of identifying criteria that distinguish benign from malignant neoplasms of the renal tubules. This problem has been exacerbated by the fact that surgery cures some renal cell carcinomas and a cured cancer cannot be distinguished from a cured adenoma on the basis of the patient's outcome (Bailey and Harrison, 1937; Cass, 1980; Childs and Waterfall, 1953; Cristol et al., 1950; Judd and Simon, 1927; Kretschmer and Doehring, 1929; Morris, 1911; Norman, 1893; Shimsony et al., 1963). Notwithstanding the historical problems and success of surgery, the data support the definition of a set of criteria within which the diagnosis of papillary adenoma is safe and justified (Table 23–2). The first criterion indicates that the microscopic morphology of papillary adenoma resembles that of papillary renal cell carcinoma, including lesions with both type 1 and type 2 characteristics (Delahunt and Eble, 1997a). The second criterion defines a group of tumors that appear

to be limited in growth potential. This includes more than 95% of all papillary neoplasms of the renal tubules (see below; Eble and Warfel, 1991; Reese and Winstanley, 1958). Larger ones are more worrisome because they have demonstrated a greater capacity for growth, and may have the potential for metastasis (Evins and Varner, 1979). The third criterion reflects the fact that there is no convincing evidence that very small tumors of those other cell types are not small carcinomas. Similar criteria for papillary adenoma were accepted at international consensus conferences in Heidelberg, Germany and Rochester, Minnesota (Störkel et al., 1997).

In an alternate approach, Kovacs (1994) has suggested that cytogenetic findings could be used to classify renal epithelial neoplasms. In this proposed system, papillary adenoma is defined by the presence of cytogenetic abnormalities limited to +7, +17, and −Y. In his view, the presence of additional trisomies leads to malignant biologic potential and defines papillary carcinoma. Although this approach is interesting, more outcome data are needed to validate it.

Epidemiology

Reese and Winstanley (1958) studied single kidneys from 212 autopsies and found 49 adenomas in 31 kidneys. The youngest patient was 50 years old and 46 of the adenomas were in patients aged 51 to 80 years. The frequency of small epithelial lesions in the cortices of kidneys has been found to be between 4% and 37% in autopsy patients, depending upon the patient population and study methods (Hashine et al., 1996; Hiasa et al., 1995; Newcomb, 1936; Reis et al., 1988; Xipell, 1971). Eble and Warfel (1991) reported on a series of 400 autopsies in which both kidneys were closely sectioned and examined; epithelial cortical lesions were found in 83 patients (21%) and their frequency increased with age (10% in patients

Table 23–2. Criteria for Diagnosis of Papillary Adenoma

Papillary, tubular, or tubulopapillary growth patterns

Size less than or equal to 5 mm

Does not resemble clear cell, chromophobe, or collecting duct renal cell carcinomas

21 to 40 years old versus 40% in those 70 to 90 years old). Similar lesions frequently develop in patients on long-term hemodialysis and have been reported in up to 33% of patients with acquired renal cystic disease (Hughson et al., 1986). These appear earlier than carcinoma in this patient group and are thought to be the precursor lesions of the carcinomas that also are prevalent in these patients. Ishikawa has recommended that in uremic kidneys all tumors greater than 1.0 cm be considered malignant (Ishikawa, 1985). The association between arteriosclerotic renal vascular disease and papillary adenomas has long been recognized (Bell, 1938; Cabot and Middleton, 1938). Budin and McDonnell (1984) studied autopsy material and found that the prevalence of papillary adenomas not only was much increased in kidneys with arteriosclerotic renal vascular disease but that this was independent of age. Xipell (1971) found a strong correlation between tobacco smoking and the presence of papillary adenomas; this also was observed by Bennington (1973).

That kidneys bearing renal cell carcinoma or oncocytoma are more likely to contain papillary adenomas than normal kidneys has been recognized for more than 50 years (Cristol et al., 1946). Cheng et al (1991) found 4 papillary adenomas ranging from 2 to 4 mm in diameter in 100 radical nephrectomy specimens sectioned at 3 mm intervals. They also found 5 tumors ranging from 2 to 4 mm in diameter which they considered carcinomas; the example illustrated is a clear cell renal cell carcinoma. Occasionally, more than one adenoma will be present adjacent to the carcinoma or oncocytoma, suggesting some local factor that promotes the development of the adenomas.

Morphologic Studies

Papillary adenomas are identifiable with the naked eye as well-circumscribed, yellow to grayish-white nodules as small as less than 1 mm in diameter in the renal cortex. Hashine et al. (1996) found 59 papillary adenomas in 2201 autopsies. The mean diameter of the adenomas was 1.9 mm. Most occur just below the renal capsule but those that are invisible from the cortical surface are fairly common. The smallest ones are usually spherical or ovoid (Fig. 23–1), but larger ones are sometimes roughly conical with a

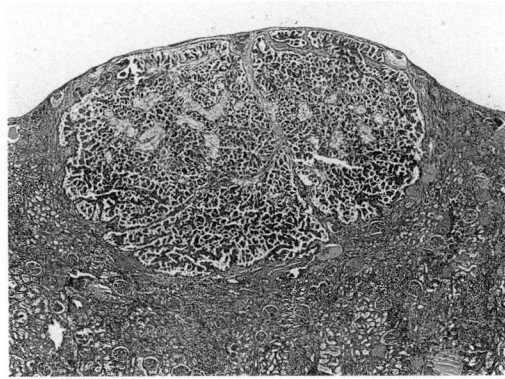

Figure 23–1. Papillary adenoma, type 1. This 4 × 2.4 mm papillary tumor was found at autopsy (hematoxylin and eosin).

wedge-shaped appearance in sections cut at right angles to the cortical surface. In an autopsy study, Budin and McDonnell (1984) found that many papillary adenomas arose within or adjacent to renal cortical scars caused by vascular insufficiency. Conversely, Reese and Winstanley (1958) found only a small minority of adenomas associated with scars. In most patients, adenomas are solitary (Reis et al., 1988), but occasionally, papillary adenomas are multiple and bilateral, rarely miliary; this condition has been called "renal adenomatosis," (Corwin, 1940; Syrjänen, 1979; Turley and Steel, 1924; Ullrich et al., 1990) analogous to renal oncocytomatosis (Katz, 1996; Warfel and Eble, 1982).

Papillary adenomas have tubular, papillary, or tubulopapillary architectures, often corresponding closely to the chromophil-basophil cell type described by Thoenes et al. (1986). Some are surrounded by thin fibrous pseudocapsules while others have none (Reese and Winstanley, 1958). The cells have round to oval nuclei with stippled to clumped chromatin and inconspicuous nucleoli (Fig. 23–2A); nuclear grooves may be present. Mitotic figures are usually absent (Reese and Winstanley, 1958). In most, the cytoplasm is scant and pale, amphophilic to basophilic (Fig. 23–2B). Occasionally, it is slightly more voluminous and appears clear or filled with minute vacuoles (Reese and Winstanley, 1958). Less frequently, the cytoplasm is voluminous and eosinophilic, resembling type 2 papillary renal cell carcinoma (Fig. 23–3; Delahunt and Eble,

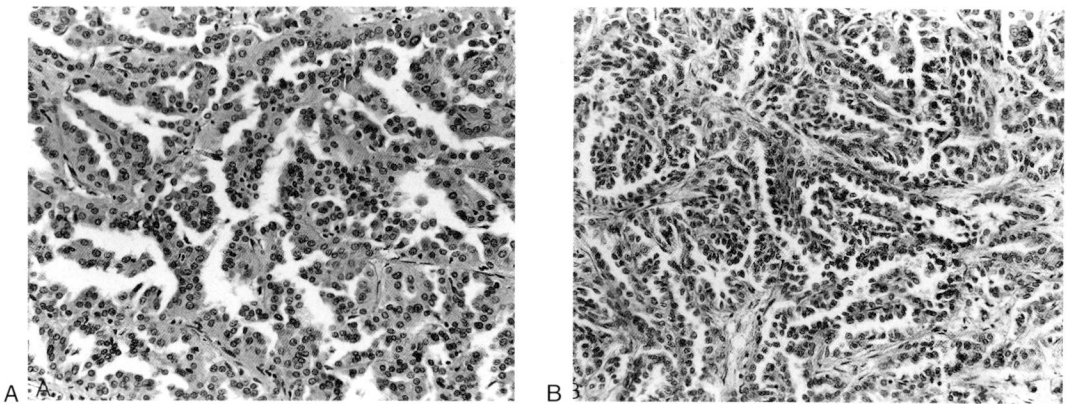

Figure 23–2. *A*: Papillary adenoma, type 1. Papillary architecture consisting of delicate stromal cores covered by cuboidal cells with small nuclei and small cytoplasmic volume (hematoxylin and eosin, original magnification ×40). *B*: Papillary adenoma, type 1. Note very high nuclear/cytoplasmic ratio but small nuclei similar in size to those of fibroblasts in the stroma (hematoxylin and eosin, original magnification ×40).

1997a). Psammoma bodies are often present, as are foamy macrophages (Reese and Winstanley, 1958).

Histochemical and Immunohistochemical Studies

Cohen et al. (1995) found that almost all papillary adenomas react with antibodies to epithelial membrane antigen (EMA) and low-molecular-weight cytokeratin, and most react with antibody to high-molecular-weight cytokeratin. Neuron-specific enolase and α-1-antitrypsin occasionally were present and carcinoembryonic antigen (CEA) could not be detected (Cohen et al., 1995). Hiasa et

al. (1995) studied 65 adenomas ranging from 1 to 5 mm in diameter and found 52 to be positive for peanut agglutinin and EMA and negative for both Leu M1 and *Lotus tetragonolobus* lectin, a pattern similar to that in the normal distal tubule. Thirteen had the opposite pattern and were similar to the lining cells of the normal proximal tubule (Hiasa et al., 1995). Farnsworth et al. (1994) found both diploid and aneuploid papillary adenomas by image cytometry.

The search for a definition that absolutely distinguishes papillary adenoma from papillary renal cell carcinoma has been futile. However, data from the autopsy studies cited

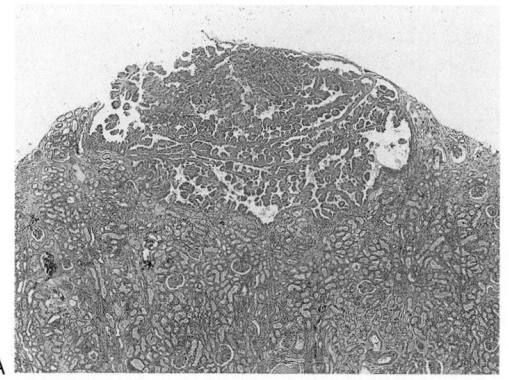
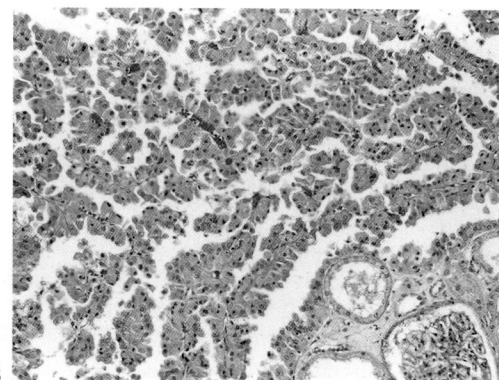

Figure 23–3. *A*: Papillary adenoma, type 2. This 3.4 × 1.7 mm tumor was found at autopsy (hematoxylin and eosin). *B*: Papillary adenoma, type 2. The cytoplasm is abundant and eosinophilic (hematoxylin and eosin, original magnification ×40).

above show that renal epithelial neoplasms meeting the criteria in Table 23–1 occur in more than 20% of adults between the ages of 20 and 40 years, while surgical series show that papillary renal cell carcinoma accounts for only about 4500 new cases of renal cell carcinoma diagnosed each year. This means that almost all papillary epithelial neoplasms that arise will show benign behavior and are probably incapable of progression without some further transforming event. Thus, the great majority of papillary epithelial neoplasms of the renal cortex are adenomas. It would have been helpful if nuclear characteristics could help to define benign from malignant among small papillary tumors. However, Brooks et al. (1993) found no difference in nuclear volume between small papillary neoplasms and large and more aggressive ones, and Delahunt and Eble (1997a) found that most papillary carcinomas are of low nuclear grade. This returns attention to size as an objective parameter, which can give insight into the tumor's capacity for growth. More than 90% of the papillary tumors found in autopsy studies are smaller than 5 mm. This indicates that larger ones have shown a greater capacity for growth than the other 90%. While by no means an absolute, a greater capacity for growth is worrisome, so excluding tumors larger than 5 mm seems a logical part of the definition. In the end, the definition proposed in Table 23–2 defines a large group of tumors with no or vanishingly little potential for further growth or metastasis and we recommend that these be diagnosed as adenomas.

RENAL ONCOCYTOMA

Morphologic Studies

Although these are potentially large tumors with growth rate indices similar to those of low-grade renal cell carcinomas (Delahunt et al., 1989), *renal oncocytomas* are benign neoplasms of the renal cortex (Davis et al., 1991) and make up approximately 5% of clinically apparent renal cell neoplasms (Thoenes et al., 1990). The architecture usually consists of solid sheets or island clusters in a background of loose edematous connective tissue (Fig. 23–4). Tubular or microcystic architectures are seen occasionally.

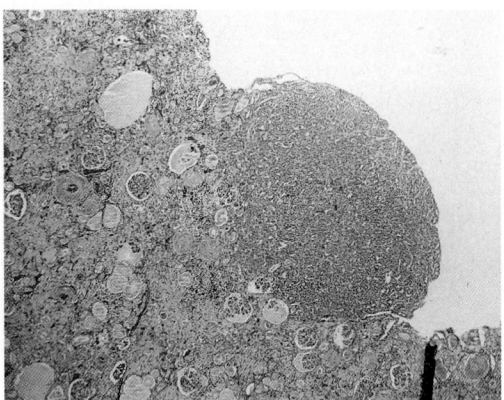

Figure 23–4. Renal oncocytoma. This 1.5 mm tumor protrudes from the renal cortex and has a compact architecture (hematoxylin and eosin).

Cytologically, renal oncocytomas are characterized by cytoplasm filled with intensely eosinophilic fine granules. While the cytoplasm ranges in quantity from moderate to abundant, its tinctorial qualities remain the same (Fig. 23–5). The nuclei are usually spheroidal with inconspicuous nucleoli, but variability in nuclear appearance is acceptable. Mitotic figures are not visible in oncocytoma cells. Since the cells of the proximal tubule also have abundant finely granular eosinophilic cytoplasm, early investigators posited an origin in the proximal tubule for renal oncocytoma (Klein and Valensi, 1976).

Ultrastructurally, the cytoplasm is filled

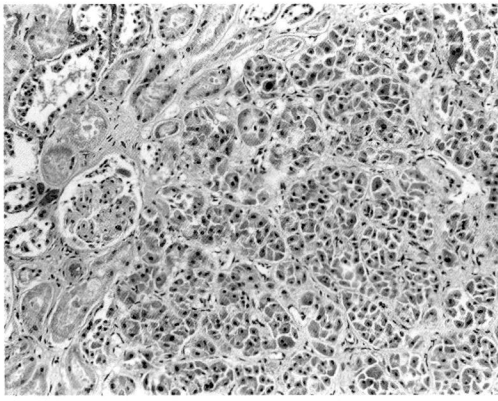

Figure 23–5. Renal oncocytoma. Note the abundant eosinophilic cytoplasm, compact architecture, and slight anisonucleosis in this small tumor (hematoxylin and eosin, original magnification ×40).

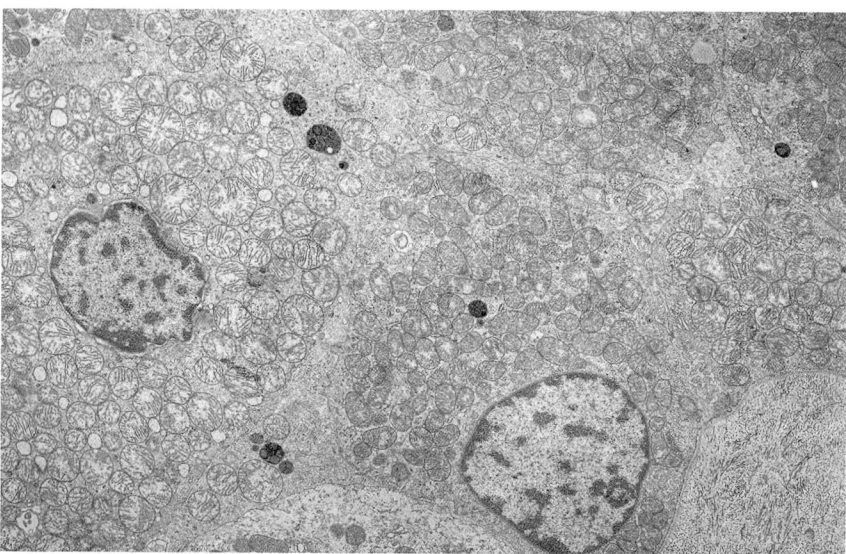

Figure 23–6. Renal oncocytoma. The cytoplasm is filled with mitochondria and other organelles are scarce. Microvilli are absent (original magnification ×19,500).

with mitochondria and other organelles are sparse (Fig. 23–6). The mitochondria of renal oncocytomas are larger than those of papillary renal cell carcinomas (Thoenes et al., 1986). Microvilli are uncommon and well-formed brush borders are absent, while basal cell surfaces and basal lamina are irregular and complex (Eble and Hull, 1984). In some cases there are amorphous and lamellated structures consisting of invaginations of basal lamina material protruding into the basal plasmalemma (Kragel et al., 1990). These features do not support origin in the proximal tubule but are suggestive of origin in the distal tubule.

Histochemical and Immunohistochemical Studies

Following the ultrastructural observations that renal oncocytomas have few features specific for the proximal tubule and more in common with the distal tubule (Eble and Hull, 1984), immunohistochemical and lectin histochemical techniques have been applied to the problem of the origin of renal oncocytomas. The results have been mixed. Nine of ten oncocytomas contained *anion exchanger band 3* and six of ten contained *carbonic anhydrase C*, markers for intercalated cells of the collecting ducts (Störkel et al., 1988). In one study of 13 on-

cocytomas and a case of oncocytomatosis, two lectin-staining patterns predominated, one with the lectins of *Dolichos biflorus* and *Glycine max*, suggesting distal tubular or collecting duct origin, and one of staining with the lectin of *Lotus tetragonolobus*, a marker for the proximal tubule (Eble and Hull, 1988). Another study also showed frequent staining with the lectin of *D. biflorus* but did not use the lectin of *L. tetragonolobus* (Ortmann et al., 1988a).

Immunohistochemical studies using antibodies to *cytochrome C oxidase* (EC 1.9.3.1) as markers for mitochondria have identified single oncocytes, oncocytic tubules, and microscopic oncocytomas in the renal cortex of rats treated with chemical carcinogens and have localized these lesions in the collecting ducts (Mayer et al., 1989). In human renal tumors, a polyclonal antibody to cytochrome C oxidase found strong immunoreactivity in 10 oncocytomas but much weaker reactivity in 43 renal cell carcinomas and small tubulopapillary basophil lesions (Ortmann et al., 1988b). Comparison with 19 chromophil (granular cell) carcinomas found markedly weaker staining than in the oncocytomas.

In a study including six renal oncocytomas, vimentin was absent, cytokeratins were absent to moderately positive, while

EMA was weakly to strongly positive (Medeiros et al., 1988). Cytokeratin positivity is typically seen in a distinctive discrete punctate pattern in renal oncocytomas (Bonsib et al., 1991). Epithelial membrane antigen is often present (Ortmann et al., 1988a).

Genetic Studies

Renal oncocytomas lack the 3p deletion and trisomy of 7 and 17, which are characteristic of clear cell and papillary renal cell carcinomas (Kovacs et al., 1994; Presti et al., 1991; Psihramis et al., 1986; Weaver et al., 1988). While the renal oncocytomas studied have had a variety of chromosomal aberrations (Kovacs et al., 1987; Psihramis et al., 1986), no consistent cytogenetic abnormality has been found. Translocations involving 11q13 are common (Dal Cin et al., 1996; Füzesi et al., 1998; Neuhaus et al., 1997; Sinke et al., 1997; van den Berg et al., 1995). Losses of chromosomes 1 and Y are fairly frequent (Presti et al., 1996). Loss of heterozygosity in 14q is common (Presti et al., 1996; Schwerdtle et al., 1997). Some oncocytomas have complex genetic abnormalities (Dujkhuizen et al., 1997). Studies of oncocytomas occurring in families may give further insight into the genetics of oncocytoma (Weirich et al., 1998). Flow cytometric analyses have generally found these tumors to be euploid (Eble and Sledge, 1986; Jow et al., 1991).

Restriction fragment analysis of mitochondrial DNA from oncocytomas has shown an additional 40 bp band in the *Hin*fI restriction pattern (Welter et al., 1989). This alteration of mitochondrial DNA was localized to the cytochrome C oxidase subunit I gene. The band was found in all of the six oncocytomas studied and was absent from the adjacent renal tissue in each case and from two renal cell carcinomas.

METANEPHRIC ADENOMA

In 1980, Pagès and Granier drew attention to a previously unrecognized renal neoplasm which they called "néphrome néphronogène" (nephronogenic nephroma) and considered to be a purely epithelial neoplasm arising from persistent blastema. Since that time, almost 100 cases have been described individually or in aggregated studies (Grignon and Eble, 1998). In 1992, Hennigar and Beckwith (1992) described five cases of a composite neoplasm in which an epithelial component identical to metanephric adenoma was combined with a proliferation of spindle cells; they proposed the name "nephrogenic adenofibroma" for this tumor. Since that report, two additional cases have been described (Bigg and Bari, 1997; Comerci et al., 1996). However, Beckwith now favors the name "metanephric adenofibroma" for these tumors to emphasize their close relationship with metanephric adenoma (B. Beckwith, personal communication); that terminology will be followed in this chapter.

Morphologic Studies

Histologically, metanephric adenoma is typically a highly cellular tumor composed of tightly packed small, uniform, round acini (Fig. 23–7). Since the acini and their lumens are so small, at low magnification this pattern may be mistaken for a solid sheet of cells. Long branching and angulated tubular structures are also common. The stroma ranges from inconspicuous to a loose paucicellular edematous stroma. Hyalinized scar and focal osseous metaplasia of the stroma are present in 10%–20% of tumors (Davis et al., 1995). Approximately 50% of tumors contain papillary structures, usually consisting of minute cysts into which have grown short, blunt papillae reminiscent of immature glomeruli (Fig. 23–8). In most of these, no blood vessel can be seen. Psammoma bodies are common and may be very numerous. The junction with the kidney is usually abrupt and lacking a pseudocapsule. The areas bulging from the surface of the kidney are separated from the perirenal tissues by the renal capsule.

All of the architectural variations of metanephric adenoma are composed of similar cells with small, uniform nuclei with absent or inconspicuous nucleoli. The nuclei are only a little larger than those of lymphocytes and are round or ovoid and have delicate chromatin. The cytoplasm is scant and pale or light pink. Mitotic figures are absent or rare.

Metanephric adenofibroma is a composite tumor in which nodules of epithelium identical to metanephric adenoma are embedded in sheets of moderately cellular spindle cells. The spindle cell component consists of fibroblast-like cells that Hennigar

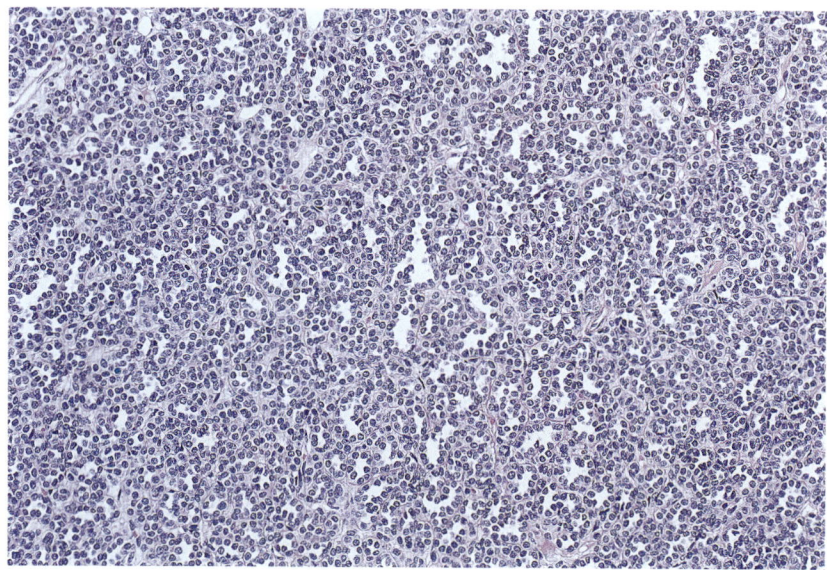

Figure 23–7. Metanephric adenoma composed of small, tubule-like spaces lined by a single layer of small cells with uniform nuclei and small volumes of cytoplasm (hematoxylin and eosin).

and Beckwith (1992) considered similar in appearance to the classical type of congenital mesoblastic nephroma. Their cytoplasm is eosinophilic but pale and the nuclei are oval or fusiform. Nucleoli are inconspicuous and mitotic figures are absent. Variable amounts of hyalinization and myxoid change are present. The relative amounts of the spindle cell and epithelial components vary from predominance of spindle cells to a minor component of spindle cells. The border of the tumor with the kidney is typically irregular and the spindle cell component may entrap renal structures as it advances. The epithelial component consists of small acini, tubules, and papillary structures, as

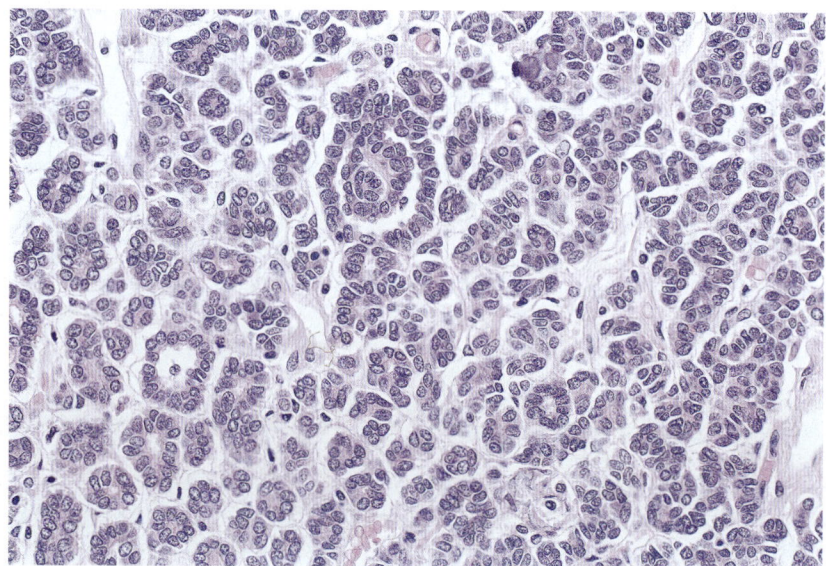

Figure 23–8. Metanephric adenoma with stubby papilla reminiscent of a glomerulus (hematoxylin and eosin).

described above in metanephric adenoma. Psammoma bodies are common and may be numerous.

Neither metanephric adenoma nor metanephric adenofibroma contains blastema nor is either associated with nephrogenic rests.

Histochemical and Immunohistochemical Studies

Immunohistochemistry and lectin histochemistry have given varied results in different laboratories and consequently do not play a large role in the differential diagnosis of metanephric adenoma. A variety of cytokeratins have been present (Davis et al., 1995; Gatalica et al., 1996; Hubert et al., 1996; Jones et al., 1995; Nonomura et al., 1995; Saint-André et al., 1992; Störkel et al., 1992), variably present (Ban et al., 1996; Hennigar and Beckwith, 1992), or absent (Gatalica et al., 1996; Nagashima et al., 1991; Renshaw et al., 1997; Störkel et al., 1992). Epithelial membrane antigen has been absent in most tumors (Davis et al., 1995; Gatalica et al., 1996; Hennigar and Beckwith, 1992; Hubert et al., 1996; Nagashima et al., 1991; Renshaw et al., 1997; Störkel et al., 1992) but some have contained it (Ban et al., 1996; Jones et al.,, 1995; Nonomura et al., 1995). Lysozyme was found in one case (Nonomura et al., 1995) but not in two others (Ban et al., 1996; Nagashima et al., 1991). Leu 7 was present in three of the seven tumors described by Jones et al. (1995) and in three others (Ban et al., 1996; Nagashima et al., 1991; Nonomura et al., 1995), while Leu M1 has not been detected (Ban et al., 1996; Jones et al., 1995; Nagashima et al., 1991; Nonomura et al., 1995). S-100 protein was present in three tumors (Ban et al., 1996; Nagashima et al., 1991; Nonomura et al., 1995) but absent from the seven cases described by Jones et al. (1995) Vimentin has frequently been found (Gatalica et al., 1996; Hubert et al., 1996; Jones et al., 1995; Nagashima et al., 1991; Störkel et al., 1992) but has been weak (Nonomura et al., 1995), or absent in others (Jones et al., 1995; Renshaw et al., 1997). Actin (Jones et al., 1995; Renshaw et al., 1997), desmin (Gatalica et al., 1996; Jones et al., 1995; Renshaw et al., 1997), neuron-specific enolase (Jones et al., 1995), and Tamm-Horsfall protein (Na-

gashima et al., 1991) have been sought but were not found.

The *Arachis hypogaea* lectin (peanut agglutinin) has often had an affinity for metanephric adenoma (Ban et al., 1996; Davis et al., 1995; Jones et al., 1995; Nagashima et al., 1991; Saint-André et al., 1992; Störkel et al., 1992), although only four of the seven cases in the series of Jones et al. (1995) reacted positively. Conversely, the reaction with *Lotus tetragonolobus* lectin has always been negative (Ban et al., 1996; Davis et al., 1995; Nagashima et al., 1991; Störkel et al., 1992). In one tumor (Ban et al.,, 1996), reactions with soybean agglutinin and *Dolichos biflorus* agglutinin were negative.

Data from metanephric adenofibromas are less extensive, but Hennigar and Beckwith (1992) found variable content of cytokeratin (A1/AE3) and no reaction for EMA, vimentin, actin, and desmin in the neoplastic epithelium.

Genetic Studies

Few metanephric adenomas have been studied genetically. A few tumors studied cytogenetically had normal karyotypes (Gatalica et al., 1996; Jones et al., 1995; Renshaw et al., 1997). However, two studies (Brown et al., 1996, 1997) including 13 tumors have found frequent gain of chromosomes 7 (9 tumors) and 17 (10 tumors) and loss of the Y chromosome (in males). These are the most common genetic abnormalities in papillary renal adenoma and papillary renal cell carcinoma. The wt1 gene protein has been found in a single tumor (Gatalica et al., 1996).

Precursor Lesions

The histologic resemblance of metanephric adenoma and metanephric adenofibroma to some appearances of Wilms' tumor and nephrogenic rests is close and Pagès and Granier (1980) considered that they were benign tumors that arose from nephrogenic rests. Brisigotti et al. (1992) held a similar view, that they are benign counterparts of Wilms' tumor, and this was shared by Davis et al. (1995) Hennigar and Beckwith (1992) concluded that metanephric adenofibromas "derive from multiple perilobar and intralobar nephrogenic rests which persist long after birth." On the other hand, some aspects of the morphology of these tumors resemble type 1 papillary renal cell carcinoma (Delahunt and Eble, 1997a). Most of the scant genetic evidence obtained to date supports the idea that metanephric adenoma is related to the common papillary neoplasms of the renal tubules.

MALIGNANT RENAL CELL NEOPLASMS

CLEAR CELL RENAL CELL CARCINOMA

Morphologic Studies

Comprising 66%–75% of clinically apparent renal cell neoplasms (Eble, 1997), clear cell renal cell carcinomas are characterized by cells with voluminous clear cytoplasm in sections stained with hematoxylin and eosin (Fig. 23–9). This clarity (Fig. 23–10) is from the large quantities of lipid and glycogen stored there and is readily demonstrable by such techniques as oil red-O and periodic acid-Schiff (PAS) staining of suitably treated specimens. Grawitz (1883) found the lipid content of clear cell renal cell carcinoma persuasive and considered them lipomas, earning the eponym *Grawitz tumor*, which appears in print even today (Govaerts et al., 1987). The superficial resemblance of clear cell renal cell carcinoma to cells of the zona fasciculata of the adrenal cortex and the frequent autopsy finding of heterotopic adrenal cortical tissue between the renal cap-

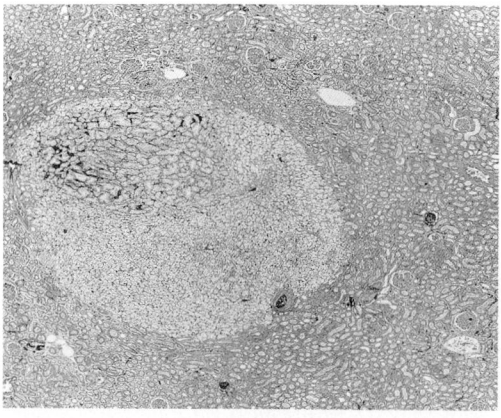

Figure 23–9. Compact and tubular clear cell renal cell carcioma 3.4 mm in diameter (hematoxylin and eosin).

sule and the renal cortex combined with the Cohnheim cell rest theory persuaded some that this was the tissue of origin and to generate the misnomer *hypernephroma* (from the *hypernephric* or *adrenal* gland) which, against all evidence, remains in usage today (Gurney et al., 1989; Tang et al., 1989).

Study of clear cell renal cell carcinomas by electron microscopy revealed well-formed brush borders on the lumenal surfaces of some cells (Oberling et al., 1960; Seljelid and Ericsson, 1965; Fig. 23–11), and this brought consensus that renal cell neoplasms arise from the epithelium of the proximal tubules of the renal cortex.

Histochemical and Immunohistochemical Studies

In one of the first studies to use immunohistochemical techniques to study the histogenesis of renal cell tumors (Wallace and Nairn, 1972), immunofluorescent methods were used to demonstrate binding of an antibody to brush border and lack of binding of an antibody to Tamm-Horsfall protein in 15 "adenomas" and 11 renal cell carcinomas. Subsequent immunohistochemical studies have consistently shown that clear cell renal cell carcinomas react with antibodies for cytokeratins and for EMA, consistent with origin from epithelium of the proximal convoluted tubule (Wick et al., 1990). Additionally, vimentin can be demonstrated in 50% to 90% of cases (Pitz et al., 1987; Waldherr and Schwechheimer, 1985). Coexpression of cytokeratins and vimentin is characteristic of clear cell renal cell carcinoma and occurs in up to 98% of cases, a property often retained in metastases (Oosterwijk et al., 1990). Neither CEA nor S-100 protein is detectable in renal cell carcinomas (Wick et al., 1990). Lectin binding varies among the segments of the normal nephron (Truong et al., 1988) and has been used to explore the histogenesis of renal cell neoplasms (Ullrich et al., 1985). The majority of clear cell renal cell carcinomas bind the *Lotus tetragonolobus* lectin, a marker for the proximal tubule (Ullrich et al., 1985).

Genetic Studies

Studies of familial clear cell renal cell carcinoma have given insight into the genetic basis of this disease (Zbar and Lerman, 1999). Early cytogenetic studies of clear cell renal

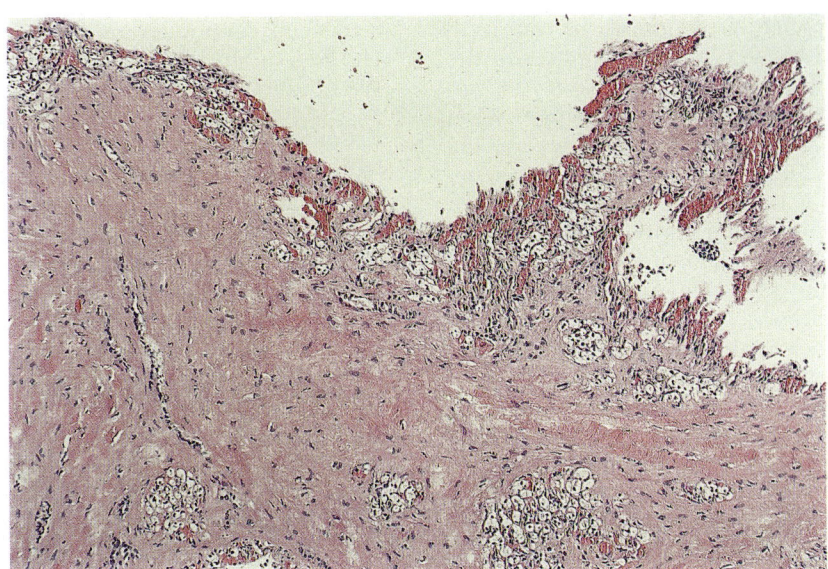

Figure 23–10. Clear cell renal cell carcinoma arising in a cyst in the kidney of a patient with von Hippel–Lindau disease (hematoxylin and eosin).

cell carcinomas found that changes leading to loss of genetic material in the short arm of chromosome 3 are the most frequent and consistent finding (Kovacs et al., 1987, 1988; Nordenson et al., 1988; Teyssier and Ferre, 1990; Walter et al., 1989; Yoshida et al., 1986). Such losses have been found in tumors as small as 11 mm (Bergerheim et al., 1990). The abnormalities range from loss of the entire chromosome, to deletions of ter-

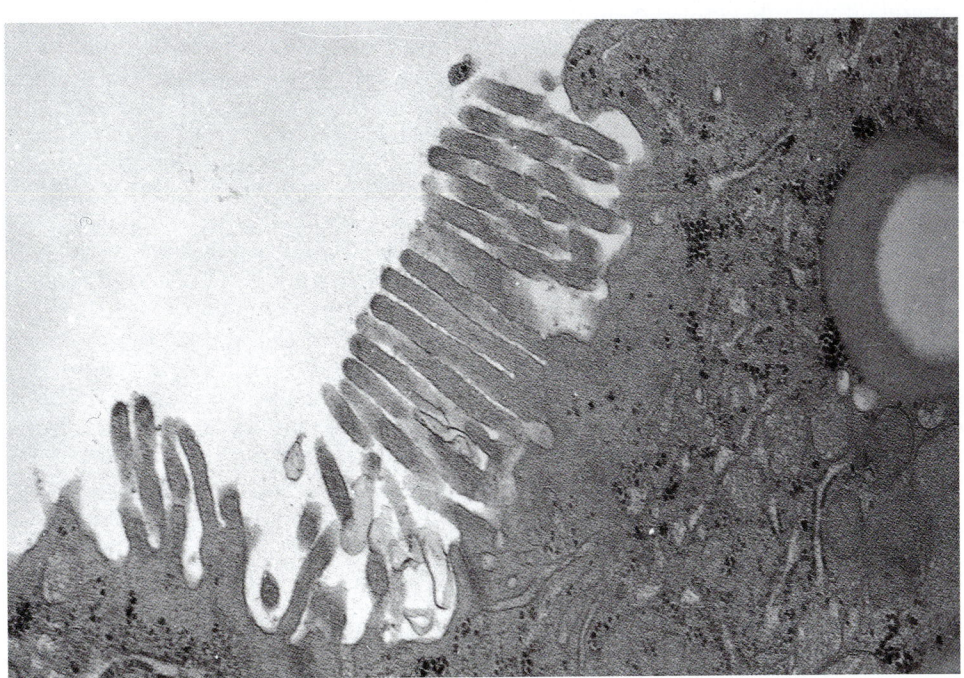

Figure 23–11. Clear cell renal cell carcinoma. Brush border at apex of cell (original magnification ×33,750).

minal or interstitial segments, to translocations, all with a net loss of sequences in the
region on 3p, which extends from p11.2 to
pter. A cluster of breakpoints in the region
of 3p13 to 3p14 has been identified and the
common fragile site in 3p14 has been implicated (Tajara et al., 1988). A study of a
family without von Hippel–Lindau disease
with 10 cases of renal cell carcinoma found
that 10 of the 22 family members had a balanced reciprocal translocation between
chromosomes 3 and 8 (Cohen et al., 1979).
This abnormality was present in all eight
members who had renal cell carcinoma and
whose karyotypes were known, while no family member without the translocation had a
renal cancer. Renal cell carcinomas arising
in patients with von Hippel–Lindau disease
also commonly have deletion or partial deletion of chromosome 3p (Goodman et al.,
1990; Jordan et al., 1989; King et al., 1987)
with a breakpoint in the proximal short arm,
near the location of the von Hippel–Lindau
(VHL) gene (Seizinger et al., 1988). The
VHL gene is a tumor suppressor gene of
great importance in the genesis of familial
and sporadic clear cell renal cell carcinoma
(Decker et al., 1997; Latif et al., 1993; Linehan et al., 1995). Loss or mutation of the
VHL tumor suppressor gene is common in
sporadic clear cell renal cell carcinoma, and
inactivation by such subtle means as hypermethylation may silence the gene (Gnarra et
al., 1994; Herman et al., 1994). While the
frequent role of mutations of the VHL gene
is well established, mutations in other genes
on chromosome 3 also appear to be important in the development of clear cell renal
cell carcinoma, particularly 3p21 and 3p12-
3p14 (Lovell et al., 1999; van den Berg and
Buys, 1997; van den Berg et al., 1996, 1997).

Additional losses of heterozygosity have
been found on chromosomes 11 and 17 and
others in advanced renal cell carcinomas,
suggesting that other suppressor genes are
involved in the progression of this cancer
(Auglard et al., 1991; Morita et al., 1991).
The finding that increasing immunohistochemical positivity for the c-*myc* gene product correlates with increasing nuclear grade
in renal cell carcinomas suggests that activation of c-*myc* plays a role in progression
(Kinouchi et al., 1989). Loss of 14q also correlates with higher stage and grade, and
poorer outcome for patients with clear cell

renal cell carcinoma (Béroud et al., 1996;
Herbers et al., 1997; Schullerus et al., 1997;
Wu et al., 1996).

Precursor Lesions

As early as 1938, Bell recognized that among
lesions with the histologic appearance of
clear cell renal cell carcinoma, "the size of
the tumor is not a certain criterion as to its
malignancy." Subsequent investigations and
case reports of small clear cell renal cell carcinomas with metastases have reinforced this
conclusion (Eschwege et al., 1996; Talamo
and Shonnard, 1980). While hyperplastic or
dysplastic epithelial proliferations in cysts in
von Hippel–Lindau disease and in other
cystic diseases, such as tuberous sclerosis
(Al-Saleem et al., 1998), may be precursors
to clear cell renal cell carcinomas in those
settings, there is little credible evidence
(Yörükoglu et al., 1999) for a morphologically identifiable precursor lesion for the vast
majority of clear cell renal cell carcinomas.

PAPILLARY RENAL CELL CARCINOMA

Morphologic Studies

Papillary renal cell carcinoma includes two
major subcategories, type 1 and type 2 (Delahunt and Eble, 1997a), and makes up approximately 10%–15% of large series of
clinically apparent renal cell carcinomas
(Eble, 1997). Type 1 is characterized by a
blue appearance in sections stained with
hematoxylin and eosin because the cells
have high nuclear/cytoplasmic ratios on account of small cytoplasmic volume (Fig.
23–12). Type 2 has pseudostratified nuclei
and often has abundant eosinophilic cytoplasm in sections stained with hematoxylin
and eosin (Fig. 23–13). A papillary or tubulopapillary architecture is typical of both
types, but compact architecture is also common in papillary renal cell carcinomas.

Ultrastructurally, type 1 papillary renal
cell carcinoma contains mitochondria,
rough endoplasmic reticulum, and other organelles in a small cytoplasmic volume
(Thoenes et al., 1986). The apical pole of
the cells often contains lipid and hemosiderin pigment. Type 2 contains abundant
mitochondria in larger cytoplasmic volume
than that of the basophil cells. The mitochondria are smaller than those of renal oncocytomas (Thones et al., 1986).

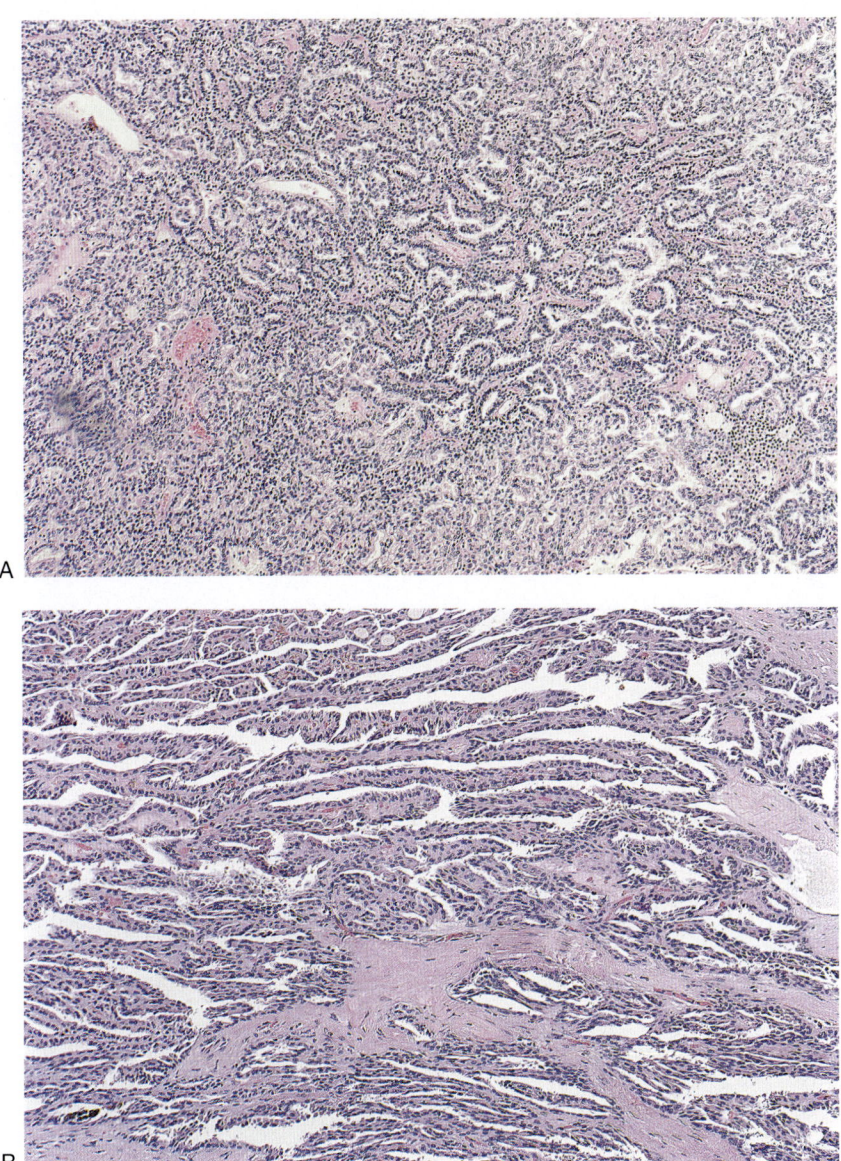

Figure 23–12. *A*: Papillary renal cell carcinoma, type 1. Complex papillary structures covered by a single layer of small cells with nuclei near the basement membrane (hematoxylin and eosin). *B*: Papillary renal cell carcinoma type 1. Trabecular growth pattern of parallel papillae (hematoxylin and eosin).

Histochemical and Immunohistochemical Studies

Both types 1 and 2 express cytokeratins and vimentin (Pitz et al., 1987).

Delahunt and Eble (1997a) found that 53 of 61 type 1 papillary renal cell carcinomas reacted with antibody to cytokeratin 7 and 43 reacted with antibody to vimentin. None of the type 1 papillary renal cell carcinomas re-

acted with *Ulex europaeus* lectin, a marker for collecting duct carcinoma. In the same study, only (20%) of type 2 papillary renal cell carcinomas reacted with antibody to cytokeratin 7 and 50% with antibody to vimentin. None reacted with *Ulex europaeus* lectin.

Genetic Studies

Studies of familial papillary renal cell carcinoma have been useful in elucidating the ge-

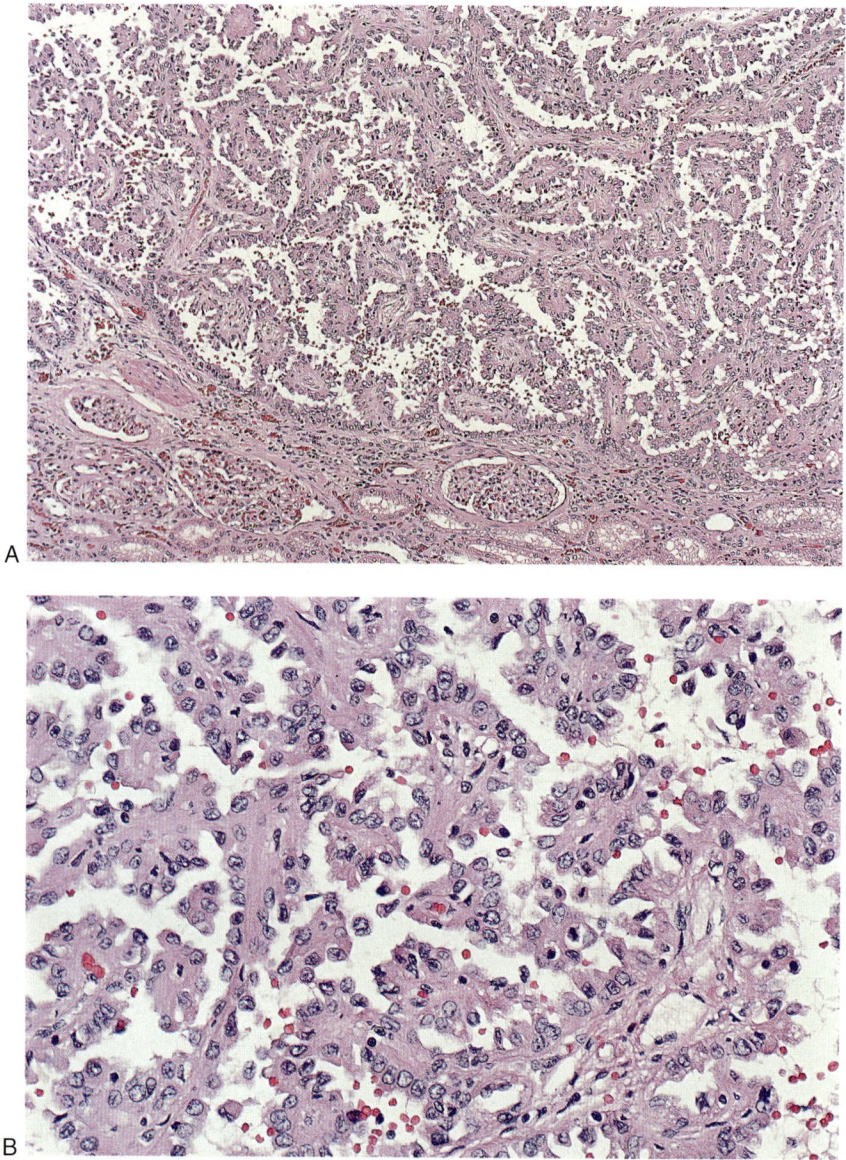

Figure 23–13. *A*: Papillary renal cell carcinoma, type 2. Papillae covered by cells with pseudostratified nuclei and eosinophilic cytoplasm (hematoxylin and eosin). *B*: Papillary renal cell carcinoma, type 2. Moderate nuclear pleomorphism and nuclei located randomly in cytoplasm (hematoxylin and eosin).

netic basis of this disease (Zbar et al., 1999). Papillary renal cell carcinomas do not have the 3p deletion characteristic of clear cell renal cell carcinoma (Kovacs et al., 1989) but instead frequently have trisomy of chromosomes 7 and 17, and of 16 (Carroll et al., 1987; Dal Cin et al., 1989; Kovacs, 1989; Presti et al., 1991). Trisomy 17 was found in two out of three papillary tumors smaller than 10 mm in diameter, leading to the con-

clusion that this cytogenetic abnormality occurs very early in the development of these neoplasms (Kovacs, 1989). Loss of the Y chromosome may play an important role in the development of papillary renal cell carcinoma (Kovacs et al., 1994). Studies of hereditary papillary renal cell carcinoma have linked its development to mutations in the *MET* proto-oncogene on 7q (Fischer et al., 1998; Schmidt et al., 1997, 1998, 1999;

Zhuang et al., 1998). In addition to the characteristic trisomies, loss of heterozygosity on chromosomes 6, 9, and 14 may play a role in the development of papillary renal cell carcinoma (Thrash-Bingham et al., 1995). Losses of Xp have correlated with poor survival (Jiang et al., 1998).

That type 1 and type 2 papillary renal cell carcinoma differ genetically as well as morphologically is supported by the observations of Jiang et al. (1998) that gains of 7p and 17p are more common in type 1 tumors ($p = 0.01$). Lubensky et al. (1999) have shown that type 1 papillary renal cell carcinomas frequently have c-*met* mutations. A subset of papillary renal cell carcinoma occurring in children and young adults and with unusual morphology of cells with abundant pale-to-clear cytoplasm has been linked to Xp11.2 translocations (Dijkhuizen et al., 1998; Sidhar et al., 1996).

Precursor Lesions

Papillary adenomas appear to be the precursors of most papillary renal cell carcinomas.

CHROMOPHOBE CELL RENAL CELL CARCINOMA

Morphologic Studies

It was not until 1985 that chromophobe renal cell carcinoma was recognized (Thoenes et al., 1985). Chromophobe renal cell carcinomas comprise approximately 5% of large series of clinically apparent renal cell neoplasms (Eble, 1997). In sections stained with hematoxylin and eosin, these tumors typically consist of large polygonal cells arranged in sheets or glandular structures, with well-defined cytoplasmic membranes and lightly staining cytoplasm with a flocculent appearance (Fig. 23–14). The cytoplasm stains strongly with the Hale's colloidal iron stain; this property is important in the diagnosis and distinguishes chromophobe cell carcinomas from other variants of renal cell carcinoma. A variant with strongly eosinophilic cytoplasm has been recognized (Thoenes et al., 1988). This eosinophilic variant of chromophobe renal cell carcinoma resembles renal oncocytoma in sections stained with hematoxylin and eosin (Bonsib and Layer, 1990) but also stains positively with Hale's colloidal iron stain.

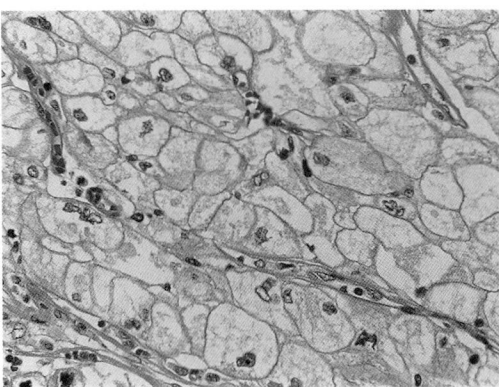

Figure 23–14. Chromophobe renal cell carcinoma. The cytoplasm is lightly staining and reticular, while the cell membranes are sharply defined (hematoxylin and eosin, original magnification ×63).

Ultrastructurally, both the typical chromophobe cells and the eosinophilic variants contain an abundance of 150-300 nm irregularly shaped cytoplasmic vesicles (Bonsib and Lager, 1990; Erlandson and Reuter, 1988; Thoenes et al., 1985, 1988; Fig. 23–15). These often contain an inner "vesicle" that suitably oriented sections show to be a cytoplasmic invagination. The origin of the vesicles is obscure and detailed studies have failed to demonstrate origin from cytoplasmic or nuclear membranes or from endoplasmic reticulum or Golgi apparatus

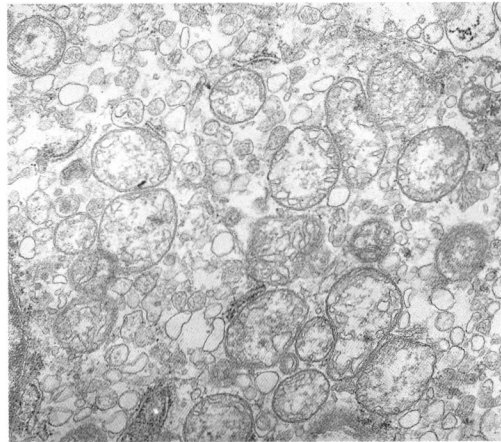

Figure 23–15. Chromophobe renal cell carcinoma. The cytoplasm contains a myriad of small vesicles, some with cytoplasmic invaginations (original magnification ×25,000).

(Bonsib and Lager, 1990). Structurally, the vesicles are similar to the vesicles seen in the intercalated cells of the normal human collecting duct (Störkel et al., 1989). The eosinophilic variant differs in containing more abundant mitochondria.

Histochemical and Immunohistochemical Studies

In addition to the distinctive cytoplasmic staining with Hale's colloidal iron mentioned above, chromophobe renal cell carcinomas exhibit diffuse strong cytoplasmic staining with antibodies to EMA, a pattern distinct from the apical and cell surface staining characteristic of clear cell and papillary renal cell carcinomas and found only in the collecting duct of the normal nephron (Störkel et al., 1989). Lectin histochemical studies also support the concept that chromophobe renal cell carcinoma originates from the epithelium of collecting ducts (Ortmann et al., 1991). Unlike clear cell and papillary renal cell carcinomas, chromophobe tumors express cytokeratin but not vimentin (Pitz et al., 1987). Immunohistochemical reactions for carbonic anhydrase C are also strong and diffuse in the cytoplasm of chromophobe cells, but negative in clear cell and papillary cell renal cell carcinomas (Störkel et al., 1989). Carbonic anhydrase is abundant in the intercalated cells of collecting duct. Chromophobe cell tumors do not express anion exchanger band 3, a marker for intercalated cells that is found in renal oncocytomas (Störkel et al., 1989).

Genetic Studies

Chromophobe renal cell carcinoma is characterized by remarkable losses of multiple whole chromosomes, to the extent that aneuploidy has been demonstrated by flow cytometry (Bonsib and Lager, 1990; Kovacs and Kovacs, 1992). Losses of chromosomes 1, 2, 6, 10, 13, and 17 are most frequent (Bugert et al., 1997; Gunawan et al., 1999; Marras et al., 1997; Schwerdtle et al., 1996; Speicher et al., 1994). Loss of the Y and X chromosomes is also common. Kinoshita et al. (1998) found that telomerase activity is uncommon in chromophobe renal cell carcinomas (Kinoshita et al., 1998).

Collecting Duct Carcinoma

Morphologic Studies:

In addition to chromophobe cell renal cell carcinoma and renal oncocytoma, diagnostically well-defined neoplasms that probably originate in the distal nephron, there is a more heterogeneous group of uncommon carcinomas arising in the renal medulla that have been categorized as *carcinomas of the collecting ducts of Bellini* or, more simply, as *collecting duct carcinomas* and make up less than 1% of large series of clinically apparent renal cell neoplasms (Srigley and Eble, 1998).

Typical collecting duct carcinoma has a tubular or tubulopapillary growth pattern. Irregular angulated tubules infiltrate a desmoplastic stroma (Figs. 23–16 and 23–17). Often, the edge of the tumor is ill defined and there is an extensive permeative pattern of growth. Microcystic change may be seen (Rumpelt et al., 1991) and the cysts are irregular in contour. Solid cord-like patterns of growth may be seen. Sarcomatoid elements may be a dominant feature of the tumor (Baer et al., 1993). The sarcomatoid change is a pattern of de-differentiation similar to that seen in other histologic types of renal carcinoma (Störkel et al., 1997).

In addition to a desmoplastic stroma, there is commonly a brisk inflammatory reaction. In many cases a neutrophilic infiltrate is seen within and around the tumor

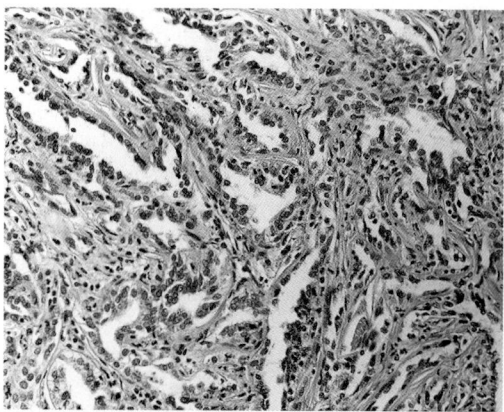

Figure 23–16. Carcinoma of the collecting ducts of Bellini. The glands and ducts have very irregular profiles and there is an abundant stroma. This 2 mm example was found at autopsy (hematoxylin and eosin, original magnification ×40).

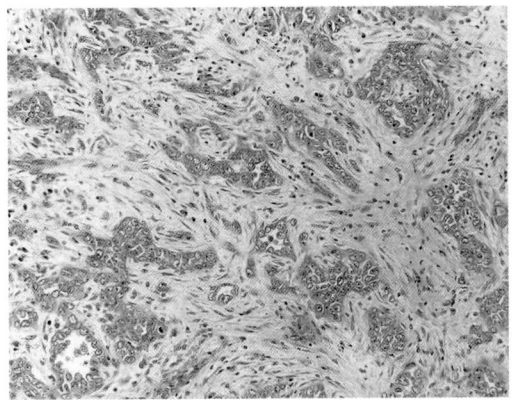

Figure 23–17. Carcinoma of the collecting ducts of Bellini. There is abundant faintly basophilic stroma surrounding the irregular glands and ducts (hematoxylin and eosin, original magnification ×40).

(Rumpelt et al., 1991). Extensive destruction of renal, medullary, and cortical tissue is often present (Rumpelt et al., 1991). Vascular and lymphatic space invasion is common (Rumpelt et al., 1991) and there is often permeation of hilar fat. The renal pelvic urothelium adjacent to the tumor may be undermined but urothelial carcinoma *in situ* is not present.

Collecting duct carcinoma is usually composed of cells with lightly eosinophilic cytoplasm and some tumors would have been classified as "granular cell carcinoma" in the older classification systems. Often, cells with a hobnail pattern are present, sometimes only focally, lining the tubules and microscopic cysts. These are diagnostically helpful since hobnial cells are not seen in clear cell, papillary, or chromophobe renal cell carcinomas. Most collecting duct carcinomas have high-grade nuclear features.

As mentioned earlier, a number of reports of collecting duct carcinoma have described predominantly papillary tumors. Many of the published photomicrographs show carcinomas that appear very similar to the common papillary renal cell carcinoma (Fig. 23–18). Other than central location and associated dysplasia of collecting duct epithelium that may distinguish these tumors from the usual papillary renal cell carcinoma, the minor criteria that have been offered to distinguish these have included lack of cir-

cumscription, broad stalks that contain fibrous and sometimes inflamed stroma, high nuclear grade, and association with areas of typical collecting duct carcinoma as defined above.

The presence of dysplastic features (nuclear enlargement, hyperchromasia, chromatin irregularity, nuclear membrane notching, and nucleolar prominence) in the epithelium of collecting ducts nearby a tumor has been taken as evidence that the tumor originated in the epithelium of the collecting ducts (Kennedy et al., 1990; Nørgaard and Skaarup, 1985). Epithelial dysplasia has occasionally been reported in renal tubules adjacent to other types of renal cell carcinoma, including clear cell renal cell carcinoma (Mourad et al., 1994), and in collecting ducts in transplanted kidneys after several years of immunosuppression (Mittal and Cotton, 1987). The presence of epithelial dysplasia in collecting ducts remote from the tumor would be better evidence of a premalignant condition in the collecting ducts than abnormalities in nearby ducts, which might be either growth of the tumor into the ducts or reactive changes caused by the inflammation associated with the carcinoma.

There are few electron microscopic studies of collecting duct carcinoma. These have usually found typical features of adenocarci-

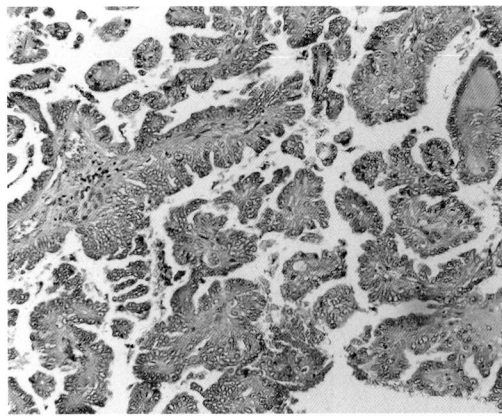

Figure 23–18. Carcinoma of the collecting ducts of Bellini. This tumor resembles a papillary renal cell carcinoma and only its medullary location enables it to be diagnosed as a collecting duct carcinoma (hematoxylin and eosin, original magnification ×40).

noma, including intracellular and extracellular lumina. Desmosomes, tight junctions, and basal lamina are common. Sometimes tonofilament-like collections of intermediate filaments may be present, correlating with the high-molecular-weight cytokeratin shown by immunohistochemistry. Additionally, complex infolding of lateral cell borders may be noted.

Histochemical and Immunohistochemical Studies

Glycogen is usually inconspicuous. In some cases, mucin is identified with the PAS, alcian blue, or mucicarmine stains (Halenda et al., 1993; Kennedy et al., 1990). Both intracytoplasmic and intraluminal mucin may be demonstrated (Kennedy et al., 1990).

The tumor cells usually react with antibodies to broad-spectrum and low-molecular-weight keratins. High-molecular-weight keratin (CK19, 34βE12) is commonly present and vimentin may be present. Variable immunostaining for EMA and lysozyme have been noted and Leu M1 (CD15) is usually absent. Importantly, lectins such as peanut lectin and *Ulex europaeus* agglutinin-1 (UEA-1) commonly have affinity for collecting duct carcinoma. The staining pattern of collecting duct carcinoma recapitulates normal distal tubular epithelium, which commonly contains high-molecular-weight cytokeratin and reacts with UEA-1.

Genetic Studies

Genetic studies of collecting duct carcinoma have been hampered by the lack of generally agreed upon criteria for the diagnosis and by lack of pathologic detail and illustration. Füzesi et al. (1992) found monosomy of chromosomes 1, 6, 14, 15, and 22 in all three cases in their series. However, the diagnosis appears to be based largely upon the central location of the tumors and the photomicrographs illustrate a papillary neoplasm indistinguishable from the common type 1 papillary renal cell carcinoma. Gregori-Romero et al. (1996) found diverse clonal chromosome abnormalities in three carcinomas which they did not illustrate. One of their cases had trisomies of chromosomes 7, 12, 16, 17, and 20, a cytogenetic abnormality typical of papillary renal cell carcinoma (Kovacs, 1993). In the case report by Cavazzana et al. (1996), a collecting duct

carcinoma demonstrated trisomies for chromosomes 4, 7, 8, 17, and 20. Using polymorphic microsatellite markers, Schoenberg et al. (1995) found frequent loss of heterozygosity in chromosome arms 8p and 13q in three of six tumors that they considered to be collecting duct carcinomas but did not illustrate. No loss of heterozygosity for 3p was found in this study. These data suggest that tumor suppressor genes on 8p and 13q may be involved in the pathogenesis of collecting duct carcinoma. Fogt et al. (1997), however, found mutaions in the VHL gene in about 50% of a series of 18 collecting duct carcinomas. Another report demonstrated loss of heterozygosity of the retinoblastoma gene in two collecting duct carcinomas (Brooks et al., 1993). Steiner et al. (1996) have found frequent loss of 1q in collecting duct carcinomas.

CYSTIC DISEASES AND RENAL CELL CARCINOMA

While most renal cell carcinomas arise sporadically in otherwise normal kidneys, a minority arise in kidneys that are grossly cystic. *Acquired cystic disease* is the most important antecedent, but *autosomal dominant polycystic disease of kidneys* (*adult polycystic disease*) and a few other cystic conditions may also predispose to the development of renal cell carcinomas.

ACQUIRED CYSTIC DISEASE

This condition arises in the native kidneys of patients with chronic renal failure, especially those treated with hemodialysis for long periods of time (Dunnill et al., 1977; Matson and Cohen, 1990). Acquired cystic disease may be defined as the presence of multiple cysts, mainly in the cortex but also in the medulla, in the native kidneys of uremic patients (Fallon and Williams, 1989). In a seven-year longitudinal study of hemodialysis patients, computerized tomography showed acquired cysts present in 87% of patients by the end of the study (Levine et al., 1991). Typically the kidneys are small, or of roughly normal size (Fig. 23–19), and most of the cysts are from 1 to 10 mm in diameter. Occasionally, larger cysts, in the range of 30–40 mm, are present. While acquired cys-

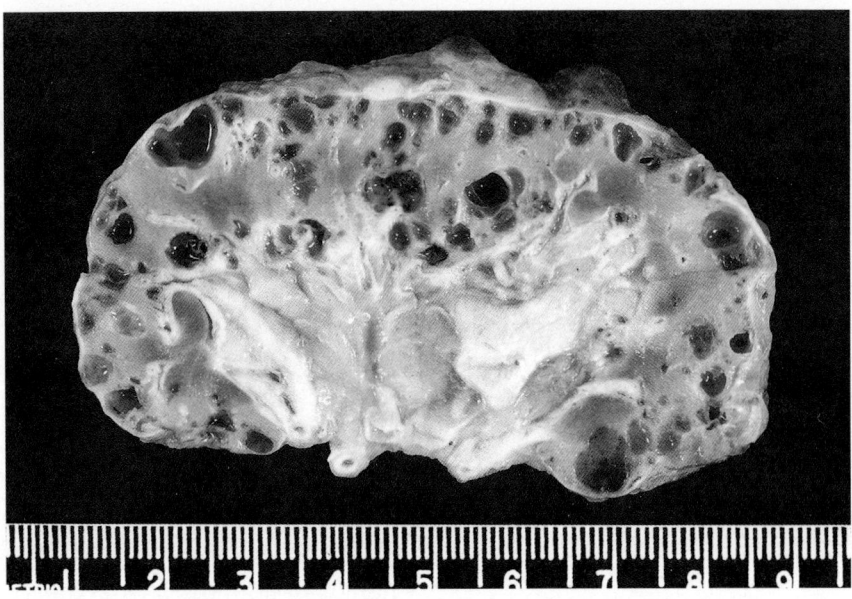

Figure 23–19. Acquired cystic disease of the kidney in a long-term hemodialysis patient. Note the small size of the kidney and the range in a size of the cysts from 1 to 10 mm.

tic disease may occur in patients with chronic renal failure before hemodialysis or in patients who are treated without hemodialysis, most of the cases studied have been patients with long histories of hemodialysis. There is some evidence that reversal of the chronic renal failure and discontinuation of dialysis when transplantation is done may induce regression of the acquired cystic disease (Minar et al., 1984). Acquired cystic disease was quickly recognized to have a strong association, on the order of 10%, with renal cell carcinomas (Bretan et al., 1986; Fayemi and Ali, 1980; Ishikawa et al., 1990). These tumors have a significant risk of metastasis (Fujimoto et al., 1988; O'Donnell et al., 1988) and approximately a 40% 3-year survival (Matson and Cohen, 1990).

Histologically, the cysts begin as dilated tubules and grow into microcysts or larger cysts. They may be lined by bland-looking cuboidal epithelium or dysplastic epithelium with enlarged, hyperchromatic nuclei (Fig. 23–20; Fayemi and Ali, 1980). In some lesions, the epithelium grows inward as polyps or papillary fronds (Figs. 23–20 and 23–21). Oxalate crystals are frequently seen in tubules and cysts (Fig. 23–22) and less frequently in the interstitium (Fayemi and Ali,

1980). The neoplasms in these kidneys have been oncocytomas (Fallon and Williams, 1989; Fayemi and Ali, 1980; Makita et al., 1991), papillary renal cell carcinomas (Fig. 23–23; Dunnill et al., 1977; Fallon and Williams, 1989), clear cell renal cell carcinomas (Fig. 23–24; Dunnill et al., 1977; Ishikawa, 1987; Krempien and Ritz, 1980), and sarcomatoid (Fujimoto et al., 1998; Hida et al., 1988). From the illustrations in the published accounts, high-grade lesions are

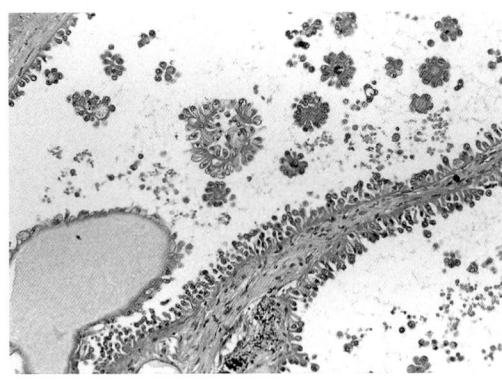

Figure 23–20. Acquired cystic disease of the kidney. Epithelial polyps within a cyst lined by dysplastic epithelium (hematoxylin and eosin, original magnification ×40.

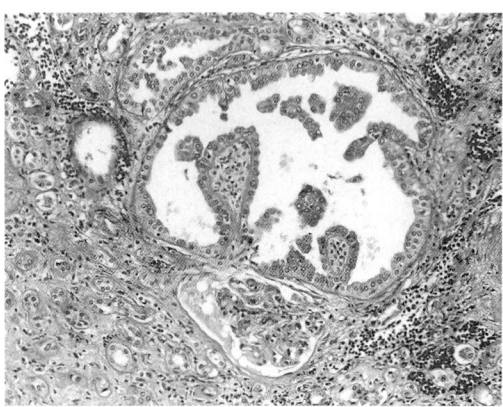

Figure 23–21. Acquired cystic disease of the kidney. Dilated tubule with polypoid ingrowth of the hyperplastic lining epithelium (hematoxyln and eosin, original magnification ×40).

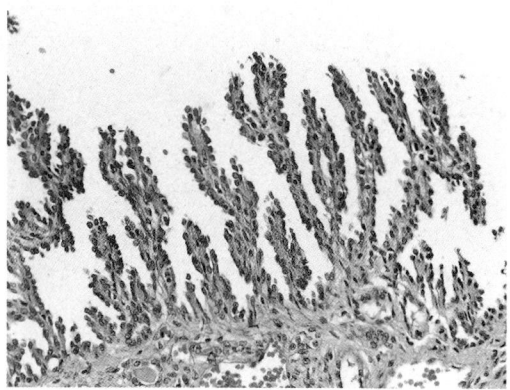

Figure 23–23. Acquired cystic disease of the kidney. Papillary renal cell carcinoma, type 1 (hematoxyln and eosin, original magnification ×40).

common. Lectin histochemical and immunohistochemical study of cysts and tumors from nine specimens of acquired cystic disease showed a predominance of characteristics consistent with proximal tubular origin in both the cysts and tumors (Kikuchi, 1989).

AUTOSOMAL DOMINANT POLYCYSTIC KIDNEY DISEASE

Renal cell carcinomas may be found in kidneys affected by autosomal dominant polycystic kidney disease (Fig. 23–25). In a study of the kidneys of 87 patients with autosomal

dominant polycystic kidney disease, 42 renal cell neoplasms, almost all of which the authors characterized as small "adenomas," were found in 24% of the patients (Gregoire et al., 1987). Based on larger populations, it is estimated that the incidence of renal cell carcinoma is 10 times greater in patients with autosomal dominant polycystic kidney disease than in the general population (Bernstein et al., 1987). Bilateral renal cell carcinoma is also more common in this population.

Epithelial proliferation is common in the tubules and cysts of these kidneys (Fig. 23–26), frequently forming papillary or polypoid projections (Fig. 23–27). These struc-

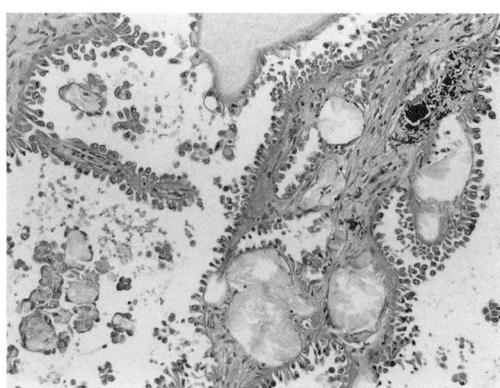

Figure 23–22. Acquired cystic disease of the kidney. Cysts lined by atypical epithelium forming papillae. Note abundant oxalate crystals in papillae and septa (hematoxylin and eosin, original magnification ×40).

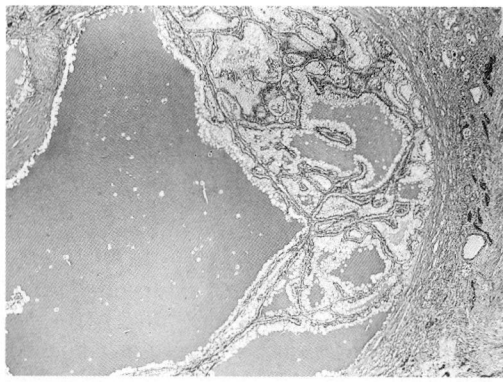

Figure 23–24. Acquired cystic disease of the kidney. Clear cell renal cell carcinoma, 1 mm in diameter (hematoxylin and eosin, original magnification ×10).

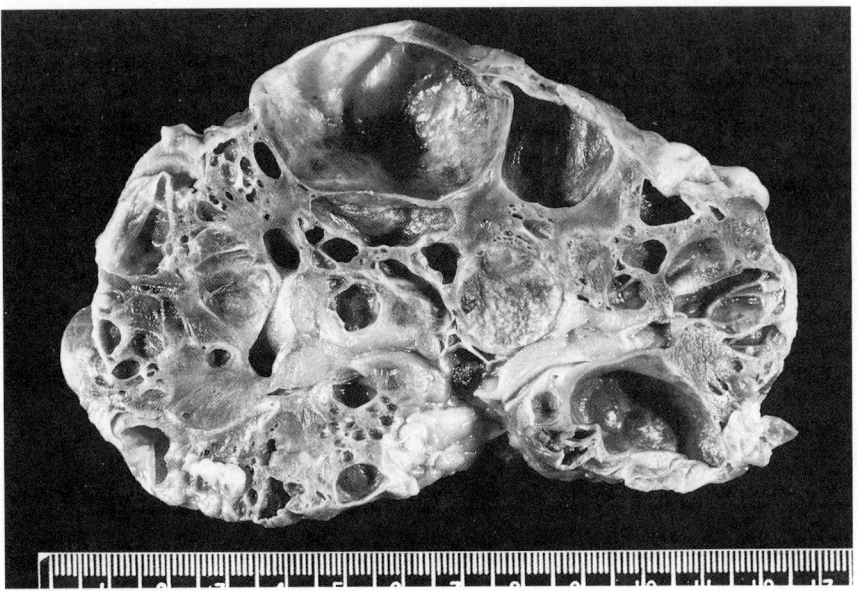

Figure 23–25. Autosomal dominant cystic disease of kidney with an 18 mm spheroidal clear cell renal carcinoma in a central location.

tures are found in more than 90% of patients (Gregoire et al., 1987), even when renal function was not much impaired and the kidneys were little enlarged. The cells of these lesions are often basophil, but clear cell and other types may be found. Most authors consider these proliferations to be hyperplastic (Bernstein et al., 1987; Gregoire et al., 1987), but at the cytologic level, their cells resemble those of recognized types of renal cell carcinomas.

OTHER CYSTIC DISEASES

Patients with von Hippel–Lindau disease often have multiple renal cysts and renal cell carcinomas. While the cysts are usually lined by benign-appearing epithelium, in some cases, the lining has consisted of clear cytoplasm resembling the cells of the carcinomas (Christenson et al., 1982). The associated

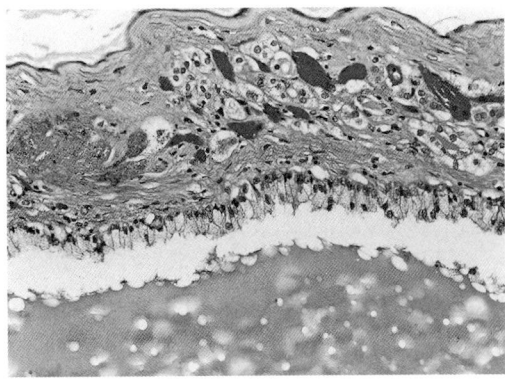

Figure 23–26. Autosomal dominant cystic disease of kidney. Atypical hyperplastic cells lining a cyst (hematoxylin and eosin, original magnification ×40).

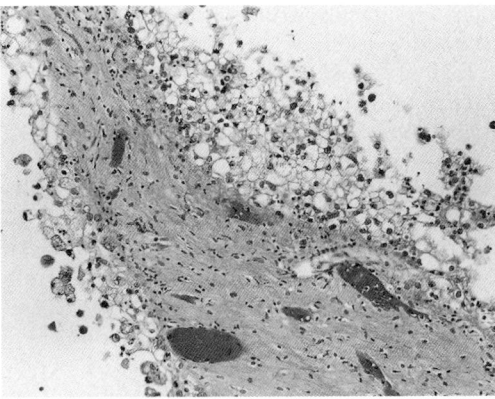

Figure 23–27. Autosomal dominant cystic disease of kidney. Clear cells with slightly pleomorphic and hyperchromatic nuclei line both sides of an intercystic septum. The cells form a lining of multiple layers and form a small papilla (hematoxylin and eosin, original magnification ×40).

carcinomas may be cystic, appearing to be an outgrowth of these cysts (Christenson et a l., 1982). In tuberous sclerosis and von Hippel–Lindau disease, atypical cysts have been found adjacent to renal cell carcinomas (Ibrahim et al., 1989). The cells in the cysts and the cells in the carcinomas are cytologically identical and have similar, essentially euploid, DNA indices. In von Hippel–Lindau disease, lectin histochemistry has identified atypical cysts and carcinomas with staining patterns characteristic of distal and proximal tubules (Kragel et al., 1991). Renal cell carcinoma has also been reported in association with multicystic dysplastic kidneys (Birken et al., 1985). There is evidence that tuberous sclerosis predisposes to renal cell carcinoma, and that this is linked to the renal cysts that are common in tuberous sclerosis (Al-Saleem et al., 1998).

The investigations of the origins of human renal cell neoplasms presented above can be synthesized into an overview in which the various types of renal cell neoplasms arise in different parts of the nephron through the accumulation of different genetic defects that correlate to a great extent with their morphologies. Clear cell renal cell carcinomas appear to arise in the proximal tubule, and loss of genes in the region of 3p appears to be an important event in this process. This picture of the origin of clear cell carcinoma will be further refined in the future as the results of more studies are available. Interestingly, serial-section studies of clear cell tumors chemically induced in rats have shown that they originate in the collecting ducts (Nogueira et al., 1989). Papillary renal cell carcinomas appear also to arise in the proximal tubule but through an adenoma–carcinoma sequence involving the progressive development of multiple trisomies. Neoplasms apparently of distal nephron origin are chromophobe cell carcinoma, renal oncocytoma, and carcinoma of the collecting ducts of Bellini. Chromophobe renal cell carcinoma arises through remarkable losses of multiple whole chromosomes. Oncocytomas commonly have translocations. The genetic defects important in the genesis of collecting duct carcinoma remain to be discovered.

While cystic diseases predispose to the development of renal cell carcinomas and intratubular and intracystic polyps are likely progenitors of the clinical cancers, most renal cell carcinomas arise in largely normal kidneys, leaving no trace of their earliest forms. Thus, with the exception of papillary renal cell carcinoma, information about the precursors of most renal cell carcinomas is largely inferential from studies of the smallest examples of each type, and there does appear to be a progression from tubules lined by atypical epithelium through nodules of millimeter size to clinical carcinoma. What little evidence is available suggests that these small lesions are often aneuploid and their morphology and immunophenotypes have much in common with their clinically apparent counterparts.

REFERENCES

Al-Saleem T, Wessner LL, Scheithauer BW, Patterson K, Roach ES, Dreyer SJ, Fujikawa K, Bjornsson J, Bernstein J, Henske EP. (1998) Malignant tumors of the kidney, brain, and soft tissues in children and young adults with the tuberous sclerosis complex. *Cancer* 83:2208–2216.

Anglard P, Tory K, Brauch H, Weiss GH, Latif F, Merino MJ, Lerman MI, Zbar B, Linehan WM. (1991) Molecular analysis of genetic changes in the origin and development of renal cell carcinoma. *Cancer Res* 51:1071–1077.

Aso Y, Homma Y. (1992) A survey on incidental renal cell carcinoma in Japan. *J Urol* 147:340–343.

Baer SC, Ro JY, Ordonez NG, Maiese RL, Loose JH, Grignon DJ, Ayala AG. (1993) Sarcomatoid collecting duct carcinoma: a clinicopathologic and immunohistochemical study of five cases. *Hum Pathol* 24:1017–1022.

Bailey OT, Harrison JH. (1937) Large benign renal neoplasms: their pathology and clinical behavior, with report of five cases. *J Urol* 38:509–529.

Ban S-I, Yoshii S, Tsuruta A, Gotoh Y, Shimizu Y, Shibata T. (1996) Metanephric adenoma of the kidney: ultrastructural, immunohistochemical and lectin histochemical studies. *Pathol Int* 46:661–666.

Béroud C, Fournet J-C, Jeanpierre C, Droz D, Bouvier R, Froger D, Chrétien Y, Maréchal J-M, Weissenbach J, Junien C. (1996) Correlations of allelic imbalance of chromosome 14 with adverse prognostic parameters in 148 renal cell carcinomas. *Genes Chromosom Cancer* 17:215–224.

Bell ET. (1938) A classification of renal tumors with observations on the frequency of the various types. *J Urol* 39:238–243.

Bennington JL. (1973) Cancer of the kidney—etiology, epidemiology, and pathology. *Cancer* 32:1017–1029.

Bennington JL, Beckwith JB. (1975) *Atlas of Tumor Pathology*, Second Series, Fasicle 12, *Tumors of the Kidney, Renal Pelvis, and Ureter*. Armed Forces Institute of Pathology, Washington, DC.

Bergerheim USR, Frisk B, Stellan B, Collins VP, Zech L. (1990) del(3p)(p13p21) in renal cell adenoma and del(4p)(p14) in bilateral renal cell carcinoma in two unrelated patients with von Hippel-Lindau disease. *Cancer Genet Cytogenet* 49:125–131.

Bernstein J, Evan AP, Gardner KD Jr. (1987) Epithelial hyperplasia in human polycystic kidney diseases, its role in pathogenesis and risk of neoplasia. *AM J Pathol* 129:92–101.

Bigg SW, Bari WA. (1997) Nephrogenic adenofibroma: an unusual renal tumor. *J Urol* 157:1835–1836.

Birken G, King D, Vane D, Lloyd T. (1985) Renal cell carcinoma arising in a multicystic dysplastic kidney. *J Pediatr Surg* 20:619–621.

Bonsib SM, Bromely C, Lager DJ. (1991) Renal oncocytoma: diagnostic utility of cytokeratin-containing globular filamentous bodies. *Mod Pathol* 4:16–23.

Bonsib SM, Lager DJ. (1990) Chromophobe cell carcinoma: analysis of five cases. *Am J Surg Pathol* 14:260–267.

Bretan PN, Busch MP, Hricak H, Williams RD. (1986) Chronic renal failure: a significant risk factor in the development of acquired renal cysts and renal cell carcinoma, case reports and review of the literature. *Cancer* 57:1871–1879.

Brisigotti M, Cozzutto C, Fabbretti G, Sergi C, Callea F. (1992) Metanephric adenoma. *Histol Histopathol* 7:689–692.

Brooks B, Sørensen FB, Olsen S, Holm-Nielsen P. (1993) Classification of tubulo-papillary renal cortical tumours using estimates of nuclear volume. *APMIS* 101:378–386.

Brooks JD, Bova S, Marshall FF, Isaacs WB. (1993) Tumor suppressor gene allelic loss in renal cancers. *J Urol* 150:1278–1283.

Brown JA, Anderl KL, Borell TJ, Qian J, Bostwick DG, Jenkins RB. (1997) Simultaneous chromosome 7 and 17 gain and sex chromosome loss provide evidence that renal metanephric adenoma is related to papillary renal cell carcinoma. *J Urol* 158:370–374.

Brown JA, Sebo TJ, Segura JW. (1996) Metaphase analysis of metanephric adenoma reveals chromosome Y loss with chromosome 7 and 17 gain. *Urology* 48:473–475.

Budin RE, McDonnell PJ. (1984) Renal cell neoplasms, their relationship to arteriolonephrosclerosis. *Arch Pathol Lab Med* 108:138–140.

Bugert P, Gaul C, Weber K, Herbers J, Akhtar M, Ljungberg B, Kovacs G. (1997) Specific genetic changes of diagnostic importance in chromophobe renal cell carcinoma. *Lab Invest* 76:203–208.

Cabot H, Middleton AW. (1938) The relation of so-called adenoma of the kidney to carcinoma of the kidney. *Trans Am Assoc Genitourin Surg* 31:91–109.

Carroll PR, Murty VVS, Reuter V, Jhanwar S, Fair WR, Whitmore WF, Chaganti RSK. (1987) Abnormalities at chromosome region 3p12-14 characterize clear cell renal carcinoma. *Cancer Genet Cytogenet* 26:253–259.

Cass AS. (1980) Large renal adenoma. *J Urol* 124:281–282.

Cavazzana AO, Prayer-Galetti T, Tirabosco R, Macciomei MC, Stella M, Lania L, Cannada-Bartoli P, Spagnoli LG, Passerini-Glazel G, Pagano F. (1996) Bellini duct carcinoma, a clinical and in vitro study. *Eur Urol* 30:340–344.

Cheng WS, Farrow GM, Zincke H. (1991) The incidence of multicentricity in renal cell carcinoma. *J Urol* 146:1221–1223.

Childs P, Waterfall WB. (1953) Renal adenoma: a review with a report of two further cases. *Br J Urol* 25:187–194.

Christenson PJ, Craig JP, Bibro MC, O'Connell KJ. (1982) Cysts containing renal cell carcinoma in von Hippel–Lindau disease. *J Urol* 128:798–800.

Cohen AJ, Li FP, Berg S, Marchetto DJ, Tsai S, Jacobs SC, Brown RS. (1979) Hereditary renal-cell carcinoma associated with a chromosomal translocation. *N Engl J Med* 301:592–595.

Cohen C, McCue PA, DeRose PB. (1995) Immunohistochemistry of renal adenomas and carcinomas. *J Urol Pathol* 3:61–71.

Comerci SCD, Levin TL, Ruzal-Shapiro C, Berdon WE, Beckwith JB, Hibshoosh H, Hurlet-Jensen A, Sitarz AL. (1996) Benign adenomatous kidney neoplasms in children with polycythemia: imaging findings. *Radiology* 198:265–268.

Corwin WC. (1940) Multiple adenomas of the kidneys, report of a case. *J Urol* 43:249–252.

Cristol DS, Bothe AE, Grotzinger PJ. (1950) Renal adenoma: survey of reported clinical cases and another case report. *J Urol* 64:58–62.

Cristol DS, McDonald JR, Emmett JL. (1946) Renal adenomas in hypernephromatous kidneys: a study of their incidence, nature and relationships. *J Urol* 55:18–27.

Dal Cin P, Gaeta J, Huben R, Li FP, Prout GR, Jr, Sandberg AA. (1989) Renal cortical tumors, cytogenetic characterization. *Am J Clin Pathol* 92:408–414.

Dal Cin P, von Poppel H, Sciot R, de Vos R, van Damme B, Baert L, Van den Berghe H. (1996) The t(1;12)(p36;q13) in a renal oncocytoma. *Genes Chromosom Cancer* 17:136–139.

Davis CJ Jr, Barton JH, Sesterhenn IA, Mostofi FK. (1995) Metanephric adenoma, clinicopathological study of fifty patients. *Am J Surg Pathol* 19:1101–1114.

Davis CJ Jr, Mostofi FK, Sesterhenn IA, Ho CK. (1991) Renal oncocytoma, clinicopathological study of 166 patients. *J Urogenital Pathol* 1:41–52.

Decker HJH, Weidt EJ, Brieger J. (1997) The von Hippel–Lindau tumor suppressor gene: a rare and intriguing disease opening new insight into basic mechanisms of carcinogenesis. *Cancer Genet Cytogenet* 93:74–83.

Delahunt B, Eble JN. (1997a) Papillary renal cell carcinoma: a clinicopathologic and immunohistochemical study of 105 tumors. *Mod Pathol* 10:537–544.

Delahunt B, Eble JN. (1997b) Renal adenoma: an evolving concept. *J Urol Pathol* 7:99–112.

Delahunt B, Nacey JN, Hammett GD, Frater WJ. (1989) Nucleolar organizing regions in renal cell carcinoma, renal oncocytoma and renal adenoma. *Anal Cell Pathol* 1:185–190.

Dujkhuizen T, van den Berg E, Störkel S, De Vries B, van der Veen AY, Wilbrink M, van Kessel AG, de Jong B. (1997) Renal oncocytoma with t(5;12;11), DER(1)t(1;8) and ADD(19): "true" oncocytoma or chromophobe adenoma? *Int J Cancer* 73:521–524.

Dijkhuizen T, van den Berg E, Störkel S, Terpe H-J, Bürger H, de Jong B. (1998) Distinct features for chromophilic renal cell cancer with Xp11.2 breakpoints. *Cancer Genet Cytogenet* 104:74–76.

Dunnill MS, Millard PR, Oliver D. (1977) Acquired cystic disease of the kidneys: a hazard of long-term intermittent maintenance haemodialysis. *J Clin Pathol* 30:868–877.

Eble JN. (1997) Neoplasms of the kidney. In: *Urologic Surgical Pathology* (Bostwick DG, Eble JN, eds.) pp. 82–147. Mosby-Year Book, St. Louis.

Eble JN, Hull MT. (1984) Morphologic features of renal oncocytoma: a light and electron microscopic study. *Hum Pathol* 15:1054–1061.

Eble JN, Hull MT. (1988) Glycoconjugate expression in human renal oncocytomas. *Arch Pathol Lab Med* 112: 805–808.

Eble JN, Sledge G. (1986) Cellular deoxyribonucleic acid content of renal oncocytomas: flow cytometric analysis of paraffin-embedded tissues from eight tumors. *J Urol* 136:522–524.

Eble JN, Warfel K (1991) Early human renal cortical epithelial neoplasia. *Mod Pathol* 4:45A.

Erlandson RA, Reuter VE. (1988) Renal tumor in a 62-year-old male. *Ultrastruct Pathol* 12:561–567.

Eschwege P, Saussine C, Steichen G, Delepaul B, Drelon L, Jacqmin D. (1996) Radical nephrectomy for renal cell carcinoma 30 mm. or less: long-term followup results. *J Urol* 155:1196–1199.

Evins SC, Varner W. (1979) Renal adenoma—a misnomer. *Urology* 13:85–86.

Fallon B, Williams RD. (1989) Renal cancer associated with acquired cystic disease of the kidney and chronic renal failure. *Semin Urol* 7:228–236.

Farnsworth WV, Cohen C, McCue PA, DeRose PB. (1994) DNA analysis of small renal cortical neoplasms, comparison with renal carcinomas. *J Urol Pathol* 2:65–79.

Fayemi AO, Ali M. (1980) Acquired renal cysts and tumors superimposed on chronic primary kidney diseases. *Pathol Res Pract* 168:73–83.

Fischer J, Palmedo G, Von Knobloch R, Bugert P, Prayer-Galetti T, Pagano F, Kovacs G. (1998) Duplication and overexpression of the mutant allele of the *MET* proto-oncogene in multiple hereditary papillary renal cell tumours. *Oncogene* 17:733–739.

Fogt F, Zhuang Z, Linehan WM, Merino MJ. (1999) Collecting duct carcinomas of the kidney: a comparative loss of heterozygosity study with clear cell renal cell carcinoma. *Oncol Rep* 5:923–926.

Füzesi L, Cober M, Mittermayer C. (1992) Collecting duct carcinoma: cytogenetic characterization. *Histopathology* 21:155–160.

Füzesi L, Gunawan B, Braun S, Bergmann F, Brauers A, Effert P, Mittermayer C. (1998) Cytogenetic analysis of 11 renal oncocytomas: further evidence of structural rearrangements of 11q13 as a characteristic chromosomal anomaly. *Cancer Genet Cytogenet* 107: 1–6.

Fujimoto S, Sumiyoshi A, Yamamoto Y, Tanaka K. (1988) Renal cell carcinoma associated with acquired renal cystic disease. *Int Urol Nephrol* 20:347–352.

Gatalica Z, Grujic S, Kovatich A, Petersen RO. (1996) Metanephric adenoma: histology, immunophenotype, cytogenetics, ultrastructure. *Mod Pathol* 9:329–333.

Gnarra JR, Tory K, Weng Y, Schmidt L, Wei MH, Li H, Latif F, Liu S, Chen F, Duh F-M, Lubensky I, Duan DR, Florence C, Pozzatti R, Walther MM, Bander NH, Grossman HB, Brauch H, Pomer S, Brooks JD, Issacs WB, Lerman MI, Zbar B, Linehan WM. (1994) Mutations of the *VHL* tumour suppressor gene in renal carcinoma. *Nature Genet* 7:85–90.

Goodman MD, Goodman BK, Lubin MB, Braunstein G, Rotter JI, Schreck RR. (1990) Cytogenetic characterization of renal cell carcinoma in von Hippel Lindau syndrome. *Cancer* 65:1150–1154.

Govaerts JJL, van Gooswilligen JC, Vooys GP, Ramaekers FCS, Herman CJ, Debruyne FMJ. (1987) Renal hamartoma associated with renal cell (Grawitz) tumor: another indication that Grawitz tumors are carcinosarcomas. *Eur Urol* 13:276–280.

Grawitz P. (1883) Die sogenannten Lipome der Niere. *Virchows Arch Pathol Anat Physiol Klin Med* 93:39–63.

Gregoire JR, Torres VE, Holley KE, Farrow GM. (1987) Renal epithelial hyperplastic and neoplastic proliferation in autosomal dominant polycystic kidney disease. *Am J Kidney Dis* 9:27–38.

Gregori-Romero MA, Morell-Quadreny L, Llombart-Bosch A. (1996) Cytogenetic analysis of three primary Bellini duct carcinomas. *Genes Chromosom Cancer* 15:170–172.

Grignon DJ, Eble JN. (1998) Papillary and metanephric adenomas of the kidney. *Semin Diagn Pathol* 15: 41–53.

Gunawan B, Bergmann F, Braun S, Hemmerlein B, Ringert RH, Jakse G, Füzesi L. (1999) Polyploidization and losses of chromosomes 1, 2, 6, 10, 13, and 17 in three cases of chromophobe renal cell carcinomas. *Cancer Genet Cytogenet* 110:57–61.

Gurney H, Larcos G, McKay M, Kefford R, Langlands A. (1989) Bone metastases in hypernephroma, frequency of scapular involvement. *Cancer* 64:1429–1431.

Halenda G, Sees JN Jr, Belis JA, Rohner TJ Jr. (1993) Atypical renal adenocarcinoma with features suggesting collecting duct origin and mimicking a mucinous adenocarcinoma. *Urology* 41:165–168.

Hashine K, Sumiyoshi Y, Kagawa S. (1996) A morphological study of renal adenoma and latent renal cell carcinoma in autopsy cases. *Nippon Hinyokika Gakkai Zasshi* 87:667–675.

Hennigar RA, Beckwith JB. (1992) Nephrogenic adenofibroma, a novel kidney tumor of young people. *Am J Surg Pathol* 16:325–334.

Herbers J, Schullerus D, Müller H, Kenck C, Chudek J, Weimer J, Bugert P, Kovacs G. (1997) Significance of chromsome arm 14q loss in nonpapillary renal cell carcinomas. *Genes Chromosom Cancer* 19:29–35.

Herman JG, Latif F, Weng Y, Lerman MI, Zbar B, Liu S, Samid D, Duan DR, Gnarra JR, Linehan WM, Baylin SB. (1994) Silencing of the *VHL* tumor-suppressor gene by DNA methylation in renal carcinoma. *Proc Natl Acad Sci USA* 91:9700–9704.

Hiasa Y, Kitamura M, Nakaoka S, Ohshima M, Konishi N, Kitahori Y, Hirao K,Fukushima Y, Tho Y, Hayashi I, and Ichijima K. (1995) Antigen immunohistochemistry of renal cell adenomas in autopsy cases: relevance to histogenesis. *Oncology* 52:97–105.

Hida M, Takamiya T, Iida T, Kitamura M, Kitajima N, Hiraga S, Satoh T. (1988) Four cases of acquired cystic disease of the kidney complicated with renal cell carcinoma in long-term hemodialysis. *Nippon Hinyokika Gakkai Zasshi* 79:164–170.

Hubert J, Lemella J-L, Grignon Y, Nodari F, Mangin P. (1996) Le néphrome néphrogène: tumeur bénigne du rein de l'adulte. A propos de deux cas. *Prog Urol* 6:98–102.

Hughson MD, Buchwald D, Fox M. (1986) Renal neoplasia and acquired cystic kidney disease in patients receiving long-term dialysis. *Arch Pathol Lab Med* 110:592–601.

Ibrahim RE, Weinberg DS, Weidner N. (1989) Atypical cysts and carcinomas of the kidneys in the phacomatoses, a quantitative DNA study using static and flow cytometry. *Cancer* 63:148–157.

Ishikawa I. (19850 Uremic acquired cystic disease of kidney. *Urology* 26:101–108.

Ishikawa I. (1987) Development of adenocarcinoma and acquired cystic disease of the kidney in hemodialysis patients. *Int Symp Princess Takamatsu Cancer Res Fund* 18:77–86.

Ishikawa I, Saito Y, Shikura N, Kitada H, Shinoda A, and Suzuki S. (1990) Ten-year prospective study on the development of renal cell carcinoma in dialysis patients. *Am J Kidney Dis* 16:452–458.

Jamis-Dow CA, Choyke PL, Jennings SB, Linehan WM, Thakore KN, Walther MM. (1996) Small (<3-cm) renal masses: detection with CT versus US and pathologic correlation. *Radiology* 198:785–788.

Jiang F, Richter J, Schraml P, Bubendorf L, Gasser T, Sauter G, Mihatsch MJ, Moch H. (1998) Chromosomal imbalances in papillary renal cell carcinoma: genetic differences between histologic subtypes. *Am J Pathol* 153:1467–1473.

Jones EC, Pins M, Dickersin GR, Young RH. (1995) Metanephric adenoma of the kidney, a clinicopathological, immunohistochemical, flow cytometric, cytogenetic, and electron microscopic study of seven cases. *Am J Surg Pathol* 19:615–626.

Jordan DK, Patil SR, Divelbiss JE, Vemuganti S, Headley C, Waziri MH, Gurll NJ. (1989) Cytogenetic abnormalities in tumors of patients with von-Hippel–Lindau disease. *Cancer Genet Cytogenet* 42:227–241.

Jow WW, Zeid MY, Cowan D, Malin B, Deberry JL III. (1991) Renal oncocytoma: long-term follow-up and flow cytometric DNA analysis. *J Surg Oncol* 46:53–59.

Judd ES, Simon HE. (1927) Benign adenoma of the kidney, report of a case. *Surg Gynecol Obstet* 44:169–172.

Katz DS, Gharagozloo AM, Peebles TR, Oliphant M. (1996) Renal oncocytomatosis. *Am J Kidney Dis* 27:579–582.

Kennedy SM, Merino MJ, Linehan WM, Roberts JR, Robertson CN, Neumann RD. (1990) Collecting duct carcinoma of the kidney. *Hum Pathol* 21:449–456.

Kikuchi Y. (1989) Lectin and immunohistochemical studies on acquired cystic kidney and associated renalcell carcinoma. *Acta Pathol Jpn* 39:373–380.

King CR, Schimke RN, Arthur T, Davoren B, Collins D. (1987) Proximal 3p deletion in renal cell carcinoma cells from a patient with von Hippel–Lindau disease. *Cancer Genet Cytogenet* 27:345–348.

Kinoshita H, Ogawa O, Mitsomori K, Kakehi Y, Terachi T, Yoshida O. (1998) Low frequency of positive telomerase activity in a chromophobe subtype of renal cell carcinoma. *J Urol* 159:245–251.

Kinouchi T, Saiki S, Naoe T, Uenaka A, Kotake T, Shiku H, Nakayama E. (1989) Correlation of c-myc expression with nuclear pleomorphism in human renal cell carcinoma. *Cancer Res* 49:3627–3630.

Klein MJ, Valensi QJ. (1976) Proximal tubular adenomas of kidney with so-called oncocytic features, a clinicopathologic study of 13 cases of a rarely reported neoplasm. *Cancer* 38:9096–914.

Kovacs A, Kovacs G. (1992) Low chromosome number in chromophobe renal cell carcinomas. *Genes Chromosom Cancer* 4:267–268.

Kovacs G. (1989) Papillary renal cell carcinoma, a morphologic and cytogenetic study of 11 cases. *Am J Pathol* 134:27–34.

Kovacs G. (1993) Molecular differential pathology of renal cell tumours. *Histopathology* 22:1–8.

Kovacs G. (1994) The value of molecular genetic analysis in the diagnosis and prognosis of renal cell tumours. *World J Urol* 12:64–68.

Kovacs G, Erlandsson R, Boldog F, Ingvarsson S, Müller-Brechlin R, Klein G, Sümegi J. (1988) Consistent chromosome 3p deletion and loss of heterozygosity in renal cell carcinoma. *Proc Natl Acad Sci USA* 85:1571–1575.

Kovacs G, Szücs S, De Riese W, Baumgärtel H. (1987) Specific chromosome aberration in human renal cell carcinoma. *Int J Cancer* 40:171–178.

Kovacs G, Szücs S, Eichner W, Maschek H-J, Wahnschaffe U, De Riese W. (1987) Renal oncocytoma, a cytogenetic and morphologic study. *Cancer* 59:2071–2077.

Kovacs G, Tory K, Kovacs A. (1994) Development of papillary renal cell tumours is associated with loss of Y-chromosome-specific DNA sequences. *J Pathol* 173:39–44.

Kovacs G, Wilkens L, Papp T, De Riese W. (1989) Differentiation between papillary and nonpapillary renal cell carcinomas by DNA anaysis. *J Natl Cancer Inst* 81:527–530.

Kragel PJ, Walther MM, Pestaner JP, Filling-Katz MR. (1991) Simple renal cysts, atypical renal cysts, and renal cell carcinoma in von Hippel–Lindau disease: a lectin and immunohistochemical study in six patients. *Mod Pathol* 4:210–214.

Kragel PJ, Williams J, Emory TS, Merino MJ. (1990) Renal oncocytoma with cylindromatous changes: pathologic features and histogenetic significance. *Mod Pathol* 3:277–281.

Krempien B, Ritz E. (1980) Acquired cystic transformation of the kidneys of haemodialysed patients. *Virchows Arch A Anat Pathol Histopathol* 386:189–200.

Kretschmer HL, Doehring C. (1929) Adenoma of the kidney. *Surg Gynecol Obstet* 48:629–635.

Latif F, Tory K, Gnarra J, Yao M, Duh F-M, Orcutt ML, Stackhouse T, Kuzmin I, Modi W, Geil L, Schmidt L, Zhou F, Li H, Wei MH, Chen F, Glenn G, Choyke P, Walther MM, Weng Y, Duan DR, Dean M, Glavac D, Richards FM, Crossey PA, Ferguson-Smith MA, Le Paslier D, Chumakov I, Cohen D, Chinault AC, Maher ER, Linehan WM, Zbar B, Lerman MI. (1993) Identification of the von Hippel–Lindau disease tumor suppressor gene. *Science* 260:1317–1320.

Levine E, Huntrakoon M, Wetzel LH. (1989) Small renal neoplasms: clinical, pathologic, and imaging features. *AJR Am J Roentgenol* 153:69–73.

Levine E, Slusher SL, Grantham JJ, Wetzel LH. (1991) Natural history of acquired renal cystic disease in dialysis patients: a prospective longitudinal CT study. *AJR Am J Roentgenol* 156:501–506.

Lineham WM, Lerman MI, Zbar B. (1995) Identification of the von Hippel–Lindau (VHL) gene, its role in renal cancer. *JAMA* 273:564–570.

Lovell M, Lott ST, Wong P, El-Naggar A, Tucker S, and Killary AM. (1999) The genetic locus *NRC-1* within chromosome 3p12 mediates tumor suppression in renal cell carcinoma independently of histological type, tumor microenvironment, and *VHL* mutation. *Cancer Res* 59:2182–2189.

Lubensky I, Schmidt L, Zhuang Z, Weirich G, Pack S, Zambrano N, Walther MM, Choyke P, Linehan WM, Zbar B. (1999) Hereditary and sporadic papillary renal carcinomas with c-*MET* mutations share a distinct morphologic phenotype. *Am J Pathol* 155:517–526.

Makita Y, Inenaga T, Kinjo M, Komatsu K, Onoyama K, Fujishima M. (1991) Renal oncocytoma developed in a long-term hemodialysis patient. *Nephron* 57: 355–357.

Marras S, Faa G, Scarpa R, Valdes E, Vanni R. (1997) Diagnosis of chromophobe renal cell carcinoma by chromosomal analysis. *Tumori* 83:753–755.

Matson MA, Cohen EP. (1990) Acquired cystic kidney disease: occurrence, prevalence and renal cancers. *Medicine* 69:217–226.

Mayer D, Weber E, Kadenbach B, Bannasch P. (1989) Immunocytochemical demonstration of cytochrome c oxidase as a marker for renal oncocytes and oncocytomas. *Toxicol Pathol* 17:46–49.

Medeiros LJ, Michie SA, Johnson DE, Warnke RA, Weiss LM. (1988) An immunoperoxidase study of renal cell carcinomas: correlation with nuclear grade, cell type, and histologic pattern. *Hum Pathol* 19:980–987.

Minar E, Tscholakoff D, Zazgornik J, Schmidt P, Marosi L, Czembirek H. (1984) Acquired cystic disease of the kidneys in chronic hemodialyzed and renal transplant patients. *Eur Urol* 10:245–248.

Mittal BV, Cotton RE. (1987) Severely atypical changes in renal epithelium in biopsy and graft nephrectomy specimens in two cases of cadaver renal transplantation. *Histopathology* 11:833–841.

Morita R, Ishikawa J, Tsutsumi M, Hikiji K, Tsukada Y, Kamidono S, Maeda S, Nakamura Y. (1991) Allelotype of renal cell carcinoma. *Cancer Res* 51:820–823.

Morris H. (1911) Renal adenomata. *Practitioner* 87:1–7.

Mostofi FK, Sesterhenn IA, Sobin LH. (1981) *Histological Typing of Kidney Tumours*, pp. 1–23. Geneva.

Mourad WA, Nestok BR, Saleh GY, Solez K, Power RF, Jewell LD. (1994) Dysplastic tubular epithelium in "normal" kidney associated with renal cell carcinoma. *Am J Surg Pathol* 18:1117–1124.

Murphy WM, Beckwith JB, Farrow GM. (1994) *Atlas of Tumor Pathology*, Third Series, Fascicle 11, *Tumors of the Kidney, Bladder, and Related Urinary Structures*. Armed Forces Institute of Pathology, Washington, DC.

Nagashima Y, Arai N, Tanaka Y, Yoshida S, Sumino K, Ohaki Y, Matsushita K, Morita T, Misuga K. (1991) Two cases of a renal epithelial tumour resembling immature nephron. *Virchows Arch A Pathol. Anat. Histopathol.* 418:77–81.

Neuhaus C, Dijkhuizen T, van den Berg E, Störkel S, Stöckle M, Mensch B Huber C, Decker H-J. (1997) Involvement of the chromosomal region 11q13 in renal oncocytoma: case report and literature review. *Cancer Genet Cytogenet* 94:95–98.

Newcomb WD. (1936) The search for truth, with special reference to the frequency of gastric ulcer cancer and the origin of Grawitz tumours of the kidney. *Proc R Soc Med* 30:113–136.

Nogueira E, Klimek F, Weber E, Bannasch P. (1989) Collecting duct origin of rat renal clear cell tumors. *Virchows Arch B* 57:275–283.

Nonomura A, Mizukami Y, Hasegawa T, Ohkawa M. (1995) Metanephric adenoma of the kidney: an electron microscopic and immunohistochemical study with quantitative DNA measurement by image analysis. *Ultrastruct Pathol* 19:481–488.

Nordenson I, Ljungberg B, Roos G. (1988) Chromosomes in renal carcinoma with reference to intratumor heterogeneity. *Cancer Genet Cytogenet* 32:35–41.

Nørgaard T, Skaarup P. (1985) Infiltrating renal collecting duct carcinoma associated with epithelial dysplasia of the renal pelvis. *Scand J Urol Nephrol* 19:69–70.

Norman C. (1893) Adenoma of the kidney in the adult. *Trans R Acad Med Ireland* 11:377–386.

Oberling C, Rivière M, Hagueneau F. (1960) Ultrastructure of the clear cells in renal carcinomas and its importance for the demonstration of their renal origin. *Nature* 186:402–403.

O'Donnell CO, Cutner A, Williams G. (1988) Metastatic native renal carcinoma in renal transplant recipients. *Nephrol Dial Transplant* 3:690–693.

Oosterwijk E, Van Muijen GNP, Oosterwijk-Wakka JC, Warnaar SO. (1990) Expression of intermediate-sized filaments in developing and adult human kidney and in renal cell carcinoma. *J Histochem Cytochem* 38:385–392.

Ortmann M, Vierbuchen M, Fischer R. (1988a) Renal oncocytoma II. Lectin and immunohistochemical features indicating an origin from the collecting duct. *Virchows Arch B Cell Pathol Incl Mol Pathol* 56: 175–184.

Ortmann M, Vierbuchen M, Fischer R. (1991) Sialylated glycoconjugates in chromophobe cell renal carcinoma compared with other renal cell tumors, indication of its development from the collecting duct epithelium. *Virchows Arch B Cell Pathol Incl Mol Pathol* 61:123–132.

Ortmann M, Vierbuchen M, Koller G, Fischer R. (1988b) Renal oncocytoma I. Cytochrome oxidase in normal and neoplastic renal tissue as detected by immunohistochemistry—a valuable aid to distinguish oncocytomas from renal cell carcinomas. *Virchows Arch B* 56:165–173.

Pagès A, Granier M. (1980) Le néphrome néphronogène. *Arch Anat Cytol Pathol* 28:99–103.

Pitz S, Moll R, Störkel S, Thoenes W. (1987) Expression of intermediate filament proteins in subtypes of renal cell carcinoma and in renal oncocytomas, distinction of two classes of renal cell tumors. *Lab Invest* 56:642–653.

Presti JC Jr, Moch H, Reuter VE, Huynh D, Waldman RM. (1996) Comparative genomic hybridization for genetic analysis of renal oncocytomas. *Genes Chromosom Cancer* 17:199–204.

Presti JC Jr, Rao PH, Chen Q, Reuter VE, Li FP, Fair WR, Jhanwar SC. (1991) Histopathological, cytogenetic, and molecular characterization of renal cortical tumors. *Cancer Res* 51:1544–1552.

Psihramis KE, Althausen AF, Yoshida MA, Prout GR Jr, Sandberg AA. (1986) Chromosome anomalies suggestive of malignant transformation in bilateral renal oncocytoma. *J Urol* 136:892–895.

Reese AJM, Winstanley DP. (1958) The small tumor-like lesions of the kidney. *Br J Cancer* 12:507–516.

Reis M, Faria V, Lindoro J, Adolfo A. (1988) The small cystic and noncystic noninflammatory renal nodules: a postmortem study. *J Urol* 140:721–724.

Renshaw AA, Maurici D, Fletcher JA. (1997) Cytologic and fluorescence in situ hybridization (FISH) examination of metanephric adenoma. *Diagn Cytopathol* 16:107–111.

Rumpelt HJ, Störkel S, Moll R, Schärfe T, Thoenes W. (1991) Bellini duct carcinoma: further evidence for this rare variant of renal cell carcinoma. *Histopathology* 18:115–122.

Saint-André JP, Guyetant S, Croué A, Rousselet MC, Fabiani B, Coupris L. (1992) Le néphrome néphrogène. *Arch Anat Cytol Pathol* 40:266–271.

Schmidt L, Duh F-M, Chen F, Kishida T, Glenn G, Choyke P, Scherer SW, Zhuang Z, Lubensky I, Dean M, Allikmets RL, Chidambaram A, Bergerheim UR, Feltis JT, Casadevall C, Zámarrón A, Bernues M, Richard S, Lips CMJ, Walther MM, Tsui L-C, Geil L, Orcutt ML, Stackhouse T, Lipan J, Slife L, Brauch H, Decker J, Niehans G, Hughson MD, Moch H, Störkel S, Lerman M, Linehan WM, Zbar B. (1997) Germline and somatic mutations in the tyrosine kinase domain of the *MET* proto-oncogene in papillary renal carcinomas. *Nat Genet* 16:68–73.

Schmidt L, Junker K, Nakaigawa N, Kinjerski T, Weirich G, Miller M, Lubensky I, Neumann HPH, Brauch H, Decker J, Vocke C, Brown JA, Jenkins R, Richard S, Bergerheim U, Gerrard B, Dean M, Linehan WM, Zbar B (1999) Novel mutations of the MET proto-oncogene in papillary renal carcinomas. *Oncogene* 18:

Schmidt L, Junker K, Weirich G, Glenn G, Choyke P, Lubensky I, Zhuang Z, Jeffers M, Woude GV, Neumann H, Walther MM, Linehan WM, Zbar B. (1998) Two North American families with hereditary papillary renal carcinoma and identical novel mutations in the MET proto-oncogene. *Cancer Res* 58:1719–1722.

Schoenberg M, Cairns P, Brooks JD, Marshall FF, Epstein JI, Isaacs WB, Sidransky D. (1995) Frequency loss of chromosome arms 8p and 13q in collecting duct carcinoma (CDC) of the kidney. Genes Chromosom. *Cancer* 12:76–80.

Schullerus D, Herbers J, Chudek J, Kanamaru H, Kovacs G. (1997) Loss of heterozygosity at chromosomes 8p, 9p, and 14q is associated with stage and grade of non-papillary renal cell carcinomas. *J Pathol* 183:151–155.

Schwerdtle RF, Störkel S, Neuhaus C, Brauch H, Weidt E, Brenner W, Hohenfellner R, Huber C, Decker H-J. (1996) Allelic losses at chromosome 1p, 2p, 6p, 10p, 13q, 17p, and 21q significantly correlate with the chromophobe subtype of renal cell carcinoma. *Cancer Res* 56:2927–2930.

Schwerdtle RF, Winterpacht A, Störkel S, Brenner W, Hohenfellner R, Zabel B, Huber C, Decker H-J. (1997) Loss of heterozygosity studies and deletion mapping identify two putative chromosome 14q tumor suppressor loci in renal oncocytomas. *Cancer Res* 57:5009–5012.

Seizinger BR, Rouleau GA, Ozelius LJ, Lane AH, Farmer GE, Lamiell JM, Haines J, Yuen JWM, Collins D, Majoor-Krakauer D, Bonner T, Mathew C, Rubenstein A, Halperin J, McConkie-Rosell A, Green JS, Trofatter JA, Ponder BA, Eierman L, Bowmer MI, Schimke R, Oostra B, Aronin N, Smith DI, Drabkin H, Waziri MH, Hobbs WJ, Martuza RL, Conneally PM, Hsia YE, Gusella JF. (1988) Von Hippel–Lindau disease maps to the region of chromosome 3 associated with renal cell carcinomas. *Nature* 332:268–269.

Seljelid R, Ericsson JLE. (1965) Electron microscopic observations on the specializations of the cell surface in renal clear cell carcinoma. *Lab Invest* 14:435–447.

Shimsony Z, Merimsky E, Suprun H. (1963) Adenoma of the kidney. *Br J Urol* 35:256–260.

Sidhar SK, Clark J, Gill S, Hamoudi R, Crew AJ, Gwilliam R, Ross M, Linehan WM, Birdsall S, Shipley J, Cooper CS. (1996) The t(x;1)(p11.2;q21.2) translocation in papillary renal cell carcinoma fuses a novel gene *PRCC* to the *TFE3* transcription factor gene. *Hum Mol Genet* 5:1333–1338.

Sinke RJ, Dijkhuizen T, Janssen B, Weghuis DO, Merkx G, van den Berg E, Schuuring E, Meloni AM, de Jong B, van Kessel AG. (1997) Fine mapping of the human renal oncocytoma-associated translocation (5;11)(q35;q13) breakpoint. *Cancer Genet Cytogenet* 96:95–101.

Speicher MR, Schoell B, du Manoir S, Schröck E, Ried T, Cremer T, Störkel S, Kovacs A, Kovacs G. (1994) Specific loss of chromosomes 1, 2, 6, 10, 13, 17, and 21 in chromophobe renal cell carciomas revealed by comparative genomic hybridization. *Am J Pathol* 145:356–364.

Srigley JR, Eble JN. (1998) Collecting duct carcinoma of kidney. *Semin Diagn Pathol* 15:54–67.

Steiner G, Cairns P, Polascik TJ, Marshall FF, Epstein JI, Sidransky D, Schoenberg M. (1996) High-density mapping of chromosomal arm 1q in renal collecting duct carcinoma: region of minimal deletion at 1q32.1-32.2. *Cancer Res* 56:5044–5046.

Störkel S, Eble JN, Adlakha K, Amin M, Blute ML, Bostwick DG, Darson M, Delahunt B, Iczkowski K. (1997) Classification of renal cell carcinoma, workgroup 1. *Cancer* 80:987–989.

Störkel S, Husman G, Thoenes W. (1992) Zur Diagnose und Differential diagnose des metanephroiden Nierentumors des Erwachsenen—ein unbekannter Nierentumor. *Verh Dtsch Ges Pathol* 76:306–306.

Störkel S, Pannen B, Thoenes W, Steart PV, Wagner S, Drenckhahn D. (1988) Intercalated cells as a probable source for the development of renal oncocytoma. *Virchows Arch B* 56:185–189.

Störkel S, Steart PV, Drenckhahn D, Thoenes W. (1989) The human chromophobe cell renal carcinoma: its probable relation to intercalated cells of the collecting duct. *Virchows Arch B* 56:237–245.

Syrjänen KJ. (1979) Renal adenomatosis, report of an autopsy case. *Scand J Urol Nephrol* 13:329–334.

Tajara EH, Berger CS, Hecht BK, Gemmill RM, Sandberg AA, Hecht F. (1988) Loss of common 3p14 fragile site expression in renal cell carcinoma with deletion breakpoint at 3p14. *Cancer Genet Cytogenet* 31:75–82.

Talamo TS, Shonnard JW. (1980 Small renal adenocarcinoma with metastases. *J Urol* 124:132–134.

Tang AL, Davies DR, Wing AJ. (1989) Remission of nephrotic syndrome in amyloidosis associated with hypernephroma. *Clin Nephrol* 32:225–228.

Teyssier JR, Ferre D. (1990) Chromosomal changes in renal cell carcinoma, no evidence for correlation with clinical stage. *Cancer Genet Cytogenet* 45:197–205.

Thoenes W, Störkel S, Rumpelt H-J. (1986) Histopathology and classification of renal cell tumors (adenomas, oncocytomas and carcinomas) the basic cytological and histopathological elements and their use for diagnostics. *Pathol Res Pract* 181:125–143.

Thoenes W, Störkel S, Rumpelt H-J. (1985) Human chromophobe cell renal carcinoma. *Virchows Arch B* 48:207–217.

Thoenes W, Störkel S, Rumpelt HJ, Moll R. (1990) Cytomorphological typing of renal cell carcinoma—a new approach. *Eur Urol* 18(suppl):6–9.

Thoenes W, Störkel S, Rumpelt H-J, Moll R, Baum H-P, Werner S. (1988) Chromophobe cell renal carcinoma and its variants—a report on 32 cases. *J Pathol* 155:277–287.

Thompson IM, Peek M. (1988) Improvement in survival of patients with renal cell carcinoma—the role of the serrendipitously detected tumor. *J Urol* 140:487–490.

Thrash-Bingham CA, Salazar H, Freed JJ, Greenberg RE, Tartof KD. (1995) Genomic alterations and instabilities in renal cell carcinomas and their relationship to tumor pathology. *Cancer Res* 55:6189–6195.

Truong LD, Phung VT, Yoshikawa Y, Mattioli CA. (1988) Glycoconjugates in normal human kidney, a histochemical study using 13 biotinylated lectins. *Histochemistry* 90:51–60.

Turley LA, Steel J. (1924) Multiple miliary adenomas of the kidney cortex, with special reference to histogenesis. *JAMA* 82:857–859.

Ullrich R, Susani M, Schuster FX, Porpáczy P, Asboth F. (1990) Multiple Adenome beider Nieren—"renale Adenomatose?". *Pathologe* 11:120–124.

Ulrich W, Horvat R, Krisch K. (1985) Lectin histochemistry of kidney tumours and its pathomorphological relevance. *Histopathology* 9:1037–1050.

van den Berg A, Buys CHCM. (1997) Involvement of multiple loci on chromosome 3 in renal cell cancer development. *Genes Chromosom Cancer* 19:59–76.

van den Berg A, Dijkhuizen T, Draaijers TG, Hulsbeek MMF, Maher ER, van den Berg E, Störkel S, Buys CHCM. (1997) Analysis of multiple renal cell adenomas and carcinomas suggests allelic loss at 3p21 to be a prerequisite for malignant development. *Genes Chromosom Cancer* 19:228–232.

van den Berg A, Hulsbeek MMF, de Jong D, Kok K, Veldhuis PMJF, Roche J, Buys CHCM. (1996) Major role for a 3p21 region and lack of involvement of the t(3;8) breakpoint region in the development of renal cell carcinoma suggested by loss of heterozygosity analysis. *Genes Chromosom Cancer* 15:64–72.

van den Berg E, Dijkhuizen T, Störkel S, de la Rivière B, Dam A, Mensink HJA, Oosterhuis JW, de Jong B. (1995) Chromosomal changes in renal oncocytomas. Evidence that t(5;11)(q35;q13) may characterize a second subgroup of oncocytomas. *Cancer Genet Cytogenet* 79:164–168.

Waldherr R, Schwechheimer K. (1985) Co-expression of cytokeratin and vimentin intermediate-sized filaments in renal cell carcinoma, a comparative study of the intermediate-sized filaments in renal cell carcinoma and normal human kidney. *Virchows Arch Pathol Anat Physiol Klin Med* 408:15–27.

Wallace AC, Nairn RC. (1972) Renal tubular antigens in kidney tumors. *Cancer* 29:977–981.

Walter TA, Berger CS, Sandberg AA. (1989) The cytogenetics of renal tumors, where do we stand, where do we go? *Cancer Genet Cytogenet* 43:15–34.

Warfel KA, Eble JN. (1982) Renal oncocytomatosis. *J Urol* 127:1179–180.

Weaver DJ, Michalski K, Miles J. (1988) Cytogenetic analysis in renal cell carcinoma: correlation with tumor aggressiveness. *Cancer Res* 48:2887–2889.

Weirich G, Glenn G, Junker K, Merino M, Störkel S, Lubensky I, Choyke P, Pack S, Amin M, Walther MM, Linehan M, Zbar B. (1998) Familial renal oncocytoma: clinicopathological study of 5 families. *J Urol* 160:335–340.

Welter C, Kovacs G, Seit G, Blin N. (1989) Alteration of mitochondrial DNA in human oncocytomas. *Genes Chromosom Cancer* 1:79–82.

Wick MR, Cherwitz DL, Manivel JC, Sibley R. (1990) Immunohistochemical findings in tumors of the kidney. In: *Tumors and Tumor-like Conditions of the Kidneys and Ureters* (JN Eble, ed.) pp. 207–247. Churchill Livingstone, New York.

Wu S-Q, Hafez GR, Xing W, Newton M, Chen X-R, Messing E. (1996) The correlation between the loss of chromosome 14q with histologic tumor grade, pathologic stage, and outcome of patients with nonpapillary renal cell carcinoma. *Cancer* 77:1154–1160.

Xipell JM. (1971) The incidence of benign renal nodules (a clinicopathologic study). *J Urol* 106:503–506.

Yoshida MA, Ohyashiki K, Ochi H, Gibas Z, Pontes JE, Prout GR Jr, Huben R, Sandberg AA. (1986) Cytogenetic studies of tumor tissue from patients with nonfamilial renal cell carcinoma. *Cancer Res* 46:2139–2147.

Yörükoglu K, Aktas S, Mungan MU, Kirkali Z. (1999) Tubular dysplasia and carcinoma in situ: precursors of renal cell carcinoma. *Urology* 53:684–689.

Zbar B, Lerman M. (1999) Inherited carcinomas of the kidney. *Adv Cancer Res* 75:163–201.

Zhuang Z, Park W-S, Pack S, Schmidt L, Vortmeyer AO, Pak E, Pham T, Weil RJ, Candidus S, Lubensky IA, Linehan WM, Zbar B, Weirich G. (1998) Trisomy 7–harbouring non-random duplication of the mutant *MET* allele in hereditary papillary renal carcinomas. *Nat Genet* 20:66–69.

24

WILMS' TUMOR

KEVIN E. BOVE

Embryonal neoplasms have a primitive cell component able to simulate the differentiation of structures characteristic of an organ or body region. These primitive cells have persisted beyond the normal developmental program and, at some point, have undergone neoplastic transformation. Embryonal neoplasms are uncommon in the newborn period and tend to appear later in childhood, suggesting that latency followed by activation is the rule rather than linear growth.

The best-characterized association of an embryonal neoplasm with persistent blastema-containing embryonic rests is Wilms' tumor (WT), which occurs without sex predilection in about 1 in 8000 live births at a mean age of 3 years and rarely beyond 10 years (Breslow et al., 1988). The molecular events that characterize WT have been elaborated in great detail but are not completely understood (Charles et al., 1998). The story of the evolution of WT will remain incomplete until it is understood how these molecular events or steps relate to the pathogenesis of nephrogenic rests from which most WT are thought to arise (Beckwith et al., 1990; Bove and McAdams, 1976).

NORMAL KIDNEY DEVELOPMENT

As background to discussion of WT, it is helpful to review normal developmental anatomy of the kidney (Murphy et al., 1994). The ureteric bud ascends from the pelvis to contact aggregates of primitive mesenchyme in the paraspinal urogenital ridge of the developing embryo. By a process involving mutual induction, blastemal cells cause the ureteric bud to elongate and branch, forming the collecting system of the kidney; the ureteric bud induces the metanephric blastema to form epithelial and stromal elements of the nephrons. Proliferation is regulated in such a way that blastema is supplied without accumulating and differentiates continuously into nephrons. At any stage of development of the kidney, the peripheral portions of the renal lobules are those most recently formed and the juxtamedullary nephrons are the oldest ones. The most rapid rate of nephrogenesis occurs between 15 and 25 weeks of gestation, when more than half of all glomeruli are formed (Hinchcliffe et al., 1991). The normal kidney consists of 12–14 lobules that begin to fuse along the lateral margins during development. In the mature human kidney, lateral lobular fusion produces columns of cortical tissue that extend from the surface to the pericalyceal soft tissue deep within the kidney. The nephrons in each lobule are derived from blastemal cells that separate early in development from progenitors in neighboring lobules. Thus it is possible for a postzygotic mutation of blastemal cells to involve a limited or an extensive area of the kidney, depending upon when the mutation occurs and when it is expressed. Although the process of glomerular and tubular maturation continues after birth, nephrogenesis is essentially complete by 35 weeks gestation, after which blastemal cells normally disappear (Potter et al., 1943).

NEPHROGENIC RESTS, WILMS' TUMOR, AND NEPHROBLASTOMATOSIS

Approximately 40% of kidneys removed for WT are now known to contain independent lesions that have been assigned various names by different authors. Potter (1961), and later, Shanklin et al. (1969) both used the term "nephroblastoma *in situ*" for abnormal nests of superfluous blastema in infants and speculated on a relationship to WT. Bove and McAdams (1976, 1978) established the concurrence of these embryonic rests with WT (Bove et al., 1969) and classified focal lesions independent of the main WT (Figs. 24–1 and 24–2) as potentially neoplastic (nodular renal blastema, metanephric hamartoma, and Wilms' tumorlet) and malformative (glomerular immaturity and cortical cysts). To simplify matters, all lesions whose origin in persistent blastema can be reasonably inferred are conveniently grouped under the generic term "nephrogenic rest" (Beckwith et al., 1990). *Nephrogenic rests* (NR) are local lesions derived from persistent blastema cells with potential for proliferation to lesions of macroscopic size, including WT, and also for partial maturation to dysplastic nephron-like structures, often accompanied by sclerosis and atrophy. Beckwith (1990) observed that NR are located either at the periphery of renal lobules (perilobar) or centrally within lobules (intralobar); these two types of NR differ to some extent in morphological characteristics, clinical associations, and molecular genetic findings. The blastemal cells in NR are considered to be lineal descendents of cells that were involved in the generation of nephrons during development and are the source of most, if not all WT. The absence of significant concurrence between NR and any of the other tumor types that may present as congenital or childhood re-

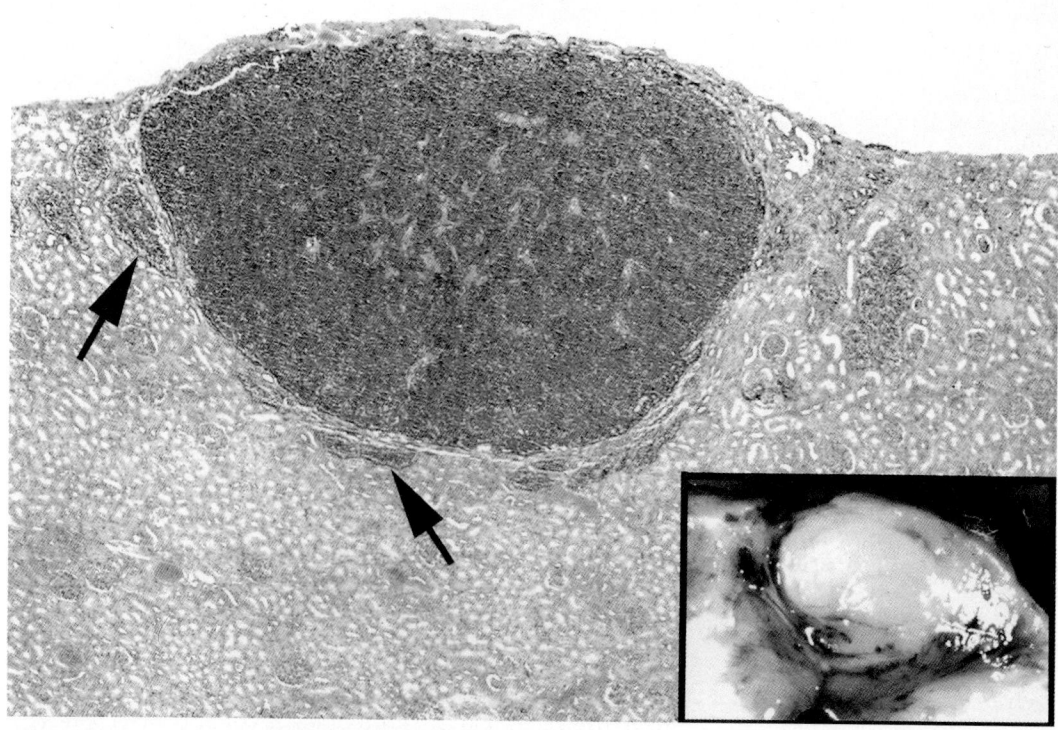

Figure 24–1. Hyperplastic perilobar nephrogenic rest (PLNR) in Wilms' tumor (WT) specimen is flanked by dormant nodules of blastema (arrows). Expansion causes compression of parenchyma around expanding NR (*inset*) in WT specimen.

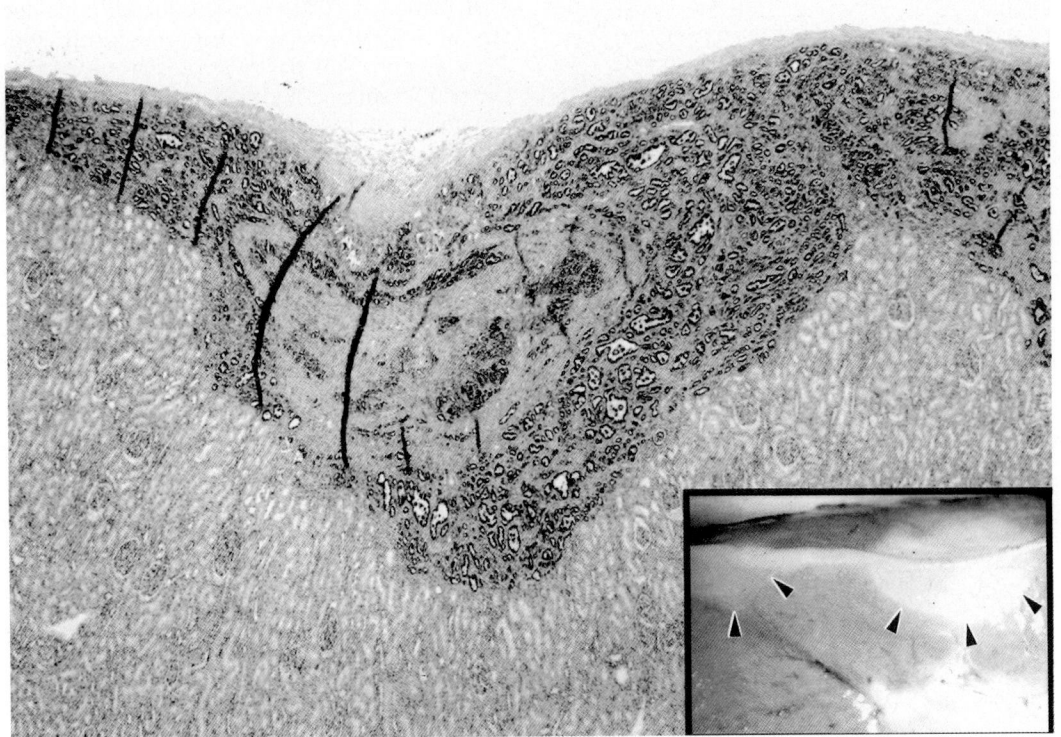

Figure 24–2. Ageing, plaque-like perilobar nephrogenic rest contains adenoma-like tubules and sclerotic collagen. In a similar lesion in a Wilms' tumor specimen, surface pallor and indentation were visible (*inset*).

nal tumors is evidence that only WT is derived from totipotential renal blastema. An alternative explanation for the rare conjunction of a NR with mesoblastic nephroma or sporadic renal dysplasia is a nongenetic pathway to NR, such as a physical effect of an expanding congenital tumor or a dysplastic cyst on nephrogenic blastema (Charles, 1996).

The modern appreciation of NR as precursors to WT is derived from study of the entire kidney in which WT arises and from careful inspection and sampling of the contralateral kidney, thereby providing an exceptional opportunity, compared with other tumor sites, for assessing the tumorgenic environment. Modern imaging methods have verified these concepts and provide invaluable tools for study of the natural history of NR/WT. The condition in which a WT is accompanied by independent NR is now known as *nephroblastomatosis*. Bove and McAdams (1976) defined nephroblastomatosis as a spectrum of morphological lesions that range from frankly benign (malformed

nephrons and immature glomeruli) to possibly neoplastic (nodular renal blastema and blastema-containing metanephric hamartoma) to probably neoplastic (expanding blastema-containing lesions of variable size) to frankly neoplastic. Minor manifestations of nephroblastomatosis are common in children with unilateral WT and are almost universal in those with bilateral WT.

Microscopic nodules of blastema (Fig. 24–3a) may be encountered in random sections of as many as 1% of full-term infants at autopsy (Beckwith, 1986) and for some time have been suspected to be forerunners of WT, but these are far too common to be considered *in situ* neoplasms in the sense that the process of neoplastic transformation is complete. It is not known whether the kidneys of all newborn infants contain a few NR or if the presence of even one NR is a marker for a subclass of infants with increased potential for developing WT. Because the incidence of NR is much higher in infant autopsies than the incidence of WT in later childhood, it seems likely that most NR

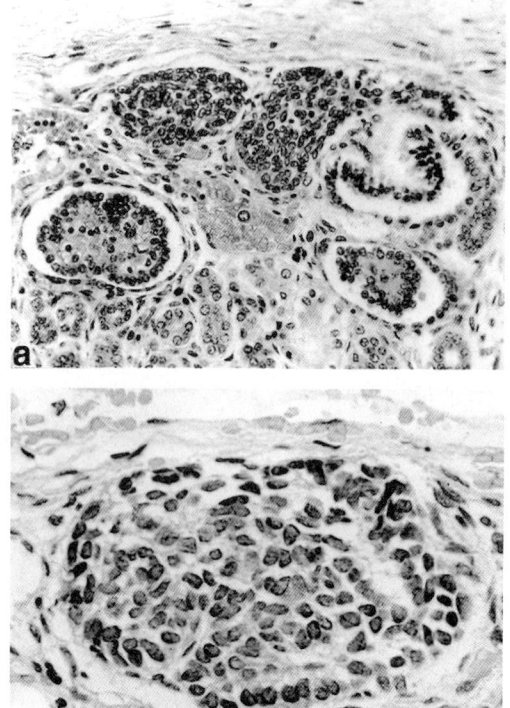

Figure 24–3. *a*: This perilobar nephrogenic rest (PLNR) was an incidental finding in an infant autopsy. *b*: This PLNR was an incidental finding in a multicystic dysplastic kidney (upper renal pole with obstructed duplicated drainage system).

regress and eventually disappear. Incidental NR associated with congenital heart disease have an uncertain relationship with WT. No link between WT and congenital heart disease has been found in large studies of WT. However, a report of a 10-fold increase of the incidence of septal defects in patients with WT compared with other childhood neoplasms (Stiller et al., 1987) suggests that events predisposing to WT may be teratogenic for the heart as well. Superficial and deep NR are found in 1%–2% of kidneys removed for common sporadic unilateral renal dysplasia (Craver et al., 1986; Vogler et al., 1988). The disturbed lobular architecture in dysplastic kidneys makes topographical classification difficult, but most NR in dysplastic kidneys surgically removed during early childhood are perilobar (Fig. 24–3b). Such observations indicate an important link between NR and renal maldevelopment. The

risk of WT in a frankly dysplastic kidney is extremely small and is considered insufficient to warrant prophylactic nephrectomy of unilateral dysplastic kidneys or a surveillance program of imaging for early detection of WT. Nephrogenic rests are also found with increased frequency in kidneys of infants with trisomy syndromes, particularly in infants of greater than 35 weeks gestational age who have trisomy 18 (Fig. 24–4). Perilobar NR are most prevalent in trisomy 18, but intralobar NR may occur. In dysplastic kidneys and in trisomy 18, NR seem to arise from a late gestational disturbance of proliferation and maturation without having undergone the genetic changes that are necessary for neoplasia. Genuine risk is established in the rare children with trisomy 18 who survive beyond infancy, in whom at least six examples of WT are known (Olson et al., 1995).

Beyond infancy, persistence of renal blastema is abnormal and potentially tumorgenic. Some NR may expand sufficiently by hyperplasia before or during the process of maturation and regression to permit detection by modern imaging technology. At the time of detection, some NR are histologically indistinguishable from small WT, whereas others display less aggressive qualities or sufficient maturation or regression to be of less concern. Beckwith et al. (1990) subclassified NR as dormant, maturing or sclerosing, hyperplastic, and neoplastic in an insightful effort to relate morphological properties to biological behavior. This classification is based upon evaluation of both gross and microscopic features of each lesion. Dormant NR are usually microscopic but may attain macroscopic size. Detectable mitoses make dormancy unlikely. In the perilobar location, hyperplastic NR are usually visible to the naked eye and may be round, oval, or embedded in a plaque-like lesion. Any NR that is grossly visible, nodular in shape, compresses surrounding renal tissue (Fig. 24–1, inset), and enlarges over time is presumed to be neoplastic. Needle biopsy of such lesions is not helpful for determining whether evolution to WT has occurred. Further refinement may be achieved by using methods to assess proliferation rates (Figs. 24–5 and 24–6). Using a proliferation marker and counting Silver-associated nucleolar organizing regions (AgNors), Bove et al. (1995) determined that some micro-

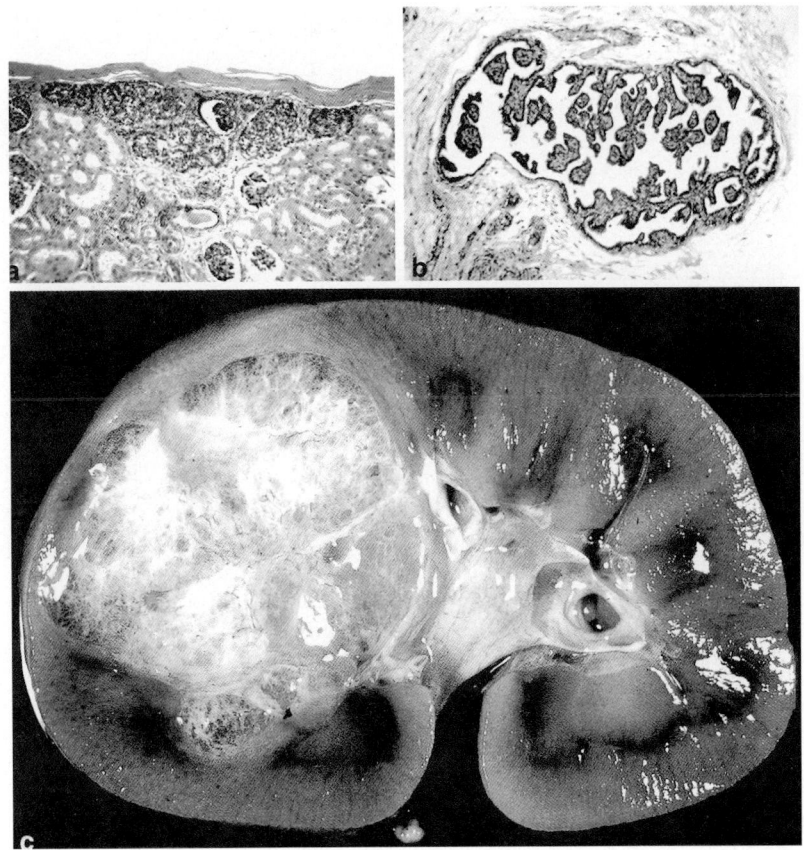

Figure 24–4. All panels are renal lesions in tri-somy 18 syndrome. *a:* Perilobar nephrogenic rest (PLNR) with focal glomerular immaturity. *b:* Intralobar nephrogenic rest (ILNR) in severe renal dysplasia. *c:* Wilms' tumor-like solitary ILNR in older infant.

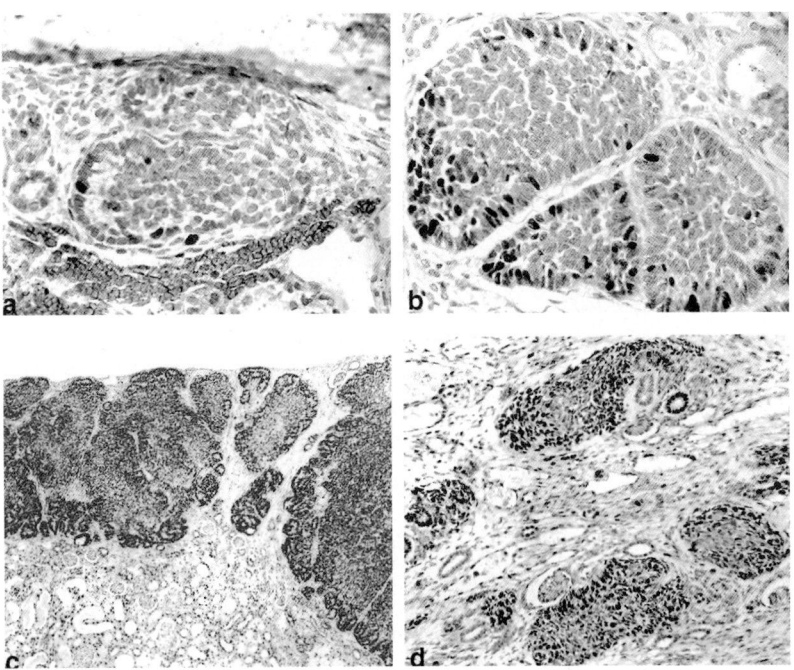

Figure 24–5. Immunohistology of nephrogenic rests (NR) using anti-PCNA. Dark-staining nuclei are positive for proliferation marker. *a:* Dormant PLNR in renal dysplasia. *b:* Focal proliferation in PLNR. *c:* Marked proliferation in PLNR. *d:* Marked proliferation in ILNR. (*b–d* in Wilms' tumor specimens).

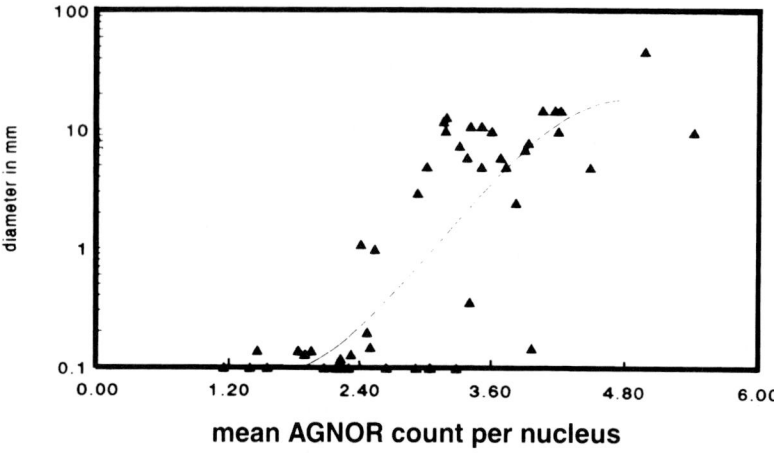

Figure 24–6. AgNOR count in nephrogenic rest (NR) is related to diameter of rest. Mean count in nuclei of 49 Wilms' tumors (about 4.0) overlaps with large NR.

scopic and small macroscopic NR resembled WT, whereas most were truly dormant or slowly proliferating pure blastemal lesions that lacked morphological evidence of neoplastic transformation. Unequivocal histological determination of the neoplastic potential of a suspect NR awaits development of markers either for loss of ability to mature or for a change that signals molecular genetic progression to malignancy, or perhaps both.

Perilobar and Intralobar Nephrogenic Rests

Perilobar nephrogenic rests (PLNR) and intralobar nephrogenic rests (ILNR) differ in intrarenal location, histologic features, and syndromic associations. Awareness of this is extremely helpful in the interpretation of renal images, findings at surgery, and evaluation of renal tissue specimens. Perilobar NR are found at the periphery of a renal lobule under the renal capsule or along the lateral fused margins of adjacent lobules and are demarcated from surrounding renal tissue by a thin capsule (Fig. 24–7). They tend to be oval to rounded when composed entirely of blastema, no matter how small, and retain rounded contour during periods of expansion due to hyperplasia or transition to WT. Perilobar NR tend to become angulated or flattened, presumably because of loss of volume, as they mature or regress and sclerose

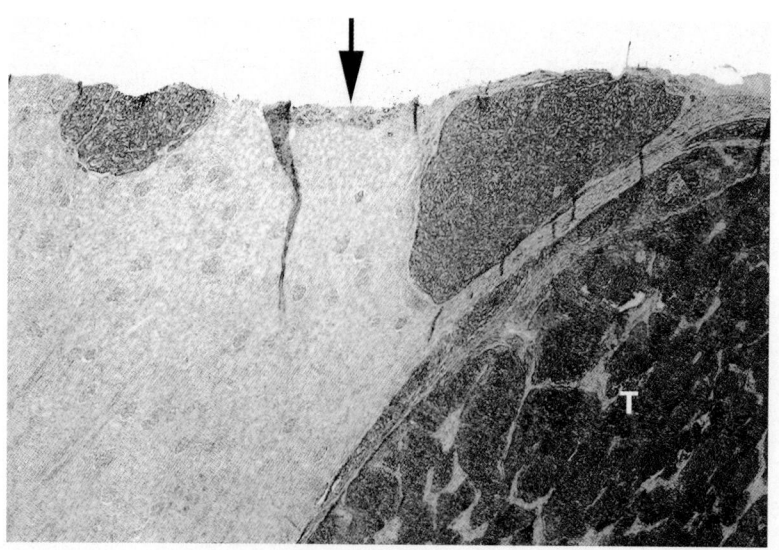

Figure 24–7. Cluster of independent nephrogenic rest (NR) in Wilms' tumor (WT) specimen, from left to right contain differentiating blastema, tubulopapillary profiles with sclerosis (arrow), and differentiating blastema. Near-by 1.5 cm neoplasm (T) is a small WT, or arguably, a hyperplastic NR.

(Fig. 24–2b). They are more common in sporadic WT, in Beckwith-Wiedemann syndrome (BWS), and with hemihypertrophy. Intralobar NR typically are found centrally within renal lobules and are unencapsulated, appearing as a cluster of nests of blastema intermingled with surrounding dysplastic and normal nephrons (Figs. 24–8 to 24–10).

Both PLNR and ILNR can occur as local or extensive lesions within a kidney and may coexist (Fig. 24–11). Most kidneys with WT have only a few NR identified. The distribution of NR within nephrectomy specimens has not been studied systematically. It seems, however, that in many cases of WT, NR are limited to one lobule or region in proximity to the tumor. This suggests that in cases of WT lacking NR, the NR that gave rise to the tumor may have been destroyed in the process. The seemingly common topographic limitation of NR to one or several adjacent lobules may be a marker for a somatic cell mutation occurring in one precursor cell early in gestation and resulting in a cluster of NR, any one of which could be triggered by subsequent events to develop into a WT.

The topograhic distinction between PLNR and ILNR raises questions regarding relative neoplastic potential and biological significance. From the time of their recognition, PLNR have evinced speculation that they

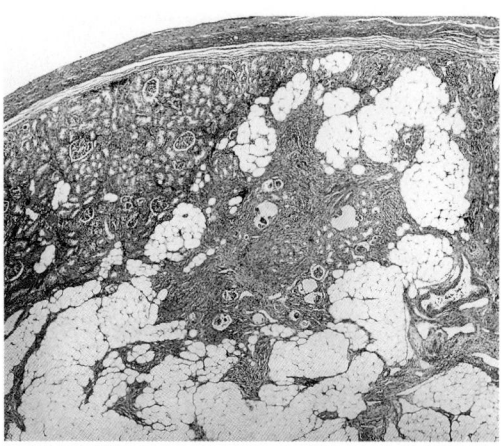

Figure 24–9. This large maturing/sclerosing intralobar nephrogenic rest was the sole kidney lesion in a child with hemihypertrophy. It contains collagen, fat, dysplastic glomeruli, and tubules, plus adenoma-like nodules.

were late-evolving by-products of terminal nephrogenic activity. In contrast, deep-lying ILNR may evolve earlier in gestation when the first generations of glomeruli are forming. Perilobar NR are delicately encapsulated, rich in blastema exhibiting subtle signs of differentiation along the margins, and often surrounded by cortex containing abnormal, immature-appearing glomeruli (Figs. 24–11 and 24–12). Many PLNR undergo maturation and atrophy when still of microscopic size. In contrast, most ILNR lack capsules and interdigitate with dysgenetic glomeruli and tubules plus significant

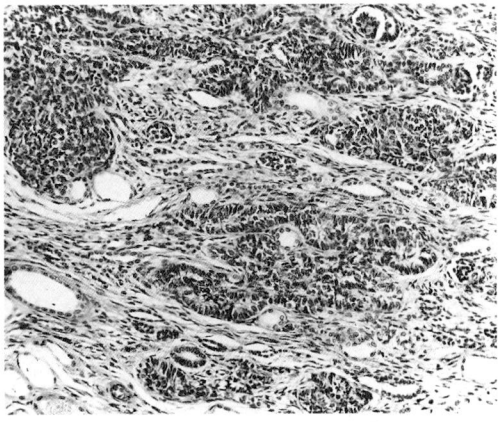

Figure 24–8. This intralobar nephrogenic rest has typical complexity, containing nodules of blastema, partially differentiated tubules, immature glomeruli, excess stroma, and trapped normal nephrons.

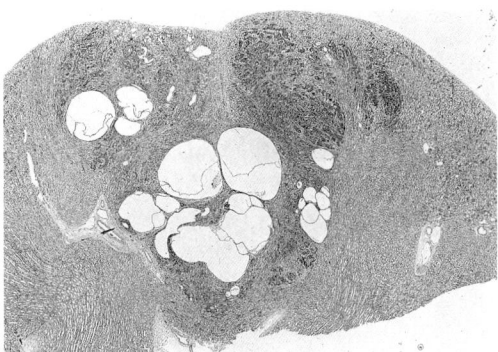

Figure 24–10. This large intralobar nephrogenic rest in Wilms' tumor specimen has dominant component of blastema and cysts that may be derivatives or trapped normal nephron segments.

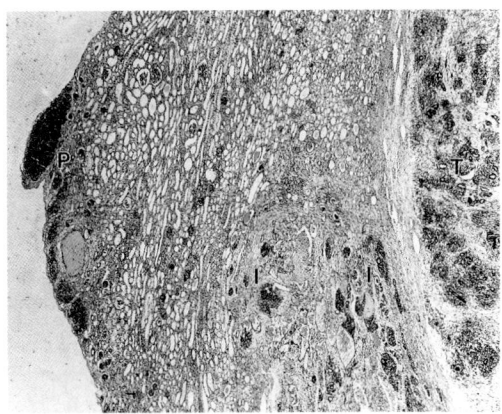

Figure 24–11. Perilobar nephrogenic rest (P) and intralobar nephrogenic rest (I) coexist on the flank of a Wilms' tumor (T).

cellular stroma (Fig. 24–8). Both PLNR and ILNR contain undifferentiated or partly differentiated blastema and both may achieve considerable size as maturation occurs (Figs. 24–2 and 24–9). ILNR may mimic the triphasic histological complexity of WT when small. It remains uncertain whether WT more commonly arise in perilobar or intralobar precursor lesions. Data from the National Wilms' Tumor Study suggest that PLNR are more common in sporadic WT, BWS, and hemihypertrophy, whereas ILNR are more apt to be found in WAGR syndrome (Wilm's tumor, aniridia, genitourinary anomalies, mental retardation) and in Denys-Drash syndrome, both of which are associated with constitutional abnormalities in 11p (see below).

DIFFUSE NEPHROBLASTOMATOSIS

Nephroblastomatosis is a term that has engendered some confusion. It was originally applied to the extremely rare, bilateral pancortical renal lesion described by Hou and Holman (1961) [with citation to Nicholson (1931)], in which the kidneys were enlarged and exhibited an unusual hyperplastic dysplasia characterized by extensive superfluous metanephric blastema intermixed with and actively generating partially mature nephrons. Cortical disorganization with absence of a discrete nephrogenic zone and lack of orderly maturation of nephrons completed the description of this condition in which renal function was impaired, leading

to death in early infancy. Somewhat similar cases continue to be reported as nephroblastomatosis (Hsueh et al., 1987; Murata et al.,1989). Gaulier et al.'s (1993) case appears to be a frankly dysplastic kidney, which is unusual because of prevalence of deep nests of blastema interpreted as ILNR. Because all kidneys, dysplastic or not, arise from metanephric blastema, and this particular kidney, as illustrated, lacked lobar organization, it may not be appropriate to class such foci as ILNR. Paucity or absence of normal renal tissue, lack of discrete hyperplastic nodules containing blastema, unproven neoplastic potential, and absence of molecular genetic data that provides a link to WT in these cases contrast with nephroblastomatosis of neoplastic type, for which it is preferable to reserve the term.

The most common form of neoplastic nephroblastomatosis is WT in the presence of NR, which includes about 40% of all cases of WT. The most spectacular, although least common, form of neoplastic nephroblastomatosis is a multifocal confluent nodular lesion composed of hyperplastic blastema that extensively involves one or both kidneys. The patients are usually infants with bilateral NR overlying or interspersed with normal kidney. The diffuse form, like the multifocal form, may also be unilateral. In such cases, NR may be either perilobar (FIgs. 24–12 and 24–13) or intralobar (Figs. 24–14 and 24–15), but the perilobar type seems to be much more common. Extensive intralobar nephroblastomatosis has been reported by Machin and McGaughy (1984) and extensive combined

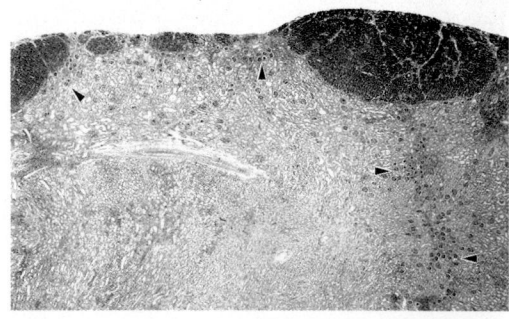

Figure 24–12. Extensive multifocal perilobar nephrogenic rests overlie clusters of immature glomeruli (arrowheads) indicating maldevelopment prior to emergence of NR in nephroblastomatosis.

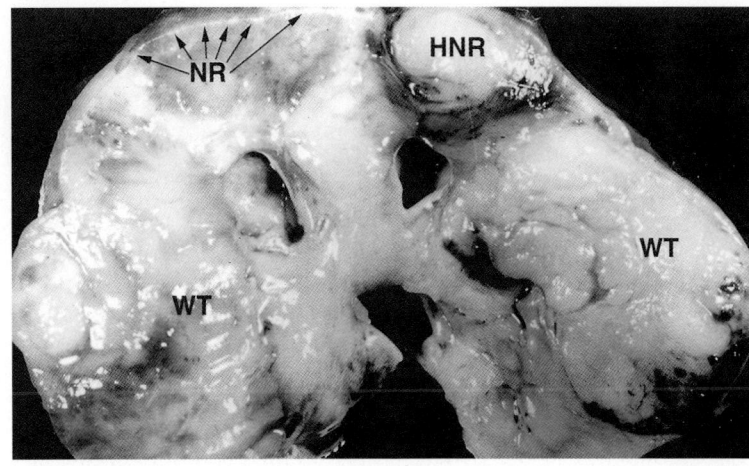

Figure 24–13. Kidney with diffuse superficial nephroblastomatosis has two separate Wilms' tumors (WT) and a hyperplastic nephrogenic rest (HNR). Arrows designate zone of multifocal small perilobar nephrogenic rests.

perilobar and intralobar nephroblastomatosis is discussed by Walford (1990). Neoplastic transformation of hyperplastic blastema may be unifocal or multifocal and conceivably may not have occurred in all of the lesions at the time a diagnosis of WT is made during an investigation for unexplained nephromegaly. Lack of a marker for transformation underscores the practical difficulty of distinguishing hyperplastic and neoplastic NR. A surprisingly large number of infants with extensive multifocal or diffuse nephroblastomatosis have no extrarenal abnormalities (deChadarevian et al., 1977; Machin and McGaughy, 1984; Walford, 1990). A few of these cases show phenotypic overlap with syndromic forms of WT (Perlman et al., 1975;

Greenberg et al., 1986). In a unique case classified as diffuse nephroblastomatosis, all of the nodules were composed of hyperplastic tubules resembling the adenoma-like derivatives of PLNR, but no blastema was present (Regalado et al., 1996); such cases defy rationalization because it is impossible to determine whether the nodules arose from blastema or directly from mature epithelium.

SPORADIC WILMS' TUMOR AND NEPHROGENIC RESTS

The common sporadic form of WT accounts for more than 90% of cases of WT, is occasionally associated with hemihypertrophy or

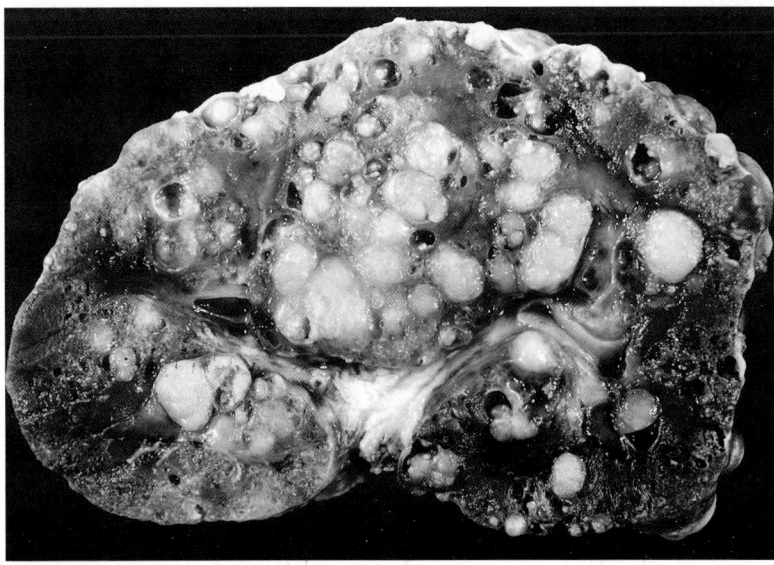

Figure 24–14. Kidney with diffuse panlobar nephroblastomatosis contains cystic and nodular perilobar nephrogenic rests and intralobar nephrotic rests. The central cluster of confluent nodules is a Wilms' tumor.

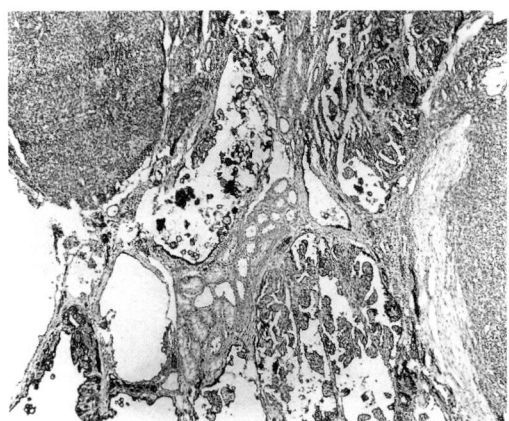

Figure 24–15. Most nodules in the specimen illustrated were hyperplastic nephrogenic rests (NR) or maturing NR with adenoma-like papillary fronds and psammoma bodies.

extrarenal anomalies (Miller et al., 1964), and is bilateral in about 5% of cases. Patients with bilateral WT display a slight excess of associated extrarenal anomalies (Bond, 1975). Among sporadic cases, 30%–40% have NR in the ipselateral kidney (Beckwith et al., 1990; Bove and McAdams, 1976, 1978) and 1 in 4 of these have NR in the contralateral kidney at the time of nephrectomy. Experience has repeatedly demonstrated that the presence of even one independent NR in a nephrectomy specimen is an indicator for a potential metachronous contralateral primary WT (Warner et al., 1988). When this happens in a nonsyndromatic case of WT, one may hypothesize that a postzygotic event affects blastema cells in both kidneys. About half of patients with WT, including many sporadic cases, have loss of heterozygosity (LOH) for alleles located on 11p in tumor tissue compared to normal somatic control tissue such as kidney or blood leukocytes. In the largest group of WT studied for LOH (Grundy et al., 1996), 286 WT and associated NR were analyzed. About 40% of the NR studied had LOH for alleles on 11p. In ILNR, LOH usually involved alleles at both 11p13 and 11p5, whereas in PLNR, LOH was at 11p13 only. This is further evidence that the pathogenesis of these two classes of NR differs. Moreover, LOH for alleles on 11p in many WT more commonly maps to 11p15, which is the region involved in BWS, than to 11p13. This locus, named

WT2, may have great importance for the pathogenesis of WT and other forms of childhood cancer. A cluster of genes at this locus includes that for insulin-like growth factor 2 (ILGF-2), overproduction of which is involved in the pathogenesis of BWS, a generalized tissue overgrowth disorder (Hedborg et al., 1994; Reeve, 1996). Studies of regulation of the expression of ILGF-2 indicate a critical role for normal parental imprinting, loss of which occurs in BWS, and which has emerged as a novel mutational mechanism in human cancer (Feinberg, 1996; Reik and Surani, 1989). Another tumor suppressor gene, *H19*, also located at 11p15, is expressed in developing nephrons, and inactivated in WT and NR, and may influence expression and imprinting of ILGF-2 (Cui et al., 1997). It now seems likely that the pathway to sporadic WT is extraordinarily complex, involving multiple interactive gene abnormalities, not all of which have been identified.

SYNDROMIC WILMS' TUMOR AND NEPHROGENIC RESTS

About 7% of patients with WT have congenital anomalies that represent significant associations rather than incidental findings. These include hemihypertrophy, aniridia, hypospadias, cryptorchidism, somatic overgrowth, macroglosia, and omphalocele. Wilms' tumor also has important recognizable syndromic associations accounting for about 5% of cases. These include WAGR syndrome, Denys-Drash syndrome, Frasier syndrome, Beckwith-Wiedemann syndrome, Perlman syndrome, and possibly several other somatic overgrowth disorders such as Simpson-Golabi-Behmel syndrome, Sotos syndrome and Bloom syndrome, and familial WT without syndromic stigmata. Syndromic and familial WT tend to occur at a younger age than sporadic cases and are more often bilateral (Beckwith et al., 1990; Knudson and Strong, 1972).

WAGR SYNDROME
(WILMS' TUMOR, ANIRIDIA, GENITOURINARY ANOMALIES, MENTAL RETARDATION)

About 1% of patients with WT have aniridia of the sporadic type (often unilateral) and ambiguous external genitalia. The dominant type of aniridia is bilateral, one parent is also involved, and no association with WT exists (Miller et al., 1964). Almost all patients with sporadic aniridia have an interstitial deletion at 11p13 (Riccardi et al., 1978; Shannon et al., 1982). The cause of WAGR syndrome is now recognized as a germline mutation of a gene at 11p13 that is designated *WT1*, establishing the first major link between WT and a particular region of the genome. Because only one-third of patients with WAGR develop WT, it is clear that other factors influence the expression of this defect; it is not known whether additional mutations are required or some sort of host–resistance factors are at work (Matsunaga, 1981). The incidence of bilateral WT in WAGR is increased to 10%–20%. Nephrectomy specimens in WAGR syndrome are more likely to have ILNR than PLNR but may have neither (Beckwith et al., 1990; Kobayashi and Nagahara, 1990). Wilms' tumors in WAGR tend to be more complex than usual WT, often displaying polymorphous mesenchymal differentiation, particularly to skeletal muscle.

DENYS-DRASH SYNDROME

Denys-Drash syndrome (DDS) is rare and consists of mesangial glomerulopathy, both internal and external abnormal sex differentiation in males, and a high incidence of WT (Drash et al., 1970; Manivel et al., 1987). Gonadoblastoma is common in the dysgenetic gonads. The glomerulopathy is progressive, typically precedes the appearance of WT, and may be congenital. Both complete and incomplete forms exist, and the syndrome may be difficult to recognize in females. When fully developed, DDS includes male pseudohermaphroditism and gonadal dysgenesis with cryptorchidism. Karyotype is normal and the syndrome is sporadic. Almost all of the patients studied have germline point mutations in the *WT1* gene (Pelletier et al., 1991), a tumor suppressor gene that is required for normal kidney and gonadal development in mice. The risk for a patient with DDS developing WT is at least 50%, but a clinical variant, Frasier syndrome, has a much lower risk. Several different WT1 mutations have been described that may relate to the difference in risk for WT among patients with DDS and Frasier syndromes (Klamt et al., 1998). In complete and incomplete DDS, ILNR are extremely common and PLNR may not occur (Heppe et al., 1991). It is reasonable to speculate that in DDS, ILNR and glomerulopathy are a consequence of a mutation that occurs very early in gestation. It would be of interest to compare the structure of immature glomeruli that are associated with ILNR and PLNR with the generalized glomerulopathy of DDS. Glomeruloid structures produced by WT are usually poorly vascularized or avascular (Payton et al., 1988).

BECKWITH-WIEDEMANN SYNDROME

Beckwith-Wiedemann syndrome (BWS) consists of generalized somatic and visceral overgrowth with liability to neonatal hypoglycemia due to islet cell hyperplasia, and increased risk for several childhood neoplasms, including WT (Beckwith, 1969; Wiedemann, 1983). External features include gigantism, omphalocele, macroglossia, and craniofacial dysmorphia. Hemihypertrophy may be present. Visceromegaly is manifest in the kidney as bilateral renal hypertrophy caused by what appears to be increased numbers of nephrons alone or in combination with medullary dysplasia and, in many cases, PLNR. All infants with BWS do not have nephromegaly, but, when present, it may be a risk factor for WT (DeBaun et al., 1998). Microscopic evidence of hyperplasia is found in the islets of Langerhans, Leydig cells, and adrenals, where fetal zone cytomegaly is a spectacular, though not specific, feature. In BWS, the risk of developing a neoplasm during childhood (WT, hepatoblastoma, adrenal carcinoma, rhabdomyosarcoma, and glioma) is between 7% and 21%, with about half of the tumors being WT (Schneid et al., 1997; Weidemann, 1983). Incomplete forms of BWS are relatively common and may be difficult to recognize (Sotelo-Avila et al., 1980). This has implications for so-called sporadic forms of WT, which tend to develop in infants whose birthweights are slightly excessive (Leisenring et al., 1994).

Most examples of BWS are sporadic. A few families have autosomal dominant BWS that is sex-linked with transmission through the maternal lineage. Discordancy for BWS in monozygotic twins is the rule (similar to familial WT), suggesting that postzygotic somatic recombination may be involved (Cote and Gyftodimou, 1991). The gene for BWS, unlike *WT1*, has not been cloned. Referred to as *WT2*, it is located at 11p15.5 with a cluster of other genes that are normally maternally imprinted, including those for ILGF-2 and H19, which may regulate its expression (Weksberg and Squire, 1996).

Perlman Syndrome

Perlman syndrome (PS) is a rare neonatal overgrowth syndrome associated with multiple congenital anomalies that resembles BWS in several important respects (Perlman et al., 1975) but differs in others (Fahmy et al., 1998; van der Stege et al., 1998). The principal shared features are macrosomia, islet cell hyperplasia with liability to neonatal hypoglycemia, abnormal kidneys, and a strong predisposition to WT, but not to other childhood tumors. The facies is abnormal in a distinctive manner, consisting of a depressed nasal bridge and anteverted upper lip. The kidneys are abnormally large and are the seat of extensive nephroblastomatosis consisting of partially to completely mature NR, the latter having been referred to as *hamartomas,* combined with hyperlobulation and variable renal cortical and medullary dysplasia. Associated anomalies differ from those in BWS and include hypoplasia of abdominal wall muscles, volvulus, intestinal atresia, diaphragmatic hernia, heart defects, and cryptorchidism. Perlman syndrome has been described in siblings and is thought to be a recessive trait. Thus far, genetic abnormalities in 11p have been described but are not well characterized.

Other Congenital Syndromes with Possible Linkage to Wilms' Tumor

The Simpson-Golabi-Behmel syndrome consists of gigantism with a bulldog face, stocky physique, skeletal anomalies, heart defects, enlarged kidneys, and genitourinary anomalies. There is minor overlap with BWS and PS. Inheritance is X-linked and maps to Xq26. Neoplasia is not increased but there

is one report of familial WT (Hughs-Benzie et al., 1992). The Sotos syndrome features macrocephaly, increased body length, and an increased incidence of neoplasms of many types at all ages. Most cases are sporadic but inheritance in an autosomal dominant pattern is reported. Two examples of WT are known (Hersh et al., 1992). Bloom syndrome (BS) is a form of congenital constitutional dwarfism inherited as an autosomal recessive trait with the gene mapped to 15q26.1. Anomalies are not major features. About 25% of patients with BS develop malignancy, most commonly, leukemia. Among the solid tumors reported are three patients with WT, one of them bilateral (Cairney et al., 1987). Chromosome breakage and exchange in BS result in high recombination rates, predisposing to pangenomic loss of heterozygosity, making it likely that WT results from one or more random events. Two cases of WT have been reported in 2q37 deletion syndrome, which includes craniofacial dysmorphia, mental retardation, stocky build, propensity to genital anomalies, and contralateral renal "dysplasia" in one case (Viot-Szoboszlai et al., 1998). The WT in this case had normal *WT1* coding sequences, information that adds perspective. In the Brachmann–de Lang syndrome, another form of constitutional growth deficiency tentatively mapped to 3q26, minor renal dysgenesis is common, and both NR and a single example of WT are separately reported (Charles et al., 1997). In most of the above syndromes, the occurrence of NR is not known to be a regular feature and NR are rarely mentioned in the descriptions of the nephrectomy specimens.

FAMILIAL WILMS' TUMOR

Familial Wilms' tumor (FWT) is rare, accounting for 1%–2% of all cases (Breslow et al., 1996). Most examples are in siblings and a few families exhibit vertical transmission through either the paternal or maternal line as an autosomal dominant trait with reduced expression. Penetrance and age at diagnosis do not depend on the gender of the transmitting parent. Excluding cases of overgrowth syndromes, FWT is not associated with congenital anomalies, with the exception of hemihypertrophy (Meadows et al.,

1974). Familial WT tends to occur at a younger mean age and is more often bilateral than sporadic WT (Knudson and Strong, 1972), two features that are shared with WAGR and DDS syndromes. It is surprising that the incidence of bilaterality is not much higher in FWT than in sporadic WT (16% vs. 7%), given the likelihood of germline mutation in FWT. Furthermore, all three reported monozygotic twins in such families are disconcordant for WT.

The frequency of associated NR in FWT is the same as in sporadic WT, but ILNR are more common than PLNR (Breslow et al., 1996), a finding that supports the thesis that intralobar NR may be a marker for germline mutation. No association has been found between FWT and abnormalities of 11p. Recent evidence mapping a FWT gene to 17q (Rahman et al., 1996) could not be confirmed in other families (Huff et al., 1997). Strong evidence for a locus at 19q in five families (McDonald et al., 1998) suggests multiple pathways to FWT. The two genes linked to FWT are known as *FWT1* and *FWT2*, respectively.

KARYOTYPE

Numerous analyses of karyotype in WT have been reported, whereas the karyotype of NR have only rarely been described. Nonrandom abnormalities reported in WT include 11p13-15 deletions (Riccardi et al., 1978), abnormalities of 16q, 1q/1p rearrangements, and trisomies 6, 8, 12, 13, and 18. Linkage of WT to chromosome 7 abnormalities has been suggested (Peier et al., 1995; Wilmore et al., 1994). Karyotype abnormalities in WT are usually not prominent and are often absent. A large series based on short-term culture of mainly nonsyndromatic WT, with follow-up in nude mouse implants in most cases (Wang-Wuu et al., 1990), has recently been updated to 54 cases, including 51 without nuclear anaplasia (Soukup et al., 1997). Only 4 (7%) of these cases had detectable 11p deletions. Their data show that 75% of WT cells that enter mitosis have abnormal karyotypes, with modal chromosome number increased from 47 to 57 in half of the cases. Flow cytometry detects these slightly hyperdiploid cells (Sheng et al., 1990). Mild hyperdiploidy was related to the prevalence of trisomy in this series, specifically for chromosomes 12, 8, 18,20, 13, 7, and 6, in order of incidence. Some of these abnormalities probably result from clonal progression and/or may be ubiquitous to neoplasia (1q/1p). Others are of interest when seen as the sole abnormality in a WT and/or in association with similar germline abnormality. In one instance, a NR shared constitutional mosaicism for 8q with the WT as the only abnormality (Betts et al., 1997).

Karyotype data on NR in conjunction with associated normal somatic cells and WT would be useful for recognizing changes related to clonal progression and for identifying changes related to timing of early molecular events that predispose to the development of WT. The paucity of data on NR is understandable. Obstacles to obtaining this information are the need for pathologists to recognize these lesions and sample them prior to fixation, plus the likelihood that many NR are mitotically dormant. Preoperative imaging studies that demonstrate the existence of NR will facilitate efforts to obtain this kind of data.

MOLECULAR GENETICS OF WILMS' TUMOR

The genetic events that determine progression of NR to WT are currently of great interest, as are the factors, largely unknown, that determine regression or maturation of these precursor lesions. Less than 5% of WT occur in patients with germline mutations (Li et al., 1996). Included in this group are WAGR syndrome, Denys-Drash syndrome, a small minority of patients with Beckwith-Wiedemann syndrome, Perlman syndrome, and FWT without extrarenal anomalies. With the exception of FWT, current data point to chromosome 11p as a major locus for genes involved in the pathogenesis of WT. About 10% of all WT carry a point mutation involving a gene *WT1*, which maps to 11p13. This gene has been identified as a tumor suppressor gene that has a demonstrable anti-tumor effect in embryonal tumor cell lines (Haber et al., 1996). *WT1* has a critical role in the development of the metanephric kidney and the gonad (Kreidberg et al., 1993) and in the developmental evolution of mesothelium from mesenchyme (Armstrong et al., 1992). Among neoplasms of childhood, *WT1* is commonly expressed only in WT and possibly in rare tumors of mesothelial cell origin (Thorner et al., 1999). Despite the significant association between ILNR and syndromatic WT, it is clear that NR are not a consistent marker for germline mutation. Therefore it is likely that many and perhaps most NR arise as a consequence of postzygotic mutation. Data on the presence and type of genetic abnormalities in WT, associated NR, normal renal tissue, and extrarenal tissue of patients with WT are provocative, but fragmentary. Some NR, more commonly intralobar NR, exhibit some of the same genetic abnormalities as the WT and the kidneys in which they occur (Charles et al., 1998; Park et al., 1993). Similar genetic changes also have been observed in the normal kidney tissue and tissue from extrarenal sites in a few cases of WT (Chao et al., 1993; Charles et al., 1998; Ogawa et al., 1993). This may be the basis for the presence of subtle gross and/or microscopic structural abnormalities in many kidneys bearing WT, particularly in proximity to NR, and for the association of WT with several forms of somatic overgrowth disorder.

Using bilateral occurrence of WT and young age at diagnosis as a marker for a presumably genetic susceptibility factor, Knudson and Strong (1972) predicted that 38% of all WT are inherited in an autosomal dominant pattern, with reduced penetrance accounting for the relatively low incidence of clinically apparent tumors. The ever-increasing complexity of the genetic abnormalities associated with WT will inevitably require some modification of Knudson's one-locus, two-hit hypothesis as it applies to most WT. At least four genetic loci may be involved (WT1, WT2, FWT1, and FWT2). The cytogenetic data from WT suggest the possibility of other sites in the genome where early, if not primary, alterations regularly occur (Huff, 1998). It is now recognized that one or more of the genes suspected to be involved in the pathogenesis of WT are also involved in genitourinary development, influence both renal and generalized tissue growth, may be involved in the pathogenesis of other childhood tumors, and are normally subject to parental imprinting. Preferential loss of maternal alleles and retention of paternal alleles is

common in WT and is a consistent feature in BWs. In both, the heterogeneous combination of overgrowth, malformations, and tumor predisposition would fit a model in which imbalance between maternal and paternal growth-promoting genes that control renal development modify other genes that may contain mutations predisposing to NR and WT (Li et al., 1998). The existence of particular germline mutations in WAGR syndrome and DDS, or late gestational overexpression of ILGF-2 in BWS, may determine whether NR are mainly intralobar or extralobar as well as the risk of WT. In many cases, NR probably are not a consequence of a single event or first hit, but, similar to most WT, result from multiple genetic events, which are not sufficient, even in those with a germline mutation, to consistently result in a WT. Additional factors that favor clonal expansion and neoplastic progression may determine evolution to clinical tumors. Presumably, it is the absence of these as-yet unspecified factors that is responsible for the regression of most NR to adenoma-like foci or minute undistinguished scars during early postnatal life. Study of genetic heterogeneity among NR is important because available data indicate that some NR possess the same genetic abnormalities as the associated WT, whereas other NR do not (Charles et al., 1998; Park et al., 1993).

General acceptance of the hypothesis that WT arise from NR does not obviate exceptions. Extrarenal NR, for which no frequency estimates are available, occur outside the renal capsule, in the renal sinus and in the retroperitoneum and pelvic soft tissue along the pathway of the developing urinary tract, and are a postulated source of rare extrarenal WT, which theoretically also could arise from mesonephric remnants or germ cells. Rarely, WT occurs in adults, in whom the absence of associated NR has been commented upon (Huser et al., 1990). Yet NR are capable of persisting in adults, although rarely described (Scharfenberg and Beckman, 1984). It is probable that at all ages WT in the absence of NR reflects either insufficient sampling or destruction by tumor expansion of a small loci cluster of NR. It is most unlikely that a differentiated cell of a mature nephron could dedifferentiate and give rise to a neoplasm displaying embryonal characteristics, although recent success cloning mammals from mature somatic cells suggests a need for caution in this regard.

REFERENCES

Armstrong JF, Pritchard-Jones K, Bickmore WA, et al. (1992) The expression of the Wilms tumor gene, WT1, in the developing mammalian embryo. *Mech Dev* 40:85–97.

Beckwith JB. (1969) Macroglossia, omphalocele, adrenal cytomegaly, gigantism and hyperplastic visceromegaly. *Birth Defects* 5:188–196.

Beckwith JB. (1986) Wilms' Tumor and other renal tumors of childhood: an update. *J Urol* 136:32–34.

Beckwith JB, Kiviat NB, Bonadio JF. (1990) Nephrogenic rests, nephroblastomatosis, and the pathogenesis of Wilms' tumor. *Pediatr Pathol* 10:1–36.

Betts DR, Koesters R, Pluss HJ, et al. (1997) Routine karyotyping in Wilms tumor. *Cancer Genet Cytogenet* 96:151–156.

Bond JV. (1975) Bilateral Wilms' tumor. *Lancet* 2:482–484.

Bove KE, Koffler H, McAdams AJ. (1969) Nodular renal blastema: definition and possible significance. *Cancer* 24:323–332.

Bove KE, Lewis C, Kiser-Debrosse B. (1995) Proliferation and maturation indices in nephrogenic rests and Wilms tumor: the emergence of heterogeneity from dormant nodular blastema. *Pediatr Pathol Lab Med* 15:223–244.

Bove KE, McAdams AJ. (1976) The nephroblastomatosis complex and its relationship to Wilms' tumor: a clinicopathologic treatise. *Perspect Pediatr Pathol* 3:185–223.

Bove KE, McAdams AJ. (1978) Multifocal nephroblastic neoplasia. *J Natl Cancer Inst* 61:285–294.

Breslow NE, Beckwith JB, Ciol M, et al. (1988) Age distribution of Wilms' tumor: Report from the National Wilms' Tumor Study. *Cancer Res* 48:1653–1657.

Breslow NE, Olson J, Moksness J, et al. (1996) Familial Wilms' tumor: a descriptive study. *Med Pediatr Oncol* 27:398–403.

Cairney AEL, Andrews M, Greenberg M, et al. (1987) Wilms' tumor in three patients with Bloom syndrome. *J Pediatr* 111:414–416.

Chao LY, Huff V, Tomlinson G, et al. (1993) Genetic mosaicism in normal tissues of Wilms' tumor patients. *Nat Genet* 3:127–131.

Charles A. (1996) Nephrogenic rest and mesoblastic nephroma (letter). *Pediatric Pathology Lab Med* 16:695–696.

Charles AK, Brown KW, Berry PJ. (1998) Microdissecting the genetic events in nephrogenic rests and Wilms' tumor development. *Am J Pathol* 153:991–1000.

Charles AK, Porter HJ, Sams V, et al. (1997) Nephrogenic rests and renal abnormalities in Braachmann-de Lang syndrome. *Pediatr Pathol Lab Med* 17:209–219.

Cote GB, Gyftodimou J. (1991) Twinning and mitotic crossing-over: some possibilities and their implications. *Am J Hum Genet* 46:672–681.

Craver R, Dimmick J, Johnson H, et al. (1986) Congenital obstructive uropathy and nodular renal blastema. *J Urol* 136:305–307.

Cui H, Hedborg F, He L, et al. (1997) Inactinactivation of H19, an imprinted and putative tumor suppressor gene, is a preneoplastic event during Wilms' tumorgenesis. *Cancer Res* 57:4469–4473.

DeBaun M, Siegle MJ, Choyke PL. (1998) Nephromegaly in infancy and early childhood: a risk factor for Wilms' tumor in Beckwith-Wiedemann syndrome. *J Pediatr* 132:401–404.

deChadarevian JP, Fletcher BD, Chatten J, et al. (1977) Massive infantile nephroblastomatosis: a clinical, radiological and pathological analysis of four cases. *Cancer* 39:2294–2305.

Drash A, Sherman F, Hartman WH, et al. (1970) A syndrome of pseudohermaphroditism Wilms' tumor, hypertension and degenerative renal disease. *J Pediatr* 786:585–593.

Fahmy J, Kaminsky CK, Parisi MT. (1998) Perlman syndrome: a case report emphasizing its similarity to and distinction from Beckwith-Wiedemann and prune-belly syndrome. *Pediatr Radiol* 28:179–182.

Feinberg AP. (1996) Multiple genetic abnormalities in Wilms' Tumor. *Med Pediatr Oncol* 27:484–489.

Gaulier A, Boccon-Gibod L, Sabatier P, et al. (1993) Panlobar nephroblastomatosis with cystic dysplasia; an unusual case with diffuse renal involvement studied by immunohistochemistry. *Pediatr Pathol* 13:741–749.

Greenberg F, Stein F, Gresik VV, et al. (1986) The Perlman familial nephroblastomatosis syndrome. *Am J Med Genet* 24:101–110.

Grundy P, Telzerow P, Moksness J, et al. (1996) Clinicopathologic correlates of loss of heterozygosity in Wilms' tumor. *Med Pediatr Oncol* 27:429–433.

Haber D, Englert C, Maheswaren S. (1996) Functional properties of WT1. *Med Pediatr Oncol* 27:453–455.

Hedborg F, Holmgren L, Sandstedt B, et al. (1994) The cell type-specific IGF2 expression during human development correlates to the pattern of overgrowth and neoplasia in the Beckwith-Wiedemann syndrome. *Am J Pathol* 145:802–817.

Heppe RK, Koyle MA, Beckwith BJ. (1991) Nephrogenic rests in Wilms' tumor patients with Drash syndrome. *J Urol* 145:1225–1228.

Hersh JH, Cole TRP, Bloom AS, et al. (1992) Risk of malignancy in Sotos syndrome. *J Pediatr* 120:572–574.

Hinchcliffe SA, Sargent PH, Howard CW, et al. (1991) Human intrauterine renal growth expressed in absolute number of glomeruli assessed by the "dissector" method and Cavalieri principle. *Lab Invest* 64:777–784.

Hou LT, Holman RL. (1961) Bilateral nephroblastomatosis in a premature infant. *J Pathol Bacteriol* 82:249–255.

Hsueh C, Hseu W, Gonzalez-Crussi F. (1987) Bilatreal renal dysplasia with features of nephroblastomatosis. *Pediatr Pathol* 7:437–446.

Huff V. (1998) Wilms tumor genetics. *Am J Med Genet* 79:260–267.

Huff V, Amos CI, Douglass EC, et al. (1997) Evidence for genetic heterogeneity in familial Wilms' tumor. *Cancer Res* 57:1859–1862.

Hughs-Benzie RM, Hunter AG, Allanson JE, et al. (1992) Simpson-Golabi-Behmel syndrome associated with renal dysplasia and embryonal tumors: localization of gene to Xqcen-q21. *Am J Med Genet* 43:428–435.

Huser J, Grignon DJ, Ro JY, et al. (1990) Adult Wilms' tumor: a clinicopathologic study of 11 cases. *Mod Pathol* 3:321–326.

Klamt B, Koziell A, Poulat F, et al. (1998) Frasier syndrome is caused by defective alternative splicing of WT1 leading to an altered ratio of WT1$^+$/WT1$^-$ isoforms. *Hum Mol Genet* 7:707–714.

Knudson AG, Strong LC. (1972) Mutation and cancer: a model for Wilms tumor of the kidney. *J Natl Cancer Inst* 48:313–324.

Kobayashi Y, Nagahara H. (1990) A pathological study of Wilms' tumor with congenital aniridia. *Acta Pathol Jpn* 40:417–424.

Kreidberg JA, Sariola H, Loring JM, et al. (1993) WT1 is required for early kidney development. *Cell* 74:679–691.

Leisenring WM, Breslow NE, Evans IE, et al. (1994) Increased birth weights of National Wilms' Tumor Study patients suggest a growth factor excess. *Cancer Res* 54:4680–4683.

Li FP, Breslow NE, Morgan JM, et al. (1996) Germline WT1 mutations in Wilms' tumor patients: preliminary results. *Med Ped Oncol* 27:404–407.

Li M, Squiare JA, Weksberg R. (1998) Molecular genetics of Widemann-Beckwith syndrome. *Am J Med Genet* 79:253–259.

Machin GA, McGaughy WTE. (1984) A new precursor lesion for Wilms' tumour (nephroblastoma): intralobar nephroblastomatosis. *Histopathology* 8:35–53.

Manivel JC, Sibley RK, Dehner LP. (1987) Complete and incomplete Drash syndrome: A clinicopathologic study of five cases of a dysontogenetic-neoplastic complex. *Hum Pathol* 18:80–89.

Matsunaga E. (1981) Genetics of Wilms' tumor. *Hum Genet* 57:231–246.

McDonald JM, Douglass EC, Fisher R, et al. (1998) Linkage of familial Wilms' tumor predisposition to chromosome 19 and a two-locus model for the etiology of familial tumors. *Cancer Res* 58:1387–1390.

Meadows AT, Licntenfeld JL, Coop CE. (1974) Wilms' tumor in three children of a woman with congenital hemihypertrophy. *N Engl J Med* 291:23–24.

Miller RW, Fraumeni JF, Manning MD. (1964) Association of Wilms' tumor with anaridia, hemihypertrophy and other congenital anomalies. *N Engl J Med* 270:922–927.

Murata T, Yoshida T, Takanari H, et al. (1989) Bilateral diffuse nephroblastomatosis, pancortical type: a case report with immunohistochemical investigations. *Arch Pathol Lab Med* 113:729–734.

Murphy WW, Beckwith JB, Farrow WM. (1994) Tumors of the kidney, bladder and related urinary structures. In: *Atlas of Tumor Pathology*, 3rd Series, Fascicle 11. Armed Forces Institute of Pathology, Washington DC.

Nicholson GW. (1931) An embryonic tumor of the kidney in a foetus. *J Pathol Bacteriol* 34:711–730.

Ogawa O, Becroft DM, Morriso IM, et al. (1993) Constitutional relaxation of insulin-like growth factor II gene imprinting associated with Wilms' tumor and gigantism. *Nature Genet* 5:408–412.

Olson JM, Hamilton A, Breslow NE. (1995) Non-11p constitutional chromosome abnormalities in Wilms' tumor patients. *Med Pediatr Oncol* 24:305–309.

Park S, Bernard A, Bove KE, et al. (1993) Inactivation of WT1 in nephrogenic rests, genetic precursors to Wilms' tumor. *Nat Genet* 5:563–567.

Payton D, Thorner P, Baumal R, et al. (1988) Characterization of glomeruli by immunohistochemistry and electronmicroscopy in a case of Wilms' tumor. *Arch Pathol Lab Med* 112:536–539.

Peier AM, Meloni AM, Erling MA, et al. (1995) Involvement of chromosome 7 in Wilms tumorl. *Cancer Genet Cytogenet* 79:92–94.

Pelletier J, Bruning W, Kashtan CE, et al. (1991) Germline mutations in the Wilms' tumor suppressor gene are associated with abnormal urogenital development in Denys-Drash syndrome. *Cell* 67:437–447.

Perlman M, Goldberg GM, Bar-Ziv J, et al. (1975) Renal hamartomas and nephroblastomatosis with fetal gigantism. *J Pediatr* 83:414–418.

Potter EI, Thierstein ST. (1943) Glomerular development in the kidney as an index of fetal maturity. *J Pediatr* 22:695–706.

Potter EL. (1961) *Pathology of the Fetus and Newborn.* Year Book Medical Publishers, Chicago.

Rahman N, Arbour L, Tonin P, et al. (1996) Evidence for a familial Wilms' tumor gene on chromosome 17q12-21. *Nat Genet* 13:461–463.

Reeve AE. (1996) Role of genetic imprinting in Wilms' tumor and overgrowth disorders. *Med Pediatr Oncol* 27:470–475.

Regalado JJ, Rodriguez MM, Beckwith JB. (1996) Multinodular hyperplastic pannephric nephroblastomatosis with tubular differentiation; a new morphological variant. *Pediatr Pathol Lab Med* 16:961–972.

Reik W, Surani MA. (1989) Genomic imprinting and embryonal tumors. *Nature* 338:112–113.

Riccardi VM, Sujansky E, Smith AC, et al. (1978) Chromosomal inbalance inthe aniridia-Wilms' tumor association: 11p interstitial deletion. *Pediatrics* 61:604–610.

Scharfenberg JC, Beckman EN. (1984) Persistent renal blastema in an adult. *Hum Pathol* 15:791–793.

Schneid H, Vazquez MP, Vacher C, et al. (1997) The Beckwith-Wiedemann syndrome phenotype and the risk of cancer. *Med Pediatr Oncol* 28:411–415.

Shanklin DR, Sotelo-Avila C. (1969) In situ tumors in fetuses, newborns and young infants. *Biol Neonate* 14:286–316.

Shannon RS, Mann JR, Harper E, et al. (1982) Wilms' tumor and aniridia: clinical and cytogenetic features. *Arch Dis Child* 57:685–690.

Sheng WW, Jacobs D, Soukup S, et al. (1990) Comparison of flow chromosome analysis to DNA content by flow cytometry for pediatric tumors. *Pediatr Pathol* 10:761–769.

Sotelo-Avila C, Gonzalez-Crussi F, Fowler JW. (1980) Complete and incomplete forms of Beckwith-Wiedemann syndrome: their oncogenic potential. *J Pediatr* 96:47–50.

Soukup S, Gotwals B, Blough R, et al. (1997) Wilms tumor: summary of 54 cytogenetic analysis. *Cancer Genet Cytogenet* 97:169–171.

Stiller CA, Lennon EL, Wilson LM. (1987) Incidence of cardiac septal defects in children with Wilms' tumor and other malignant diseases. *Carcinogen* 8:129–132.

Thorner P, Squire J, Plavsic N, et al. (1999) Expression of WT1 in pediatric small cell tumors: report of two cases with a possible mesothelial cell origin. *Peditr Dev Pathol* 2:33–41.

van der Stege JG, van Eyck J, Arabin B. (1998) Prenatal ultrasound observations in subsequent pregnancies in Perlman syndrome. *Ultrasound Obstet Gynecol* 11:149–151.

Viot-Szoboszlai G, Amiel J, Doz F, et al. (1998) Wilms' tumor and gonadal dysgenesis in a child with the 2q37.1 deletion syndrome. *Clin Genet* 53:278–270.

Vogler CA, Sotila-Avila C, Ramon-Garcia G, et al. (1988) Nodular renal blastema and metanephric hamartomas in children with urinary malformations: a morphologic specturm of abnormal metanephric differentiation. *Semin Diagn Pathol* 5:122–131.

Walford N. (1990) Panlobar nephroblastomatosis: a distinct form of renal dysplasia associated with Wilms' tumor. *Histopathology* 17:37–44.

Wang-Wuu S, Soukup S, Bove K, et al. (1990) Chromosome analysis of 31 Wilms' tumors. *Cancer Res* 50:2786–2793.

Warner BW, Bove KE, Kaufman RA, et al. (1988) Multicentric Wilms tumor with contralateral recurrence; comments on management. *Am J Pediatr Hematol Oncol* 10:129–133.

Weksberg R, Squire J. (1996) Molecular biology of Beckwith-Wiedemann syndrome. *Med Pediatr Oncol* 27: 462–469.

Wiedemann HR. (1983) Tumours and hemihypertrophy associated with Wiedemann-Beckwith syndrome. *Eur J Pediatr* 141:129.

Wilmore HP, White GFJ, Howell RT, et al. (1994) Germline and somatic abnormalities of chromosome 7 in Wilms tumor. *Cancer Genet Cytogenet* 77: 93–98.

25

NEUROBLASTOMA AND RELATED TUMORS

J. BRUCE BECKWITH

Neuroblastomas are embryonal neoplasms derived from neural crest cells, usually arising in the sympathetic nervous system and paraganglia. They rank fourth in frequency among childhood malignancies, behind leukemias, lymphomas, and tumors of the central nervous system (Gurney et al., 1995). The peak incidence is in the first year of life, with a median age at diagnosis of 22 months (Brodeur and Castleberry, 1997).

Neuroblastomas exhibit a diverse spectrum of differentiation toward neural or neuroendocrine cell types. Undifferentiated tumors are designated *neuroblastomas*. Tumors composed entirely of ganglion cells or other differentiated cells of neural crest origin are *ganglioneuromas*, and those containing both mature and undifferentiated cellular elements are *ganglioneuroblastomas*. Increasing differentiation in neuroblastic tumors usually correlates with decreasing malignancy potential, and ganglioneuromas are clinically benign neoplasms. In this chapter, the term "neuroblastoma" will be used as a generic designation for the entire series of neuroblastic tumors, unless specified otherwise. While most emphasis is placed upon neuronal differentiation in neuroblastomas, maturation in extra-adrenal neuroblastomas is often characterized by markers of an extra-adrenal chromaffin cell lineage (Hoehner et al., 1996). Schwann cells are a commonly observed component of differentiating neuroblastomas, and their relative prominence in neuroblastomas is recognized as a key marker of less aggressive tumor biology in current histological grading systems (Shimada et al., 1984).

Interestingly, Schwann cells in neuroblastomas have been found to lack the cytogenetic abnormalities seen in other cellular components of the tumor, which suggests they are a reactive population of host cells invading the tumor (Ambros et al., 1996). About 40% of neuroblastomas arise within the adrenal medulla. Most of the remainder originate from paraxial autonomic ganglia in the neck, thorax, abdomen, and pelvis. Although neuroblastomas are usually assumed to arise from sympathetic ganglia or adrenergic neuroendocrine cells of the adrenal medulla, other candidate sites include parasympathetic and cranial nerve ganglia, extra-adrenal paraganglia, and dorsal root ganglia of the spinal cord (Beckwith and Martin, 1968). The potential relationship of neuroblastic neoplasms of the peripheral nervous system to those of the neuraxis and to peripheral primitive neuroepithelial tumors (PNET) remains somewhat controversial, although molecular, immunohistochemical, and ultrastructural features can usually distinguish PNET from neuroblastomas in the diagnostic laboratory (Dehner 1985, 1986, 1998).

The natural history of neuroblastoma presents one of the most intriguing and elusive challenges in human oncology. The spontaneous maturation of a malignant undifferentiated neuroblastoma to benign ganglioneuroma, reported by Cushing and Wolbach in 1927, stimulated early investigators to search for nutritional or other biochemical methods of facilitating this process of maturation. Additional impetus to research into the natural history of neuroblastoma was provided by the observation that neuroblastomas diagnosed in the first year of life were often associated with a favorable outcome, while those diagnosed later in childhood generally proved lethal. This suggested that some immunological or biochemical peculiarity of immature infants might be utilized to favorably influence the clinical biology of undifferentiated neuroblastoma in older children. However, despite these provocative clues, neuroblastoma remains one of the most lethal neoplasms of childhood, and only in the past few years have studies of the cytogenetic and molecular features of neuroblastomas begun to reveal some of the fundamental secrets of this elusive neoplasm.

Undifferentiated neuroblastomas comprise a biologically heterogeneous spectrum, with cases destined for spontaneous regression or maturation at one end and inexorably progressive tumors at the other (Pahlman and Grotta, 1982). This heterogeneity is closely correlated with molecular and cytogenetic features, as discussed below (Brodeur et al., 1998).

An intriguing category of patients with a generally favorable prognosis is those who present, usually in early infancy, with multifocal undifferentiated neuroblastic tumors limited to the adrenals, skin, liver, and bone marrow, without radiologically demonstrable bony metastases. This pattern of presentation has been designated *stage IV-S*, or *D(S)*, and has a propensity for spontaneous regression without the need for aggressive adjuvant therapy (Evans et al., 1981). However, a subset of approximately 30% of infants within this group have been found to have histological and biological markers of adverse prognostic significance, with clinically aggressive and unresponsive tumors (Katzenstein et al., 1998).

Comprehensive reviews of the clinical, pathological, and biological aspects of neuroblastoma are available (Askin and Perlman 1998; Brodeur and Castleberry 1997; Kelly and Joshi, 1996).

EMBRYOLOGICAL CONSIDERATIONS

Neuroblastomas have long been assumed to originate from cells of the embryonic neural crests, and share numerous molecular and phenotypic features with those cells (Tsokos et al., 1987). These tumors are included among a diverse group of disorders that have been termed *neurocristopathies* (Bolande, 1997). Neural crest cells in the human embryo first become recognizable at about day 18, along both sides of the neural groove at its junction with surface ectoderm. They occur along the entire length of the neural groove, including its cranial and caudal ends. These cells migrate, sometimes over considerable distances, to their ultimate destinations in the developing body. It has been known for many years that neural crest cells are progenitors of most neural, neuroendocrine, and supporting cells of the peripheral nervous system, including autonomic and dorsal root ganglia, as well as adrenal medulla and related paraganglia. More recently, it was recognized that they also participate in the development of many other organs and tissues, as listed in Table 25–1.

Table 25–1. Derivatives of the Neural Crest

Neurons

Autonomic ganglia

Dorsal root ganglia

Some neurons in cranial nerve ganglia (V, VII, IX, X)

Neural support cells

Schwann cells, nerve sheath cells

Satellite cells of autonomic and spinal ganglia

Glial and satellite cells of cranial nerve ganglia VII, VIII, X, XI

Pigment cells

Melanocytes of skin and internal organs

Melanophores of ocular iris

Endocrine and paraendocrine cells

Adrenal medulla, other adrenergic paraganglia

Thyroid C cells

Type I and II cells of carotid body

Mesectodermal cells

Bone and cartilage of facial and visceral skeleton

Dermis of face and ventral neck region

Connective tissue of salivary glands, thyroid, parathyroids

Corneal cells

Connective tissue of thymus

Musculoconnective tissue of large arteries derived from aortic arches

Ciliary muscles, certain other muscles of facial and visceral region

Modified from Le Douarin (1980).

This expanded role of the neural crests in somatic development was revealed primarily by a classical series of studies by Le Douarin and colleagues (1980). These investigators performed transplants of neural crest cells between chicken and quail embryos and were able to maintain the chimeric recipient birds to maturity. Structural differences in nuclear morphology between these species can be readily recognized with the light microscope, enabling these investigators to follow the migration and distribution of engrafted neural crest cells in recipient birds. These studies established that engrafted cells from the donor neural crest populated many organs and tissues. This expanded view of the role of neural crest cells in development helps to explain the occasional association of neuroblastoma with a variety of abnormalities, including cardiovascular malformations (Beckwith, 1989), Hirschsprung disease (Clausen et al., 1989; Michna et al., 1988; Roshkow et al., 1988), and neurofibromatosis (Clausen et al., 1989).

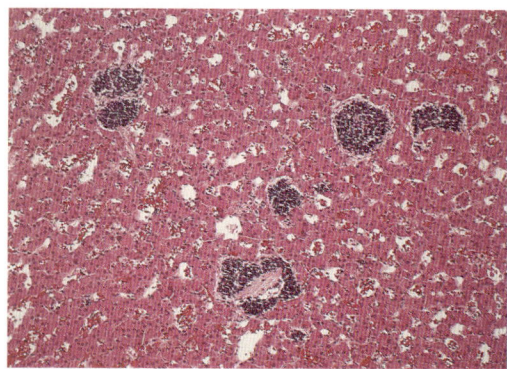

Figure 25–1. Fetal adrenal gland at 16 weeks gestation. Normal neuroblastic clusters migrate through fetal cortex.

NEUROBLASTIC MIGRATION AND DEVELOPMENT IN THE ADRENAL MEDULLA

Although neuroblastomas arise in multiple sites in the body, the putative early stages in tumor development discussed in this chapter have been described only in the adrenal glands. The adrenals have a dual embryological origin. The cortex develops from dorsal coelomic mesodermal condensations adjacent to the genital ridge, whereas the medulla is derived from neural crest cells originating at the level of the future upper abdominal region (Le Douarin, 1980). Beginning in the seventh week of gestation, migrating neuroblasts, usually in groups, are found throughout the adrenal cortex (Fig. 25–1). By mid-gestation most cells have arrived in the region of the future medulla, where they are destined to differentiate into both neuroendocrine and ganglion cell populations. These immature neural crest cells tend to aggregate into clusters, usually 60 to 80 μm in diameter, which were termed *neuroblastic nodules* by Turkel and Itabashi (1974). These authors reported that neuroblastic nodules attained their maximum

size between weeks 15 and 17. After this gestational age, the nodules diminished rapidly in size as individual neuroblasts dispersed through the medulla and began to mature. Ikeda et al. (1981) found a few neuroblastic nodules larger than those of Turkel and Itabashi, but confirmed that their maximum size was reached between weeks 15 and 18, and rapidly declined after that gestational age. Scattered single neuroblasts may persist beyond intrauterine life, and perhaps even until puberty in some individuals (Wiesel, 1902). However, persistence of larger neuroblastic nodules into the latter half of gestation was not observed by Turkel and Itabashi, nor by Ikeda et al. This is an important point, because neuroblastic nodules are in general distinctly smaller, and occur at a much earlier period in development, than the *in situ* neuroblastomas described in the next section. Considerable misunderstanding exists in the literature concerning this point, and many authors suggest erroneously that neuroblastic nodules are indistinguishable from *in situ* neuroblastoma.

IN SITU ADRENAL NEUROBLASTOMA

In 1963, we reported a series of 13 small neuroblastic tumors that had been found incidentally during routine postmortem examinations of young infants (Beckwith and Perrin, 1963). Seven of these small tumors were encountered retrospectively in the adrenals of 1571 infants dying between birth and 3 months of age. The tumors formed discrete, homogenous nodules, and most were invasive, with mitotic activity. On the basis of their microscopic appearances, it was presumed that they represented early neuroblastomas, discovered accidentally because the infants harboring them had died of unrelated causes. In addition to these smaller tumors, all of which were 1 cm or less in maximum diameter, the same population also included three infants with macroscopically obvious but clinically undetected neuroblastomas, presumably unrelated to the cause of death. Thus, the prevalence of the smaller *in situ* neuroblastomas was 1/224 infant autopsies. When the three larger incidentally encountered tumors are included, the proportion increased to 1/157 autopsies. We calculated that only 1 in 10,000 liveborn infants was destined to develop clinically overt adrenal neuroblastoma, so the apparent prevalence of early neuroblastomas in routine infant postmortems was difficult to ascribe to chance alone. This finding suggested that early neuroblastomas have a propensity to disappear, and that most are not destined to become clinically overt.

The relative frequency of *in situ* neuroblastomas in infant autopsies was confirmed in subsequent studies by others (Guin et al., 1969; Hasegawa et al., 1982; Ikeda et al., 1981; Shanklin and Sotelo-Avila, 1969). Prevalence data from these studies are summarized in Table 25–2. These *in situ* neuroblastomas have to date been recognized only in the adrenals, and not, to our knowledge, in sympathetic ganglia or other sites of neural crest migration. This limited distribution is probably due to the fact that adrenals are consistently sampled during routine pediatric autopsies, whereas other potential sites of neuroblastoma development are rarely examined systematically. As shown in Table 25–2, careful prospective search for small or *in situ* neuroblastomas revealed their presence in more than 1% of infant autopsies. If these are in fact early neuroblastomas, as suggested by their morphological and cytological features, it would appear that most neuroblastomas do not evolve into clinically apparent tumors.

It must be emphasized that the *in situ* neuroblastomas reported by us (Beckwith and Perrin, 1963) were all diagnosed in term or near-term infants. The smallest measured 0.7 mm in diameter, 11 of 13 were over 1 mm, and 1 was 9.5 mm. Although Turkel and Itabashi (1974) suggested that *in situ* neuroblastomas might represent mere persistence of neuroblastic nodules, the size range of *in situ* neuroblastomas is not consistent with their suggestion. Their largest lesion was 0.4 mm in diameter, and most were less that 0.08 mm. None of their larger nodules were encountered in the last half of gestation. While it has not been proven that *in situ* neuroblastomas are identical except in size to clinically diagnosed neuroblastomas,

Table 25–2. Prevalence of Adrenal *in situ* Neuroblastoma in Postmortem Series

Reference	Study Population	Prevalence	Comments
Retrospective Reviews			
Beckwith and Perrin (1963)	9051 children (all ages)	9 (1 / 1005)	Cincinnati
	3569 children (all ages)	7 (1 / 510)	Los Angeles
	1571 Infants < 3 months	7 (1 / 224)	Los Angeles
Guin et al. (1969)	2596 children (all ages)	6 (1 / 432)	
Shanklin and Sotelo-Avila (1969)	2059 children (all ages)	5 (1 / 412)	
	471 infants < 4 months	5 (1 / 95)	
Prospective Search			
Guin et al. (1969)	155 infants < 6 months	3 (1 / 52)	Step sections of entire gland
Beckwith (unpublished)	262 SIDS cases < 12 months	4 (1 / 66)[a]	Careful search of 1 mm slices All suspicious foci embedded

[a]Includes 2 *in situ* adrenal neuroblastomas, one 1.5 cm adrenal neuroblastoma with early liver metastases, and one small neuroblastoma in the parasacral region.

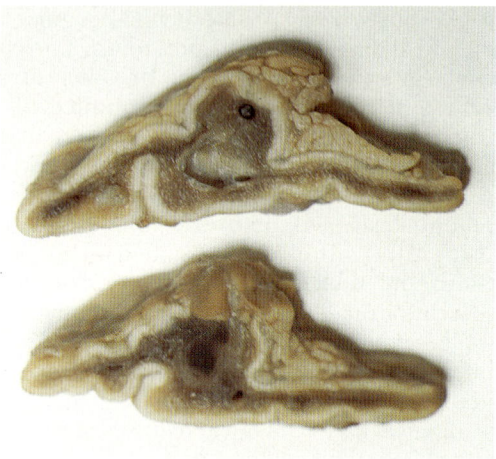

Figure 25–2. *In situ* neuroblastoma found in adrenal gland of infant dying at 2 months of sudden infant death syndrome.

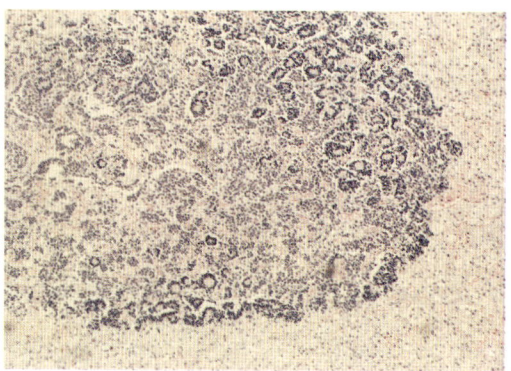

Figure 25–4. Portion of *in situ* neuroblastoma from infant aged 1 month with congenital heart disease. Homer Wright rosettes are prominent.

they certainly represent abnormal lesions and not mere persistence of normal cellular elements. Their possible significance will be discussed below.

Even the smallest *in situ* neuroblastomas can usually be detected by careful gross examination. Their recognition is facilitated by fixing the adrenals intact, then sectioning them at approximately 1 mm intervals with a sharp blade. This procedure renders the lesions easily recognizable, although it obviously limits their usefulness for biological studies. As shown in Figure 25–2, *in situ* neuroblastomas usually present as rounded gray or hemorrhagic masses, and occasionally

they appear cystic. Hemorrhagic tumors sometimes appear grossly similar to adrenal hemorrhage from another cause, and all suspicious nodules should be embedded for microscopic examination.

Figures 25–3 to 25–5 show some of the microscopic features of *in situ* neuroblastomas. These lesions are composed of uniform populations of neuroblasts, sometimes forming Homer Wright rosettes (Fig. 25–4). Ganglion cell differentiation is found rarely within them. Degenerative changes, including cyst formation (Fig. 25–5), hemorrhage, calcification, and apoptosis, are common, and suggest that spontaneous degenerative changes could account for the disappearance of most of these lesions. *In situ* neuroblastomas usually appear expansile, and invade adjacent adrenal cortex. Mitotic figures were readily demonstrated in 7 of 13 cases in our study (Beckwith and Perrin, 1963).

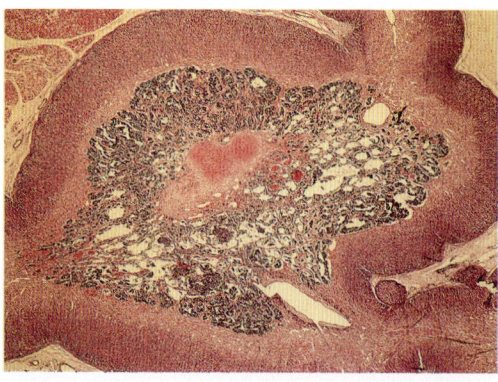

Figure 25–3. *In situ* neuroblastoma in adrenal gland of infant aged 3 months, who died with multiple malformations.

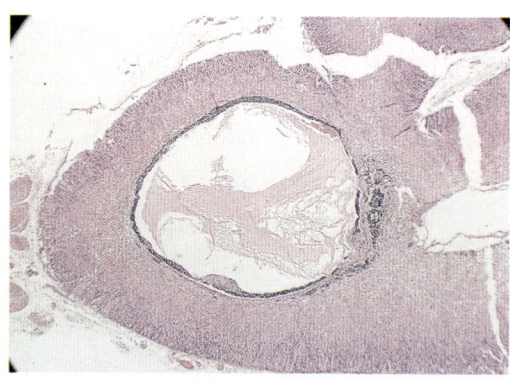

Figure 25–5. Cystic *in situ* neuroblastoma.

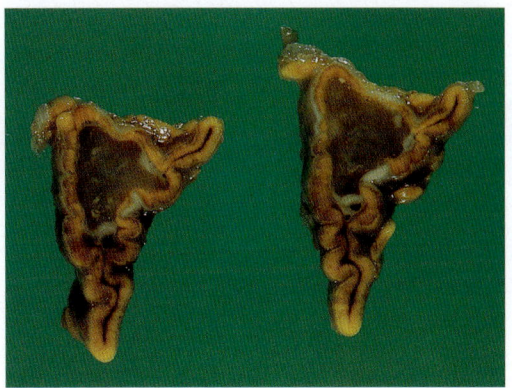

Figure 25–6. Gross appearance of nodular lesion in adrenal gland of a child aged 2.5 years who died of congenital heart disease.

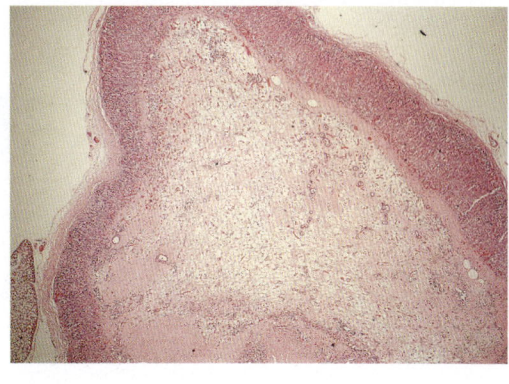

Figure 25–7. Microscopic appearance of lesion shown in Figure 25–5, interpreted as completely necrotic *in situ* neuroblastoma.

Lesions suggestive of necrotic or calcific *in situ* neuroblastomas are sometimes encountered in older infants and children. Figures 25–6 and 25–7 show a translucent, pale nodule in the adrenal medulla of a child 2.5 years old who died of congenital heart disease. Microscopically the mass was necrotic, without evidence of prior hemorrhage. Some of the nodular calcifications found at autopsy, or in imaging studies, in the adrenals of infants and children may represent spontaneously regressed neuroblastomas, though the majority of such calcifications are assumed to be relics of prior adrenal hemorrhages.

Nine of the 13 infants in our original series (Beckwith and Perrin, 1963) had major congenital malformations, 7 of which included the cardiovascular system. Other large retrospectively collected series of incidentally encountered *in situ* neuroblastomas included a high proportion of infants with malformations, as summarized in Table 25–3. Single case reports are not included in this table because of potential selection bias. The high prevalence of malformations, especially of the cardiovascular system, in these series has generated speculation that *in situ* neuroblastomas, and perhaps neuroblastomas in general, might have a teratogenic basis. Shanklin and Sotelo-Avila (1969) proposed that the apparent association with cardiovascular malformations might represent a response on the part of adrenomedullary precursor cells to fetal hypoxia. Another potential connection between cardiovascular malformations and neuroblastic tumors is the relatively recent recognition that the neural crest plays a major role in development of the heart and great vessels (Le Douarin, 1980), suggesting that this association might represent another form of neurocristopathy (Bolande, 1997). An infant dying at 2 days of age with severe congenital microcephaly was reported to have small *in situ* neuroblastomas in both adrenals (Park and Chi, 1993). However, the high proportion of malformations in most infant autopsy

Table 25–3. Prevalence of Major Malformations in Infants with *In Situ* Neuroblastomas

Reference	Cases	Total Malformations n (%)	Cardiovascular n (%)	Controls[a] (%)
Beckwith and Perrin (1963)	13	9 (69)	7 (54)	48
Shanklin and Sotelo-Avila (1969)	14	7 (50)	6 (43)	42–48
Guin et al. (1969)	11	7 (64)	4 (36)	62
Hasegawa et al. (1982)	8	1 (13)	0	Unknown
Total	46	24 (52)	17 (34)	

[a]Age-matched autopsies without neuroblastic tumors.

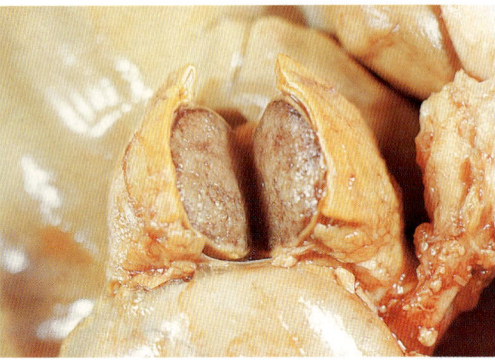

Figure 25–8. Small adrenal neuroblastoma from infant dying at 2.5 months of sudden infant death syndrome. Several small liver metastases up to 0.8 cm in diameter were also present.

series renders uncertain the significance of this association, and a relationship between *in situ* neuroblastomas and malformations remains unproven (Beckwith, 1989).

In situ neuroblastoma occurred within a sibship that included four infants with neuroblastoma (Chatten and Voorhess, 1969). Numerous other examples of familial neuroblastoma have been reported, but, with the exception of certain neurocristopathies as noted above, clinical neuroblastoma shows no strong association with malformation syndromes or cardiovascular malformations (Kushner et al., 1986).

Some of the early neuroblastomas encountered incidentally at autopsy in infants are larger and clearly represent neoplastic masses. Figure 25–8 shows a 1.5 cm adrenal neuroblastoma that was associated with several small metastatic lesions in the liver, which was discovered incidentally during the autopsy of an infant aged 4 months who died of sudden infant death syndrome.

IN SITU NEUROBLASTOMAS: HYPERPLASTIC OR NEOPLASTIC?

We and other authors reporting *in situ* neuroblastomas in previous decades assumed, from their microscopic appearances, that they represented small malignant neuroblastomas. However, subsequent studies on precursor lesions of another embryonal neoplasm, Wilms tumor (nephroblastoma),

have suggested an alternative interpretation. It is now known that *hyperplastic* proliferation of undifferentiated precursor cells can produce large masses that closely mimic their neoplastic counterpart. Nephrogenic rests, a recognized precursor lesion of Wilms tumors, sometimes undergo hyperplastic overgrowth, producing bulky masses of embryonal cells resembling those of Wilms tumor (Beckwith 1993; Beckwith et al., 1990; Chapter 24, this volume). In the light of these observations, it is tempting to speculate that many *in situ* neuroblastomas might represent abnormal *hyperplastic* proliferation of undifferentiated neuroblastic cells, analogous to hyperplastic nephrogenic rests in the kidney. Subsequent molecular events within such a lesion would be required for neoplastic induction.

A somewhat analogous suggestion was made by Knudson and Meadows (1980), who postulated that the majority of neuroblastomas in the first year of life, and those presenting with stage IV-S disease, might reflect the first event in a two-mutation concept of embryonal tumor formation. Subsequent loss or mutation of the remaining allele would be required for acquisition of neoplastic characteristics. They postulated that the infantile and IV-S subgroups might represent defective maturation, coupled with persistent proliferative activity, resulting in undifferentiated polyclonal tumors with a high likelihood of regression or maturation. Molecular studies of *in situ* specimens will be required to settle the question of whether these lesions represent preneoplastic hyperplasia, or are already committed neoplasms.

CYTOGENETIC AND MOLECULAR CORRELATES OF NEUROBLASTOMA

It has long been known that some neuroblastomas have a relatively low degree of biological aggressiveness, with a propensity for disappearance or maturation, while others pursue a notoriously aggressive clinical course with a high mortality rate. These observations have stimulated many investigators to search for molecular and cytogenetic determinants of neuroblastoma biology. After many years of disappointing results, a number of powerful cytogenetic and molec-

Table 25–4. Neuroblastoma: Cytogenetic and Molecular Markers of Biological Behavior[a]

Marker	Favorable	Unfavorable
N-*myc*	Not amplified	Amplified
1p36	Present	Deleted or mutated
TRK-A	Expressed	Not expressed
TRK-B	Not expressed	Expressed
DNA content	Triploid	Diploid, tetraploid
DM, HSRs[b]	Absent	Present
bcl-2 expression	Absent	Present

[a]Unfavorable prognostic factors often are associated with one another. Independent prognostic significance is not necessarily proven.

[b]Double minutes (DM) and homogeneous staining regions (HSRs) on karyotype studies.

ular markers have been found to be associated with the degree of aggressiveness of neuroblastomas. Table 25–4 lists some of the more important of these prognostic determinants. Space does not permit complete discussion of this rapidly changing field of knowledge; the reader is referred to recent reviews that include more extended discussions of this topic (Ambros et al., 1996; Askin and Perlman, 1998; Brodeur and Castleberry, 1997; Brodeur et al., 1998; Kelly and Joshi, 1996).

The first important molecular prognostic feature to be recognized was the association of numerous copies of the N-*myc* oncogene with advanced stage disease (Brodeur et al., 1984) and with rapid progression of neuroblastoma (Seeger et al., 1985). Recent studies have suggested that N-*myc* amplification is a powerful indicator of adverse prognosis in patients over 1 year of age, but is not predictive of outcome in infants (Bordow et al., 1998). Cytogenetic studies have revealed the presence of extrachromosomal chromatin bodies known as *double minutes*, which often represents amplification of a large region on chromosome 2 containing the N-*myc* locus (Kelly and Joshi, 1996). Amplification of other oncogenes in some neuroblastomas is suggested by the presence of *homogeneous staining regions* on various chromosomes in a small proportion of primary neuroblastoma specimens. Both double minutes and homogenous staining regions are considered to be markers of aggressiveness in neuroblastoma (Kelly and Joshi, 1996).

Karyotypic studies have yielded other important results that are correlated with tumor biology (Brodeur and Castleberry,

1997). An important prognostic marker in neuroblastoma is deletion of portions of the short arm of chromosome 1, which consistently includes region 1p36. This same region is abnormal in other human malignancies. A candidate tumor suppressor gene in this region, currently designated *p73*, has recently been identified (Jost et al., 1997; Kaghad et al., 1997). This gene shares considerable structural and functional similarity with the more familiar p53.

Ploidy is a significant prognostic indicator in neuroblastomas. Diploid DNA content is an adverse prognostic feature, and hyperdiploid karyotypes have been associated with less aggressive tumor biology (Brodeur and Castleberry, 1997). Within the hyperdiploid category of neuroblastomas, tetraploidy is usually associated with numerous structural chromosome anomalies and tends to be associated with a more adverse prognosis, whereas triploidy is usually associated with fewer structural anomalies and less aggressive tumor biology (Ambros et al., 1996).

As reviewed recently by Nakagawara (1998), nerve growth factor (NGF or neurotrophin), a potent promoter of sympathetic neuronal maturation, was long suspected of playing a role in the biology of neuroblastoma. During the 1960s, several patients were treated unsuccessfully with this substance in an effort to stimulate maturation of malignant neuroblasts. Interest in NGF was rekindled by the discovery of tyrosine kinase receptor A (TRK-A) a high-affinity receptor for NGF. TRK-A is preferentially expressed in early-stage neuroblastomas and in infants under 1 year of age, and is downregulated in advanced tumors with N-*myc* amplification. An inverse effect is seen with TRK-B, a receptor for brain-derived neurotrophin 4. The presence of high levels of TRK-B in neuroblastomas promotes cell proliferation, invasion, and metastasis. These markers of favorable or unfavorable prognosis usually occur together, making it difficult to distinguish their effects independently of one another. Most congenital or early onset neuroblastomas, and those with stage IV-S disease, have been found to have hyperdiploid (usually triploid) DNA content, intact 1p36, and no amplification of N-*myc*, and express high levels of TRK-A. Most undifferentiated neuroblastomas diagnosed beyond infancy and presenting with nonlocalized disease have diploid or near-diploid DNA content, deletions of 1p36, N-*myc* amplification, and high expression of TRK-B (Nakagawara et al., 1993). Molecular and cytogenetic studies for these prognostic markers is now a fundamental part of the prognostic evaluation of newly diagnosed neuroblastomas. Some of them clearly lead to malignant progression of neuroblastomas, and it is hoped that various steps in this progression pathway can become better understood by studying the molecular pathology of early and *in situ* neuroblastomas.

SCREENING FOR NEUROBLASTOMA

The concept of biochemical screening of young infants for urinary or blood metabolites of neuroblastoma was first popularized in Japan in the 1970s. While this procedure resulted in a fivefold increase in the rate of detection of neuroblastomas in infancy (Bessho, 1998), there was little if any decrease in the death rate from neuroblastoma. Presumably most of the tumors detected by early screening represented neuroblastomas that would have disappeared spontaneously had they not been detected by screening. This result led to efforts in several countries to screen at 6 months or at 12 months, but similar results were obtained (Bessho, 1998; Kerbl et al., 1998). A special issue of *Medical and Pediatric Oncology* (November 1998, Volume 38) was devoted entirely to this subject, and covers all aspects of this complex and controversial topic in detail. While consensus about the value of

screening at later ages has not yet been achieved, it is agreed by most workers that screening at or before 6 months of age produces more problems than benefits. False-positive results and detection of biologically less aggressive cases are the principal causes for problems.

In summary, early screening detects about five times as many neuroblastomas as were detected by clinical presentation as tumors. The rate of incidental discovery of *in situ* and early neuroblastomas during infant autopsies is well over 10 times the incidence detected by screening. These results, along with the high cure rate for neuroblastomas diagnosed clinically in the first year of life, demonstrate that incipient neuroblastic tumors are in general destined to disappear, unless specific genetic events, including 1p36 loss, N-*myc* amplification, and loss of TRK-A expression, occur within the tumor. Some *in situ* neuroblastomas are likely to represent hyperplastic proliferative lesions comparable to hyperplastic nephrogenic rests in the kidney.

REFERENCES

Ambros IM, Zellner A, Roald B, et al. (1996) Role of ploidy, chromosome 1p, and Schwann cells in the maturation of neuroblastoma. *N Engl J Med* 334:1505–1511.

Askin FB, Perlman EJ. (1998) Neuroblastoma and peripheral neuroectodermal tumors. *Am J Clin Pathol* 109:S23–30.

Beckwith JB. (1989) One the preceding paper: cardiovascular malformations and the neural crest. *Pediatr Radiol* 19:122–123.

Beckwith JB. (1993) Precursor lesions of Wilms tumor: clinical and biological implications. *Med Pediatr Oncol* 21:158–168.

Beckwith JB, Kiviat NB, Bonadio JF. (1990) Nephrogenic rests, nephroblastomatosis, and the pathogenesis of Wilms tumor. *Pediatr Pathol* 10:1–36.

Beckwith JB, Martin RF. (1968) Observations on the histopathology of neuroblastoma. *J Pediatr Surg* 3:106–110.

Beckwith JB, Perrin EV. (1963) *In situ* neuroblastoma. A contribution to the natural history of neural crest tumors. *Am J Pathol* 43:1089–1104.

Bessho F. (1998) Colloquy on neuroblastoma screening: is there a future for neuroblastoma mass screening? *Med Pediatr Oncol* 31:106–110.

Bolande RP. (1997) Neurocristopathy: its growth and development in 20 years. *Pediatr Pathol and Lab Med* 17:1–25.

Bordow SB, Norris MDS, Haber PS, et al. (1998) Prognostic significance of N-*Myc* oncogene expression in childhood neuroblastomas. *J Clin Oncol* 16:3286–3294.

Brodeur GM, Castleberry RP. (1997) Neuroblastoma. In: *Principles and Practice of Pediatric Oncology, 3rd ed.*

(Pizzo PA, Poplack, DG, eds.) pp. 761–797. Lippincott-Raven, Philadelphia.

Brodeur GM, Seeger RC, Schwab M, Varmus HE, Bishop JM. (1984) Amplification of N-*myc* in untreated human neuroblastomas correlates with advanced disease stage. *Science* 224:1121–1124.

Brodeur GM, Ambros PF, Favrot MC. (1998) Biological aspects of neuroblastoma screening. *Med Pediatr Oncol* 31:394–400.

Chatten J, Voorhess ML. (1969) Familial neuroblastoma. Report of a kindred with multiple disorders including neuroblastoma in four siblings. *N Engl J Med* 277:1230–1236.

Clausen N, Andersson P, Tommerup N. (1989) Familial occurrence of neuroblastoma, Von Recklinghausen's neurofibromatosis, Hirschsprung's agangliosis, and jaw-winking syndrome. *Acta Paediatr Scand* 78:736–741.

Cushing H, Wolbach SB. (1927) The transformation of a malignant paravertebral sympathicoblastoma into a benign ganglioneuroma. *Am J Pathol* 3:203–216.

Dehner LP. (1985) Will the real neuroblastoma please stand up? *Arch Pathol Lab Med* 109:794.

Dehner LP. (1986) Peripheral and central peripheral neuroectodermal tumors. A nosologic concept seeking consensus. *Arch Pathol Lab Med* 110:997–1005.

Dehner LP. (1998) The evolution of the diagnosis and understanding of primitive and embryonic neoplasms in children: living through an epoch. *Mod Pathol* 11:669–685.

Evans AE, Baum E, Chard R. (1981) Do infants with stage IV-S neuroblastoma need treatment? *Arch Dis Child* 56:271–274.

Guin GH, Gilbert EF, Jones B. (1969) Incidental neuroblastoma in infants. *Am J Clin Pathol* 51:126–136.

Gurney JG, Severson RK, Davis S, Robison LL. (1995) Incidence of cancer in children in the United States. Sex-, race-, and 1-year age-specific rates by histologic type. *Cancer* 75:2186–2195.

Hasegawa R, Tatematsu M, Imaida K, et al. (1982) Neuroblastoma *in situ*. *Acta Pathol Jpn* 32:537–546.

Hoehner JC, Gestblom C, Hedborg F, et al. (1996) A developmental model of neuroblastoma: differentiating stroma-poor tumors progress along an extraadrenal chromaffin lineage. *Lab Invest* 75:659–675.

Ikeda Y, Lister J, Bouton JM, Buyukpamucku M. (1981) Congenital neuroblastoma, neuroblastoma *in situ* and the normal fetal development of the adrenal. *J Pediatr Surg* 16:636–644.

Jost CA, Marin MC, Kaelin WG Jr. (1997) p73 is a human p53-related protein that can induce apoptosis. *Nature* 389:191–194.

Kaghad M, Bonnet H, Yang A, et al. (1997) Monoallelically expressed gene related to p53 at 1p36, a region frequently deleted in neuroblastoma and other human cancers. *Cell* 90:809–819.

Katzenstein HM, Bowman LC, Brodeur GM, Thorner PS, et al. (1998) Prognostic significance of age, MYCN oncogene amplification, tumor cell ploidy, and histology in 100 infants with stage D(S) neuroblastoma: the pediatric oncology group experience. *J Clin Oncol* 16:2007–2017.

Kelly DR, Joshi VV. (1996) Neuroblastoma and related tumors. In: *Pediatric Neoplasia, Morphology and Biology* (Parham DM, ed.) pp. 105–152. Lippincott-Raven, Philadelphia.

Kerbl R, Urban CE, Ambros IM, Ambros PF. (1998) Neuroblastoma screening for children: delay, repeat, or delete? *Med Pediatr Oncol* 31:111–112.

Knudson AG. (1971) Mutation and cancer: statistical study of retinoblastoma. *Proc Natl Acad Sci* 68:820–823.

Knudson AG, Meadows AT. (1980) Regression of neuroblastoma IV-S: a genetic hypothesis. *N Engl J Med* 302:1254–1256.

Kushner BH, Gilbert F, Helson L. (1986) Familial neuroblastoma: case report, literature review, and etiologic considerations. *Cancer* 57:1887–1893.

Le Douarin N. (1980) Migration and differentiation of neural crest cells. *Curr Top Devel Biol* 16 (2):31–85.

Michna BA, McWilliams NB, Krummel TM, et al. (1988) Multifocal ganglioneuroblastoma coexistent with total aganglionosis. *J Pediatr Surg* 23:57–59.

Nakagawara A. (1998) The NGF story and neuroblastoma. *Med Pediatr Oncol* 31:113–115.

Nakagawara A, Arima-Nakagawara M, Scavarda NJ, et al. (1993) Association between high levels of expression of the TRK gene and favorable outcome in human neuroblastoma. *N Engl J Med* 328:847–854.

Pahlman S, Grotte Z. (1982) Are there two different types of neuroblastoma? *Z Kinderheilk* 35:62–63.

Park WS, Chi JG. (1993) Bilateral neuroblastoma in situ associated with microcephaly. *J Korean Med Sci* 8:99–103.

Roshkow JE, Haller JO, Berdon WE, Sane SM. (1988) Hirschsprung's disease, Ondine's curse, and neuroblastoma—manifestations of neurocristopathy. *Pediatr Radiol* 19:45–49.

Seeger RC, Brodeur GM, Sather H, et al. (1985) Association of multiple copies of the N-*myc* oncogene with rapid progression of neuroblastomas. *N Engl J Med* 313:1111–1116.

Shanklin DR, Sotelo-Avila C. (1969) *In situ* tumors in fetuses, infants, newborns, and young infants. *Biol Neonat* 14:2286–316.

Shimada H, Chatten J, Newton WA Jr, et al. (1984) Histopathologic prognostic factors in neuroblastic tumors: definition of subtypes of ganglioneuroblastoma and an age-linked classification of neuroblastomas. *J Natl Cancer Inst* 73:405–416.

Tsokos M, Scarpa S, Ross RA, Triche TJ. (1987) Differentiation of human neuroblastoma recapitulates neural crest development: study of morphology, neurotransmitter enzymes, and extracellular matrix proteins. *Am J Pathol* 128:484–496.

Turkel SB, Itabashi HH. (1974) The natural history of neuroblastic cells in the fetal adrenal gland. *Am J Pathol* 76:225–244.

Wiesel J. (1902) Beiträge zur Anatomie und Entwickelung der menschlichen Nebenniere. *Anat Hefte* 19:481–522.

26

ENDOCRINE ORGANS: PITUITARY, THYROID, PARATHYROID, ADRENAL GLAND, PARAGANGLIA, AND PANCREAS

A number of genetically determined endocrine syndromes involve multiple organs, as summarized in Table 26–1. The most common syndromes are multiple endocrine neoplasia (MEN) I (Wermer, 1954), characterized most often by parathyroid hyperplasia, pituitary adenoma, and pancreatic endocrine tumor or islet cell hyperplasia; MEN IIA (Sipple, 1961), which typically consists of medullary thyroid carcinoma, parathyroid hyperplasia, and pheochromocytoma; and MEN IIB (Gorlin et al., 1968; Williams and Pollack, 1966), whose hallmarks are medullary thyroid carcinoma, pheochromocytoma, intestinal ganglioneuromatosis (mucosal neuromas), and marfanoid body habitus. These syndromes have autosomal dominant transmission with a high degree of penetrance and variable expression. Other combinations and mixed patterns have been reported (Carney et al., 1980; Griffiths et al., 1983; Larraza-Hernandez et al., 1982; Morris and Tymms, 1980; Nathan et al., 1980; Tateishi et al., 1978). Recognition of these is important to manage optimally all the manifestations in the individual patient, who is at risk for multifocal synchronous or metachronous lesions. Even more important is to identify preinvasive or early invasive neoplasms in family members, ideally by genetic testing at a time when surgical excision is curative.

The neoplasms in these syndromes involve neuroendocrine organs. Neuroendocrine cells have diverse embryologic origins, including neural crest, endoderm, and mesoderm, but all are involved in the production and secretion of peptide hormones or amines. Neuroendocrine cells may be argyrophilic or argentaffinic (Fig. 26–1), and they contain dense core secretory granules that by electron microscopy are generally round or elongated and pleomorphic (Figs. 26–2 and 26–3). However, ultrastructural granule morphology is usually not specific for individual hormones. Chromogranin, synaptophysin, and neuron-specific enolase can be demonstrated by immunohistochemistry in most neuroendocrine cells (Fig. 26–4). With some exceptions, most of these cells produce only a single peptide hormone, which can act systemically (endocrine function) or locally on adjacent cells (paracrine function). Although the biologic effects of most peptide hormones are known, some, such as pancreatic polypeptide and bombesin, have no clear physiologic function in humans. In some cases, peptide hormones or prohormones are deposited in the tumor stroma as amyloid. Immunohistochemical staining for specific hormones has enhanced our understanding of endocrine hyperplasia and neoplasia, but synthesis of hormones without intracellular storage, altered hormone structure, or fixation and sampling problems may contribute to negative results.

646

Table 26–1. Multiple Endocrine Neoplasia Syndromes

	MEN I (%)	MEN IIa (%)	MEN IIb (%)
Parathyroid			
Chief cell hyperplasia	85–90	10–25	Rare
Endocrine pancreas			
Hyperplasia/neoplasm	75–80		
Pituitary			
Adenoma	60		
Adrenal			
Cortical hyperplasia/nodule	40		
Pheochromocytoma/medullary hyperplasia		50	50
Thyroid			
Medullary carcinoma/C-cell hyperplasia		100	100
Carcinoid			
(Gastrointestinal tract, lung, thymus)	5		
Ganglioneuromatosis			
(Mucosal neuromas)			100
Marfanoid habitus			100

Through genetic analysis the abnormalities responsible for some hereditary endocrine syndromes have been detected. For example, the genetic defect responsible for the MEN I syndrome has been mapped to the long arm of chromosome 11 at the 11q 13 locus (Chandrasekharappa et al; 1997; Skogsied et al., 1992). Familial medullary thyroid carcinoma, MEN IIa, and MENIIb syndromes have been linked to mutations of the tyrosine kinase receptor RET protooncogene, which is located at the chromosome 10q 11.2 region (Hofstra et al., 1994).

PITUITARY GLAND

The master gland of the endocrine system is largely under control of the hypothalamus and homeostatic feedback inhibition loops. Adenoma is the most common pituitary tumor. Any cell type may proliferate, and any normal hormone may be produced in excess, most frequently prolactin, growth hormone, or adrenocorticotropic hormone (ACTH). Hypopituitarism or local mass ef-

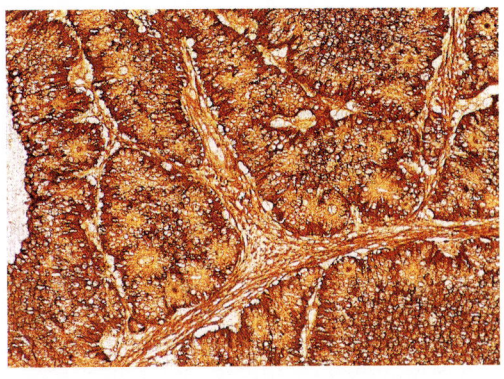

Figure 26–1. Carcinoid tumor showing intense and diffuse argyrophilia with the Grimelius stain.

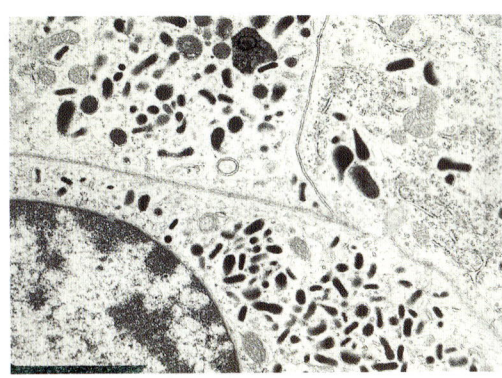

Figure 26–2. Pheochromocytoma of adrenal gland. The cells show numerous pleomorphic, cytoplasmic, membrane-bound neurosecretory granules with dense cores and halos.

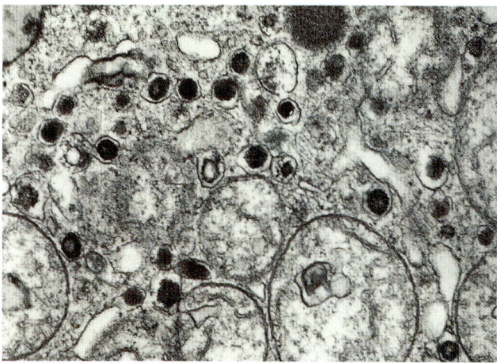

Figure 26–3. Chief cell of a carotid body paraganglioma containing relatively uniform, round, electron-dense, cytoplasmic granules.

fects may be presenting manifestations of clinically nonfunctional adenomas. About 60% of patients with MEN I have pituitary adenomas, most often prolactinomas, but most of these are clinically silent (Levine et al., 1979; Scheithauer et al., 1987).

Hyperplasia

Hyperplasia of anterior pituitary cell lines is difficult to diagnose owing to regional variation in the density of normal cell types, poorly defined histologic criteria for hyperplasia, fragmentation of surgical specimens, and the necessity of immunohistochemistry for its recognition (Horvath and Kovacs, 1988; Saeger and Ludecki, 1983). Hyperplasia may be unifocal or multifocal, nodular or diffuse. It may involve any cell type and give rise to

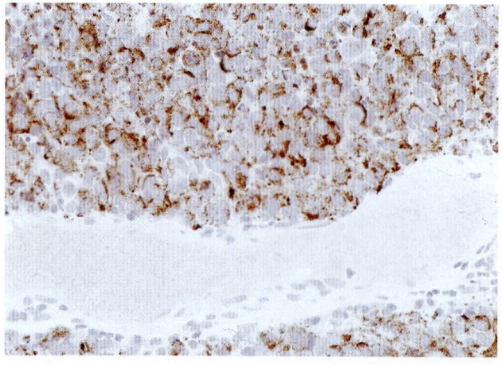

Figure 26–4. Large cell neuroendocrine carcinoma of the uterine cervix showing intense immunoreactivity for chromogranin.

clinical syndromes similar to those produced by adenomas (Khalil et al., 1984; Kubota et al., 1992; Moran et al., 1990). Hyperplasia is characterized by preservation of the normal adenohypophyseal reticulin network, as opposed to adenomas, in which scant reticulin is confined to perivascular zones (Kovacs and Horvath, 1986). Hyperplasia may coexist with an adenoma, though this is considered uncommon (Horvath and Kovacs, 1991; Lloyd et al., 1986). Prolactin cell hyperplasia is physiologic during the second half of pregnancy and lactation, and hyperplasia of thyrotrope cells containing cytoplasmic periodic acid-Schiff (PAS)–positive globules is typical in hypothyroid patients (Scheithauer et al., 1985). Gonadotroph hyperplasia that can progress to adenoma has been reported in association with long-standing primary hypogonadism (Nicolis et al., 1988). Occasionally, idiopathic hypothalamic overstimulation or ectopic production of releasing hormones causes hyperplasia of an anterior pituitary cell line, which clinically mimics an adenoma, as reported in cases of Cushing's syndrome or acromegaly (Lamberts et al., 1980; McKeever et al., 1982; Thorner et al., 1984). Bronchial and pancreatic carcinoids that produce growth hormone–releasing hormone have caused somatotroph hyperplasia and acromegaly (Berger et al., 1984; Ezzat et al., 1994).

Adenoma

Pituitary adenomas are found in 3% to 20% of autopsies, depending on the criteria and method of detection (McComb et al., 1983). Through computed tomography or magnetic resonance imaging approximately 20% of normal pituitary glands are noted to harbor a microadenoma (Elster, 1993). The high rate of incidental microadenomas in the general population and the low incidence of symptomatic pituitary adenomas (2 per 100,000 population) (Gold, 1981) suggest that most microadenomas remain stable and do not progress to clinically manifest tumors. Microadenomas are tumors less than 10 mm in diameter; their detection may allow more successful surgical treatment, with preservation of normal pituitary tissues. However, most microadenomas are asymptomatic and represent incidental autopsy findings (Fig. 26–5A, B). Symptomatic pituitary adenomas represent 20% to 25% of all intracranial neoplasms

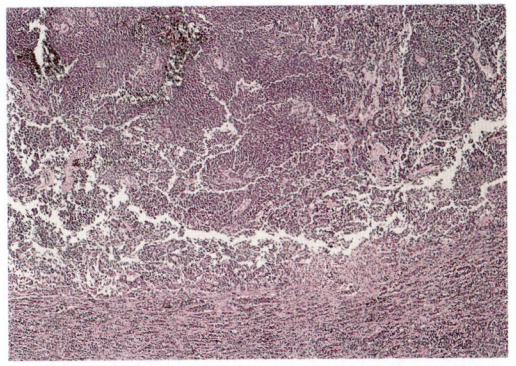

A

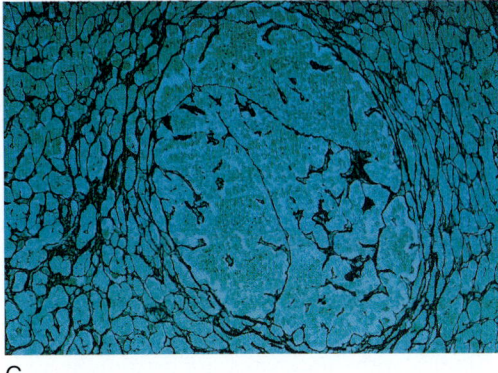

C

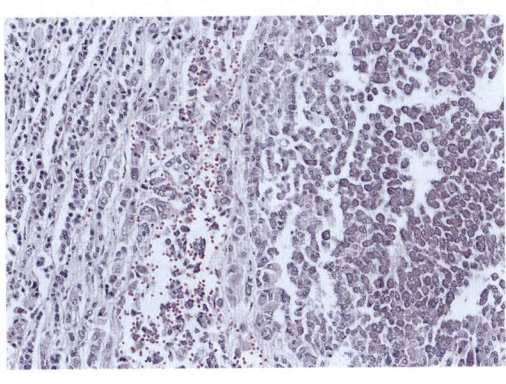

B

Figure 26–5. *A*: Low-power view of pituitary microadenoma. *B*: The tumor is compressing the normal pituitary tissue. *C*: Reticulin fibers are noted around blood vessels but not among tumor cells.

(Scheithauer, 1984) and in children they seem to follow a less aggressive clinical course than in adults (Kane et al., 1994). Although typically circumscribed, only large adenomas have a pseudocapsule. Reticulin is virtually absent within adenomas, except adjacent to blood vessels (Fig. 26–5C).

Ideally, classification of adenomas should be based on routine histologic sections, special stains, hormonal identification by immunohistochemistry, and ultrastructural features. By light microscopy, relatively uniform polygonal acidophilic, chromophobic, or basophilic cells are arranged in trabecular, sinusoidal, papillary, or diffuse patterns. By electron microscopy, secretory granules vary greatly in size, shape, number, and location. Granule density is a useful feature for the classification of adenomas (Horvath and Kovacs, 1991). Stromal amyloid, calcification, and extrusion of secretory granules on lateral cell membranes ("misplaced exocytosis") are features of prolactinomas, the most common type of pituitary adenomas. Somatotroph adenomas may be acidophilic, densely granulated, and slow growing, or

they may be chromophobic, sparsely granulated, invasive, and aggressive. There is a roughly equal incidence of each type. Basophilia with PAS positivity, peripheral cytoplasmic localization of secretory granules, and perinuclear type I microfilaments are typical of corticotrope cell adenomas. Gonadotroph and thyrotroph cell adenomas are less common. About 56% of pituitary adenomas are in the above categories. Occasional tumors (about 6%) contain well-differentiated cells resembling corticotroph or prolactin cells but are clinically silent. About 25% of pituitary adenomas are poorly differentiated by electron microscopy. Two-thirds of these are null cell adenomas, and the remainder are oncocytomas, both showing decreased rough endoplasmic reticulum and Golgi complexes, with greater than 15% volume density of mitochondria in the latter. Approximately 13% of pituitary adenomas are plurihormonal, showing immunohistochemical and/or clinical evidence of production of multiple hormones normally produced by one or more cell lines. Usually a single hormonal syndrome is dominant.

Some pituitary adenomas show infiltrative destructive growth and invade the dura, brain, bone, and cavernous sinus. Others invade the sphenoid bone and present as nasopharyngeal masses. The vast majority of invasive adenomas are large and difficult to resect. A recent study concludes that the Ki-67 labeling index is a useful marker in determining the invasive behavior of pituitary adenomas (Mastronardi et al., 1999). By immunohistochemistry most invasive adenomas are thyrotroph and corticotroph cell adenomas. Pituitary carcinomas with metastases are extremely rare (Kovacs and Horvath, 1986); only 36 cases had been reported through 1989, 44% of which were associated with hypersecretion of either growth hormone or corticotropin (Mountcastle et al., 1989). Since then, 28 additional cases have been published (Pernicone et al., 1997). Of these, 64 cases, 74% were hormone-producing. MIB-1 and PCNA labeling indices are higher in carcinomas than in adenomas. Likewise, p53 expression is seen in nearly all carcinomas, but not in adenomas (Thapar et al., 1996). This p53 immunoreactivity, however, does not correlate with genetic mutation. It is not known whether adenomas progress to carcinomas or if these neoplasms are malignant from their inception.

There are a few studies dealing with the molecular abnormalities involved in the pathogenesis of pituitary neoplasms. *Ras* mutations are uncommon in adenomas (Cai et al., 1994) but relatively frequent in carcinomas (Cai et al., 1994; Pei et al., 1994), suggesting that these mutations are important in malignant transformation. Mutations of the *p53* gene have not been detected in pituitary neoplasms.

THYROID—FOLLICULAR CELLS

Hyperplasia and Papillary Carcinoma

Hyperplasia of the thyroid may be diffuse (Graves disease) or nodular. Histologically, Graves disease consists of follicles with scant colloid and prominent papillary infolding of columnar cells with pale cytoplasm. The stimulus for hyperplasia and hyperthyroidism is provided by immunoglobulin G (IgG) autoantibodies, which bind to thyroid-stimulating hormone (TSH) receptors on follicular cells. Although small, incidental papillary carcinomas are present in 1% to 9% of thyroidectomy specimens for Graves disease (Farbota et al., 1985), no causal relationship is suspected. Radiation to the thyroid gland for Graves disease may produce hyperplasia, nuclear atypia, and a slight increase in the incidence of papillary carcinoma (Ozaki et al., 1994; Schneider et al., 1980). Nodular hyperplastic colloid goiters show marked histologic variability, frequently with degenerative changes and papillae. Papillary structures in these goiters lack the nuclear features of papillary carcinoma (Fig. 26–6). The cellular hyperplastic nodules of sporadic or endemic goiters may develop a capsule and be indistinguishable from adenomas. Moreover, trabecular and insular growth patterns are occasionally seen, complicating even more the histologic interpretation. Several studies have shown that most of these hyperplastic thyroid nodules are monoclonal (Apel et al., 1994; Chung, et al., 1999; Kopp et al., 1994). Thyroid-stimulating hormone is the stimulus for hyperplasia in goiters, whether due to dietary iodine insufficiency (endemic or sporadic), administration of antithyroid drugs such as propylthiouracil, or genetic defects in thyroid hormone synthesis (dyshormonogenetic). Colloid or adenomatous thyroid nodules (parasitic nodules) may become detached from the thyroid gland and grow in skeletal muscle and adipose tissue near the thyroid. They should not be confused with carcinoma.

Populations with endemic goiters have a higher incidence of follicular and anaplastic carcinomas, whereas the proportion of papillary carcinomas increases as supplemental dietary iodine is introduced (Harach et al., 1985; Hofstadter, 1980).

Dyshormonogenetic Goiter and Carcinoma

Dyshormonogenetic goiters are genetically determined thyroid disorders due to an inherited error in the metabolism of thyroid hormones (Barsano and De Groot, 1979; Matos et al., 1994). The patients are usually children, adolescents or young adults with hypothyroidism. The thyroid glands are enlarged and multinodular, weighing up to 500 g. Microscopically, there is marked dif-

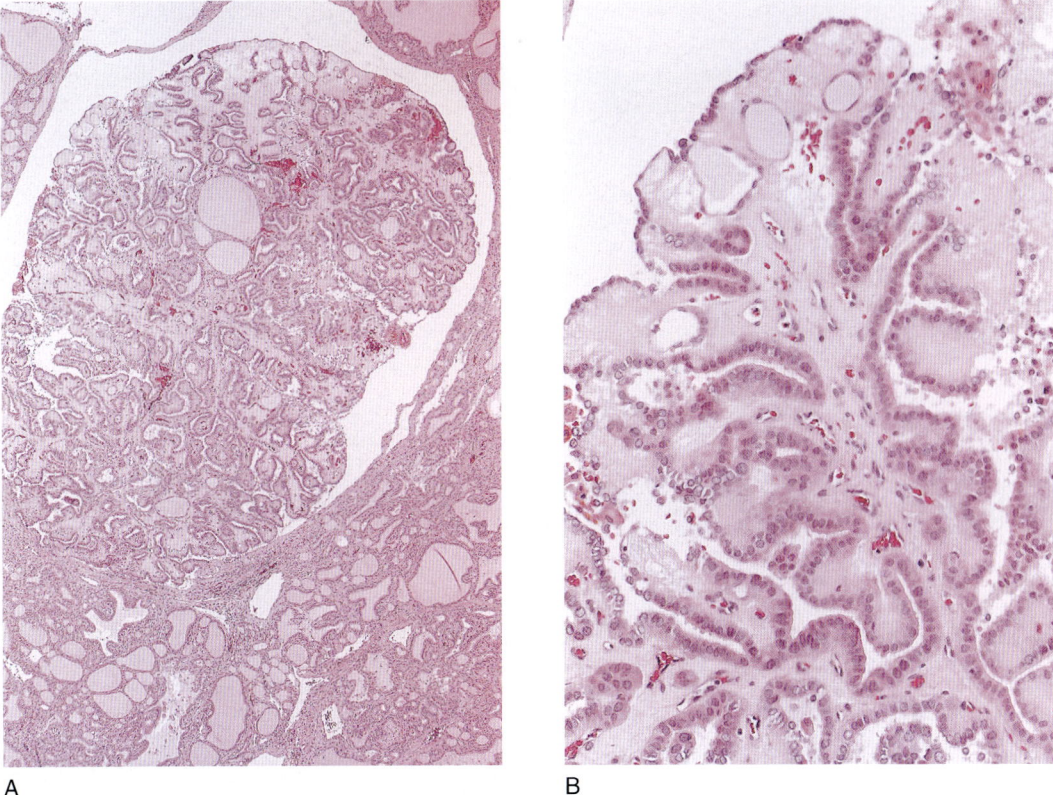

A   B

Figure 26–6. *A*: Complex papillary structure projecting into a large distended follicle in a multinodular colloid goiter. *B*: Higher magnification of the papillary structure showing hyperchromatic nuclei.

fuse hyperplasia of follicular thyroglobulin-positive cells that grow in nodules, trabeculae or nesting (insular) patterns (Fig. 26–7A). The follicles contain little or no colloid, and the hyperplastic process involves the entire gland. The follicular cells are enlarged and contain large, round, clear nuclei similar to those of papillary carcinoma. In contrast to papillary carcinoma nuclei, however, dyshormonogenetic goiter cell nuclei show few or no grooves or pseudoinclusions (Fig. 26–7B). In other cases, the cells contain round hyperchromatic nuclei and are arranged in trabeculae and nests mimicking follicular carcinoma (Fig. 26–7C). Marked cytologic atypia is commonly seen. Because of these cytologic and architectural features, dyshormonogenetic goiters are often confused with papillary and follicular carcinomas. However, the incidence of cancer in dyshormonogenetic goiters is low (5%) (Ghossein et al., 1998), and most tumors are papillary carcinomas.

Hashimoto's Thyroiditis, Papillary, Squamous, and Mucoepidermoid Carcinoma

Hashimoto's thyroiditis has been linked to an increased incidence of papillary carcinoma in several studies. Whether there is only a statistical association or a causal relationship remains controversial (Ott et al., 1985; Vickery et al., 1985). In some cases of Hashimoto's thyroiditis, the follicular cells have clear nuclei. This nuclear change is usually focal but may be diffuse and can lead to an erroneous interpretation of papillary carcinoma in both histologic sections and cytologic preparations (Fig. 26–8). Activation of the RET/PTC1 and 3 oncogenes thought to be specific of papillary thyroid carcinoma is found in 95% of cases of Hashimoto's thyroiditis (Wirtschafter et al., 1997). These findings suggest that the abnormalities in these oncogenes lack specificity for papillary thyroid carcinoma. Well-

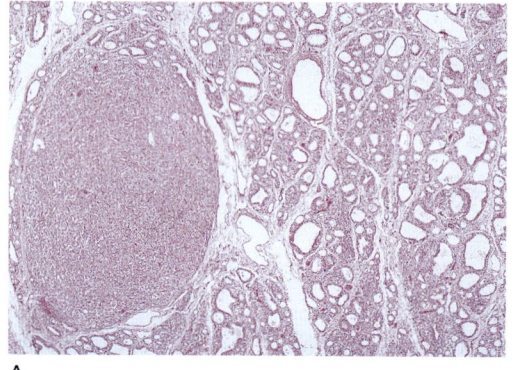

A

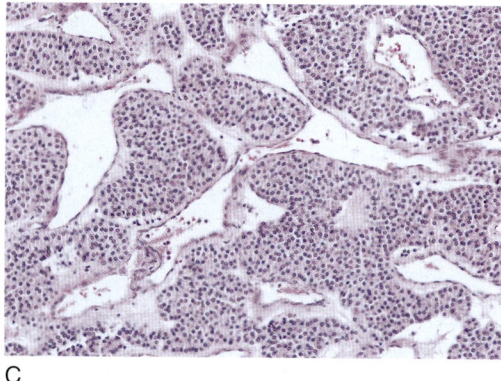

C

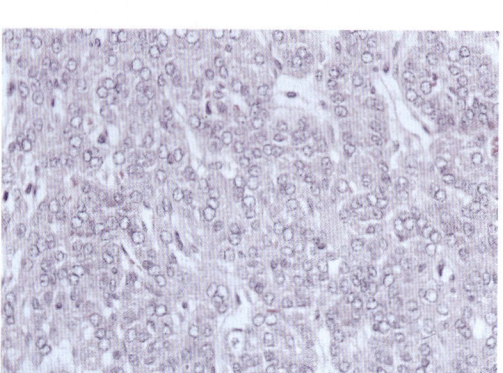

B

Figure 26–7. *A*: Dyshormonogenetic goiter. A well-defined nodule and empty follicles are seen. *B*: The nuclei of the follicular cells are large and clear, mimicking papillary carcinoma. *C*: Insular pattern in dyshormonogenetic goiter resembling follicular carcinoma. (Tissue courtesy of Dr. C. Heffes).

demarcated and even encapsulated hyperplastic Hürthle cell nodules, which may show considerable cytologic atypia, should not be confused with Hürthle cell carcinomas (Mizukami et al., 1992). Likewise, small nodules detached from the thyroid gland often

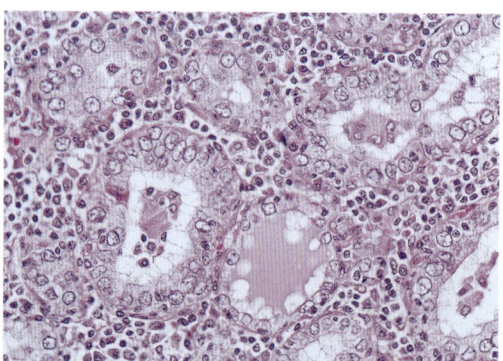

Figure 26–8. Hashimoto's thyroiditis. Follicular cells with large clear nuclei mimicking those of papillary carcinoma. In contrast to papillary carcinoma nuclei, however, the clear nuclei of Hashimoto's thyroiditis lack grooves and pseudoinclusions.

contain abundant lymphoid tissue with follicles and germinal centers resembling a lymph node. The small thyroid follicles embedded in the lymphoid tissue of these nodules should not be confused with metastatic follicular carcinoma. Some papillary carcinomas that arise in a background of Hashimoto's thyroiditis consist predominantly of cells with oxyphilic (oncocytic) cytoplasm and contain a prominent lymphoplasmacytic infiltrate in the stroma (Fig. 26–9; Apel et al., 1995). Low-grade sclerosing mucoepidermoid carcinoma nearly always is associated with the sclerosing variant of Hashimoto's thyroiditis (Fig. 26–10). In fact, this tumor may arise from foci of squamous metaplasia often seen in this autoimmune inflammatory thyroid condition (Chan et al., 1991; Sim et al., 1997; Wenig et al., 1995) (Fig. 26–11). An alternative histogenetic explanation is that the mucoepidermoid differentiation may represent a recapitulation of the solid cell nests of ultimobranchial body remnants. Some of these tumors lack the mucinous component and should be regarded as low-grade sclerosing squamoid tu-

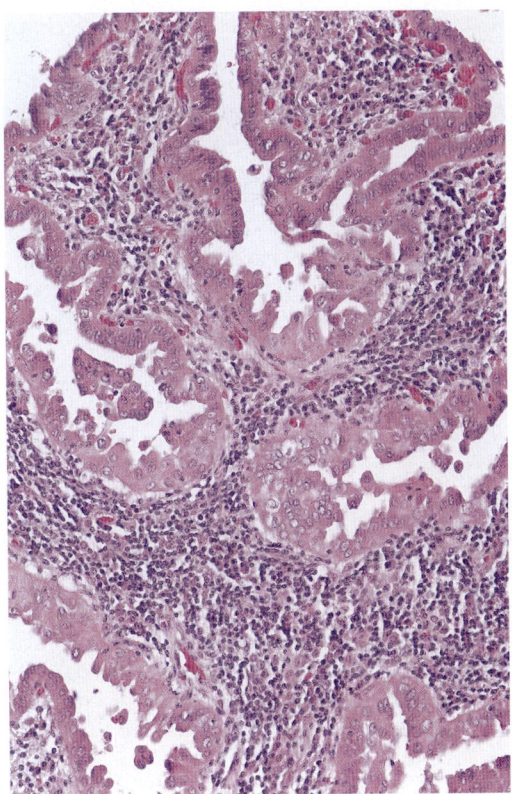

Figure 26–9. Papillary carcinoma that arose in a background of Hashimoto's thyroiditis. The cytoplasm of the tumor cells is eosinophilic, and the stroma contains lymphocytes and plasma cells.

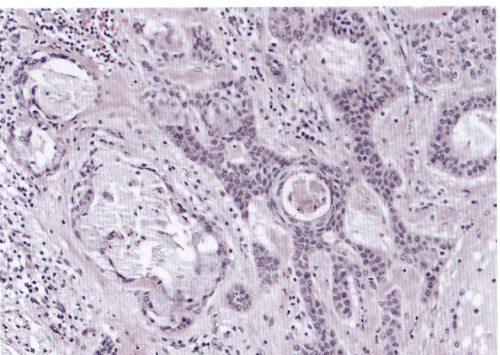

Figure 26–10. Low-grade mucoepidermoid carcinoma. Both the squamous and mucinous components are depicted. This neoplasm, which often has a sclerotic stroma containing numerous eosinophils, usually arises in a background of Hashimoto's thyroiditis.

mors with numerous eosinophils (Rosai et al., 1987) or as low-grade squamous carcinomas; others coexist with papillary carcinomas. High-grade squamous carcinomas occurring in association with Hashimoto's thyroiditis have been documented (Harada et al., 1994). Rarely, Hürthle cell and medullary carcinomas arise from Hashimoto's thyroiditis. Tumors showing dual follicular and C-cell differentiation may also be derived from ultimobranchial tissue (Albores-Saavedra et al., 1990; Williams, 1989).

In contrast to Hashimoto's thyroiditis, invasive fibrous thyroiditis (Reidel's disease) is not associated with malignant epithelial or lymphoid neoplasms. It is mentioned here because clinically it is often confused with malignant tumors. Invasive fibrous thyroiditis appears as a localized, fixed, hard mass that shows extracapsular extension. Microscopically, the thyroid follicles are not lined by oxyphil (Hürthle) cells. The inflammatory cells consists of lymphocytes, plasma cells, and eosinophils that extend beyond the capsule and infiltrate soft tissues. Lymphoid follicles with germinal centers are not numerous whereas dense keloid-like fibrous bands are abundant. The fibrotic process may be localized or be part of a systemic disease such as retroperitoneal fibrosis. Autoimmune mechanisms have been postulated in the pathogenesis of invasive fibrous thyroiditis (Heufelder and Hay, 1994; Zimmermann et al., 1994).

RADIATION-INDUCED THYROID CARCINOMA

Radiation exposure has long been known to induce thyroid carcinoma in humans

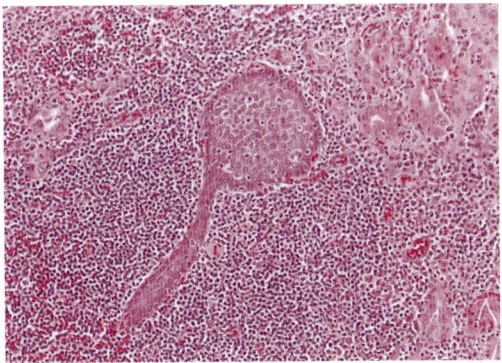

Figure 26–11. Focus of squamous metaplasia in a case of Hashimoto's thyroiditis from which squamous and mucoepidermoid tumors may arise.

(Schneider et al., 1980; Winship and Rosvoll, 1970). The vast majority of radiation-induced malignant thyroid tumors are papillary carcinomas and occur in children and adolescents. The latent period is between 4 and 20 years and is probably dose related (Baverstock et al., 1992; Kazakov et al., 1992; Nikiforov and Gnepp, 1994; Winship and Rosvall, 1970). Radiation-induced follicular and medullary carcinomas are quite rare (Nikiforov and Gnepp, 1994). As a result of the recent accident at the Chernobyl nuclear power station, large segments of the populations of the Republic of Belarus were exposed to radiation (Baverstock, et al., 1992; Kazakov et al., 1992).

Radioiodines, mainly I-131, were abundant in the fallout and were specifically responsible for the radiation dose to the thyroid gland. The histologic changes of radiation-induced thyroid lesions in children and adolescents from Belarus varied (Nikiforov et al., 1995). The most common lesion was the adenomatoid nodule or multinodular goiter often with papillary structures lined by cuboidal or columnar cells with hyperchromatic nuclei. Less frequently there was diffuse hyperplasia with nodularity and marked cytologic atypia. Follicular adenomas were also induced. These adenomas were usually hypercellular, and some exhibited cytologic atypia. It is possible that these adenomas are precursors of follicular carcinoma.

Papillary Carcinoma

Papillary carcinoma is the most common malignant tumor of the thyroid. Geographic variations in the prevalence of papillary carcinoma have been reported. Familial forms rarely occur. Twelve morphologic variants have been described. The mortality rate for this tumor is less than 1%. Adverse prognostic factors in all variants of papillary carcinoma include large size, advanced age, extrathyroidal extension, distant metastases, and certain histologic types (Coburn and Wanebo, 1995; Hay et al., 1993). The vast majority of papillary carcinomas are thyroglobulin positive by immunohistochemistry. The RET proto-oncogene is activated by gene rearrangements in papillary thyroid carcinoma (Lloyd, 1995). By in situ hybridization techniques, an incidence of 43% activated RET mRNA in 40 patients with pap-

illary thyroid carcinoma was detected (Lam et al., 1998). Since none of the follicular carcinomas, follicular adenomas, nodular hyperplasias, and normal thyroids studied expressed the RET mRNA, RET staining was considered a useful marker for papillary carcinoma (Lam et al., 1998). Immunostains for thyroglobulin are useful in the diagnosis of metastatic papillary carcinoma, especially in those patients with occult tumors. Traditionally, papillary carcinomas have been termed "occult" when less than 1.5 cm in diameter, though such a mass may be palpable clinically (Woolner et al., 1960).

Papillary Microcarcinoma

The World Health Organization (WHO) defines *papillary microcarcinomas* as those papillary cancers 1 cm or less in diameter (Hedinger et al., 1988). These lesions usually do not produce a mass clinically and are often discovered incidentally by the pathologist upon sectioning the gland. In Finland, for example, microcarcinomas are found in 35% of all autopsies (Harach et al., 1985b). There is no conclusive evidence that papillary microcarcinomas progress to clinically evident papillary carcinomas, though it would seem logical, since many histologic features are similar, and the propensity for regional lymph node metastases is shared. We have seen examples of nonencapsulated sclerosing papillary microcarcinomas composed almost entirely of tall cells. The high frequency (5% to 35%) of papillary microcarcinoma in autopsy series (Fukunaga and Yatani, 1975; Harach et al., 1985a; Lang et al., 1988) and the low incidence (<0.1% lifetime risk) of clinically manifest papillary carcinoma (Waterhouse et al., 1976) suggest that most papillary thyroid carcinomas never become clinically evident.

The earliest recognizable papillary microcarcinomas consist of small clusters of follicles or a single follicle with irregular contours or papillary infolding, showing enlarged crowded irregular nuclei with ground glass chromatin, grooves, or intranuclear cytoplasmic pseudoinclusions (Sampson et al., 1971; Fig. 26–12A,B). In larger microcarcinomas, additional features are seen, such as encapsulation, stromal fibrosis, psammoma bodies, and lymphatic invasion (Fig. 26–12C,D). In a series of 408 consecutive autopsies from Japan

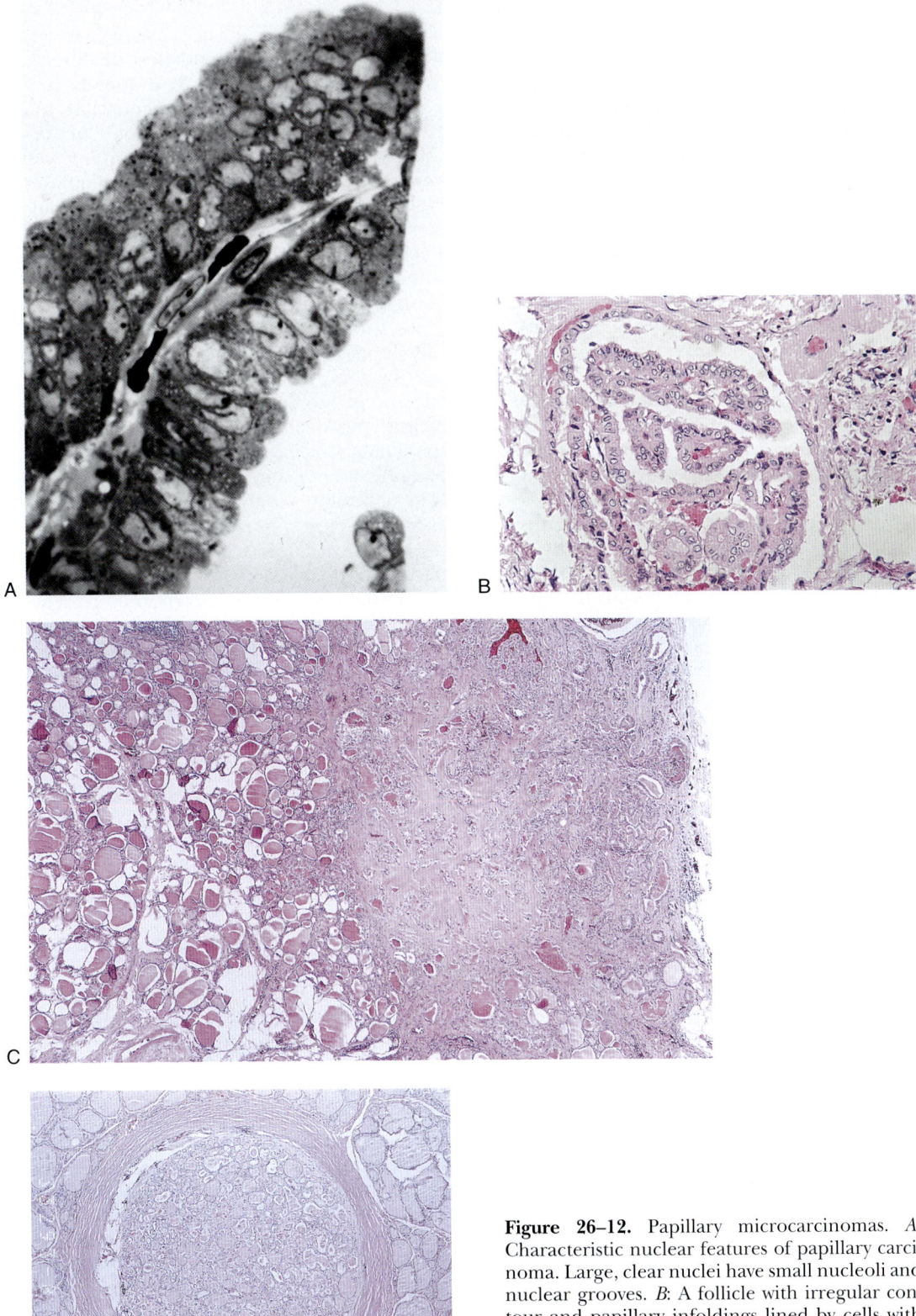

Figure 26–12. Papillary microcarcinomas. *A*: Characteristic nuclear features of papillary carcinoma. Large, clear nuclei have small nucleoli and nuclear grooves. *B*: A follicle with irregular contour and papillary infoldings lined by cells with large clear nuclei. *C*: Nonencapsulated, sclerosing papillary microcarcinoma. *D*: Encapsulated follicular variant of papillary microcarcinoma.

(Yamamoto et al., 1990), 64 papillary carcinomas under 8 mm in diameter were found in 46 patients whose ages ranged from 16 to 82 years. The tumors showed characteristics of papillary carcinomas, including large ground-glass overlapping nuclei with grooves and pseudoin-clusions. Only 1 in 23 (4.3%) tumors under 1 mm in diameter showed papillae, compared with 9 of 13 (69%) larger than 3.1 mm in diameter. The tumors were classified into three groups on the basis of the presence or absence of a capsule and stromal fibrosis. On average, the smallest lesions (26 cases) were nonsclerosing tumors that had neither a fibrous capsule nor stromal fibrosis and averaged 0.9 mm in diameter. Intermediate in size were 28 nonencapsulated sclerosing tumors averaging 2.1 mm in diameter, which always showed interstitial fibrosis without encapsulation; most lesions invaded adjacent thyroid parenchyma. The largest lesions, averaging 4.6 mm, were 10 cases of encapsulated tumors, which also had the highest average age of onset (no patient under age 50; mean, 68.6 years). These were the lesions most likely to show calcification (80%) and a papillary growth pattern (70%), with 60% showing invasion through the capsule into surrounding parenchyma (Fig. 26–12C). In this series, metastatic thyroid carcinoma was found in cervical lymph nodes in 2 of 42 autopsies in which an intensive search was made, and in both of these cases the primary thyroid tumors were of the nonencapsulated sclerosing type with psammoma bodies and intrathyroidal metastatic foci. Fibrosclerotic nodules composed of fibrous connective tissue with calcification or focal ossification were identified in the thyroids of 26 patients (1 with 2 lesions), with a mean diameter of 3.6 mm. No epithelial components were identified originally in fibrosclerotic nodules, although serial sections showed minute foci of papillary carcinoma in two lesions. Six cases had small foci of benign follicular epithelial tissue within fibrotic scars, and 19 lesions showed no epithelial component on serial sections. Yamamoto et al. (1990) postulated that most fibrosclerotic nodules represent the end result of involution of occult papillary carcinomas. They further documented no significant difference in the incidence of microcarcinomas between sexes (10.5% of males, 12.4% of females), despite the markedly higher incidence of clinical thyroid carcinomas in Japanese women, 6 to 7 times that of men (Waterhouse et al., 1976). If TSH serves as a promoter of thyroid cancer progression, the TSH levels known to occur in females would explain the higher likelihood of clinically manifest cancers in women (Williams, 1979). Elevation of TSH may also contribute to the increased incidence of microcarcinomas in goiters (Yamashita et al., 1985).

The first step in the development of clinically apparent papillary thyroid carcinoma may be the formation of microscopic nonsclerosing, nonencapsulated lesions, which typically have a follicular architecture but "papillary" nuclear features. With TSH stimulation, under appropriate conditions of host immune status, the tumors may progress, most often to nonencapsulated sclerosing carcinomas and less often to encapsulated tumors, usually acquiring papillary architecture as the lesions enlarge. The so-called papillary adenoma is now considered an encapsulated papillary carcinoma and carries an even more favorable prognosis than other papillary carcinomas (Evans, 1987; Vickery et al., 1985). Carcinomas with mixed follicular and papillary architecture and those with entirely follicular architecture but nuclear features of papillary carcinoma (follicular variant of papillary carcinoma) have the same biologic behavior as ordinary papillary carcinoma (Chen and Rosai, 1977; Lindsay, 1960; Rosai et al., 1983).

Most primary papillary thyroid carcinomas do not represent diagnostic problems for the pathologist. However, metastatic deposits of papillary carcinoma with unusual cytologic and architectural features (with clear cells, a focal cribriform pattern or foci of squamous cell carcinoma) may be difficult to recognize. In these cases, immunostains for thyroglobulin are useful in solving the diagnostic problem (Fig. 26–13).

Multifocality of papillary carcinomas has been recognized for many years, ranging from 30% to 80% in various series. Multiple tumor foci within the gland represent either multicentricity or intraglandular lymphatic metastases (Russell et al., 1963), with the extreme example being the diffuse sclerosing variant of papillary carcinoma (Vickery et al., 1985).

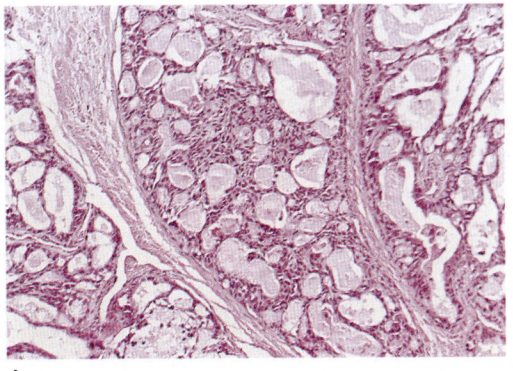

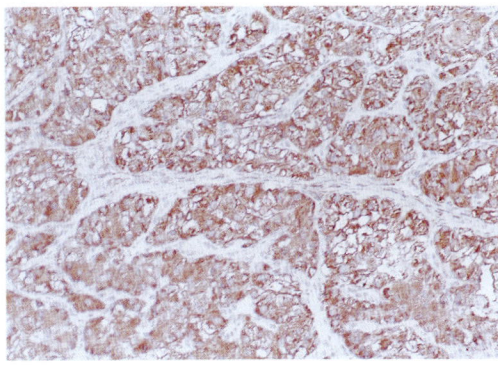

A

C

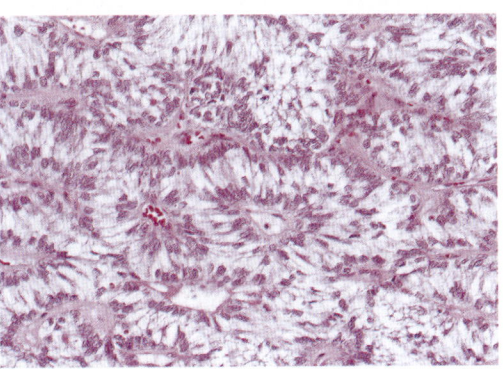

B

Figure 26–13. Metastatic papillary carcinomas showing unusual cytologic and architectural features: *A*: with focal cribriform features; *B*: containing clear cells; *C*: thyroglobulin-positive metastatic follicular variant of papillary carcinoma with clear cell features.

Macrofollicular Variant of Papillary Carcinoma

The macrofollicular variant of papillary carcinoma (Albores-Saavedra et al., 1991) probably represents the most advanced phase of differentiation of papillary carcinoma with relatively low proliferative activity (Galuzzi et al., 1994; Nakamura et al., 1998). This variant is usually encapsulated and composed of colloid-filled macrofollicles over 200 μm in diameter, which constitute more than 50% of the cross-sectional area of the tumor, resembling a colloid nodule or goiter (Fig. 26–14). Many of the large and small follicles are lined by cells with clear nuclei typical of papillary carcinoma. Other follicles are lined by cuboidal cells with hyperchromatic nuclei. Regional lymph node metastases were documented in 2 of 17 cases, and more recently, pulmonary metastases in 2 of 6 patients. The overall appearance of the metastatic deposits resembles benign thyroid tissue in lymph nodes and lung. Macrofollicular papillary carcinomas are diploid (Gamboa-Dominguez et al., 1996) and may

have a minor insular component that does not alter the excellent prognosis associated with these tumors (Albores-Saavedra et al., 1997).

Diffuse Sclerosing Variant

As its name implies, this unusual variant of papillary carcinoma may involve diffusely one or both thyroid lobes because of lymphatic permeation without forming a discrete mass (Carcangiu and Bianchi, 1989; Fujimoto et al., 1990; Vickery et al., 1985). In fact, in most cases the tumor cells that line small papillary structures are seen predominantly within dilated vascular spaces. Characteristically there is extensive squamous differentiation, and numerous psammoma bodies are present (Fig. 26–14B). These psammoma bodies may induce a foreign-body reaction. Two additional features are lymphocytic infiltration and stromal fibrosis. A dominant nodule is seen in more than 50% of cases. Rarely, the dominant nodule shows histologic features of the follicular variant of papillary carcinoma and

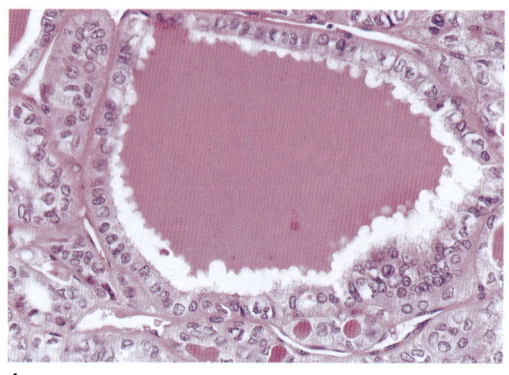

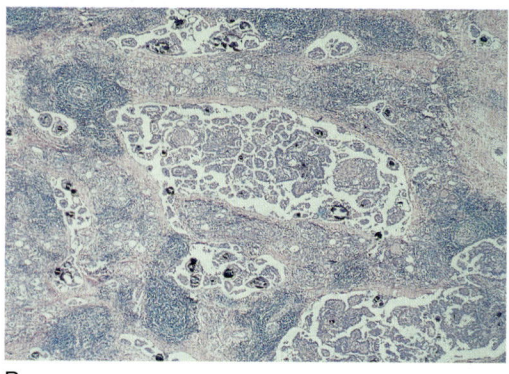

A   B

Figure 26–14. *A*: Macrofollicular variant of papillary thyroid carcinoma. A macrofollicle and a few microfollicles are lined by cells with large, clear nuclei. *B*: Diffuse sclerosing variant of papillary thyroid carcinoma. Most of the tumor is within vascular spaces. There are numerous psammoma bodies and a prominent lymphocytic infiltrate.

may contain numerous clear cells. This follicular variant of papillary carcinoma has no resemblance to the intravascular component of the tumor. We have seen cases in which the lymphocytic infiltration is minimal or absent. The tumor occurs predominantly in adult females, but we have observed three cases in children.

Ectopic Thyroid Follicles in Cervical Lymph Nodes

Most thyroid follicles seen in cervical lymph nodes lateral to the medial borders of the sternocleidomastoid muscles represent metastatic papillary carcinoma. Such foci are diagnostic if the follicles are located in lymph node sinuses, contain psammoma bodies, show papillary structure, or have the typical nuclear morphology of papillary carcinoma. Even if no clinically evident thyroid mass is present, ipsilateral thyroid lobectomy will usually reveal papillary microcarcinoma. However, most pathologists accept rare examples of "lateral aberrant thyroid," which are represented by a few ectopic thyroid follicles lined by cells with bland nuclei lacking features of papillary carcinoma, present within or immediately beneath the lymph node capsule (Meyer and Steinberg, 1969). These ectopic thyroid follicles are often incidental findings in radical lymph node dissections for squamous carcinomas of the head and neck. Ectopic thyroid tissue has also been documented in the mediastinum, stomach, duodenum, gallbladder, adrenal

gland, and liver (Albores-Saavedra et al., 1999; Shiraishi et al., 1999). In contrast to papillary carcinomas, follicular carcinomas rarely metastasize to cervical lymph nodes but preferentially metastasize to lung and bone.

Columnar Cell Variant of Papillary Carcinoma

Although the columnar cell variant of papillary carcinoma has been considered to be poorly differentiated with an aggressive clinical course (Evans, 1986), there have been recent reports indicating that clinical staging is the most important prognostic factor in these tumors (Wenig et al., 1998). In fact, the encapsulated columnar cell variant as well as the tumors that are confined to the thyroid rarely metastasize (Evans, 1996; Ferreiro et al., 1996; Wenig et al., 1998; Fig. 26–15A). The columnar variant of papillary thyroid carcinoma has a broad morphologic spectrum. It is composed predominantly of pseudostratified columnar cells, some with cytoplasmic vacuoles (Fig. 26–15B,C). Cells with large clear nuclei characteristic of conventional papillary carcinoma are focally seen in some tumors. The neoplastic cells show variable thyroglobulin reactivity. Squamoid morules are less common than in conventional papillary thyroid carcinoma. The growth patterns include papillary, solid, microfollicular, and trabecular. In some tumors the follicles are empty and elongated, resembling gland-like structures (Fig.

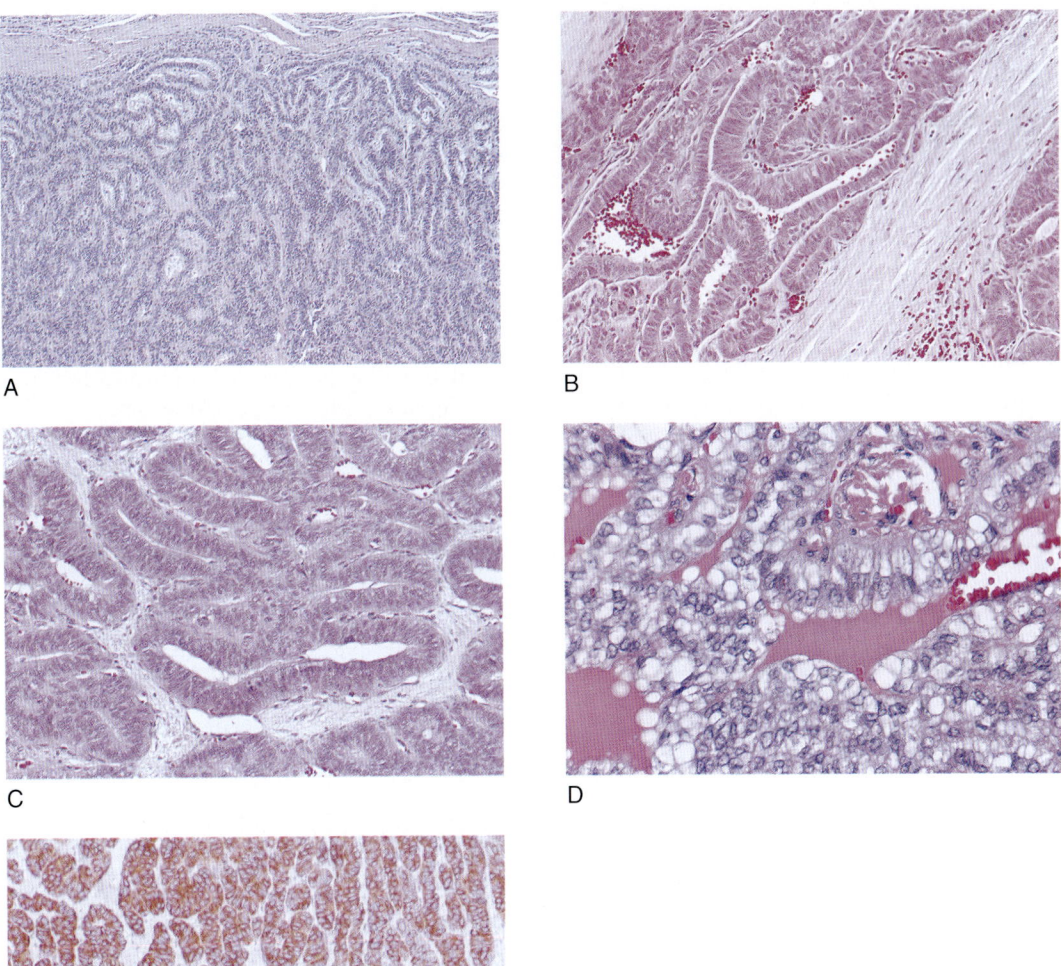

Figure 26–15. *A*: Encapsulated (incipient) columnar cell variant of papillary carcinoma. *B*: Papillary structures lined by pseudostratified columnar cells. *C*: Empty follicles resembling gland-like structures. *D*: Cytoplasmic vacuoles. *E*: Encapsulated columnar cell variant of papillary carcinoma showing diffuse positivity for thyroglobulin.

26–15D). When these structures predominate in metastatic deposits, the tumor can be confused with adenocarcinomas of the lung or gastrointestinal tract.

Tall Cell Variant of Papillary Carcinoma

When cells whose height are at least twice their width predominate (>50%) in a papillary thyroid neoplasm, the tall cell variant should be diagnosed. This variant of papil-

lary carcinoma is poorly defined because a significant proportion of tall cells are seen in different types of papillary carcinomas, and the average width of the columnar cell of conventional papillary carcinoma is variable. We believe that cell height alone is not enough to regard this papillary tumor as poorly differentiated carcinoma. Papillary and trabecular growth patterns are common in most tumors (Fig. 26–16). The cytoplasm of the neoplastic cells is abundant and

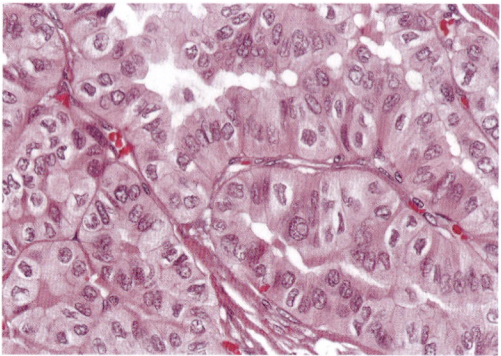

Figure 26–16. Tall cell variant of papillary carcinoma. The tall neoplastic cells have abundant eosinophilic cytoplasm.

oxyphilic, and the nuclear features are similar to those of conventional papillary carcinoma. A number of studies have shown that the prognosis of this variant of papillary carcinoma is worse than that of conventional papillary carcinoma. In some series, however, most of the tumors showed extrathyroidal extension, which is a well-known adverse prognostic factor (Johnson et al., 1988; Ostrowski and Merino, 1996). The tall cell variant of papillary carcinoma may progress to anaplastic carcinoma.

Papillary and Follicular Carcinomas with Insular Component

There has been controversy regarding the terminology, histologic features, and biologic behavior of these tumors. Some authors have expressed the opinion that tumors with an insular component are a distinctive type of poorly differentiated thyroid carcinoma with an aggressive clinical course (50% mortality rate) and have proposed the term "insular carcinoma" (Carcangiu et al., 1984; Sasaki et al., 1996). Others believe that these tumors are cytologically and architecturally heterogenous and variants of follicular and papillary carcinomas (Ashfaq et al., 1994). The insular and trabecular patterns may be focal or may predominate in the tumor. Microscopically, all the tumors that we have studied showed areas of conventional follicular and papillary carcinoma. A few contained predominantly clear cells. The trabeculae, insulae, or cell nests are composed of cells with either hyperchromatic nuclei similar to those of follicular carcinoma—large, clear nuclei

having grooves and pseudoinclusions similar to those of papillary carcinoma—or nuclei with features intermediate between follicular and papillary-type nuclei (Figs. 26–17A,B). The nuclei seen in the cell nests are similar to those seen in the differentiated follicular or papillary areas. The biologic behavior appears to correlate with stage rather than with the insular pattern. In a series of 41 cases, the 5-year survival rate was 85% (Ashfaq et al., 1994). In our experience, minimally invasive follicular carcinomas with predominant insular pattern behave as minimally invasive conventional follicular carcinomas (Fig. 26–17C). Moreover, in follicular and papillary carcinomas, a minor (focal) insular component does not alter the prognosis of these tumors (Albores-Saavedra et al., 1997). We have seen papillary carcinomas with a predominant insular component metastasize as purely papillary carcinoma. Follicular and papillary carcinomas with an insular component, on the other hand, may become anaplastic and behave aggressively. We have seen follicular carcinomas with an insular component in which the neoplastic cells had large, vesicular nuclei with prominent nucleoli and showed numerous mitotic figures and areas of necrosis. We classified these tumors as poorly differentiated follicular carcinomas.

FOLLICULAR ADENOMA AND CARCINOMA

Most pathologists currently believe follicular carcinomas arise *de novo* rather than representing progression from follicular adenomas (Franssila et al., 1985; Lang et al., 1980). However, follicular adenomas have been proven to be monoclonal and may be precursors of carcinoma (Hicks et al., 1989; Namba and Fagin, 1989). Follicular carcinomas are now divided into two major types: minimally invasive and widely invasive. The minimally invasive tumors show definite microscopic breaching of the capsule or blood vessel invasion, usually within the capsule or immediately outside the capsule, and fall into the category of incipient neoplasia of low malignant potential (Wieneke et al., 1999) (Fig. 26–18). Historically, minimally invasive follicular carcinomas were called "angioinvasive follicular adenomas" (Hazard and Kenyon, 1954), in recognition of their good prognosis. Widely invasive follicular

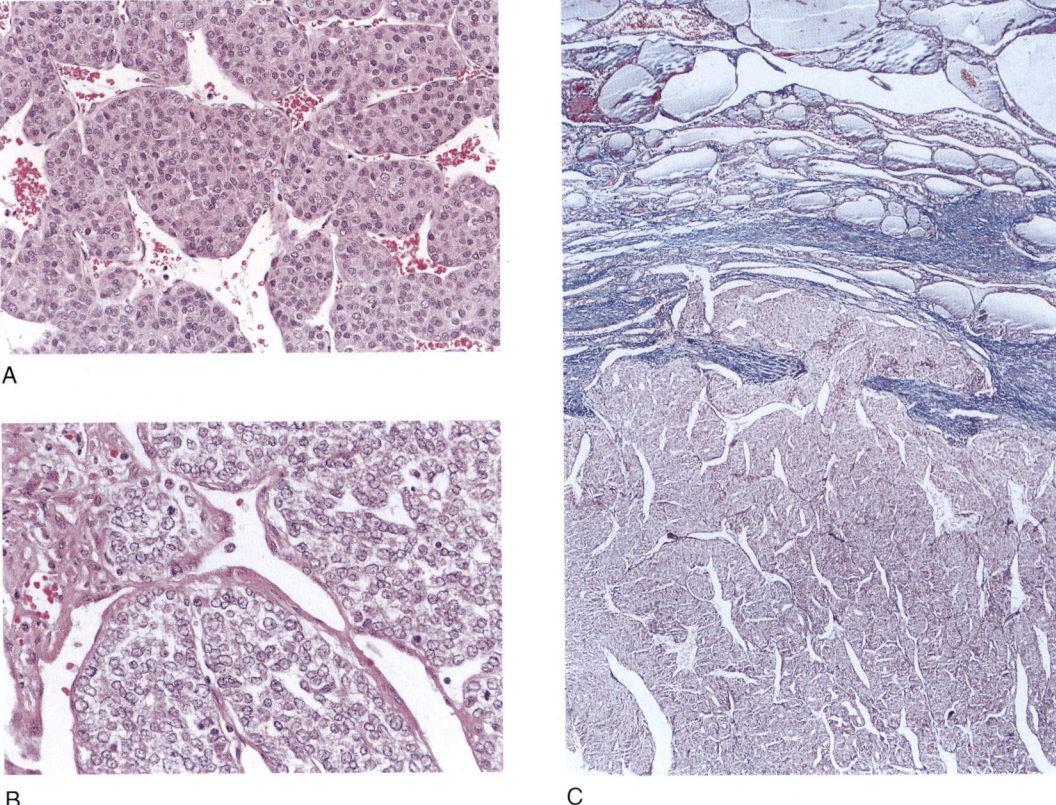

Figure 26–17. *A*: Follicular carcinoma with insular pattern. *B*: Papillary carcinoma with insular pattern. Cells with large, clear nuclei are forming nests separated by capillaries. *C*: Minimally invasive follicular carcinoma with predominant insular pattern.

carcinomas with incomplete encapsulation or abundant vascular invasion are associated with a much higher risk of metastasis—60% to 80% versus 3% to 15% for minimally invasive tumors (Evans and Vassilopoulon, 1998; Lang et al., 1986; Wieneke et al., 1999). Some follicular neoplasms show marked cytologic atypia but do not invade the capsule or vascular channels. Such tumors are usually termed "atypical adenomas" (Lang et al., 1980), but some believe they represent encapsulated follicular carcinomas (Koss et al., 1984). Indeed, some patients presenting with documented metastatic follicular carcinoma have shown primary thyroid neoplasms in which neither capsular nor vascular invasion was found. Admittedly, pathologists might relax their histologic criteria for capsular or vascular invasion when faced with a follicular neoplasm showing extreme nuclear pleomorphism,

abundant mitotic figures, or known visceral metastases. Some pathologists accept invasion into but not through the capsule as sufficient for a diagnosis of carcinoma (Kahn and Perzin, 1983; LiVolsi, 1990). The capsule of follicular carcinoma tends to be thick and irregular, in contrast to the thin, delicate capsule of an adenoma (Evans, 1984).

HÜRTHLE CELL CARCINOMA

Hürthle (oxyphil) cell neoplasms are variants of follicular neoplasms (Franssila et al., 1985; Rosai and Carcangiu, 1984) composed predominantly of oxyphil (mitochondrion-rich) cells (Fig. 26–19). In some tumors the mitochondria become distended and the cytoplasm appears clear under the light microscope (Fig. 26–20A). Glycogen and, rarely, mucin accumulation may also be responsible for the clear cell change in other

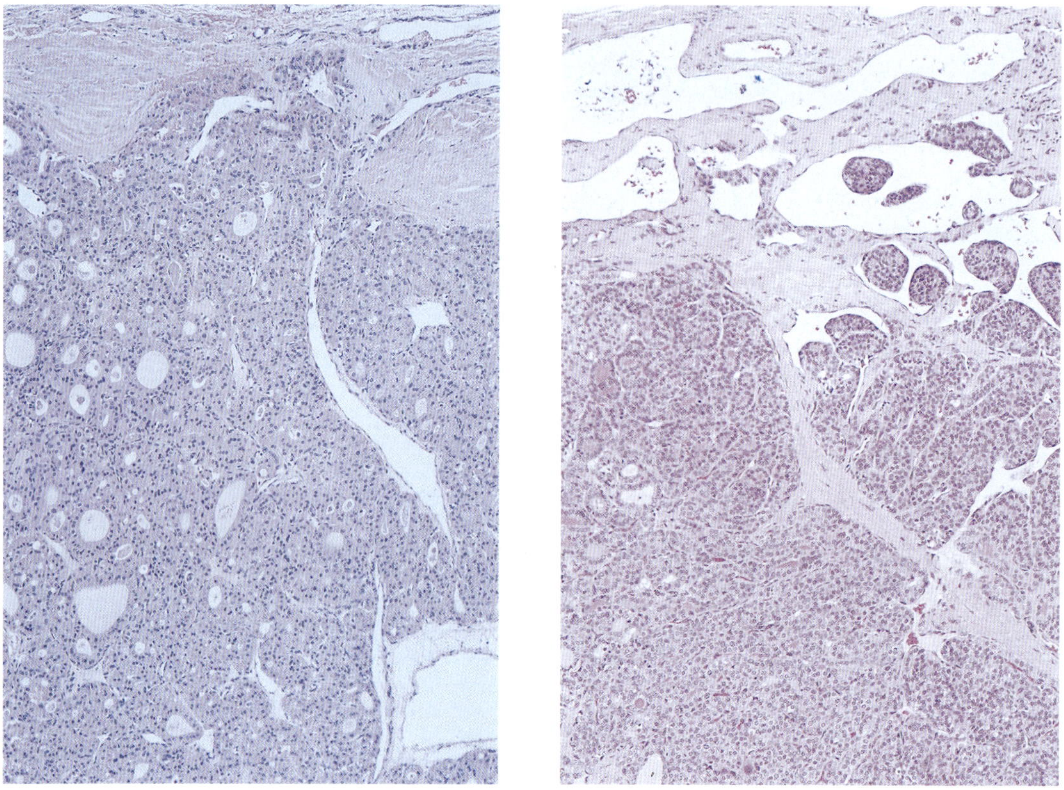

A

B

Figure 26–18. *A:* Minimally invasive follicular carcinoma. Low-power view shows capsular invasion. *B:* Small dilated blood vessels present in the capsule contain tumor thrombi.

tumors (Carcangiu et al., 1985a; Civantos et al., 1984). The neoplastic cells may form follicles or show trabecular or solid growth patterns. A focal papillary pattern is occasionally seen. Hürthle cell carcinomas composed predominantly of clear cells and with a trabecular growth pattern can be confused with metastatic renal cell carcinoma. Thyroglobulin immunostains are helpful in the differential diagnosis because they are focally positive in follicular carcinoma and negative in metastatic renal cell carcinoma (Civantos et al., 1984). Clear cells are not unique to Hürthle cell tumors; they are also seen in non-neoplastic thyroid lesions such as goiters as well as in a variety of thyroid tumors, including follicular adenomas, and papillary and medullary carcinomas. Capsular and blood vessel invasion enable separation of benign from malignant Hürthle cell neoplasms (Carcangiu et al., 1991). A number of studies have shown that Hürthle cell

carcinomas follow a more aggressive clinical course than conventional follicular carcinomas (Carcangiu et al., 1991; McDonald et al., 1996; Shaha et al., 1996). However, a recent

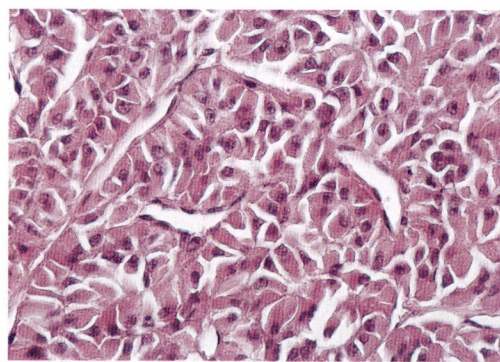

Figure 26–19. Hürthle cell carcinoma. Cells with abundant eosinophilic cytoplasm are arranged in trabecular structures.

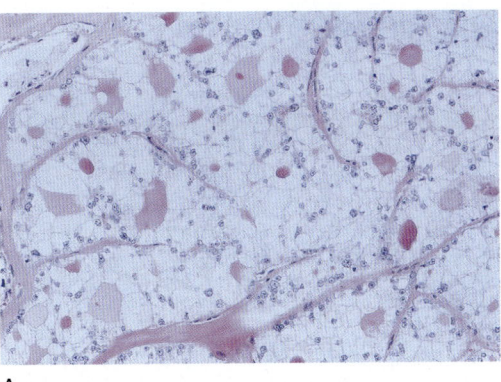
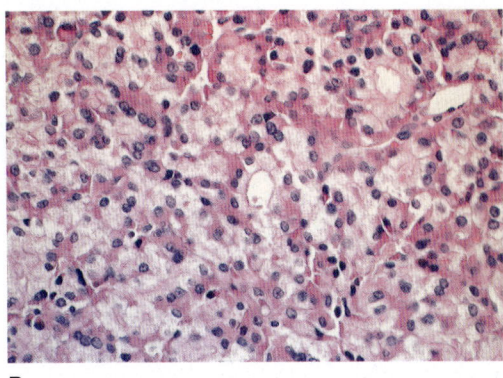

A

B

Figure 26–20. *A*: Hürthle cell carcinoma with a predominance of clear cells. Some small follicles still contain colloid. *B*: Higher magnification of tumor showing cells with cytoplasm that is both eosinophilic and clear.

well-conducted study concluded that the biologic behavior of follicular and Hürthle cell carcinomas is essentially the same when patients are stratified by extent of tumor invasion (Evans and Vassilopoulu-Sellen, 1998). In this series, Hürthle cell carcinomas that lacked extracapsular extension (incipient carcinomas) did not metastasize and caused no deaths (Evans and Vassilpoulou, 1998). In contrast, only 50% of the patients with widely invasive Hürthle cell carcinomas survived 5 years or longer.

Hyalinizing Trabecular Adenoma and Carcinoma

A distinctive type of adenoma with trabecular and nesting patterns resembling medullary carcinoma and with cytologic features similar to those of papillary carcinoma has been designated *hyalinizing trabecular adenoma* (Carney et al., 1987). The presence of extracellular hyaline basal lamina material resembling amyloid has been the source of confusion with medullary carcinoma (Fig. 26–21). Cytoplasmic yellow bodies consistent with giant lysosomes are a constant feature (Rothenberg et al., 1999). Some of these yellow bodies are often pale and poorly defined. Because tumor cells contain nuclei with grooves and pseudoinclusions, hyalinizing trabecular adenomas are often confused with papillary carcinoma by fine-needle aspiration (FNA) (Rothenberg et al., 1999; Fig. 26–22). Occasionally, papillary carcinoma can arise within or immediately adjacent to hyalinizing trabecular adenoma

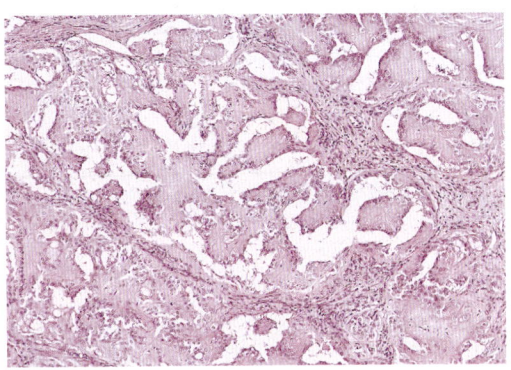

Figure 26–21. Hyalinizing trabecular adenoma with abundant basal lamina among tumor cells.

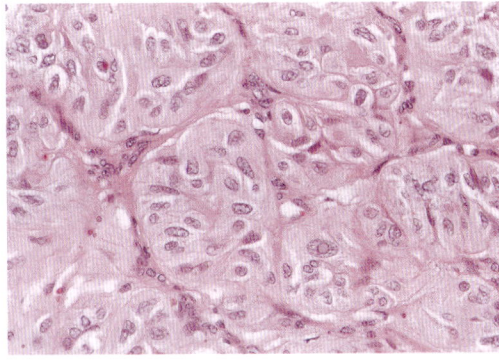

Figure 26–22. Hyalinizing trabecular adenoma. The cells have nuclear grooves and pseudoinclusions.

(Molberg and Albores-Saavedra, 1994). Because of these features, some authors have suggested that these tumors are variants of papillary carcinoma (Li et al., 1997), an opinion we do not share because the trabecular adenomas follow a benign clinical course (Rothenberg et al., 1999). Rarely, similar tumors extend into the capsule and invade blood vessels; therefore, they should be regarded as hyalinizing trabecular carcinomas (Molberg and Albores-Saavedra, 1994). So far, none of the reported minimally invasive hyalinizing trabecular carcinomas has metastasized. Thyroid adenomas with a trabecular pattern but without the cytologic features of the hyalinizing type also occur in the thyroid.

Anaplastic Spindle and Giant Cell Carcinoma

A small proportion of papillary and follicular carcinomas (1% to 2%), including those with insular components, progress to anaplastic spindle and giant cell carcinoma and show aggressive clinical behavior. Similarly, extensive sectioning of anaplastic spindle and giant cell carcinomas of the thyroid has shown the frequent association of these usually fatal malignancies with residual foci of papillary or follicular neoplasms (Fig. 26–23A,B), which presumably are the precursors (Aldinger et al., 1978; Carcangiu et al., 1985b; Ibanez et al., 1966). Occasional patients have only focal anaplastic transformation in differentiated carcinomas and may be cured surgically (Aldinger et al., 1978; Rosai et al., 1985). However, the vast majority of patients with anaplastic thyroid carcinomas die shortly after diagnosis. We have seen examples of early spindle and giant cell anaplastic transformation of papillary and follicular carcinoma in which the anaplastic spindle cells lose cohesion and show a pseudovascular pattern (Fig. 26–23C). Foci of squamous cell carcinoma are present in 15% to 20% of anaplastic carcinomas. The spindle cells usually overexpress p53 protein, whereas the adjacent differentiated neoplastic follicular cells are p53 negative (Fig. 26–23D). However, p53 positivity by immunohistochemistry does not necessarily correlate with genetic mutation. In one study of 40 p53-positive anaplastic carcinomas, only 5 had detectable *p53* gene muta-

tions (Zedenius et al., 1996). In contrast, the follicular cells express thyroglobulin whereas the spindle cells are usually thyroglobulin negative. The dedifferentiation seen in anaplastic carcinomas should be distinguished from squamous metaplasia or solid growth occurring in papillary thyroid carcinomas, frequent occurrences without prognostic significance.

THYROID C CELLS

During embryologic development, C cells migrate from the neural crest to the ultimobranchial body and then to the thyroid. The presence of C cells in thyroids from the DiGeorge anomaly, which affects derivatives of the third and fourth bronchial pouches, suggests that a subset of C cells is of endodermal derivation (Burke et al., 1987; Pueblitz et al., 1993). The greatest concentration of C cells is found at the junction between the upper and middle thirds of the right and left lobes, in the vicinity of solid cell nests, which represent remnants of the ultimobranchial body (Williams et al., 1989). In humans, normal C cells are present within thyroid follicles, not in the interfollicular stroma. Ultrastructural studies have shown that these cells are within and abut the follicular basement membranes, but they do not reach the colloid because of interposed follicular cell cytoplasm. By light microscopy using hematoxylin-eosin stains, C cells are almost indistinguishable from follicular cells, possessing pale, clear, or granular cytoplasm and round or oval nuclei with granular chromatin. The cells may be identified by argyrophil stains, by immunohistochemistry for general neuroendocrine markers (chromogranin, neuron specific enolase), by secretory products (calcitonin, calcitonin gene related peptide, somatostatin, gastrin releasing peptide), or by electron microscopic identification of dense core neurosecretory granules.

C-Cell Hyperplasia and Medullary Microcarcinoma

There are two types of C-cell hyperplasia: one represents a reactive or physiologic process with very low malignant potential and the other is neoplastic and is associated

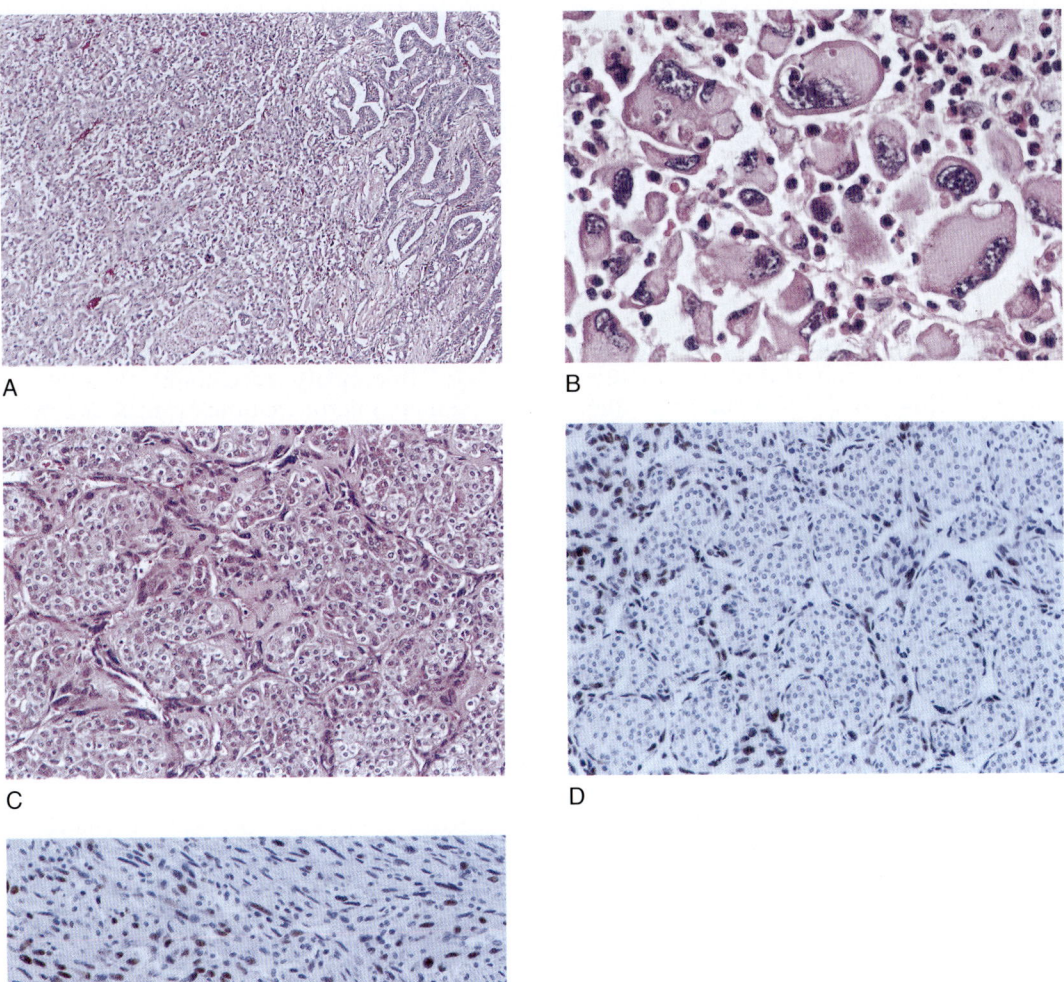

Figure 26–23. Anaplastic spindle and giant cell carcinomas. *A*: With papillary carcinoma. *B*: The anaplastic giant cell component is shown. *C*: Early anaplastic spindle cell transformation in follicular carcinoma with insular pattern. *D*: The anaplastic spindle cells are p53 positive whereas the differentiated follicular cells are negative. *E*: Most anaplastic spindle cells are p53 positive.

with familial medullary carcinoma and the MEN IIa and MEN IIb syndromes (Kotzmann et al., 1999; Perry et al., 1996). The preoperative diagnosis of physiologic C-cell hyperplasia is seldom made because it is nearly always asymptomatic. It has `been reported in association with Hashimoto's thyroiditis, and hyperparathyroidism, in residual thyroid following resection of sporadic medullary carcinoma, and adjacent to follicular cell neoplasms, (Albores-Saavedra,

et al., 1988; Biddinger et al., 1991; Libby et al., 1989; Ulbright et al., 1981). Few patients have shown elevated serum levels of calcitonin. Physiologic C-cell hyperplasia has also been documented in newborns and is probably related to TSH overstimulation (Thorpe-Beeston et al., 1991). Animals receiving an iodine-deficient diet or propylthiouracil develop C-cell hyperplasia, probably because of TSH stimulation (Peng et al., 1977; Yasumura et al., 1967). Hyperplastic C-cell nodules found at autopsy in elderly subjects are presumed to be physiologic and perhaps related to osteoporosis (Gibson et al., 1980; O'Toole et al., 1985). There are at least two mechanisms of physiologic C-cell hyperplasia: TSH overstimulation and hypercalcemia. Since not all examples of physiologic C-cell hyperplasia can be explained by these two mechanisms, other factors must be involved in its pathogenesis. Because of the complex interactions between follicular and C cells, it is possible that the number of C cells varies in many pathologic processes affecting follicular cells, including inflammatory, metabolic, and neoplastic conditions. Histologically, physiologic C-cell hyperplasia usually involves only part of the follicle (focal) or replaces the entire follicle (diffuse) in a ring-like fashion. Focal and diffuse C-cell hyperplasia usually coexist in the same thyroid. Rarely, the follicle is completely obliterated by C cells (nodular). Because of close morphologic similarities between non-neoplastic C cells, follicular cells, and histiocytes, immunohistochemical

stains are imperative for identification of C cells (Fig. 26–24). Although the definition of physiologic C-cell hyperplasia has been controversial, most pathologists agree that at least 50 calcitonin-positive cells per one low-power field are required for the diagnosis (Albores-Saavedra, et al., 1988).

It has now been established that neoplastic C-cell hyperplasia (medullary carcinoma *in situ*) preceeds the development of medullary thyroid carcinoma. The preoperative diagnosis of neoplastic C-cell hyperplasia (medullary carcinoma *in situ*) or medullary microcarcinoma can be made by the detection of germline mutations of the RETE proto-oncogene by genetic analysis, which is a highly reliable and specific test for the diagnosis of familial medullary carcinoma and the MEN IIa and MEN IIb syndromes. Genetic analysis can identify patients who have C-cell hyperplasia or medullary microcarcinoma but who do not have a positive pentagastrin stimulation test (Lips et al., 1994). Microscopically, neoplastic C-cell hyperplasia may show focal, diffuse, or

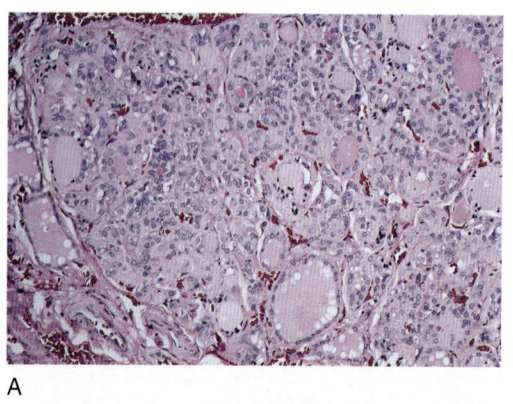

A

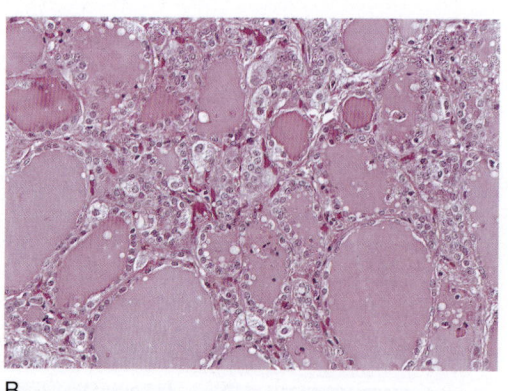

B

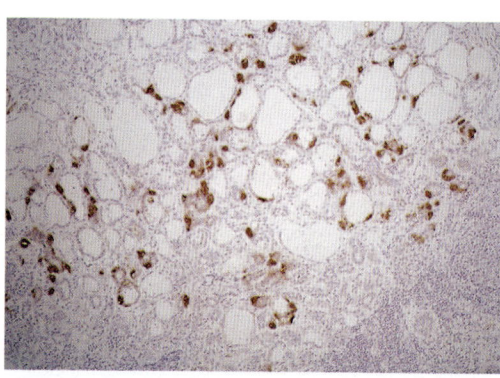

C

Figure 26–24. *A*: Physiologic C-cell hyperplasia. In this microscopic field the C cells are impossible to distinguish from follicular cells. *B*: Physiologic C-cell hyperplasia in a case of Hashimoto's thyroiditis. The C cells have abundant clear cytoplasm. *C*: Numerous calcitonin-positive cells in physiologic C-cell hyperplasia of Hashimoto's thyroiditis.

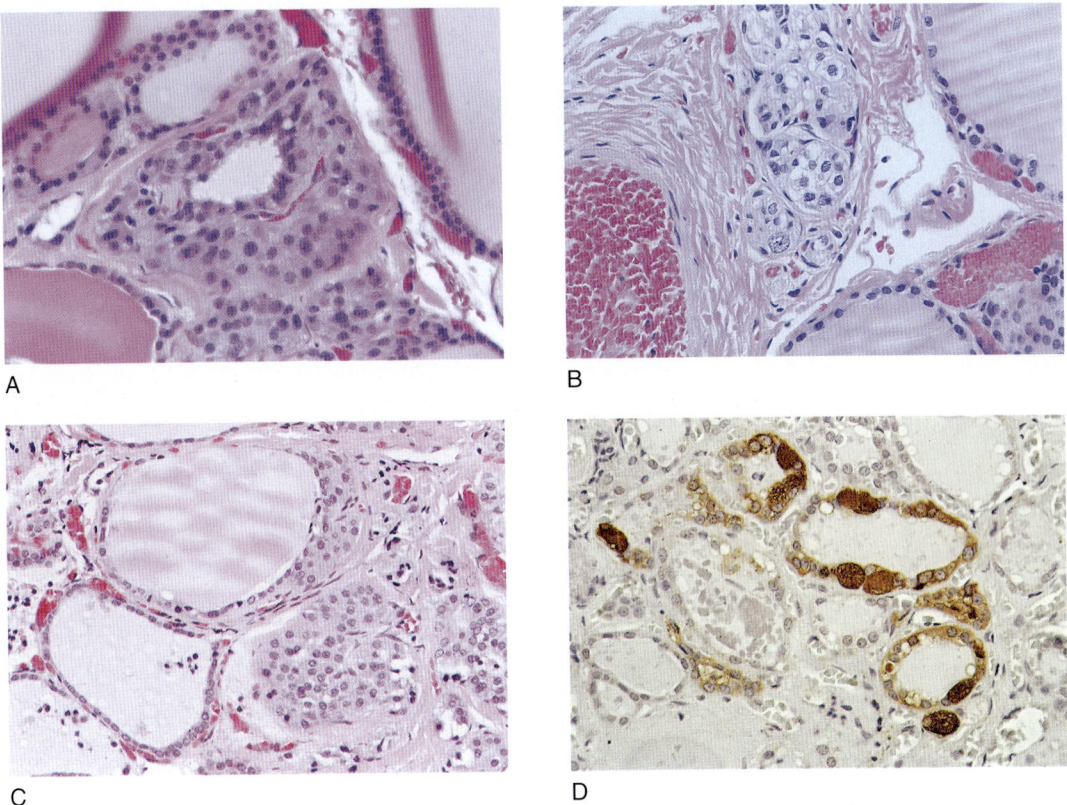

Figure 26–25. *A*: Diffuse neoplastic C-cell hyperplasia (medullary carcinoma *in situ*) associated with MEN IIa. The cells can easily be distinguished from adjacent follicular cells. *B*: Nodular C-cell hyperplasia in a patient with MEN IIa. *C*: Focal and nodular neoplastic C-cell hyperplasia in a patient with MEN IIa. *D*: Large calcitonin-positive cells have replaced the follicular cells.

nodular growth patterns (Fig. 26–25A–C). It may be the only pathologic finding, especially in children with the MEN IIa and MEN IIb syndromes, or may appear at the periphery of familial medullary thyroid carcinoma in adult patients. Occasionally C-cell hyperplasia is seen in association with sporadic medullary thyroid carcinoma (Kasener et al., 1998; Perry et al., 1996). The C cells in the neoplastic form of C-cell hyperplasia are mildly to moderately atypical but confined within the basement membrane of thyroid follicles. The detection of similar genetic abnormalities in C-cell hyperplasia and medullary thyroid carcinoma provides additional support for the neoplastic nature of C-cell hyperplasia (Xu et al., 1998). Moreover, these C cells, which stain intensely for calcitonin and weakly for carcinoembryonic antigen (CEA), can be identified with hematoxylin and eosin stains and are indistin-

guishable from those of invasive medullary thyroid carcinoma. Consequently, the number of C cells is irrelevant for the diagnosis of neoplastic C-cell hyperplasia. Medullary carcinoma is characterized by neoplastic C cells extending beyond the bounds of follicles and infiltrating the stroma, which may be desmoplastic and may contain amyloid (Fig. 26–26). Medullary microcarcinoma is defined as a tumor measuring less than 1 cm (Guyetant et al., 1999) These microcarcinomas are calcitonin-positive; some however, are multihormonal and immunoreactive for a variety of peptide hormones, including somatostatin, ACTH, gastrin-releasing peptide, and serotonin.

The importance of distinguishing medullary microcarcinoma from C-cell hyperplasia (medullary carcinoma *in situ*) is based on the metastatic potential of the former. We have seen regional lymph node metastases in one

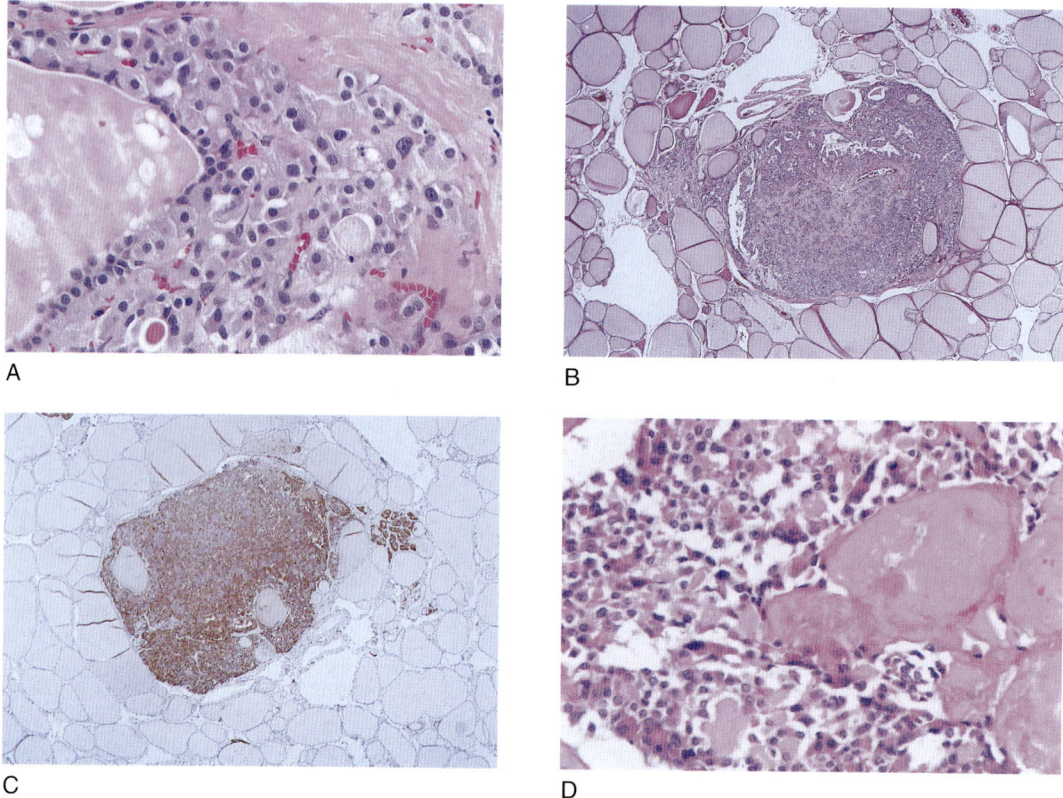

Figure 26–26. *A*: Incipient medullary carcinoma in a patient with MEN IIa. The C cells infiltrate the fibrous stroma adjacent to a follicle which contains C cells. *B*: Incipient nodular medullary carcinoma associated with MEN IIa. *C*: Same tumor showing immunoreactivity for calcitonin. *D*: Classic medullary carcinoma with amyloid stroma.

adult patient with medullary microcarcinoma measuring only a few millimeters in diameter. Bilateral neoplastic C-cell hyperplasia and/or medullary carcinomas occur in 80% of familial cases (Block et al., 1980). Total thyroidectomy is the treatment of choice for these patients. Neoplastic C-cell hyperplasia and incipient medullary thyroid carcinoma (medullary microcarcinoma) detected by genetic analysis have an excellent prognosis (Krueger et al., 2000). None of the eleven patients reported by Krueger et al. died as a result of the tumor. Palpable medullary carcinomas in MEN IIa patients tend to be indolent. Approximately 50% of the patients with symptomatic medullary carcinomas die as a result of the tumor (Albores-Saavedra et al., 1985; Kakudo et al., 1985). Age of the patients, size of the tumors and stage of the disease appear to be the most imporatnt independent prognostic factors (Bergholm et

al., 1997). Some investigators have recommended calcitonin screening for all patients with nodular thyroid disease to detect sporadic medullary carcinoma in early stages and thereby improve its prognosis (Kasener et al., 1998).

PARATHYROID GLAND

The superior parathyroids develop from the fourth branchial pouch and migrate with the ultimobranchial body and C cells, while the inferior parathyroids develop from the third branchial pouch, migrate with the thymus, and are more variable in their final location. About 13% of humans have more than four glands. Total weight averages 120 mg, with parenchyma accounting for 50% to 75% of the weight and adipocytes accounting for the remainder. Chief cells are the dominant parenchymal functional component, with numerous cytoplasmic fat droplets in normal and suppressed cells. Oxyphil and transitional oxyphil cells increase in number with advancing age and may form nodules, which can be mistaken for adenomas.

HYPERPLASIA

Most pathologists regard primary parathyroid hyperplasia as a proliferative process involving all glands (usually four), though involvement may be asymmetric and even asynchronous. In most cases no more than two glands are grossly enlarged (Grimelius et al., 1991). Patients may have microscopic ectopic deposits of parathyroid tissue in adipose tissue (spontaneous or surgically implanted) that participate in hyperplasia, termed "parathyromatosis" (Fitko et al., 1990). About 15% to 20% of hyperparathyroidism is due to primary parathyroid hyperplasia, which can be familial and is found in 90% of MEN I patients but in only 10% to 25% of MEN II patients. The monoclonality and the high rate of 11q13 LOH (100%) detected in MEN I parathyroid lesions suggests that they are neoplastic rather than hyperplastic (Friedman et al., 1989; Lubensky et al., 1996). However, monoclonality does not always indicate neoplastic proliferations. Parathyroid mitogenic activity has been demonstrated in the serum of these patients (Brandi et al., 1986). Primary chief cell hyperplasia affects females more often than males. It may be nodular or diffuse, usually contains admixed oxyphil and transitional oxyphil cells, and lacks nuclear pleomorphism (Fig. 26–27). These hyperplastic cells usually contain less fat than normal cells. Areas of nonhyperplastic parenchyma may simulate the rim of an adenoma and contain cytoplasmic fat droplets.

Water clear cell hyperplasia shows extreme glandular enlargement, greater superiorly, to a total weight of over 10 g. Histologically, the glands are composed of large cells with distinct cell borders and clear cytoplasm caused by vacuoles thought to be derived from the Golgi apparatus (Roth, 1970). Water clear cell hyperplasia is not associated with familial occurrence or MEN syndromes. It seems to have virtually vanished as a cause of primary hyperparathyroidism in recent decades, for unknown reasons.

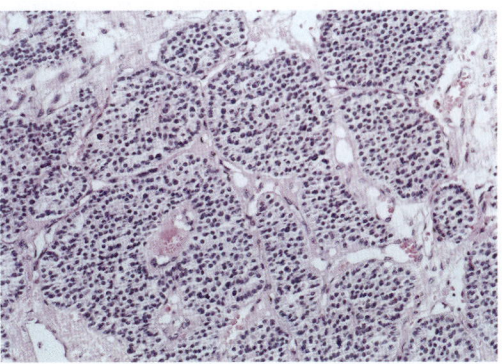

Figure 26–27. Chief cell hyperplasia in a patient with MEN I.

Secondary hyperparathyroidism represents a physiologic response to hypocalcemia and hyperphosphatemia, most often due to chronic renal failure or intestinal malabsorption. It is morphologically similar to the primary form, though all glands tend to be more uniformly involved with a diffuse pattern of hyperplasia. Tertiary hyperparathyroidism represents hypercalcemia superimposed on the secondary form. Increased asymmetry between glands, often with prominent nodularity, and an increased proportion of oxyphil cells are characteristic.

ADENOMA

Parathyroid adenoma is usually a sporadic disease that accounts for 80% of primary hyperparathyroidism, although familial cases have been reported (Allo and Thompson, 1982). For unknown reasons, females predominate (2 to 3:1), with a peak age incidence between 30 and 50 years. An inferior gland is about 5 times more likely to be involved than a superior gland. Parathyroid adenoma is a solitary enlarged hypercellular gland containing virtually no adipocytes. A remnant rim of normocellular parathyroid tissue (present in 50%) and significant nuclear pleomorphism (present in 20%) are regarded as features strongly suggestive of adenoma (Fig. 26–28A) rather than hyperplasia. The diagnosis of adenoma is assured when biopsy of a second grossly normal gland shows normal cellularity with cytoplasmic fat droplets in the chief cells (Bondeson et al., 1985). Usually, adenomas are dominated by chief cells but contain ad-

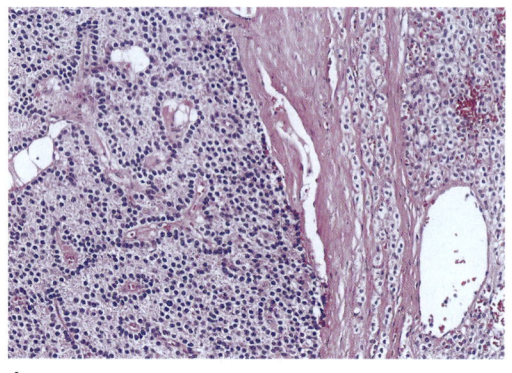
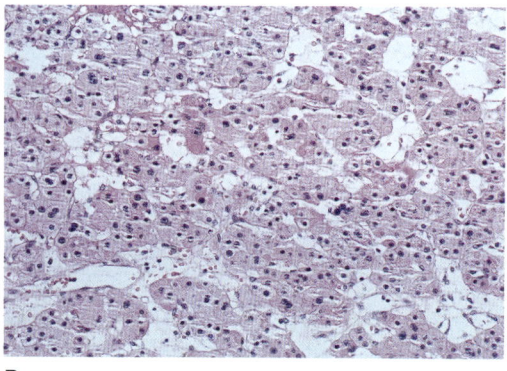

A   B

Figure 26–28. *A*: Parathyroid adenoma. This chief cell adenoma is encapsulated and compresses a rim of normal parathyroid gland. *B*: Parathyroid adenoma, oncocytic type with cytologic atypia.

mixed oxyphil and transitional oxyphil cells; 5% of adenomas are composed entirely of oxyphil cells (Fig. 26–28B). Rarely, adenomas are surrounded by a thick capsule which contains entrapped chief cells that should not be interpreted as a minimally invasive carcinoma. Parathyroid adenomas are considered to be monoclonal.

Ghandur-Mnaymneh and Kimura (1984) have suggested that parathyroid adenoma should be defined by encapsulation, a monomorphic cell population, lack of nodularity, and lack of entrapped adipocytes. Following these criteria, they found that only 6% of cases of primary hyperparathyroidism were caused by adenomas, while 75% of cases were regarded as single-gland hyperplasia. Persistent or recurrent hyperparathyroidism occurred in 44% of cases diagnosed as single-gland hyperplasia in this series, attributed to asynchronous hyperplasia of additional glands. This series contradicts traditional concepts of parathyroid adenoma and hyperplasia and thus deserves additional study.

ATYPICAL ADENOMA AND CARCINOMA

A category of "atypical parathyroid adenomas" has been proposed for neoplasms that are large (up to 2 g), may be adhesive to but do not invade adjacent organs, and have cytoarchitectural features of carcinoma, including mitoses and focal necrosis (Levin et al., 1987; LiVolsi, 1990). Most of these tumors seem to have benign clinical behavior on relatively short follow-up, although an occasional case has metastasized (San-Juan et al., 1989). Whether "atypical adenomas" are benign neoplasms with atypical features, adenomas progressing into carcinoma, or well-differentiated carcinomas is controversial. Longer follow-ups are needed to learn more about the natural history of these atypical adenomas.

It has recently been shown that cell cycle regulatory proteins, including Ki-67 and p27, are useful in the evaluation of parathyroid proliferations (Abbona et al., 1995; Lloyd et al., 1995). In one study a threefold higher expression of Ki-67 was detected in parathyroid carcinomas compared to adenomas and hyperplasias (Erickson et al., 1999). In contrast, a threefold decrease in p27 expression was found in parathyroid carcinomas compared to adenomas and hyperplasias (Erickson et al., 1999).

A recent case of hyperparathyroidism in our laboratory showed a 0.980 g trilobar parathyroid gland containing typical chief cell hyperplasia in one lobe, oxyphil cell hyperplasia in the second lobe, and well-differentiated carcinoma in the third portion. The carcinoma was characterized by fibrotic bands, vascular invasion, and numerous mitotic figures, including atypical forms. A second biopsied gland was normal. Others have reported parathyroid carcinoma arising in association with primary and secondary hyperplasia and adenomas (Haghighi et al., 1983; Kramer, 1970; Mallette et al., 1974), although most carcinomas do not have an identifiable precursor lesion. However, it is possible that most parathyroid carcinomas overgrow and obliterate their precursors by the time of diagnosis.

Often accompanied by severe hypercalcemia, parathyroid carcinomas are usually large (over 2 g) and adherent to or invasive into adjacent structures. A preoperative diagnosis is rarely made. Histologically, the cells are arranged in trabeculae of variable thickness, with lobules separated by dense fibrous bands (Schantz and Castleman, 1973; Fig. 26–29A). The cells show either marked atypia or paradoxical uniformity, though the relatively uniform small cells in some carcinomas have an increased nuclearcytoplasmic ratio (Fig. 26–29B). Mitotic figures (usually one or more per 10 high-power fields) and blood vessel invasion are usually identified (McKeown et al., 1984), while perineural invasion is an uncommon feature (Fig. 26–29C). As a note of caution, a detailed study showed mitotic figures in 80% of cases of chief cell hyperplasia and in 71% of cases of adenoma (Snover and Foucar, 1981), and fibrous bands may be identified

in parathyroid adenomas, often associated with hemosiderin deposition. DNA ploidy analysis does not reliably identify parathyroid carcinomas. It is noteworthy that 60% of primary and 100% of metastatic parathyroid carcinomas were aneuploid, but so were 50% of the cases of primary hyperplasia and 9% of the cases of adenoma (Obara et al., 1990). The overall 5-year and 10-year relative survival rates are 85.5% and 49.1%, respectively (Hundahl et al., 1999).

ADRENAL CORTEX

The adrenal cortex develops from the mesoderm of the urogenital ridge. Zona glomerulosa cells produce aldosterone, the primary mineralocorticoid, under renin-angiotensin feedback control, largely independent of ACTH. Clear cells of the zona fasciculata and compact eosinophilic cells of the zona reticularis produce and secrete corticosteroid and sex hormones under pituitary control. Corticotropin stimulation causes lipid de-

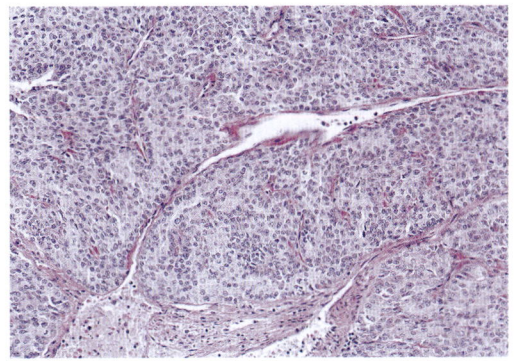

A

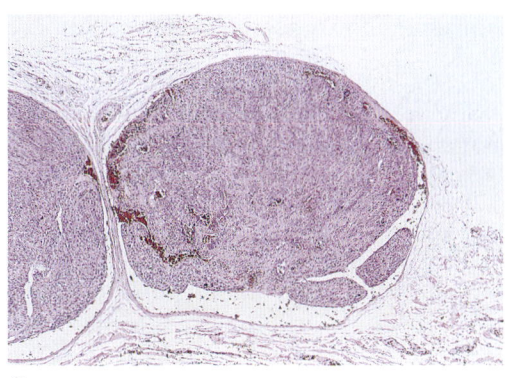

C

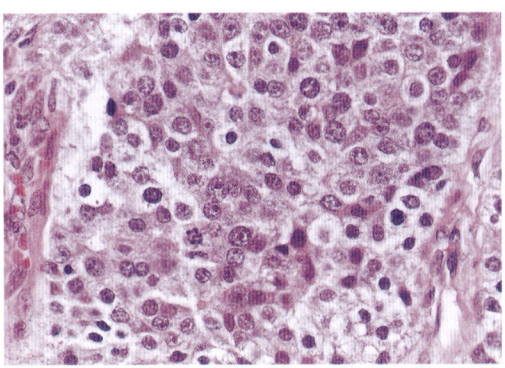

B

Figure 26–29. *A*: Parathyroid carcinoma with a trabecular growth pattern. *B*: The neoplastic cells have large atypical vesicular nuclei with prominent nucleoli. *C*: Blood vessels filled with tumor thrombi.

pletion of clear cells, which then appear more compact and eosinophilic.

Hyperplasia

Hyperplasia of the adrenal cortex is either nodular or diffuse, primary or secondary, functional or nonfunctional, and nearly always bilateral. The hyperplastic glands usually show an increase in size and weight. Nodular hyperplasia is subdivided into macro- and micronodular types. Macronodules measure more than 1 cm. Nodular hyperplasia with a dominant nodule may simulate an adenoma. In many glands nodular and diffuse hyperplasia coexist, suggesting a morphologic continuum. With com-puted tomography and magnetic resonance imaging, adrenal cortical nodules less than 1 cm can be visualized. The morphologic and functional classifications of adrenal cortical hyperplasia appear in Tables 26–2 and 26–3, respectively.

Cytomegaly of the adrenal cortex is usually an incidental finding in otherwise normal glands of newborns or premature stillborns. Affected cells show large hyperchromatic nuclei. These cytomegalic cells contain over 50 times the normal amount of nuclear DNA (Favara et al., 1991).

In the Beckwith-Wiedemann syndrome, characterized by exomphalos, macroglossia, and giantism, there is adrenal gland enlargement with marked cytomegaly.

Congenital adrenal hyperplasia is caused by a genetic defect in a synthetic enzyme for cortisol, usually 21-hydroxylase, with precursors shunted predominantly into androgen

Table 26–2. Morphologic Classification of Adrenal Cortical Hyperplasia

Bilateral adrenal cortical hyperplasia

Diffuse hyperplasia

Nodular hyperplasia
  Micronodular (less than 1 cm in diameter)
  Macronodular (greater than 1 cm)
  Combined micronodular and macronodular

Combined diffuse and nodular hyperplasia
  Dominant cortical nodule with diffuse hyperplasia
  Multiple nodules with diffuse hyperplasia

Macronodular hyperplasia with marked adrenal enlargement

Primary pigmented nodular adrenocortical disease

Incidental pigmented nodules

Unilateral adrenal cortical hyperplasia

Diffuse and/or nodular hyperplasia

Incidental pigmented nodule(s)

From Lack EE. (1997) *Tumors of the Extra-Adrenal Gland and Extra-Adrenal Paraganglia. Atlas of Tumor Pathology,* Fascicle 19, Third Series. Armed Forces Institute of Pathology, Washington, DC.

synthetic pathways (White et al., 1987). There is bilateral diffuse adrenocortical hyperplasia, up to 30 g each, often with a cerebriform appearance. Excessive androgens are produced by compact cells under ACTH stimulation in the absence of feedback inhibition by cortisol, resulting in virilization (adrenogenital syndrome). Hyperplasia with hyperaldosteronism shows triangular collections of zona glomerulosa cells, with the triangle apex oriented toward the central vein, with or without nodules or an aldosteronoma (Neville and O'Hare, 1985). Simple diffuse or micronodular cortical hyperplasia

Table 26–3. Clinical Endocrine Syndromes Associated with Diffuse or Nodular Hyperplasia

Endocrine Syndrome	Adrenal Cortical Hyperplasia
Hypercortisolism	
Cushing's syndrome	
Pituitary-dependent (Cushing's disease)	Diffuse and/or nodular
Ectopic ACTH production	Predominantly diffuse
Primary pigmented nodular adrenocortical disease	Predominantly micronodular
Macronodular hyperplasia with marked adrenal enlargement	Macronodular
Ectopic secretion of corticotropin-releasing factor	Macronodular
Hyperaldosteronism	Predominantly diffuse
Virilization (congenital adrenal hyperplasia)	Diffuse and/or micronodular
Eucorticalism	Predominantly diffuse Diffuse and/or nodular

From Lack EE. (1997) *Tumors of the Extra-Adrenal Gland and Extra-Adrenal Paraganglia. Atlas of Tumor Pathology,* Fascicle 19, Third Series. Armed Forces Institute of Pathology, Washington, DC.

most often results from a pituitary corti-cotrope adenoma (Cushing's disease), with each gland up to double its normal weight of 6 g. Diffuse cortical hyperplasia with weights up to 30 g each may occur if ectopic ACTH is produced by an autonomous neo-plasm. Multinodular bilateral hyperplasia with hypercortisolism is associated with chronically elevated ACTH levels and shows macronodules with adrenal weights of 30 to 100 g each (Smals et al., 1984). Adrenocor-tical function seems autonomous, since there is resistance to high-dose dexametha-sone suppression (Hermus et al., 1988). Residual cortex is difficult to identify be-tween the nodules, which are composed of mixed clear, compact, and intermediate cells, and nuclear pleomorphism may be marked. Rare cases of adrenocortical carci-noma have arisen in association with the Beckwith-Wiedemann syndrome (Wiede-mann, 1983), congenital adrenal hyperpla-sia (Bauman and Bauman, 1982), and hyperplasia secondary to pituitary corti-cotrope adenoma (Anderson et al., 1978).

Primary pigmented nodular adrenocorti-cal disease (dysplasia) is a rare cause of Cush-ing's syndrome, which is characterized by low ACTH levels and normal-sized adrenals with bilateral brown to black, 1 to 5 mm nod-ules of predominantly compact eosinophilic cells (Iseli and Hedinger, 1985; Shenoy et al., 1984). The pigmentation is the result of cy-toplasmic accumulation of lipofuscin. Some nodules occupy the entire thickness of the cortex and may even extend into the peria-drenal fat. Occasionally, the nodules project into the lumen of veins, suggesting malig-nancy. Some cases are familial, and an asso-ciation with cardiac myxoma, myxoid mammary fibroadenoma, spotty cutaneous pigmentation, large cell calcifying Sertoli cell tumor, or psammomatous melanocytic schwannoma has been noted (Carney et al., 1985). The etiology of the disease is un-known, but an autoimmune pathogenesis for the adrenocortical hyperfunction has been suggested. The hyperfunction is be-lieved to be due to circulating immuno-globulins reactive against ACTH receptors (Wulffraat et al., 1988), analogous to the sit-uation in Graves' disease. Nonhyperfunc-tioning nodules and cortical adenomas may also be pigmented, containing lipofuscin and neuromelanin (Damron et al., 1987).

Hypercortisolism is relatively uncommon in MEN syndromes, since most pituitary ade-nomas in MEN I do not produce ACTH (Miyagawa et al., 1988), and few medullary thyroid carcinomas or pheochromocytomas in MEN IIa or IIb produce ectopic ACTH. Although adrenocortical nodules are found in 40% of MEN I patients (Ballard et al., 1964), solitary hyperfunctioning adenomas are very rare. An aldosteronoma in MEN I has been reported (Gould et al., 1987).

ADENOMA

Adrenal cortical adenoma is usually a small, solitary, well-demarcated mass that com-monly gives rise to a clinical syndrome due to excessive secretion of adrenal steroids. The most common syndrome associated with adrenocortical adenoma is primary aldosteronism, followed by Cushing's syn-drome, virilization, and feminization. Adreno-cortical neoplasms weighing 50 g or less are usually adenomas, although weight alone does not always predict biologic behavior. There is no evidence that adrenocortical adenomas become malignant. Computed to-mography and magnetic resonance imaging identify small (1 cm or less), asymptomatic adrenal nodules in 1% of patients. Scintig-raphy for uptake of a steroid analogue ra-dionuclide shows that these nodules are usually neither nonfunctional nor hyper-functional and are analogous to nodular eu-thyroid goiter (Gross et al., 1987). It is preferable to regard small nonhyperfunc-tioning cortical masses as "nodules," reserv-ing the diagnosis of adenoma for solitary unilateral benign neoplasms usually associ-ated with an endocrine syndrome (Lack et al., 1990).

If nonhyperfunctional nodules are ex-cluded, cortical neoplasms are uncommon. Adrenocortical adenomas are solitary, func-tionally autonomous, benign neoplasms. The morphology of adenomas does not cor-relate well with functional type, so that it is difficult to predict function from histologic features alone (Fig. 26–30A,B). Aldos-teronomas are most common, and 80% of hyperaldosteronism is caused by adenomas, which are bright yellow, average 1.5 cm in diameter, and show adjacent normal cortex or hyperplastic zona glomerulosa. Aldos-teronomas most often have a predominant

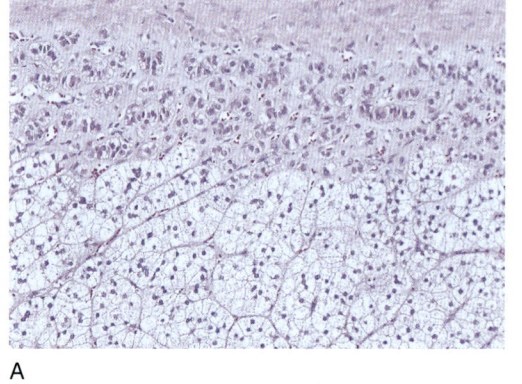

A

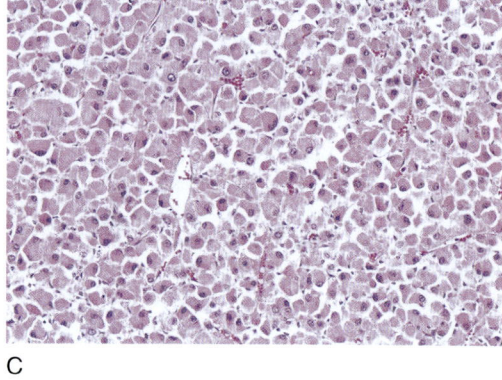

C

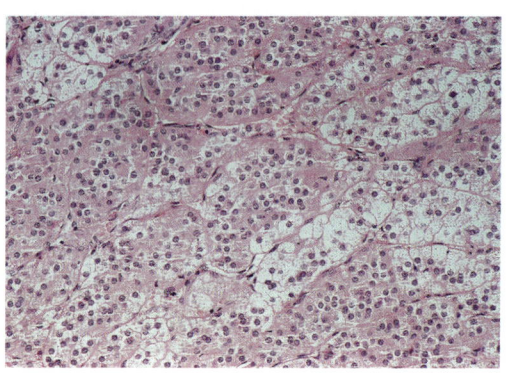

B

Figure 26–30. Adrenal cortical adenomas. *A:* The atrophic cortex is compressed by the adenoma, which is composed of lipid-rich cells. *B:* In this adenoma associated with Cushing's syndrome, cells with lipid-rich and compact eosinophilic cytoplasm are seen. *C:* Oncocytic type of adrenocortical adenoma with cytologic atypia.

population of large, lipid-rich, fasciculata-type cells and hybrid cells with clear cytoplasm showing mixed features of fasciculata and glomerulosa cells without nuclear pleomorphism. Spironolactone bodies are cytoplasmic inclusions found within tumor cells of aldosterone-producing adenomas. These inclusions stain with the Luxol fast blue stain.

Cortisol-producing adenomas are responsible for less than 20% of cases of Cushing's syndrome and are associated with low serum levels of ACTH and atrophy of adjacent zona fasciculata and reticularis. Some black adenomas can give rise to Cushing's syndrome or primary aldosteronism (Cohen et al., 1991; Kovacs et al., 1976). Adenomas producing the adrenogenital syndrome tend to be large (over 5 cm) and are relatively more common in children, but they are difficult to distinguish from virilizing carcinomas, which tend to be well differentiated. Feminizing adrenal neoplasms are rare and are usually malignant, even if histologically bland (Neville and O'Hare, 1985). Onco-

cytic adenomas are usually nonfunctioning tumors.

In general, adenomas have mild nuclear pleomorphism and a thin fibrous pseudocapsule, weigh under 50 g with a diameter less than 5 cm, and lack necrosis and significant mitotic activity. Oncocytic adenomas are often large, show considerable nuclear pleomorphism, and are composed of mitochondrion-rich cells (Lin et al., 1998; Sasano et al., 1991; Fig. 26–30A). Black adenomas are quite rare and microscopically similar to other adenomas that do not contain excessive lipochrome pigment. Grossly, these black adenomas can be confused with melanoma or hematomas.

CARCINOMA

Cortical carcinomas are usually large, nearly all weighing over 100 g and frequently extending into adjacent structures. Microscopically, they often show trabecular architecture with broad fibrous bands and geographic necrosis. The neoplastic cells

may show multivacuolated or compact cytoplasm and anaplastic nuclei or a paradoxically uniform appearance in which the small
cells have an increased nuclear/cytoplasmic
ratio (Hough et al., 1979; King and Lack,
1979; Lack et al., 1990; Van Slooten et al.,
1985; Weiss, 1984). Rarely, adrenocortical
carcinomas are composed predominantly of
oncocytic cells. Mitotic figures greater than
2 per 10 high-power fields are found in most
tumors. When present, blood vessel invasion
is diagnostic of malignancy. Marked variation of histologic appearance within carcinomas is common, with abrupt transitions
from well-differentiated to poorly differentiated areas, necessitating extensive histologic
sampling for diagnosis (Fig. 26–31). No single criterion, such as weight, tumor size, cytologic atypia, or mitotic rate, distinguishes
all benign from malignant lesions (Gandour
and Grizzle, 1986; Lack, 1990). In some cases
the use of the term "adrenal cortical neoplasm of indeterminate malignant potential"
seems appropriate (Lack, 1990). Immunohistochemical stains for the expression of

MiB-1 and p53 protein are useful to distinguish cortical adenomas from carcinomas.
Carcinomas contain many more MiB-1- and
p53-positive nuclei than adenomas (Vargas
et al., 1997). DNA flow cytometry has shown
that most carcinomas are aneuploid whereas
most adenomas are diploid (Bowlby et al.,
1986; Hosaka et al., 1987; Joensuu and
Klemi, 1988). Other studies, however, have
found no correlation between aneuploidy
and biologic behavior in both children and
adults (Bugg et al., 1994; Haak et al., 1993).
Genetic analysis appears to be a useful tool
to distinguish adenomas from adrenal cortical carcinomas. In one study, genetic
changes were observed in 61% of the carcinomas while none of the hyperplastic lesions
and adenomas tested showed genetic abnormalities. The most common genetic
changes observed in carcinomas were LOH
at the p53 locus, 1p and 9p (Fogt, et al.,
1998). In children, especially those under 5
years of age, favorable outcomes are more
common with large adrenocortical neoplasms that have mitoses, necrosis, broad fi-

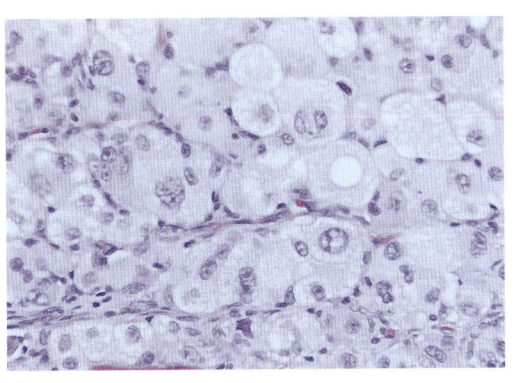

A

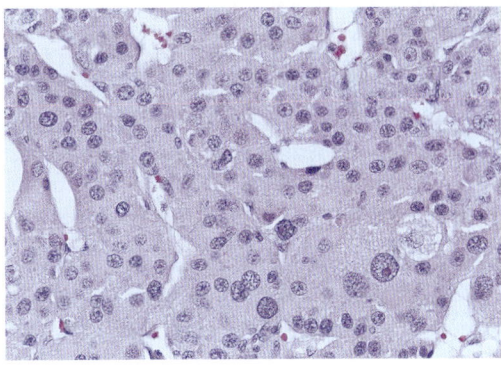

C

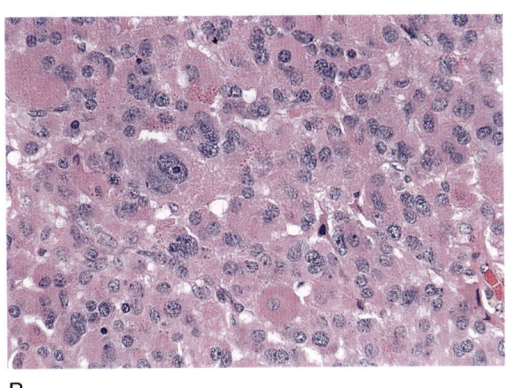

B

Figure 26–31. Adrenocortical carcinoma. *A:* The
neoplastic cells show lipid-rich cytoplasm and
vesicular nuclei with prominent nucleoli. Mild
nuclear pleomorphism is also present. *B:* In this
example of adrenocortical carcinoma, the cells
have compact eosinophilic cytoplasm. *C:* A prominent trabecular pattern is illustrated here.

brous bands, and significant nuclear pleo-morphism (Lack et al., 1992).

Most series of adrenocortical neoplasms have 10% or more cases that are difficult to classify as clearly adenoma or carcinoma us-ing histologic criteria. In one series (Hough et al., 1979), 7 of 41 tumors were considered indeterminate for malignancy; 4 of these tu-mors metastasized. A review of 23 tumors in children showed malignant behavior in 6 of 14 diagnosed as malignant, in 1 of 7 that were borderline, and in neither of 2 adeno-mas (Cagle et al., 1986). The borderline cat-egory suggests the possibility that an adenoma may be a precursor lesion that can progress to carcinoma in some cases. Alter-natively, certain neoplasms may be malig-nant from inception, with the borderline tumors representing the most well-differen-tiated end of the spectrum (Lack et al., 1990). Because adrenocortical carcinoma has a high mortality rate, which is related to tumor stage and histologic grade, early di-agnosis is desirable. However, to resect suc-cessfully one small (under 6 cm) carcinoma identified by computed tomography, which would probably be nonhyperfunctional, more than 60 operations would have to be performed on patients with incidental be-nign nodules (Copeland, 1983).

Adrenocortical carcinomas are slightly more common in females and have bimodal age peaks in the fifth decade and in children under 5 years. Rare familial cases have been reported (Hartley et al., 1987), some associ-ated with sarcomas in addition to breast or lung carcinomas (Lynch et al., 1985). Bilat-eral carcinomas are exceedingly rare but should not be confused with metastasis to the contralateral adrenal gland. A palpable abdominal mass without evidence of an en-docrine syndrome characterizes 20% to 40% of cases. Functioning carcinomas most often produce Cushing's syndrome with mixed features of virilism. The cells are often rela-tively deficient in 11-β-hydroxylase and demonstrate a blunted response *in vitro* to ACTH compared with the response seen in adenomas (O'Hare et al., 1979). Hypo-glycemia and hypercalcemia have been re-ported in patients with adrenocortical carcinomas (Orland et al., 1968). Electron microscopy shows that carcinomas differ from adenomas in having disrupted or ab-sent basement membrane around cell clus-ters (Tannenbaum, 1973). Carcinomas may have cytoplasmic lipid, mitochondria with shelf-like and tubular or tubulovesicular cristae, rough and smooth endoplasmic reticulum, primitive intercellular junctions, and endothelial fenestrations (Silva et al., 1982).

ADRENAL MEDULLA

The *adrenal medulla* is a neuroendocrine or-gan, a paraganglion of the sympathetic ner-vous system derived from embryologic migration of neural crest cells. The normal adrenal medulla is composed of compact nests of polyhedral cells with amphophilic granular cytoplasm and vesicular nuclei, among which are scattered ganglion cells and autonomic nerve fibers. In normal hu-man adrenal glands, all medullary tissue is confined to the head and body, without ex-tension into the tail or ala. The neural ele-ments of the adrenal medulla give rise to neural neoplasms, most commonly gan-glioneuroma, which is an encapsulated mass of histologically mature ganglion cells, with mixed, randomly arranged nerve fibers and fibrous stroma resembling neurofibroma. Binucleate and multinucleate ganglion cells are frequent, without satellite cells, but mi-totic figures are not seen.

HYPERPLASIA

Adrenal medullary hyperplasia is a precur-sor of pheochromocytomas in MEN syn-dromes (Carney et al., 1976). It is characterized by an increased number of chromaffin cells with expansion of the medullary region of the gland. Adrenal medullary hyperplasia can produce exces-sive secretion of catecholamines and give rise to symptoms similar to those seen in pa-tients with pheochromocytoma. Sporadic cases of adrenal medullary hyperplasia have also been reported, especially in children (Bialestock, 1961). In sporadic cases, adrenomedullary hyperplasia may be unilat-eral. The diagnosis of adrenal medullary hy-perplasia based on morphometric analysis of increased medullary weight or volume (DeLellis et al., 1976) is considered prefer-able to that based solely on abnormal corti-comedullary ratios of random adrenal sections. The gland is weighed, serially sectioned, and embedded, with sections from each block analyzed by point counting on a lattice to determine the cortical/medullary ratio (normally 10:1) and calculated medullary weight (normally 0.47 ± 0.15 g per gland). Cases of adrenal medullary hyperplasia not associated with multiple endocrine neoplasia or neurocutaneous phakomatosis syndromes have been reported (Rudy et al., 1980; Visser and Axt, 1975). Victims of sudden infant death syndrome and patients with cystic fibrosis have been noted to have adrenal medullary hyperplasia.

Histologically, adrenal medullary hyperplasia is characterized by an exaggeration of the organoid architecture of the normal medulla. The cells show increased size with pleomorphism, as well as occasional mitotic figures. Nodularity may even be seen grossly (Fig. 26–32A). There are no histologic criteria that distinguish medullary nodular hyperplasia from small pheochromocytomas (Carney et al., 1976). Both contain nests or trabeculae of polyhedral cells with amphophilic granular cytoplasm and vesicular nuclei surrounded by a dense network of capillaries (Fig. 26–32B,C). A diffuse pattern has also been described in adrenal medullary hyperplasia. It has been proposed that lesions less than 1 cm in diameter should be called nodular hyperplasia, while those 1 cm or larger should be regarded as pheochromocytomas (Carney et al., 1978).

The presence of a discrete capsule with compression of the adjacent tissue favors a diagnosis of pheochromocytoma. The DNA content in adrenomedullary hyperplasia is diploid or euploid while the DNA content of pheochromocytomas is usually nondiploid or aneuploid (Padberg et al., 1990).

PHEOCHROMOCYTOMA

Familial pheochromocytoma syndromes are often divided into those with a high frequency of pheochromocytoma (MEN IIa and IIb, 30% to 70%) and those with a lower risk (neurocutaneous phakomatosis syndromes, such as the von Hippel–Lindau syndrome, von Recklinghausen's neurofibromatosis, and Sturge-Weber syndrome, 5% or less). Diffuse or nodular adrenal medullary hyperplasia is commonly seen in kindreds with a high frequency of pheochromocytomas and may also be found in the contralateral adrenal or in the adrenal medulla adjacent to a pheochromocytoma. Adrenal medullary hyperplasia may produce excess catecholamines, with the same symptoms as seen in pheochromocytomas.

Patients with familial pheochromocytomas usually have multifocal tumors; 66% are bilateral, compared with less than 10% bilaterality in sporadic cases, which constitute more than 80% of all cases (Webb et al., 1980). Pheochromocytomas are reported to occur in 0.005% to 0.1% of unselected autopsies and associated with about 0.5%

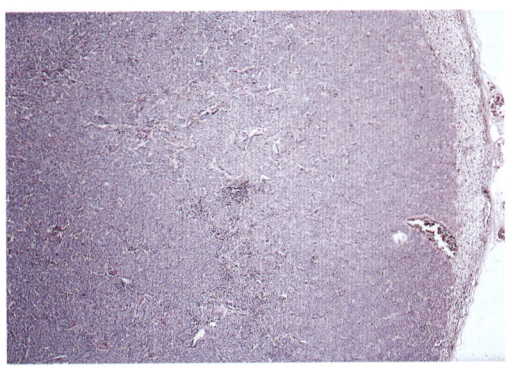

A

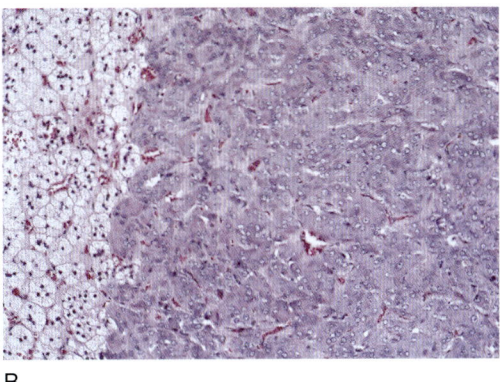

B

Figure 26–32. Nodular adrenal medullary hyperplasia associated with MEN IIa. *A*: An 8 mm, well-defined nodule expands the adrenal medulla and compresses the adrenal cortex. *B*: Sheets of uniform adrenomedullary cells compress the clear cells of the cortex. *C*: Higher magnification of adrenal medullary hyperplasia to depict cell detail.

of cases with significant clinical hypertension. Most pheochromocytomas appear soft, rounded, and encapsulated, with an organoid (*Zellballen*) architecture of polyhedral cells with finely granular amphophilic cytoplasm and coarse chromatin (Fig. 26–33A,B). Occasionally, clear to vacuolated PAS-positive cytoplasm, intranuclear cytoplasmic pseudoinclusions, and pseudoglandular, trabecular, or solid architecture are noted. Prominent spindling, marked pleomorphism, interstitial hyalinization, vascular invasion, and necrosis are features of larger pheochromocytomas, especially those greater than 5 cm. Some pheochromocytomas contain ganglion cells and are designated "composite pheochromocytoma ganglioneuroma" (Fig. 26–33C). Areas resembling neuroblastoma have also been documented in pheochromocytomas. Malignancy is suggested by capsular invasion, necrosis, mitotic figures, small cell size, and large tumor size, but can be proven only by metastases (Lack, 1990). Metastatic deposits must be distinguished from concurrent extra-adrenal para-gangliomas and, in MEN IIa and IIb patients, from metastatic medullary thyroid carcinoma. In one series, benign pheochromocytomas averaged 156 g, compared to 759 g for malignant tumors (Medeiros et al., 1985). Recent studies with DNA flow cytometry suggest that tetraploidy and aneuploidy correlate with malignancy (Hosaka et al., 1986), although another study found aneuploidy to be frequent in clinically benign pheochromocytomas (Amberson et al., 1987).

PARAGANGLIA

Paraganglia are classified as sympathetic (adrenal medulla, organ of Zuckerkandl, and paraspinal homologues) or parasympathetic (carotid body, aortic body, and other head and neck and visceral sites). Chief cells are the catecholamine-producing neuroendocrine component, present in nests, surrounded by supporting sustentacular cells that are S-100 protein positive, and separated by a plexiform vascular network.

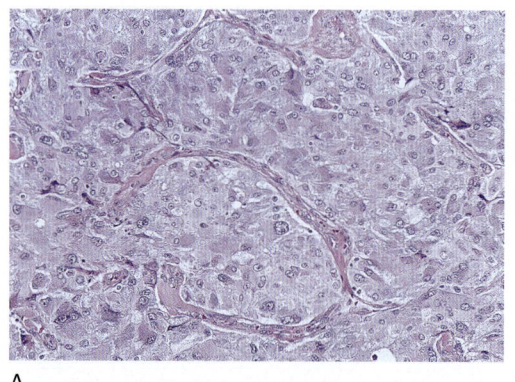

A

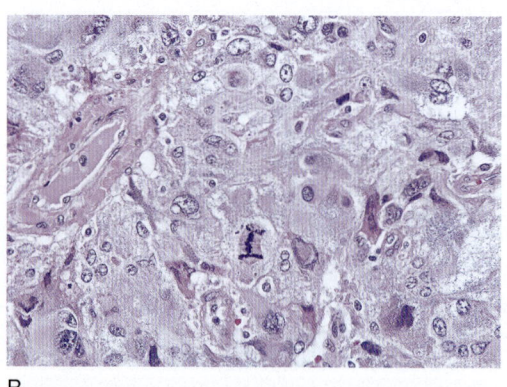

B

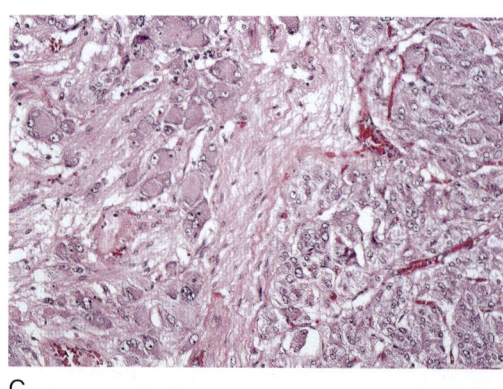

C

Figure 26–33. Pheochromocytoma of adrenal gland. *A*: Nests of polygonal cells with abundant amphophilic cytoplasm. *B*: Abnormal mitotic figure in a benign pheochromocytoma. *C*: Pheochromocytoma with ganglioneuroma (composite pheochromocytoma).

HYPERPLASIA

The carotid bodies are chemoreceptor organs for homeostasis of blood oxygenation. Carotid body hyperplasia, the precursor of paraganglioma, is considered a physiologic response to high altitudes and anoxia (Arias-Stella and Valcarcel, 1976; Lack, 1978). Hyperplasia of carotid bodies has also been reported in patients with obstructive pulmonary disease and hypertension (Lack, 1978). Chronic hypoxemia caused by cystic fibrosis and cyanotic heart disease has led to carotid body hyperplasia (Lack, 1977). Hyperplasia of vagal paraganglia has been documented in patients with chronic hypoxemia due to chronic obstructive pulmonary disease and cyanotic heart disease (Lack, 1978). This hyperplasia tends to support a chemoreceptor role for vagal paraganglia (Lack, 1978). Hyperplasia of the organs of Zuckerkandl is poorly understood and rarely seen as an incidental microscopic finding in retroperitoneal node dissections. Some of these hyperplastic organs of Zukerkandl may consist entirely of clear cells. It is important not to confuse them with metastatic carcinomas, especially when they are seen adjacent to lymph nodes.

PARAGANGLIOMA

Benign carotid body paragangliomas are found 10 times more frequently in high-altitude populations than in those living at sea level (Rodriguez-Cuevas et al., 1986; Saldana et al., 1973). Rarely paragangliomas have been reported in association with obstructive pulmonary disease and cyanotic heart disease (Chedid and Jao, 1974; Nissenblatt, 1978). These tumors show prominent cords and organoid *(Zellballen)* nests of slightly pleomorphic amphophilic chief cells, occasionally with spindling and stromal sclerosis. Cytologic atypia with marked hyperchromatism does not correlate with malignant behavior. The nests are surrounded by sustentacular cells, with interposed delicate blood vessels (Fig. 26–34). A significant proportion of carotid body paragangliomas are

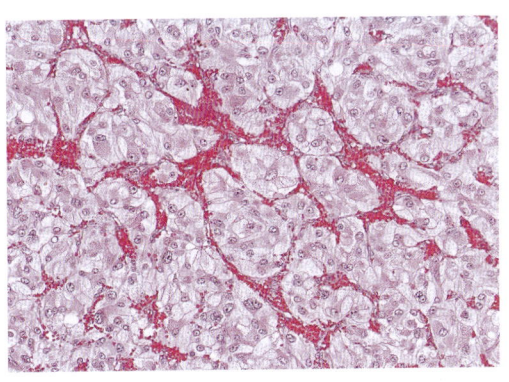

A

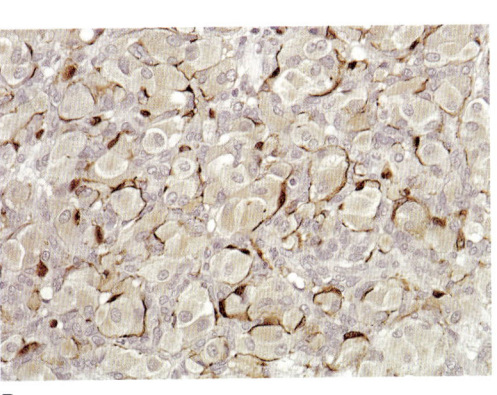

B

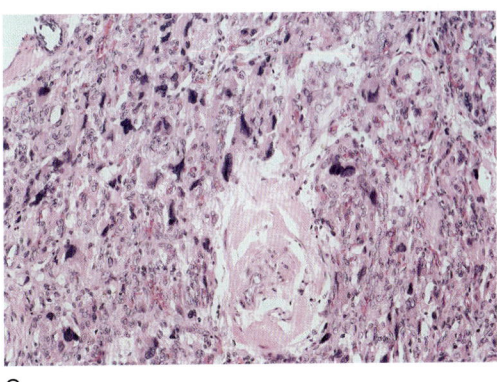

C

Figure 26–34. Paraganglioma of carotid body. *A*: The characteristic *Zellballen* pattern is seen. *B*: The peripheral sustentacular cells are highlighted with S-100 protein stain. *C*: Cytologic atypia in benign carotid body paraganglioma.

immunoreactive for serotonin but lack reactivity for peptide hormones. Most of these tumors occur in women and behave in a benign fashion. Some investigators have expressed the view that these tumors represent exuberant hyperplasia of the carotid bodies rather than neoplasms.

Familial cases of head and neck paragangliomas, as well as individuals with multifocal paragangliomas, are well documented (Chedid and Jao, 1974), constituting approximately 10% of cases. Patients with familial carotid body parangliomas often have bilateral tumors and may develop paragangliomas in other sites. Bilateral carotid body paragangliomas have also been described as part of a genetically determined MEN syndrome in which the pituitary gland and the thyroid are also involved (Larraza-Hernandez et al., 1982). A syndrome affecting young women, characterized by extra-adrenal paraganglioma, gastric leiomyosarcoma, and pulmonary chondroma, has also been reported (Carney et al., 1977; Raafat et al., 1986). Of children with sympathetic paragangliomas, 35% have multicentric tumors without familial syndromes. Patients with MEN IIa and IIb usually have adrenal medullary disease without involvement of the carotid bodies.

Thoracic, abdominal, and retroperitoneal paragangliomas resemble pheochromocytomas grossly and microscopically. Most tumors show a prominent *Zellballen* or trabecular pattern. Bizarre nuclei and vascular invasion are not criteria for malignancy, and benign tumors may be locally invasive. In one study, numerous mitotic figures, decreased neuropeptide immunoreactivity, and lack of sustentacular cells correlated with malignancy (Linnoila et al., 1988). Other investigators have found lack of correlation between the presence of sustentacular cells and biologic behavior. In fact, paragangliomas with a benign histologic appearance and numerous sustentacular cells may metastasize. Pigmented paragangliomas have been reported in several anatomic sites but not in the carotid bodies (Moran et al., 1997). Multicentricity should be considered before metastases are diagnosed (Capella et al., 1988). Approximately 10% of paragangliomas of the head, neck, and thorax and 30% of intra-abdominal extra-adrenal paragangliomas have been considered malignant, but longer follow-up

has shown a higher proportion of malignancy, at least in some locations (Olson and Salyer, 1978).

ENDOCRINE PANCREAS

The islets of Langerhans develop from pancreatic ductular cells in humans, as do the acinar cells, rather than by migration from the neural crest (Rutter, 1980). Although the endocrine cells of the pancreas are found predominantly in the islets, some are present among the ductal cells. Normal islets measure 50 to 250 μm in diameter, showing rounded contours with organoid and trabecular cytoarchitecture. Glucagon-containing A cells, somatostatin-containing D cells, and pancreatic polypeptide (PP) cells are found at the periphery of the islets, while the more numerous insulin-containing B cells are located in the central zone. The adult pancreas contains no gastrin (G) or vasoactive intestinal peptide (VIP) cells (Mukai, 1983). Endocrine cells are not disproportionately localized to the pancreatic tail, as was previously thought (Klöppel et al., 1991).

HYPERPLASIA AND NESIDIOBLASTOSIS

Considerable variation in the size and number of islets is seen in normal human subjects, a finding that complicates the diagnosis of islet cell hyperplasia. Ideally, the diagnosis of islet cell hyperplasia should be made by quantitative studies. Islet cell hyperplasia and hypertrophy with B-cell pleomorphism is well documented in infants born of diabetic mothers as a homeostatic response to hyperglycemia. Islet cell hyperplasia has also been documented in erythroblastosis fetalis, hereditary tyrosinemia of hepatorenal type, and the Beckwith-Wiedemann syndrome (Stefan et al., 1985). Islet cell hyperplasia is most commonly associated with advanced chronic pancreatitis (Bartow et al., 1981; Klöppel et al., 1978). Immunohistochemical analysis has shown that all normal islet cell types participate in the hyperplastic process (Bartow et al., 1981), but no hyperfunctional endocrine abnormality has been identified; rather, diabetes mellitus often develops. In some cases the endocrine cells show pseudoinvasive

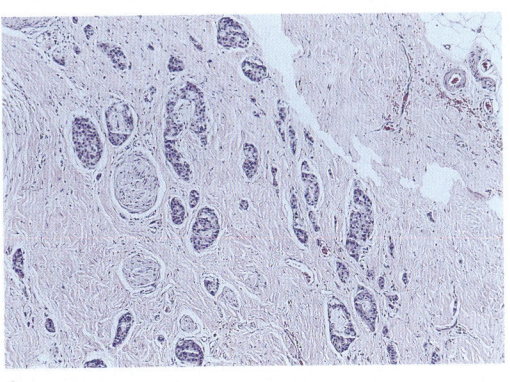
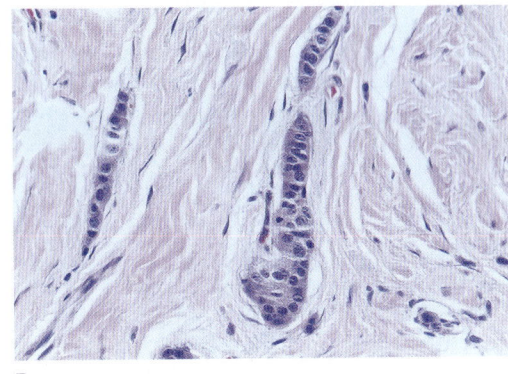

A   B

Figure 26–35. *A*: Hyperplasia of endocrine cells in chronic fibrosing pancreatitis. The cells grow in nests and cords simulating an endocrine neoplasm. *B*: Higher magnification showing the cords of endocrine cells lying in fibrous stroma.

properties and grow in cords simulating a neoplasm (Fig. 26–35). Perineural invasion is occasionally found in these cases. Rarely, this hyperplastic process evolves into a small endocrine tumor.

Nesidioblastosis (also called "endocrine-cell dysplasia" and other terms) is a type of B-cell hyperplasia that causes persistent hyperinsulinemic hypoglycemia in infants. Histologically, nesidioblastosis represents recruitment by budding of ductular cells, which proliferate with the phenotype of insulin-producing neuroendocrine cells, termed "ductuloinsular complexes" (Dahms et al., 1980; Gould et al., 1983; Jaffe et al., 1980). Focal mass lesions, which may be unifocal, adenomatosis-like, adenoma-like, or multifocal, show enlarged islets containing all normal cell types but with increased number and size of B cells. These cases respond to surgical excision of the mass (Goossens et al., 1989). The diffuse adenomatosis form of nesidioblastosis shows hyperplasia or hyperfunction of B cells in all islets. It is treated by near-total pancreatectomy (Goossens et al., 1989; Lloyd et al., 1981). Occasional childhood cases are familial (Vance et al., 1969). However, there is no evidence that either neonatal islet cell hyperplasia or nesidioblastosis progresses to pancreatic endocrine tumors. Rarely, nesidioblastosis occurs in adults, but is usually not functioning and histologic criteria are controversial (Goossens, et al., 1989; Gould et al., 1984).

Islet cell hyperplasia adjacent to endocrine tumors of the pancreas has been reported and may represent a precursor lesion (Larsson, 1978).

MEN I AND SPORADIC PANCREATIC TUMORS

Genetic linkage analysis has located the MEN I gene between D11S480 and D11S460 on chromosome 11q13 (Fujimani et al., 1992). In patients with MEN I, multiple small (0.5 cm or less), clinically silent endocrine pancreatic tumors are common and termed "microadenomatosis" (Thompson et al., 1984). Most of these microadenomas are glucagon and pancreatic polypeptide secreting. If multiple small tumors are found in a patient, MEN I should be suspected (Klöppel et al., 1986). More frequently, in 80% of MEN I cases, a single neoplastic mass of endocrine cells develops whose clinical presentation is determined by the dominant polypeptide hormone secreted or by mass effects if the lesion is nonfunctional. A high rate of 11q13 LOH has been detected in MEN I pancreatic endocrine tumors (Lubensky et al., 1996). In contrast, *Ras* mutations have not been detected in these tumors, suggesting that such mutations do not play a role in the pathogenesis of endocrine pancreatic tumors (Pellegata et al., 1994). Although Zollinger-Ellison syndrome is common in MEN I, the gastrinoma is often duodenal rather than pancreatic. (Padberg et al., 1995; Pipeleers-Marichal et al., 1993). The most common pancreatic endocrine tumor in MEN I is a polypeptide-secreting tumor (Ppoma), followed by glucagonoma, gastrinoma, and insulinoma (Klöppel and Heitz, 1988). Patients with combined clinical syndromes, especially Zollinger-Ellison syndrome and Cushing's syndrome, often have MEN I (Klöppel et al., 1986; Maton et al., 1986; Miyagawa et al., 1988). Pancreatic endocrine tumors have been recorded in patients with the von Hippel–Lindau (VHL) syndrome (Probst et al., 1978) and familial pheochromocytoma (Carney et al., 1980). However, the VHL tumor suppressor gene does not appear to play a pathogenetic role in the development of sporadic endocrine pancreatic tumors (Chung et al., 1997). Allelic deletions and mutations of the MEN I gene have been detected in 15% to 30% of sporadic endocrine pancreatic tumors, suggesting a role in the development of these tumors, especially VIPomas, somatostatinomas, and glucagonomas (Görtz et al., 1999). An allelic loss at chromosome 3p25 may help to distinguish benign from malignant tumors (Chung et al., 1997).

Endocrine tumors of the pancreas are uncommon, accounting for 1% of all pancreatic tumors. Approximately 30% of sporadic tumors show loss of heterozygosity (LOH) at 11q13, supporting the hypothesis that the genetic abnormalities are similar in sporadic and MEN I endocrine pancreatic tumors (Eubanks et al., 1993). Their biologic behavior is often challenging for the pathologist and difficult to predict on histologic grounds alone. Our approach to these tumors is to consider them all as potentially malignant. The two best predictors of clinical behavior are size and functional status. Tumors measuring less than 2 cm seldom metastasize, as exemplified by the clinically nonfunctioning microadenomas of the MEN 1 syndrome and the insulin-producing tumors. On the other hand, pancreatic endocrine tumors greater than 5 cm metastasize more frequently than small tumors. However, one should keep in mind that size is not an absolute criterion of malignancy. Microscopic features that correlate with malignant behavior are extension beyond the pancreas, blood vessel invasion, tumor necrosis, and a high mitotic rate. As a rule, nonfunctioning endocrine tumors are malignant. There have been many studies correlating biologic behavior, with other parameters such as DNA content, proges-

terone receptors, expression of the α-subunit of human chorionic gonadotropin, proliferating cell index, etc., with variable results. In some studies these parameters correlate poorly with prognosis (Bordi et al., 1988; Heitz et al., 1983; Pelosi et al., 1996).

Insulin-secreting B-cell tumors (insulinomas) are the most common functioning pancreatic tumors, followed by gastrinomas, VIPomas, glucagonomas, PPomas, and somatostatinomas.

Pancreatic endocrine tumors are generally circumscribed masses composed of mildly pleomorphic cells with granular amphophilic cytoplasm arranged in cords, sheets, organoid nests, or gyriform or glandular patterns. They frequently have sclerotic stroma, which may contain amyloid (Fig. 26–36). Occasional cases show clear cell or oncocytic changes or mucin production. We have seen two functioning B-cell tumors that contained clusters of goblet cells, representing dual differentiation. Pancreatic endocrine tumors containing acinar cells have also been reported (Klimstra et al., 1994; Schron and Mendelsohn, 1984; Ulich et al., 1982).

Although pancreatic endocrine tumors are usually dominated by a population of cells producing a single hormone, immunohistochemical analysis frequently shows occasional cells that may be neoplastic or entrapped normal cells containing other hormones (Bordi et al., 1987; Fig. 26–37). Occasionally, the clinical syndrome of a patient changes during the course of disease, as when a metastatic focus produces a hormone different from the resected primary (Wynick et al., 1988).

An unusual feature of pancreatic endocrine tumors is the remarkably different risk of malignant behavior (metastasis or extrapancreatic invasion) in tumors producing different hormones: 10% of insulinomas, 60% of gastrinomas, 70% of glucagonomas, and 80% of VIPomas. This difference is partially related to the severity of endocrine symptoms. Insulinomas tend to become clinically manifest at a smaller size on average than the other tumors: 90% are solitary, 70% are less than 1.5 cm in diameter. Glucagonomas that cause the glucagonoma syndrome are usually solitary, large, malignant, and poorly reactive by immunohistochemistry (Hamid et al., 1986), while those not asso-

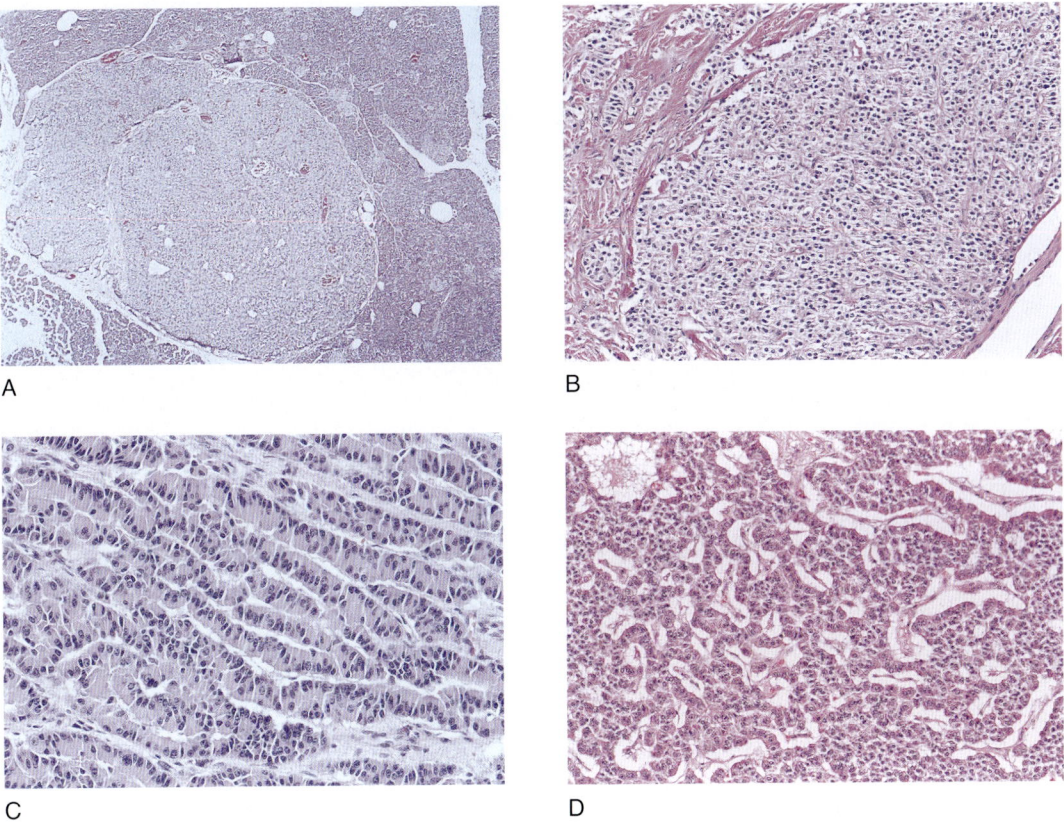

Figure 26–36. Endocrine tumors of the pancreas. *A*: Glucagon-producing microadenoma that gave rise to the glucagonoma syndrome, an exceedingly rare occurrence. *B*: Insulin-producing tumor with a nodular pattern. The nodules recapitulate the structure of the islets. *C*: Somatostatin-producing neoplasm with a cord-like pattern. *D*: Gastrin-producing tumor with anastomosing cell cords.

ciated with the syndrome are often multiple, small, benign, and strongly immunoreactive. However, we have seen a glucagon-producing microadenoma that was associated with the glucagonoma syndrome (Fig. 26–36A).

Gastrinomas associated only with the Zollinger-Ellison syndrome are usually solitary and often malignant, in contrast to the higher likelihood of multifocal benign tumors when MEN I is present (Zollinger, 1985). Occasional gastrinomas are present within peripancreatic lymph nodes. Whether they arise within ectopic islet tissue or represent metastases from occult primary tumors in the pancreas, duodenum, or gastric antrum was controversial until recently (Bhagavan et al., 1986). However, the absence of primary tumors in the pancreas or gastrointestinal tract at autopsy and the return of serum gastrin levels to normal fol-

lowing surgical removal of the lymph nodes strongly supports the view that these gastrin-producing tumors are primary in peripancreatic lymph nodes (Bhagavan et al., 1986). Pancreatic somatostatinomas are usually large and malignant, and they produce the somatostatinoma syndrome. In contrast, somatostatinomas of the duodenum and ampulla of Vater are non-functioning, small and less aggressive and histologically contain gland-like structures and psammoma bodies (Burke et al., 1990; Dayal et al., 1983).

CARCINOID TUMOR AND SMALL CELL CARCINOMA

Carcinoid tumor is defined here as the serotonin-producing neoplasm of the pancreas (Fig. 26–38). Usually no peptide hormones

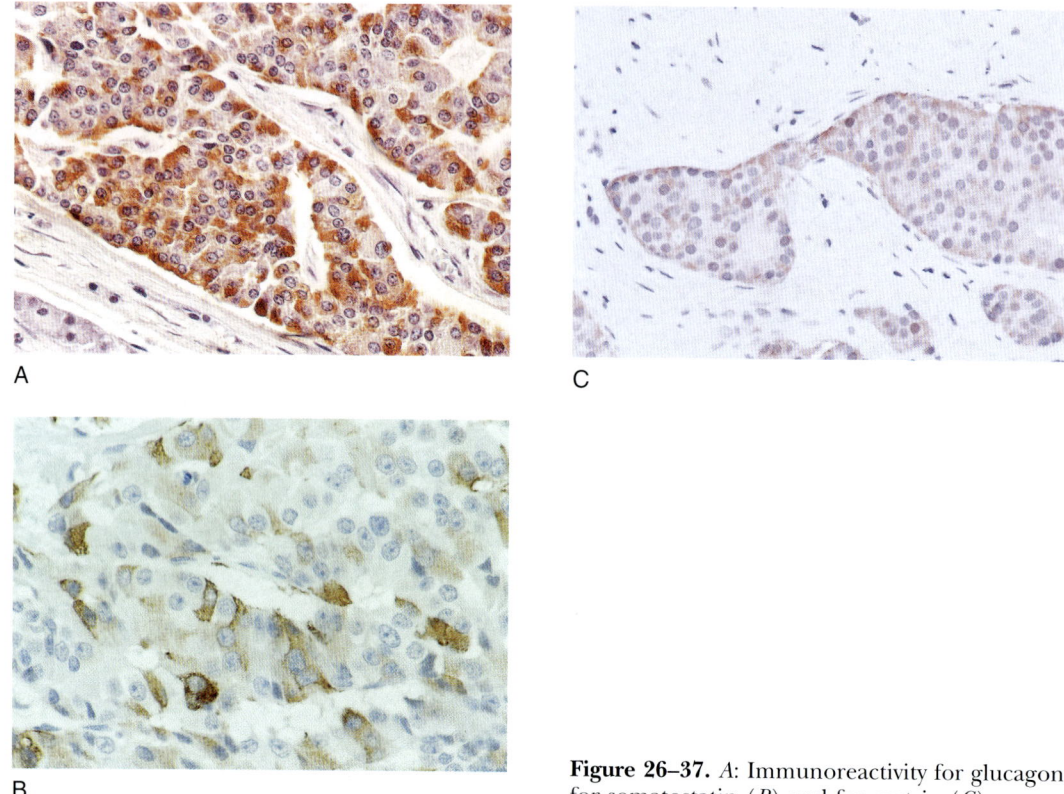

Figure 26–37. *A*: Immunoreactivity for glucagon, for somatostatin (*B*) and for gastrin (*C*).

are demonstrated in tumor cells by immunohistochemistry. Forty-five cases have been reported (Mao et al., 1998). Carcinoid tumors are usually diagnosed late, after they have metastasized (Ordonez et al., 1985). Occasionally, these tumors arise from the main pancreatic duct. Histologically, they

are difficult to separate from other endocrine tumors of the pancreas. The carcinoid syndrome has been reported in patients with liver metastases. In some carcinoid tumors, however, ectopic hormone production has been reported (Berger et al., 1984).

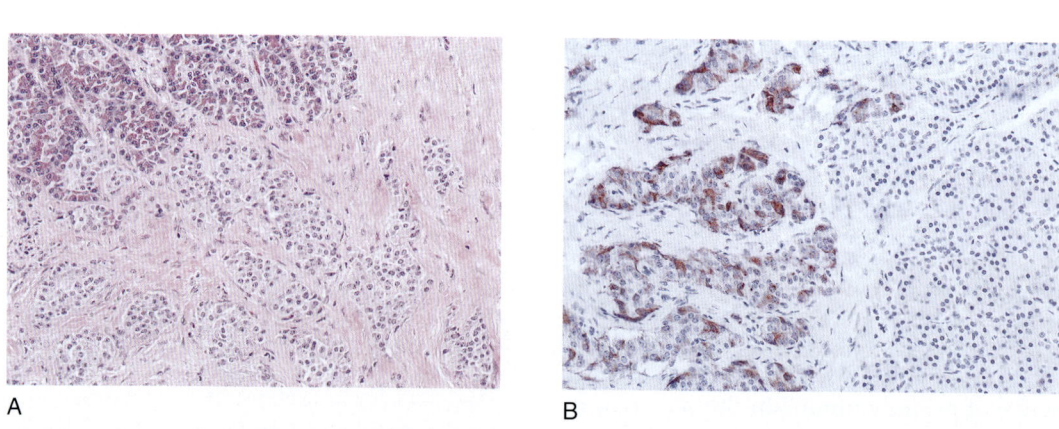

Figure 26–38. Carcinoid tumors that arose in the main pancreatic duct. *A*: Cords of tumor cells are separated by a desmoplastic stroma. *B*: The neoplastic cells are immunoreactive for serotonin.

Small cell carcinomas have been described in the pancreas (O'Connor et al., 1992). They are exceedingly rare, representing 1% of all pancreatic malignant tumors. Their biologic behavior and histologic structure are similar to those of pulmonary small cell carcinoma. Focal positivity for neuron-specific enolase and synaptophysin is seen in most tumors. A case of small cell carcinoma of the pancreas that produced ACTH and another associated with hypercalcemia have been reported (Corrin et al., 1973; Hobbs et al., 1984). We have seen an example of a large cell neuroendocrine carcinoma primary in the pancreas.

REFERENCES

Abbona GC, Papotti M, Gasparri G, Bussolati G. (1995) Proliferative activity in parathyroid tumors as detected by Ki-67 immunostaining. *Hum Pathol* 26:125–138.

Albores-Saavedra J. (1989) Letter to the editor. *Am J Surg Pathol* 13:987–988.

Albores-Saavedra J, Gorraez de la Mora T, De la Torre F, et al. (1990) Mixed medullary papillary carcinoma of the thyroid. *Hum Pathol* 21:1151–1155.

Albores-Saavedra J, Gould E, Vardaman C, Vuitch F. (1991) The macrofollicular variant of papillary thyroid carcinoma. *Hum Pathol* 22:1195–1205.

Albores-Saavedra J, Henson DE, Klimstra D. (2000) *Tumors of the Gallbladder, Extrahepatic Bile Ducts and Ampulla of Vater*, Fascicle 25, Third Series. Armed Forces Institute of Pathology, Washington, DC.

Albores-Saavedra J, Housini I, Vuitch F, Snyder WH. (1997) Macrofollicular variant of papillary thyroid carcinoma with minor insular component. *Cancer* 80:1110–1116.

Albores-Saavedra J, LiVolsi VA, Williams ED. (1985) Medullary carcinoma. *Semin Diagn Pathol* 2:137–150.

Albores-Saavedra J, Monforte H, Nadji M, et al. (1988) C-cell hyperplasia in thyroid tissue adjacent to follicular cell tumors. *Hum Pathol* 19:795–799.

Aldinger KA, Samann NA, Ibanez M, Hill CS Jr. (1978) Anaplastic carcinoma of the thyroid. A review of 84 cases of spindle and giant cell carcinoma of the thyroid. *Cancer* 41:2267–2275.

Allo MD, Thompson NW. (1982) Familial hyperparathyroidism caused by solitary adenomas. *Surgery* 92:486–490.

Amberson JB, Vaughan ED Jr, Gray GF, Naus GJ. (1987) Flow cytometric determination of nuclear DNA content in benign adrenal pheochromocytomas. *Urology* 30:102–104.

Anderson DC, Child DF, Sutcliffe CH, et al. (1978) Cushing's syndrome, nodular adrenal hyperplasia and virilizing carcinoma. *Clin Endocrinol* 9:1–14.

Apel RL, Asa SL, LiVolsi VA. (1995) Papillary Hürthle cell carcinoma with lymphocytic stroma. "Warthin-like" tumor of the thyroid. *Am J Surg Pathol* 19:810–814.

Apel RL, Ezzat S, Bapat BV, et al. (1994) Clonality of thyroid nodules in sporadic goiter. *Diagn Mol Pathol* 4;113–121.

Arias-Stella J, Valcarcel J. (1976) Chief cell hyperplasia in the human carotid body at high altitudes. Physiologic and pathologic significance. *Hum Pathol* 7:361–373.

Asa SL, Kovacs K. (1991) Pathogenesis of endocrine tumors. In: *Functional Endocrine Pathology*, Vol. 2. (Kovacs K, Asa SL, eds.) 1005–1113. Blackwell Scientific Publications, Oxford.

Asa SL, Singer W, Kovacs K, et al. (1987) Pancreatic endocrine tumour producing growth hormone-releasing hormone associated with multiple endocrine neoplasia type I syndrome. *Acta Endocrinol* 115:331–337.

Ashfaq R, Delgado R, Vuitch F, Albores-Saavedra J. (1994) Papillary and follicular thyroid carcinomas with insular component. *Cancer* 73:416–423.

Ballard HS, Frame B, Hartsock RJ. (1964) Familial multiple endocrine adenoma–peptic ulcer complex. *Medicine* 43:481.

Barsano CP, De Groot LJ. (1979) Dyshormonogenetic goiter. *Clin Endocrinol Metab* 8:145–165.

Bartow S, Mukai K, Rosai J. (1981) Pseudoneoplastic proliferation of endocrine cells in pancreatic fibrosis. *Cancer* 47:2627–2633.

Bauman A, Bauman CG. (1982) Virilizing adrenocortical carcinoma. *JAMA* 248:3140–3141.

Baverstock K, Egloff B, Pinchara A, et al. (1992) Thyroid cancer after Chernobyl. *Nature* 359:21–22.

Bergholm U, Bergstrom R, Ekbom A. (1997) Long term follow-up of patients with medullary carcinoma of the thyroid. *Cancer* 79:132–138.

Berger G, Trouillas J, Block B, et al. (1984) Multihormonal carcinoid tumor of the pancreas secreting growth hormone-releasing factor as a cause of acromegaly. *Cancer* 54:2097–2108.

Bhagavan BS, Slavin RE, Goldberg J, et al. (1986) Ectopic gastrinoma and Zollinger-Ellison syndrome. *Hum Pathol* 17:584–592.

Bialestock D. (1961) Hyperplasia of the adrenal medulla in hypertension of children. *Arch Dis Child* 36:465–473.

Biddinger PW, Brennan MF, Rosen PP. (1991) Symptomatic C-cell hyperplasia associated with chronic lymphocytic thyroiditis. *Am J Surg Pathol* 15:599–604.

Bigner SH, Mendelsohn G, Wells SA Jr, et al. (1981) Medullary carcinoma of the thyroid in the multiple endocrine neoplasia IIA syndrome. *Am J Surg Pathol* 5:459–472.

Block MA, Jackson CE, Greenawald KA, et al. (1980) Clinical characteristics distinguishing hereditary from sporadic medullary thyroid carcinoma. Treatment implications. *Arch Surg* 115:142–148.

Bondeson A-G, Bondeson L, Ljungberg O, Tibblin S. (1985) Fat staining in parathyroid disease—diagnostic value and impact on surgical strategy: clinicopathologic analysis of 191 cases. *Hum Pathol* 16:125–126.

Bordi C, De Vita O, Pilato FP, et al. (1987) Multiple islet cell tumors with predominance of glucagon-producing cells and ulcer disease. *Am J Clin Pathol* 88:153–161.

Bordi C, Pilato FP, D'Adda T. (1988) Comparative study of seven neuroendocrine markers in pancreatic endocrine tumours. *Virchows Archiv A Pathol Anat Histopathol* 413:387–398.

Bowlby LS, DeBault LE, Abraham SR. (1986) Flow cytometric analysis of adrenal cortical tumor DNA.

Relationship between cellular DNA and histopathologic classification. *Cancer* 58:1499–1505.

Brandi ML, Aurbach GD, Fitzpatrick LA, et al. (1986) Parathyroid mitogenic activity in plasma from patients with familial endocrine neoplasia, type 1. *N Engl J Med* 314:1287–1293.

Bugg MF, Ribeiro RC, Robertson PK, et al. (1994) Correlation of pathologic features with clinical outcome in pediatric adrenocortical neoplasia. *Am J Clin Pathol* 101:625–629.

Burke AP, Sobin LH, Federspiel BH, et al. (1990) Carcinoid tumors of the duodenum. A clinicopathologic study of 99 cases. *Arch Pathol Lab Med* 114:700–704.

Burke BA, Johnson J, Gilbert E, et al. (1987) Thyrocalcitonin containing cells in the DiGeorge anomaly. *Hum Pathol* 18:355–360.

Burrow GN, Wartzman G, Rewcastle NB, et al. (1981) Microadenomas of the pituitary and abnormal sellar tomograms in an unselected autopsy series. *N Engl J Med* 304:156–158.

Cagle PT, Hough AJ, Pysher TJ, et al. (1986) Comparison of adrenal cortical tumors in children and adults. *Cancer* 57:2235–2237.

Cai WY, Alexander JM, Hedley-White ET, et al. (1994) *Ras* mutations in human prolactinomas and pituitary carcinomas. *J Clin Endocrinol Metab* 78:89–93.

Capella C, Riva C, Cornaggia M. (1988) Histopathology, cytology and cytochemistry of pheochromocytomas and paragangliomas including chemodectomas. *Pathol Res Pract* 183:176–187.

Carcangiu ML, Bianchi S. (1989) Diffuse sclerosing variant of papillary thyroid carcinoma. Clinicopathologic study of 15 cases. *Am J Surg Pathol* 13:1041–1049.

Carcangiu ML, Bianchi S, Savino D, et al. (1991) Follicular Hürthle cell tumors of the thyroid gland. *Cancer* 68:1944–1953.

Carcangiu ML, Sibley RK, Rosai J. (1985a) Clear cell change in primary thyroid tumors. A study of 38 cases. *Am J Surg Pathol* 9:705–722.

Carcangiu ML, Steeper T, Zampi G, Rosai J. (1985b) Anaplastic thyroid carcinoma. A study of 70 cases. *Am J Clin Pathol* 83:135–158.

Carcangiu ML, Zampi G, Rosai J. (1984) Poorly differentiated ("insular") thyroid carcinoma. A reinterpretation of Langhans' "wuchernde struma." *Am J Surg Pathol* 8:655–668.

Carney JA, Go VLW, Gordon H, et al. (1980) Familial pheochromocytoma and islet cell tumor of the pancreas. *Am J Med* 68:515–521.

Carney JA, Gordon H, Carpenter PC, et al. (1985) The complex of myxomas, spotty pigmentation and endocrine overactivity. *Medicine* 64:270–283.

Carney JA, Ryan J, Goellner JR. (1987) Hyalinizing trabecular adenoma of the thyroid gland. *Am J Surg Pathol* 11:583–591.

Carney JA, Sheps SG, Go VLW, Gordon H. (1977) The triad of gastric leiomyosarcoma, functioning extraadrenal paraganglioma and pulmonary chondroma. *N Engl J Med* 296:1517–1518.

Carney JA, Sizemore GW, Hales AB. (1978) Multiple endocrine neoplasia, type 2b. *Patholobiol Annu* 8:105–153.

Carney JA, Sizemore GW, Sheps SG. (1976) Adrenal medullary disease in multiple endocrine neoplasia, type 2. Pheochromocytoma and its precursors. *Am J Clin Pathol* 66:279–290.

Chan JKC, Albores-Saavedra J, Battifora H, et al. (1991) Sclerosing mucoepidermoid thyroid carcinoma with eosinophilia. *Am J Surg Pathol* 15:438–448.

Chandrasekharappa SC, Guru SC, Manickam P, et al. (1997) Positional cloning of the gene for multiple endocrine neoplasia-type I. *Science* 276:404–407.

Chedid A, Jao W. (1974) Hereditary tumors of the carotid bodies and chronic obstructive pulmonary disease. *Cancer* 33:1635–1641.

Chen KTK, Rosai J. (1977) Follicular variant of thyroid papillary carcinoma: a clinicopathologic study of six cases. *Am J Surg Pathol* 1:123–130.

Chung DC, Smith AP, Louis DN, et al. (1997) A novel pancreatic endocrine tumor suppressor gene locus on chromosome 3p with clinical prognostic implications. *J Clin Invest* 100:404–410.

Chung DH, Kang GH, Kim WH, Ro JY. (1999) Clonal analysis of a solitary follicular nodule of the thyroid with the polymerase chain reaction method. *Mod Pathol* 12:265–271.

Civantos F, Albores-Saavedra J, Nadji M, et al. (1984) Clear cell variant of thyroid carcinoma. *Am J Surg Pathol* 8:187–192.

Coburn MC, Wanebo HJ. (1995) Age correlates with increased frequency of high risk factors in elderly patients with thyroid cancer. *Am J Surg* 170:471–475.

Cohen RJ, Brits R, Phillips JI, et al. (1991) Primary hyperaldosteronism due to a functional black (pigmentned) adenoma of the adrenal cortex. *Arch Pathol Lab Med* 115:813–815.

Cooper DS, Axelrod L, DeGroot LJ, et al. (1981) Congenital goiter and the development of metastatic follicular carcinoma with evidence for a leak of nonhormonal iodide. Clinical, pathological, kinetic, and biochemical studies and a review of the literature. *J Clin Endocrinol Metab* 52:294–306.

Copeland PM. (1983) The incidentally discovered adrenal mass. *Ann Intern Med* 98:940–945.

Corrin B, Gilby ED, Jones NF, Patrick J. (1973) Oat cell carcinoma of the pancreas with ectopic ACTH secretion. *Cancer* 31:1523–1527.

Costello RT. (1936) Subclinical adenoma of the pituitary gland. *Am J Pathol* 12:205–215.

Dahms BB, Landing BH, Blaskovics M, Roe TF. (1980) Nesidioblastosis and other islet cell abnormalities in hyperinsulinemic hypoglycemia of childhood. *Hum Pathol* 11:641–649.

Damron TA, Schelper RL, Sorensen L. (1987) Cytochemical demonstration of neuromelanin in black pigmented adrenal nodules. *Am J Clin Pathol* 87:334–341.

Dayal Y, Doos WG, O'Brien MJ, et al. (1983) Psammomatous somatostatinomas of the duodenum. *Am J Surg Pathol* 7:653–665.

DeLellis RA, Wolfe HJ. (1981) Pathobiology of the human calcitonin (C) cell: a review. *Pathol Annu* 16:(part 2):25–52.

DeLellis RA, Wolfe JH, Gagel RF, et al. (1976) Adrenal medullary hyperplasia: a morphometric analysis of patients with familial medullary thyroid carcinomas. *Am J Pathol* 83:177–196.

Driman D, Murray D, Kovacs K, et al. (1991) Encapsulated medullary carcinoma of the thyroid. A morphologic study including immunocytochemistry, electron microscopy, flow cytometry, and in situ hybridization. *Am J Surg Pathol* 15:1089–1095.

Elstar AD. (1993) Modern imaging of the pituitary. *Radiology* 187:1–14.

Erickson LA, Jin L, Wollan P, et al. (1999) Parathyroid hyperplasia, adenomas, and carcinomas. Differential expression of p27^{Kip1} protein. *Am J Surg Pathol* 23:288–295.

Evans H. (1986) Columnar-cell carcinoma of the thyroid. A report of two cases of an aggressive variant of thyroid carcinoma. *Am J Clin Pathol* 85:77–80.

Evans HL. (1984) Follicular neoplasms of the thyroid. *Cancer* 54:535–540.

Evans HL. (1987) Encapsulated papillary neoplasms of the thyroid. A study of 14 cases followed for a minimum of 10 years. *Am J Surg Pathol* 11:592–597.

Evans HL. (1996) Encapsulated columnar-cell neoplasms of the thyroid. A report of four cases suggesting favorable outcome. *Am J Surg Pathol* 20:1205–1211.

Evans HL, Vassilopoulou-Sellin R. (1998) Follicular and Hürthle cell carcinomas of the thyroid. A comparative study. *Am J Surg Pathol* 22:1512–1520.

Ezzat S, Asa SL, Stefaneanu L, et al. (1994) Somatotroph hyperplasia without pituitary adenoma associated with a long standing growth hormone-releasing hormone-producing bronchial carcinoid. *J Clin Endocrinol Metab* 78:555–560.

Favara BE, Steele A, Grant JH, et al. (1991) Adrenal cytomegaly: quantitative assessment by image analysis. *Pediatr Pathol* 11:521–536.

Farbota LM, Calandra DB, Lawrence AM, Paloyan E. (1985) Thyroid carcinoma in Graves' disease. *Surgery* 98:1148–1152.

Ferreiro JA, Hay ID, Lloyd RV. (1996) Columnar cell carcinoma of the thyroid: report of three additional cases. *Hum Pathol* 27:1156–1160.

Fialkow PJ, Jackson CE, Block MA, Greenwald KA. (1977) Multicellular origin of parathyroid "adenomas." *N Engl J Med* 297:696–698.

Fink M, Weinhäusel A, Niederle B, et al. (1996) Distinction between sporadic and medullary thyroid carcinoma by mutation analysis of the RET protooncogene. *Int J Cancer* 69:312–316.

Fitko R, Roth SI, Hines JR, et al. (1990) Parathyromatosis in hyperparathyroidism. *Hum Pathol* 21: 234–237.

Fogt F, Vargas P, Zhuang Z, et al. (1998) Utilization of molecular genetics in the differentiation between adrenal cortical adenomas and carcinomas. *Hum Pathol* 28:518–521.

Franssila KO, Ackerman LV, Brown CL, Hedinger CE. (1985) Follicular carcinoma. *Semin Diagn Pathol* 2:101–122.

Friedman E, Sakaguchi K, Bale AE, et al. (1989) Clonality of parathyroid tumors in familial multiple endocrine neoplasia type I. *N Engl J Med* 321:213–218.

Fujimari M, Wells SA Jr, Nakamura Y. (1992) Fine scale mapping of the gene responsible for multiple endocrine neoplasia type I (MEN1) *Am J Hum Genet* 50:399–403.

Fujimoto Y, Obata T, Ito Y, et al. (1990) Diffuse sclerosing variant of papillary carcinoma of the thyroid. *Cancer* 66:2306–2312.

Fukunaga FH, Yatani R. (1975) Geographic pathology of occult thyroid carcinomas. *Cancer* 36:1095–1099.

Galluzzi MC, Kwan P, DeLlelis RA. (1994) Proliferative activity of papillary carcinoma of the thyroid. An immunohistochemical study. *Lab Invest* 70:53A.

Gamboa-Dominguez A, Candenado F, Vieitz-Martinez J, et al. (1996) Macrofollicular variant of papillary thyroid carcinoma. *Endocr Pathol* 7:303–308.

Gandour MJ, Grizzle WE. (1986) A small adrenocortical carcinoma with aggressive behavior. An evaluation of criteria for malignancy. *Arch Pathol Lab Med.* 110:1076–1079.

Ghandur-Mnaymneh L, Kimura N. (1984) The parathyroid adenoma: a histopathologic definition with a study of 172 cases of primary hyperparathyroidism. *Am J Pathol* 115:70–83.

Ghossein RA, Rosai J, Heffess C. (1998) Dyshormonogenetic goiter: a clinicopathologic study of 56 cases. *Endocrine Pathol* 4:283–292, 1998.

Gibson WCH, Peng TC, Croker BP. (1980) C cell nodules in adult human thyroid: a common autopsy finding. *Am J Clin Pathol* 73:347–351.

Gold EB. (1981) Epidemiology of pituitary adenomas. *Epidemiol Rev* 3:163–183.

Goossens A, Gepts W, Saudubray J-M, et al. (1989) Diffuse and focal nesidioblastosis: a clinicopathological study of 24 patients with persistent neonatal hyperinsulinemic hypoglycemia. *Am J Surg Pathol* 13:766–775.

Gorlin RJ, Sedano HO, Vickers RA, Cervenka J. (1968) Multiple mucosal neuromas, pheochromocytoma and medullary carcinoma of thyroid. A syndrome. *Cancer* 22:293–299.

Görtz B, Roth J, Krähenmann A, et al. (1999) Mutations and allelic deletions of the MEN I gene are associated with a subset of sporadic endocrine pancreatic and neuroendocrine tumors and not restricted to foregut neoplasms. *Am J Pathol* 154:429–436.

Gould E, Albores-Saavedra J, Shuman J. (1987) Pituitary prolactinoma, pancreatic glucagonoma, aldosterone-producing adrenal cortical adenoma: a suggested variant of multiple endocrine neoplasia type I. *Hum Pathol* 18:1290–1293.

Gould VE, Chejfec G, Shah K, et al. (1984) Adult nesidiodysplasia. *Semin Diagn Pathol* 1:43–52.

Gould VE, Memoli VA, Dardi LE, Gould NS. (1983) Nesidiodysplasia and nesidioblastosis of infancy: structural and functional correlations with the syndrome of hyperinsulinemic hypoglycemia. *Pediatr Pathol* 1: 7–31.

Grant CS. (1995) Operative and postoperative management of the patient with follicular and Hürthle cell carcinoma. Do they differ? *Surg Clin North Am* 75:395–403.

Griffiths DFR, Williams GT, Williams ED. (1983) Multiple endocrine neoplasia associated with von Recklinghausen's disease. *BMJ* 287:1341–1343.

Grimelius L, Åkerström G, Johansson H, Juhlin C, Rastad J. (1991) The parathyroid glands. In: *Functional Endocrine Pathology*, Vol. 1 (Kovacs K, Asa SL, eds.) pp. 375–395. Blackwell Scientific Publications, Oxford.

Grimelius L, Hultquist G, Stenquist B. (1975) Cytological differentiation of asymptomatic pancreatic islet cell tumors in autopsy material. *Virchows Arch A Pathol Anat Histopathol* 365:275–288.

Gross MD, Wilton GP, Shapiro B, et al. (1987) Functional and scintigraphic evaluation of the silent adrenal mass. *J Nucl Med* 28:1401–1407.

Guyetant S, et al. (1999) Medullary thyroid microcarcinoma. A clinicopathologic retrospective study of 38 patients with no prior familial disease. *Hum. Pathol.* 30:957–963.

Haak HR, Cornelisse CJ, Hermaus J, et al. (1993) Nuclear DNA content and morphologic characteristics in the prognosis of adrenocortical carcinoma. *Br J Cancer* 68:151–155.

Haghighi P, Astartia R, Wepsic H, et al. (1983) Concurrent primary parathyroid hyperplasia and parathyroid carcinoma. *Arch Pathol Lab Med* 107:349–350.

Hamid QA, Bishop AE, Sikri KL, et al. (1986) Immunocytochemical characterization of 10 pancreatic tumours, associated with the glucagonoma syndrome, using antibodies to separate regions of the proglucagon molecule and other neuroendocrine markers. *Histopathology* 10:119–133.

Harach HR, Escalante DA, Onativia A, et al. (1985a) Thyroid carcinoma and thyroiditis in an endemic goitre region before and after iodine prophylaxis. *Acta Endocrinol* 108:55–60.

Harach HR, Franssila KO, Wasenius V. (1985b) Occult papillary carcinoma of the thyroid: a "normal" finding in Finland. A systematic autopsy study. *Cancer* 56:531–538.

Harada T, Shimoaka K, Katagin M, et al. (1994) Rarity of squamous cell carcinoma of the thyroid. *World J Surg* 18:542–546.

Hartley AL, Birch JM, Marsden HB, et al. (1987) Adrenal cortical tumours: epidemiological and familial aspects. *Arch Dis Child* 62:683–689.

Hawkins E, Singer DB. (1976) The adrenal cortex in cystic fibrosis in the pancreas. *Am J Clin Pathol* 66:710–714.

Hay ID, Bergstralh EJ, Ebersold JR, et al. (1993) Predicting outcome in papillary thyroid carcinoma. Development of a reliable prognostic scoring system in a cohort of 1779 patients surgically treated at one institution during 1940 through 1989. *Surgery* 114:1050–1058.

Hazard B, Kenyon R. (1954) Encapsulated angioinvasive carcinoma (angioinvasive adenoma) of thyroid gland. *Am J Clin Pathol* 24:755.

Hedinger C, Williams ED, Sobin LH. (1988) *Histological Typing of Thyroid Tumors*. World Health Organization. Springer-Verlag, Berlin.

Heitz PU, Kasper M, Klöppel G, et al. (1983) Glycoprotein-hormone alpha-chain production by pancreatic endocrine tumours: a specific marker for malignancy. Immunocytochemical analysis of tumours of 155 patients. *Cancer* 51:277–278.

Hermus AR, Pieters GF, Smals AG, et al. (1988) Transition from pituitary-dependent to adrenal-dependent Cushing's syndrome. *N Engl J Med* 318:966–970.

Heufelder AE, Hay ID. (1994) Evidence of autoimmune mechanisms in the evolution of invasive fibrous thyroiditis (Reidel's struma). *Clin Invest* 72:788–793.

Hicks DG, LiVolsi VA, Neidich JA, et al. (1989) Solitary follicular nodules of the thyroid are monoclonal proliferations. *Lab Invest* 60:40A.

Hobbs RD, Stewart AF, Ravin ND, Carter D. (1984) Hypercalcemia in small cell carcinoma of the pancreas. *Cancer* 53:1552–1553.

Hofstadter F. (1980) Frequency and morphology of malignant tumours of the thyroid before and after the introduction of iodine prophylaxis. *Virchows Arch A Pathol Anat Histopathol* 385:263–270.

Hofstra RMW, Landsvater RM, Ceccherine I, et al. (1994) A mutation in the RET protooncogene associated with multiple endocrine neoplasia type 2b and sporadic medullary thyroid carcinoma. *Nature* 367:375–376.

Horvath E, Kovacs K. (1988) Pituitary gland. *Pathol Res Pract* 183:129–142.

Horvath E, Kovacs K. (1991) The adenohypophysis. In: *Functional Endocrine Pathology*, Vol. 1. (Kovacs K, Asa SL, eds.) pp. 245–281. Blackwell Scientific Publications, Oxford.

Hosaka Y, Rainwater LM, Grant CS, et al. (1986) Pheochromocytoma: nuclear deoxyribonucleic acid patterns studied by flow cytometry. *Surgery* 100:1003–1010.

Hosaka Y, Rainwater LM, Grant CS, et al. (1987) Adrenocortical carcinoma: nuclear deoxyribonucleic acid ploidy studied by flow cytometry. *Surgery* 102:1027.

Hough AJ, Holifield JW, Page DL, et al. (1979) Prognostic factors in adrenal cortical tumors. *Am J Clin Pathol* 72:390–399.

Hundahl SA, Fleming ID, Gremgen AM, Menck HR. (1999) Two hundred eighty-six cases of parathyroid carcinoma treated in the US between 1985–1995. *Cancer* 86:538–544.

Ibanez ML, Russell WO, Albores-Saavedra J, et al. (1966) Thyroid carcinoma. Biologic behavior and mortality. *Cancer* 19:1039–1052.

Iseli BE, Hedinger CE. (1985) Histopathology and ultrastructure of primary adrenocortical nodular dysplasia with Cushing's syndrome. *Histopathology* 9:1171–1193.

Jaffe R, Hashida Y, Yunis EJ. (1980) Pancreatic pathology in hyperinsulinemic hypoglycemia of infancy. *Lab Invest* 42:356–365.

Joensuu H, Klemi PJ. (1988) DNA aneuploidy in adenomas of endocrine organs. *Am J Pathol* 132:145–151.

Johnston TL, Lloyd RV, Thompson NW, et al. (1988) Prognostic implications of the tall cell variant of papillary thyroid carcinoma. *Am J Surg Pathol* 12:22–27.

Kahn N, Perzin KH. (1983) Follicular carcinoma of the thyroid: an evaluation of the histologic criteria used for diagnosis. *Pathol Annu* 18(Part 1):221–253.

Kakudo K, Carney JA, Sizemore GW. (1985) Medullary carcinoma of thyroid. Biologic behavior of the sporadic and familial neoplasm. *Cancer* 55:2818–2821.

Kane LA, Leinung MC, Scheithauer BW, et al. (1994) Pituitary adenomas in childhood and adolescence. *J Clin Endocrinol Metab* 79:1135–1140.

Kaserer K, Scheuba C, Neuhold N, et al. (1998) C-cell hyperplasia and medullary thyroid carcinoma in patients routinely screened for serum calcitonin. *Am J Surg Pathol* 22:722–728.

Kazakov VS, Demidchik EP, Astakhova LN. (1992) Thyroid cancer after Chernobyl. *Nature* 359:21.

Khalil A, Kovacs K, Sima AA, Burrow GN, Horvath E. (1984) Pituitary thyrotroph hyperplasia mimicking prolactin-secreting adenoma. *J Endocrinol Invest* 7:399–404.

King DR, Lack EE. (1979) Adrenal cortical carcinoma. A clinical and pathologic study of 49 cases. *Cancer* 44:239–244.

Klimstra DS, Rosai J, Heffess CS. (1994) Mixed acinar endocrine carcinomas of the pancreas. *Am J Surg Pathol* 18:765–778.

Klöppel G, Bommer G, Commandeur G, Heitz PU. (1978) The endocrine pancreas in chronic pancreatitis. Immunocytochemical and ultrastructural studies. *Virchows Arch A Pathol Anat Histopathol* 377: 157–174.

Klöppel G, Heitz PU. (1988) Pancreatic endocrine tumors. *Path Res Pract* 183:155–168.

Klöppel G, In't Veld PA, Stamm B, Heitz PU. (1991) The endocrine pancreas. In: *Functional Endocrine Pathology*, Vol. 1 (Kovacs K, Asa SL, eds.) pp. 396–457. Blackwell Scientific Publications, Oxford.

Klöppel G, Willemer S, Stamm B, et al. (1986) Pancreatic lesions and hormonal profile of pancreatic tumors in multiple endocrine neoplasia type I. An immunocytochemical study of nine patients. *Cancer* 57:1824–1832.

Kopp P, Kimura ET, Aeschimann S, et al. (1994) Polyclonal and monoclonal thyroid nodules coexist within human multinodular goiter. *J Clin Endocrinol Metal* 79:90134–90139.

Koss LG, Woyke W, Olszewski W. (1984) The thyroid. In: *Aspiration Biopsy, Cytologic Interpretation and Histologic Bases* (Koss LG, ed.) pp. 154–190. Igaku-Shoin, New York.

Kovacs K, Horvath E. (1986) Tumors of the pituitary gland. Atlas of Tumor Pathology. 2nd series. Fascicle 21. Washington DC. Armed Forces Institute of Pathology.

Kotzman H, Schmidt A, Scheuba C et al. (1999) Based calcitonin levels and the response to pentagastrin stimulation in patients after kidney transplantation or on chronic hemodialysis as indicators of medullary carcinoma. Thyroid 9:943–947.

Kovacs K, Horvath E, Feldman PS. (1976) Pigmented adenoma of adrenal cortex associated with Cushing's syndrome: light and electron microscopic study. *Urology* 7:641–645.

Kramer WM. (1970) Association of parathyroid hyperplasia with neoplasia. *Am J Clin Pathol* 53:275–283.

Krueger JE, Martra A, Albores-Saavedra J. (2000) Inherited medullary microcarcinoma of the thyroid. *Am J Surg Pathol*. In press.

Kubota T, Hayashi M, Kabuto M, et al. (1992) Cortocotroph cell hyperplasia in a patient with Addison disease: case report. *Surg Neurol* 37:441–447.

Lack EE. (1977) Carotid body by putrophy in patients with cystic fibrosis and cyanotic congenital heart disease. Hum. Pathol. 8:39–51.

Lack EE. (1978) Hyperplasia of vagal and carotid body paraganglia in patients with chronic hypoxemia. *Am J Pathol* 91:497–516.

Lack EE. (1990) Adrenal medullary hyperplasia and pheochromocytoma. In *Pathology of the Adrenal Glands. Contemporary Issues in Surgical Pathology*, Vol. 14 (Lack EE, ed.) pp. 173–236. Churchill Livingstone, New York.

Lack EE. (1997) Tumors of the adrenal gland and extra-adrenal paraganglia. In: *Atlas of Tumor Pathology*, Fascicle 19, Third series. Armed Forces Institute of Pathology, Washington, DC.

Lack EE, Mulvihill JJ, Travis WD, Kozakewich HPW. (1992) Adrenal cortical neoplasms in the pediatric and adolescent age group. Clinicopathologic study of 30 cases with emphasis on epidemiological and prognostic factors. *Pathol Annu* 27(part 1):1–53.

Lack EE, Travis WD, Oertel JE. (1990) Adrenal cortical nodules, hyperplasia, and hyperfunction. Adrenal cortical neoplasms. In: *Pathology of the Adrenal Glands and Contemporary Issues in Surgical Pathology*, Vol. 14 (Lack EE, ed.), pp. 75–113 and 115–171. Churchill Livingstone, New York.

Lam AKY, Montone KT, Nolan KA, et al. (1998) Ret oncogene activation in papillary thyroid carcinoma: prevalence and implication on the histological parameters. *Hum Pathol* 29:565–568.

Lambers SWJ, Stefanko SZ, deLange SA, et al. (1980) Failure of clinical remission after transsphenoidal removal of a microadenoma in a patient with Cushing's disease: multiple hyperplastic and adenomatous cell nets in surrounding pituitary tissue. *J Clin Endocrinol Metab* 50:793–795.

Lang W, Borrusch H, Bauer L. (1988) Occult carcinomas of the thyroid: evaluation of 1,020 sequential autopsies. *Am J Clin Pathol* 90:72–76.

Lang W, Choritz H, Hundeshagen H. (1986) Risk factors in follicular thyroid carcinomas: a retrospective follow-up study covering a 14-year period with emphasis on morphological findings. *Am J Surg Pathol* 10:246–255.

Lang W, Georgii A, Stauch G, Kienzle E. (1980) The differentiation of atypical adenomas and encapsulated follicular carcinomas in the thyroid gland. *Virchows Arch A Pathol Anat Histopathol* 385:125–141.

Larraza-Hernandez O, Albores-Saavedra J, Benavides G, et al. (1982) Pituitary adenoma, multicentric papillary thyroid carcinoma, bilateral carotid body paraganglioma, parathyroid hyperplasia, gastric leiomyoma, and systemic amyloidosis. *Am J Clin Pathol* 78:527–532.

Larsson LI. (1978) Endocrine pancreatic tumors. *Hum Pathol* 9:401–411.

Levin KE, Galante M, Clark OH. (1987) Parathyroid carcinoma versus parathyroid adenoma in patients with profound hypercalcemia. *Surgery* 101:649–660.

Levine JH, Sagel J, Rosebrock G et al. (1979) Prolactin-secreting adenoma as part of the multiple endocrine neoplasia type I (MEN-I) syndrome. *Cancer* 43:2492–2496.

Li M, Carcangiu ML, Rosai J. (1997) Abnormal intracellular and extracellular distribution of basement membrane material in papillary carcinoma and trabecular tumors of the thyroid. Implications for deregulation of secretory pathways. *Hum Pathol* 28:1366–1372.

Libbey NP, Nowakowski KJ, Tucci JR. (1989) C cell hyperplasia of the thyroid in a patient with goitrous hypothyroidism and Hashimoto's thyroiditis. *Am J Surg Pathol* 13:71–77.

Lin BTY, Bonsib SM, Mierau GW, et al. (1998) Oncocytic adrenocortical neoplasms. *Am J Surg Pathol* 22:603–614.

Lindsay S. (1960) *Carcinoma of the Thyroid Gland. A Clinical and Pathologic Study of 293 Patients at the University of California Hospital*. Charles C. Thomas, Springfield, IL.

Linnoila RI, Lack EE, Steinberg SM, Keiser HR. (1988) Decreased expression of neuropeptides in malignant paragangliomas. An immunohistochemical study. *Hum Pathol* 19:41–50.

Lips CJM, Landsvater RM, Höppener JWM, et al. (1994) Clinical screening as compared with DNA analysis in families with multiple endocrine neoplasia type IIa. *N Engl J Med* 331:828–835.

Lips CJM, Leo JR, Berends MJ, et al. (1987) Thyroid C cell hyperplasia and micronodules in close relative of MEN-2A patients: pitfalls in early diagnosis and reevaluation of criteria for surgery. *Henry Ford Hosp Med J* 35:133–138.

LiVolsi VA. (1990) Follicular lesions of the thyroid. In:

Surgical Pathology of the Thyroid (LiVolsi VA, ed.) pp. 173–212, W.B. Saunders, Philadelphia.

Lloyd RV. (1995) Ret proto-oncogene mutations and rearrangements in endocrine diseases. *Am J Pathol* 147:1539–1544.

Lloyd RV, Caceres V, Warner TFCS, Gilbert EF. (1981) Islet cell adenomatosis. A report of two cases and review of the literature. *Arch Pathol Lab Med* 105:198–202.

Lloyd RV, Carney JA, Ferreiro JA, et al. (1995) Immunohistochemical analysis of the cell cycle–associated protein in parathyroid carcinomas and adenomas. *Endocr Pathol* 6:279–287.

Lloyd RV, Chandler WF, McKeever PE, Schteingart DE. (1986) The spectrum of ACTH-producing pituitary lesions. *Am J Surg Pathol* 10:618–626.

Lubensky IA, Debelenko LV, Zhuang Z, et al. (1996) Allelic deletions on chromosome 11q13 in multiple tumors from individuals MEN1 patients. *Cancer Res* 56:5272–5278.

Lynch HT, Katz DA, Bogard PJ, et al. (1985) The sarcoma, breast cancer, lung cancer and adrenocortical carcinoma syndrome revisited. Childhood cancer. *Am J Dis Child* 139:134–136.

Mallette LE, Bilezikian JP, Ketcham AS, Aurbach GD. (1974) Parathyroid carcinoma in familial hyperparathyroidism. *Am J Med* 57:642–648.

Mao C, et Attar A, Domenico DR, et al. (1998) Carcinoid tumors of the pancreas. Status report based on two cases and review of the world's literature. *Int J Pancreatol* 23:153–164.

Mastronardi L, Guiducci A, Spera C, et al. (1999) Ki-67 labelling index and invasiveness among anterior pituitary adenomas: analysis of 103 cases using MIB-1 monoclonal antibody. *J Clin Pathol* 52:107–111.

Mathew CGP, Chin KS, Easton DF, et al. (1987) A linked genetic marker for multiple endocrine neoplasia type 2A on chromosome 10. *Nature* 328:527–528.

Maton PN, Gardner JD, Jensen RT. (1986) Cushing's syndrome in patients with the Zollinger-Ellison syndrome. *N Engl J Med* 315:1–5.

Matos PS, Bisi H, Medeiros-Neto GS. (1994) Dyshormonogenetic goiter: a morphological and immunohistochemical study. *Endocr Pathol* 5:49–58.

McComb DJ, Ryan N, Horvath E, et al. (1983) Subclinical adenomas of the human pituitary. New light on old problems. *Arch Pathol Lab Med* 107:488–491.

McDonald MP, Sanders LE, Silverman ML, et al. (1996) Hürthle cell carcinoma of the thyroid. *Surgery* 120:1000–1005.

McKeever PE, Koppelman MCS, Metcalf D, et al. (1982) Refractory Cushing's disease caused by multinodular ACTH-cell hyperplasia. *J Neuropathol Exp Neurol* 41:490–499.

McKeown PP, McGarity WC, Sewell CW. (1984) Carcinoma of the parathyroid gland: is it overdiagnosed? A report of three cases. *Am J Surg* 147:292–298.

Medeiros LJ, Wolf B, Balogh K, Federman M. (1985) Adrenal pheochromocytoma: a clinicopathologic review of 60 cases. *Hum Pathol* 16:580–589.

Mendelsohn G, Oertel JE. (1981) Encapsulated medullary thyroid carcinoma. *Lab Invest* 44:43A.

Mendelsohn G, Wells SA, Baylin SB. (1984) Relationship of tissue carcinoembryonic antigen and calcitonin to tumor virulence in medullary thyroid carcinoma. An immunohistochemical study in early, localized and virulent disseminated stages of disease. *Cancer* 54:657–662.

Meyer JS, Steinberg LS. (1969) Microscopically benign thyroid follicles in cervical lymph nodes. Serial section study of lymph nodes inclusions and entire thyroid gland in 5 cases. *Cancer* 24:302–311.

Miyagawa K, Ishibashi M, Kasuga M, et al. (1988) Multiple endocrine neoplasia type 1 with Cushing's disease, primary hyperparathyroidism and insulinglucagonoma. *Cancer* 61:1232–1236.

Mizukami Y, Michigishi T, Kawato M, et al. (1992) Chronic thyroiditis: thyroid function and histologic correlations in 601 cases. *Hum Pathol* 23:980–988.

Molberg K, Albores-Saavedra J. (1994) Hyalinizing trabecular carcinoma of the thyroid gland. *Hum Pathol* 26:192–197.

Moran CA, Albores-Saavedra J, Wenig BM, Mena H. (1997) Pigmented extraadrenal paragliomas. A clinicopathologic and immunohistochemical study of five cases. *Cancer* 79:398–402.

Moran A, Asa SL, Kovacs K, et al. (1990) Gigantism due to pituitary mammosomatotroph hyperplasia. *N Engl J Med* 323:322–327.

Morris TA, Tymms DJ. (1980) Oat cell carcinoma, pheochromocytoma and carcinoid tumors—multiple APUD cell neoplasia—a case report. *J Pathol* 313:107–115.

Mountcastle RB, Roof BS, Mayfield RK, et al. (1989) Case report: pituitary adenocarcinoma in an acromegalic patient. Response to bromocriptine and pituitary testing. A review of the literature on 36 cases of pituitary carcinoma. *Am J Med Sci* 298:109–118.

Mukai K. (1983) Functional pathology of pancreatic islets. Immunocytochemical exploration. *Pathol Annu* 18(Part 2):87–107.

Naeye RL. (1976) Brain-stem and adrenal abnormalities in the sudden infant-death syndrome. *Am J Clin Pathol* 66:526–530.

Nakamura T, Mariyama S, Sano K, et al. (1998) Macrofollicular variant of papillary thyroid carcinoma. *Pathol Int* 48:467–470.

Namba H, Fagin JA. (1989) Clonal origin of human thyroid tumors. Determination by X-chromosome inactivation analysis. *Clin Res* 37:108A.

Nathan DM, Daniels GH, Ridgway EC. (1980) Gastrinoma and phaeochromocytoma: is there a mixed multiple endocrine adenoma syndrome? *Acta Endocrinol* 93:91–93.

Neville AM, O'Hare MJ. (1985) Histopathology of the human adrenal cortex. *Clin Endocrinol Metab* 14:791–820.

Nicolis E, Shimshi M, Allen C, et al. (1988) Gonadotropin-producing pituitary adenoma in a man with long-standing primary hypogonadism. J Clin Endocrinol Metab 66:237–241.

Nikiforov Y, Gnepp DR. (1994) Pediatric thyroid cancer after the Chernobyl disaster: pathomorphologic study of 84 cases (1991–1992) from the Republic of Belarus. *Cancer* 74:748–766.

Nikiforov YE, Heffess CS, Korzenko AV, et al. (1995) Characteristics of follicular tumors and nonneoplastic thyroid lesions in children and adolescents exposed to radiation as a result of the Chernobyl disaster. *Cancer* 76:900–909.

Nissenblatt MJ. (1978) Cyanotic heart disease: low altitude risk from carotid body tumor. *J Hosp Med J* 142:12–21.

Obara T, Fujimoto Y, Kanaji Y, et al. (1990) Flow cytometric DNA analysis of parathyroid tumors. *Cancer* 66:1555–1562.

O'Connor TP, Wade TP, Sunwoo YC, et al. (1992) Small

cell undifferentiated carcinoma of the pancreas. Report of a patient with tumor marker studies. *Cancer* 70:1514–1519.

O'Hare MJ, Monaghan P, Neville AM. (1979) The pathology of adrenocortical neoplasia: a correlated structural and functional approach to the diagnosis of malignant disease. *Hum Pathol* 10:137–154.

Olson JL, Salyer WR. (1978) Mediastinal paragangliomas (aortic body tumor). A report of four cases and a review of the literature. *Cancer* 41:2405–2412.

Ordonez NG, Manning JT, Raymond AK. (1985) Argentaffin endocrine carcinoma (carcinoid) of the pancreas with concomitant breast metastasis: an immunohistochemical and electron microscopic study. *Hum Pathol* 16:746–751.

Orland SM, Stewart AF, LiVolsi VA, et al. (1968) Detection of the hypercalcemic hormone of malignancy in adrenal cortical carcinoma. *J Urol* 136: 1000–1002.

Ostrowski ML, Merino MJ. (1996) Tall cell variant of papillary thyroid carcinoma. *Am J Surg Pathol* 20: 964–974.

O'Toole K, Fenoglio-Preiser C, Pushparaj N. (1985) Endocrine changes associated with the human aging process. III. Effect of age on the number of calcitonin immunoreactive cells in the thyroid gland. *Hum Pathol* 16:991–1000.

Ott RA, Calandra DB, McCall A, et al. (1985) The incidence of thyroid carcinoma in patients with Hashimoto's thyroiditis and solitary cold nodules. *Surgery* 98:1202–1206.

Ozaki O, Ito K, Mimura T, et al. (1994) Thyroid carcinoma after radioactive iodine therapy for Graves' disease. *World J Surg* 18:518–521.

Padberg BC, Garbe E, Achilles E, et al. (1990) Adrenomedullary hyperplasia and pheochromocytoma. DNA cytophotometric findings in 47 cases. *Virchows Arch A Pathol Anat Histopathol* 416:443–446.

Padberg B, Schröder S, Capella C, et al. (1995) Multiple endocrine neoplasia type 1 (MEN 1) revisited. *Virchows Arch* 426:541–548.

Parent AD, Brown B, Smith EE. (1982) Incidental pituitary adenomas: a retrospective study. *Surgery* 92: 880–883.

Pei L, Melmed S, Schithauer B, et al. (1994) H-ras mutations in human pituitary carcinoma metastases. *J Clin Endocrinol Metab* 78:842–846.

Pelosi G, Bresaola E, Bogina G, et al. (1996) Endocrine tumors of the pancreas. Ki-67 immunoreactivity on paraffin sections is an independent predictor for malignancy: a comparative study with proliferating-cell nuclear antigen and progesterone receptor protein immunostaining, mitotic index, and other clinicopathologic variables. *Hum Pathol* 27:1124–1134.

Pellegata NS, Sissa F, Renault B, et al. (1994) K ras and p53 gene mutation in pancreatic cancer: ductal and nonductal tumors progress through different genetic lesions. *Cancer Res* 54:1556–1560.

Peng TC, Cooper CW, Elks ML, et al. (1977) Thyrocalcitonin (TCT) in rats chronically treated with propylthiouracil (PTU). *Fed Proc* 36:985.

Pernicone PJ, Scheithauer BW, Sebo TJ, et al. (1997) Pituitary carcinoma. A clinicopathologic study of 15 cases. *Cancer* 79:804 812.

Perry A, Molberg K, Albores-Saavedra J. (1996) Physiologic versus neoplastic C-cell hyperplasia of the thyroid. *Cancer* 77:750–756.

Pipeleers-Marichal M, Donow C, Heitz PU, Klöppel G. (1993) Pathologic aspects of gastrinomas in patients with Zollinger-Ellison syndrome with and without multiple endocrine neoplasia type I. *World J Surg* 17:481–488.

Probst A, Lotz M, Heitz PU. (1978) Von Hippel–Lindau's disease, syringomyelia and multiple endocrine tumors: a complex neuroendocrinopathy. *Virchows Arch. A Pathol Anat Histopathol* 378:265–272.

Puebltz S, Weinberg AG, Albores-Saavedra J. (1993) Thyroid C-cells in the DiGeorge anomaly. A quantitative study. *Pedriat Pathol* 13:463–473.

Raafat F, Salman WD, Roberts K, et al. (1986) Carney's triad. Gastric leiomyosarcoma, pulmonary chondroma and extra-adrenal paraganglioma in young females. *Histopathology* 10:1325–1333.

Rodriguez-Cuevas H, Lau I, Rodriguez HP. (1986) High-altitude paragangliomas. Diagnostic and therapeutic considerations. *Cancer* 57:672–676.

Rosai J, Carcangiu ML. (1984) Pathology of thyroid tumors: some recent and old questions. *Hum Pathol* 15:1008–1012.

Rosai J, Albores-Saavedra J, Battifora H. (1987) Sclerosing squamous tumor of the thyroid with eosinophilic infiltration arising in Hashimoto's thyroiditis. Report of 4 cases of a distinct tumor entity. *Lab Invest* 56:66A.

Rosai J, Saxén EA, Woolner L. (1985) Undifferentiated and poorly differentiated carcinoma. *Semin Diagn Pathol* 2:123–136.

Rosai J, Zampi G, and Cargangiu ML. (1983) Papillary carcinoma of the thyroid: a discussion of its several morphological expressions, with particular emphasis on the follicular variant. *Am J Surg Pathol* 7: 809–817.

Roth SI. (1970) The ultrastructure of primary water-clear cell hyperplasia of the parathyroid glands. *Am J Pathol* 61:233–240.

Rothenberg HJ, Goellner JR, Carney JA. (1999) Hyalinizing trabecular adenoma of the thyroid gland. Recognition and characterization of its cytoplasmic yellow body. *Am J Surg Pathol* 23:118–125.

Rudy FR, Bates RD, Cimorelli AJ, et al. (1980) Adrenal medullary hyperplasia: a clinicopathologic study of four cases. *Hum Pathol* 11:650–657.

Russell WO, Ibanez ML, Clark RL. (1963) Thyroid carcinoma. Classification, intraglandular dissemination, and clinicopathology study based upon whole organ sections of 80 glands. *Cancer* 16:1425.

Rutter WJ. (1980) The development of the endocrine and exocrine pancreas. In: *The Pancreas* (Fitzgerald PJ, Morrison AB, eds.) pp. 30–38, Williams and Wilkins, Baltimore.

Saeger W, Ludecke DK. (1983) Pituitary hyperplasia. Definition, light and electron microscopic structures and significance in surgical specimens. *Virchows Arch A Pathol Anat Histopathol* 399:277–287.

Saldana MJ, Salem LE, Travezan R. (1973) High altitude hypoxia and chemodectomas. *Hum Pathol* 4: 251–263.

Sampson RJ, Key CR, Buncher CR, Iijma S. (1971) Smallest forms of papillary carcinoma of the thyroid. *Arch Pathol* 91:334–339.

San-Juan J, Monteagudo C, Fraker D, et al. (1989) Significance of mitotic activity and other morphologic parameters in parathyroid adenomas, and their correlation with clinical behavior. *Am J Clin Pathol* 92:523.

Sasano H, Suzuki T, Sano T, et al. (1991) Adrenocortical oncocytoma. A true non-functioning adrenocortical tumor. *Am J Surg Pathol* 15:949–956.

Sasaki A, Daa T, Kashima K, et al. (1996) Insular component as a risk factor of thyroid carcinoma. *Pathol Int* 46:939–946.

Schantz A, Castleman B. (1973) Parathyroid carcinoma. A study of 70 cases. *Cancer* 31:600–605.

Scheithauer BW. (1984) Surgical pathology of the pituitary: the adenomas. *Pathol Ann* Part I, 19:317–374.

Scheithauer BW, Kovacs K, Randall RV, Ryan N. (1985) The pituitary gland in hypothyroidism: histologic and immunocytologic study. *Arch Pathol Lab Med* 109:499–504.

Scheithauer BW, Laws ER, Jr, Kovacs, K, et al. (1987) Pituitary adenomas of the multiple endocrine neoplasia type I syndrome. *Semin Diag Pathol* 4:205–211.

Schneider AB, Pinsky S, Bekerman C, Ryo UY. (1980) Characteristics of 108 thyroid cancers detected by screening in a population with a history of head and neck irradiation. *Cancer* 46:1218–1227.

Schron DS, Mendelsohn G. (1984) Pancreatic carcinoma with duct, endocrine, and acinar differentiation. *Cancer* 54:1766–1770.

Scopsi L, DiPalma S, Ferrari C, et al. (1991) C-cell hyperplasia accompanying thyroid diseases other than medullary carcinomas: an immunocytochemical study by means of antibodies to calcitonin and somatostatin. *Mod Pathol* 4:297–304.

Shamma AH, Goddard JW, Sommers SC. (1958) A study of the adrenal status in hypertension. *J Chronic Dis* 8:587.

Shenoy BV, Carpenter PC, Carney JA. (1984) Bilateral primary pigmented nodular adrenocortical disease. Rare cause of the Cushing syndrome. *Am J Surg Pathol* 8:335–344.

Shiraishi T, Imai H, Fukutome K, et al. (1999) Ectopic thyroid in the adrenal gland. *Hum Pathol* 30:105–108.

Silva EG, MacKay B, Samaan NA, et al. (1982) Adrenocortical carcinomas: an ultrastructural study of 22 cases. *Ultrastruct Pathol* 3:1–7.

Sim SJ, Ro JY, Ordóñez NG, et al. (1997) Sclerosing mucoepidermoid carcinoma with eosinophilia of the thyroid. *Hum Pathol* 28:1091–1096.

Sipple JH. (1961) The association of pheochromocytoma with carcinoma of the thyroid gland. *Am J Med* 31:163.

Skogzeid B, Larsson C, Lindgren PG, et al. (1992) Clinical and genetic features of adrenocortical lesions in multiple endocrine neoplasia type I. *J Clin Endocrinol Metab* 75:76–81.

Smals AGH, Pieters GFFM, Van Haelst UJG, et al. (1984) Macronodular adrenocortical hyperplasia in long-standing Cushing's disease. *J Clin Endocrinol Metab* 58:25–31.

Snover DC, Foucar K. (1981) Mitotic activity in benign parathyroid disease. *Am J Clin Pathol* 75:345–347.

Stefan Y, Bordi C, Grasso S, et al. (1985) Beckwith-Wiedermann syndrome: a quantitative, immunohistochemical study of pancreatic islet cell populations. *Diabetologia* 28: 914–919.

Tannenbaum M. (1973) Ultrastructural pathology of the adrenal cortex. *Pathol Annu* 8:109–156.

Tateishi R, Wada A, Ishiguro S, et al. (1978) Coexistence of bilateral pheochromocytoma and pancreatic islet cell tumor. *Cancer* 42:2928–2934.

Terada T, Kovacs K, Stefaneanu L, et al. (1995) Incidence, pathology and recurrence of pituitary adenomas: study of 647 unselected surgical cases. *Endocr Pathol* 6:301–310.

Thapar K, Scheithauer BW, Kovacs K, et al. (1996) p53 expression in pituitary adenomas and carcinomas: correlation with invasiveness and tumor growth fractions. *Neurosurgery* 38:765–777.

Thompson N.W, Lloyd R.V, Nishiyama R.H, et al. (1984). MEN 1 pancreas: A histological and immunohistochemical study. *World J Surg* 8:561–574.

Thorner MO, Frohman LA, Leong DA, et al. (1984) Extrahypothalamic growth-hormone-releasing factor (GRF) secretion is a rare cause of acromegaly: plasma GRF levels in 177 acromegalic patients. *J Clin Endocrinol Metab* 59:846–849.

Thorpe-Beeston JG, Nicolaides KH, Felton CV, et al. (1991) Maturation of the secretion of thyroid hormone and thyroid-stimulating hormone in the fetus. *N Engl J Med* 324:532–536.

Ulbright TM, Kraus FT, O'Neal LW. (1981) C-cell hyperplasia developing in residual thyroid following resection of sporadic medullary carcinoma. *Cancer* 48:2076–2079.

Ulich T, Cheng L, Lewin K. (1982) Acinar-endocrine cell tumor of the pancreas. *Cancer* 50:2099–2105.

Vance J, Stoll RW, Kitabchi AE, et al. (1969) Nesidioblastosis in familial endocrine adenomatosis. *JAMA* 207:1679–1682.

Van Slooten H, Schaberg A, Smeenk D, Moolenaar AJ. (1985) Morphologic characteristics of benign and malignant adrenocortical tumors. *Cancer* 55:766–773.

Vargas MP, Vargas HI, Kleiner DE, et al. (1997) Adrenocortical neoplasms: role of prognostic markers MiB-1 p53 and RB. *Am J Surg Pathol* 21:556–562.

Vickery AL, Jr. (1983) Thyroid papillary carcinoma: pathological and philosophical controversies. *Am J Surg Pathol* 7:777–807.

Vickery AL Jr, Carcangiu ML, Johannessen JV, Sobrinho-Simoes M. (1985) Papillary carcinoma. *Semin Diagn Pathol* 2:90–100.

Visser JW, Axt R. (1975) Bilateral adrenal medullary hyperplasia: a clinicopathological entity. *J Clin Pathol* 28:298–304.

Waterhouse J, Muir C, Correa P, Powell J. (1976) *Cancer Incidence in Five Countries,* Vol. 3, pp. 268–279. IARC Scientific Publications, Lyon, France.

Webb TA, Sheps SG, Carney JA. (1980) Differences between sporadic pheochromocytoma and pheochromocytoma in multiple endocrine neoplasia type 2. *Am J Surg Pathol* 4:121–126.

Weiss LM. (1984) Comparative histologic study of 43 metastasizing and nonmetastasizing adrenocortical tumors. *Am J Surg Pathol* 8:163–163.

Weiss LM, Medeiros LJ, Vickery AL. (1989) Pathologic features of prognostic significance in adrenocortical carcinoma. *Am J Surg Pathol* 13:202–206.

Wenig BM, Adair CF, Heffess CS. (1995) Primary mucoepidermoid carcinoma of the thyroid gland. A report of six cases and a review of the literature of a follicular epithelial-derived tumor. *Hum Pathol* 26:1099–1108.

Wenig BM, Thompson LDR, Adair CF, et al. (1998) Thyroid papillary carcinoma of columnar cell type. A clinicopathologic study of 16 cases. *Cancer* 82:740–753.

Wermer P. (1954) Genetic aspects of adenomatosis of endocrine glands. *Am J Med* 16:363–371.

White PC, New MI, Dupont B. (1987) Congenital adrenal hyperplasia. *N Engl J Med* 316:1519 and 1580–1586.

Wiedemann HR. (1983) Tumours and hemihypertrophy associated with Wiedemann-Beckwith syndrome. *Eur J Pediatr* 141:129.

Wieneke JA, Thompson LDR, Frommelt RA, et al. (1999) Minimally invasive follicular carcinoma of the thyroid gland: a clinicopathologic study of 132 cases. *Lab Invest* 79:70A.

Williams ED. (1979) The aetiology of thyroid tumours. *Clin Endocrinol Metab* 8:193–207.

Williams ED. (1984) C cell hyperplasia. *Bull Cancer (Paris)* 71:122–124.

Williams ED, Pollack DJ. (1966) Multiple mucosal neuromata with endocrine tumors—a syndrome allied to Von Recklinghausen's disease. *J Pathol Bacteriol* 91:71–80.

Williams ED, Toyn CE, Harach HR. (1989) The ultimobranchial gland and congenital thyroid abnormalities in man. *J Pathol* 159:135–141.

Winship T, Rosvoll RV. (1970) Thyroid carcinoma in childhood: final report on a 20 year study. *Clin Proc Child Hosp Washington, DC* 26:327–349.

Wirtschafter A, Schmidt R, Rosen D, et al. (1997) Expression of the RET/PTC fusion gene as a marker for papillary carcinoma in Hashimoto's thyroiditis. *Laryngoscope* 107:95–100.

Wolfe HJ, Voelkel EF, Tashjian AH. (1974) Distribution of calcitonin containing cells in the normal adult human thyroid gland: a correlation of morphology and peptide content. *J Clin Endocrinol Metab* 38:688–694.

Woolner LB, Lemmon ML, Beahrs OH, et al. (1960) Occult papillary carcinoma of the thyroid gland: a study of 140 cases observed in a 30 year period. *J Clin Endocrinol Metab* 20:89.

Wulffraat NM, Drexhage HA, Wiersinga, WM, et al. (1988) Immunoglobulins of patients with Cushing's syndrome due to pigmented adrenocortical micronodular dysplasia stimulate in vitro steroidogenesis. *J Clin Endrocinol Metab* 66:301–307.

Wynick D, Williams SJ, Bloom SR. (1988) Symptomatic secondary hormone syndromes in patients with established malignant pancreatic endocrine tumors. *N Engl J Med* 319:605–607.

Xu B, Diaz-Cano SJ, Wolfe HJ. (1998) Is C-cell hyperplasia in MEN II A a preneoplastic lesion or carcinoma in situ. *Lab Invest* 60A.

Yamamoto Y, Maeda T, Izumi K, Otsuka H. (1990) Occult papillary carcinoma of the thyroid. A study of 408 autopsy cases. *Cancer* 65:1173–1179.

Yamashita H, Nakayama I, Noguchi S, et al. (1985) Thyroid carcinoma in benign thyroid diseases: an analysis from minute carcinoma. *Acta Pathol Jpn* 35:781–788.

Yashiro T, Ito K, Akiba M, et al. (1987) Papillary carcinoma of the thyroid arising from dyshormonogenetic goiter. *Endocrinol Jpn* 34:955–964.

Yashiro et al. (1993)

Yasumura S, Burk M, Chausmer A, et al. (1967) Thyroidal content of thyrocalcitonin in hypothyroid and hyperthyroid rats. *Endocrinology* 81:256–260.

Zedenius J, Larsson C, Wallin G, et al. (1996) Alterations of p53 and expression of WAF1/p21 in human thyroid tumors. *Thyroid* 6:1–9.

Zimmermann-Belsing T, Feldt-Rasmussen U. (1994) Reidel's thyroiditis: an autoimmune or primary fibrotic disease. *J Intern Med* 235:271–274.

Zollinger RM. (1985) Gastrinoma. Factors influencing prognosis. *Surgery* 97:49–54.

27

GUT ENDOCRINE SYSTEM

CHARLES R. LASSMAN AND KLAUS J. LEWIN

The endocrine cells of the gastrointestinal tract are widely distributed throughout its entire length. Numerically, they constitute the largest endocrine organ in the body. As is true for other endocrine organs, the gastrointestinal endocrine cells can undergo hyperplasia and neoplasia (Brown et al., 1986; Gardiner et al., 1985; Godwin, 1975; Kuiper et al., 1970; Lewin, 1992; Lewin et al., 1986; Lundqvist and Wilander, 1987; Norheim et al., 1987; Solcia et al., 1989a).

Endocrine cells are found individually or in small, isolated clusters wedged between the epithelial cells and basement membrane. The majority communicate with the glandular lumen by apical microvilli. In the stomach, the endocrine cells are found predominantly between the parietal and chief cells in the fundus, and in the antrum, they lie at the junction of the foveolae and the glands. In the small intestine, appendix, and large intestine, they are found in the base of intestinal crypts.

There are many different types of endocrine cells in the gastrointestinal tract (Table 27–1). Although some specific types, such as the serotonin-producing enterochromaffin cells and the somatostatin D cells, occur throughout the length of the intestine, most endocrine cells are restricted in distribution (Lewin, 1992). Thus, gastrin cells are confined to the gastric antrum and upper duodenum, and endocrine cells containing secretin, cholecystokinin (CCK), gastric inhibitory polypeptide (GIP), motilin, and substance P are restricted to the upper small intestine. Cells containing enteroglucagon, neurotensin, peptide YY, and substance P are found in the lower small intestine and in the colon. Accurate quantitation of the absolute number of endocrine cells or the cellular content of peptide is fraught with difficulty because of technical factors relating to section thickness, pretreatment of tissues, quality of antibodies, and difficulty in estimating total mucosal volume. However, comparative studies have shown, despite difficulty in obtaining normal tissues for exact comparisons, that an alteration in the number of specific endocrine cells can occur in pathologic processes.

A few endocrine cells are also found in the lamina propria, in all divisions of the intestinal tract (Masson, 1914; Stachura et al., 1981). Endocrine cells also occur in sites of ectopic tissue, such as in heterotopic mucosa and in mucosa showing metaplastic change (Albores-Saavedra et al., 1986).

The multiplicity of endocrine cells is also recognized by electron microscopy. Ultrastructurally, the endocrine cells are characterized by dense-core secretory granules, which are composed of a central core of variable density surrounded by a single membrane frequently separated from the core by a translucent halo. A correlation exists between granule morphology and the hormone product (Table 27–1). Granule morphology, however, is not always distinctive between functionally different cells, and in neoplasms there may be even greater heterogeneity of granules.

694

Table 27–1. Features of Gastrointestinal Endocrine Cells

Cell Type	Secretory Products	Granule Morphology			Limiting Membrane	
		Size (nm)	Shape	Electron Density	Close[a]	Halo[b]
D	Somatostatin	300–400	Round	Medium	+	Narrow
EC1	Serotonin, substance P, leuenkephalin	200–300	Pleomorphic	Dense		
EC2	Serotonin, motilin, and leuenkephalin	200–400	Pleomorphic	Dense	+	
ECn	Serotonin	200–300	Oval	Moderate	+	
ECL	Unknown	Variable	Round or oval	Dense eccentric core		Wide clear space
G	Gastrin, ?ACTH-like peptide	180–300	Round	Flocculent, highly variable density	+	
I	CCK	250–300	Round to slightly irregular	Medium	+	
IG	Gastrin	175–190	Round	Dense	+	
K	GIP	200–350	Irregular	Dense eccentric core		Variable
L	Enteroglucagon Peptide YY	250–300	Round to slightly irregular	Dense		
M	Motilin	180	Round	Moderate	+	
N	Neurotensin	300	Round	Moderate	+	
P	Unknown	100–150	Round	Medium	+	
PP	Pancreatic polypeptide	150–170	Round	Dense	+	
S	Secretin	180–220	Round to moderately irregular	Dense		Narrow
X	Unknown	250	Round	Medium	+	

[a]Closely applied to the core.

[b]Separated from the core by a space or halo.

Courtesy of K. J. Lewin, M.D., from *Gastrointestinal Pathology and Its Clinical Implications*, Igaku-Shoin Medical Publishers, New York, 1991, pp. 197–257, with permission.

Although endocrine cells are difficult to visualize, in sections stained by hematoxylin and eosin, two types are recognized:

1. The basigranulated cells with small subnuclear eosinophilic granules (Fig. 27–1).
2. Clear cells, which usually are harder to recognize unless they are hyperplastic, are typically rounded with a centrally located vesicular nucleus surrounded by clear cytoplasm (see Fig. 27–2).

Previously, the most common methods for the identification of endocrine cells in tissue sections were those using silver stains (Fig. 27–3). These stains depend on the reduction of ammoniacal silver nitrate to metallic sil-

ver by the endocrine cell. In the argentaffin stain, which mainly identifies serotonin-producing cells, the reduction occurs directly in the cells. In other endocrine cells, however, the addition of an exogenous reducing agent is necessary before they can reduce the ammoniacal silver to metallic silver. This is known as the *argyrophil reaction*.

A few endocrine cells, such as the gastrin-containing cells, stain inconsistently with silver stains; consequently, a number of immunhistochemical stains have been introduced, such as neuron-specific enolase, protein gene product (PGP 9.5), chromogranin, secretogranin, and synaptophysin, in search of a universal marker for endocrine cells (Gould, 1987; Lloyd et al., 1984, 1988;

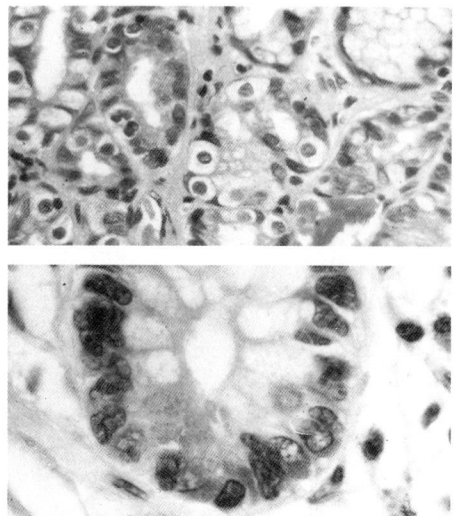

Figure 27–1. Composite photomicrograph illustrating basigranular and clear endocrine cells. A: Numerous clear-staining endocrine cells containing centrally located nuclei and surrounding clear cytoplasm. B: Base of an intestinal crypt with a basigranular cell characterized by infranuclear basophilia.

Rode et al., 1985; Weiler et al., 1988; Wiedenmann et al., 1988). Neuron-specific enolase, a soluble protein originally isolated from brain, is so nonspecific that it is of little value. PGP 9.5 is similar to neuron-specific enolase. However, chromogranins and synaptophysin can be quite specific and sensitive stains for identifying endocrine cells. The chromogranins and secretogranins are

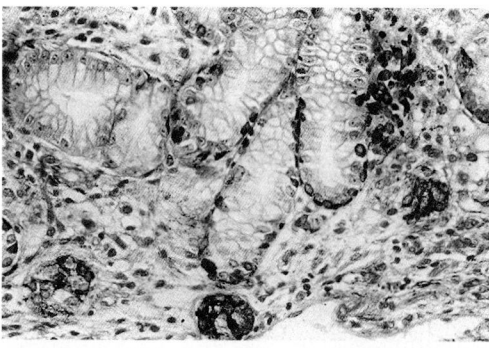

Figure 27–2. Intestinal crypts stained immunohistochemically for chromogranin A. Note the darkly staining endocrine cells, three of which clearly extend to the gland lumen (so-called open endocrine cells).

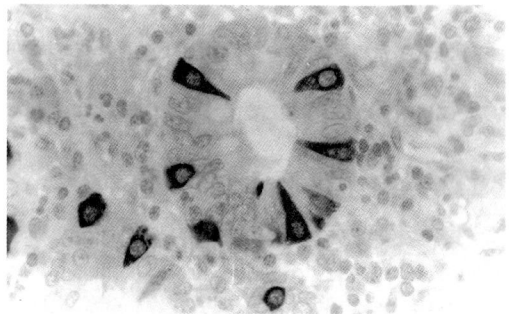

Figure 27–3. Argyrophil stain of a section of atrophic mucosa of the gastric fundus, demonstrating numerous argyrophilic endocrine cells lying between the basement membrane and the glandular epithelium. Most of these endocrine cells are enterochromaffin-like (ECL) cells, which differ from most other gastrointestinal endocrine cells in that they do not communicate with the lumen of the glands (so-called closed cells).

hydrophilic proteins present in the granule matrix (Fig. 27–2) Synaptophysin is a hydrophobic membrane glycoprotein of presynaptic vesicles, which is found in small clear vesicles in normal and neoplastic endocrine cells (Wiedenmann et al., 1988). Synaptophysin appears to be a more sensitive marker of neuroendcrine differentiation. In a recent study, all gastrointestinal and pulmonary carcinoid tumors were positive for synaptophysin whereas 88% of forgut, 100% of midgut, and 60% of hindgut tumors were positve for chromogranin (Al-Khafaji et al., 1998).

IMMUNOHISTOCHEMICAL TECHNIQUES FOR DEMONSTRATION OF ENDOCRINE CELLS

Immunohistochemical identification of the hormonal products of endocrine cells is the most definitive way to characterize these cells. To date, 18 peptides and biogenic amines have been identified; these are listed in Tables 27–1 and 27–2 (Lewin, 1992). A number of other peptides found in the gastrointestinal tract, such as growth hormone, thyrotropin-releasing hormone, gastrin-releasing peptide, and vasoactive intestinal polypeptide (VIP), have yet to be definitively localized to specific endocrine cells and may

Table 27–2. Distribution of Digestive Hormones in the Gastrointestinal Tract

Substance	Cell Type	Localization
ACTH-like peptide	G cell	Antrum
Cholecystokinin (CCK)	I cell	Duodenum and jejunum
Enteroglucagon	L cell	Small and large intestine
Gastrin	G cell	Antrum and duodenum
Gastric inhibitory polypeptide (GIP)	K cell	Duodenum and jejunum
Motilin	M cell	Duodenum and jejunum
Neurotensin	N cell	Small intestine and colon
Pancreatic polypeptide	PP/D1 cell	Duodenum
Peptide YY	L cell	Ileum and large intestine
Secretin	S cell	Duodenum and jejunum
Serotonin	EC cell	Stomach, small and large intestine
Somatostatin	D cell	Fundus, antrum, duodenum, jejunum, and colon
Substance P	EC cell	Small intestine

be limited to the ganglia and nerve fibers. In general, there is only a single peptide in each endocrine cell type, but exceptions have been noted. For example, the L cell contains glicentin and pancreatic polypeptide, and antral gastrin cells also contain immunoreactive adrenocorticotropic hormone (ACTH) (Lewin, 1992). However, these observations should be confirmed, since double staining techniques are often prone to false-positive reactions because of nonspecific immunoglobulin binding. There are a number of instances of an amine and a peptide occurring together in the same cell. For example, substance P has been localized to a subpopulation of the serotonin-containing enterochromaffin cells, enkephalin to another, and dopamine and cholecystokin have been found in single neurons. The frequency of such amine-peptide pairing is unknown, although it has been suggested that amines occur in all peptide-producing cells (Lewin, 1992).

ENDOCRINE CELL HYPERPLASIA

There is a growing awareness of the existence of endocrine cell hyperplasia, primarily in the stomach. The major significance of gastric endocrine cell hyperplasia is its association with dysplasia and carcinoid tumors. In the stomach, most hyperplasias are sec-

ondary to hypochlorhydria (Borch et al., 1987; Bordi et al., 1986; Creutzfeldt et al., 1971; Feldman et al., 1980; Hodges et al., 1981; Lehy et al., 1989; Rubin, 1973; Shimoda et al., 1983), although some cases are part of the multiple endocrine neoplasia (MEN) syndrome (Solcia et al., 1990) or related to primary hyperplasia (Frieson et al., 1972; Ganguli et al., 1973; Lewin, 1986; Lewin et al., 1984; Polak et al., 1972; Royston et al., 1978; Walsh et al., 1983). Although the latter is of interest clinically because it resembles the Zollinger-Ellison syndrome, it has not been associated with neoplastic transformation.

The incidence of endocrine cell hyperplasias in the remainder of the gastrointestinal tract is unclear. The main ones recognized are enterochromaphin and somatostatin, which are associated with celiac disease and ulcerative colitis secondary to nonspecific reaction to chronic mucosal damage (Dayal, 1994).

GASTRIC ENDOCRINE CELL HYPERPLASIA

The major stimulus for endocrine cell hyperplasia in the stomach is hypochlorhydria (Arnold et al., 1982; Borch et al., 1987; Bordi et al., 1986; Dayal, 1983; Feldman et al., 1980; Hodges et al., 1981; Lehy et al., 1989; Polak et al., 1973; Rubin, 1969, 1973;

Sjoblom et al., 1989; Shimoda et al., 1983; Stremple and Watson, 1974). Hypochlorhydria results in gastrin cell hyperplasia and hypergastrinemia by a negative feedback mechanism, since acid normally suppresses gastrin production. In most cases, there is no significant clinical symptomatology from hypergastrinemia (Bloom and Polak, 1981; Creutzfeldt, 1981).

Most cases of secondary gastrin cell hyperplasia do not progress to dysplasia or to a carcinoid tumor. Hypergastrinemia appears to be trophic for the endocrine cells in the fundus, resulting in gastric argyrophil cell hyperplasia. A number of distinctive cell types have been demonstrated by immunohistochemistry and electron microscopy, such as enterochromaffin (EC) cells, gastrin (G) cells, pancreatic polypeptide (PP), somatostatin (D) D1 cells, and enterochromaffin-like (ECL) cells, which are the most common (Bordi et al., 1986; Hodges et al., 1981; Ito et al., 1984; Ogata, 1973).

G cell hyperplasia and hypergastrinemia can occur in severe atrophic gastritis of the fundus—for example, in cases of pernicious anemia or following partial gastrectomy. Currently, the two most common causes of G-cell hyperplasia are *Helicobacter pylori* infection and esophageal reflux disease. Eradication of *H. pylori* has resulted in a decrease not only in the number of G cells but also in the level of gastrin (reviewed by Kwan et al., 1995). In patients with esophageal reflux disease, hyperplasia is induced physiologically with acid-suppressing drugs, such as histamine 2 (H_2) blockers, or the new agent omeprazole, which suppresses gastric acid secretion by specific inhibition of the H^+/K^+ ATPase enzyme system, to induce hypergastrinemia (Fig. 27–4A). In animals, omeprazole causes endocrine cell hyperplasia and even carcinoid tumors. In humans, no significant hyperplasia has been reported, probably because of the low therapeutic doses that are used (Arnold and Koop, 1989; Solcia et al., 1989b), although gastric carcinoids have been reported in patients with the Zollinger-Ellison syndrome who have been on long-term omeprazole therapy (Goldfain et al., 1989). Another cause of hypergastrinemia, albeit rare, is a gastrinoma of the gastrointestinal tract or pancreas.

HISTOLOGY

In hyperplasia, the endocrine cells proliferate in a sleeve-like manner around gastric glands and as small balls or nests budding from the base of the glands or lying within the lamina propria. Although normal gastric endocrine cell are best appreciated with silver stains (Fig. 27–5) or immunostains for chromogranin and synaptophysin, the hyperplastic cells within the gastric glands are usually prominently visible in hematoxylin and eosin sections. They are characterized as rounded cells with clear cytoplasm and central round nuclei (Fig. 27–4B). In contrast, the nodular endocrine cell proliferations within the lamina propria have a rather scant and somewhat basophilic cytoplasm and are easily confused with gastric chief cells (Fig. 27–6).

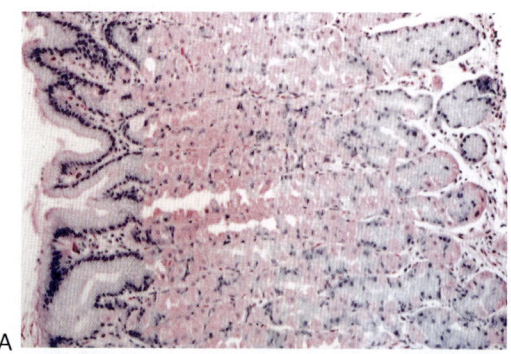 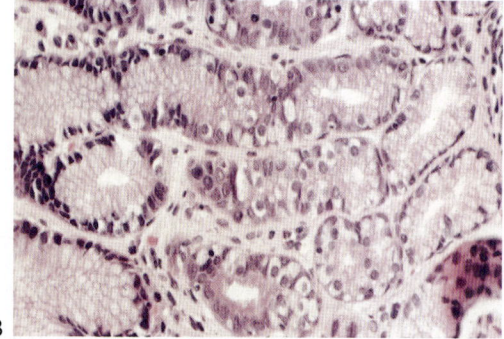

Figure 27–4. The effect of long term treatment with proton pump inhibitor. *A:* Hyperplasia and hypertrophy of gastric oxyntic cells on the gastric fundus. *B:* Hyperplasia of G cells in the gastric antrum.

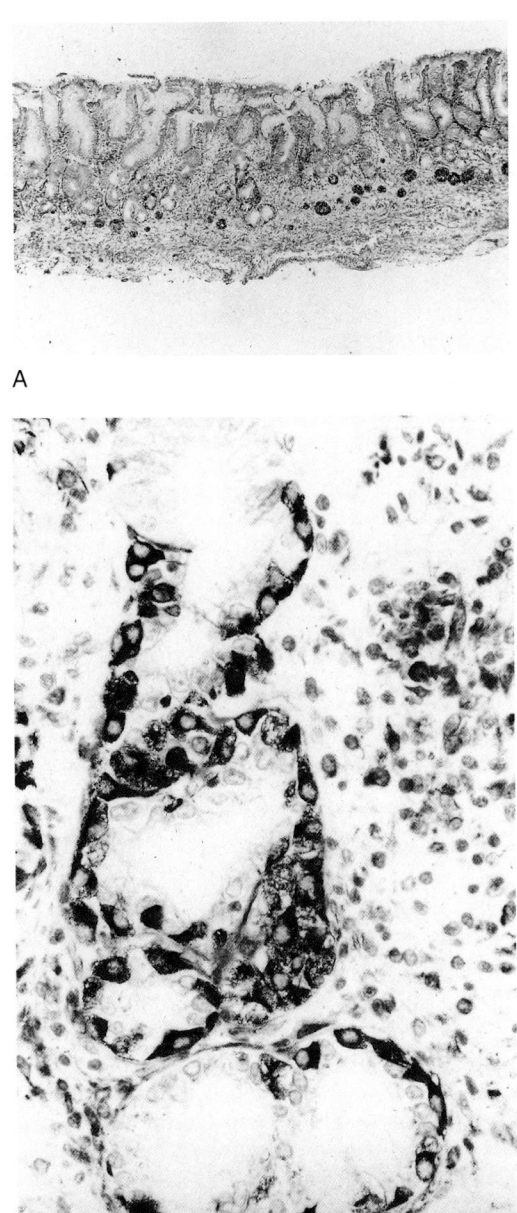

A

B

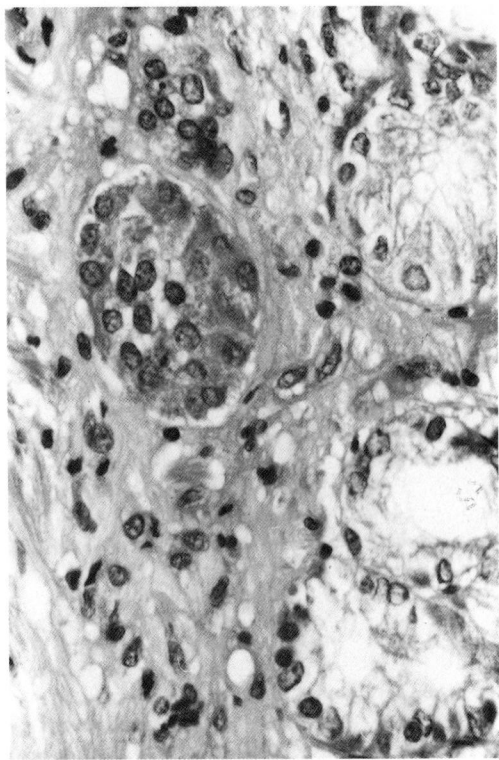

Figure 27–6. Endocrine cell hyperplasia in pernicious anemia. High-power view of fundic gastric mucosa from a patient with pernicious anemia, showing pyloric metaplasia. The proliferating endocrine cell nests appear at the base of the glands and resemble gastric chief cells.

Figure 27–5. Endocrine cell hyperplasia of the gastric fundus in severe atrophic gastritis. *A*: Low-power view of the atrophic mucosa shows hyperplasia of the endocrine cells, which appear as small, black-staining, round nests (Grimelius stain). *B*: Higher magnification of a gastric gland shows the sleeve-like proliferation of endocrine cells surrounding gastric glands (Grimelius stain).

THE HYPERPLASIA, DYSPLASIA, AND CARCINOID TUMOR SPECTRUM

In the stomach, an association between hyperplasia, endocrine cell dysplasia, and carcinoid tumor has been reported, which suggests, in some cases, progression from normal to neoplastic growth. It should be stressed, however, that the risk of neoplastic transformation in most cases of endocrine cell hyperplasia is minimal. Hypergastrinemia *per se* probably has very little, if any, neoplastic potential (Rindi et al., 1993). However, when hypergastrinemia acts on endocrine cells partially transformed by other, yet unidentified factors, such as those inherent in MEN type 1 (the gene for which has been recently cloned [Manickam et al.,

1997]) or severe atrophic gastritis in pernicious anemia, neoplasia may supervene (Solcia et al., 1988).

An association between endocrine cell hyperplasia and carcinoid tumors of the small and large intestine has also been observed. In some of these cases—for example, in celiac sprue, Crohn's disease, and ulcerative colitis—the hyperplasia has been attributed to chronic mucosal injury (Brown et al., 1986; Dodd, 1986; Gledhill et al., 1986; Miller and Sumner, 1982; Moyana and Shukoor, 1991). In other instances, the cause of the hyperplasia is unclear (Gardiner et al., 1985; Lundqvist and Wilander, 1987).

Endocrine cell proliferations have been classified into four categories: hyperplastic, adenomatoid, dysplastic, and neoplastic (Solcia et al., 1988). *Hyperplastic proliferation* is defined as micronodular clusters of five or more cells, not exceeding the diameter of gastric glands, present within either gastric glands or in the lamina propria. The clusters are surrounded by a thin basement membrane (Fig. 27–6). *Adenomatoid hyperplasia* is defined as five or more micronodules lying close to one another with an interspersed basement membrane, located deep in the mucosa (Fig. 27–7).

Endocrine cell dysplasia consists of enlargement and fusion of the micronodules (>150 μm but <0.5 mm), with disappearance of

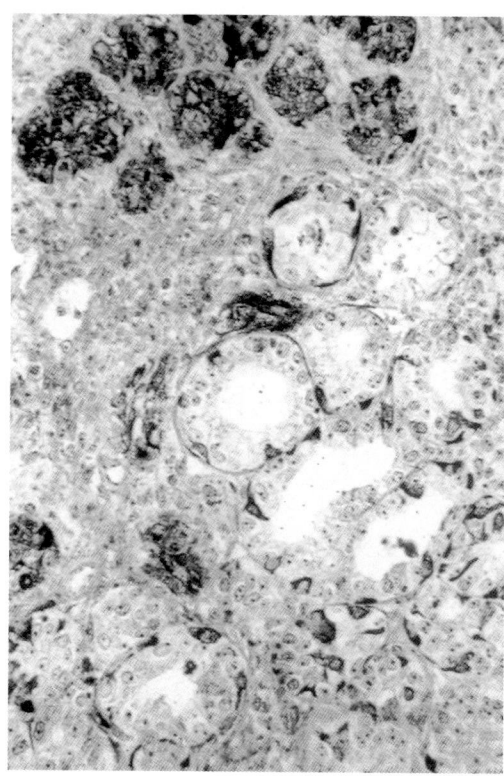

Figure 27–8. Endocrine cell dysplasia characterized by fusing endocrine cell micronodules. [Courtesy of Professors E. Solcia, M.D, and C. Bordi, M.D.]

the intervening basement membrane (Fig. 27–8). Microinvasion of the lamina propria between the glands may also occur, resulting in nodules with newly formed stroma. The cytology of these cells tends to be somewhat atypical. The cells are less regular and often exhibit reduced argyrophilia.

CARCINOID TUMORS

The gastrointestinal tract is the most frequent site of carcinoids, accounting for 74% of all tumors, followed by the brochoalveolar system, which accounts for 25% (Modlin and Sandor, 1997). In the past, the most common site of gastrointestinal carcinoids was the small intestine (29%), followed by the appendix (19%) and then the rectum (12%). Carcinoids of the esophagus are exceedingly rare (Lindberg et al., 1997).

Previously, the incidence of gastric carcinoids was about 3%, however, with the increasing use of gastric endoscopy, carcinoids

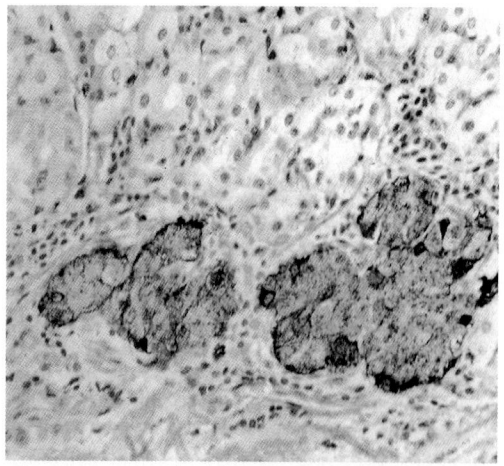

Figure 27–7. Adenomatoid hyperplasia of endocrine cells characterized by numerous micronodules of endocrine cells in excess of five. [Courtesy of Professors E. Solcia, M.D, and C. Bordi, M.D.]

of the stomach are increasingly recognized, accounting for 11% to 40% of all carcinoid tumors (Dayal, 1994). It should also be noted that the incidence of gastrointestinal carcinoids may vary from one country to another. For example, in a recent study from Taiwan, it was found that the most common carcinoid tumors occurred within the rectum. (Weng et al., 1996). However, as mentioned above, these findings may in part be a reflection of differing use of endoscopy in different nations. Lastly, it should be noted that about 15% of patients with carcinoid tumors have a second noncarcinoid tumor (Modlin and Sandor, 1997; Rivadeneira et al., 1996).

Carcinoid tumors are divided into intramucosal and invasive types. *Intramucosal* lesions consist of infiltrative or solid endocrine cell growths more than 0.5 mm in diameter but confined to the mucosa (Fig. 27–9). Endocrine cell proliferations penetrating beyond the muscularis mucosae are considered *invasive* carcinoids. Carcinoid tumors can occur anywhere in the gastrointestinal tract, including unusual sites, such as in Meckel's diverticulum (Doyle and Severance, 1966; Moyana, 1989). Identical lesions are found in virtually every organ in the body.

Grossly, the tumors are either single or multiple, occurring most frequently (as mentioned above) in the appendix and terminal ileum. Most tumors are yellow and are submucosal, measuring less than 2 cm in maximum diameter (Moertel et al., 1961). They may project into the lumen and cause attenuation of the overlying mucosa, which is rarely ulcerated. The larger lesions are generally deeply invasive and are commonly associated with extensive fibrosis and adhesions, which may produce kinking and obstruction of the viscus (Moertel et al., 1961). The larger lesions are often associated with metastases, which are frequently larger than the primary tumor (Martin and Potet, 1974; Moertel et al., 1961; Morgan et al., 1974; Teitelbaum, 1972).

Histologically, based on architecture, carcinoid tumors of the gastrointestinal tract can be divided into four major types: (*1*) insular, (*2*) tubular, (*3*) glandular and psammomatous, and (*4*) those with mixed patterns, trabecular and glandular. This classification scheme is important because there seems to be some correlation between the histologic features and immunohistochemical reactivity (Burke et al., 1990a,b). *Insular* carcinoids are usually positive for argentaffin and serotonin. *Tubular* carcinoids lack positivity for argentaffin granules and serotonin but are immunoreactive for glucagon. The *glandular and psammomatous* type is usually reactive to somatostatin, is often found in the duodenum or ampulla of Vater, and has been reported in association with neurofibromatosis and MEN type I (Burke et al., 1990c). Duodenal carcinoids may also produce gastrin and be responsible for the Zollinger-Ellison syndrome (Burke et al., 1990c). Up to 40% of cases of Zollinger-Ellison syndrome are associated with a duodenal gastrin-secreting carcinoid (Kloppel et al., 1996). Some of these gastrinomas are easily overlooked during surgical procedures or even at autopsy because of their small size, less than 0.5 cm (Thompson et al., 1989).

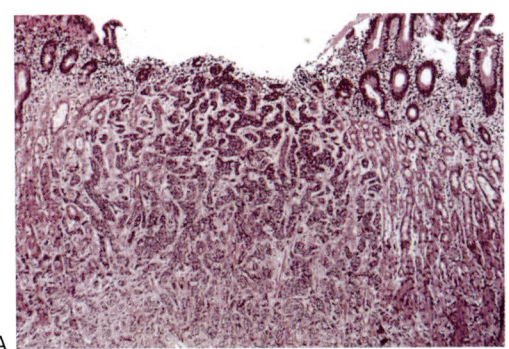
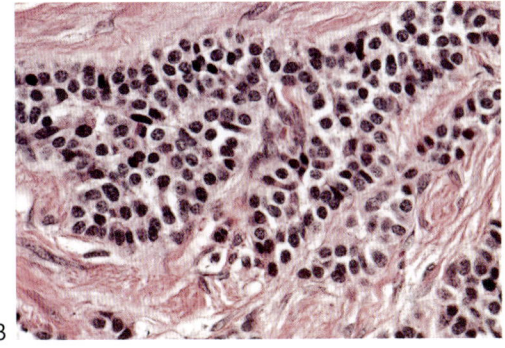

Figure 27–9. Microscopic carcinoid tumor of the stomach. *A*: Low-power view shows the small tumor within the mucosa. *B*: Higher magnification of the tumor shows the typical trabecular pattern of the carcinoid.

Duodenotomy, eversion, and palpation of the mucosa may be necessary to detect smaller tumors. Chromogranin expression in carcinoid tumors as in neuroendocrine cells is somewhat site-specific. Whereas 100% of midgut tumors were chromogranin positive only 60% of hindgut and 88% of forgut carcinoids were chromogranin positive (Al-khafaj et al., 1998).

A correlation also exists between the histologic features and anatomic location of carcinoid tumors. Insular or trabecular carcinoids are the most common type and occur anywhere along the gastrointestinal tract. Carcinoids with a mixed histologic pattern (trabecular and glandular) are the most common type of rectal carcinoid (Federspiel et al., 1990). Psammomatous carcinoids are seen almost exclusively in the duodenum and ampulla of Vater (Burke et al., 1990c).

A rare but fascinating variant of gastric carcinoid is composed entirely of clear, foamy cells. This lesion is easily confused with gastric xanthalesma, both endoscopically and histologically. The presence of a vascularized stroma and the formation of cell packets provides clues to its nonhistiocytic differentiation (Fig. 27–10). The diagnosis is confirmed by immunoperoxidase studies or by electron microscopy (Luk et al., 1997).

In addition to the morphologic patterns described above, it should be noted that a small number of carcinoid tumors are poorly-differentiated. They range from the well differentiated endocrine cell tumors to poorly differentiated tumors with severe cytologic atypia and numerous mitotic figures. They may sometimes be difficult (albeit rarely) to differentiate from other small cell tumors. (Lewin et al., 1992).

Recently, carcinoid tumors have been reclassified into four groups, according to their behavior (Klöppel et al., 1996): (1) benign; (2) tumors of uncertain behavior, i.e., tumors for which distinction between benign and low-grade malignant potential cannot be made; (3) tumors of low-grade malignancy; and (4) high-grade malignant tumors.

The main criteria are the size of the tumor, histologic differentiation, angioinvasion, invasion of adjacent organs, and the presence of metastases. The major problem that we see with these criteria is that, on the basis of endoscopy and pure morphology, it may be difficult to separate tumors into groups one to three. It would be interesting to see whether this new classification is more sensitive than the usual classification—namely, well, moderately, and poorly differentiated.

In addition to the morphologic endocrine cell features described above, it should be noted that the carcinoid tumors are often associated with fibrosis and vascular elastosis. More recently it has been shown that some of the tumors are associated with complex vascular malformations that are probably associated with the production of vascular endothelial growth factor and transforming growth factor-alpha (TGF-α). (Cai et al., 1997; Roncoroni et al., 1997; Terris et al., 1998).

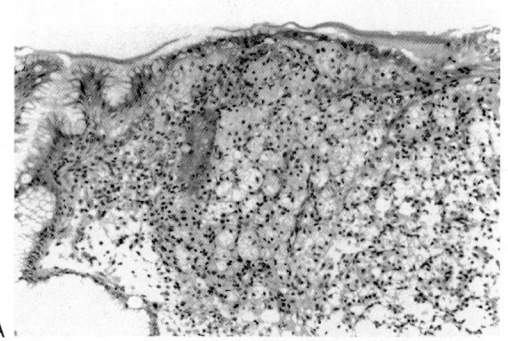
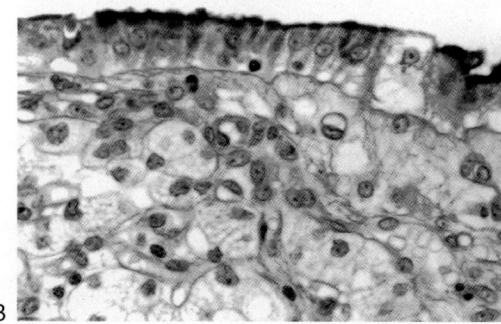

Figure 27–10. *A*: Low-power view of foamy cells filling the lamina propria. Note the architectural arangement of cells in small clusters. *B*: High-power view of carcinoid cells with abundant foamy cytoplasm but nuclei with features characteristic of carcinoid.

Carcinoid tumors grow and spread in a predictable pattern. As they grow, they extend directly into the muscle layers, serosa, and mesentery, often accompanied by extensive fibrosis. Lymphatic permeation is also present in most cases. Larger lesions metastasize both to the regional lymph nodes and to the liver, as well as to distant sites, such as bone and skin.

PROGNOSIS

In this section, some of the factors that may predict the biologic behavior of carcinoid tumors are analyzed. Our concern lies at the benign end of the spectrum: Is there indeed such a lesion as a benign carcinoid, and how does one predict the behavior of these tumors?

In assessing the prognosis, it should be noted that metastases can occur late. In studies by the Mayo Clinic, for example, the average survival of patients, who were followed from the onset of symptoms to death from metastases, was 9 years, with a range of 41 years. The average 5-year survival rate for all patients was 50% (Moertel et al., 1961). These findings have been confirmed in a recent study of 5468 cases (Modlin and Sandor 1997). Unfortunately, however, carcinoid tumors continue to recur, and after 25 years, only 23% of patients were free of recurrence. A comparison of the survival statistics of patients with small intestinal carcinoids with those of an age- and sex-matched population showed that those with localized disease had no difference in life span, and those with regionally resectable disease showed only a moderate decrease, to 15 years (Moertel, 1987).

Unfortunately, there are no absolute criteria by which to judge the malignant potential of most carcinoid tumors. Since tumors characteristically occur in the lamina propria, invasiveness *per se* cannot be used as a criterion of malignancy, as it is with most gastrointestinal carcinomas. The size of the tumor and invasiveness correlate best with the probability of metastases. Tumors associated with atrophic gastritis are rarely associated with metastases (Rindi et al., 1993).

In the Mayo Clinic study, tumors less than 0.5 cm never metastasized. Progressive increase in tumor size was associated with an increased probability of metastases. Thus, 15% of tumors less than 1 cm metastasized, 61% of tumors between 1 and 1.5 cm metastasized, and 84% of those 1.5 to 2.0 cm had spread. Of tumors more than 2.0 cm, 95% metastasized (Moertel, 1987). Others have reported similar results (Martin and Potet, 1974; Moertel et al., 1961; Morgan, et al., 1974; Teitelbaum, 1972). The previous figures reflect to a large degree the extent of tumor invasiveness. Thus, the more deeply invasive the tumor, the more guarded the prognosis. In one study, tumors confined to the bowel wall, that is, submucosa or muscle but not penetrating the serosa, had an excellent prognosis, with 5-year survival rates in excess of 85%, compared with 5% to 20% 5-year survival rates for tumors that extend to the serosa (Zakariai et al., 1975). These findings were confirmed in a more detailed recent study of 188 patients (McDermott et al., 1994); the depth of invasion was correlated with survival. Those tumors that invaded the submucosa only were associated with 100% 5-year survival, those that invaded the muscularis propria had an 81% rate of survival, those invading the submucosa had a 70% survival rate, and those that penetrated the bowel wall had a 52% survival rate. A recent review of 8305 cases of carcinoid (Modlin and Sandor, 1997) confirmed advanced stage as the worst prognostic factor.

Midgut tumors are most commonly associated with carcinoid syndrome and patients with carcinoid syndrome have a worse prognosis. This is probably a reflection of the syndrome being most common in patients with multiple metastases to the liver. Carcinoid syndrome is therefore not an independent predictor of poor prognosis. In a recent study of 301 patients with carcinoid, levels of plasma chromogranin A, urine 5-hydroxyindolacetic acid (a seratonin metabolite), and neuropeptide K and the presence of carcinoid syndrome were studied. Of these, plasma chromogranin A proved to be the only independent predictor of prognosis in patients with midgut carcinoid. The size of tumor was not assessed in this study (Janson et al., 1997).

Tumors arising in different areas may show different malignant potentials. Thus, the overall 5-year survival rates for carcinoid tumors in the stomach, ileum, rectum, and appendix are 70%, 55%, 85%, and 86%, respectively (Dockerty, 1955; Godwin, 1975; Modlin and Sandor, 1997; Morgan et al., 1974; Ritchie, 1956; Weibel et al., 1954). Carcinoid tumors of the appendix are of special interest. They infrequently metastasize, even though they frequently extend to the serosa and are commonly seen in lymphatic spaces. However, some of the larger tumors do behave in a malignant fashion. In one study, no tumors less than 2.0 cm had metastases, whereas metastases occurred with 3 of 14 tumors between 2 and 3 cm and 4 of 9 tumors larger than 3 cm (Moertel et al., 1987).

In the duodenum, features associated with metastasis include involvement of the muscularis propria, size greater than 2 cm, and the presence of mitotic figures. For tumors in the duodenum, immunohistochemical identification of somatostatin and gastrin has little prognostic value (Burke et al., 1990c). Tumors arising at or around the ampulla of Vater have an overall good prognosis because early symptoms, due to obstructive jaundice, lead to quicker diagnosis (Laura et al., 1997; the authors' experience).

Rectal carcinoids that metastasize are usually larger than 2 cm, ulcerate the overlying mucosa, and show more than 2 mitoses per 10 high-power fields (Federspiel et al., 1990). A unique immunohistochemical feature of rectal carcinoids is their reactivity for prostatic acid phosphatase (Federspiel et al., 1990). This prostatic acid phosphatase expression may be explained by the shared cloacal derivation of the rectum and prostate, resulting in the appearance of cells with dual differentiation (Azumi et al., 1991).

The histologic type of tumor may affect prognosis. In one study, tumors with an insular, trabecular, or mixed pattern behaved significantly better than those with a glandular or undifferentiated pattern (Johnson et al., 1983). Finally, women appear to have a better overall prognosis, with survival rates of 66% vs. 47% for men (McDermott et al., 1994).

Use of immunohistochemistry has not been helpful in predicting aggressive behavior. Al-khafaj et al. (1998) studied the expression of p53, Ki-67, and other immunohistochemical markers and found increased expression only in those tumors that were cytologically atypical, but not in "typical" carcinoids.

CLINICAL SIGNIFICANCE AND MANAGEMENT OF ENDOCRINE CELL HYPERPLASIA AND TUMOR

For the pathologist, there are a number of challenges in the diagnosis and workup of patients with carcinoid tumors, such as the association of gastric carcinoids with endocrine cell hyperplasia or with severe atrophic gastritis of the fundus.

The clinical significance of secondary endocrine cell hyperplasia applies primarily to gastric lesions because of its occasional association with gastric carcinoids, which are often multiple. Unfortunately, the management of endocrine cell hyperplasia and carcinoid tumors is not clearly defined in the literature.

In endocrine cell hyperplasia of the stomach with hypergastrinemia, the risk of developing carcinoid tumors is rare. Thus, regular gastroscopic screening in the search for carcinoid tumors in the stomach is not considered worthwhile, other than for high-risk patients—namely, those with sporadic carcinoids and MEN (Borch, 1987; Rindi et al., 1993; Sjoblom et al., 1988; Solcia et al., 1992).

The unpredictable behavior of carcinoid tumors makes their management difficult, especially when they are multiple. Management of these tumors is based on the following generalizations. If the tumors exceed 2 cm in diameter, the potential for metastases is significant, whereas those less than 2 cm in diameter have a very low risk for metastases. Tumors less than 1 cm in diameter remain stable for many years, often with no change in size, although exceptions may occur (Harvey et al., 1985; Janson et al., 1997; McDermott et al., 1994; Sjoblom et al., 1987; Stolte et al., 1988). Lesions in the range of 1 to 2 cm should be treated by polypectomy or circumscribed local resection (Muller et al., 1987; Sjoblom et al., 1987). Lesions larger than 2 cm in diameter should be resected. Furthermore, palliative radical resection is often recommended for patients with metastatic carcinoids because of sluggish tumor growth (Loftus et al., 1995).

For smaller multiple lesions less than 1 cm in diameter, surgery is unnecessary. These patients should be followed endoscopically and probably should have their lesions removed endoscopically, although if numerous of small lesions are present, this may not be practical or even necessary (Stolte et al., 1988). There are also reports that antrectomy, by abolishing hypergastrinemia, can cause the arrest or egression of hyperplastic lesions of the gastric fundus and, in one report, of carcinoid tumors (Borch 1987; Eckhauser et al., 1988; Kern et al., 1990). Whether the latter finding holds true for most gastric carcinoid tumors remains to be confirmed.

Recent advances in imaging technology may be of assistance in the staging and monitoring of patients with carcinoid. There are numerous reports in the literature demonstrating that positron electron transmission (PET) scanning of patients administered tryptophan precursors is a sensitive method of detecting carcinoid tumors. In addition, there have been recent advances in the treatment of some carcinoid tumors with somatostatin analogues (Orlefors et al., 1998; Shi et al., 1998).

MICROGLANDULAR GOBLET CELL CARCINOMA

Microglandular goblet cell carcinoma, also called "mucinous carcinoid," "adenocarcinoid," "crypt cell carcinoma," and "goblet cell carcinoid," is a distinctive tumor of the appendix that may extend into the cecum. It has also been reported in the stomach (Hernandez and Fernandez, 1974; Rodrigues et al., 1982). It resembles a signet ring cell carcinoma and contains variable numbers of endocrine cells. Because of its resemblance to intestinal crypts and the finding of early lesions arising within intact crypts, it has been postulated to arise from intestinal stem cells (Isaaacson, 1981).

Grossly, early tumors appear yellowish-white and mucoid and may be found incidentally during appendectomy or even in association with acute appendicitis (Rodriguez et al., 1982; Subbuswamy et al., 1974).

Histologically, the bulk of the tumor grows from the deeper portions of the mucosa into the submucosa and infiltrates through the muscularis propria to the serosa in a manner similar to carcinoid tumors, hence the name "mucinous carcinoid" (Fig. 27–9). The tumor consists of uniform nests, tubules, or a mixture of both, composed of mature goblet cells infiltrating the viscus (Figs. 27–11 to 27–13). A variable number of endocrine cells and Paneth's cells are mixed with the

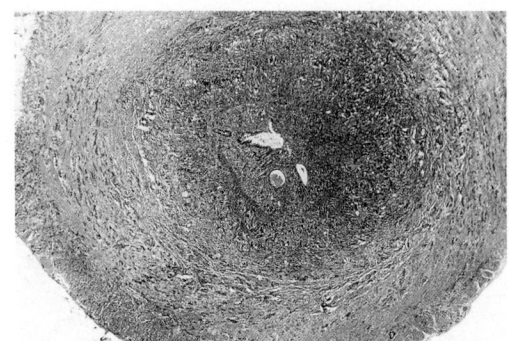

Figure 27–11. Goblet cell carcinoid of the appendix. Low-power view shows almost complete obliteration of the lumen and thickening of all coats caused by diffuse infiltration by tumor.

goblet cells (Fig. 27–14; McDonald and Hourihane, 1977; Subbuswamy et al., 1974; Watson and Alguacil-Garcia, 1987). Sometimes the glandular cords are lined by mucin-containing cuboidal cells with small

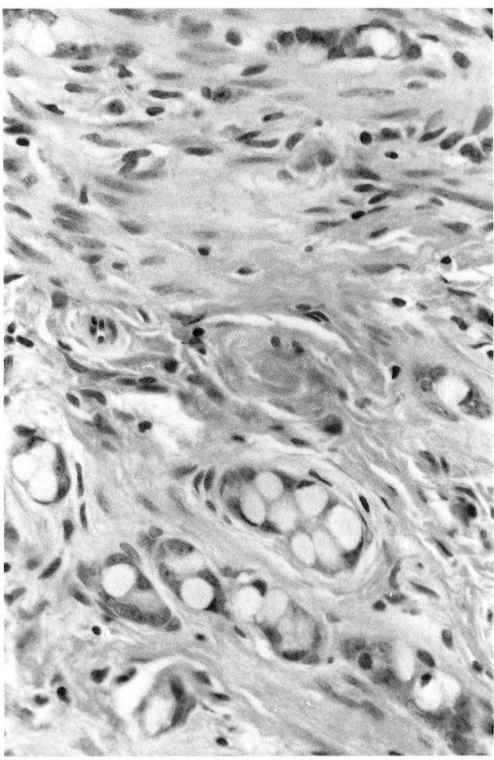

Figure 27–12. Goblet cell carcinoid of the appendix, showing the characteristic cords of mature-looking goblet cells infiltrating the wall of the appendix.

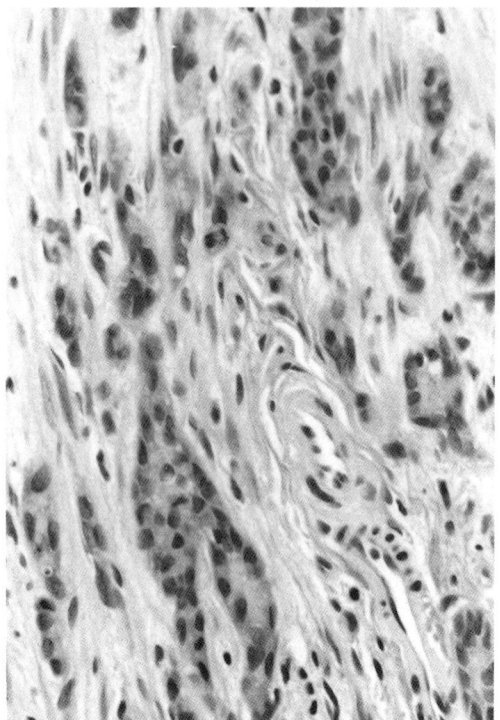

Figure 27–13. Goblet cell carcinoid of the appendix, showing invasion of the muscularis propria by attenuated glandular cords. Elsewhere in the appendix the tumor was composed of the typical goblet cell nests.

eccentric nuclei. The endocrine cells are often sparse in number and difficult to find (Isaacson, 1981). They tend to occur predominantly in the attenuated glandular cords and are usually argentaffin positive. Although a number of endocrine cell types have been described, endocrine cells usually predominate (Burke et al., 1990b; Rodriguez et al., 1982). To date, no one has convincingly demonstrated mucin and neurosecretory granules within the same cells.

These microglandular goblet cell carcinomas must be differentiated from signet-ring cell carcinoma. First, it should be noted that signet-ring cell carcinomas of the appendix are vanishingly rare. Second, in contrast to the smooth, contoured nests of tumor cells seen in goblet cell carcinoids, signet-ring cell carcinomas are usually composed of irregular glandular profiles, showing a great degree of cytologic atypia. In addition, large pools of extracellular mucin are present. In contrast to colonic carcinomas and similar to classical carcinoid tumors of the appen-

dix, goblet cell carcinoids do not show K-*ras* mutations (Ramani et al., 1999).

The overall prognosis of these tumors is significantly better than for the usual adenocarcinomas. The 5-year survival rate for all microglandular goblet cell carcinomas is 80%, in contrast to 50% for colonic adenocarcinomas (Olsson and Ljungberg, 1980; Subbuswamy et al., 1974; Watson and Alguacil-Garcia, 1987). The size of these tumors is not helpful in assessing prognosis, since some small lesions may have already invaded through the muscle layers to the serosa. Stage is the best marker for behavior. Tumors still confined to the bowel wall generally do not metastasize, whereas those that have penetrated the serosa are more likely to have metastasized, although not invariably (Warkel et al., 1978). The more aggressive lesions frequently show atypical foci of less well-differentiated glands with mitotic counts greater than 2 per 10 high-power fields. Whether the degree of atypia serves an independent prognostic factor remains to be proved.

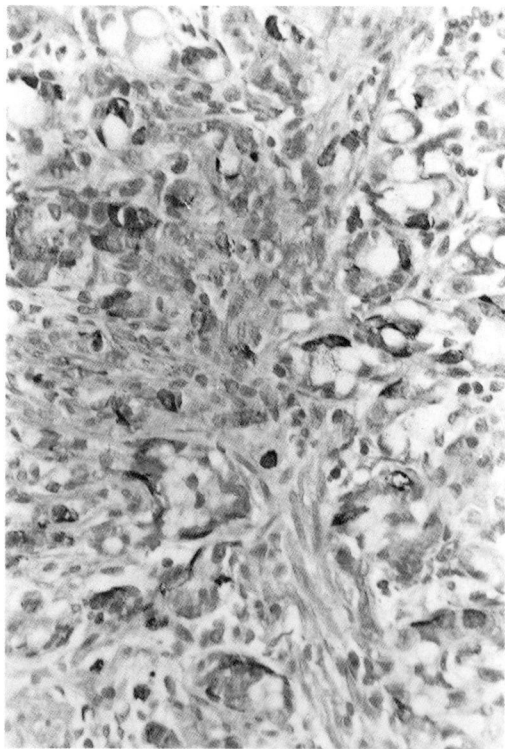

Figure 27–14. Goblet cell carcinoid of the appendix. The section has been stained with the Grimelius stain to show the scattered endocrine cells within the tumor nests.

On the basis of the above-mentioned prognostic factors, recommendations for treatment are as follows. For those tumors confined to the bowel wall without extension to the serosa, appendectomy is sufficient. If the tumor has extended to the cecum, serosa, or beyond or shows marked cytologic atypia with numerous mitoses, then a hemicolectomy is recommended (McDonald and Hourihane, 1977; Warkel et al., 1978).

MIXED ENDOCRINE AND NONENDOCRINE EPITHELIAL CELL TUMORS

Gastrointestinal epithelial cells and endocrine cells originate from a common stem cell. Therefore, it is not unusual to find tumors composed of neoplastic endocrine and nonendocrine epithelial cells. Conceptually, epithelial tumors of the gastrointestinal tract can be classified as follows:

1. Carcinomas with interspersed endocrine cells.
2. Carcinoid tumors with interspersed nonendocrine epithelial cells.
3. Composite tumors consisting of discrete areas of carcinoid tumors and discrete foci of malignant glands.
4. Amphicrine tumors composed predominantly of cells that exhibit both endocrine and nonendocrine differentiation, such as mucus and dense-core granules within the cytoplasm of the same cell. These tumors are extremely rare and have been described primarily in the pancreas and lung (Ali et al., 1984; Ulich et al., 1982).

Most of the mixed tumors—for example, adenomas (Fig. 27–15) and carcinomas (27–16) with endocrine cells, as well as carcinoid tumors with mucin—do not behave

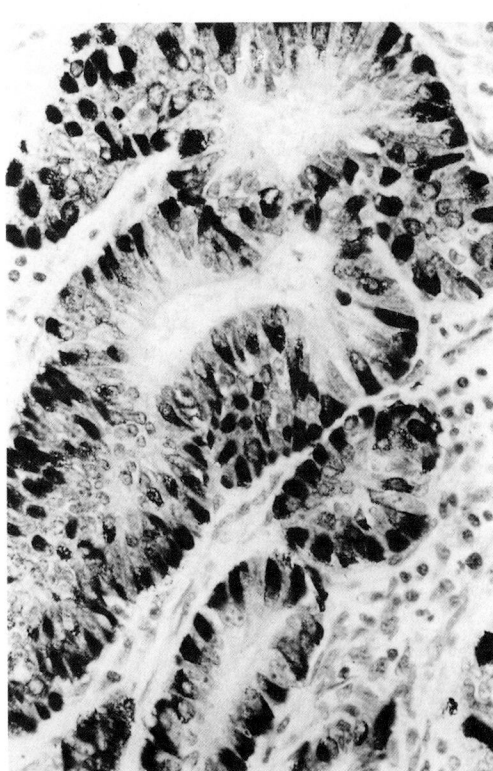

Figure 27–15. Adenoma of the colon stained by the Grimelius argyrophil stain. Note the numerous endocrine cells that make up a substantial component of the epithelial cells. [From Lewin KJ, Ulich T, Yang K, Layfield L. (1986) The endocrine cells of the gastrointestinal tract. Tumors. Part II. *Pathol Annu* 21(2):181-215, with permission of Appleton and Lange.]

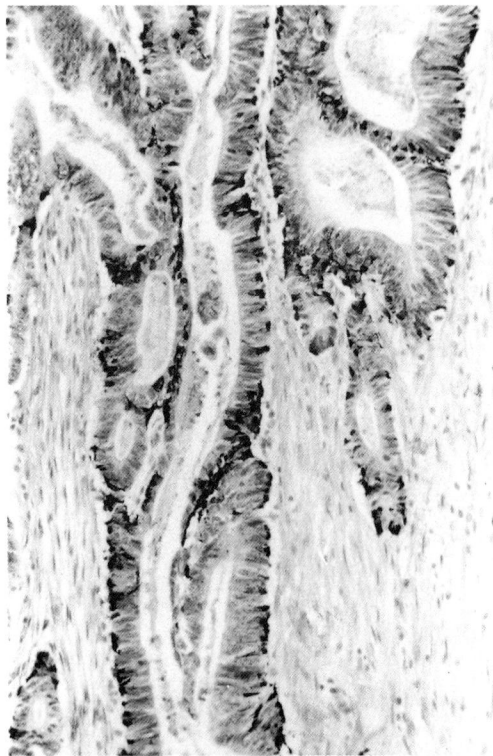

Figure 27–16. Adenocarcinoma of the colon stained by the Grimelius argyrophil stain. In this section of infiltrating tumor, a large number of tumor cells consist of endocrine cells.

differently from the corresponding pure tumors. On the other hand, some tumors (notably the goblet cell carcinoids) have a characteristic clinicopathologic behavior.

In conclusion, recent advances in our knowledge of the endocrine cells have led to a better understanding of the pathogenesis of endocrine cell proliferations and their behavior. In the stomach, for example, the pathogenesis of endocrine cell proliferations is associated in part with trophic factors such as hypergastrinemia resulting from hypochlorhydria. Furthermore, there appears to be an association between hyperplasia, dysplasia, and carcinoid tumor. Our understanding of some of the causes of endocrine cell proliferations has led to a more reasonable foundation for the management of gastric endocrine cell proliferations. The same cannot yet be said for the intestinal endocrine cell proliferations.

In the past few years, we have also come to appreciate that many epithelial tumors of the gastrointestinal tract, including those of the gallbladder and extrahepatic bile ducts, are not pure but contain mixtures of different cells, such as glandular epithelium, endocrine cells, and Paneth's cells (Albores-Saavedra and Henson, 1986). The recognition of these different cell types is important, since not all these tumors behave identically and may vary in virulence, depending on their cellular components.

REFERENCES

Albores-Saavedra J, Henson DE. (1986). *Tumors of the Gallbladder and Extrahepatic Bile Ducts. Atlas of Tumor Pathology,* 2nd Series. p. 115. Armed Forces Institute of Pathology, Washington, DC.

Albores-Saavedra J, Nadji M, Henson DE, et al. (1986) Intestinal metaplasia of the gallbladder. *Hum Pathol* 17:614–620.

Ali MH, Davidson AK, Azzopardi JG. (1984) Composite gastric carcinoid and adenocarcinoma. *Histopathology* 8:259–536.

Al-Khafaji B, Noffsinger AE, Miller MA, DeVoe G, Stemmermann GN, Fenoglio-Preiser C. (1998) Immunohistologic analysis of gastrointestinal and pulmonary carcinoid tumors. *Hum Pathol* 29:992–999.

Arnold R, Hulst MV, Neuhof CH, et al. (1982) Antral gastrin producing G-cells and somatostatin-producing D-cells in different states of gastric acid secretion. *Gut* 23:285–291.

Arnold R, Koop H. (1989) Omeprazole: long-term safety. *Digestion* 44 (Suppl):77–86.

Azumi N, Traweek T, Battifora H. (1991) Prostatic acid phosphatase in carcinoid tumors. *Am J Surg Pathol* 15:785–790.

Bloom SR, Polak JM. (1981) Hormone profiles. In: *Gut*

Hormones (Bloom SR, Polak JM, eds.) pp. 555–560. Churchill Livingstone, Edinburgh.

Borch K, Renvall H, Kullman E. (1987) Gastric carcinoid associated with the syndrome of hypergastrinemic atrophic gastritis. A prospective analysis of 11 cases. *Am J Surg Pathol* 11:435–444.

Bordi C, Ferrari C, D'Adda T, et al. (1986) Ultrastructural characterization of fundic endocrine cell hyperplasia associated with atrophic gastritis and hypergastrinemia. *Virchows Arch A Pathol Anat Histopathol* 409:335–347.

Brown GA, Kollin J, Rajan PH. (1986) The coexistence of carcinoid tumor and Crohn's disease. *J Clin Gastroenterol* 8:286–289.

Burke AP, Sobin LH, Federspiel BH, et al. (1990a) Carcinoid tumors of the duodenum. A clinicopathologic study of 99 cases. *Arch Pathol Lab Med* 114:700–704.

Burke AP, Sobin LH, Federspiel BH, et al. (1990b) Goblet cell carcinoids and related tumors of the vermiform appendix. *Am J Clin Pathol* 94:27–35.

Burke AP, Sobin LH, Shekitka KM, et al. (1990c) Somatostatin-producing duodenal carcinoids in patients with von Recklinghausen's neurofibromatosis. A predilection for black patients. *Cancer* 65:1591–1595.

Cai YC, Barnard G, Hiestand L, Woda B, Colby J, Banner B. (1997) Florid angiogenesis in mucosa surrounding an ileal carcinoid tumor expressing transforming growth factor-alpha. *Am J Surg Pathol* 21:1373–1377.

Creutzfeldt W. (1981) Gut hormones and disease: a perspective. In: *Gut Hormones,* (Bloom SR, Polak JM, eds.) pp. 533–540. Churchill Livingstone, Edinburgh.

Creutzfeldt W, Arnold R, Creutzfeldt C, et al. (1971) Gastrin and G-cells in the antral mucosa of patients with pernicious anemia, acromegaly, and hyperparathyroidism and in a Zollinger-Ellison tumor of the pancreas. *Eur J Clin Invest* 1:461–479.

Dayal Y. (1983) Endocrine cells of the gut and their neoplasms. In: *Pathology of the Colon, Small Intestine and Anus.* (Norris TH, ed.) pp. 267–302. Churchill Livingstone, New York.

Dayal Y. (1994) Hyperplastic proliferations of enteroendocrine cells. *Endocr Pathol* 5:4.

Dockerty MB. (1955) Carcinoids of the gastrointestinal tract. *Am J Clin Pathol* 25:794–796.

Dodd SM. (1986) Chronic ulcerative colitis complicated by atypical carcinoid tumor. *J Clin Pathol* 39:913–916.

Doyle JL, Severance AO. (1966) Carcinoid tymors of Meckels' diverticulum. *Cancer* 19:1591–1593.

Eckhauser FE, Lloyd RV, Thompson NW, et al. (1988) Antrectomy for multicentric, argyrophil gastric carcinoid: a preliminary report. *Surgery* 104:1046–1053.

Federspiel BH, Burke AP, Sobin LH, et al. (1990) Rectal and colonic carcinoids: a clinico-pathologic study of 84 cases. *Cancer* 65:135–140.

Feldman AJ, Weinberg M, Raess D, et al. (1980) Gastric carcinoid tumor: its occurrence with ossification and diffuse argyrophil cell hyperplasia. *Arch Surg* 116:118–121.

Frieson SR, Schimke RN, Pearse AGE. (1972) Genetic aspects of the Z-E syndrome: prospective studies in two kindred; antral gastrin cell hyperplasia. *Ann Surg* 176:370–383.

Ganguli PC, Polak JM, Pearse et al. (1973) Antral "G"

cell hyperplasia with peptic ulcer disease: a new clinical entity. *Gut* 14:822–823.

Gardiner GW, Van Patter T, Murray D. (1985) Atypical carcinoid tumor of the small bowel complicating celiac disease. *Cancer* 56:2716–2722.

Gledhill A, Hall PA, Cruse JP, Pollack DJ. (1986) Enteroendocrine cell hyperplasia, carcinoid tumors and adenocarcinoma in long-standing ulcerative colitis. *Histopathology* 10:501–508.

Godwin JD. (1975) Carcinoid tumors, an analysis of 2837 cases. *Cancer* 36:560–569.

Goldfain D, le Bodic MF, Lavergne A, et al. (1989) Gastric carcinoid tumors in patients with Zollinger-Ellison syndrome on long-term omeprazole. *Lancet* 1:776–777.

Gould VE. (1987) Synaptophysin: a new and promising pan-neuroendocrine marker (editorial). *Arch Pathol Lab Med* 111:791–794.

Gould VE, DeLellis RA. (1983) The neuroendocrine cell system: its tumors, hyperplasias and dysplasias. In: *Principles and Practice of Surgical Pathology* (Silverberge SC, ed.) pp. 1487–1501. John Wiley and Sons, New York.

Harvey RF, Bradshaw MJ, Davidson CM, et al. (1985) Multifocal gastric carcinoid tumours, achlorhydria, and hypergastrinemia. *Lancet* 1:951–954.

Hernandez FJ, Fernandez BB. (1974) Mucus-secreting colonic carcinoid tumors: Light- and electron-microscopic study of three cases. *Dis Colon Rectum* 17:387–396.

Hodges JR, Isaacson P, Wright R. (1981) Diffuse enterochromaffin-like (ECL) cell hyperplasia and multiple gastric carcinoids: a complication of pernicious anemia. *Gut* 22:237–241.

Isaacson P. (1981) Crypt cell carcinoma of the appendix (so-called adenocarcinoid tumor). *Am J Surg Pathol* 5:213–224.

Ito H, Yokozaki H, Hata J, et al. (1984) Glicentin containing cells in intestinal metaplasia, adenoma and carcinoma of the stomach. *Virchows Arch A Pathol Anat Histopathol* 404:17–29.

Janson ET, Holmberg L, Stridsberg M, Eriksson B, Theodorsson E, Wilander E, Oberg K. (1997) Carcinoid tumors: analysis of prognostic factors and survival in 301 patients from a referral center. *Ann Oncol* 8:685–690.

Johnson LA, Lavin P, Moertel CG, et al. (1983) Carcinoids: the association of histologic growth pattern and survival. *Cancer* 51:882–889.

Kern SE, Yardley JH, Lazenby AJ, et al. (1990) Reversal by antrectomy of endocrine cell hyperplasia in the gastric body in pernicious anemia: a morphometric study. *Mod Pathol* 3:561–566.

Kloppel G, Heitz PU, Capella C, Solcia E. (1996) Pathology and nomenclature of human gastrointestinal neuroendocrine (carcinoid) tumors and related lesions. *World J Surg* 20:132–141.

Kuiper DH, Gracie WA Jr, Pollard HM. (1970) Twenty years of gastrointestinal carcinoids. *Cancer* 25:1424–1430.

Kwan CP, Tytgat GN. (1995) Antral G-cell hyperplasia: a vanishing disease? *Eur J Gastroenterol Hepatol* 7:1099–1103.

Laura V, Rossi B, Paladino R, Gori A, Lugani P, Sanguineti G, Di Ciolo L, Falchero E. (1997) Carcinoid of Vater's papilla. The authors' own experience. *Minerva Chirurg* 52:1215–1222.

Lehy T, Mignon M, Cadiot G, et al. (1989) Gastric endocrine cell behavior in Zollinger-Ellison patients upon long-term potent antisecretory treatment. *Gastroenterology* 96:1029–1040.

Lewin KJ. (1986) The endocrine cells of the gastrointestinal tract. The normal endocrine cells and their hyperplasias. *Pathol. Annu.* (Part I) 21:1–27.

Lewin KJ. (1992) Endocrine cells of the gastrointestinal tract. In: *Gastrointestinal Pathology and Its Clinical Implications* (Lewin KJ, Riddell R, Weinstein WM, eds.) pp. 197–257. Igaku-Shoin, New York.

Lewin KJ, Ulich T, Yang K, Layfield L. (1986) The endocrine cells of the gastrointestinal tract. *Pathol Annu* (Tumors, Part II) 21:181–215.

Lewin KJ, Yang K, Ulich T, et al. (1984) Primary gastrin cell hyperolasia: report of five cases and a review of the literature. *Am J Surg Pathol* 8:821–832.

Lindberg GM, Molberg KH, Vuitch MF, Albores-Saavedra J. (1997) Atypical carcinoid of the esophagus: a case report and review of the literature. *Cancer* 79:1476–1481.

Lloyd RV, Cano M, Rosa P, et al. (1988) Distribution of chromogranin A, secretogranin 1 (chromogranin B) in neuroendocrine cells and tumors. *Am J Pathol* 130:296–304.

Lloyd RV, Mervak T, Schmidt K, et al. (1984) Immunohistochemical detection of chromogranin and neuron specific enolase in pancreatic endocrine neoplasm. *Am J Surg Pathol* 8:607–614.

Loftus JP, van Heerden JA. (1995) Surgical management of gastrointestinal carcinoid tumors. *Adv Surg* 28:317–336.

Luk IS, Bhuta S, Lewin KJ. (1997) Clear cell carcinoid of the stomach; a variant mimicking gastric xanthalesma. *Arch Pathol Lab Med* 121:1100–1103.

Lundqvist M, Wilander E. (1987) A study of the histopathogenesis of carcinoid tumors of the small intestine and appendix. *Cancer* 60:201–206.

Manickam P, Olufemi SE, Liotta LA, Chandrasekharappa SC, Collins FS, Spiegal AM, Burns AL, Marx SJ. (1997) Germline mutations of the MEN1 gene in familial multiple endocrine neoplasia type 1 and related states. *Hum Mol Genet* 6:1169–1175.

Martin ED, Potet F. (1974) Pathology of endocrine tumours of the GI tract. *Clin Gastroenterol* 3:511–532.

Masson P. (1914) La glande endocrine de l'intestine chez l'homme. *Comptes Rendus Acad Sci Paris* 158:59–61.

McDermott EWM, Guduric B, Brennan MF. (1994) Prognostic variables in patients with gastrointestinal carcinoid tumours. *Br J Surg* 81:1007–1009.

McDonald GSA, Hourihane DOB. (1977) Mucinous carcinoid tumor of the appendix containing Paneth cells. *Ir J Med Sci* 146:386–389.

Miller RR, Sumner HW. (1982) Argyrophilic cell hyperplasia and an atypical carcinoid tumor in chronic ulcerative colitis. *Cancer* 50:2920–2925.

Modlin IM, Sandor A. (1997) An analysis of 8305 cases of carcinoid tumors. *Cancer* 79:813–829.

Moertel CG. (1987) An odyssey in the land of small tumors. *J Clin Oncol* 5:1503–1522.

Moertel CG, Sauer WG, Dockerty MB, Baggenstoss AH. (1961) Life history of the carcinoid tumor of the small intestine. *Cancer* 14:901–912.

Moertel CG, Weiland LH, Nagornney DM, Dockerty MB. (1987) Carcinoid tumor of the appendix: treatment and prognosis. *N Engl J Med* 317:1699–1701.

Morgan JG, Marks C, Hearn D. (1974) Carcinoid tumors of the gastrointestinal tract. *Ann Surg* 180:720–727.

Moyana TN. (1989) Carcinoid tumors arising from Meckel's diverticulum. A clinical, morphologic, and immunohistochemical study. *Am J Clin Pathol* 91:52–56.

Moyana TN, Shukoor S. (1991) Gastrointestinal endocrine cell hyperplasia in celiac disease: A selective proliferative process of serotonergic cells. *Mod Pathol* 4:419–423.

Muller J, Kirchner T, Muller-Hermelink HK. (1987) Gastric endocrine cell hyperplasia and carcinoid tumors in atrophic gastritis type A. *Am J Surg Pathol* 11:909–917.

Norheim I, Oberg K, Theodorsson-Norheim E, et al. (1987) Malignant carcinoid tumors: an analysis of 103 patients with regards to tumor localization, hormone production and survival. *Ann Surg* 206:115–126.

Ogata T. (1973) An electron microscopic study on the endocrine cell sin the atypical epithelial lesion of the stomach. In: *Gastro-Entero-Pancreatic Endocrine System. A Cell-Biological Approach* (Fugita T, ed.) pp. 120–124. Igaku-Shoin, Tokyo.

Olsson B, Ljungberg O. (1980) Adenocarcinoid of the vermiform appendix. *Virchows Arch A Pathol Anat Histopathol* 386:201–210.

Orlefors H, Sundin A, Ahlstreom H, Bjurling P, Bergstreom M, Lilja A, Leangstreom B, Oberg K, Eriksson B. (1998) Positron emission tomography with 5-hydroxytryprophan in neuroendocrine tumors. *J Clin Oncol* 16:2534–2541.

Polak JM, Hoffbrand AV, Reed PI, et al. (1973) Qualitative and quantitative studies of antral and fundic G-cells in pernicious anemia. *Scand J Gastroenterol* 8:361–367.

Polak JM, Stagg B, Pearse AGE. (1972) Two types of Zollinger-Ellison syndrome: immunofluorescent, cytochemical, and ultrastructural studies of the antral and pancreatic gastrin cells in different clinical states. *Gut* 13:501–512.

Ramnani DM, Wistuba II, Behrens C, Gazdar AF, Sobin LH, Albores-Saavedra J. (1999) K-*ras* and p53 mutations in the pathogenesis of classical and goblet cell carcinoids of the appendix. *Cancer* 86:14–21.

Rindi G, Luinetti O, Cornaggia M, Capella C, Solcia E. (1993) Three subtypes of gastric argyrophil carcinoid and the gastric neuroendocrine carcinoma: a clinicopathologic study. *Gastroenterology* 104:994–1006.

Ritchie AC. (1956) Carcinoid tumors. *Am J Med Sci* 222:311–328.

Rivadeneira DE, Tuckson WB, Naab T. (1996) Increased incidence of second primary malignancy in patients with carcinoid tumors: case report and literature review. *J Nat Med Assoc* 88:310–312.

Rode J, Dhillon AP, Doran JF, et al. (1985) PGP 9.5, a new marker for human neuroendocrine tumors. *Histopathology* 9:147–158.

Rodriguez FH Jr, Sarma DP, Lunseth JH. (1982) Goblet cell carcinoid of the appendix. *Hum Pathol* 13:286–288.

Roncoroni L, Costi R, Canavese G, Violi V, Bordi C. (1997) Carcinoid tumor associated with vascular malformation as a cause of massive gastric bleeding. *Am J Gastroenterol* 92:2119–2121.

Royston CMS, Polak JM, Bloom SR, et al. (1978) G cell population of gastric antrum, plasma gastric and gastric acid secretion in patients with and without duodenal ulcer. *Gut* 19:689–698.

Rubin W. (1969) Proliferation of endocrine-like (enterochromaffin) cells in atrophic gastric mucosa. *Gastroenterology* 57:641–648.

Rubin W. (1973) A fine structural characterization of the proliferated endocrine cells in atrophic gastric mucosa. *Am J Pathol* 70:109–118.

Shi W, Buchanan KD, Johnston CF, Larkin C, Ong YL, Ferguson R, Laird J. (1998) The octreotide suppression test and [111In-DTPA-D-Phe1]-octreotide scintigraphy in neuroendocrine tumours correlate with responsiveness to somatostatin analogue treatment. *Clin Endocrinol* 48:303–309.

Shimoda T, Tanoue S, Ikegami M, et al. (1983) A histopathological study of diffuse hyperplasia of gastric argyrophil cells. *Acta Pathol Jpn* 33:1259–1267.

Sjoblom SM, Haapiainen R, Miettinen M, Jarvinen H. (1987) Gastric carcinoid tumors and atrophic gastritis. *Acta Chir Scand* 153:37–43.

Sjoblom SM, Sipponen P, Karonen SL, JaNiren HJ. (1989) Mucosal argyrophil endocrine cells in pernicious anemia and upper gastrointestinal carcinoud tumors. *J Clin Pathol* 42:371–377.

Sjoblom SM, Sippon P, Miettinen M, et al. (1988) Gastroscopic screening for gastric carcinoids and carcinoma in pernicious anemia. *Endoscopy* 20:52–56.

Solcia E, Bordi C, Creutzfeldt W, et al. (1988) Histopathological classification of nonantral gastric endocrine growths in man. *Digestion* 41:185–200.

Solcia E, Capella C, Fiocca R, et al. (1989a) The gastroenteropancreatic endocrine system and related tumors. *Gastroenterol Clin North Am* 18:671–693.

Solcia E, Capella C, Fiocca R, et al. (1990) Gastric argyrophil carcinoidosis in patients with Zollinger-ellison syndrome due to type 1 multiple endocrine neoplasia. A newly organized association. *Am J Surg Pathol* 14:503–513.

Solcia E, Rindi G, Havu N, Elm G. (1989b): Qualitative studies of gastric endocrine cells in patients treated long-term with omeprazole. *Scand J Gastroenterol Suppl.* 166:129–137.

Stachura J, Krause WJ, Ivey KJ. (1981) Ultrastructure of endocrine-like cells in lamina propria of human gastric mucosa. *Gut* 22:534–541.

Stolte M, Ebert D, Siefert E, et al. (1988) The prognosis of carcinoid tumors of the stomach. *Leber Magen Darm* 18:246–256.

Stremple JF, Watson CG. (1974) Serum calcium, serum gastrin, and gastric acid secretion before and after parathyroidectomy for hyperparathyroidism. *Surgery* 75:841–852.

Subbuswamy SG, Gibbs NM, Ross CF, Morson BC. (1974) Goblet cell carcinoid of the appendix. *Cancer* 34:338–344.

Teitelbaum SL. (1972) The carcinoid, a collective review. *Am J Surg* 123:564–572.

Terris B, Scoazec JY, Rubbia L, Bregeaud L, Pepper MS, Ruszniewski P, Belghiti J, Flejou J, Degott C. (1998) Expression of vascular endothelial growth factor in digestive neuroendocrine tumours. *Histopathology* 32:133–138.

Thompson NW, Vinik AI, Eckhauser FE. (1989) Microgastrinomas of the duodenum. A cause of failed operations for the Zollinger-Ellison syndrome. *Ann Surg* 209:396–404.

Ulich T, Cheng L, Lewin KJ. (1982) Acinar-endocrine cell tumor of the pancreas: report of a pancreatic tumor containing both zymogen and neuroendocrine granules. *Cancer* 50:2099–2105.

Walsh JH, Nair PK, Kleibeuker J, et al. (1983) Pathological acid secretion not due to gastrinoma. *Scand J Gastroenterol* 18 (Suppl. 82):45–58.

Warkel RL, Cooper PH, Helwig EB. (1978) Adenocarcinoid, a mucin-producing carcinoid tumor of the appendix. A study of 39 cases. *Cancer* 42:2781–2793.

Watson PH, Alguacil-Garcia A. (1987) Mixed crypt cell carcinoma: a clinicopathologic study of the so-called goblet cell carcinoid. *Virchows Arch A Pathol Anat Histopathol* 412:175–182.

Weibel LA, Joergenson EJ, Keasbey LE. (1954) A clinical study of small bowel tumors. Report of 165 lesions. *Am J Gastroenterol* 21:466–477.

Weiler R, Fisher-Colbrie R, Schmid KW, et al. (1988) Immunological studies on the occurrence and properties of chromogranin A and B and secretogranin II in endocrine tumors. *Am J Surg Pathol* 12:877–884.

Wiedenmann B, Waldherr R, Buhr H, et al. (1988) Identification of gastroenteropancreatic neuroendocrine cells in normal and neoplastic human tissue with antibodies against synaptophysin, chromogranin A, secretogranin I (chromogranin B) and secretogranin II. *Gastroenterology* 95:1364–1374.

Weng YJ, Wang SS, Yang WG, Chao Y, Lai CR, Lee SD. (1996) Carcinoid tumors of the gastrointestinal tract in Chinese of Taiwan: an analysis of fifty cases. *Chung-Hua I Hsueh Tsa Chih* [Chinese Medical Journal] 58(4):254-258.

Zakariai YM, Quan SHQ, Hajdu SI. (1975) Carcinoid tumors of the gastrointestinal tract. *Cancer* 35:588–591.

28

SOFT TISSUE TUMORS

Ruby Delgado, Enrique de Alava, and Jorge Albores-Saavedra

The stark contrast between the morphologic plurality and heterogeneity of soft tissue neoplasms and the seemingly limited range of cell and tissue types from which they derive is such that many of the soft tissue tumors appear not to have a normal counterpart, nor are there recognizable histologic precursor lesions for most of them. Nevertheless, the predilection exhibited by some soft tissue tumors to arise in certain topographical locations (trunk versus extremities, proximal versus distal, and superficial versus deep) may provide insights into the nature, properties, and/or capacity of the native mesenchyme at this site. Similarly, the varying behavior of a histologic tumor type according to a superficial or deep (lipomatous and fibrohistiocytic tumors), or proximal and distal (epithelioid sarcoma, extraskeletal myxoid chondrosarcoma) location is also telling. Their occurrence in certain age-groups may shed light on the operative regulatory mechanisms. More recently and of greater relevance, the events surrounding tumor-specific chromosomal translocations may provide direct insights into sarcomagenesis.

Although benign precursor lesions of soft tissue sarcomas are rare, some low-grade soft tissue sarcomas may evolve into high-grade soft tissue sarcomas (e.g., well-differentiated liposarcoma, dermatofibrosarcoma protuberans), and others frequently do so (e.g., myxofibrosarcoma). Progression of low-grade precursors may occur merely through the gradual acquisition of cellularity, pleomorphism, and mitotic activity, or by means of transformation into a different histologic

type(s), so-called dedifferentiation. Tumor progression may be noted in the primary tumor or in its subsequent recurrence(s). The percentage of high-grade or dedifferentiated components having clinical relevance may vary for each tumor type. Interestingly, in some tumor types, histologic progression may "revert"—that is, only the low-grade precursor may be present in the recurrence of a dedifferentiated sarcoma. Some soft tissue tumors may be considered precursors by means of their potential for divergent differentiation (such as malignant peripheral nerve sheath tumor giving rise to angiosarcoma). On the other hand, several tumor types may converge on a common phenotype, such as rhabdoid, epithelioid, and pleomorphic (malignant fibrous histiocytoma-like) tumors. Interestingly, the most common benign precursor among the soft tissue tumors, neurofibroma, is of neuroectodermal, and not mesenchymal, origin.

MALIGNANT TRANSFORMATION

Peripheral Nerve Sheath Tumors

Malignant Peripheral Nerve Sheath Tumors Arising in Benign Peripheral Nerve Sheath Tumors (Neurofibroma, Schwannoma)

The *malignant peripheral nerve sheath tumor* (MPNST) is a tumor arising from or differentiating toward cells intrinsic to the pe-

Table 28–1. Malignant Transformation of Peripheral Nerve

Precursor	Malignant Tumor
Peripheral nerve (NF1, sporadic)	MPNST, spindle cell sarcoma type or MPNST, epithelioid type MPNST, PNET-like (in children)

Neurofibroma (NF1,[a] sporadic)
    Plexiform
    Localized intraneural
	MPNST, spindle cell sarcoma type (85%) or
	MPNST, with divergent differentiation (15%)
	MPNST, PNET-like (in children)

Schwannoma[b] Classic	MPNST, epithelioid type or MPNST, neuroepithelial type

Ganglioneuroma
    Nonradiated
    With radiation-induced
        maturation
	MPNST

?	Perineural MPNST

MPNST, malignant peripheral nerve sheath tumor; NF1, neurofibromatosis 1; PNET, primitive neuroepithelial tumor.

[a]Neurofibroma associated with NF1 is the most common precursor of MPNSTs.

[b]A tendency for epithelioid angiosarcoma to arise in schwannoma has been reported (Menamin and Fletcher, 2000; Mentzel and Katenkamp, 1999).

ripheral nerve sheath. There are histomorphologic differences between the MPNSTs arising from neurofibromas and those arising from schwannomas, which may be related to their precursor cell(s) (Scheithauer et al., 1999; Woodruff et al., 1994; Table 28–1). In neurofibromas, the putative precursors are, in addition to Schwann cells, a range of cells of possible mesenchymal derivation, including perineurial-like cells, fibroblasts, and a cell intermediate between the perineurial-like cell and fibroblasts. This may account for most conventional malignant peripheral nerve sheath tumors, arising from neurofibromas, having the appearance of spindle cell sarcomas. This may also explain the occurrence of metaplastic malignant mesenchymal elements, such as chondrosarcoma and rhabdomyosarcoma, in these tumors. Alternatively, a genetically altered Schwann cell present in neurofibromas in the setting of neurofibromatosis 1 may be capable of multidirectional differentiation. On the other hand, the neuroectodermal-derived Schwann cell is the sole precursor of the schwannoma, which upon malignant transformation acquires epithelioid or neuroepithelial features. The vast majority of MPNSTs arise from neurofibromas—neurofibromatosis associated or sporadic.

Neurofibromatosis Type 1

Neurofibromatosis 1 (NF1) is caused by autosomal dominantly inherited or *de novo* mutations in the *NF1* gene on chromosome 17q (Feldkamp et al., 1998; Guha, 1998; Zwarthoff, 1996). The *NF1* gene has a very high mutation frequency, which may be related in part to its large size, a total length over 300 kb. Except for cases in which the whole gene appears to be deleted, no relationship has been observed between genotype and phenotype.

The *NF1* gene product, *neurofibromin,* acts as a negative regulator in the *ras* signal transduction pathway and may also act downstream of *ras*. The Ras pathway is a key signal transduction pathway that transmits mitogenic signals to the nucleus. Ras is a member of the small G protein family, characterized by being bound to GDP in the basal inactive state and being activated in the GTP bound state. Activated Ras-GTP is slowly hydrolyzed to GDP by intrinsic GTPase activity in native Ras, a process that is rapidly catalyzed by Ras-GTPase activating proteins (Ras-GAPs). Neurofibromin shares 30% homology with members of the Ras-GAP family through its GAP-related domain (GRD), and enhances the conversion of active ras-GTP to inactive-GDP. Loss of neurofibromin is postulated to lead to functional upregulation of the Ras pathway in NF1 with increased mitogenic signaling. The NF-1 neurofibromas and neurogenic sarcomas have markedly elevated levels of activated Ras (Ras bound to GTP) and lack neurofibromin.

Interestingly, no mutations that activate

Ras have been found in neural crest–derived tumors, suggesting that active *Ras* cannot transform these cells. This has led some investigators to postulate that neurofibromin can inhibit Ras-dependent growth by a mechanism other than its GTPase-accelerating function (Klose et al., 1998; Zwarthoff, 1996).

While NF1 mRNA is detectable in most tissues, the expression of the neurofibromin protein is more tightly regulated, with the highest levels found in neurons, oligodendrocytes, nonmyelinated Schwann cells, adrenal medulla, leukocytes, and testis (Feldkamp et al., 1998). Four neurofibromin isoforms that differ in their developmental and tissue expression have been identified. Type 2 is the isoform predominantly expressed in tissues derived from the neural crest, such as Schwann cells and adrenal medullary cells, in addition to glia and anterior horn cells of the adult spinal cord (Feldkamp et al., 1998). In the cell types that are affected in patients with NF1, the absence of neurofibromin leads to increased proliferation and tumor formation.

Malignant transformation of neurofibromas in neurofibromatosis 1

The MPNSTs can occur *de novo* in peripheral nerves in patients with NF1, but most are derived from neurofibromas (Scheithauer et al., 1999; Woodruff, 1999). Malignant transformation of neurofibromas occurs in approximately 2% of NF1 patients. Only two forms of neurofibroma, plexiform and localized intraneural neurofibroma, are significant precursors of MPNSTs, involving a large or medium-sized nerve or nerve plexus (McCarron and Goldblum, 1998; Woodruff, 1999; Table 28–1). Clinically, the onset of malignancy may become manifest through an increased rate of growth of a portion or all of the lesion or through the occurrence of spontaneous and unremitting pain not explained by trauma (Korf, 1999).

The MPNST arising within plexiform neurofibroma may be grossly inapparent or multifocal (Scheithauer et al., 1999). Both cross- and longitudinal sectioning of plexiform neurofibromas after malignant transformation show variation in the cellularity of nodules as individual neurofibromas are unevenly replaced by spreading MPNST. In practice, a coexisting neurofibroma is far more often apparent microscopically than grossly. When grossly apparent, the MPNST is usually firm, gray-tan, and opaque, unlike the soft translucent character of neurofibromas. Areas of necrosis are grossly apparent in approximately 60% of the cases. Given the tendency of MPNSTs arising in sizable nerves to undergo intraneural extension, it is imperative at the time of surgery to undertake frozen section assessment of proximal and distal margins. The MPNSTs are usually solitary, even when they arise from a plexiform neurofibroma. Histologically, malignant transformation may occur through abrupt change into a MPNST or through gradual acquisition of increased mitotic activity and atypia.

The minimal criteria necessary for the diagnosis of malignant change in neurofibroma are definite cell crowding, general nuclear enlargement (at least three times the size of ordinary neurofibroma nuclei), and hyperchromasia (Scheithauer et al., 1999; Woodruff, 1999). Mitotic figures may or may not be present in such cases (Fletcher, 1995). The sole finding of a few mitoses in an otherwise histologically unremarkable neurofibroma is not regarded as evidence of malignant transformation. This early, or *low-grade, MPNST* must be distinguished from two variants of neurofibroma that may exhibit worrisome histologic features, although they are clinically benign: cellular neurofibroma and atypical neurofibroma. Atypical neurofibromas lack significant cellularity but contain scattered pleomorphic cells with bizarre, often hyperchromatic nuclei. Such cells have a degenerative smudgy chromatin appearance and may feature nuclear-cytoplasmic pseudoinclusions. There is at present no evidence that such cytologic atypia is in and of itself an indication of malignant change. Atypical neurofibromas (Lin et al., 1997) lack significant mitotic activity and show no appreciable MIB-1 labeling (Lin et al., 1997). *Cellular neurofibromas* is the term given to neurofibromas showing an increased cellularity with or without a low level of mitotic activity, but lacking any of the three aforementioned features of malignancy.

Most MPNSTs arising from neurofibromas in patients with NF1 are high grade on presentation. Histologically, *high-grade MPNSTs*

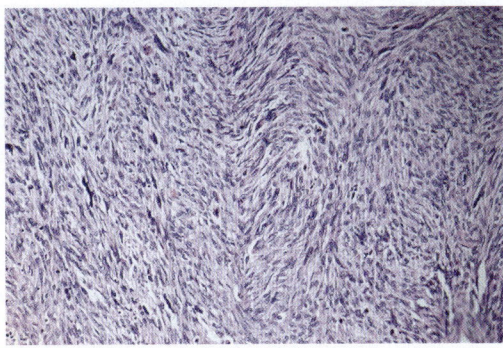

Figure 28–1. Malignant peripheral nerve sheath tumor, high grade. This cellular neoplasm, which arose from the sciatic nerve, is composed of interlacing fascicles of spindle cells and multinucleated giant cells. A herringbone pattern is seen.

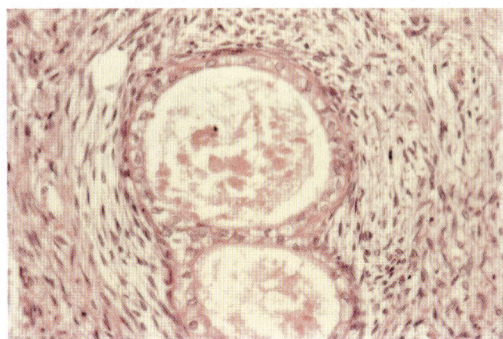

Figure 28–3. Malignant peripheral nerve sheath tumor with glandular elements.

are characterized by fasciculated growth of crowded, hyperchromatic, and mitotically active spindle cells, closely resembling fibrosarcoma (Ducatamanet al., 1986; Fletcher, 1995; Scheithauer et al., 1999; Wanebo et al., 1993; Woodruff, 1999). There is a moderate amount of eosinophilic cytoplasm but there are no clear cell outlines. Scattered multinucleated cells are sometimes present (Fig. 28–1). A geographic form of necrosis is common (Fig. 28–2). Approximately 15% of high-grade MPNSTs show divergent differentiation with formation of heterologous tissues, mainly of mesenchymal type, but also epithelial glands (Ducataman and Scheithauer, 1984). The types of mesenchymal differentiation include chondrosarcoma, rhabdomyosarcoma, osteosarcoma, and angiosarcoma.

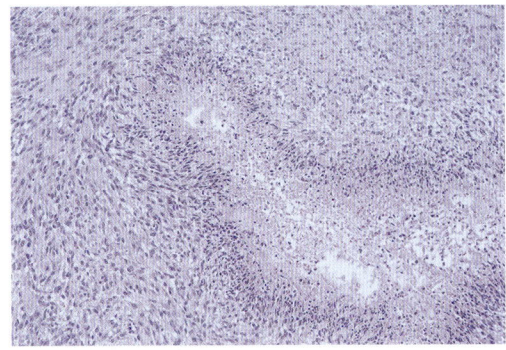

Figure 28–2. Malignant peripheral nerve sheath tumor, high grade, showing areas of necrosis with pseudopalisading of neoplastic cells.

The MPNSTs with epithelial glandular differentiation (glandular MPNSTs) frequently contain neuroendocrine cells (Fig. 28–3). A single MPNST may contain more than one heterologous tissue. Of the MPNSTs with divergent differentiation, glandular MPNST is seen predominantly in NF1 patients and MPNST with angiosarcoma is seen almost exclusively in NF1 patients (Mentzel and Katenkamp, 1999; Woodruff, 1999). It is of interest regarding the latter that the increased Ras activity noted in NF1 neurogenic sarcomas is also accompanied by transcriptional up-regulation of vascular endothelial growth factor (VEGF), the most potent and specific angiogenic factor (Guha, 1998; Mentzel and Katenkamp, 1999).

Since malignant tumors occur in only a minority of patients with NF1, it is possible that mutations in other genes, in addition to those in both alleles of the NF1 gene, are required for these tumors to develop. The immunohistochemical detection of intranuclear p53 is common in the malignant areas but is uncommon in the precursor neurofibroma. In neurofibrosarcomas from NF1 patients, loss or missense mutations in the *p53* gene are often observed. Thus it seems that a *p53* mutation might be an obligatory step for malignant transformation (Feldkamp et al., 1998; Halling et al., 1996; McCarron and Goldblum, 1998; Zwarthoff, 1996).

Characteristics of MPNSTs in NF1:
• Represent 50%–60% of patients with MPNSTs
• Most arise from neurofibromas
• Typically present at a younger age (Doorn et al., 1995; Wanebo et al., 1993)

- Show a male predominance
- About 80% are high grade
- Heterologous elements are seen most often (angiosarcoma exclusively in NF1 and glandular predominantly in NF1 patients)
  - Patients are at risk for developing a second MPNST (Doorn et al., 1995)
  - Tend to have a poorer prognosis.

Malignant Peripheral Nerve Sheath Tumors Arising in Schwannoma

Malignant transformation of schwannomas is an extremely rare event, and all acceptable cases have occurred in classical schwannoma (Rasbridge et al., 1989; Woodruff et al., 1994). The MPNSTs arising from schwannomas differ from conventional ones in that they have a purely epithelioid or neuroepithelial morphology (Table 28–1). The epithelioid tumors are composed of polygonal cells with densely eosinophilic cytoplasm and pleomorphic hyperchromatic nuclei, sometimes showing prominent eosinophilic nucleoli. Mitotic figures are readily identified. They show patchy positivity for S-100 protein as compared to strong reactivity of the precursor schwannoma, but in keeping with their epithelioid morphology, they are diffusely and strongly immunoreactive for cytokeratin (Cam 5.2). The malignant component may consist of a mitotically active, small round cell tumor akin to primitive neuroectodermal tumors (PNET). They may show Homer-Wright-like rosettes and are diffusely reactive for S-100 protein. Malignant transformation occurs abruptly within the substance of the schwannoma.

These transformed schwannomas must be distinguished from three forms of schwannoma that are clinically benign despite worrisome histologic features: cellular schwannoma, plexiform schwannoma, and a small group of schwannomas with rosette-like Verocay bodies that mimic neuroblastomatous differentiation. Also, because of their rarity, a primary tumor that might have metastasized to a schwannoma must be excluded. The tumors present at a mean age greater than that of patients with conventional MPNSTs. They are widely distributed and usually >5 cm. The outcome is poor, with metastasis to lung and a mean survival of 6 months.

Malignant Peripheral Nerve Sheath Tumors Arising in a Ganglioneuroma

The MPNSTs may arise in ganglioneuroma, either *de novo* (spontaneous) (Banks et al., 1989; Chandrosoma et al., 1986; Damiani et al., 1991; Drago et al., 1997; Fletcher et al., 1988; Ghali et al., 1992) or following irradiation-induced maturation of a neuroblastic tumor (neuroblastoma or ganglioneuroblastoma) (Keller et al., 1984; Ricci, 1984). They are regarded to be of schwannian-stroma origin (Table 28–1).

Malignant Peripheral Nerve Sheath Tumors *de novo*

The MPNSTs may also arise *de novo* from a peripheral nerve, in patients with or without NF1, and with or without a history of radiation to the nerve (Ducataman and Scheithauer, 1983; Ducataman et al., 1986). Large and medium-sized nerves are distinctly more prone to involvement than small nerves. The MPNSTs involving cranial nerves appear to arise *de novo*. Most MPNSTs *de novo* often have spindle cell sarcoma-like features but also account for the vast majority of epithelioid tumors reported (Woodruff et al., 1994). A predominantly epithelioid differentiation occurs more frequently in MPNSTs from patients without NF1 than from those with this disorder (Woodruff et al., 1994). Incidentally, a peripheral nerve origin is uncommon for the perineurial MPNSTs (Hirose et al., 1998) (Table 28–1).

Malignant Peripheral Nerve Sheath Tumors in Children

Malignant peripheral nerve tumors arising *de novo* or in a neurofibroma in children with or without NF1 show a wide histologic spectrum that, compared to the adult counterpart, features a more primitive appearance resembling that of a primitive neuroepithelial tumor (Meis et al., 1992; Table 28–1).

CHRONIC LYMPHEDEMA AND ANGIOSARCOMA

It has long been established that chronic lymphedema may lead to the development of angiosarcoma (Stewart and Treves, 1948). The most common form of chronic lymphedema–associated angiosarcoma occurs in patients subjected to radical mastectomy for breast carcinoma (Woodward et al., 1972). Among 894 women treated by mastectomy for breast carcinoma, 0.4% developed this malignant vascular tumor (Shirger, 1962). The average interval between the appearance of lymphedema and the development of the tumor is 10 years. Postmastectomy angiosarcomas can also occur in men (Manivel and Albores-Saavedra, 1993). These tumors may also arise in the setting of massive localized lymphedema in morbidly obese individuals (Farshid and Weiss, 1998; Manivel and Albores-Saavedra, 1993). There are reports of lymphangiosarcoms occurring in the lower extremities of patients with chronic lymphedema caused by filarial infection and in edematous legs following radical hysterectomy for squamous cell carcinoma of the uterine cervix (Muller et al., 1987; Sordillo et al., 1981). Angiosarcoma arising in congenital and idiopathic chronic lymphedema has also been reported.

Chronic lymphatic obstruction stimulates proliferation of lymphatic vessels in the dermis. Subsequently, some of these vascular channels are lined by atypical endothelial cells, a lesion termed *lymphangiomatosis*. Occasionally, this lesion merges imperceptibly with vascular channels that are lined by cells with obvious features of malignancy. In many cases it is difficult to draw the line between lymphangiomatosis and angiosarcoma. Some of these lymphedema-associated angiosarcomas show prominent

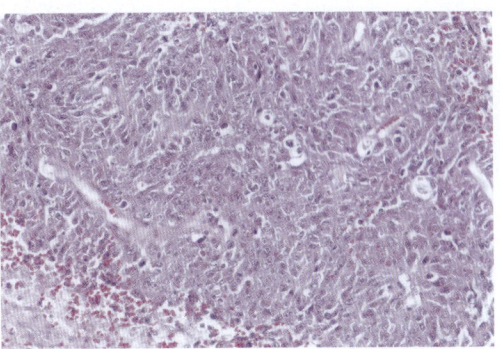

Figure 28–5. Solid areas in epithelioid angiosarcoma mimicking carcinoma.

epithelioid features, are focally cytokeratin positive, and metastasize to lymph nodes, leading to the erroneous diagnosis of carcinoma (Meis-Kindblom and Kindblom,1998; Wenig et al., 1994; Figs. 28–4 and 28–5). Immunoreactivity for CD31, CD34, and ulex europaus lectin clarifies the diagnosis (Miettinen et al, 1994; Fig. 28–6).

OTHER SOFT TISSUE TUMORS

Glomangiosarcomas may arise in the midst of its benign counterpart, glomangioma or glomus tumor. Such tumors are characterized by the presence of typical benign glomus tumor merging histologically into areas of increased cellularity and nuclear pleomorphism, showing vesicular nuclei with prominent nucleoli and variable mitotic activity (Gould et al., 1990). They behave as low-grade malignancies, being locally aggressive but rarely metastasizing.

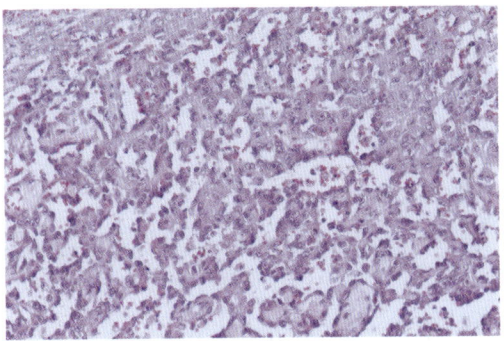

Figure 28–4. Epithelioid angiosarcoma. This tumor arose in the abdominal wall of a morbidly obese woman and shows freely anastomosing vascular channels lined by epithelioid cells.

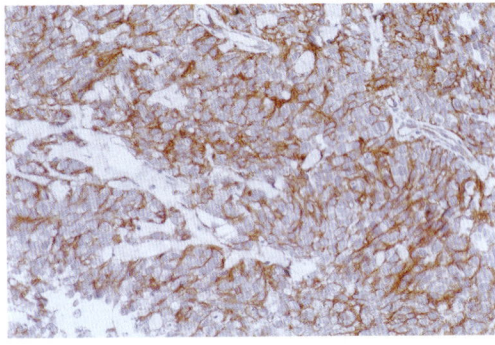

Figure 28–6. The neoplastic cells in this epithelioid angiosarcoma are CD31 positive.

There is a rare case report of sarcomatous transformation of an angiomyofibroblastoma of the vulva into a high grade sarcoma resembling a myxoid malignant fibrous histiocytoma and designated *angiomyofibrosarcoma* (Nielsen et al., 1997).

TUMOR PROGRESSION

Giant Cell Fibroblastoma– Dermatofibrosarcoma Protuberans–Fibrosarcomatous Transformation

GCF ↔ DFSP ↔ FS

Giant cell fibroblastoma (GCF) and *dermatofibrosarcoma protuberans* (DFSP) were originally described as distinct soft tissue tumors (Shmookler, 1989; Shmookler and Enzinger 1982; Taylor and Helwig, 1962), with the former occurring in infants and children and the latter in young to middle-aged adults (Figs. 28–7 and 28–8). However, on the basis of a number of observations at different levels, they are now regarded as related, overlapping, or transitional entities. Clinically, they share the same site of occurrence—the deep dermis of trunk and proximal extremities. Microscopically, (*1*) GCF may recur as DFSP (Alguacil-Garcia, 1991; Allen and Zwi, 1992; Harvell et al., 1998; Perry et al., 1993) or as a Bednar tumor (DeChadarevian et al., 1993), and conversely, recurrences of DFSP may resemble GCF (Coyne et al., 1992; Pitt et al., 1994); (*2*) combined "hybrid" lesions exhibiting features of both (Harvell et al., 1998; Maeda et al., 1998; Michal and Zámecnik, 1992), including a pigmented variant of

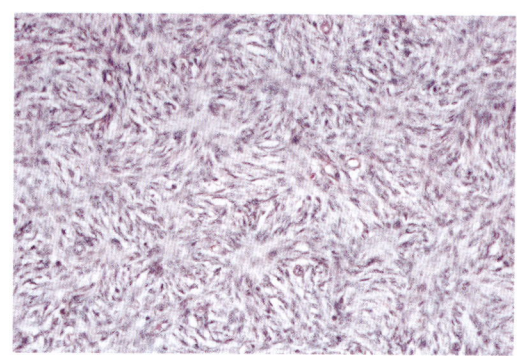

Figure 28–8. Dermatofibrosarcoma protuberans, classical type, with prominent storiform patterns.

DFSP (Zámecnik and Michall, 1994), have been described; (*3*) DFSP may contain areas resembling GCF that are often at the periphery (Beham and Fletcher, 1990; Harvell et al., 1998); and (*4*) DFSP may contain the type of giant cells that characterize GCF (Connelly and Evans, 1992). *Immunophenotypically*, both tumor types show reactivity for CD34 (Diaz-Cascajo et al., 1996; Goldblum, 1996; Harvell et al., 1998; Weiss and Nickoloff, 1993). By cytogenetic analysis, GCF and DFSP are characterized by a t(17;22)(q21;q13) translocation, a der(22), as well as supernumerary ring chromosomes and chromosome markers harboring sequences derived from chromosomes 17 and 22 (Craver et al., 1995; Dal Cin et al., 1996, 1997a; Naeem et al., 1995; Pedeutour, 1995; Pedeutour et al., 1996). Giant cell fibroblastoma was once considered a juvenile form of DFSP (Shmookler, 1989); however, both have now been reported over a wide range of ages (Annesi et al., 1993; Gardner et al., 1998; Mckee and Fletcher, 1991; Pappo et al., 1997). A main distinguishing feature between the two, however, is that while both are prone to local recurrence, virtually only DFSP has been reported to undergo morphologic tumor progression, in the form of fibrosarcomatous transformation, and acquire the capacity to metastasize.

Dermatofibrosarcoma protuberans with fibrosarcomatous transformation (DFSP-FS) (Connelly and Evans, 1992; Diaz-Cascajo, 1997; Ding et al., 1989; Mentzel et al., 1998; Wrotnowski et al., 1988) follows the distribution of DFSP, the trunk and limb girdles being the most common sites. It occurs in 9.5% to

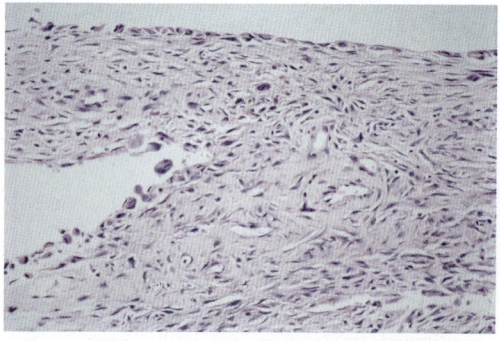

Figure 28–7. Characteristic microscopic features of giant cell fibroblastoma.

20% of cases of DFSP cases seen in consultation. Fibrosarcomatous transformation occurs more commonly in primary, *de novo* lesions but may also develop in recurrent lesions. (A DFSP has recurred as GCF with subsequent fibrosarcomatous change [Pitt et al., 1994]). It is manifested by increased cellularity, a fascicular or herringbone growth pattern rather than the usual storiform pattern, and by increased mitotic activity (10–16 mitoses/10 high power fields [hpf] in DFSP-FS compared to 2–4 mitoses/10 hpf in DFSP) (Fig. 28–9). Tumor cells in the fibrosarcomatous component have slightly more plump nuclei than those of classic DFSP but nuclear pleomorphism is usually not a prominent feature. The transition from classic to fibrosarcomatous morphology may be gradual or abrupt. In contrast to the infiltrative border of the DFSP, the fibrosarcomatous component is often circumscribed and may be pseudoencapsulated. The fibrosarcomatous component is typically in the deep portion and subcutaneous but may occasionally extend upward into the dermis. Necrosis may be seen in the fibrosarcomatous component. The DFSP component may contain melanin-pigmented dendritic cells (Bednar, FS-DFSP) or multinucleated giant cells resembling the giant cells of GCF (Connelly and Evans, 1992; Coyne et al., 1992), or may show myxoid change (Mentzel et al., 1998). Focal myofibroblastic or myoid differentiation may be present in the form of discrete bundles or nodules composed of eosinophilic spindle cells, with well-defined cytoplasmic margins and tapering vesicular nuclei. These myoid nodules often show hyalinization (Calonje

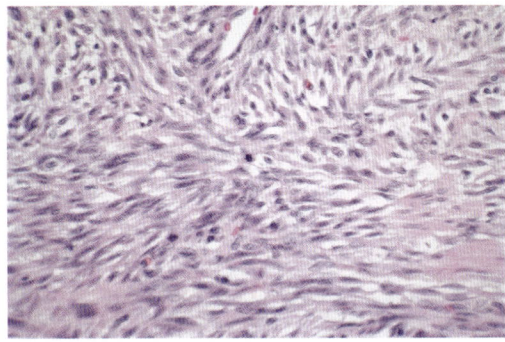

Figure 28–9. Fibrosarcomatous areas in dermatofibrosarcoma protuberans.

and Fletcher, 1996; Diaz-Cascajo, 1997; Mentzel et al., 1998; Morimitsu et al., 1998; O'Connell and Trotter, 1996). Myoid areas are negative for CD34 but positive for smooth muscle actin and muscle-specific actin; desmin is negative (Calonje and Fletcher, 1996; Mentzel et al., 1998). The presence of myoid nodules has been variably interpreted as being related to reactive hyperplasia of myofibroblasts in stroma (Morimitsu, 1998), hypertrophy/hyperplasia of vascular smooth muscle (Diaz-Cascajo, 1997), and as myofibroblastic differentiation in tumor cells (Calonje and Fletcher, 1996; O'Connell and Trotter, 1996). Immunoreactivity for CD34 is negative or patchy and less intense in fibrosarcomatous areas compared to areas of surrounding DFSPs (Goldblum, 1995).

The DFSP-FS has shown a rate (approximately 58%) and time of recurrence similar to those of ordinary DFSP but a higher rate of systemic metastases (14.7% vs. 1%) and tumor-related deaths (5.8%) (Mentzel et al., 1998). Primary DFSP-FS may recur as DFSP only or as FS only, the latter having an adverse outcome (Connelly and Evans, 1992; Mentzel et al., 1998). Ordinary DFSP may also recur as pure fibrosarcoma (Mentzel et al., 1998). Progression to an undifferentiated pleomorphic sarcoma upon recurrence has also been reported (Mentzel et al., 1998). A fibrosarcomatous component is present in the metastases, which are primarily to lung.

With regard to prognostic factors in DFSP-FS, neither the depth of the lesion nor the amount of fibrosarcomatous change appears to influence the prognosis significantly. Similarly, the minimum amount of fibrosarcomatous component that must be present in a tumor for it to have clinical significance has not been determined. Necrosis, a high mitotic rate (>10 mitotic figures per 10 hpf) and the presence of pleomorphic areas, and a short prerecurrent interval (<48 months) tend to be related with poor clinical outcome (Mentzel et al., 1998).

The juxtaposition and/or amplification of chromosomes 17 and 22 sequences (either as reciprocal translocation t(17;22) or, more commonly, as supernumerary chromosomes containing sequences derived from chromosomes 17 and 22) appears to be a cytogenetic event unique to GCF and DFSP and relevant in their pathogenesis (Dal Cin et al., 1996; Simon et al., 1997). It has been shown that these rearrangements result in fusion between the platelet-derived growth factor beta-chain gene (PDGFB), the cellular equivalent of the v-*sis* oncogene, and the collagen type 1 α-1 gene (COL1A1), the major protein constituent of the extracellular matrix in connective tissue of skin (O'Brien et al., 1998; Simon et al., 1997). The chimeric transcript places the PDGFB (located in 22q13) under the control of the COL1A1 promoter (located in 17q21-22), removing all known elements negatively controlling PDGFB transcription and translation. The DFSP not only secretes PDGFB but also possesses PDGFB receptors, providing an autocrine loop whereby the tumor cells can stimulate their own growth (Harvell et al., 1998). The cell of origin remains unknown, although dermal and periadnexal fibroblastic or dendritic cells are likely candidates (Harvell et al., 1998; O'Connell and Trotter, 1996).

Dermatofibrosarcoma Protuberans: Other Precursors

The DFSP often begins as a plaque, which progresses to become nodular or multinodular. If the tumor remains untreated, it can attain massive dimensions resulting in the large, "protuberant" nodules for which it is named. Occasionally, DFSP persists as a nonprotuberant plaque. Such lesions, termed *atrophic DFSP*, are otherwise histologically and prognostically indistinguishable from classical nodular DFSP, and may be considered the early "non-protuberant" phase (Davis and Sanchez, 1998; Fujimoto et al., 1998). In contrast, *plaque-like DFSP* (Davis and Sanchez, 1998) consists of slender fascicles of CD34-immunoreactive spindle cells arranged parallel to the epidermis, developing into a protuberant nodule with traditional storiform histology. Thus both atrophic and plaque-like variants of DFSP may be regarded as histologic precursors in the evolution of the typical DFSP.

LIPOSARCOMAS

Despite the common occurrence of lipomas, liposarcomas are regarded as *de novo* lesions. *Liposarcomas*, or soft tissue sarcomas of adipocytic lineage or differentiation, are a clinical, morphological, and cytogenetically heterogenous group of neoplasms representing different pathways of tumor genesis and evolution (Table 28–2). Myxoid liposarcoma and round cell liposarcoma are the ends of a morphologic continuum that recapitulates lipogenesis. Malignant transformation of mature adipose tissue resulting in well-differentiated liposarcoma more often follows a polyphenotypic evolution.

Table 28–2. Genesis of Liposarcomas

Lower-Grade Precursor	Tumor Progression
Myxoid liposarcoma	Mixed, myxoid and round cell liposarcoma Pure round cell liposarcoma

Well-differentiated liposarcoma	Low-grade dedifferentiation
	  Fibromatosis-like
	  Low-grade fibrosarcoma
	  DFSP-like
	  Meningioma-like

Well-differentiated and/or low-grade dedifferentiated liposarcoma	High-grade dedifferentiation
	  MFH-like
	  High-grade fibrosarcoma

Well-differentiated liposarcoma myxoid/round cell liposarcoma combined liposarcoma	? Pleomorphic liposarcoma
Atypical lipomatous tumor with mild adipocytic atypia (of superficial soft tissues)	Atypical lipomatous tumor with moderate to marked adipocytic atypia and lipoblasts (well-differentiated liposarcoma) ? Spindle cell liposarcoma

DFSP, dermatofibrosarcoma protuberans; MFH, malignant fibrous histiocytoma.

Myxoid Liposarcoma–Round Cell Liposarcoma

Myxoid liposarcoma and round cell liposarcoma are histogenetically and genetically related. They occur disproportionately in deep soft tissues of lower extremities (mainly thigh), and rarely in the retroperitoneum or intra-abdominally. Low-grade, purely myxoid liposarcoma has the potential for gradual progression to high-grade round cell liposarcoma, with purely round cell liposarcoma being rare. *Myxoid liposarcoma* has a distinct histology; it is composed of a myxoid stroma, bland spindled or stellate cells, and lipoblasts (mainly of signet-ring cell type) and has a delicate, plexiform vascular pattern. (Figs. 28–10 and 28–11) As long as cells remain spindled, separated by at least some myxoid stroma, and the plexiform vascularity is still discernible, increased cellularity per se does not seem to be a sign of significant biological progression. Such transitional areas alone do not appear to alter the prognosis of myxoid liposarcoma (Smith et al., 1996). Similarly, the percent of lipoblasts, reported to range from 10% to 90%, does not influence tumor behavior (Kilpatrick et al., 1996).

In *round cell liposarcoma*, as the name implies, the cells are round, not spindled, separated by little or no stroma, so that cells may show overlapping nuclear borders, and obscure the underlying plexiform vascular pattern (Fig. 28–12). The presence of hypercellular areas featuring unequivocally round cell or undifferentiated morphology defines a myxoid-round cell liposarcoma. In the early stage of progression toward a

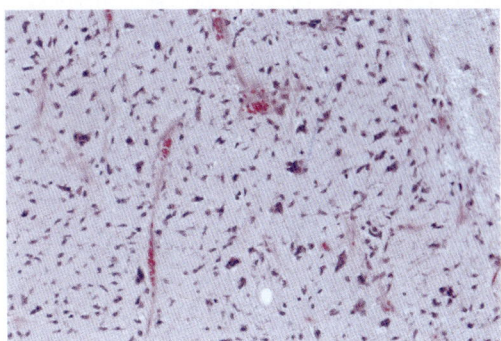

Figure 28–11. Myxoid liposarcoma with multinucleated giant cells.

round cell liposarcoma, distribution of round cells is often around blood vessels or at the edge of the tumor (Kilpatrick et al., 1996; Fig. 28–13).

A trend has been observed between increasing round cell differentiation of >5% and decreased survival in patients (Kilpatrick et al., 1996; Smith et al., 1996), but only tumors with >25% round cell differentiation are significantly associated with development of metastases and a poor prognosis (Kilpatrick et al., 1996). However, even patients with pure myxoid liposarcoma (0% round cell component) have developed metastases (Kilpatrick et al., 1996). Parenthetically, unlike most other sarcomas that metastasize preferentially to lung parenchyma, myxoid/round cell liposarcoma has a tendency to metastasize to other soft tissues (Pearlstone et al., 1999; Spillane et al., 1999). The round cell component may be absent in the

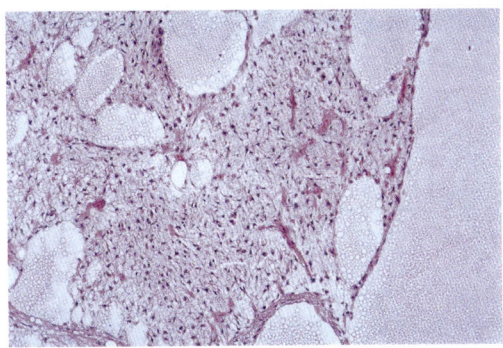

Figure 28–10. Myxoid liposarcoma. Stellate cells, a prominent capillary network, and pools of acid mucopolysaccarides characterized the tumor.

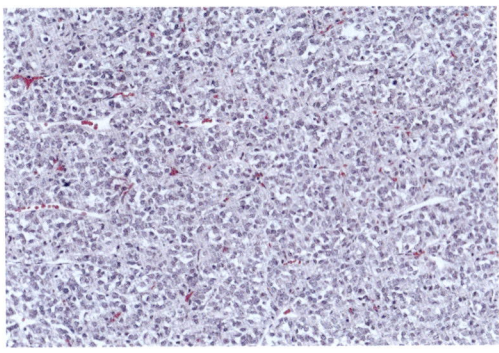

Figure 28–12. Round cell liposarcoma. The tumor is densely cellular and is composed of round cells with scant cytoplasm and small nucleoli. Numerous capillaries are still visible in the stroma.

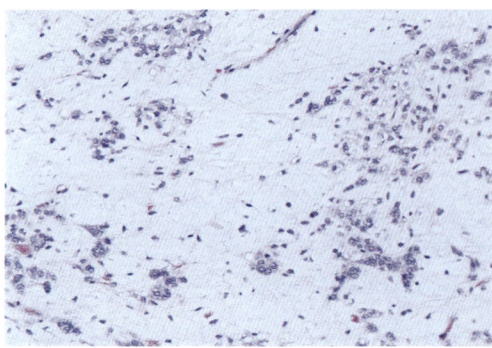

Figure 28–13. Lobule of myxoid liposarcoma with small groups of undifferentiated round cells most likely representing neoplastic progression.

primary tumor but present in recurrences or metastases (Fukuda et al., 1999; Smith et al., 1996). Clinically, a history of rapid enlargement of the lesion often signals the development of round cell areas (Mentzel and Fletcher, 1997). The mechanisms driving the biological progression in myxoid/round cell liposarcoma, cytogenetically characterized by a t(12;16)(q13;p11), are unknown. Secondary chromosomal aberrations have accompanied a high-grade histology (Altungoz et al., 1995; Orndal et al., 1990) but do not seem to be a prerequisite (Knight et al., 1995; Mrozek et al., 1997).

Once referred to as "embryonal liposarcoma," myxoid liposarcoma appears to recapitulate the actively proliferating zone of developing adipose tissue. The neoplastic cells in liposarcoma originate from a dividing population of perivascular mesenchymal cells that begins lipoblastic differentiation as it migrates away from the capillary (Erlandson, 1994). This perhaps explains the perivascular location of round cells in early round cell liposarcoma, as it might represent differentiation arrest of the precursor dividing population.

Lipoma-like and Sclerosing Liposarcoma: Dedifferentiation

Lipoma-like and sclerosing liposarcoma are intimately related and often coexisting lesions encompassed by the term *well-differentiated liposarcoma*, defined as a predominantly mature, albeit atypical, adipocytic lesion. Progression of well-differentiated liposarcoma is usually along nonlipogenic lines, so-called dedifferentiation, into sarcoma(s) of other histologic type(s) (Evans, 1979).

Well-differentiated liposarcoma has a wider anatomic distribution, involving both deep soft tissues (mainly retroperitoneum and the anatomically related inguinal region) and superficial soft tissues (extremities). Lipoma-like liposarcoma is characterized by variation in adipocyte size, adipocytic nuclear atypia, and lipoblasts. In addition to these features, sclerosing liposarcoma shows fibrous septa containing sparse atypical, hyperchromatic stromal cells, whereas lipoblasts are more difficult to find (Fig. 28–14).

Dedifferentiation is believed to be a time-dependent phenomenon occurring predominantly in, but not restricted to, locations where there is a likelihood of clinical persistence of disease. Hence, more commonly occurs it in deep-seated lesions in the retroperitoneum and inguinal region (Weiss and Rao, 1992), and it occurs infrequently in liposarcomas arising from subcutaneous tissue (Dei Tos et al., 1994; Henricks et al., 1997; McCormick et al., 1994; Yoshikawa et al., 1996). Dedifferentiation may manifest itself in recurrences, but most dedifferentiated liposarcomas are *de novo* lesions (Henricks et al., 1997). The dedifferentiation probably derives from evolution of a single clone of undifferentiated mesenchymal cells (McCormick et al., 1994).

Grossly, dedifferentiated foci appear as firm, tan-gray areas within the yellow tan masses of the precursor well-differentiated liposarcoma. Histologically, several types of interface between dedifferentiated compo-

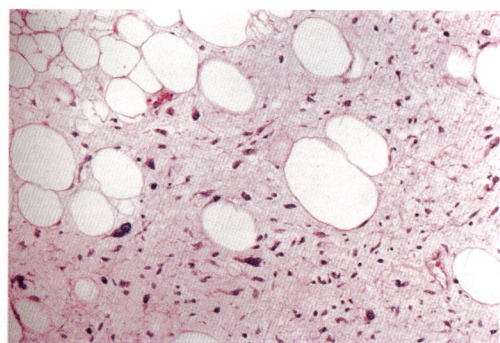

Figure 28–14. Sclerosing liposarcoma. Bands of fibrous tissue surround adipocytes, some with large hyperchromatic nuclei. Atypical cells are also present in the fibrous bands.

nent and underlying tumors have been noted: abrupt, which is the most common; gradual; co-mingling, giving an impression of mosaicism (Henricks et al., 1997); and multifocal-micronodular (McCormick et al., 1994). Transitional zones of gradual tumor progression may be seen in sclerosing liposarcomas as expansion of fibrous septa accompanied by an increased number of atypical cells and an increased number of fibrous septa, progressively coalescing into solid zones of dedifferentiation (Weiss and Rao, 1992). These transitional zones may gradually blend with areas of low-grade to high-grade dedifferentiation (Henricks et al., 1997).

Dedifferentiation may have a low- or high-grade histology or both. In its earliest form, dedifferentiation is only evident microscopically. Microscopic foci of dedifferentiation (incipient or minimal dedifferentiation) have been noted to either, evolve during a protracted period into an exclusively dedifferentiated tumor or, to be absent in recurrences (Evans, 1988; Henricks et al., 1997; Weiss and Rao, 1992).

Low-grade dedifferentiation is usually along fibroblastic lines, consisting of bland, spindled cells arranged in long or short fascicles and resembling fibromatosis, well-differentiated fibrosarcoma, or DFSP (Henricks et al., 1997). An entirely low-grade component is unusual, comprising approximately 10% of the cases (Henricks et al., 1997).

High-grade dedifferentiation is morphologically diverse. The most common patterns are that of a high-grade malignant fibrous histiocytoma (pleomorphic fibrosarcoma), con-

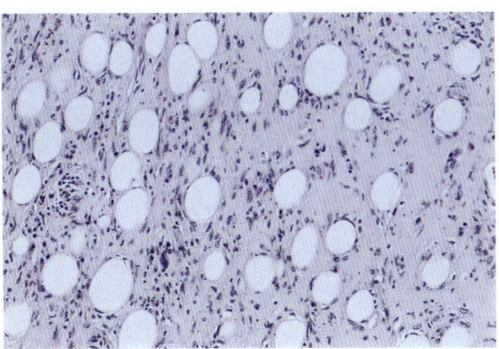

Figure 28–16. Higher magnification of the well-differentiated liposarcomatous component of the tumor shown in Figure 28–15.

sisting of atypical spindled and pleomorphic cells arranged haphazardly in short fascicles, or a high-grade fibrosarcoma (Henricks et al., 1997; McCormick et al., 1994; Weiss and Rao, 1992; Figs. 28–15 to 28–17). Other patterns include sheets of round cells with eosinophilic cytoplasm and prominent nuclei and nucleoli (carcinoma- or melanoma-like), or patterns reminiscent of palisaded myofibroblastoma. Some dedifferentiated liposarcomas are remarkable for containing large, bizarre, hibernoma-like cells (Henricks et al., 1997; McCormick et al., 1994). Dedifferentiation in liposarcomas may coincide with the emergence of heterologous elements including leiomyosarcoma, rhabdomyosarcoma, osteosarcoma, and angiosarcoma (Evans et al., 1994; Henricks et al., 1997; Tallini et al., 1993). The behavior of dedifferentiated liposarcoma is that of a high-grade sarcoma with a local recurrence

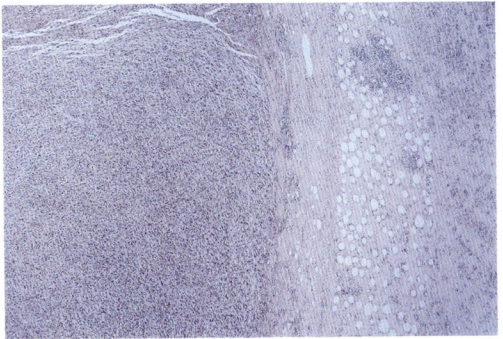

Figure 28–15. Dedifferentiated liposarcoma. Two nodules with different cell densities are clearly seen.

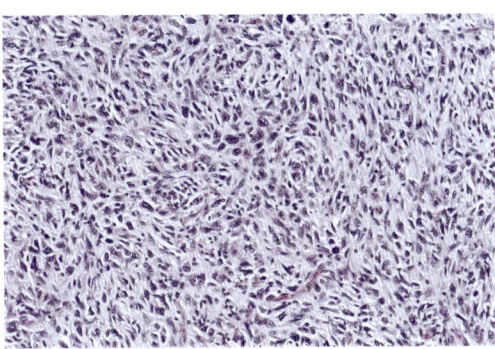

Figure 28–17. Highly cellular nodule shows a high-grade spindle cell sarcoma with astoriform pattern.

rate of 41%, a metastatic rate of 17%, and a disease-related mortality of 28% (Henricks et al., 1997). Tumors located in the retroperitoneum have a worse prognosis than those in accessible soft tissues (Henricks et al., 1997).

Most dedifferentiated liposarcomas are of a high histologic grade and represent >25% of the tumor (Henricks et al., 1997). Low-grade dedifferentiation may be coexist with, and is a likely precursor of, high-grade dedifferentiated liposarcomas (Henricks et al., 1997). Approximately 25% of high-grade dedifferentiated liposarcomas are associated with a low-grade component. Significantly, neither low-grade dedifferentiation nor a low percentage of dedifferentiation (<25%) is associated with an improved outcome. Moreover, the behavior of liposarcomas in which the dedifferentiated component is entirely low grade seems to be more similar to that of conventional (high-grade) dedifferentiated liposarcoma, having the capacity to metastasize and cause death, than to that of well-differentiated liposarcoma (Henricks et al., 1997). Dedifferentiation of either low- or high-grade histology is accompanied by metastatic capacity to lung, liver, brain, or bone. Notably, dedifferentiated liposarcomas may recur as well-differentiated liposarcomas (Henricks et al., 1997; McCormick et al., 1994). It is believed that the nonlipogenic tumor may obscure the underlying precursor, which may become apparent in the recurrence. Because of the frequency of both liposarcomas and their dedifferentiation in the retroperitoneum and inguinal region, a precursor well-differentiated liposarcoma should be suspected when confronted with a nonlipogenic sarcoma in this location.

Dedifferentiation has also been reported for morphologic variants of well-differentiated liposarcoma, so-called inflammatory or lymphocyte-rich (Argani et al., 1997; Kraus et al., 1997), and spindle cell liposarcoma (Dei Tos et al., 1994). A peculiar pattern of dedifferentiation has been recognized that consists of ovoid to spindled cells (showing plump, vesicular nuclei, eosinophilic nucleoli, and scant amphophilic cytoplasm) forming tight, concentric whorls, in a manner reminiscent of, neurothekeoma or meningioma. These lesions of unknown histogenesis are associated with peripheral metaplastic

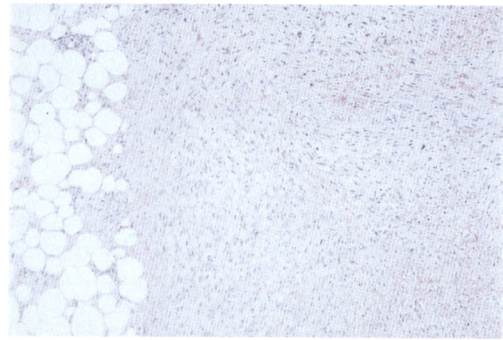

Figure 28–18. Spindle cell liposarcoma. The tumor appears well demarcated and is hypoocellular.

bone formation (Nascimento et al., 1998; Fanburg-Smith and Miettinen, 1998). The behavior of tumors having only this pattern of dedifferentiation has been as expected for well-differentiated liposarcoma (Nascimento et al., 1998). However, this pattern may also coexist with high-grade components and behave accordingly (Fanburg-Smith and Miettinen, 1998).

Spindle cell liposarcoma has been described as variant of well-differentiated liposarcoma, arising primarily from subcutaneous adipose tissue (Dei Tos et al., 1994). Morphologically, it is characterized by a bland spindle cell proliferation, organized in fascicles and whorls and set in a variably myxoid and collagenized stroma (Figs. 28–18 and 28–19). The spindle cell areas are accompanied by an adipocytic component exhibiting morphological features in keeping with a well-differentiated liposarcoma/atypical lipoma, including lipoblasts. Unlike most atypical

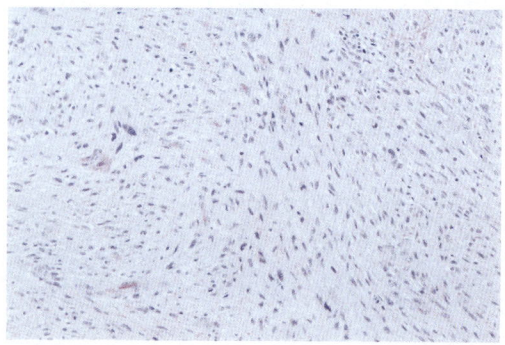

Figure 28–19. Spindle cell liposarcoma. Mild nuclear atypia is seen in the spindle cells.

lipomatous tumors located in subcutaneous tissue, which generally don't recur, spindle cell liposarcomas demonstrate a significant potential for recurrence and the capacity to dedifferentiate (to a malignant fibrous histiocytoma-like high-grade tumor). Given this unusual morphology and unlikely behavior for superficially located atypical lipomatous tumors, it is possible that spindle cell liposarcoma represents a form of low-grade dedifferentiation, akin to that occurring in deep-seated well-differentiated liposarcomas (described above).

Myxoid/Round Cell Liposarcoma: Dedifferentiation

As mentioned above, gradual progression of myxoid to round cell liposarcoma is the most common form of tumor progression for myxoid liposarcoma (Figs. 28–20 and 28–21). Rare examples of myxoid (Mentzel and Fletcher, 1995, 1997) and myxoid/round cell liposarcoma (Mentzel and Fletcher, 1997) showing *de novo* abrupt transition to nonlipogenic, high-grade sarcoma have been reported. These cases arose in retroperitoneum and in the inguinal region, unusual sites for myxoid/round cell liposarcoma but the most common sites for dedifferentiation.

Combined Liposarcomas

The occurrence, albeit rare, of combined (or mixed-type) myxoid and well-differentiated liposarcomas, with or without dedifferentiation, suggests that they are more closely related in biological terms than is generally believed (Klimstra et al., 1995; Mentzel and Fletcher, 1997; Pearlstone, 1999). This view

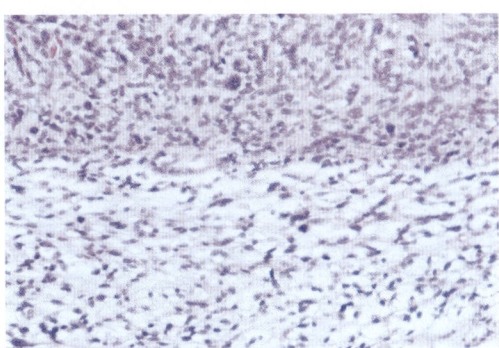

Figure 28–21. Higher magnification of the tumor shown in Figure 28–20.

is particularly supported by the vicinity of chromosomal regions involved by specific karyotypic aberrations in these tumors (Mentzel and Fletcher, 1997). Myxoid/round cell liposarcoma is associated with a t(12;16)(q13.3;p11.2). Well-differentiated liposarcomas and their superficial counterpart, so-called atypical lipomatous tumor, show ring and giant marker chromosomes composed of the q13-q15 regions of chromosome 12. A correlation has been noticed between ring and giant marker chromosomes and the presence of lipoblasts and marked cytologic adipocytic atypia. Significantly, dedifferentiated liposarcomas have shown identical supernumerary ring chromosomes (Fletcher et al., 1996).

Pleomorphic Liposarcoma

Tumor progression along lipogenic lines. *Pleomorphic liposarcoma,* containing numerous markedly atypical lipoblasts intimately admixed with the pleomorphic area is the least common subtype of liposarcomas (Fig. 28–22). It includes three variants: (*1*) pleomorphic malignant fibrous histiocytoma-like tumors with definite evidence of focal adipocytic differentiation or multivacuolated lipoblasts, perhaps the most common variant; (*2*) extensively pleomorphic high-grade tumors with prominent adipocytic differentiation, characterized by pleomorphic monovacuolated and multivacuolated lipoblasts; and (*3*) a recently described epithelioid variant that shows evidence of adipocytic differentiation but focally resembles a solid carcinoma (Miettinen and Enzinger, 1999; Fig. 28–23).

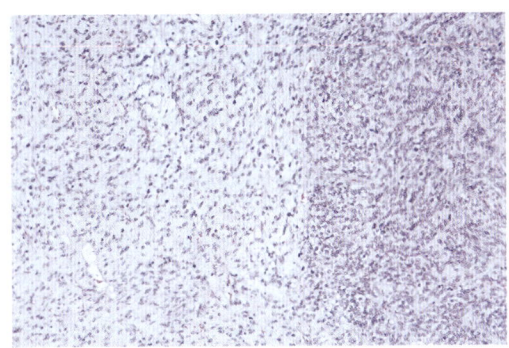

Figure 28–20. Myxoid and round cell liposarcoma. The myxoid component is less cellular than the nodule composed of round cells.

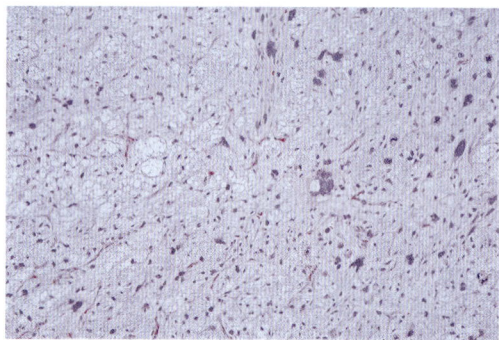

Figure 28–22. Combined myxoid liposarcoma and pleomorphic liposarcoma. The capillary network of the myxoid liposarcoma is still visible.

Pleomorphic liposarcomas have traditionally been considered a separate entity (Henricks et al., 1997). However, the possibility that pleomorphic liposarcomas could be derived from more differentiated tumors cannot be excluded (Miettinen and Enzinger, 1999). Thus, in some cases, one or all variants of pleomorphic liposarcoma could represent the culmination of tumor progression along the adipocytic lineage of a preexisting precursor. This would explain the occasional presence of ring and giant marker chromosomes or detection of the FUS-CHOP fusion transcripts—the cytogenetic signature of well-differentiated–dedifferentiated liposarcoma and of myxoid/round cell liposarcoma, respectively—in pleomorphic liposarcoma (Rosai et al., 1996; Willeke et al., 1998).

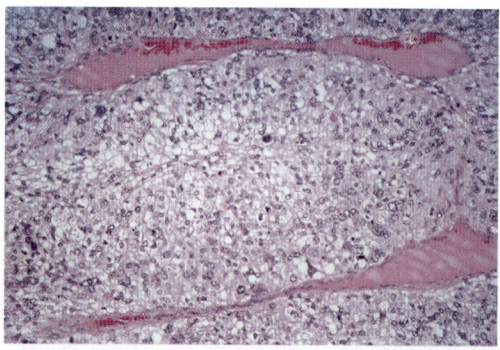

Figure 28–23. Liposarcoma composed of cohesive vacuolated epithelioid cells resembling carcinoma.

Five cases of myxoid/round cell liposarcoma mixed with pleomorphic liposarcoma have been mentioned in the literature. Also, interestingly, areas of well-differentiated lipoma-like liposarcoma and of pleomorphic liposarcoma were seen in the second recurrence of a dedifferentiated myxoid/round cell liposarcoma (Mentzel and Fletcher, 1997).

From a molecular standpoint, inactivation of p53 appears to be a critical event in the process of dedifferentiation of mesenchymal tumors (Nakayama et al., 1995). Different pathways of p53 deregulation correlate with subgroups of well-differentiated liposarcoma (Pilotti et al., 1997). In retroperitoneal well-differentiated liposarcoma this occurs through MDM2-mediated inactivation of p53. MDM2 maps to chromosome 12q14.3-15, a region that is amplified via supernumerary chromosomes (Pedetour et al., 1999) in well-differentiated liposarcoma. Therefore, MDM2 amplification is an early event in retroperitoneal well-differentiated liposarcomas that may show a progressive, possibly time-dependent increase evolving into inactivation of p53 and dedifferentiation. Thus, the grade of MDM2 amplification has been noted to correlated with the histologic grade of dedifferentiation (Nakayama et al., 1995). In nonretroperitoneal well-differentiated liposarcoma, dedifferentiation occurs through *p53* gene mutation, with or without MDM2 overexpression. *CDK4*, a flanking gene of the MDM2 amplicon, may also contribute to transformation in both retroperitoneal and nonretroperitoneal liposarcomas (Pilotti et al., 1998). Tumor progression of myxoid liposarcoma involves an undefined MDM2/p53-independent pathogenetic mechanism (Pilotti et al., 1997).

A unique finding described in retroperitoneal well-differentiated liposarcoma is the presence of atypical hyperchromatic cells within tumor blood vessel walls, which are thought to represent mural invasion by tumor cells (Weiss and Rao, 1992). Interestingly, distribution of MDM2 and p53 nuclear immunoreactivity within vessel walls of well-differentiated liposarcomas has also been noted. This has led to the speculation that these cells may represent the precursors of liposarcoma (and/or of dedifferentiated liposarcoma) (Pilotti et al., 1997).

Myxofibrosarcoma

Low-grade myxofibrosarcoma →
High-grade myxofibrosarcoma

Myxofibrosarcoma is an entity characterized by histomorphologic continuity from hypocellular, myxoid low-grade lesions to hypercellular, pleomorphic high-grade lesions, with tumors showing a tendency to become progressively higher grade in recurrences (Fukunaga and Fukunaga, 1997; Mentzel et al., 1996). Myxofibrosarcoma is one of the most common sarcomas to occur in the extremities and trunk of elderly patients (patients with high-grade lesions being older). Most tumors are superficial (dermal or subcutaneous) and less often deep (intramuscular or subfascial) (Angervall et al., 1977).

Grossly, *low-grade myxofibrosarcoma* is composed of multiple, glistening, gelatinous nodules that often spread in a longitudinal manner, whereas *high-grade myxofibrosarcoma* is more discrete and has fleshy solid areas as well as necrosis and hemorrhage. Microscopically, low-grade tumors are characterized by a multinodular growth pattern (nodules separated by fibrous septae), a myxoid matrix containing elongated, curvilinear capillaries or a plexiform capillary network similar to that seen in myxoid liposarcoma, and sparsely distributed fusiform, round or stellate cells with indistinct cell margins, slightly eosinophilic cytoplasm, and hyperchromatic atypical nuclei (Figs. 28–24 to 28–26). The cells are few in number and may show perivascular condensation. The mitotic rate may range from 0.5 to 6 mitoses/10 hpf (mean of 2 mitoses/10

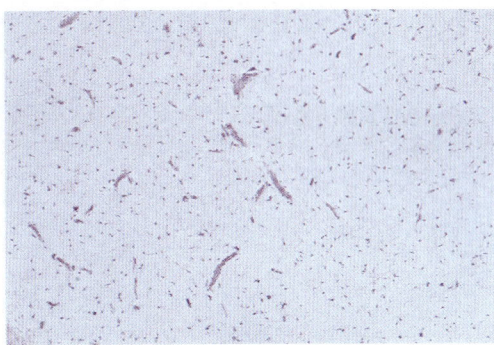

Figure 28–25. Myxofibrosarcoma, low grade. One of the myxoid nodules containing small vacuolar channels is shown.

hpf). At the other end of the spectrum, high-grade myxofibrosarcomas are hypercellular and more solid, with conspicuous cellular pleomorphism, numerous, often atypical mitotic figures, and have confluent areas of hemorrhage and necrosis (Figs. 28–27 and 28–28). The cellular areas tend to have a fascicular or storiform growth pattern or more often, may be patternless. Bizarre multinucleated giant cells with eosinophilic cytoplasm, osteoclast type giant cells, and cells reminiscent of lipoblasts (so-called pseudolipoblasts) may be present. Mitoses range from 3 to 41 mitoses/10 hpf (mean, 18 mitoses/10 hpf). Tumors lacking areas of necrosis and pronounced cellular pleomorphism but are more cellular than low-grade lesions and contain small, solid, and fascicular areas and multinucleated giant cells have been classified as intermediate grade.

Ultrastructurally, fibroblast-like and my-

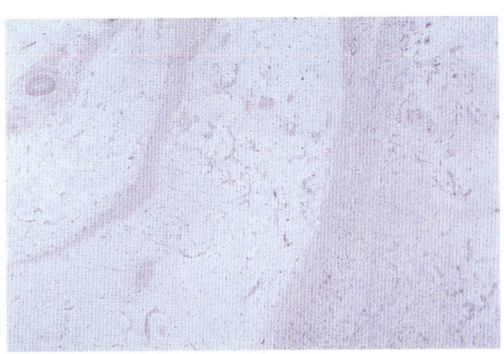

Figure 28–24. Myxofibrosarcoma, low grade, showing a multinodular pattern.

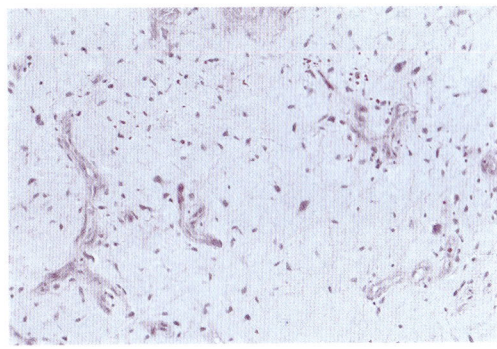

Figure 28–26. Myxofibrosarcoma, low grade, with mild cytologic atypia near the curvilinear vessels.

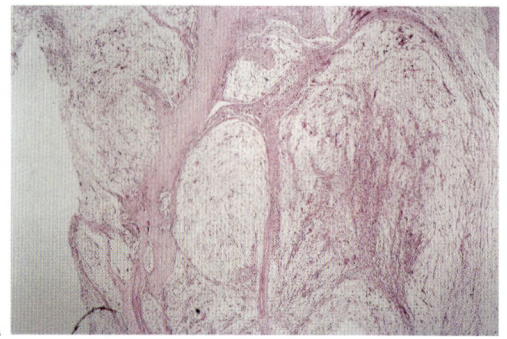
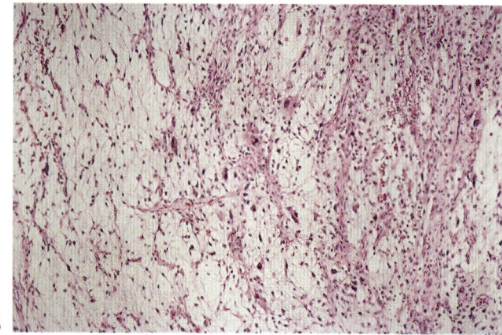

Figure 28–27. The tumor shows a nodular growth pattern (*A*) and is moderately cellular (*B*).

ofibroblast-like cells have been reported to predominate in low-grade myxofibrosarcomas, and histiocyte-like cells in high-grade lesions (Kindblom et al., 1979). In a more recent study, the ultrastructural features of low- to high-grade myxofibrosarcomas were in keeping with fibroblasts showing secretory activity (Mentzel et al., 1996).

The local recurrence rate of 55% is independent of histologic grade and of depth of tumor location, although most superficial tumors are low grade and deeply located ones are high grade (Mentzel et al., 1996). Tumor progression to a high-grade lesion with local recurrence is accompanied by the potential to metastasize and the increased occurrence of tumor-related deaths. Myxofibrosarcoma is potentially curable at its low-grade stage if complete resection is attained and local recurrence—and likely progression—is avoided. Identification of a typical low-grade myxoid component in a high-grade myxofibrosarcoma (accounting for at least 10% of the tumors) allows its distinction from a pleomorphic malignant fibrous histiocytoma, which it resembles histologically but which carries a worse prognosis. The minimum amount of a high-grade component capable of altering the tumor biology from locally aggressive to metastasizing and fatal has not been determined.

SYNOVIAL SARCOMA

Poorly differentiated synovial sarcoma, in any of its three forms—large cell or epithelioid, small cell (mimicking small, blue, round cell tumors), or high-grade spindled—is considered a variant of synovial sarcoma that appears to be associated with a poor prognosis (van de Rijn et al., 1999). "Pure" poorly differentiated synovial sarcomas have been reported as well as tumors in which areas of usual monophasic or biphasic synovial sarcoma were also present (Figs. 28–29 to 28–31). Significantly, in some of the

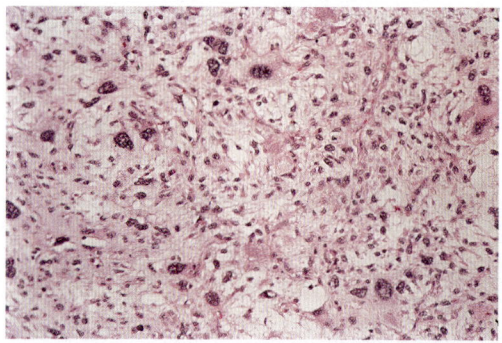

Figure 28–28. Myxofibrosarcoma, high grade, showing collections of anaplastic giant cells.

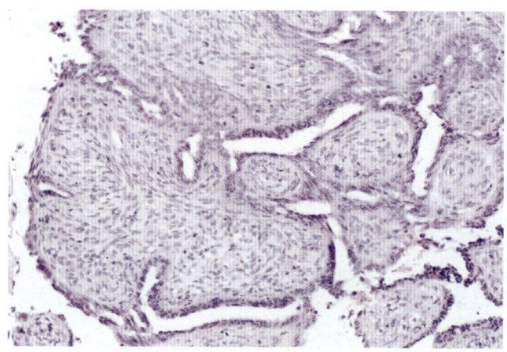

Figure 28–29. Biphasic synovial sarcomas, low grade, with papillary architecture.

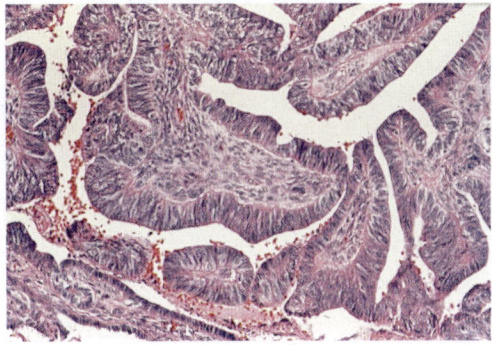

Figure 28–30. Biphasic synovial sarcoma, high grade.

cases, the poorly differentiated component was noted only in the recurrent lesions of usual biphasic (Folpe et al., 1998) or monophasic spindle cell synovial sarcomas (van de Rijn et al., 1999). We encountered a similar case of a primary biphasic synovial sarcoma showing a poorly differentiated epithelioid component in its second recurrence. Poorly differentiated synovial sarcoma probably represents the phenotypic expression of tumor progression in synovial sarcomas. Accordingly, the presence of poorly differentiated areas is associated with an adverse outcome (Machen et al., 1999). The large cell or epithelioid variant is the most common form of poorly differentiated synovial sarcoma (van de Rijn et al., 1999) and consists of large pleomorphic cells with abundant cytoplasm, irregular nuclei, and prominent nucleoli. Molecular studies of poorly differentiated tumors have yielded the same chromosomal translocations or fu-

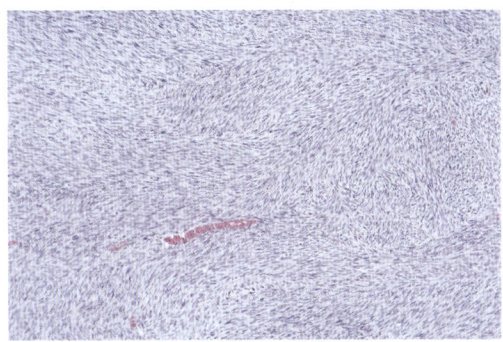

Figure 28–31. High-grade monophasic synovial sarcoma.

sion transcripts characterizing the usual types of synovial sarcoma.

OTHER SOFT TISSUE TUMORS

A less consistent tendency toward tumor progression with recurrence or metastasis has been reported for a variety of soft tissue tumors. Recurrent *solitary fibrous tumors*, now regarded to be of mesenchymal rather than mesothelial origin (Mentzel et al., 1997), have shown the acquisition of atypical histologic features, including nuclear atypia, increased cellularity, necrosis, and >4 mitoses/10 hpf (Vallat-Decouvelare et al., 1998; Yokoi et al., 1998). Foci of sarcomatoid transformation with myofibroblastic (Fukunaga et al., 1997), smooth muscle (Vallat-Decouvelaere et al., 1998), or skeletal muscle differentiation (R. Delgado, personal observation) may also occur. Histologic progression may be accompanied by loss of the diagnostic CD34 immunoreactivity and/or overexpression of p53 (Yokoi et al., 1998). High-grade transformation may occur within benign, low-grade, and intermediate-grade solitary fibrous tumors (Yokoi et al., 1998).

Ossifying fibromyxoid tumor is an unusual soft tissue tumor of uncertain histogenesis but with a unique histology. It is composed of fibromyxoid lobules of uniform oval to round cells often arranged in a cord- or lace-like pattern and a peripheral shell of lamellar bone. Areas of increased cellularity and atypia (Zámecnik et al., 1997) as well as transition toward an osteoid-forming, low-grade osteosarcoma-like lesion has been documented in recurrent tumors (Enzinger et al., 1989).

According to their microscopic features and biologic behavior, *granular cell tumors* are classified as benign, atypical, and malignant (Fanburg-Smith et al., 1998). Malignant granular cell tumors fulfill three or more of the six histologic criteria considered to be of prognostic significance: necrosis, spindling of tumor cells, vesicular nuclei with large nucleoli, increased mitotic rate (>2 mitoses/10 hpf), high nuclear-to-cytoplasmic (N:C) ratio, and pleomorphism. Atypical granular cell tumors meet one or two criteria. Benign granular cell tumors have none of the criteria or only focal pleomorphism. Malignant granular cell tumors may also contain areas indistinguishable from the benign and atyp-

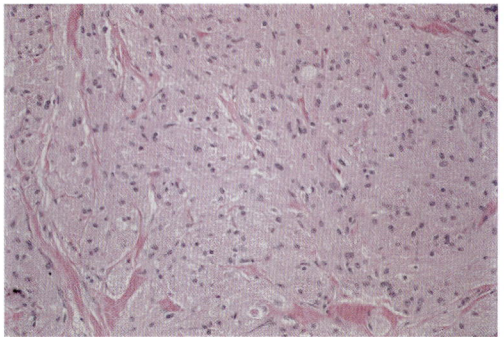

Figure 28–32. Benign granular cell tumor composed of granular cells without nuclear atypia.

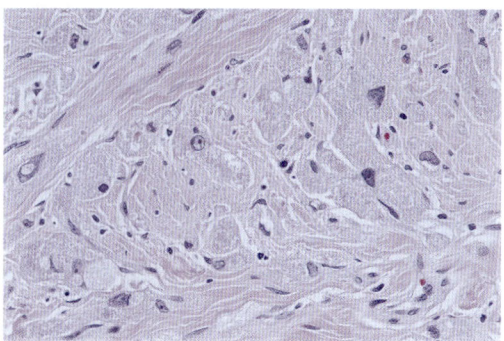

Figure 28–34. Atypical granular cell tumor. The granular cells show prominent nucleoli.

ical tumors, in the primary site as well as in the metastases (Figs. 28–32 to 28–37), findings that suggest neoplastic progression. The atypical granular cell tumors may recur locally, whereas the malignant tumors metastasize to regional lymph nodes and distant organs.

RADIATION-INDUCED SARCOMAS

The widespread anatomic distribution of soft tissues in the body probably accounts for soft tissue sarcomas being one of the most common radiation-induced malignancies, in spite of the relatively rare occurrence of primary soft tissue sarcomas. The increased survival of cancer patients because of improved therapy regimens, combined with an overall increased life expectancy of the general population, will likely result in an increased incidence of radiation-induced soft

tissue sarcomas, although this may be mitigated somewhat by the use of targeted devices (e.g., brachytherapy) that reduce the amount of normal tissue irradiated. Children with cancer are at greatest risk for developing radiation-induced sarcomas. This risk is further enhanced in the setting of genetic syndromes such as bilateral retinoblastoma, Li-Fraumeni syndrome, and NF1, among others.

The modified criteria for radiation-induced sarcomas, first described in 1948, include (*1*) a prior history of radiation; (*2*) development of a histologically confirmed sarcoma within the field of irradiation used to treat the primary tumor; (*3*) latency of several years (at least 2 to 5 years) between irradiation and sarcoma development (Spiro and Suit, 1997); and (*4*) proof that the sarcoma is histologically different from the radiated primary lesion (Laskin et al., 1988). Notably, in patients with genetic predisposition to the sarcoma, the tumors may

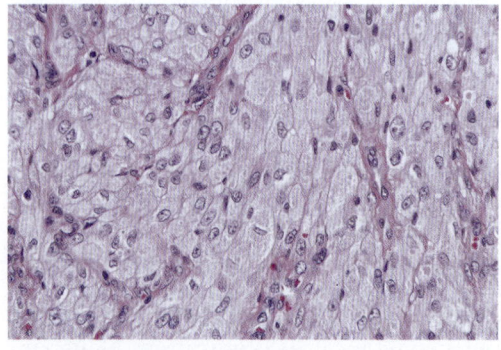

Figure 28–33. Atypical, granular cell tumor showing greater cellularity.

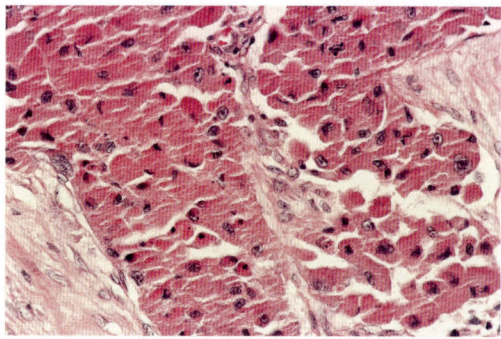

Figure 28–35. Malignant granular cell tumors with minimal nuclear atypia.

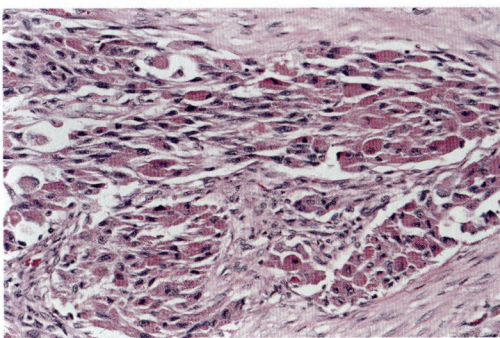

Figure 28–36. Malignant granular cell tumor with atypical spindle cells.

also arise outside of the irradiation field (Hasegawa et al., 1998; Spiro and Suit, 1997).

The frequency of histological types of radiation-induced soft tissue sarcomas differs from that of their spontaneous counterparts (Pitcher et al., 1994). The most common radiation-induced soft tissue sarcomas are malignant fibrous histiocytoma-like pleomorphic sarcomas, fibrosarcomas, extraskeletal osteosarcomas, MPNSTs, and angiosarcomas (Bloechle et al., 1995; Laskin et al., 1988; Wilklund et al., 1991); liposarcoma, the most common primary soft tissue sarcoma of adult life, is underrepresented. These histological tumor types reflect the cell types (tissues) most susceptible to radiation oncogenesis. The preponderance of malignant fibrous histiocytoma-like sarcomas and fibrosarcomas may result from the eventual malignant transformation of the stromal atypical fibroblasts, commonly seen in irradiated tissues, or from the differentiation along these lines of un-

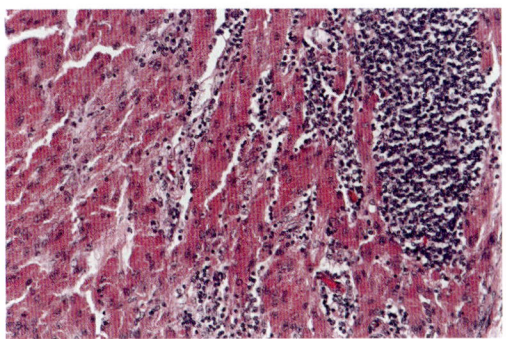

Figure 28–37. Metastatic granular cell tumor in a lymph node showing only mild cytologic atypia.

differentiated mesenchymal stem cells. The occurrence of extraskeletal osteosarcomas may be a function of fascial mesenchymal cells, which have osteogenic capability, and may modulate into osteoid-producing cells (Laskin et al., 1988).

Compared to their primary counterparts, radiation-induced sarcomas (in particular, malignant fibrous histiocytoma-like) are associated with the production of abundant collagen resulting in haphazard arrangement of neoplastic cells in a dense sclerotic or hyalinized stroma (Laskin et al., 1988). A second feature that may be noted in radiation-induced sarcomas is the presence of radiation-induced changes in non-neoplastic tissues surrounding or adjacent to the sarcoma (Laskin et al., 1988). These usually show a high-grade histology and aggressive behavior. Early detection followed by complete radical resection (the tumor must be covered three-dimensionally by uninvolved tissue), if anatomically feasible, offers the only possibility of long-term survival (Bloechle et al., 1995; Wiklund et al., 1991).

The time interval between prior radiotherapy and onset of postirradiation sarcoma ranges from 2 to 40 years, with a median of 13 years (Wilklund et al., 1991), and does not correlate with either the type of primary tumor treated or the type of postirradiation sarcoma (Bloeche et al., 1995). Latency has been reported to be the longest in brachytherapy, followed by orthovoltage and megavoltage (Bloeche et al., 1995; Wiklund et al., 1991). Megavoltage is associated with deeply located tumors (Laskin et al., 1988). Radiotherapy modality does not seem to influence histological type of sarcoma or survival (Bloeche et al., 1995). Presenting symptoms are local tension and pain in combination with a mass formation (Bloeche et al., 1995). Notably, although soft tissue sarcoma following radiotherapy for cancer is a recognized sequelae of exposure to high-dose radiation, sarcomas have not been increased in populations exposed to much lower radiation levels. The risk per gray for development of sarcoma is lower than that estimated for most other forms of radiation-induced cancer (Wong et al., 1997). Chemotherapy has also been observed to increase the rate of radiation-induced sarcomas (Spiro and Suit, 1997) and reduce the median latent interval from 14 years with radiotherapy alone to 8 years with combined therapy (Pitcher et al., 1994).

RADIATION EFFECTS ON THE GENOME

The mechanisms of radiation oncogenesis have not been established (Liber and Phillips, 1998). Radiation induces many types of DNA lesions, including single- and double-strand breaks, DNA-DNA and DNA-protein cross-links, and various types of DNA base alterations (Morgan et al., 1996). Much of the damage is induced via reactive oxygen intermediates (ROI) or other free radicals, which are derived from ionization of water. Consequently, radiation induces virtually all classes of mutations, including base pair substitutions, small insertions or deletions, larger Kb to Mb deletions, and chromosomal alterations, including DNA amplification and homologous and nonhomologous recombination. Radiation is also efficient at inducing loss of heterozygosity (LOH), which commonly occurs in cancers and arises by deletion, recombination, or gene conversion. Therefore, a direct mechanism of radiation oncogenesis would be that exposure leads to a mutation (caused by direct traversal of the critical DNA sequence by an ionizing track) in one (or more) of the steps in the oncogenic pathway, in a fraction of the target cells in the tissue (Cox, 1994). Large genes, tumor suppressor genes and transforming genes, with many mutational sites may be more sensitive to radiation-induced deletions and rearrangements than the smaller proto-oncogenes, in which the known mutations are predominantly point mutations and limited to a few codons (Sankaranarayanan and Chakraborty, 1995). However, evidence has accumulated in support of the hypothesis that radiation exposure induces a persistent genomic instability (Kronenberg, 1994; Morgan et al., 1996; Murnane, 1996).

Multiple metabolic pathways govern the accurate duplication and distribution of DNA to progeny cells; other pathways maintain the integrity of the information coded by DNA and regulate the expression of genes during growth and development. For each of these genomic stability functions there is a normal baseline frequency at which errors occur, leading to spontaneous mutations and other genomic anomalies. Genomic instability is characterized by the increased rate of acquisition of alterations in the mammalian genome (Morgan et al., 1996). Genomic instability is manifested in multiple ways, including delayed reproductive death and an increased rate of nonlethal heritable alterations such as point mutations and chromosome rearrangements. A destabilized genome in the surviving population may eventually drive the progression required for the neoplastic transformation (Morgan et al., 1996). Cancer-predisposed genotypes (already exhibiting genomic instability) may be more sensitive to radiation-induced cancers (Sankaranarayanan and Chakraborty, 1995; Wong et al., 1997).

The mechanisms of genomic instability are not known. Relaxed genomic stability could be initiated by primary alterations in genes involved in DNA replication, DNA repair, telomere stability, or chromosome segregation. Activation of signal transduction pathways and alternative gene expression may provide indirect routes leading toward destabilized genomes. Although initiation of genomic instability may be a transient process, perpetuation can be a dynamic process that persists within cells and their progeny for many generations (Morgan et al., 1996).

Cells react rapidly to irradiation, evoking a mammalian stress response that includes a plethora of biological responses, such as the initiation of signal transduction pathways, the activation of gene transcription, the repair of damaged DNA, and cell cycle–specific growth arrest. These early events are likely to be preconditions and determinants of the later fate of the irradiated cells (i.e., whether a cell will go through necrosis, senescence, or apoptosis or ultimately survive and proliferate). If a cell does survive, the initial biological response to radiation-induced insult may influence whether the cell participates in normal differentiation, exhibits a limited life span, or proliferates and begins to acquire, via genomic instability, those characteristics associated with neoplastic transformation (Morgan et al., 1996). The high percentage of cells that develop induced genetic instability after radiation exposure, and the prolonged period over which the instability occurs, indicates that the instability is not in response to residual damage in the DNA or mutations in specific genes. Instead, changes affecting most of the exposed cells, such as *epigenetic* alterations in gene expression or chain reactions of chromosome rearrangements, are a more likely explanation (Liber and Phillips, 1998; Murnane, 1996).

MOLECULAR INCIPIENT NEOPLASIA IN SOFT TISSUE SARCOMAS: CHROMOSOMAL TRANSLOCATIONS AND FUSION GENES

Many recurrent chromosomal translocations in soft tissue sarcomas resulting in fusion genes show a strict specificity for tumor type (Åman, 1999). This specificity can most likely be explained by the specific sets of target genes deregulated by the unique fusion gene product that results in reproducible patterns of aberrant differentiation (tumor phenotypes). Thus, these tumor type–specific chromosome rearrangements are believed to be involved in the early development of the soft tissue sarcomas harboring them, particularly when they are the sole cytogenetic abnormality found (Table 28–3).

The mechanisms behind chromosome rearrangements in sarcomas are largely unknown (Åman, 1999). There is evidence that some neoplasia-associated chromosomal translocations may not be random events and may be specifically promoted by the presence of certain DNA sequence motifs at or around target genes. These sequences might serve as specific recognition or bind-

Table 28–3. Genetic Translocations Leading to Tumor Development

Tumor Type	Translocation	Chimeric Transcript	Prevalence (%)
Ewing tumor	t(11;22)(q24;q12)	EWS-FLI1	95
	t(21;22)(q22;q12)	EWS-ERG	5
	t(7;22)(p22;q12)	EWS-ETV1	<1
	t(2;22)(q33;q12)	EWS-E1AF	<1
	t(1;22)(q42;q12)	EWS-?	<1
	t(2;22)(q33;q12)	EWS-FEV	<1
	t(17;22)(q12;q12)	EWS-ETV4	
DSRCT	t(11;22)(p13;q12)	EWS-WT1	100
Myxoid/round cell	t(12;16)(q13;p11)	TLS-CHOP	95
liposarcoma	t(12;22)(q13;q12)	EWS-CHOP	5
Extraskeletal myxoid	t(9;22)(q22;q12)	EWS-CHN (TEC)	75
chondrosarcoma	t(9;17)(q22;q11)	HTAFII68-CHN(TEC)	
Clear cell sarcoma	t(12;22)(q13;q21)	EWS-ATF1	
Synovial sarcoma	t(X;18)(p11.23;q11)	SYT-SSX1	65
	t(X;18)(p11.21;q11)	SYT-SSX2	35
	t(X;18)(p11;q11)	SYT-SSX4	
Alveolar RMS	t(2;13)(q35;q14)	PAX3-FKHR	75
	t(1;13)(p36;q14)	PAX7-FKHR	10
DFSP	t(17;22)(q22;q13)	COL1A1-PDGFB	
Congenital fibrosarcoma	t(12;15)(p13;q25)	ETV6-NTRK3	

CCS, clear cell sarcoma of soft tissues; DFSP, dermatofibrosarcoma protuberans; DSRCT, desmoplastic small round cell tumor; RMS, rhabdomyosarcoma.

EWS, TLS/FUS, and *hTAF1168* (in bold) are genes with RNA-binding domains that are replaced by DNA-binding domains of their translocation partners encoding transcription factors FLI1, ERG, ETV1, E1AF, ETV4 , WT1, CHOP, CHN, and ATF1. EWS, TLS/FUS, and hTAF1168 are believed to mediate the enhanced transcriptional activation of the fusion protein. *SYT* contains a transcriptional activation domain that replaces an *SSX* transcriptional repressor domain. *PDGFB,* a growth factor gene (c-sis proto-oncogene), is placed under the control of the *COL1A1* (a collagen gene) promoter. The PAX3 or PAX7 DNA-binding domain is fused to the COOH-terminal FKHR transcriptional activation domain. The protein dimerization domain of ETV6 fuses to the protein kinase domain of NTRK3. Some transcription factors such as FLI1, WT1, and PAX are developmentally regulated and are thought to confer target specificity (i.e., site, tissue, age) to the transcriptional activity generated by the fusion protein (Ladanyi, 1995).

ing sites for enzymes or proteins with recombinogenic properties (Ishida et al., 1998; Kanoe et al., 1999; Panagopoulos et al., 1997). Furthermore, it has been suggested that endogenous mobile elements or an endogenous retrovirus may take part in gene rearrangements. On the other hand, chromosomal translocations may involve an illegitimate recombination mechanism in which individual processing of single-stranded DNA occurs before joining (Zucman-Rossi et al., 1998). It is possible that certain cell type–specific processes are more vulnerable to the translocation mechanism, regardless of whether DNA recombination is illegitimate or based on site-specific signals. The outcome of the translocation may be influenced by the cell type in which it occurs, by differentiation stages, tissue locations, or microenvironments. It is noteworthy to point out the developmental character (either in presentation and/or appearance) of most translocation-bearing soft tissue sarcomas.

Molecular heterogeneity of tumor-specific chromosomal translocations may determine a distinct tumor morphology (synovial sarcoma), clinical behavior (alveolar rhabdomyosarcoma, Ewing tumors, synovial sarcoma), or both (synovial sarcoma) (de Alava et al., 2000; de Alava, 1998a; Kawai et al., 1998; Kelly et al., 1997).

The chromosomal translocations result in the formation of chimeric genes (rearranged constructs of the interrupted genes) encoding hybrid transcripts and novel fusion proteins. Many of these fusion proteins contain juxtaposed functional domains usually found in separate proteins and function as potent and/or aberrant oncogenic transcriptional activators, with unique downstream effector functions.

The fusion genes found in sarcomas are dominated by the Ewing sarcoma (*EWS*) and *TLS/FUS* family of genes and by genes encoding transcription factors. The *EWS* gene, which maps to band q12 of human chromosome 22, has been found to be the 5′ partner together with alternative 3′ partners in fusion genes in Ewing tumors, desmoplastic round cell tumor, clear cell sarcoma, and extraskeletal myxoid chondrosarcoma. The amino terminal domain of EWS functions as a regulatory domain for the transcriptional activation properties of the fusion proteins (Ohno et al., 1994).

The Ewing family tumors result from the effects of chromosomal translocations that fuse the *EWS* gene to various genes encoding transcription factors. At least five different fusion partners for *EWS* have been reported in Ewing tumors: *FLI1, ERG, FEV, ETV1,* and *E1AF/ETV4,* all belonging to the Ets family of transcription factors. The resulting chimeric EWS fusion proteins are transcriptional activators with transforming potential.

The most frequent translocations found in Ewing tumors (Ewing's sarcoma/PNET) are t(11;22)(q24;q12), resulting in fusion of *EWS* and *FLI1* genes (Delattre et al., 1994) and t(21;22)(q22;q12) involving *EWS* and *ERG* genes (Sorensen et al., 1994). (Figs. 38 and 39) There are several other less frequent fusion types (Table 28–3; de Alava et al., 2000). EWS encodes a 68 kDa protein that bears an RNA-binding carboxyl-terminal domain (Burd and Dreyfuss, 1994). The amino-terminal domain of EWS transactivates the carboxyl-terminal domain. The function of EWS is unknown, although it may play a role in transcription control, probably through its interaction with RNA polymerase II complex (Bertolotti et al., 1998) or with transcription regulators—that is, modulating interaction of transcription factors with the basal transcription complex (Bennicelli and Barr, 1999). FLI1, in contrast, is a transcription factor (May et al., 1993), a protein able to bind specific regions of DNA that control gene transcription. The reason for this feature is the presence of a carboxyl-terminal domain in FLI1 that binds DNA (May et al., 1993). This domain is called ETS, and gives the name to the whole family of transcription factors. The breakpoints of the translocation t(11;22) are located within EWS (chromosome 22) and FLI1 (chromosome 11). The result of the translocation is therefore the fusion of the amino-terminal domain of EWS to the carboxyl-terminal domain of FLI1. This structure is maintained in other similar fusions, such as EWS-ERG.

Recent studies have evaluated the contribution of molecular heterogeneity in the Ewing tumor family to prognosis. Gene fusions in Ewing's sarcoma and PNET show molecular variability, with at least 18 different structural possibilities. There are two sources of variability: the fusion partner (*FLI1, ERG, ETV1, E1A,* or *FEV*) and the breakpoint location within the genes. A better outcome has been reported for patients with localized tumors expressing the most common *EWS-FLI1* chimeric transcript (EWS exon 7 fused to FLI1 exon 6) than for those with other EWS-FLI1 fusion types (de Alava, 1998a; Zoubek et al., 1996). This raises the possibility that heterogeneity in chimeric transcript structure may reliably define clinically distinct risk groups. The biologic basis for the prognostic difference between EWS fusion types is unknown, but recent reports have shown functional differences among the various fusion genes (de Alava et al., 2000; Lin et al., 1999). Direct comparison between treatment response and EWS fusion type may reveal a role of certain chimeras in therapy resistance. Thus far, *EWS-FLI1* gene fusions and *EWS-ERG* gene fusions result in similar clinical phenotypes in EWS (Ginsberg et al., 1999).

In desmoplastic small round-cell tumor (DSRCT), the *EWS* gene is fused to *WT1*. *WT1* was originally isolated as a tumor suppressor gene involved in Wilm's tumor and the *EWS-WT1* fusion is the first instance of a recurrent rearrangement of a tumor suppressor gene. The EWS-WT1 chimeric transcript has been found in 97% of studied cases. (Fig. 40) This consistency is useful for diagnosis of this entity, especially when appearing at unusual sites or age-groups (Gerald et al., 1998). The consistent presence of the fusion gene also suggests that this genetic event is of importance in the development of DSRCT. In fact, the fusion protein functions as an aberrant transcription factor, modulating the expression of genes that overlap with those normally regulated by WT1. Interestingly, one of those genes is *PDGFA*, a potent fibroblast growth factor that contributes to the characteristic reactive fibrosis associated with this unique tumor (Lee et al., 1997). Furthermore, the serosal lining of the body cavities, the most usual site for DSRCT, is a structure that has an intense transient fetal expression of the *WT1* gene. This gene could then be related to the normal development of specific mesodermal tissues close to the serosal lining. Inappropriate activation of *WT1*-responsive genes due to the EWS-WT1 fusion protein could explain why DSRCT commonly arises in the coelomic cavities (Gerald et al., 1998).

EWS is fused to *ATF1* in clear cell sarcoma (malignant melanoma) of soft parts (Zucman et al., 1993). The *ATF1* gene, a transcription factor that is normally regulated by cAMP, contains a leucine zipper domain (bZIP) to which the amino-terminal domain of EWS is fused. Therefore, as in Ewing tumors, EWS is linked to a DNA-binding domain of a transcription factor. EWS-ATF1 functions as an efficient constitutive transcriptional activator, unlike the normal ATF-1 protein, which needs to be induced (Fujimura et al., 1996). This novel gene may well alter the transcriptional regulation of genes normally controlled by ATF1. Also as in Ewing tumors, breakpoints may vary and different fusion proteins can occur (Speleman et al., 1997). A new type of chimeric fusion product between EWS and ATF1 was associated with unusually aggressive behavior (Pellin et al., 1998).

An *EWS-CHN* fusion, originating through a t(9;22), is observed in extraskeletal myxoid chondrosarcoma. This fusion is absent in skeletal myxoid chondrosarcoma (Antonescu et al., 1998; Brody, 1997). CHN (or TEC) encodes a novel orphan nuclear receptor with a zinc finger DNA-binding domain (Brody et al., 1997). The fusion protein contains the amino-terminal domain of the EWS protein that is fused to the whole coding sequence of the orphan nuclear receptor and is more active than the native receptor (Labelle et al., 1999). These receptors are involved in the control of cell proliferation and differentiation by modulating the response to growth factors and retinoic acid. This fusion results in the oncogenic conversion of a nuclear receptor and is the first to involve the orphan subfamily (Labelle et al., 1995). A recently reported novel translocation, t(9;17), results in the fusion of the entire coding region of CHN to the N-terminal transactivation domain of *RBP56/hTAFII68* or *TAF2N*, a third member of the *EWS*, *TLS/FUS* gene family (Attwooll et al., 1999; Panagopoulos et al., 1999; Sjogren et al., 1999). Thus the N-terminal domain of EWS and RBP56 have similar oncogenic potential, making them pathogenetically equivalent as partners in fusion genes.

In addition, an *EWS*-like gene, *TLS/FUS*, is involved in tumor-associated gene fusions in about 90% of myxoid and round cell liposarcoma (*TLS/FUS-CHOP*) (Rabbitts et al., 1993). TLS (translocated in liposarcoma) is a novel nuclear RNA-binding protein with extensive sequence homology to EWS (Crozat et al., 1993). *CHOP* encodes a transcription factor belonging to the C/EBP family of basic leucine zipper group of transcription factors. In TLS-CHOP, the RNA-binding domain of TLS is replaced by the DNA-binding and leucine zipper dimerization domain of CHOP. The targeting of a conserved effector domain of RNA-binding proteins to DNA may play a role in tumor formation. CHOP, by having a DNA-binding domain, can inhibit transcription of other transcription factors that regulate adipocyte differentiation. It is suggested that CHOP may play a role in an inducible growth arrest pathway that is triggered by metabolic cues (stress) and is of particular importance in adipose tissue, an organ that undergoes marked changes in its metabolic activity. TLS-CHOP fails to induce growth arrest, hence establishing a mechanistic role in the genesis of myxoid liposarcoma (Barone et al., 1994). Significantly, the cellular distribution of TLS-CHOP fusion protein differs from that of both the parent proteins and appears to be localized to distinct nuclear structures. The histogenetic relationship between myxoid and round cell liposarcoma has been confirmed by the finding of TLS-CHOP fusions in tumors composed entirely or partially of round cells (Knight et al., 1995; Mrozek et al., 1997). It appears that the presence of secondary cytogenetic aberrations is not a prerequisite for the development of round cell histology. A small proportion of cases (5%–10%) of myxoid liposarcoma shows *EWS-CHOP* fusions as t(12;22) (Panagopoulos et al., 1996), in which the N-terminal part of EWS replaces the N-terminal part of FUS, having an apparently similar oncogenic effect (Dal Cin et al., 1997b). Thus, the RNA-binding proteins, TLS and EWS, appear to be functionally interchangeable, whereas the transcription factor component, CHOP, specifies tumor type (Zinsner et al., 1994).

Alveolar rhabdomyosarcomas are associated with a common chromosomal translocation t(2;13) and a variant t(1;13), which result in an in-frame fusion of the genes for the paired box proteins PAX3 and PAX7, respectively, to the *FKHR* (forkhead in rhabdomyosarcoma) gene on chromosome 13q14 (Davis et al., 1995; Galili et al., 1993). These translocations result in the tumor-specific expression of chimeric transcripts encoding the N-terminal PAX DNA-binding domain fused to the C-terminal FKHR transcriptional activation domain (Bennicelli et al., 1996; Davis et al., 1995). *PAX* genes consist of a family of developmentally regulated transcription factors that are essentially required for the genesis of a variety of tissues and organs (Mansouri, 1998). PAX3 and PAX7 are specifically expressed in the dorsal neural tube and the developing somite. PAX 3 is necessary for the proper formation of caudal neural crest derivatives and for the migration of myoblasts into the limb. FKHR is a member of the forkhead family of transcription factors. Experimental studies suggest that PAX3 may suppress the terminal differentiation of migrating limb myoblasts (Epstein et al., 1995). PAX3-FKHR fusion protein is a more potent transcriptional activator than PAX3 (Fredericks et al., 1995) and may contribute to the phenotype of alveolar rhabdomyosarcoma by maintaining cells in a deregulated undifferentiated and proliferative state (Epstein et al., 1995; Mansouri, 1998). This increased function results from the insensitivity of the COOH-terminal FKHR activation domain to the inhibitory effects of the NH$_2$-terminal PAX3 domains (Barr, 1999). Amplification of the fusion genes has been noted in some of PAX7-FKHR fusion–positive tumors, indicating that translocation and amplification can occur sequentially in a cancer, altering both the structure and copy number of a gene and thereby activating oncogenic activity by complimentary mechanisms (Barr et al., 1996; Davis et al., 1995). Transcription of PAX3-FKHR is increased relative to wild-type PAX3 by a copy number–independent process. These gene-specific, distinct mechanisms of overexpression ensure a critical level of gene product for the oncogenic effects of these fusions (Davis, 1997). The differences in overexpression strategies suggest important differences between the mechanisms regulating PAX3 and PAX7 expression. These differences extend to the clinical level: PAX7-FKHR tumors tend to occur in the extremities of younger patients, are more often localized, metastasize to only a few sites, and have an overall improved survival, compared to PAX3-FKHR tumors

(Barr, 1999; Kelly et al., 1997). These distinct clinical phenotypes share the same morphology in rhabdomyosarcoma. Of special interest is the up-regulation of the platelet-derived growth factor α receptor in PAX3-FKHR–carrying cells.

The characteristic translocation t(X;18) (p11;q11) of synovial sarcoma originates in the fusion gene *SYT-SSX* (Clark et al., 1994). The *SSX* gene is actually duplicated, with two copies, *SSX1* and *SSX2*, located within two subregions of Xp11 (23 and 21, respectively). The *SSX1* and *SSX2* genes encode closely related proteins (Crew et al., 1995). SYT-SSX1 or SYT-SSX2 transcripts can be detected in about 95% of synovial sarcomas by reverse-transcription polymerase chain reaction (RT-PCR) (Fligman et al., 1995). *SYT* contains a predicted glutamine-proline-glycine–rich region suggestive of a transcriptional activation domain, which replaces a region of the 5′ end of *SSX* genes that has homology with Kruppel-associated box (KRAB), a transcriptional repressor domain. The substitution of a repressor domain by a transactivation domain suggests that the chimeric products in synovial sarcoma most likely function as abnormal transcription factors. Interestingly, a correlation between transcript type and tumor phenotype has been noted (Kawai et al., 1998; Renwick et al., 1995). Biphasic synovial sarcoma is associated with SYT-SSX1 fusion transcript, present in both epithelial and spindle cell elements (Birdsall et al., 1999), and monophasic synovial sarcoma with the SYT-SSX2. Furthermore, at the clinical level, patients with SYT-SSX2 tumors have had a low risk of relapse and significantly better metastasis-free survival (Kawai et al., 1998), whereas an association between the SYT-SSX1 variant and a high tumor proliferation rate and poor clinical outcome has been noted (Nilsson et al., 1999). A variant *SYT-SSX1* fusion has been detected in a predominantly epithelioid synovial sarcoma (Sanders et al., 1999), as has a novel fusion gene, *SYT-SSX4* (Skytting et al., 1999).

The recurrent t(17;22) in DFSP and its related entity, GCF, generates a fusion gene involving *COL1A1*, a collagen gene, and *PDGFB*, a growth factor gene, also known as oncogene *sis* (Simon et al., 1997). The chimeric transcript places the PDGFB under the control of the COL1A1 promoter, removing all known elements that control PDGFB transcription negatively. In congenital fibrosarcoma, the recurrent t(12;15) fuses the *ETV6* (*TEL*) gene to the *NTRK3* neurotrophin-3 receptor (*TRKC*) gene (Knezevich et al., 1998c).

The last two examples represent exceptions to the general rule that gene fusions in soft tissue sarcomas result in novel transcription factors. ETV6-NTRK3 is a chimeric tyrosine kinase that may contribute to oncogenesis by dysregulation of NTRK3 signal transduction pathways, and PDGFB-COL1A1 probably acts as an autocrine growth factor. Interestingly, *ETV6-NTRK3* gene fusions described in congenital fibrosarcoma are also found in cellular congenital mesoblastic nephroma (Knezevich et al., 1998a; Rubin, 1998).

Isolated case reports of other polyphenotypic tumors have been recently published. These tumors had morphological features similar to those of DSRCT or were mixed embryonal and alveolar rhabdomyosarcomas, but showed different chimerical transcripts (EWS-FLI1 and EWS-ERG), characteristic of Ewing tumors (Gerald, personal communication; Katz et al., 1997; Ordi et al., 1998; Thorner et al., 1996). These findings suggest that classification of this group of primitive tumors is not yet fully established, and new entities could be described within the next years.

Rare cases of simultaneous expression of transcripts corresponding to different tumor types have been reported. A biphenotypic sarcoma showing muscle and neuroectodermal differentiation simultaneously expressed both EWS-FL1 and PAX3-FKHR transcripts, which are specific to Ewing family tumors and alveolar rhabdomyosarcoma (de Alava et al., 1998b). Interestingly, a der(16)t(1;16) (q21;q13) has been identified as the most common secondary structural aberration in EWS, alveolar rhabdomyosarcoma and extraskeletal myxoid chondrosarcoma (Day et al., 1997; Douglass et al., 1990; McManus et al., 1996). A der(16)t(12;16) was identified in a metastasis of a myxoid liposarcoma (Schneider-Stock et al., 1999). Additional rearrangements involving chromosomes 1, 12, and 16 accompanied areas of histologic progression in a myxoid liposarcoma (Orndal et al., 1990). In EWS, specific secondary chromosomal aberrations appear to be associated with disease progression (Kullendorf et al., 1999; Stark et al., 1996). It has also been suggested that loss of fusion transcripts may be associated with tumor differentiation (Knezevich et al., 1998b).

Expression of *ALK*, the anaplastic lymphoma kinase gene at chromosome 2p23, appears to be of relevance in the pathogenesis of inflammatory myofibroblastic tumors (Coffin et al., 2000; Rubin et al., 2000). Inflammatory myofibroblastic tumors have been shown to contain rearrangements of *ALK* with the tropomyosin 4 (*TPM4*) gene on chromosome 19p13 and with its highly homologous gene, tropomyosin 3 (*TPM3*) (Rubin et al., 2000).

REFERENCES

Alguacil-Garcia A. (1991) Giant cell fibroblastoma recurring as dermatofibrosarcoma protuberans. *Am J Surg Pathol* 15:798–801.

Allen PW, Zwi J. (1992) Giant cell fibroblastoma transforming into dermatofibrosarcoma protuberans [letter]. *Am J Surg Pathol* 16:1127–1129.

Altungoz O, Meloni AM, Peier A, Zalupski M, Spanier S, Brooks JS, Sandberg AA. (1995) Deletion 6q in three cases of mixed-type liposarcoma in addition to t(12;16). *Cancer Genet Cytogenet* 79:104–110.

Åman P. (1999) Fusion genes in solid tumors. *Cancer Biol* 303–318.

Angervall L, Kindblom LLG, Merck C. (1977) Myxofibrosarcoma: a study of 30 cases. *Acta Pathol Microbiol Scand A* 85:127–140.

Annessi G, Cimitan A, Girolomoni G, Giannetti A. (1993) Congenital dermatofibrosarcoma protuberans. *Pediatr Dermatol* 10:40–42.

Antonescu CR, Argani P, Eerlandson RA, Healey JH, Ladanyi M, Huvos AG. (1998) Skeletal and extraskeletal myxoid chondrosarcoma: a comparative clinicopathologic, ultrastructural, and molecular study. *Cancer* 83:1504–1521.

Argani P, Facchetti F, Inghirami G, Rosai J. (1997) Lymphocyte-rich well-differentiated liposarcoma: report of nine cases. *Am J Surg Pathol* 2:884–895.

Attwooll C, Tariq M, Harris M, Coyne JD, Telford N, Varley JM. (1999) Identification of a novel fusion gene involving hTAFII68 and CHN from a t(9;17)(q22;q11.2) translocation in an extraskeletal myxoid chondrosarcoma. *Oncogene* 18:7599–7601.

Banks E, Yum M, Brodhecker C, Goheen M. (1989) A malignant peripheral nerve sheath tumor in association with a paratesticular ganglioneuroma. *Cancer* 64:1738–1742.

Barone MV, Crozat A, Tabaee A, Philipson L, Ron D. (1994) CHOP (GADD153) and its oncogenic variant, TLS-CHOP, have opposing effects on the induction of G!/S arrest. *Genes Dev* 8:453–464.

Barr FG. (1999) The role of chimeric paired box transcription factors in the pathogenesis of pediatric rhabdomyosarcoma. *Cancer Res* 59:1711s–1715s.

Barr FG, Nauta LE, Davis RJ, Schafer BW, Nycum LM, Biegel JA. (1996) In vivo amplification of the PAX3-FKHR and PAX7-FKHR fusion genes in alveolar rhabdomyosarcoma. *Hum Mol Genet* 5:15–21.

Beham A, Fletcher CDM. (1990) Dermatofibrosarcoma protuberans with areas resembling giant cell fibroblastoma: report of two cases. *Histopathology* 17:165–182.

Bennicelli JL, Barr FG. (1999) Genetics and the biologic basis of sarcomas. *Curr Opin Oncol* 11:267–274.

Bennicelli JL, Edwards RH, Barr FG. (1996) Mechanism for transcriptional gain of function resulting from chromosomal translocation in alveolar rhabdomyosarcoma. *Proc Natl Acad Sci USA* 93:5455–5459.

Bertolotti A, Melot T, Acker J, Vigneron M, Delattre O, Tora L. (1998) EWS, but not EWS-FLI-1, is associated with both TFIID and RNA polymerase II: interactions between two members of the TET family, EWS and hTAFII68, and subunits of TFIID and RNA polymerase II complexes. *Mol Cell Biol* 18:1489–1497.

Birdsall S, Osin P, Lu YJ, Fisher C, Shipley J. (1999) Synovial sarcoma specific translocation associated with both epithelial and spindle cell components. *Int J Cancer* 82:605–608.

Bloechle C, Peiper M, Schwarz R, Schroeder S, Zornig C. (1995) Post-irradiation soft tissue sarcoma. *Eur J Cancer* 31A:311–334.

Brody RI, Ueda T, Hamelin A, et al. (1997) Molecular analysis of the fusion of EWS to an orphan nuclear receptor gene in extraskeletal myxoid chondrosarcoma. *Am J Pathol* 150:1049–1058.

Burd CG, Dreyfuss G. (1994) Conserved structures and diversity of functions of RNA-binding proteins. *Science* 265:615–621.

Calonje E, Fletcher CDM. (1996) Myoid differentiation in dermatofibrosarcoma protuberans and its fibrosarcomatous variant: clinicopathologic analysis of 5 cases. *J Cutan Pathol* 23:30–36.

Chandrosoma P, Shibata D, Radin R, Brown LP, Koss M. (1986) Malignant peripheral nerve sheath tumor arising in an adrenal ganglioneuroma in an adult male homosexual. *Cancer* 57:2022–2025.

Clark J, Rocques PJ, Crew AJ, et al. (1994) Identification of novel genes SYT and SSX, involved in t(X;18)(p11.2;q11.2) translocation found in human synovial sarcoma. *Nat Genet* 7:502–508.

Coffin CM, Hussong J, Perkins S, Griffin CA, Perlman EJ. (2000) ALK and p80 expression in inflammatory myofibroblastic tumor (IMT) [abstract]. *Mod Pathol* 8A.

Connelly JH, Evans HL. (1992) Dermatofibrosarcoma protuberans. A clinicopathologic review and emphasis on fibrosarcomatous areas. *Am J Surg Pathol* 16:921–925.

Cox R. (1994) Molecular mechanisms of radiation oncogenesis. *Int J Radiat Biol* 65:57–64.

Coyne J, Kaftan SM, Craig RDP. (1992) Dermatofibrosarcoma protuberans recurring as a giant cell fibroblastoma. *Histopathology* 21:184–187.

Craver RD, Correa H, Kao YS, Van Brunt T, Golladay ES. (1995) Aggressive giant cell fibroblastoma with a balanced 17;22 translocation. *Cancer Genet Cytogenet* 80:20–22.

Crew AJ, Clark J, Fisher C, Gill S, Grimer R, Chand A, Shipley J, Gusterson BA, Cooper CS. (1995) Fusion of SYT to two genes, SSX1 and SSX2, encoding proteins with homology to the Kruppel-associated box in human synovial sarcoma. *EMBO J* 14:2333–2340.

Crozat A, Aman P, Mandahl N, Ron D. (1993) Fusion of CHOP to a novel RNA-binding protein in human myxoid liposarcoma. *Nature* 363:640–644.

Dal Cin P, Polito P, Van Eyken P. (1997a) Anomalies of chromosomes 17 and 22 in giant cell fibroblastoma. *Cancer Genet Cytogenet* 97:165–166.

Dal Cin P, Sciot R, de Wever I, Brock P, casteels-Van Daele M, Van Damme B, Van Den Berghe H. (1996) Cytogenetic and immunohistochemical evidence that giant cell fibroblastoma is related to dermatofibrosarcoma protuberans. *Genes Chromomosomes Cancer* 15:73–75.

Dal Cin P, Sciot R, Panagopoulos I, Aman P, Samson I, Mandahl N, Mitelman F, Van den Berghe H, Fletcher CD. (1997b) Additional evidence of a variant translocation t(12;22) with EWS/CHOP fusion in myxoid liposarcoma: clinicopathological features. *J Pathol* 182:437–441.

Damiani S, Manetto V, Carrillo G, Di Blasi A, Nappi O, Eusebi V. (1991) Malignant peripheral nerve sheath tumor arising in a "de novo" ganglioneuroma. A case report. *Tumori* 77:90–93.

Davis DA, Sanchez RL. (1998) Atrophic and plaque like dermatofibrosarcoma protuberans. *Am J Dermatopathol* 20:498–501.

Davis RJ, Bennicelli JL, Macina RA, Nycum LM, Biegel JA, Barr FG. (1995) Structural characterization of the FKHR gene and its rearrangement in alveolar rhabdomyosarcoma. *Hum Mol Genet* 4:2355–2362.

Day SJ, Nelson M, Rosenthal H, Vergara GG, Bridge JA. (1997) Der (16)t(1;16)(q21;q13) as a secondary structural aberration in yet a third sarcoma, extraskeletal myxoid chondrosarcoma. *Genes Chromosomes Cancer* 20:425–427.

de Alava E, Gerald WL. (2000) Biology of neoplasia. Ewing's sarcoma and related tumors. Tumor biology and clinical applications. *J Clin Oncol* 18:204–213.

de Alava E, Kawai A, Healey JA, Fligman I, Meyers PA, Huvos AG, Gerald WL, Jhanwar SC, Argani P, Antonescu CR, Pardo-Mindan FJ, Ginsberg J, Womer R, Lawlor EER, Wunder J, Andrulis I, Sorensen PH, Barr FG, Ladanyi M. (1998a) EWS-FLI1 fusion transcript structure is an independent determinant of prognosis in Ewing's sarcoma. *J Clin Oncol* 16:1248–1255.

de Alava E, Lozano MD, Sola JJ, Panizo A, Idoata MA, Martinez-Isla C, Forteza J, Sierrasesumaga L, Pardo-Mindan FJ. (1998b) Molecular features in a biphenotypic small cell sarcoma with neuroectodermal and muscle differentiation. *Hum Pathol* 29:181–184.

de Alava E, Panizo A, Antonescu C, Huvos AG, Pardo-Mindan FJ, Barr FG, Ladanyi M. (2000) Association of EWS-FLI1 type I fusion with lower proliferative rate and lower expression of IGF1 receptor in Ewing's sarcoma. *Am J Pathol.* 156:849–855.

DeChadarevian J-P, Coppola D, Billmire DF. (1993) Bednar tumor pattern in recurring giant cell fibroblastoma. *Am J Clin Pathol* 100:164–166.

Dei-Tos AP, Mentzel T, Newman PL, Fletcher CDM. (1994) Spindle cell liposarcoma, a hitherto unrecognized variant of liposarcoma. Analysis of six cases. *Am J Surg Pathol* 18:913–921.

Delattre O, Zucman J, Melot T, Garau XS, Zucker JM, Lenoir GM, Ambros PF, Sheer D, Turc-Carel C, Triche TJ. (1994) The Ewing family of tumors—a subgroup of small-round-cell tumors defined by specific chimeric transcripts. *N Engl J Med* 331:294–299.

Diaz-Cascajo C. (1997) Myoid differentiation in dermatofibrosarcoma protuberans and its fibrosarcomatous variant. *J Cutan Pathol* 24:197–198.

Diaz-Cascajo C, Borrego L, Bastida-Inarrea J, Borghi S. (1996) Giant cell fibroblastoma: new histological observations. *Am J Dermatopathol* 18:403–408.

Ding J, Hashimoto H, Enjoji M. (1989) Dermatofibrosarcoma protuberans with fibrosarcomatous areas. A clinicopathologic study of nine cases and a comparison with allied tumors. *Cancer* 64:721–729.

Doorn PF, Molenaar WM, Buter J, Hoekstra HJ (1995). Malignant peripheral nerve sheath tumors in patients with an without neurofibromatosis. *Eur J Surg Oncol* 21:78–82.

Douglass EC, Rowe ST, Valentine M, Parham D, Meyer WH, Thompson EI. (1990) A second nonrandom translocation, der (16)t(1;16)(q21;q13), in Ewing sarcoma and peripheral neuroectodermal tumor. *Cytogenet Cell Genet* 53:87–90.

Drago G, Pasquier B, Pasquier D, Pinel N, Rouault-Plantaz V, Dyon JF, Durand C, Amari-Alla C, Plantaz D. (1997) Malignant peripheral nerve sheath tumor arising in a "de novo" ganglioneuroma: a case report and review of the literature. *Med Pediatr Oncol* 28:216–222.

Ducatman BS, Scheithauer BW. (1983) Post-irradiation neurofibrosarcoma. *Cancer* 51:1028–1033.

Ducatman BS, Scheithauer BW. (1984) Malignant peripheral nerve sheath tumors with divergent differentiation. *Cancer* 54:1049–1057.

Ducatman BS, Scheithauer BW, Piepgras DG, Reiman HM, Ilstrup DM. (1986) Malignant peripheral nerve sheath tumors. A clinicopathologic study of 120 cases. *Cancer* 57:2006–2021.

Enzinger FM, Weiss SW, Liang CY. (1989) Ossifying fibromyxoid tumor of soft parts. A clinicopathological analysis of 59 cases. *Am J Surg Pathol* 13:817–827.

Epstein JA, Lam P, Jepeal L, Maas RL, Shapiro DN. (1995) Pax3 inhibits myogenic differentiation of cultured myoblast cells. *J Biol Chem* 270:11719–11722.

Erlandson RA. (1994) Ultrastructural features of specific human neoplasms. In: *Diagnostic Transmission Electron Microscopy of Tumors*, pp. 475–481. Lippincott-Raven, Philadelphia.

Evans HL. (1979) Liposarcoma. A study of 55 cases with a reassessment of its classification. *Am J Surg Pathol* 3:507–523.

Evans HL. (1988) Liposarcomas and atypical lipomatous tumours: a study of 66 cases followed for a minimum of 10 years. *Surg Pathol* 1:41–54.

Evans HL, Khurana KK, Kemp BL, Ayala AG. (1994) Heterologous elements in the dedifferentiated component of dedifferentiated liposarcoma. *Am J Surg Pathol* 18:1150–1157.

Fanburg-Smith JC, Meis-Kindblom JM, Fante R, Kindblom LG. (1998) Malignant granular cell tumor of soft tissue: diagnostic criteria and clinicopathologic correlation. *Am J Surg Pathol* 22:779–794.

Fanburg-Smith JC, Miettinen M. (1998) Liposarcoma with meningothelial-like whorls: a study of 17 cases of a distinctive histological pattern associated with dedifferentiated liposarcoma. *Histopathology* 33:414–424.

Farshid G, Weiss SW. (1998) Massive localized lymphedema in the morbidly obese. A histologically distinct reactive lesion simulating liposarcoma. *Am J Surg Pathol* 22:1277–1283.

Feldkamp MM, Gutmann DH, Guha A. (1998) Neurofibromatosis type 1. Piecing the puzzle together. *Can J Neurol Sci* 25:181–191.

Fletcher CDM. (1995) Malignant peripheral nerve sheath tumors. *Curr Top Pathol* 89:333–354.

Fletcher CDM, Akerman M, Dal Cin P, de Wever I, Mandahl N, Mertens F, Mitelman F, Rosai J, Rydholm A, Sciot R, Tallini G, van den Berghe H, van de Ven W, Vanni R, Willen H. (1996) Correlation between clinicopathological features and karyotype in lipomatous tumours. A report of 178 cases from the Chromosomes and Morphology (CHAMP) Collaborative Study Group. *Am J Pathol* 148:623–630.

Fletcher CDM, Fernando IN, Braimbridge MV, McKee PH, Lyall JR. (1988) Malignant nerve sheath tumor arising in a ganglioneuroma. *Histopathology* 12:445–448.

Fligman I, Lonardo F, Jhanwar SC, Jhanwar SC, Gerald WL, Woodruff J, Ladanyi M. (1995) Molecular diagnosis of synovial sarcoma and characterization of a variant SYT-SSX2 fusion transcript. *Am J Pathol* 147:1592–1599.

Folpe AL, Schmidt RA, Chapman D, Gown AM. (1998) Poorly differentiated synovial sarcoma. *Am J Surg Pathol* 22:673–682.

Fredericks WJ, Galili N, Mukhopadhyay S, Rovera G, Bennicelli J, Barr FG, Rauscher FJ 3rd. (1995) The PAX3-FKHR fusion protein created by the t(2;13) translocation in alveolar rhabdomyosarcomas is a more potent transcriptional activator than PAX3. *Mol Cell Biol* 15:1522–1535.

Fujimoto M, Kikuchi K, Okochi H, Furue M. (1998) Atrophic dermatofibrosarcoma protuberans: a case report and review of the literature. *Dermatology* 196:422–424.

Fujimura Y, Ohno T, Siddique H, Lee L, Rao VN, Reddy ES. (1996) The EWS-ATF-1 gene involved in malignant melanoma of soft parts with t(12;22) chromosome translocation, encodes a constitutive transcriptional activator. *Oncogene* 12:159–167.

Fukuda T, Oshiro Y, Yamamoto I, Tsuneyoshi M. (1999) Long-term follow up of pure myxoid liposarcomas with special reference to local recurrence and progression to round cell lesions. *Pathol Int* 49:710–715.

Fukunaga M, Fukunaga N. (1997) Low-grade myxofibrosarcoma: progression in recurrence. *Pathol Int* 47:161–165.

Fukunaga M, Naganuma H, Nikaido T, Harada T, Ushigome S. (1997) Extrapleural solitary fibrous tumor: a report of seven cases. *Mod Pathol* 10:443–450.

Galili N, Davis RJ, Fredericks WJ, Mukhopadhyay S, Fauscher FJ 3d, Emanuel BS, Rovera G, Barr FG. (1993) Fusion of a fork head domain gene to PAX3 in the solid tumour alveolar rhabdomyosarcoma. *Nat Genet* 5:230–235.

Gardner TL, Elston DM, Wotowic PJ. (1998) A familial dermatofibrosarcoma protuberans. *J Am Acad Dermatol* 39:504–505.

Gerald WL, Ladanyi M, de Alava E, Cuatrecasas M, Kushner B, LaQuaglia MP, Rosai J. (1998) Clinical, pathologic and molecular spectrum of tumors associated with t(11;22)(p13;q12): desmoplastic small round cell tumor and its variants. *J Clin Oncol* 16:3028–3036.

Ghali VS, Gold JE, Vincent RA, Cosgrove JM. (1992) Malignant peripheral nerve sheath tumor arising spontaneously from retroperitoneal ganglioneuroma: a case report, review of the literature, and immunohistochemical study. *Hum Pathol* 23:72–75.

Ginsberg JP, de Alava E, Ladanyi M, et al. (1999) EWS-FLI1 and EWS-ERG gene fusions are associated with similar clinical phenotypes in Ewing's sarcoma. *J Clin Oncol* 17:1809–1814.

Goldblum JR. (1995) CD-34 positivity in fibrosarcomas which arise in dermatofibrosarcoma protuberans. *Arch Pathol Lab Med* 119:238–241.

Goldblum JR. (1996) Giant cell fibroblastoma: a report of three cases with histologic and immunohistochemical evidence of a relationship to dermatofibrosarcoma protuberans. *Arch Pathol Lab Med* 120:1052–1055.

Gould EW, Manivel JC, Albores-Saavedra J, Monforte H. (1990) Locally infiltrative glomus tumors and glomangiosarcomas. A clinical, ultrastructural, and immunohistochemical study. *Cancer* 65:310–318.

Guha A. (1998) Ras activation in astrocytomas and neurofibromas. *Can J Neurol Sci* 25:267–281.

Halling KC, Scheithauer BW, Halling AC, Nascimento AG, Ziesmer SC, Roche PC, Wollan PC. (1996) P53 expression in neurofibroma and malignant peripheral nerve sheath tumor. An immunohistochemical study of sporadic and NIF1-associated tumors. *Am J Clin Pathol* 106:282–288.

Harvell JD, Kilpatrick SE, White WL. (1998) Histogenetic relations between giant cell fibroblastoma and dermatofibrosarcoma protuberans. *Am J Dermatopathol* 20:339–345.

Hasegawa T, Matsuno Y, Niki T, Hirohashi S, Shimoda T, Takayama J, Watanabe C, Kaneko A, Sano T, Sato M, Suzuki J. (1998) Second primary rhabdomyosarcomas in patients with bilateral retinoblastoma. *Am J Surg Pathol* 22:1351–1360.

Henricks WH, Chu YC, Goldblum JR, Weiss SW. (1997) Dedifferentiated liposarcoma. A clinicopathological analysis of 155 cases with a proposal for an expanded definition of dedifferentiation. *Am J Surg Pathol* 21:271–281.

Hirose T, Scheithauer BW, Sano T. (1998) Perineurial malignant peripheral nerve sheath tumor (MPNST). A clinicopathologic, immunohistochemical, and ultrastructural study of seven cases. *Am J Surg Pathol* 22:1368–1378.

Ishida S, Yoshida K, Kaneko Y, Tanaka Y, Sasaki Y, Urano F, Umezawa A, Hata J, Fujinaga K. (1998) The genomic breakpoint and chimeric transcripts in the EWSR1-ETV4/E1AF gene fusion in Ewing sarcoma. *Cytogenet Cell Genet* 82:278–283.

Kanoe H, Nakayama T, Hosaka T, Murakami H, Yamamoto H, Nakashima Y, Tsuboyama T, Nakamura T, Ron D, Sasaki MS, Toguchida J. (1999) Characteristics of genomic breakpoints in TLS-CHOP translocations in liposarcomas suggest the involvement of Translin and topoisomerase II in the process of translocation. *Oncogene* 18:721–729.

Katz RL, Quezado M, Senderowicz AM, Villalba L, Laskin WB, Tsokos M. (1997) An intra-abdominal small round cell neoplasm with features of primitive neuroectodermal and desmoplastic round cell tumor and a EWS/FLI-1 fusion transcript. *Hum Pathol* 28:502–509.

Kawai A, Woodruff J, Healey JH, Brennan MF, Antonescu CR, Ladanyi M. (1998) SYT-SSX gene fusion as a determinant of morphology and prognosis in synovial sarcoma. *N Engl J Med* 338:153–160.

Keller SM, Papazoglou S, McKeever P, Baker A, Roth JA. (1984) Late occurrence of malignancy in a ganglioneuroma 19 years following radiation therapy to a neuroblastoma. *J Surg Oncol* 25:227–231.

Kelly KM, Womer RB, Sorensen PH, Xiong QB, Barr FG. (1997) Common and variant gene fusions predict distinct clinical phenotypes in rhabdomyosarcoma. *J Clin Oncol* 15:1831–1836.

Kilpatrick SE, Doyon J, Choong PFM, Sim FH, Nascimento AG. (1996) The clinicopathologic spectrum of myxoid and round cell liposarcoma. A study of 95 cases. *Cancer* 77:1450–1458.

Kindblom L-G, Merck C, Angervall L. (1979) The ultrastructure of myxofibrosarcoma. A study of 11 cases. *Virchows Arch A Pathol Anat Histol* 381:121–139.

Klimstra DS, Moran CA, Perino G, Koss MN, Rosai J. (1995) Liposarcoma of the anterior mediastinum and thymus. A clinicopathologic study of 28 cases. *Am J Surg Pathol* 19:782–791.

Klose A, Ahmadian MR, Schuelke M, Scheffzek K, Hoffmeyer S, Gewies A, Schmitz F, Kaufmann D, Peters H, Wittinghofer A, Nurnberg P. (1998) Selective disactivation of neurofibromin GAP activity in neurofibromatosis type 1 (NF1). *Hum Mol Genet* 7: 1261–1268.

Knezevich SR, Garnett MJ, Pysher TJ, Beckwith JB, Grundy PE, Sorensen PH. (1998a) ETV6-NTRK3 gene fusions and trisomy 11 establish a histogenetic link between mesoblastic nephroma and congenital fibrosarcoma. *Cancer Res* 58:5046–5048.

Knezevich SR, Hendson G, Mathers JA, Carpenter B, Lopez-Terrada D, Brown KL, Sorensen PH. (1998b) Absence of detectable EWS/FLI1 expression after therapy-induced neural differentiation in Ewing sarcoma. *Hum Pathol* 29:289–294.

Knezevich SR, McFadden DE, Tao W, Lim JF, Sorensen PH. (1998c) A novel ETV6-NTRK3 gene fusion in congenital fibrosarcoma. *Nat Genet* 18:184–187.

Knight JC, Renwick PJ, Cin PD, Van Den Berge H, Fletcher CDM. (1995) Translocation t(12;16) (q13;p11) in myxoid liposarcoma and round cell liposarcoma: molecular and cytogenetic analysis. *Cancer Res* 55:24–27.

Korf BR. (1999) Plexiform neurofibromas. *Am J Med Genet (Semin Med Genet)* 89:31–37.

Kraus MD, Guillou L, Fletcher CDM. (1997) Well-differentiated inflammatory liposarcoma: an uncommon and easily overlooked variant of a common sarcoma. *Am J Surg Pathol* 21:518–527.

Kronenberg A. (1994) Radiation-induced genomic instability. *Int J Radiat Biol* 66:603–609.

Kullendorff CM, Mertens F, Donner M, Wiebe T, Akerman M, Mandahl N. (1999) Cytogenetic aberrations in Ewing sarcoma: are secondary changes associated with clinical outcome? *Med Pediatr Oncol* 32:79–83.

Labelle Y, Bussieres J, Courjal F, Goldring MB. (1999) The EWS/TEC fusion protein encoded by the t(9;22) chromosomal translocation in human chondrosarcomas is a highly potent transcriptional activator. *Oncogene* 18:3303–3308.

Labelle Y, Zucman J, Stenman G, Kindblom LG, Knight J, Turc-Carel C, Dockhorn-Dworniczak B, Mandahl N, Desmaze C, Peter M. (1995) Oncogenic conversion of a novel orphan nuclear receptor by chromosome translocation. *Hum Mol Genet* 4:2219–2226.

Ladanyi M. (1995) The emerging molecular genetics of sarcoma translocations. *Diagn Mol Pathol* 4:162–173.

Laskin WB, Silverman TA, Enzinger FM. (1988) Postradiation soft tissue sarcomas. An analysis of 53 cases. *Cancer* 62:2330–2340.

Lee SB, Kolquist KA, Nichols K, Englert C, Maheswaran S, Ladanyi M, Gerald WL, Haber DA. (1997) The EWS-WT1 translocation product induces PDGFA in desmoplastic small round-cell tumour. *Nat Genet* 17: 309–313.

Liber HL, Phillips EN. (1998) Interrelationships between radiation-induced mutations and modifications in gene expression linked to cancer. *Eukaryotic Gene Expressions* 8:257–276.

Lin BT, Weiss LM, Medeiros LJ. (1997) Neurofibroma and cellular neurofibroma with atypia: a report of 14 tumors. *Am J Surg Pathol* 21:1443–1449.

Lin PP, Brody RI, Hamelin A, Bradner JE, Healey JH, Ladanyi M. (1999) Differential transactivation by alternative EWS-FLI1 fusion proteins correlates with clinical heterogeneity in Ewing's sarcoma. *Cancer Res* 59:1428–1432.

Machen SK, Easley KA, Goldblum JR. (1999) Synovial sarcoma of the extremities. A clinicopathologic study of 34 cases, including semi-quantitative analysis of spindled, epithelial, and poorly differentiated areas. *Am J Surg Pathol* 23:268–275.

Maeda T, Hirose T, Furuya K, Shirakawa K, Kobayashi K. (1998) Giant cell fibroblastoma associated with dermatofibrosarcoma protuberans: a case report. *Mod Pathol* 11:491–495.

Manivel JC, Albores-Saavedra J. (1993). Soft tissue. In: *Pathology of Incipient Neoplasia* (Henson DE, Albores-Saavedra J, eds.) pp. 489–507. W.B. Saunders Co, Philadelphia.

Mansouri A. (1998) The role of PAX3 and PAX7 in development and cancer. *Crit Rev Oncogene* 9:141–149.

May WA, Gishizky ML, Lessnick SL, Lunsford LB, Lewis BC, Delattre O, Zucman J, Thomas G, Denny CT. (1993) Ewing sarcoma 11;22 translocation produces a chimeric transcription factor that requires the DNA-binding domain encoded by FLI1 for transformation. *Proc Natl Acad Sci USA* 90:5752–5756.

McCarron KF, Goldblum JR. (1998) Plexiform neurofibroma with and without associated malignant peripheral nerve sheath tumor: A clinicopathologic and immunohistochemical analysis of 54 cases. *Mod Pathol* 11:612–617.

McCormick D, Mentzel T, Beham A, Fletcher CDM. (1994) Dedifferentiated liposarcoma. Clinicopathologic analysis of 32 cases suggesting a better prognostic subgroup among pleomorphic sarcomas. *Am J Surg Pathol* 18:1213–1223.

McKee PH, Fletcher CDM. (1991) Dermatofibrosarcoma protuberans presenting in infancy and childhood. *J Cutan Pathol* 18:241–246.

McManus AP, Min T, Swansbury GJ, Gusterson BA, Pinkerton CR, Shipley JM. (1996) der (16)t(1;16) (q21;q13)0 as a secondary change in alveolar rhabdomyosarcoma. A case report and review of the literature. *Cancer Genet Cytogenet* 87:179–181.

McMenamin ME and Fletcher CDM. (2000) Epithelioid malignant change in benign schwannomas [abstract]. *Mod Pathol* 13A.

Meis JM, Enzinger FM, Martz KL, Neal JA. (1992) Malignant peripheral nerve sheath tumors (malignant schwannomas) in children. *Am J Surg Pathol* 16: 694–707.

Meis-Kindblom JM, Kindblom LG. (1998) Angiosarcoma of soft tissue: a study of 80 cases. *Am J Surg Pathol* 22:683–697.

Mentzel T, Bainbridge TC, Katenkamp D. (1997) Solitary fibrous tumour; clinicopathological, immunohistochemical, and ultrastructural analysis of 12 cases arising in soft tissues, nasal cavity and nasopharynx, urinary bladder and prostate. *Virchows Arch* 430:445–453.

Mentzel T, Beham A, Katenkamp, Dei Tos AP, Fletcher CDM. (1998) Fibrosarcomatous("high-grade") dermatofibrosarcoma protuberans. Clinicopathologic and immunohistochemical study of a series of 41 cases with emphasis on prognostic significance. *Am J Surg Pathol* 22:576–587.

Mentzel T, Calonje E, Wadden C, Camplejohn RS, Beham A, Smith MA, Fletcher CD. (1996) Myxofibrosarcoma. Clinicopathologic analysis of 75 cases with emphasis on the low-grade variant. *Am J Surg Pathol* 20:391–405.

Mentzel T, Fletcher CDM. (1995) Lipomatous tumours of soft tissues: an update. *Virchows Arch* 427:353–363.

Mentzel T, Fletcher CDM. (1997) Dedifferentiated myxoid liposarcoma: a clinicopathological study suggesting a closer relationship between myxoid and well-differentiated liposarcoma. *Histopathology* 30: 457–463.

Mentzel T, Katenkamp MT. (1999) Intraneural angiosarcoma and angiosarcoma arising in benign and malignant peripheral nerve sheath tumours: clinicopathological and immunohistochemical analysis of four cases. *Histopathology* 35:114–120.

Michal M, Zámecni M. (1992) Giant cell fibroblastoma with a dermatofibrosarcoma protuberans component. *Am J Dermatopathol* 14:549–552.

Miettinen M, Enzinger FM. (1999) Epithelioid variant of pleomorphic liposarcoma: a study of 12 cases of a distinctive variant of high-grade liposarcoma. *Mod Pathol* 12:722–728.

Miettinen M, Lindenmayer AE, Chaubal A. (1994) Endothelial cell markers CD31, CD34, and BNH9 antibody to H- and Y-antigens: evaluation of their specificity and sensitivity in the diagnosis of vascular tumors and comparison with von Willebrand factor. *Mod Pathol* 7:82–90.

Morgan WF, Day JP, Kaplan MI, McGhee EM, Limoli CL. (1996) Genomic instability induced by ionizing radiation. *Radiat Res* 146:247–258.

Morimitsu Y, Hisaoka M, Okamoto S, Hashimoto H, Ushijima M. (1998) Dermatofibrosarcoma protuberans and its fibrosarcomatous variant with areas of myoid differentiation: a report of three cases. *Histopathology* 32:547–551.

Mrozek K, Szumigala J, Brooks JS, Crossland DM, Karakousis CP, Bloomfield CD. (1997) Round cell liposarcoma with the insertion (12;16)(q13;p11.2p13). *Am J Clin Pathol* 108:35–39.

Muller R, Hajdu SI, Brennan MF. (1987) Lymphangiosarcoma associated with chronic filaria lympedema. *Cancer* 59:179–183.

Murnane JP. (1996) Role of induced genetic instability in the mutagenic effects of chemicals and radiation. *Mutat Res* 367:11–23.

Naeem R, Lux ML, Huang S-F, Naber SP, Corson JM, Fletcher JA. (1995) Ring chromosomes in dermatofibrosarcoma protuberans are composed of interspersed sequences from chromosomes 17 and 22. *Am J Pathol* 147:1553–1558.

Nakayama T, Toguchida J, Wadayama B, Kanoe H, Kotoura Y, Sasaki MS. (1995) MDM2 gene amplification in bone and soft-tissue tumors: association with tumor progression in differentiated adipose-tissue tumors. *Int J Cancer* 64:342–346.

Nascimento AG, Kurtin PJ, Guillou L, Fletcher CDM. (1998) Dedifferentiated liposarcoma. A report of nine cases with a peculiar neurallike whorling pattern associated with metaplastic bone formation. *Am J Surg Pathol* 22:945–955.

Nielsen GP, Young RH, Dickersin GR, Rosenberg AE. (1997) Angiomyofibroblastoma of the vulva with sarcomatous transformation ("angiomyofibrosarcoma"). *Am J Surg Pathol* 21:1104–1108.

Nilsson G, Skytting B, Xie Y, Brodin B, Perfekt R, Mandahl N, Lundeberg J, Uhlen M, Larsson O. (1999) The SYT-SSX1 variant of synovial sarcoma is associated with a high rate of tumor cell proliferation and poor clinical outcome. *Cancer Res* 59:3180–3184.

O'Brien KP, Seroussi E, Dal Cin P, Sciot R, Mandahl N, Fletcher JA, Turc-Carel C, Dumanski JP. (1998) Various regions within the alpha-helical domain of the COLIAI gene are fused to the second exon of the PDGFB gene in dermatofibrosarcomas and giant-cell fibroblastomas. *Genes Chromosomes Cancer* 23: 187–193.

O'Connell JX, Trotter MJ. (1996) Fibrosarcomatous dermatofibrosarcoma protuberans: a variant. *Mod Pathol* 9:273–278.

Ohno T, Ouchida M, Lee L, Gatalica Z, Rao VN, Reddy ES. (1994) The EWS gene, involved in Ewing family of tumors, malignant melanoma of soft parts and desmoplastic small round cell tumors, codes foro an RNA binding protein with novel regulatory domains. *Oncogene* 9:3087–3097.

Ordi J, de Alava E, Torne A, Mellado B, pardo-Mindan J, Iglesias X, Cardesa A. (1998) Intraabdominal desmoplastic small round cell tumor with EWS/ERG fusion transcript. *Am J Surg Pathol* 22:1026–1032.

Orndal C, Mandahl N, Rydholm A, Nilbert M, Heim S, Akerman M, Mitelman F. (1990) Chromosomal evolution and tumor progression in a myxoid liposarcoma. *Acta Orthop Scand* 61:99–105.

Panagopoulos I, Hoglund M, Mertens F, Mandahl N, Mitelman F, Aman P. (1996) Fusion of the EWS and CHOP genes in myxoid liposarcoma. *Oncogene* 12: 489–494.

Panagopoulos I, Lassen C, Isaksson M, Mitelman F, Mandahl N, Aman P. (1997) Characteristic sequence motifs at the breakpoints of the hybrid genes FUS/CHOP, EWS/CHOP and FUS/ERG in myxoid liposarcoma and acute myeloid leukemia. *Oncogene* 11:1357–1362.

Panagopoulos I, Mencinger M, Dietrich CU, Bjerkehagen B, Saeter G, Mertens F, Mandahl N, Heim S. (1999) Fusion of the RBP56 and CHN genes in extraskeletal myxoid chondrosarcomas with translocation t(9;17)(q22;q11). *Oncogene* 18:7594–7598.

Pappo AS, Rao BN, Cain A, Bodner S, Pratt CB. (1997) Dermatofibrosarcoma protuberans: the pediatric experience at St. Jude Children's Research Hospital. *Pediatr Hematol Oncol* 14:563–568.

Pearlstone DB, Pisters PW, Bold RJ, Feig BW, Hunt KK, Yasko AW, Patel S, Pollack A, Benjamin RS, Pollock RE. (1999) Patterns of recurrence in extremity liposarcoma: implications for staging and follow-up. *Cancer* 85:85–92.

Pedeutour F, Forus A, Coindre JM, Berner JM, Nicolo G, Michiels JF, Terrier P, Ranchere-Vince D, Collin F, Myklebost O, Turc-Carel C. (1999) Structure of the supernumerary ring and giant rod chromosomes in adipose tissue tumors. *Genes Chromosomes Cancer* 1:30–41.

Pedeutour F, Simon MP, Minoletti F, Barcelo G, Terrier-Lacombe MJ, Combemale P, Sozzi G, Ayraud N, Turc-Carel C. (1996) Translocation t(17;22) (q22;q13) in dermatofibrosarcoma protuberans. A new tumor associated chromosome rearrangement. *Cytogenet Cell Genet* 72:171–174.

Pellin A, Monteagudo C, Lopez-Gines C, Carda C, Boix J, Llombart-Bosch A. (1998) New type of chimeric fusion product between the EWS and ATFI genes in clear cell sarcoma (malignant melanoma of soft parts). *Genes Chromosomes Cancer* 23:358–360.

Perry DA, Schultz LR, Dehner LP. (1993) Giant cell fibroblastoma with dermatofibrosarcoma protuberans-like transformation. *J Cutan Pathol* 20:451–454.

Pilotti S, Della Torre G, Lavarino C, Di Palma S, Sozzi G, Minoletti F, Rao S, Pasquini G, Azzarelli A, Rilke F, Pierotti MA. (1997) Distinct mdm2/p53 expression patterns in liposarcoma subgroups: implications for different pathogenetic mechanisms. *J Pathol* 181:14–24.

Pilotti S, Della Torre G, Lavarino C, Sozzi G, Minoletti F, Vergani B, Azzarelli A, Rilke F, Pierotti MA. (1998) Molecular abnormalities in liposarcoma: role of MDM2 and CDK4-containing amplicons at 12q13–22. *J Pathol* 185:188–190.

Pitcher ME, Davidson TI, Fisher C, Thomas JM. (1994) Post irradiation sarcoma of soft tissue and bone. *Eur J Surg Oncol* 20:53–56.

Pitt MA, Coyne JD, Harris M, McWilliam LJ. (1994) Dermatofibrosarcoma protuberans recurring as a giant cell fibroblastoma with subsequent fibrosarcomatous change. *Histopathology* 24:197–202.

Rabbits TH, Forster A, Larson R, Nathan P. (1993) Fusion of the dominant negative transcription regulator CHOP with a novel gene FUS by translocation t(12;16) in malignant liposarcoma. *Nat Gen* 4:175–180.

Rasbridge SA, Browse NL, Tighe JR, Fletcher CDM. (1989) Malignant nerve sheath tumor arising in a benign ancient schwannoma. *Histopathology* 14:525–528.

Renwick PJ, Reeves BR, Dal Cin P, Fletcher CD, Kempski H, Sciot R, Kazmierczak B, Jani K, Sonobe H, Knight JC. (1995) Two categories of synovial sarcoma defined by divergent chromosome translocation breakpoints in Xp11.2, with implications for the histologic sub-classification of synovial sarcoma. *Cytogenet Cell Genet* 70:58–63.

Ricci A Jr, Parham DM, Woodruff JM, Callihan T, Green A, Erlandson RA. (1984) Malignant peripheral nerve sheath tumors arising from ganglioneuromas. *Am J Surg Pathol* 8:19–29.

Rosai J, Akerman M, Dal Cin P, DeWever I, Fletcher CD, Mandahl N, Mertens F, Mitelman F, Rydholm A, Sciot R, Tallini G, Van den Berghe H, Van de Ven W, Vanni R, Willen H. (1996) Combined morphologic and karyotypic study of 59 atypical lipomatous tumors. Evaluation of their relationship and differential diagnosis with other adipose tissue tumors (a report of the CHAMP Study Group). *Am J Surg Pathol* 20:1182–1189.

Rubin BP. (1998) Congenital mesoblastic nephroma t(12;15) is associated with ETV6-NTRK3 gene fusion: cytogenetic and molecular relationship to congenital (infantile) fibrosarcoma. *Am J Pathol* 153:1451–1458.

Rubin BP, Lawrence BD, Perez-Atayde A, Xiao S, Yi ES, Fletcher CDM, Fletcher JA. (2000) *TMP-ALK* fusion genes and ALK expression in inflammatory myofibroblastic tumor. *Mod Pathol* (abstract) 15A.

Sanders ME, van de Rijn M, Barr FG. (1999) Detection of a variant SYT-SSX1 fusion in a case of predominantly epithelioid synovial sarcoma. *Mol Diagn* 4:65–70.

Sankaranarayanan K, Chakraborty R. (1995) Cancer predisposition, radiosensitivity and the risk of radiation-induced cancers. I. Background. *Radiat Res* 143:121–143.

Scheithauer BW, Woodruff JM, Erlandson RA. (1999) Tumors of the peripheral nervous system. In: *Atlas of Tumor Pathology*, Third Series, Fascicle 24. Armed Forces Institute of Pathology, Washington, D.C.

Schneider-Stock R, Rys J, Walter H, Limon J, Iliszko M, Niezabitowski A, Roessner A. (1999) A rare chimeric TLS/FUS-CHOP transcript in a patient with multiple liposarcomas: a case report. *Cancer Genet Cytogenet* 111:130–133.

Shirger A. (1962) Postoperative lymphedema. Etiologic and diagnostic factors. *Med Clin North Am* 46:1045–1050.

Shmookler BM, Enzinger FM. (1982) Giant cell fibroblastoma: a peculiar childhood tumor [abstract] *Lab Invest* 46:76A.

Shmookler BM, Enzinger FM, Weiss SW. (1989) Giant cell fibroblastoma: a juvenile form of dermatofibrosarcoma protuberans. *Cancer* 64:2154–2161.

Simon M-P, Pedeutour F, Sirvent N, Grossgeorge J, Minoletti F, Coindre JM, Terrier-Lacombe MJ, Mandahl N, Craver RD, Blin N, Sozzi G, Turc-Carel C, O'Brien KP, Kedra D, Fransson I, Guilbaud C, Dumanski JP. (1997) Deregulation of the platelet-derived growth factor B-chain gene via fusion with collagen gene COL1A1 in dermatofibrosarcoma protuberans and giant-cell fibroblastoma. *Nat Genet* 15:95–98.

Sjogren H, Meis-Kindblom J, Kindblom LG, Aman P, Stenman G. (1999) Fusion of the EWS-related gene TAF2N to TEC in extraskeletal myxoid chondrosarcoma. *Cancer Res* 59:5064–5067.

Skytting B, Nilsson G, Brodin B, Xie Y, Lundeberg J, Uhlen M, Larsson O. (1999) A novel fusion gene, *SYT-SSX4*, in synovial sarcoma. *J Natl Cancer Inst* 91:974–975.

Smith TA, Easley KA, Goldblum JR. (1996) Myxoid/round cell liposarcoma of the extremities. A clinicopathologic study of 29 cases with particular attention to extent of round cell liposarcoma. *Am J Surg Pathol* 20:171–180.

Sordillo PP, Hadju SI, Good RA. (1981) Lymphangiosarcoma after filarial infection. *J Dermatol Surg Oncol* 7:235–249.

Sorensen PHB, Lessnick SL, Lopez-Terrada D, Liu XF, Triche TJ, Denny CT. (1994) A second Ewing's sarcoma translocation, t(21;22), fuses the EWS gene to another ETS-family transcription factor, ERG. *Nat Genet* 6:146–151.

Speleman F, Delattre O, Peter M, Hauben E, Van Roy N, Van Marck E. (1997) Malignant melanoma of the soft parts (clear-cell sarcoma): confirmation of EWS and ATF-1 gene fusion caused by a t(12;22) translocation. *Mod Pathol* 10:496–499.

Spillane AJ, Fisher C, Thomas JM. (1999) Myxoid liposarcoma—the frequency and the natural history of nonpulmonary soft tissue metastases. *Ann Surg Oncol* 6:389–394.

Spiro IJ, Suit HD. (1997) Radiation-induced bone and soft tissue sarcomas: clinical aspects and molecular biology. In: *Soft Tissue Sarcomas: Present Achievements and Future Prospects* (Verweij J, Pinedo HM, Suite HD, eds.) Kluwer Academic Publishers, Boston.

Stark B, Zoubek A, Hattinger C, Jeison M, Gobuzov R, Mor C, Cohen I, Yaniv I, Ambros PF, Kovar H, Zaizov R. (1996) Metastatic extraosseous Ewing tumor. Association of the additional translocation der (16)t(1;16) with the variant EWS/ERG rearrangement in a case of cytogenetically inconspicuous chromosome 22. *Cancer Genet Cytogenet* 87:161–166.

Stewart FM, Treves N. (1948) Lymphangiosarcoma in post-mastectomy lymphedema: a report of six cases of elephantiasis chururgica. *Cancer* 1:64–73.

Tallini G, Erlandson RA, Brennan MF, Woodruff JM. (1993) Divergent myosarcomatous differentiation in retroperitoneal liposarcoma. *Am J Surg Pathol* 17:546–556.

Taylor HB, Helwig EB. (1962) Dermatofibrosarcoma protuberans: a study of 115 cases. *Cancer* 15:717.

Thorner P, Squire J, Chilton-MacNeil S, Marrano P, Bayani J, Malkin D, Greenberg M, Lorenzana A, Zielenska M. (1996) Is the EWS/FLI-1 fusion transcript specific for Ewing sarcoma and peripheral primitive neuroectodermal tumor? A report of four cases showing this transcript in a wider range of tumor types. *Am J Pathol* 148:1125–1138.

Wanebo JE, Malik JM, VandenBerg SR, Wanebo HJ, Driesen N, Persing JA. (1993) Malignant peripheral nerve sheath tumors. A clinicopathologic study of 28 cases. *Cancer* 71:1247–1253.

Weiss SW, Nickoloff BJ. (1993) CD-34 is expressed by a distinctive cell population in peripheral nerve, nerve sheath tumors, and related lesions. *Am J Surg Pathol* 17:1039–1045.

Weiss SW, Rao VK. (1992) Well-differentiated liposarcoma (atypical lipoma) of deep soft tissue of the extremities, retroperitoneum, and miscellaneous sites. A follow-up study of 92 cases with analysis of the incidence of "dedifferentiation". *Am J Surg Pathol* 16:1051–1058.

Wenig BM, Abbondanzo SL, Heffess CS. (1994) Epithelioid angiosarcoma of the adrenal glands. A clinicopathologic study of nine cases with a discussion of the implications of finding "epithelial-specific" markers. *Am J Surg Pathol* 18:62–73.

Wiklund TA, Blomqvist CP, Räty J, Elomaa I, Rissanen P, Miettinen M. (1991) Postirradiation sarcoma. Analysis of a nationwide cancer registry material. *Cancer* 68:524–531.

Willeke F, Ridder R, Mechtersheimer G, Schwarzbach M, Duwe A, Weitz J, Lehnert T, Herfarth C, von Knebel Doeberitz M. (1998) Analysis of FUS-CHOP fusion transcripts in the different types of soft tissue liposarcoma and their diagnostic implications. *Clin Cancer Res* 4:1779–1784.

Wong FL, Boice JD, Jr, Abramson DH, Tarone RE, Kleinerman RA, Stovall M, Goldman MB, Seddon JM, Tarbell N, Fraumeni JF Jr, Li FP. (1997) Cancer incidence after retinoblastoma. Radiation dose and sarcoma risk. *JAMA* 278:1262–1267.

Woodruff JM. (1999) Pathology of tumors of the peripheral nerve sheath in type 1 neurofibromatosis. *Am J Med Genet (Semin Med Genet)* 89:23–30.

Woodruff JM, Selig AM, Crowley K, Allen PW. (1994) Schwannoma (neurilemoma) with malignant transformation. A rare distinctive peripheral nerve tumor. *Am J Surg Pathol* 18:882–895.

Woodward AH, Ivings JJ, Soule EH. (1972) Lymphangiosarcoma arising in chronic lymphedematous extremities. *Cancer* 30:562–572.

Wrotnowski U, Cooper PH, Shmookler BM. (1988) Fibrosarcomatous change in dermatofibrosarcoma protuberans. *Am J Surg Pathol* 12:287–293.

Yokoi T, Tsuzuki T, Yatabe Y, Suzuki M, Kurumaya H, Koshikawa T, Kuhara H, Kuroda M, Nakamura N, Nakatani Y, Kakaudo K. (1998) Solitary fibrous tumour: significance of p53 and CD34 immunoreactivity in its malignant transformation. *Histopathology* 32:423–432.

Yoshikawa H, Takafumi U, Mori S, Araki N, Myoui A, Uchida A, Fukuda H. (1996) Dedifferentiated liposarcoma of the subcutis. *Am J Surg Pathol* 20:1525–1530.

Zámecnik M, Michal M. (1994) Giant-cell fibroblastoma with pigmented dermatofibrosarcoma protuberans component. *Am J Surg Pathol* 18:736–740.

Zámecnik M, Michal M, Simpson RHW, Lamovec J, Hlavcak P, Kinkor Z, Mukensnabl P, Matejovsky Z, Betlach J. (1997) Ossifying fibromyxoid tumor of soft parts: a report of 17 cases with emphasis of unusual histological features. *Ann Diagn Pathol* 1:73–81.

Zinszner H, Albalat R, Ron D. (1994) A novel effector domain from the RNA-binding protein TLS or EWS is required for oncogenic transformation by CHOP. *Genes Dev* 8:2513–2526.

Zoubek A, Dockhorn-Dworniczak B, Delattre O, Christiansen H, Niggli F, Gatterer-Menz I, Smith TL, Jurgens H, Gadner H, Kovar H. (1996) Does expression of different EWS chimeric transcripts define clinically distinct risk groups of Ewing tumor patients? *J Clin Oncol* 14:1245–1251.

Zucman J, Melot T, Desmaze C, Ghysdael J, Plougastel B, Peter M, Zucker JM, Triche TJ, Sheer D, Turc-Carel C (1993) Combinatorial generation of variable fusion proteins in the Ewing family of tumours. *EMBO J* 12:4481–4487.

Zucman-Rossi J, Legoix P, Victor JM, Lopez B, Thomas G. (1998) Chromosome translocation based on illegitimate recombination in human tumors. *Proc Natl Acad Sci USA* 95:11786–11791.

Zwarthoff EC. (1996) Neurofibromatosis and associated tumour suppressor genes. *Path Res Pract* 192:647–657.

29

BONES AND JOINTS

K. Krishnan Unni and Carrie Y. Inwards

Neoplasms and neoplasm-like conditions of the skeleton are extremely uncommon. Very few centers see significant numbers of these lesions. Hence, information about clinical features, pathologic aspects, treatment, and prognosis comes from a small number of studies. There probably is no one single cause for malignancies in general; almost surely the etiology is multifactorial. Information about causative agents in neoplasms of bone is sparse.

Evidence has been accumulating that at least some sarcomas of bone are related to genetic abnormalities. Although osteosarcoma arising in retinoblastoma was first reported following exposure to radiation, it was soon recognized that osteosarcomas are relatively frequent in patients with familial bilateral retinoblastoma, although they are uncommon in those with unilateral retinoblastoma (Berg and Weiland, 1978; Schimke et al., 1974). There is an estimated 15% to 20% incidence of second malignancies in patients who survive bilateral retinoblastoma. The most common type has been osteosarcoma of long bones. In the Mayo Clinic files, bone sarcoma developed in two patients with bilateral retinoblastoma, one an osteosarcoma and one a Ewing's tumor. The gene responsible for the development of retinoblastoma and osteosarcoma is located on chromosome 13 (Benedict et al., 1988). There are a few genetic disorders in which patients are prone to malignancies, and in some of these sarcomas of bone also develop. Rothmund-Thomson syndrome is

an autosomal dominant hereditary disease with variable expression. The syndrome is associated with various clinical features, including short stature, small hands and feet, small dystrophic nails, and prematurely gray hair. Patients generally have atrophy of the skin and absent or hypoplastic thumbs and immune deficiencies. Various types of malignancies have been described in patients with Rothmund-Thomson syndrome, including visceral and skin tumors. Cumin and co-authors (1996) reported on three patients with osteosarcoma and Rothmund-Thomson syndrome. Of the approximately 2000 cases of osteosarcoma seen at the Mayo Clinic, two patients had Rothmund-Thomson syndrome. One, a 15-year-old girl, presented with multicentric osteosarcoma involving the proximal tibia, distal fibula, and proximal humerus. Several years later, the patient's brother presented with osteosarcoma of the proximal tibia.

Another genetic syndrome associated with malignancy is Bloom's syndrome. Until 1996, several instances of malignancies have been reported in patients with this syndrome (German, 1995). Patients have short stature, photosensitivity, and a predisposition to malignancy. The Mayo Clinic files include two patients with osteosarcoma and Bloom's syndrome. One patient presented with multicentric osteosarcoma involving several bones of one leg. Several years later, his brother presented with an osteosarcoma involving the distal ulna.

The Li-Fraumeni syndrome is also well

recognized as being associated with the development of malignancies. There is one example of an osteosarcoma arising in a patient with Li-Fraumeni syndrome in the Mayo Clinic files.

Trauma has also been invoked in the causation of sarcomas of bone. The relationship between the two is not very clear. It is much more likely that the trauma draws attention to a preexisting neoplasm than that it is the cause. Osteosarcoma arising at the site of a prior fracture has been reported (Berry et al., 1980). The Mayo Clinic files contain only one patient with osteosarcoma who had a clear history of trauma to the site several years previously—a 37-year-old man who suffered from a bullet wound to the leg 11 years before an osteosarcoma developed at exactly the same site.

SARCOMA RELATED TO A DEFINITE ANTECEDENT PROCESS

An approach to the problem is to study well-documented examples of sarcoma in which there has been a definite antecedent neoplasm or non-neoplastic condition.

CHONDROSARCOMA

Of the more than 900 cases of chondrosarcomas on file at the Mayo Clinic, 150 can be considered secondary to another condition. Osteochondroma, either solitary (70) or multiple (41), was the single most common preexisting condition. Whether enchondromas can give rise to chondrosarcoma is debatable. There are very few well-documented examples of enchondroma undergoing malignant change. There are, however, several instances of malignant change in patients with "multiple chondromas." Multiple chondromas probably are dysplastic conditions rather than neoplasms. Seventeen of the chondrosarcomas arose in multiple chondromas—Ollier's disease (11), Maffucci's syndrome (4), and multiple chondromas (2). Three chondrosarcomas arose in patients with fibrous dysplasia. One of these patients had been treated with radiation therapy. Five chondrosarcomas were considered to be postradiation occurrences, one of them being a clear cell chondrosarcoma.

One patient with chondrosarcoma of the hyoid bone had Gardner's syndrome. Three patients had chondrosarcomas arising in preexisting synovial chondromatosis.

OSTEOSARCOMA

The Mayo Clinic files contain more than 1700 examples of osteosarcoma. Of these, 173 can be considered secondary to a preexisting condition. Prior radiation therapy accounted for the largest single group, with 89 cases. Fifty-five osteosarcomas arose in Paget's disease; fibrous dysplasia accounted for 12; the remaining conditions were infarct of bone (2), osteomyelitis (2), osteochondroma (3) (1 patient had multiple exostosis), melorheostosis (1), osteopoikilosis (1), bullet wound (1), bilateral retinoblastoma (1), Bloom's syndrome (2), Rothmund-Thomson syndrome (2), and Li-Fraumeni syndrome (1).

MALIGNANT FIBROUS HISTIOCYTOMA

Our files contain more than 83 cases of malignant fibrous histiocytoma. Of these, 19 are considered to be secondary. Thirteen arose in a field of prior radiation, three were associated with Paget's disease, two appeared in infarcts of bone, and one occurred at the site of a prior total hip arthroplasty.

FIBROSARCOMA

Of the approximately 260 fibrosarcomas in the Mayo Clinic files, 61 were considered secondary. Forty-five fibrosarcomas arose in the field of prior radiation, six were associated with Paget's disease, and three were related to infarcts. Four fibrosarcomas arose in a preexisting giant cell tumor without prior radiation. Two ameloblastic fibromas underwent malignant change to ameloblastic fibrosarcomas, and one tumor arose in fibrous dysplasia. Four patients with von Recklinghausen's disease had fibrosarcomas of the skeleton; whether the two conditions were related is unclear.

CHORDOMA

It is very unusual to see chordoma in a preexisting condition. Of the more than 360 examples of chordoma in our files, only 2 were considered to be associated with a preexisting condition. Both patients had multiple "chondromas," including one patient with Ollier's disease.

EWING'S TUMOR

Ewing's tumor is also infrequently associated with a preexisting condition. Of our more than 550 cases of Ewing's sarcoma, 1 patient had a history of bilateral retinoblastoma and 1 patient had prior radiotherapy.

MYELOMA

Myeloma is by far the most common malignant neoplasm of bone. More than 3000 patients with myeloma have been treated at the Mayo Clinic. However, only some 900 patients had surgical material for the diagnosis of myeloma. In three the myeloma may be considered secondary—in one patient who had long-standing osteomyelitis, in one with systemic mastocytosis, and in one with an associated chondroma, though this probably was an incidental finding.

MALIGNANT LYMPHOMA

Among the more than 700 examples of malignant lymphoma in the Mayo Clinic files, only one patient could be considered to have had a preexisting condition, long-standing osteomyelitis.

ADAMANTINOMA

There is controversy in the literature about the relationship between adamantinoma and osteofibrous dysplasia. We believe that several adamantinomas have areas simulating the appearance of osteofibrous dysplasia. We have not, however, seen clear-cut examples of adamantinoma becoming superimposed on osteofibrous dysplasia.

PREMALIGNANT LESIONS OF BONE

Premalignant lesions of bone can be broadly divided into three groups (Table 29–1).

Table 29–1. Premalignant Lesions of Bone

Premalignant non-neoplastic conditions

Radiation effect

Paget's disease

Chronic osteomyelitis

Infarct of bone

Osteogenesis imperfecta

Melorheostosis

Osteopoikilosis

Metal implants

Premalignant tumor-like conditions

Osteochondroma
 Solitary
 Multiple

Chondroma
 Solitary
 Multiple

Fibrous dysplasia
 Monostotic
 Polyostotic

Synovial chondromatosis

Pigmented villonodular synovitis

Premalignant tumors

Giant cell tumor

Chondroblastoma

Chondromyxoid fibroma

Osteoblastoma

POSTRADIATION SARCOMA

Cahan and co-authors (1948) suggested the following criteria for diagnosis of postradiation sarcoma of bone: (*1*) microscopic or roentgenographic evidence of the benignity of the primary condition; (*2*) radiation in any of its forms must have been given and a sarcoma that later developed must have arisen in the area included within the radiotherapeutic beam; (*3*) a relatively long symptom-free latent period; and (*4*) all the sarcomas were confirmed histologically. At least two of these criteria need modification. More and more patients are now being recognized who acquire a postradiation sarcoma after surviving a prior malignancy of bone, especially Ewing's sarcoma (Fig. 29–1). It is also questionable whether a latent period of 5 years or more is always necessary. It is possible that the addition of chemotherapy to radiation therapy decreases the latent period. Several large series have confirmed the occurrence of bone sar-

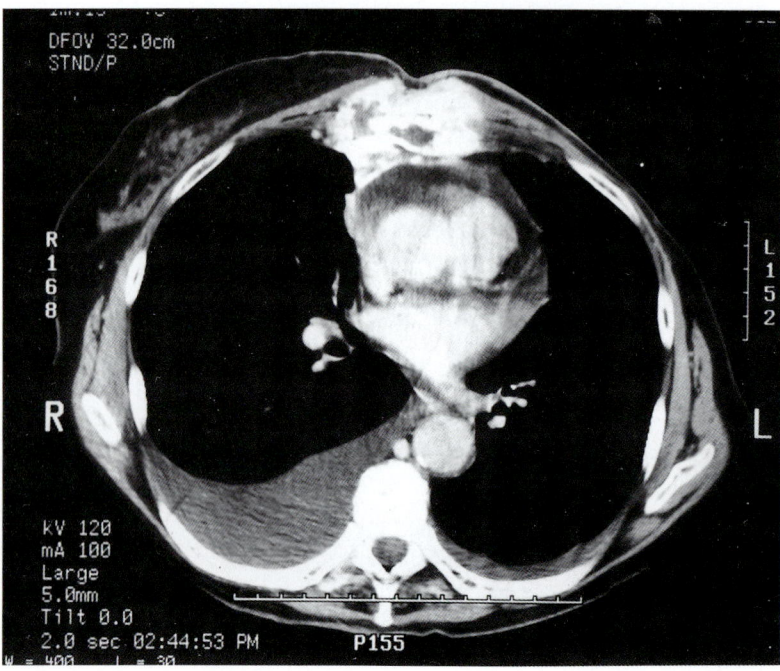

Figure 29–1. Large postradiation osteosarcoma with soft tissue extension involving the left scapula in a 23-year-old man following radiation therapy for Ewing's sarcoma 9 years earlier.

coma after irradiation (Fig. 29–2; Arlen et al., 1971; Weatherby et al., 1981). Soft tissue sarcomas following irradiation are less common (Laskin et al., 1988). Tucker and co-authors (1987) have demonstrated a sharp dose–response gradient in the development of sarcoma of bone after irradiation, reaching a 40-fold risk after doses to the bone of more than 6000 rads.

There were 156 examples of postradiation sarcoma in the Mayo Clinic files until the beginning of 1994. Unlike most bone sar-

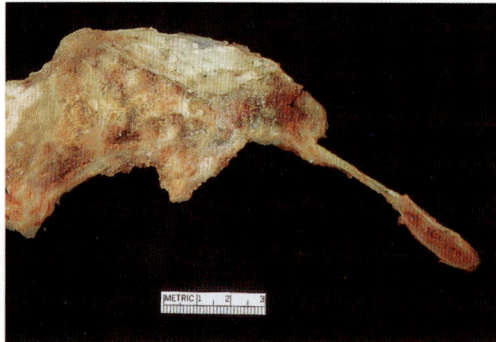

Figure 29–2. Postradiation osteosarcoma involving the sternum in a 73-year-old woman after a left mastectomy for breast carcinoma 18 years earlier.

comas, these showed a definite female predilection: 98 females, 58 males. The patients were generally older than those with sarcomas of bone, the greatest incidence being in the fourth, fifth, sixth, and seventh decades of life. There was also a tendency for unusual skeletal sites to be involved. The most common single bone involved was the sacrum (17 tumors), the second most common was the scapula (15 tumors). The latent period between radiation therapy and the development of sarcoma varied considerably, from 1 year to 55 years. Less than 8% of patients had a latent period of less than 5 years. Almost one-third of the patients had a latent period of between 5 and 10 years, the average being just over 15 years.

Radiation therapy was employed for a large variety of conditions. Giant cell tumor of bone was the single most common neoplasm that underwent malignant change after radiation therapy. The conditions for which irradiation was given are shown in Table 29–2.

A variety of sarcomas were included in the group of postradiation sarcoma. The single most common type was osteosarcoma, which accounted for 89 tumors. The types of sarcomas developing after radiation therapy are given in Table 29–3.

Table 29–2. Conditions for Which Radiation Therapy Was Given

Conditions	No. of Cases
Giant cell tumor of bone	24
Fibrous dysplasia	12
Aneurysmal bone cyst	3
Brain tumors	7
Soft tissue tumors	7
Malignant lymphoma	7
Hodgkin's disease	7
Ewing's sarcoma of bone	5
Miscellaneous malignancies	21
Carcinoma of breast	17
Miscellaneous bone lesions	25
Miscellaneous other conditions	26

It is obvious that most sarcomas arising after irradiation were spindle cell sarcomas. Most of these were also of high grade. It is unusual to see low-grade sarcomas arising after radiation therapy.

The overall prognosis in patients with postradiation sarcoma tends to be poor. However, these results should be viewed in the context of involvement of unusual and difficult-to-treat skeletal sites such as the sacrum, pelvis, and bones of the chest wall. If only lesions of the long bones are considered, the prognosis in postradiation sarcoma seems to be identical to that of sarcomas arising *de novo*.

PAGET'S DISEASE

Sir James Paget, in 1877, described a disease that he called "osteitis deformans." It has since been commonly called "Paget's disease

Table 29–3. Types of Tumors Developing After Radiation Therapy

Diagnosis	No. of Cases
Osteosarcoma	89
Fibrosarcoma	45
Malignant fibrous histiocytoma	13
Chondrosarcoma	5
Hemangioendothelioma	2
Ewing's sarcoma	1
Malignant lymphoma	1

of bone." He discussed five cases, and in two of these the disease was complicated by sarcoma. He later described 23 cases of Paget's disease; 5 patients died of sarcoma.

As with many other conditions, it is difficult to establish the true incidence of sarcomatous change in Paget's disease. Haibach and associates (1985) reported on 82 cases of sarcomas arising in Paget's disease. The majority were osteosarcomas, with a small number of fibrosarcomas, chondrosarcomas, and giant cell tumors. Only 18% of patients were less than 51 years old. The femur and the humerus were involved in almost equal numbers of cases. In the series described from Memorial Hospital (Huvos et al., 1983), the most common skeletal site was the pelvic bones, followed by the humerus. In the Mayo Clinic files until the end of 1993, there were 54 examples of sarcomas arising in Paget's disease, which accounted for 3.3% of all osteosarcomas. In this series, too, the pelvic bones were most commonly affected. Even in the Mayo Clinic files, there appears to be a peculiar predilection for involvement of the humerus. In both the series described by Haibach and associates (1985) and the Mayo Clinic files, there was a 2:1 male-to-female ratio. In the Memorial Hospital series, however, men outnumbered women only slightly. In all large series of Paget's sarcoma, the patients are older than is usual in cases of osteosarcoma. Patients with Paget's disease often complain of pain, especially when the disease is associated with fractures. However, the presence of unrelenting localized pain should alert one to the development of sarcoma. Roentgenographic features of Paget's disease are practically diagnostic. There is thickening of cortical bone and medullary trabeculae. A sharp demarcation is seen between the involved segment of bone and the uninvolved marrow, a feature that has been termed the "flame" sign. Paget's disease almost invariably extends to the end of the bone. Roentgenograms usually show areas of lysis and sclerosis. If there are large areas of lysis in an otherwise typical appearance of Paget's disease, sarcomatous change should be suspected (Fig. 29–3). The histologic features of sarcoma arising in Paget's disease are not different from those of the respective sarcomas arising *de novo*. Almost all of the sarcomas are high grade (Fig. 29–4). For some reason, the

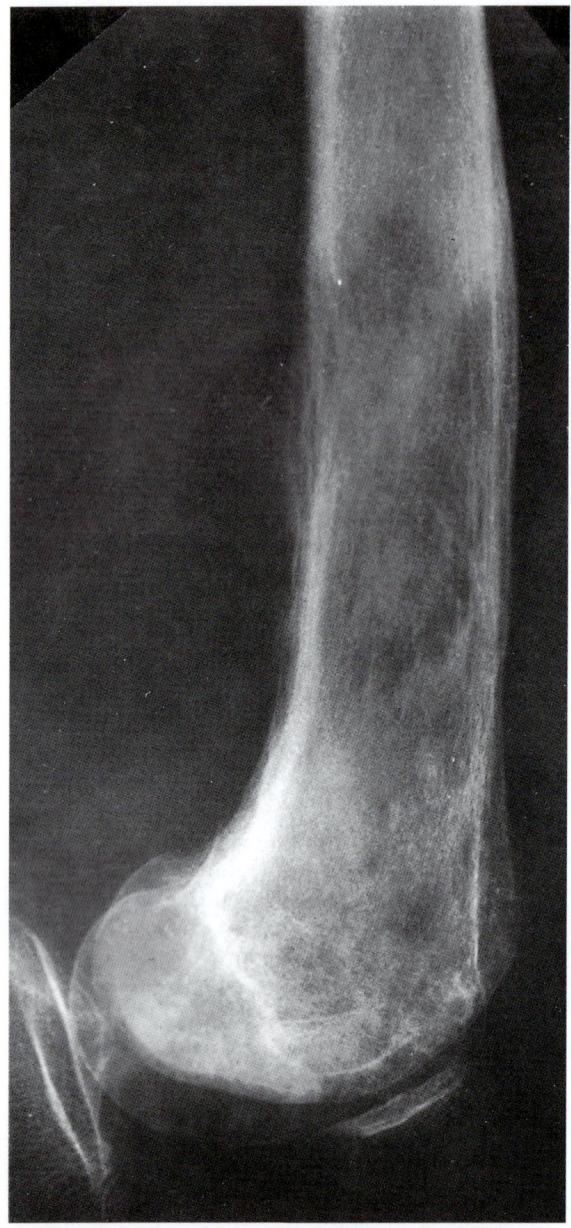

Figure 29–3. Osteosarcoma forming a destructive lesion in the distal femur which exhibits radiographic changes of Paget's disease.

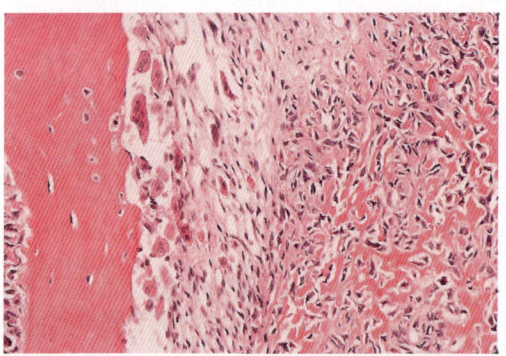

Figure 29–4. Paget's disease, with thickened osseous trabeculae and osteoblastic rimming, merging with high-grade osteosarcoma.

prognosis in Paget's sarcoma has been poor. In the series of Haibach and associates (1985), only 5% of patients had survived after 5 years; in the series from Memorial Hospital, only 3 of 65 patients were alive after 5 years; and in the Mayo Clinic files, 4 patients survived for more than 10 years.

CHRONIC OSTEOMYELITIS

It is well recognized in orthopedic oncology that osteomyelitis can simulate a neoplasm. Clinical features, roentgenographic characteristics, and even the gross appearance of osteomyelitis and Ewing's tumor can be identical. Long-standing chronic osteomyelitis can simulate an indolent bone neoplasm, such as myeloma or even a giant cell tumor (Cabanela et al., 1974).

Less common is the development of a malignancy in chronic osteomyelitis associated with a draining sinus, although such an association has been known for a long time (Fig. 29–5). The estimated incidence has varied from 0.2% to 1.7% (Fitzgerald et al., 1976). Although most malignancies arising in the draining sinus of chronic osteomyelitis are squamous cell carcinomas, sarcomas have also been described (Akbarnia et al., 1976). McGrory and co-authors (1999) have recently updated the Mayo Clinic experience with malignancies in the sinus tract of osteomyelitis. It has generally been considered that involvement of bone with squamous epithelium is necessary to make a diagnosis of squamous cell carcinoma in this clinical setting. However, in this study of 53 patients, 12 did not have involvement of the bone with proliferating squamous epithelium. Only the sinus tract was involved.

Patients generally present with chronic osteomyelitis of long standing with a draining sinus, which itself has usually been present for decades. The patients note increasing pain, increasing discharge that may become foul smelling, or a mass lesion. Rarely, a patient presents with a pathologic fracture. Only 5 of 41 patients with involvement of bone were women. In 24 of the 41 patients, the tibia was involved, in 10, the femur. It is obviously very rare to see malignancy associated with chronic osteomyelitis in any other skeletal site. Fifty-one of the 53 malignancies were squamous cell carcinoma. There was one case of myeloma and one of

lymphoma involving the skeleton. When a squamous cell carcinoma arises in the setting of osteomyelitis, it usually is well differentiated, with features of verrucous carcinoma. Of the 39 squamous cell carcinomas with involvement of bone, 25 were considered grade 1, 6 were grade 2, 6 were grade 3, and 2 were grade 4. Of the squamous cell carcinomas arising only in the sinus tract, eight were grade 1, three were grade 2, and one was grade 3. The distinction between pseudoepitheliomatous hyperplasia associated with the sinus tract and a verrucous squamous cell carcinoma can be difficult. If the squamous cells permeate bone, diagnosis of squamous cell carcinoma is definite. In the setting of only a sinus tract, the diagnosis is more subtle and has to be based on recognition of the characteristic features of verrucous carcinoma arising in other sites, such as mucous membranes. Among the patients with involvement of bone, follow-up was available in 38 patients, and 19 died. However, only five patients died from the effects of the tumor. In the small series of patients with involvement of the sinus tract, only two experienced local recurrences and one died with nodal metastasis. In addition, two osteosarcomas arose in the setting of chronic osteomyelitis.

INFARCT OF BONE

The first association between infarct of bone and sarcoma was reported by Furey and co-workers (1960). There have been sporadic reports of this association since. Mirra and co-authors (1974) reported on four patients with malignant fibrous histiocytoma and osteosarcoma arising in association with bone infarcts. Two of the patients were caisson workers. Although avascular necrosis of the femoral head is a type of infarct, it is rarely associated with sarcoma. This paucity may be explained by the fact that avascular necrosis of the femoral head is quite symptomatic and hence the patients are treated. Infarcts of other sites in bone are not usually symptomatic and are incidental findings on X-ray. Although most infarcts of bone are considered idiopathic, there are several known causes. The most common are working under conditions of compressed air (caisson workers and divers), steroid therapy, alcoholism, and vasculitis, such as systemic lupus erythematosus. The roentgenographic ap-

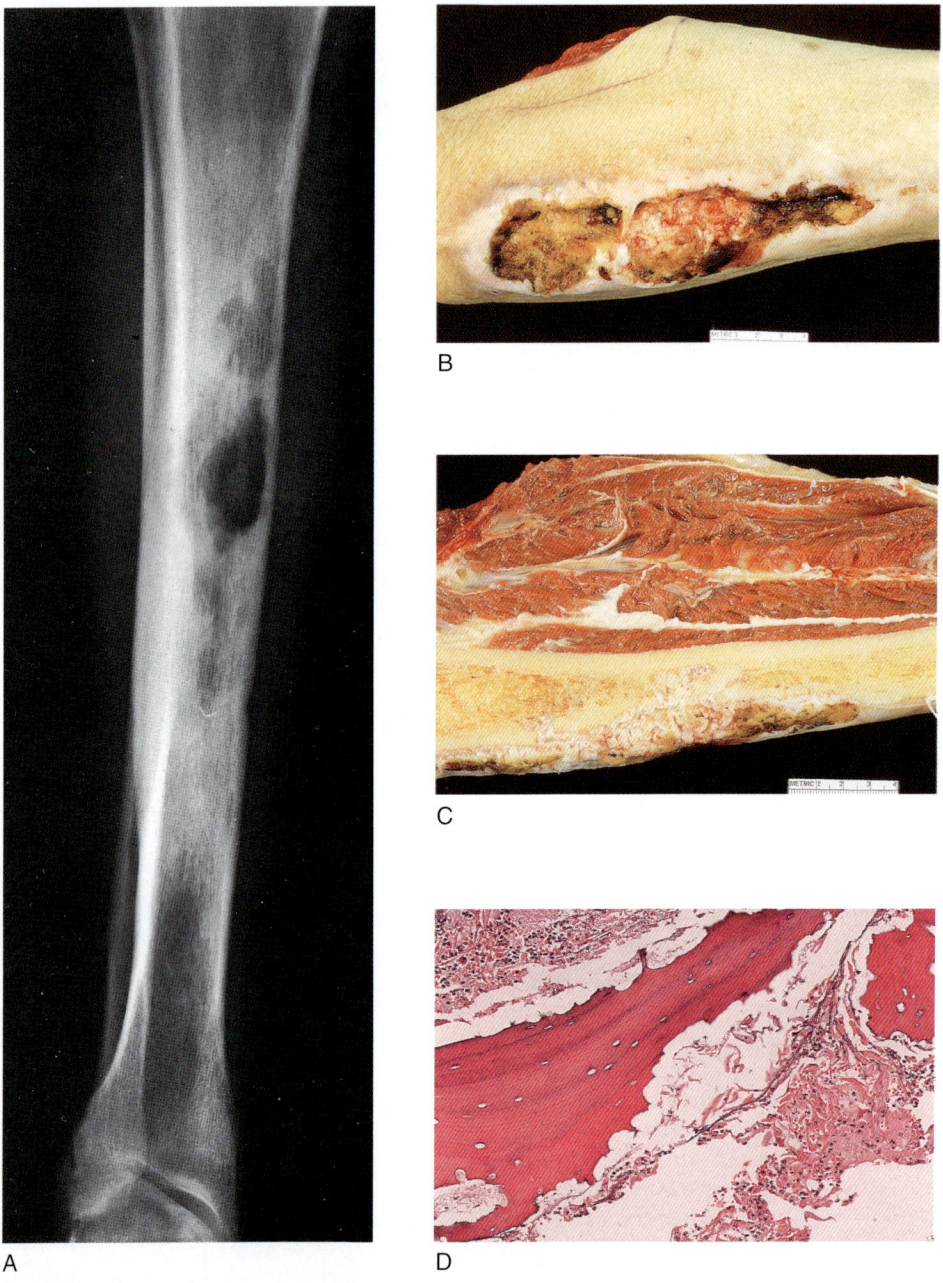

Figure 29–5. Squamous cell carcinoma arising in the tibia of a 69-year-old man with a 61-year history of chronic osteomyelitis. Radiograph (*A*) shows irregular lucency and sclerosis in the diaphysis of the tibia, consistent with osteomyelitis. Within this area is a destructive lesion corresponding to the underlying squamous cell carcinoma. The lesion breaks through overlying skin, forming a large ulcer (*B*) and eroding into the underlying cortex (*C*). There is abundant gray-white keratinous material. Microscopically (*D*), well-differentiated squamous cell carcinoma permeates osseous trabeculae.

pearance of an infarct of bone is quite typical. It tends to involve the metaphyseal region of long bones and may be bilateral and symmetric. The lesion appears as an area of lucency surrounded by an area of calcifica-

tion. When a sarcoma arises, an area of destruction is usually seen adjacent to the infarct (Fig. 29–6).

Grossly, infarcts appear as irregular areas of calcification with central necrosis (Fig.

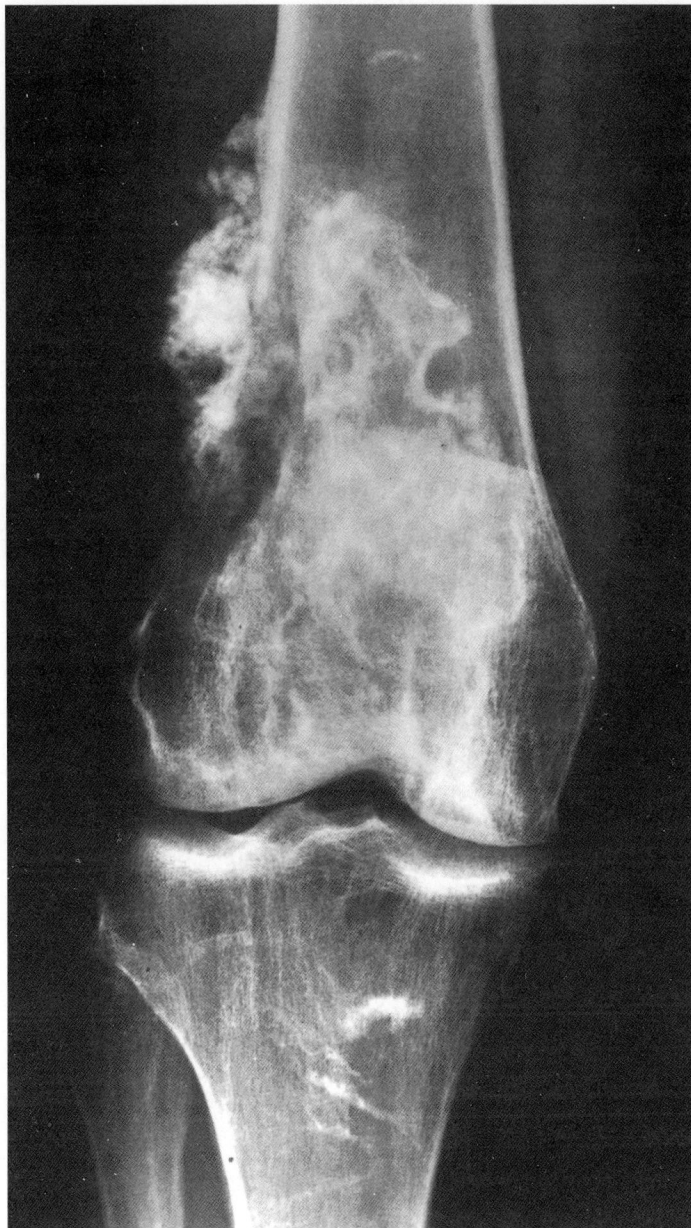

Figure 29–6. Osteosarcoma associated with an infarct. Mineral appears in the metaphysis of the distal femur, which shows the characteristic peripheral calcification of an infarct. Lateral to the infarct are cortical destruction and flocculent soft tissue mineral corresponding to the osteosarcoma.

29–7). Microscopically, an infarct is identified by lack of nuclei in the osteocytic lacunae and fat necrosis in medullary bone. The necrotic fat is usually replaced by amorphous calcification.

The Mayo Clinic files include seven instances of sarcoma in association with infarcts. Three tumors were considered to be fibrosarcomas, two were malignant fibrohistiocytomas, and two were osteosarcomas. Other examples of sarcomas arising in infarcts may remain unrecognized. It is possible that the antecedent infarct is destroyed by the tumor and hence is not recognized at the time of treatment; however, the incidence of sarcomatous change is low and therefore this consideration should not be a major factor in managing patients with infarcts of bone.

OSTEOGENESIS IMPERFECTA

Osteogenesis imperfecta is a complex developmental anomaly characterized by alter-

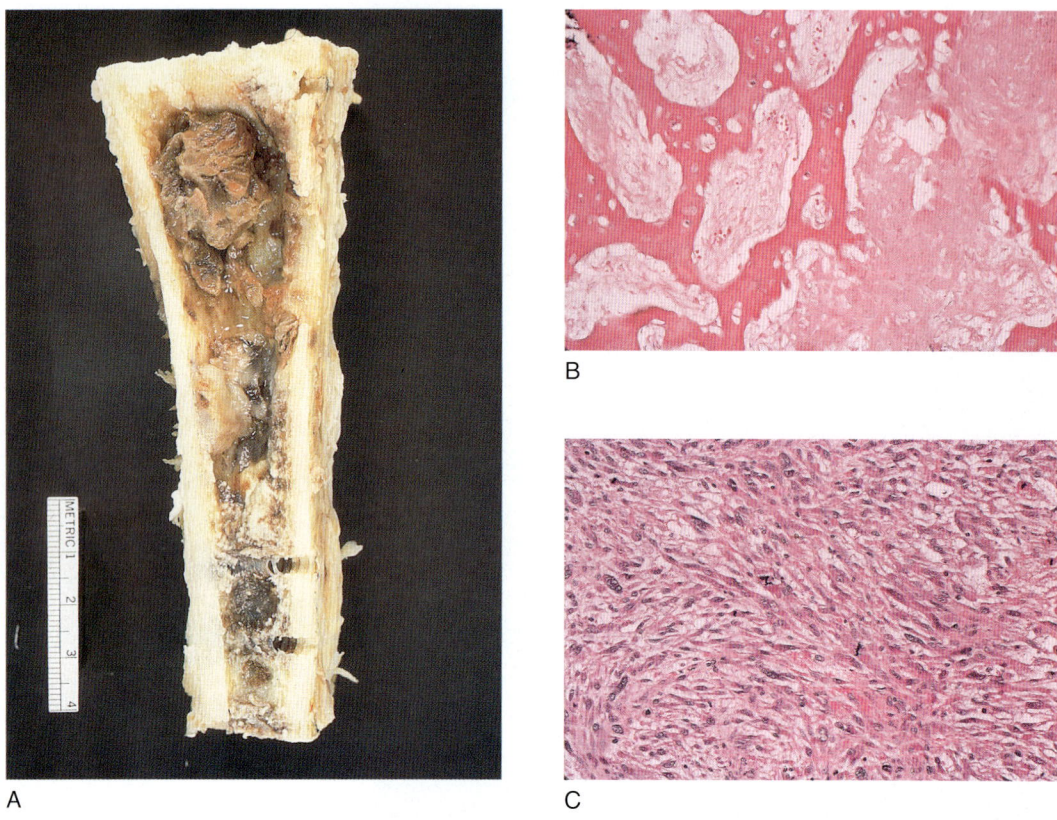

Figure 29–7. Fibrosarcoma associated with an infarct in the proximal tibia of a 75-year-old man. Gross photo (*A*) shows the calcified yellow-white infarct associated with the lobulated sarcoma extending proximally. Microscopic studies show the infarct (*B*) and the high-grade fibrosarcoma (*C*).

ations in bone, the eye (sclera), and the skin. Patients have multiple fractures, blue sclerae, deafness, and loose-jointedness. There is a form of osteogenesis imperfecta in which skeletal manifestations may be delayed (osteogenesis imperfecta tarda). The most common presentation is multiple skeletal fractures. These fractures are usually associated with hyperplastic callus, a condition that may be mistaken for a sarcoma. There have been few instances of true sarcomatous change in association with osteogenesis imperfecta, and hence it is possible that they are not causally related. Klenerman and associates (1967) reported on two patients with osteosarcoma arising in osteogenesis imperfecta. Rutkowski and co-authors (1979) reported a single case. There are no examples in the Mayo Clinic files; we have seen a small number of cases in consultation. The differentiation between a hyperplastic callus and a sarcoma may be difficult. The callus is typically associated with large amounts of

cartilage, which may be quite cellular with enlarged nuclei. However, the nuclei do not show hyperchromasia, and there is orderly maturation into trabecular-appearing bone. The loose arrangement of the spindle cells between the trabeculae of bone also helps to distinguish hyperplastic callus from true sarcoma.

MELORHEOSTOSIS

Melorheostosis is a rare monostotic or polyostotic bone disease of unknown etiology. It is characterized by a slowly progressing linear hyperostosis and fibrosis of the skin and subcutaneous tissues. The bone condition is usually asymptomatic. Roentgenograms generally show thickening of the cortical surface of bone. The appearance has been described as wax dripping from a candle. Bostman and co-authors (1987) described one example of osteosarcoma arising in melorheostosis. There is only one example of sarcoma arising in melorheostosis in the Mayo Clinic files. It involved the tibia of a 43-year-old man in whom a chondroblastic osteosarcoma arose in the midportion of the tibia.

Osteopoikilosis

Osteopoikilosis is an unusual abnormality in which symmetric bone islands occur in many parts of the skeleton. The condition is asymptomatic and is usually detected as an incidental roentgenographic finding. Roentgenograms show discrete, round lesions of increased density involving many portions of the skeleton. Mindell and co-authors (1978) described an example of osteosarcoma arising in osteopoikilosis. There has been only one case in the Mayo Clinic files, that of an osteosarcoma arising in the sacrum of a 43-year-old woman who was known to have had osteopoikilosis since 14 years previously.

Metal Implants

Metal implants have been used extensively in recent years for the treatment of fractures and in the management of joint diseases. Rare examples of sarcomas arising at the site of a metal implant have been reported. Lee and co-authors (1984) described the development of a malignant fibrous histiocytoma at the site of a metal plate used for fixation of a fracture 14 years previously. Hughes and associates (1987) described a malignant fibrous histiocytoma arising in the proximal femur at the site of a hip screw that had been placed 30 years previously. Brien and co-authors (1990) reported an example of osteosarcoma arising at the site of a prior total hip replacement. There has been only one example of such an association in the Mayo Clinic files. It involved the proximal femur of a 79-year-old man in whom a high-grade malignant fibrous histiocytoma developed at the site of a prior total hip arthroplasty.

PREMALIGNANT TUMOR-LIKE CONDITIONS

Osteochondroma

Osteochondromas are probably not true neoplasms but rather growths of displaced epiphyseal plates that produce a mass of car-tilage and bone, either sessile or with a stalk, usually in the metaphyseal portion of long bones. The roentgenographic appearance is quite typical, with the cortex of the involved bone sweeping out into the cortex of the osteochondroma and the medullary cavity of the bone being continuous with the inner aspect of the osteochondroma. The tumor may be solitary or multiple. Multiple osteochondromas are inherited as an autosomally dominant trait. Osteochondromas are usually incidental findings but can cause symptoms by the sheer size of the tumor, impingement on nearby structures, especially nerves, or a pathologic fracture of the stalk.

Although it has been recognized that chondrosarcomas may arise in osteochondroma, there is controversy about the incidence. Because most osteochondromas are asymptomatic, and hence do not come to surgery, it is difficult to know their true incidence. Patients with a secondary malignancy are more likely to be seen in a medical center. Tan and co-authors (Tan TS, Unni KK, Collins MS, Wenger DE, Sim FH, unpublished data) recently studied 107 patients from the Mayo Clinic files with secondary chondrosarcoma. There were 61 patients with solitary osteochondroma and 46 with multiple hereditary exostosis. During the same period, 802 patients with solitary exostosis and 120 patients with multiple exostosis were treated at our institution. Hence, in this surgical series, the incidence of malignant change was 7.6% in patients with solitary exostosis and 36.3% in those with multiple hereditary exostosis. Patients usually complained of a swelling, which may have been present from weeks to months before diagnosis. Pain was less frequent. Occasionally, the tumors were incidental findings on roentgenograms. The most frequent sites of involvement were the ilium and the pubis. There was a slight male predominance, and patients ranged in age from 15 to 77 years. Roentgenographic features are critical in differentiating osteochondroma from secondary chondrosarcoma (Fig. 29–8). Osteochondromas tend to show a smooth surface of the cartilage cap and uniform mineralization of the interior. When a chondrosarcoma supervenes, the cartilage cap becomes thicker and irregular. Inhomogeneous mineralization within the cap and the presence of a soft tissue mass with punctate calcification are also features of malignancy. With

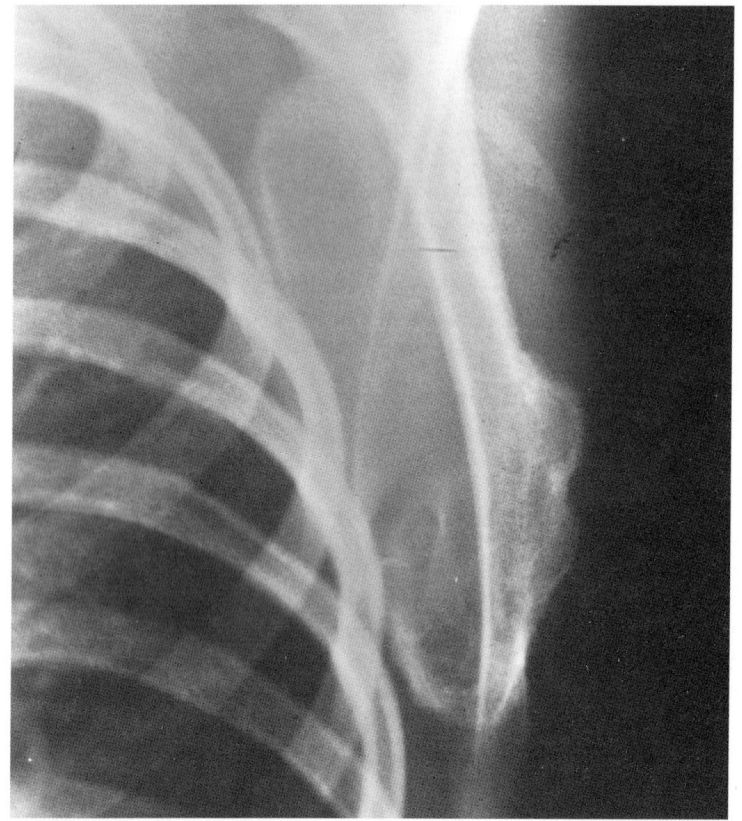

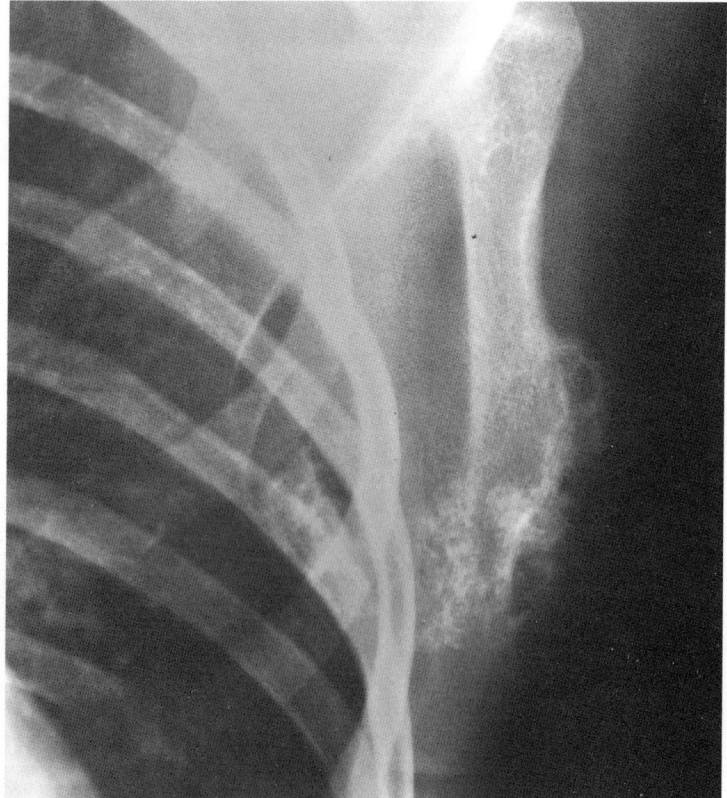

Figure 29–8. Osteochondroma arising in the scapula of a 15-year-old boy. *A*: Typical radiographic appearance of osteochondroma in a flat bone. *B*: Three years later an X-ray of the area shows a chondrosarcoma arising in the osteochondroma. The margin is irregular and there is cartilaginous mineral in surrounding soft tissue.

modern imaging techniques such as magnetic resonance imaging and computed tomography, the thickness of the cartilage cap can be evaluated more precisely.

The gross appearance of the lesion is also important. Osteochondromas generally tend to show a smooth surface of the cartilage cap. The cap itself is usually quite thin, no more than 4 or 5 mm in thickness. When the cap becomes lobulated and thick, usually more than 2 cm, secondary chondrosarcoma should be suspected (Fig. 29–9). Cystic change within the cartilage is also a sign of malignancy.

Histologically, secondary chondrosarcomas tend to be well differentiated; hence, distinction between osteochondroma and chondrosarcoma cannot be made purely on cytologic grounds. Under low power, permeation into soft tissue, manifested as nodules of cartilage separated from the main tumor mass, is a worrisome sign. It is unusual to see permeation into the stalk or the un-

derlying bone. Marked myxoid change of the matrix giving rise to cystic spaces and nuclear atypia are also important signs. Of the 107 tumors studied, 97 were considered to be grade 1, and only 10 were grade 2. There were no grade 3 chondrosarcomas. Secondary chondrosarcoma is generally associated with a good prognosis because surgery is quite effective. Only 18 of the 107 patients died of the effects of tumor, usually from local disease.

CHONDROMA

Chondromas probably are not true neoplasms. They may be solitary or multiple. Solitary chondromas are usually incidental findings on X-rays, except in the small bones, where they may give rise to pathologic fracture and hence pain. They are usually hot on a bone scan and are frequently identified in patients undergoing bone scan for some other kind of malignancy. Roentgenographically, enchondromas present as well-demarcated nodules in the metaphyseal or diaphyseal region of long bones, associated with a uniform mineralization pattern. A sign of malignancy is destruction of surrounding tissues, especially the cortex. It has been well recognized that the distinction between an enchondroma and a well-differentiated chondrosarcoma is almost impossible on the basis of histologic features alone. We depend heavily on the roentgenographic appearance in making this distinction. Hence, it becomes almost impossible to prove the existence of areas of enchondroma in a newly diagnosed chondrosarcoma. There are indeed rare examples of enchondroma followed for a number of years in which chondrosarcoma subsequently developed. Since these instances are so uncommon, there is no justification for the treatment of enchondromas for fear that a chondrosarcoma will later develop.

Rarely, patients will present with multiple "chondromas." Most of these patients probably have a dysplastic condition such as Ollier's disease or Maffucci's syndrome. These almost surely do not represent neoplasms. There remains a small number of patients who do not have dysplastic conditions but purely multiple chondromas.

Ollier's disease is a rare nonhereditary disorder characterized by cartilaginous masses

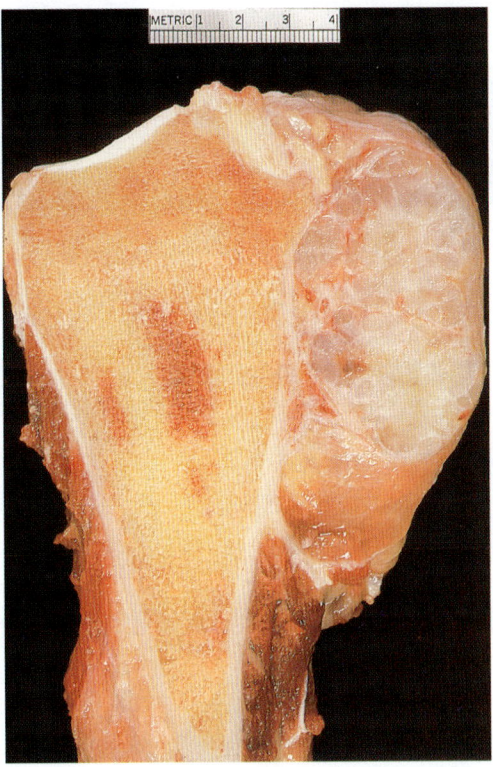

Figure 29–9. Secondary chondrosarcoma in a patient with multiple hereditary exostoses forming a large, lobulated, cartilaginous mass.

persisting in the metaphysis and diaphysis. The disease process may involve the entire skeleton or be limited to half of the body. Roentgenograms show masses of cartilage in the metaphyseal and diaphyseal regions of long bones, associated with longitudinal striations. There may be chondroid masses on the surface of the bone, also similar to a periosteal chondroma. Histologically, Ollier's disease presents with nodules of hypercellular cartilage within the medullary cavity and sometimes on the surface of bone. The cartilage tends to be quite hypercellular, and the nuclei are enlarged. Out of context these features may suggest a diagnosis of chondrosarcoma, and so the distinction from that tumor can be quite difficult. Roentgenographically, the development of chondrosarcoma is manifested as destruction of cortex and a soft tissue mass (Fig. 29–10). Grossly, the chondrosarcomatous area looks quite distinctly different from the benign preexisting condition. The matrix in dysplastic cartilage is quite firm and has the typical blue-gray appearance of cartilage. When chondrosarcoma supervenes, there is a marked myxoid change of the matrix that may lead to cystification. Histologically, it is important to compare the suspicious area with the benign counterparts. Marked myxoid change in the matrix and permeation with entrapment of preexisting structures are features of malignancy. Liu and co-authors (1987) reported on the Mayo Clinic experience with sarcomas in Ollier's disease. In this study, of 55 patients with a diagnosis of Ollier's disease, 16 had sarcomas. The majority were conventional chondrosarcomas, whereas two patients had dedifferentiated chondrosarcoma.

Maffucci's syndrome is a very unusual condition in which multiple chondroid lesions of the bones are associated with soft tissue hemangiomas. Roentgenograms show chondroid masses similar to those seen in Ollier's disease. Soft tissue hemangiomas are usually identified by the calcified phleboliths in the vascular malformations. Nine patients with Maffucci's syndrome and a surgical biopsy have been seen at the Mayo Clinic. In five of these patients, chondrosarcoma developed (Sun et al., 1985).

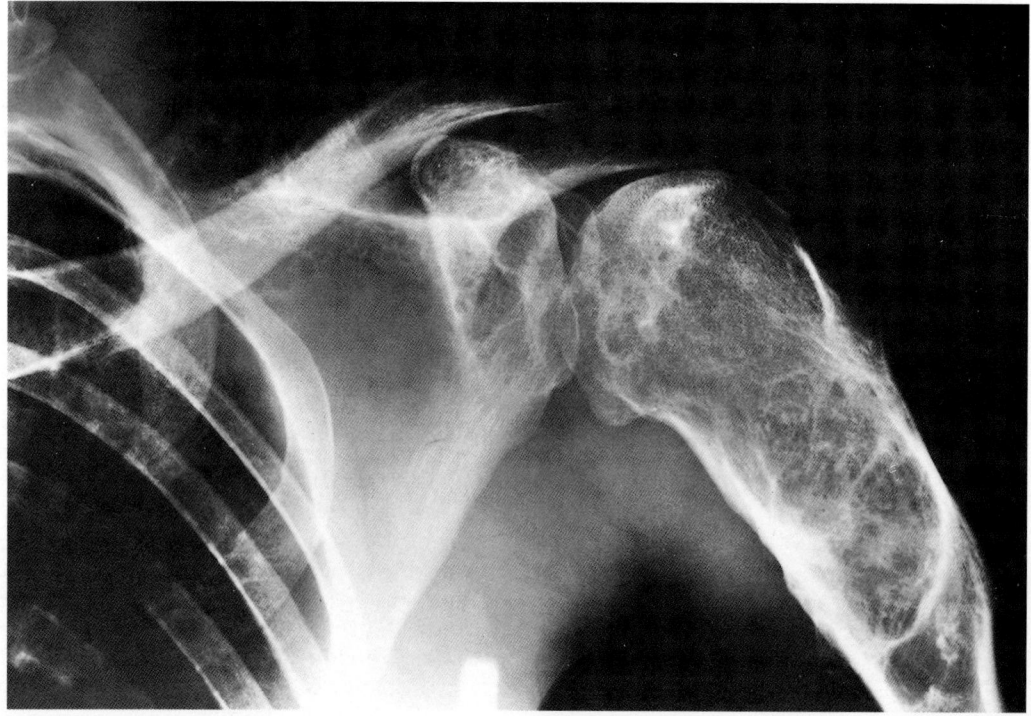

A

Figure 29–10. Ollier's disease in a 40-year-old man. *A*: Radiograph shows the typical features of enchondromatosis. A large enchondroma occupies the proximal humerus. (*Continued*)

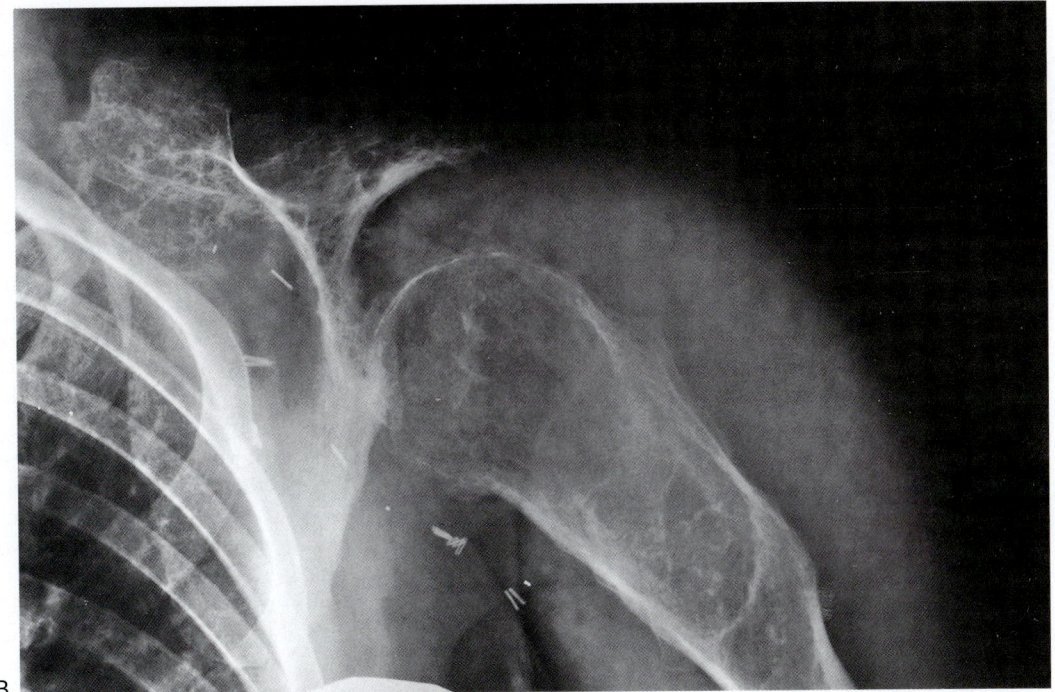

B

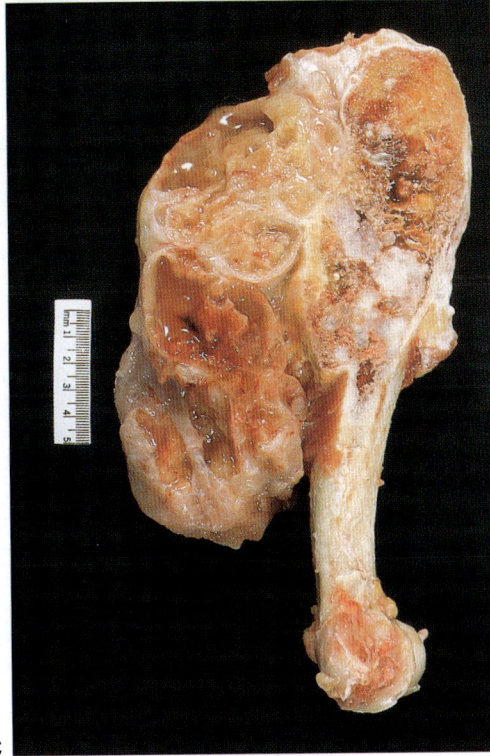

C

Figure 29–10. (*Continued*) Ollier's disease in a 40-year-old man. *B*: Radiograph taken 7 years later shows chondrosarcoma secondary to Ollier's disease involving the proximal humerus. There is destruction of the bone with a large soft tissue mass. The corresponding gross specimen. *C*: shows extensive myxoid change of the matrix.

FIBROUS DYSPLASIA

Fibrous dysplasia is not a neoplasm but a defect in ossification in bone. It may be polyostotic or, more commonly, monostotic. Monostotic fibrous dysplasia is often asymptomatic but may present with a pathologic fracture, especially in the femoral neck. When it involves the skull or facial skeleton, it can produce deformities. Fibrous dysplasia frequently involves the femoral neck, the ribs, the jaw bones, and the skull. Patients with polyostotic fibrous dysplasia may have associated skin pigmentation, endocrine abnormalities, and precocious puberty (Albright's syndrome).

It is difficult to calculate the incidence of sarcomatous change in fibrous dysplasia because the condition is so often asymptomatic. There are few reports of large series of sarcomatous change in fibrous dysplasia. In 1972 Huvos and co-authors reported on 15 patients with sarcoma arising in fibrous dysplasia; only 1 patient had prior radiation. Ruggieri and co-authors (1994) reported 28 cases of sarcoma arising in fibrous dysplasia among the 1122 cases of fibrous dysplasia in the Mayo Clinic files. Sixteen of these patients were seen at the Mayo Clinic, and 12 were from our consultation files. Nineteen patients had monostotic and nine had polyostotic fibrous dysplasia. In almost half the patients (13) the craniofacial bones were involved. The second most common site was the proximal femur, with seven cases. Only one patient had Albright's syndrome. Of the 28 patients, 13 had had radiation treatment either for fibrous dysplasia or for an unrelated condition, and fibrous dysplasia involved a bone in the field of radiation. The interval between radiation therapy and the occurrence of sarcoma ranged from 3 to 52 years, with a mean of 19 years. Roentgenograms generally showed areas of destruction with poor margination, typical of a malignancy, associated with typical areas of fibrous dysplasia (Fig. 29–11). Of the 28 sarcomas, 19 were classified as osteosarcoma, and there was 1 malignant fibrous histiocytoma. Five were considered to be fibrosarcomas, and three were chondrosarcomas, including a clear cell chondrosarcoma. Of the 28 patients, 15 had died of tumor, 4 were lost to follow-up, and 9 were alive. Two of the surviving patients had persistent disease; three had a short follow-up. Only four patients were alive without disease for more than 5 years.

SYNOVIAL CHONDROMATOSIS

Synovial chondromatosis is a rare disorder of major joints in which nodules of cartilage are found within synovium. The process is almost always monoarticular and may involve any joint, although the knee and the hip predominate. Smaller joints such as the temporomandibular joint and the facet joints of the spine may also be involved. The cause is unknown, and there is controversy over whether or not the process is a neoplasm. Histologic examination shows nodules of cartilage within the synovial membrane with chondrocytes in a very typical clustering arrangement. The chondrocytes frequently show cytologic features of malignancy, such as enlarged size, hyperchromasia, irregularity, and double nucleation. Taken out of context, these features may lead to a mistaken diagnosis of chondrosarcoma. The process can be quite extensive and erode surrounding structures, including bone. Synovial chondromatosis has to be separated from osteocartilaginous loose bodies, which are secondary to an underlying process such as degenerative joint disease. The cartilage present in loose bodies does not show the clustering arrangement and cytologic atypia usually seen in synovial chondromatosis. There have been sporadic case reports of chondrosarcoma arising in synovial chondromatosis (Hamilton et al., 1987; Perry et al., 1988). Bertoni and co-authors (1991) described 10 cases from the Mayo Clinic files. Four of these patients had been treated at the Mayo Clinic, and the remainder were from our consultation files. The 10 patients consisted of 6 women and 4 men ranging in age from 30 to 70 years. Five lesions involved the knee joint, three were in the hip, and one each involved the elbow and the ankle. Of the 10 cases, 5 had definite evidence of preexisting synovial chondromatosis either at the time of diagnosis of malignancy or in the past. In three cases, there were features suggestive of synovial chondromatosis, and the two others were considered to be primary chondrosarcoma of the synovium.

As indicated previously, synovial chondro-

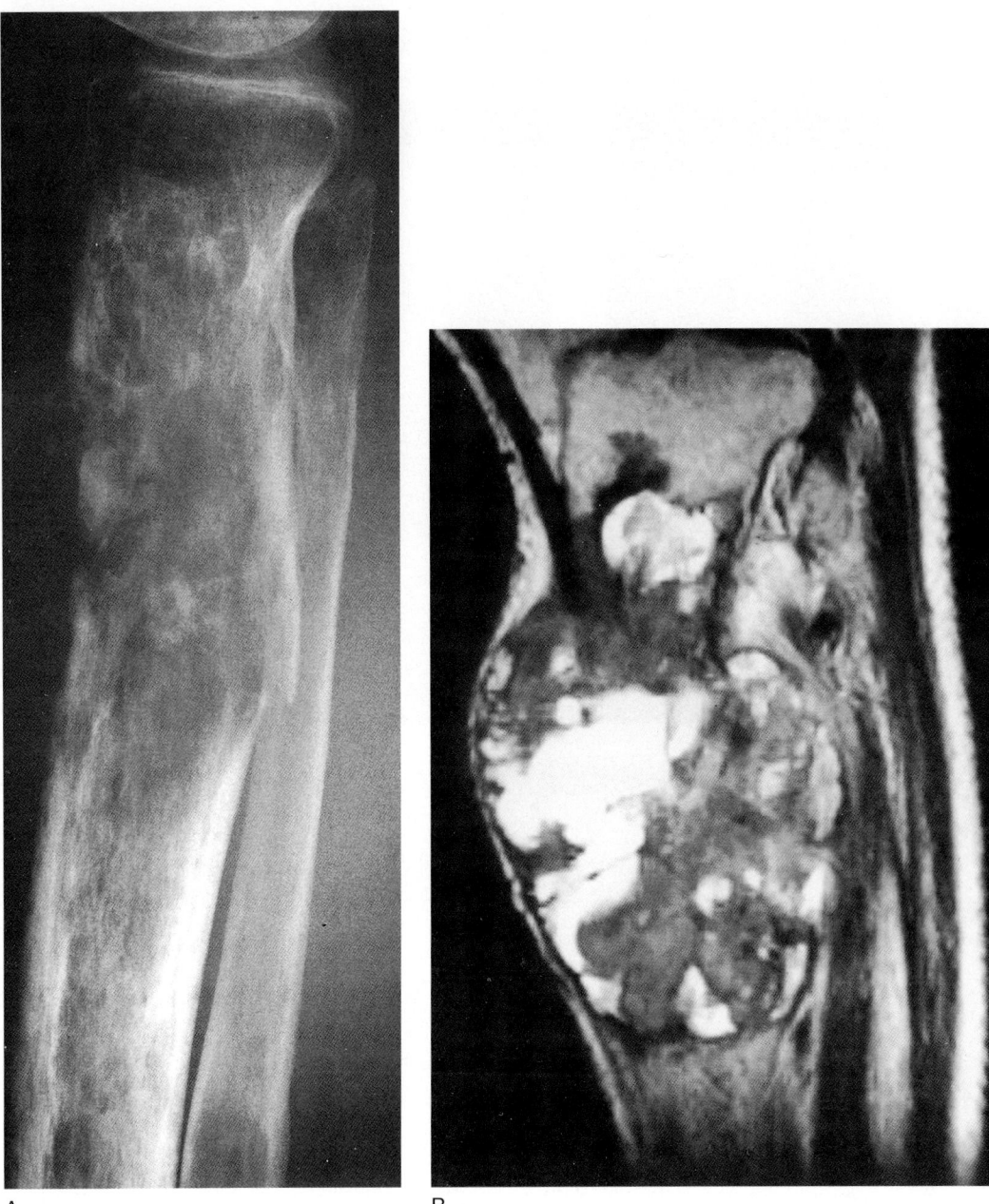

A B

Figure 29–11. Osteosarcoma involving the proximal femur of a 41-year-old man with Albright's syndrome. Plain film (*A*) and magnetic resonance imaging (*B*) show a permeative, destructive lesion with cortical breakthrough and soft tissue mass. Corresponding gross photo. (*Continued*)

matosis can appear malignant histologically. Hence, recognition of malignant change in this condition can be very difficult. Grossly, synovial chondromatosis has the appearance of firm hyaline cartilage. Marked myxoid quality of the chondroid nodules manifested as a mucoid appearance of the cartilage or even cystic change is a worrisome sign. As mentioned, synovial chondromatosis has a very characteristic clustering arrangement of chondrocytes. When chondrosarcoma supervenes, this clustering arrangement is lost,

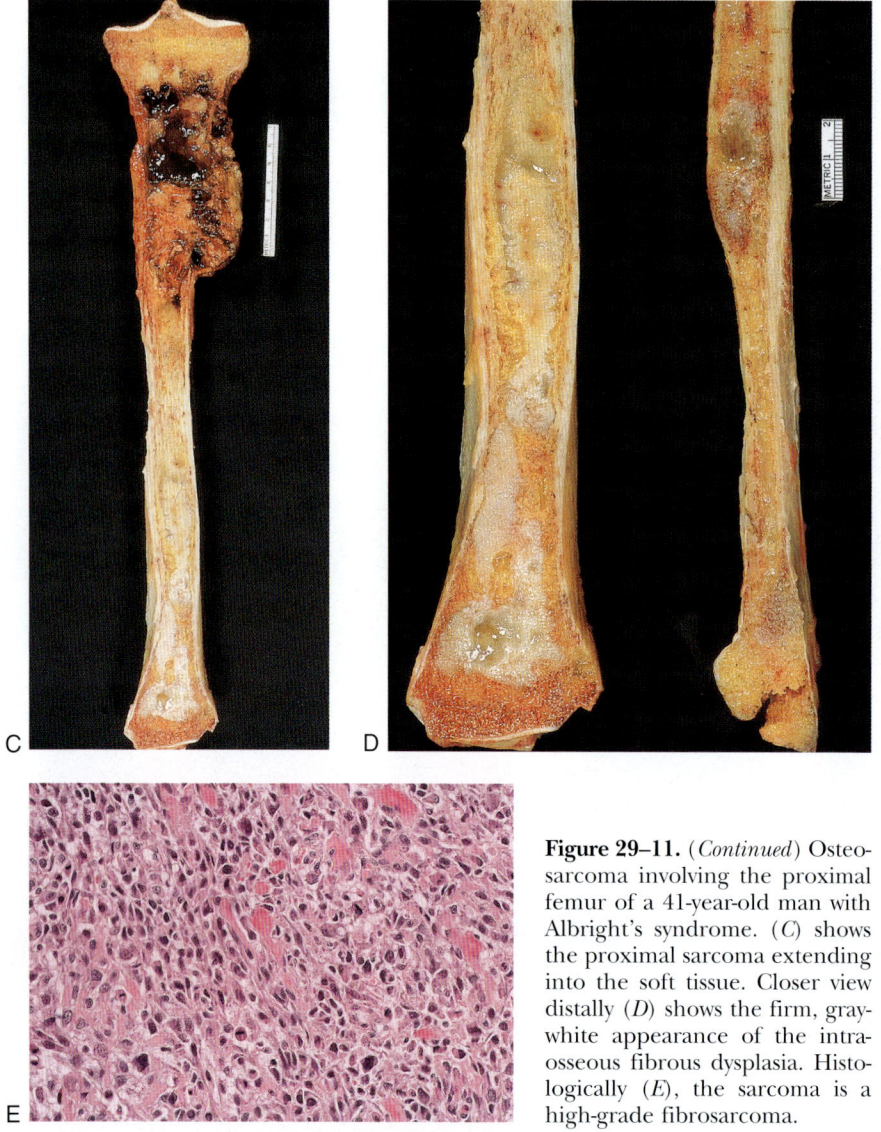

Figure 29–11. (*Continued*) Osteosarcoma involving the proximal femur of a 41-year-old man with Albright's syndrome. (*C*) shows the proximal sarcoma extending into the soft tissue. Closer view distally (*D*) shows the firm, graywhite appearance of the intraosseous fibrous dysplasia. Histologically (*E*), the sarcoma is a high-grade fibrosarcoma.

and the cartilage cells appear to be in sheets. Peripheral condensation of nuclei, especially with spindling, is also a sign of malignancy. The malignant behavior of the secondary chondrosarcomas is evident in the follow-up. In 5 of the 10 patients pulmonary metastasis developed, and 4 of these died.

PIGMENTED VILLONODULAR SYNOVITIS

Pigmented villonodular synovitis is a proliferative condition of synovial lining of un-

certain etiology, usually involving major joints. The disease is characterized by villous hyperplasia of synovium which in areas may form nodules. The hyperplastic villi are populated with proliferating mononuclear synovial cells and benign giant cells. Hemosiderin pigment is almost always found, and other changes such as collections of foam cells are common. Most examples of pigmented villonodular synovitis show diffuse involvement of the synovial lining, although a rare example of localized pigmented villonodular synovitis can be found. The disease is locally aggressive and may invade surrounding structures, especially bones. Recurrences are common unless a total synovectomy can be performed. In a review of the Mayo Clinic experience with pigmented villonodular synovitis (Schwartz et al., 1989), the knees were found to be involved most commonly, followed by the hip joints. Shoulders and elbows were involved only rarely. The disease may also be found in unusual sites, such as the spine.

There have been only rare examples of malignancy arising in pigmented villonodular synovitis (Fig. 29–12). Enzinger and Weiss (1995) defined malignant pigmented villonodular synovitis as a lesion in which it is possible to identify pigmented villonodular synovitis and malignancy or a malignant lesion occurring at the site of previously documented pigmented villonodular synovitis. Bertoni and co-authors (1997) reported on eight examples of malignant pigmented villonodular synovitis. The distinction between this disorder and malignancy of the synovium can be extremely difficult. The features found in the study from the Mayo Clinic were a nodular configuration of the tumor without prominent villi. The tumor cells are small, round, uniform, and crowded together. Cytologic features of malignancy are subtle. Benign giant cells and xanthomatous cells are less evident than in pigmented villonodular synovitis. Although small foci of necrosis may be seen in pigmented villonodular synovitis, large geographic areas of necrosis should arouse suspicion of malignancy. Four of our eight patients died with metastatic disease.

PREMALIGNANT TUMORS

There are a few "benign" neoplasms of bone that may undergo change to a malignant tumor. One may argue about classifying some of these neoplasms, especially giant cell tumor, as benign. Both giant cell tumors and chondroblastomas are known to metastasize in an occasional case. In giant cell tumor, the incidence is about 2%; in chondroblastoma, it is considerably less. It might be argued that a neoplasm that metastasizes to distant sites should not be considered benign. The histologic features of those few tumors that metastasize are no different from those of the vast majority that do not metastasize. The

metastatic deposits also do not have cytologic features of malignancy. Most importantly, only a small percent of patients with metastasis will die of the effects of the tumor. There have even been documented examples of spontaneous regression of metastases from these lesions.

GIANT CELL TUMOR

Giant cell tumors typically occur at the ends of long bones in skeletally mature persons. In the Mayo Clinic files, giant cell tumors constituted approximately 5% of all bone tumors. Seventeen patients had benign metastasis to the lungs.

Thirty-five tumors were considered to be "malignant giant cell tumors." In order to make a diagnosis of a malignant giant cell tumor, one must be able to demonstrate zones of typical benign giant cell tumor in the malignant neoplasm or in previous tissue obtained from the same site. There is much confusion in the literature about the term "malignant giant cell tumor." It has been employed indiscriminantly for all kinds of malignancies, including osteosarcomas and malignant fibrous histiocytomas with a large number of giant cells. For a diagnosis of a malignant giant cell tumor to be valid, the lesion obviously has to occur at the site where giant cell tumors occur—that is, in an epiphysis or an apophysis. A giant cell continuing tumor occurring in the metaphysis or a diaphysis is probably not a malignant giant cell tumor.

Using this criterion, malignant giant cell tumor may be divided into primary and secondary types. The secondary type is by far the more common. Thirty of the 35 tumors were considered to be secondary in the sense that they occurred after treatment of a typical benign giant cell tumor. Twenty-four of these 30 tumors occurred after treatment of a benign giant cell tumor which included radiation (Fig. 29–13). Hence, these 24 sarcomas would also be included in the group of postradiation sarcoma, and they are considered to be malignant giant cell tumors only because the lesion for which radiation therapy was given was a typical giant cell tumor. Six giant cell tumors underwent malignant change after only surgical treatment. The interval from the diagnosis of giant cell tumor to the diagnosis of sarcoma varied from 1 to

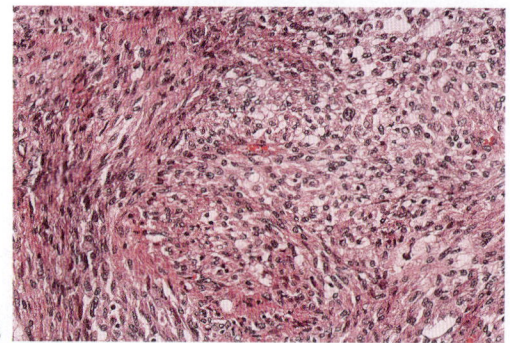

A

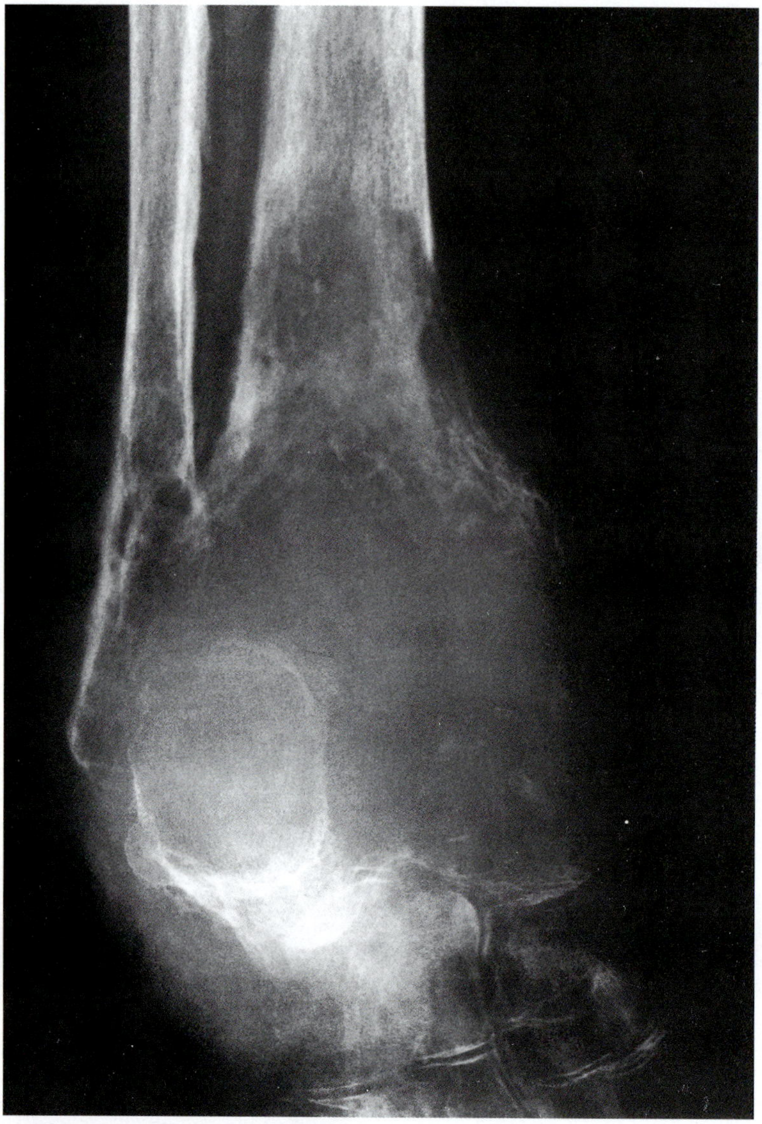

B

Figure 29–12. Malignancy in pigmented villonodular synovitis in an 85-year-old woman who had surgical removal of pigmented villonodular synovitis involving the right ankle 57 years earlier. Radiograph (*A*) shows an aggressive lytic and infiltrative lesion involving soft tissues around the ankle, with destruction of the distal tibia and fibula. Microscopically (*B*), the tumor contains compact sheets of malignant round to oval-shaped cells with areas of spindling.

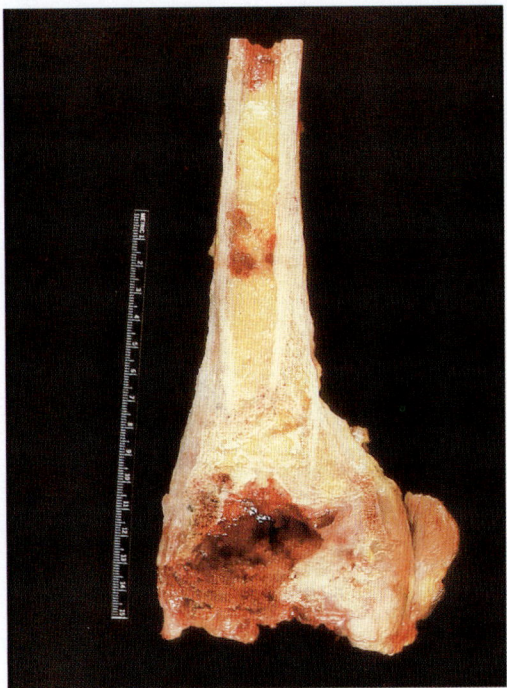

Figure 29–13. Malignancy in a giant cell tumor destroying the distal femur in a 44-year-old man who was treated with radiation to the area 10 years earlier.

42 years. The last five cases, which may be referred to as primary malignant giant cell tumor, presented with all the characteristics of a giant cell tumor, including typical X-ray appearance. On histologic examination, typical areas of giant cell tumor were juxtaposed with high-grade spindle cell sarcoma.

Patients with malignant giant cell tumor tend to be somewhat older than those with typical giant cell tumor. There is a slight female predilection, as with benign giant cell tumor. The location is very similar to that of a benign giant cell tumor, with the distal femur and proximal tibia being the most common sites. Histologically, the sarcomatous component is usually high grade, hence distinction from a spindling area in an otherwise typical giant cell tumor should not be difficult. Of the sarcomas, 21 were considered to be fibrosarcomas, 11 were osteosarcomas, and 3 were malignant fibrous histiocytomas. The treatment and prognosis of these sarcomas are similar to those in high-grade sarcomas arising *de novo*.

CHONDROBLASTOMA OF BONE

Chondroblastomas are considered to be benign neoplasms of cartilaginous origin. They also occur in the ends of long bones, in the epiphysis or apophysis. They tend to involve patients who have open epiphysial plates. Chondroblastoma accounts for less than 1% of all bone tumors in the Mayo Clinic files.

There are rare but well-documented examples of benign metastasizing chondroblastoma. The Mayo Clinic files contain two such cases. *Aggressive chondroblastoma* is a term used for a chondroblastoma that behaves aggressively locally but does not metastasize. No examples of malignant change in chondroblastoma appear in the Mayo Clinic files. In the large series of cases reported by Kurt and associates (1989), none was considered to be malignant. There are a few reported cases of postradiation sarcoma arising at the site of a previous chondroblastoma (Steiner, 1965). Sirsat and Doctor (1970) reported on an example of a chondroblastoma that underwent malignant change over a period of approximately 10 years. The initial surgical specimens clearly showed chondroblastoma. The lesion recurred several times and eventually became a high-grade spindle cell sarcoma.

CHONDROMYXOID FIBROMA

Chondromyxoid fibroma is one of the rarest of bone tumors. It accounts for less than 0.5% of all bone tumors in the Mayo Clinic files. It tends to involve the metaphyseal region of long bones in young patients. The lesion typically has a benign appearance on roentgenograms with a lytic defect surrounded by sclerosis. Histologically, it is unusual to see well-developed cartilage. The tumor is lobulated and consists of spindle to stellate cells, which may appear epithelioid in a myxoid background. Because the lesion is well demarcated, it is easily removed surgically. Recurrences are uncommon. However, recurrences may involve soft tissues and may create problems in management. Malignant transformation of chondromyxoid fibroma is extremely unusual. There has been only one such instance in the Mayo Clinic files. This patient had a chondromyxoid fibroma of the pubis, as confirmed by biopsy.

The patient died suddenly, before definitive treatment, and at autopsy a typical chondromyxoid fibroma of the pubis was found to be juxtaposed to a high-grade histiocytic-appearing sarcoma. The tumor had metastasized widely, the immediate cause of death having been metastasis to the heart. Zillmer and Dorfman (1989) described one case of chondromyxoid fibroma that underwent malignant change to a high-grade sarcoma after radiation therapy.

Osteoblastoma

Osteoblastoma is a rare, benign, bone-forming neoplasm. The tumor is composed of proliferating osteoblasts with uniform, trabecular-appearing bone formation. The osteoblasts tend to rim bony trabeculae, and the intertrabecular spaces show a loose arrangement. The roentgenographic appearance of an osteoblastoma can simulate that of a malignant neoplasm. Unfortunately, osteosarcomas share many histologic features with osteoblastoma. This problem has been referred to as *osteoblastoma-like osteosarcoma* (Bertoni et al., 1985).

There have been several case reports of osteosarcoma arising in osteoblastoma, but it is very difficult to evaluate the authenticity of these reports because of the difficulty of separating osteoblastoma from osteosarcoma initially. Most of these lesions were probably osteosarcomas to start with. Two instances of sarcoma arising in osteoblastoma appear in the Mayo Clinic files. One was a postradiation sarcoma involving cervical vertebrae in a patient who had removal of an osteoblastoma 10 years previously followed by radiation therapy. In the second instance, an osteosarcoma developed at the site of a well-documented osteoblastoma in the proximal tibia in a 16-year-old boy. The tumor recurred twice within 40 months, and at the time of the second occurrence it was considered to be an osteosarcoma. Review of the original slide still suggests that the original diagnosis of osteoblastoma was correct. The patient experienced pulmonary metastasis after an above-knee amputation. The metastases were resected surgically, and the patient is alive and free of disease 23 years later. In the large series reported by Lucas and coauthors (1994), one additional case of malignant transformation without radiation therapy was documented.

REFERENCES

Akbarnia BA, Wirth CR, Colman N. (1976) Fibrosarcoma arising from chronic osteomyelitis. Case report and review of literature. *J Bone Joint Surg Am* 58:123–125.

Arlen M, Higinbotham NL, Huvos AG, Marcove RC, Miller T, Shah IC. (1971) Radiation-induced sarcoma of bone. *Cancer* 28:1087–1099.

Benedict WF, Fung YK, Murphree AL. (1988) The gene responsible for the development of retinoblastoma and osteosarcoma. *Cancer* 62 (Suppl):1691–1694.

Berg HL, Weiland AJ. (1978) Multiple osteogenic sarcoma following bilateral retinoblastoma. A case report. *J Bone Joint Surg Am* 60:251–253.

Berry MP, Jenkin RD, Fornasier VL, Rideout DF. (1980) Osteosarcoma at the site of previous fracture. A case report. *J Bone Joint Surg Am* 62:1216–1218.

Bertoni F, Unni KK, Beabout JW, Sim FH. (1991) Chondrosarcomas of the synovium. *Cancer* 67:155–162.

Bertoni F, Unni KK, Beabout JW, Sim FH. (1997) Malignant giant cell tumor of the tendon sheaths and joints (malignant pigmented villonodular synovitis). *Am J Surg Pathol* 21:153–163.

Bertoni F, Unni KK, McLeod RA, Dahlin DC. (1985) Osteosarcoma resembling osteoblastoma. *Cancer* 55: 416–426.

Bostman OM, Holmstrom T, Riska EB. (1987) Osteosarcoma arising in a melorheostotic femur. A case report. *J Bone Joint Surg Am* 69:1232–1237.

Brien WW, Salvati EA, Healey JH, Bansal M, Ghelman B, Betts F. (1990) Osteogenic sarcoma arising in the area of a total hip replacement. A case report. *J Bone Joint Surg Am* 72:1097–1099.

Cabanela ME, Sim FH, Beabout JW, Dahlin DC. (1974) Osteomyelitis appearing as neoplasms. A diagnostic problem. *Arch Surg* 109:68–72.

Cahan WG, Woodard HQ, Higinbotham NL, Stewart FW, Coley BL. (1948) Sarcoma arising in irradiated bone. Report of eleven cases. *Cancer* 1:3–29.

Cumin I, Cohen JY, David A, Mechinaud F, Avet-Loiseau H, Harousseau JL. (1996) Rothmund-Thomson syndrome and osteosarcoma. *Med Pediatr Oncol* 26: 414–416.

Enzinger FM, Weiss SW. (1995) *Soft Tissue Tumors.* third ed., pp. 749–751. Mosby, St. Louis.

Fitzgerald RH Jr, Brewer NS, Dahlin DC. (1976) Squamous-cell carcinoma complicating chronic osteomyelitis. *J Bone Joint Surg Am* 58:1146–1148.

Furey JG, Ferrer-Torells M, Reagan JW. (1960) Fibrosarcoma arising at the site of bone infarcts. A report of two cases. *J Bone Joint Surg Am* 42:802–810.

German J. (1995) Bloom's syndrome. *Dermatol Clin* 13: 7–18.

Haibach H, Farrell C, Dittrich FJ. (1985) Neoplasms arising in Paget's disease of bone: a study of 82 cases. *Am J Clin Pathol* 83:594–600.

Hamilton A, Davis RI, Hayes D, Mollan RA. (1987) Chondrosarcoma developing in synovial chondromatosis. A case report. *J Bone Joint Surg Br* 69:137–140.

Hughes AW, Sherlock DA, Hamblen DL, Reid R. (1987)

Sarcoma at the site of a single hip screw. A case report. *J Bone Joint Surg Br* 69:470–472.

Huvos AG, Butler A, Bretsky SS. (1983) Osteogenic sarcoma associated with Paget's disease of bone. A clinicopathologic study of 65 patients. *Cancer* 52:1489–1495.

Huvos AG, Higinbotham NL, Miller TR. (1972) Bone sarcomas arising in fibrous dysplasia. *J Bone Joint Surg Am* 54:1047–1056.

Klenerman L, Ockenden BG, Townsend AC. (1967) Osteosarcoma occurring in osteogenesis imperfecta. Report of two cases. *J Bone Joint Surg Br* 49:314–323.

Kurt AM, Unni KK, Sim FH, McLeod RA. (1989) Chondroblastoma of bone. *Hum Pathol* 20:965–976.

Laskin WB, Silverman TA, Enzinger FM. (1988) Postradiation soft tissue sarcomas. An analysis of 53 cases. *Cancer* 62:2330–2340.

Lee YS, Pho RW, Nather A. (1984) Malignant fibrous histiocytoma at site of metal implant. *Cancer* 54:2286–2289.

Liu J, Hudkins PG, Swee RG, Unni KK. (1987) Bone sarcomas associated with Ollier's disease. *Cancer* 59:1376–1385.

Lucas DR, Unni KK, McLeod RA, O'Connor MI, Sim FH. (1994) Osteoblastoma: clinicopathologic study of 306 cases. *Hum Pathol* 25:117–134.

McGrory JE, Pritchard DJ, Unni KK, Ilstrup D, Rowland CM. (1999) Malignant lesions arising in chronic osteomyelitis. *Clin Orthop* 362:181–189.

Mindell ER, Northup CS, Douglass HO Jr. (1978) Osteosarcoma associated with osteopoikilosis. *J Bone Joint Surg Am* 60:406–408.

Mirra JM, Bullough PG, Marcove RC, Jacobs B, Huvos AG. (1974) Malignant fibrous histiocytoma and osteosarcoma in association with bone infarcts; report of four cases, two in caisson workers. *J Bone Joint Surg Am* 56:932–940.

Paget J. (1889) Remarks on osteitis deformans. *Illust Med News (Lond)* 2:181–182.

Perry BE, McQueen DA, Lin JJ. (1988) Synovial chondromatosis with malignant degeneration to chondrosarcoma. Report of a case. *J Bone Joint Surg Am* 70:1259–1261.

Ruggieri P, Sim FH, Bond JR, Unni KK. (1994) Malignancies in fibrous dysplasia. *Cancer* 73:1411–1424.

Rutkowski R, Resnick P, McMaster JH. (1979) Osteosarcoma occurring in osteogenesis imperfecta. A case report. *J Bone Joint Surg Am* 61:606–608.

Schimke RN, Lowman JT, Cowan AB. (1974) Retinoblastoma and osteogenic sarcoma in siblings. *Cancer* 34:2077–2079.

Schwartz HS, Unni KK, Pritchard DJ. (1989) Pigmented villonodular synovitis. A retrospective review of affected large joints. *Clin Orthop* 247:243–255.

Sirsat MV, Doctor VM. (1970) Benign chondroblastoma of bone. Report of a case of malignant transformation. *J Bone Joint Surg Br* 52:741–745.

Steiner GC. (1965) Postradiation sarcoma of bone. *Cancer* 18:603–612.

Sun TC, Swee RG, Shives TC, Unni KK. (1985) Chondrosarcoma in Maffucci's syndrome. *J Bone Joint Surg Am* 67:1214–1219.

Tucker MA, D'Angio GJ, Boice JD Jr, Strong LC, Li FP, Stovall M, Stone BJ, Green DM, Lombardi F, Newton W, Hoover RN, Fraumeni JF Jr. (1987) Bone sarcomas linked to radiotherapy and chemotherapy in children. *N Engl J Med* 317:588–593.

Weatherby RP, Dahlin DC, Ivins JC. (1981) Postradiation sarcoma of bone: review of 78 Mayo Clinic cases. *Mayo Clin Proc* 56:294–306.

Zillmer DA, Dorfman HD. (1989) Chondromyxoid fibroma of bone: thirty-six cases with clinicopathologic correlation. *Hum Pathol* 20:952–964.

30

THE CENTRAL NERVOUS SYSTEM

Elisabeth J. Rushing and Dennis K. Burns

The topic of central nervous system (CNS) neoplasia embraces a clinically and morphologically diverse group of neoplasms that affect patients of all ages. Recent advances in radiographic imaging techniques, including computed tomography (CT), magnetic resonance imaging (MRI), and positron emission tomography (PET) scanning, have revolutionized the approach to the diagnosis and management of intracranial and intraspinal tumors. Such imaging techniques have enabled the accurate identification and localization of lesions at much earlier stages than was possible one or two decades ago. Advances in imaging procedures have been paralleled by refinements in neurosurgical techniques, so that such lesions are not only identified at earlier stages but are also subject to earlier surgical intervention (Dohrmann and Rubin, 1985; Moore et al., 1989). Certain types of CNS tumors e.g., anaplastic oligodendrogliomas, may respond quite favorably to specific therapeutic regimens (Cairncross et al., 1994, 1998), an indication that the treatment of CNS tumors has become increasingly sophisticated in recent years. Such continuing refinements in the diagnosis and treatment of neoplasms of the CNS have, in turn, placed increasing demands on anatomic pathologists for accurate classification and histological grading of these lesions.

The clinical manifestations of CNS neoplasms are influenced by a number of different factors, including the size of the neoplasm, its rate of growth, and its location. In the case of tumors situated in certain strategic locations, such as the motor cortex, clinical manifestations may bring the neoplasm to attention at a comparatively early stage. At the other extreme, slowly growing neoplasms arising in clinically "silent" areas, such as cortical association areas, may reach considerable size before being recognized clinically.

The etiology and pathogenesis of most CNS neoplams remain elusive. In some instances, CNS neoplasms may develop in the context of a hereditary disorder associated with dysplastic or malformative lesions, such as neurofibromatosis and tuberous sclerosis. Specific chromosomal and genetic aberrations have now been identified in a number of these conditions, the presence of which may ultimately provide important insights into the pathogenesis of associated CNS tumors. Table 30–1 summarizes the genetic and chromosomal abnormalities, and corresponding nervous system neoplasm(s), associated with major inherited cancer syndromes. Certain environmental factors, notably radiation, have also been implicated in the development of a variety of CNS tumors (Anderson and Treip, 1986; Liwnicz et al., 1985; Zucarello et al, 1986). Finally, conditions such as trauma, multiple sclerosis, and progressive multifocal leukoencephalopathy have been investigated as possible precursors to CNS neoplasms with intriguing but inconclusive results (Anderson et al., 1980;

Table 30–1. Genetic Profiles and Central Nervous System Manifestations of Major Inherited Syndromes

Syndrome	Gene	Chromosome	Nervous System Neoplasms
Neurofibromatosis 1	NF1	17q11	Neurofibroma; optic glioma; astrocytoma; malignant peripheral nerve sheath tumor
Neurofibromatosis 2	NF2	22q12	Bilateral acoustic schwannomas, meningioma, spinal ependymoma, astrocytoma, meningoangiomatosis
von Hippel–Lindau	VHL	3p25	Hemangioblastoma
Tuberous sclerosis	TSC1	9p24	Subependymal giant cell astrocytoma
	TSC2	16p13	
Li-Fraumeni	TP53	17p13	Astrocytoma, primitive neuroectodermal tumor
Turcot	APC	5q21	Medulloblastoma
	HMLH1	3p21	
	HPSM2	7p22	Glioblastoma
Cowden	PTEN (MMAC1)	10q23	Dysplastic gangliocytoma of the cerebellum
Gorlin	PTCH	9q31	Medulloblastoma

Modified from Kleihues and Cavanee (1993) *Pathology and Genetics: Tumors of the Nervous System*, with permission from Springer-Verlag.

Perez-Diaz et al., 1985; Sima et al., 1983). Such conditions are associated with only a small percentage of primary CNS tumors.

Recent observations have shed light on our understanding of some of the molecular events associated with the induction and progression of CNS tumors. It is now apparent that the sequential evolution of histological changes from normal to overtly malignant morphology likely occurs as a result of specific genetic alterations that activate oncogenes and/or inactivate tumor suppressor genes (Arnoldus et al., 1992; Eppenberger and Mueller, 1994; von Deimling et al., 1995; Westermark and Nister, 1995). In any given tumor type, a characteristic combination of activated oncogenes and inactivated tumor suppressor genes appears to influence histological and biological progression of the neoplasm. The specific genetic alterations involved vary considerably, as might be expected from the morphological and biological heterogeneity of these neoplasms. In general, oncogenes directly encode for autocrine and paracrine growth factors and their receptors, which modulate the proliferative activity of target cells. It appears that aberrant expression or overexpression of proteins encoded by certain oncogenes disturbs normal signal transduction pathways, leading to abnromal cell growth and differentiation. The protein products of tumor suppressor genes, in contrast, inhibit cell growth and regulate programmed cell death, or apoptosis. It now

appears that a disruption of the homeostasis established by normal interactions between oncogenes and tumor suppressor genes culminates in the development of neoplasia. Identification of specific genetic and phenotypic subsets among CNS tumors may be important predictors of clinical behavior. In the case of glioblastoma multiforme, for example, at least two distinct molecular pathways have been identified that correspond to unique clinical subsets of this tumor. Primary, or *de novo* glioblastomas typically occur in older patients, are highly aggressive, and are associated with epidermal growth factor receptor (EGFR) amplification. In contrast, so-called secondary glioblastomas evolving from preexisting lower-grade tumors have a more protracted clinical course and frequently contain p53 mutations, but are not associated with EGFR amplification (Ng and Lam, 1998).

With the exception of the malformative and/or dysplastic lesions associated with neurofibromatosis and tuberous sclerosis, the microscopic hemangioblastomas encountered in the von Hippel–Lindau syndrome, and the polymporphous B cell proliferations associated with some cases of lymphoma, the morphological "precursors" of most CNS neoplasms remain undefined. A retrospective study by Cavanaugh (1958) suggested that small glial malformations in some patients with long-standing epilepsy might serve as precursors to more conventional gliomas. Alternatively, the possibility that many neoplasms of the CNS might develop in the absence of a preneoplastic precursor lesion was suggested in a study of early neoplasms of the central and peripheral nervous systems; these neoplasms were identified in a retrospective review of over 2000 neuropathological accessions (Iglesias-Rozas and Collia-Fernandez, 1980). In this study, minute neoplastic proliferations measuring less than 2 mm in diameter were identified in 16 cases. In all of these minute, and presumably early lesions, the microscopic features were identical to those of larger lesions, which suggests that in these cases, neoplasms of the nervous system developed in the absence of a specific precursor lesion. Accordingly, in contrast to the situation in other organ systems in which dysplastic or preneoplastic precursor lesions are reasonably well defined, a discussion of incipient neoplasia in the CNS requires some discussion of the morphology of established neoplasms in this site. Neoplasms that are not unique to the CNS, such as lymphomas, germ cell tumors, and certain soft tissue tumors, are discussed in chapters dedicated to those entities.

MENINGIOMAS

Meningiomas account for approximately 15% of primary intracranial neoplasms and 25% of primary intraspinal neoplasms (Kepes, 1982; Sloof et al., 1964). Clinically symptomatic meningiomas occur predominantly in adults, with a peak incidence in the fifth and sixth decades. Children may also be affected and have a higher frequency of intraventricular and aggressive papillary tumors (Hope et al., 1992). A consistent female predominance has been observed in menigiomas occurring in adults, particularly in the case of intraspinal lesions; this likely reflects the expression of progesterone receptors by these neoplasms and a positive trophic influence by this hormone (Cahill et al., 1984; Ironside et al., 1986; Tilzer et al, 1982).

Meningiomas are derived from the arachnoid cap cells that populate the leptomeninges and, in some cases, from the stroma of the choroid plexus. Factors responsible for the neoplastic transformation of these cells remain incompletely defined,

but almost certainly include advancing age and, as noted above, hormonal influences. Radiation exposure has been associated with an increase in the frequency of meningiomas in a number of retrospective studies (Modun et al., 1974; Ron et al., 1988; Sznajder et al., 1996). Multifocality and atypical histological features have been noted more frequently in cases of meningiomas arising in the context of prior radiation exposure (Harrison et al., 1991; Mack and Wilson, 1993). The roles played by trauma and viral infection in the development of these tumors, if any, remain controversial (Choi et al., 1970; Rachlin and Rosenblum, 1991). Patients with the central form of neurofibromatosis (NF2) are at increased risk for the development of both solitary and multifocal meningiomas (Louis et al., 1995; Rachlin and Rosenblum, 1991; Riccardi, 1987). Deletions or mutations in the NF2 gene located on chromosome 22 occur in most meningiomas exhibiting a transitional or fibroblastic histology (discussed below). NF2 abnormalities are far less common in meningiomas with a syncitial (menigotheliomatous) histology, however, which suggests that other genetic factors play a role in the development of this variant (Wellenreuther et al., 1995, 1997). Allelic losses on chromosomal arms 10q, 14q, and, on occasion, 1p have been associated with the process of malignant transformation in meningiomas (Peters et al., 1998; Simon et al., 1995). In particular, allelic losses on chromosome 10 are found in anaplastic (malignant) meningiomas but have never been encountered in benign tumors (Peters et al., 1998).

Grossly, the typical meningioma presents as a lobulated, discrete mass with a firm dural attachment, although an occasional lesion may proliferate in a more flattened, plaque-like fashion (meningioma *en plaque*). Favored sites of origin include the parasagittal cerebral convexities, falx cerebri, sphenoid wings, olfactory grooves, and cerebellopontine angle, where differentiation from eighth nerve schwannoma becomes an important diagnostic consideration. Less common intracranial sites include the foramen magnum, the ventricular cavities, and, exceptionally, the intraparenchymal compartment. Within the spinal canal, meningiomas occur most frequently in the thoracic intradural compartment. In contrast to schwannomas in this site, which tend to arise dorsally, most spinal meningiomas arise ventrally or laterally near nerve root exit zones, where meningothelial cells are most highly concentrated. Meningiomas may invade contiguous structures, including bone and dural sinuses, but typically remain well demarcated from the underlying CNS parenchyma in the absence of malignant change (Fig. 30–1).

A variety of histological patterns are encountered in meningiomas, some of which recapitulate the structure of the meningothelial nests commonly encountered in the leptomeninges of adults (Fig. 30–2). In many instances, these different patterns have no biological significance, although knowledge of their existence is important to the pathologist in recognizing the meningothelial nature of these microscopically diverse lesions. Common histological subtypes include the *syncitial* (menigotheliomatous)

(Fig. 30–3), *fibroblastic* (Fig. 30–4), and the so-called *transitional* (Fig. 30–5) variants, the last comprising a mixture of syncitial and fibroblastic elements. Concentric whorls, often accompanied by laminated, calcified psammoma bodies, are common. A variety of regressive and metaplastic changes may also occur, adding to the histological diversity of meningiomas. The accumulation of fluid in the extracellular space can impart a delicate, fibrillar architecture to some tumors, which are designated *microcystic* meningiomas. Ultrastructural studies have confirmed the meningothelial character of such microcystic lesions, which may be confused with other lesions, including hemangioblastomas and even gliomas (Kleinman et al., 1980). *Chordoid* meningiomas represent another uncommon histological variant of meningioma, which may be confused with the more aggressive chordoma (Kepes et al., 1988).

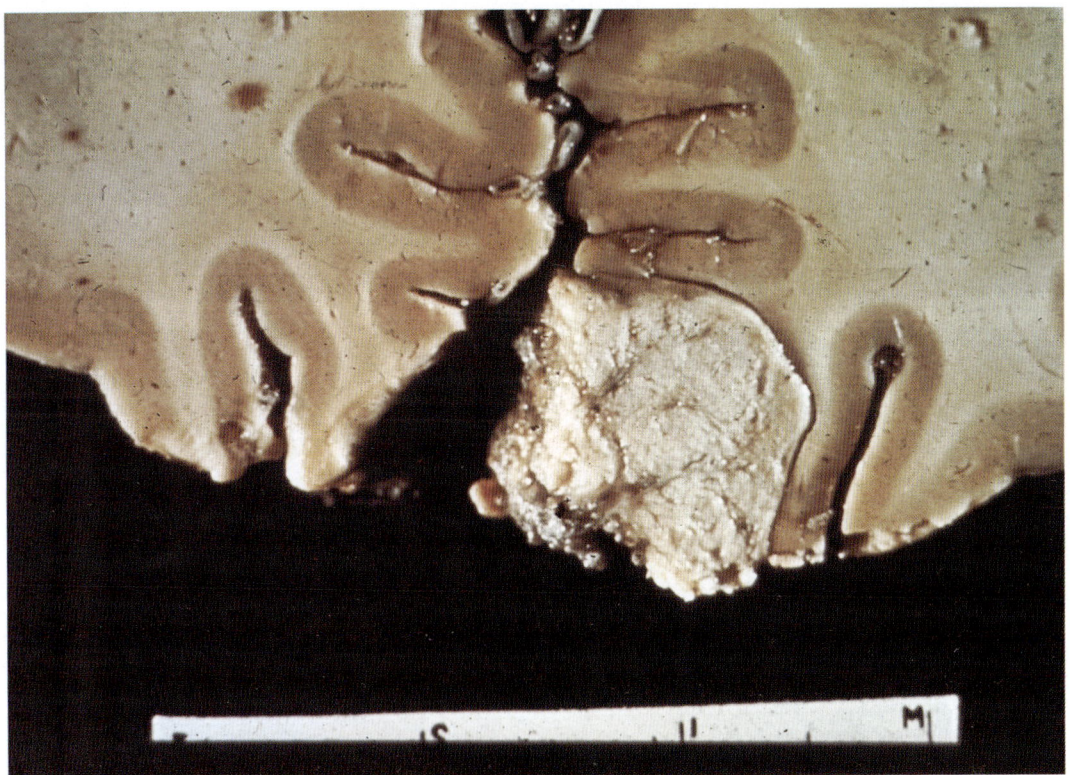

Fig. 30–1. Gross photograph of a meningioma arising in the olfactory region, demonstrating a well-defined interface between the tumor and adjacent brain parenchyma. By virtue of the slow growth, such lesions may reach a considerable size before coming to clinical attention. Gross invasion of brain parenchyma is unusual in meningiomas and, if present, usually indicates a biologically aggressive lesion.

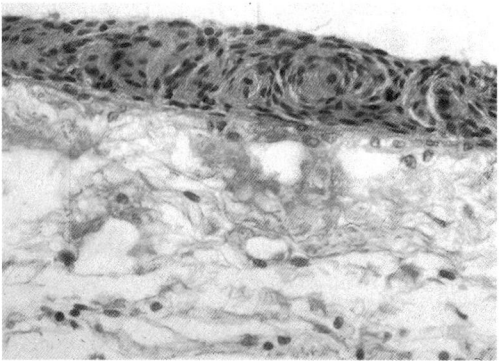

Fig. 30–2. Photomicrograph of arachnoid cell nest, a common incidental finding in the leptomeninges of adults. Such nests are the likely site of origin of meningiomas.

In other instances, histological patterns may have prognostic significance. The glycogen-rich *clear cell* meningioma, for example, is an additional distinct subtype noted both for its resemblance to metastatic renal cell carcinoma and for its aggressive biological behavior. In the first reported series of this particular variant of meningioma, over 61% of cases recurred, and 23% of patients died of their disease, despite gross total excision of the tumor (Zorludemir et al., 1995). *Pap-*

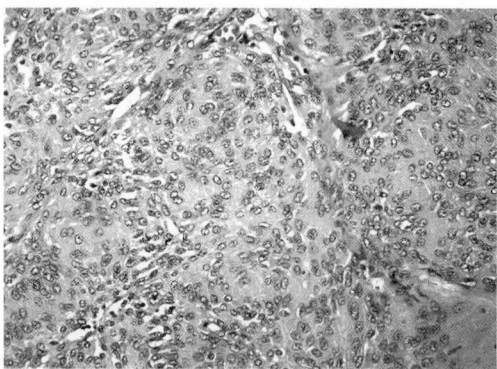

Fig. 30–3. Photomicrograph of a syncitial variant of meningioma, demonstrating bland nuclei and perikarya with indistinct cell borders. At an ultrastructural level, such foci contain complex, interdigitating cell processes that are difficult to resolve in routine histological sections, resulting in a "syncitial" appearance. Such meningiomas are less likely to be associated with abnormalities in the NF2 gene than other histological variants.

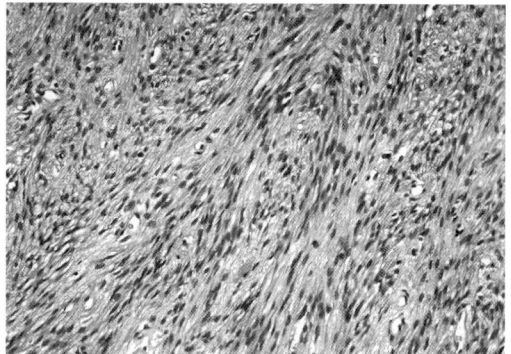

Fig. 30–4. Light microscopic appearance of a fibroblastic meningioma, characterized by elongated, fibroblast-like cells arrayed in interlacing fascicles. An abundant collagenous stroma is often present in these tumors, which are less likely to express epithelial membrane antigen than other types of meningioma. Fibroblastic lesions of this type may be difficult to distinguish from schwannomas in certain locations, such as the cerebellopontine angle.

illary meningiomas, discussed below, are also notable for their higher frequency of recurrence and locally aggressive growth.

The prognosis of meningioma is influenced by several factors, including size, location, and adequacy of excision of the primary tumor. Surgical accessibility, in particular, appears to be of major prognostic significance (Jaaskelainen, 1986). In addition, certain histological features have been asso-

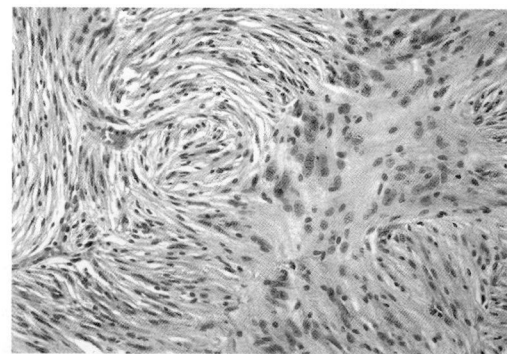

Fig. 30–5. Photomicrograph of a so-called transitional variant of meningioma, containing a mixture of fibroblastic and syncitial patterns. Whorl formation, sometimes accompanied by calcified psammoma bodies, is usually conspicuous in such lesions.

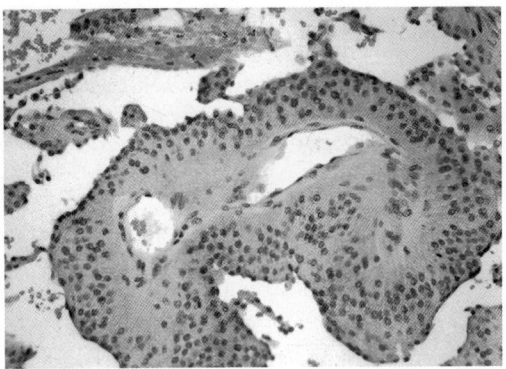

Fig. 30–6. Histological appearance of incipient papillary change in a meningioma, characterized by radial orientation of neoplastic cells around a central vascular core, and loss of cohesion between adjacent cells. Papillary change may be encountered in any histological variant of meningioma and is frequently associated with other "aytpical" histological features. A significant number of papillary meningiomas behave in an aggressive fashion.

ciated with more aggressive behavior (de la Monte et al., 1986; Kepes, 1982). These include hypercellularity, the presence of "active" nuclei with prominent nucleoli, mitotic activity, microscopic areas of necrosis, the development of a sheet-like growth pattern with loss of whorl formation, and irregular invasion of the underlying brain parenchyma. Papillary change (Fig. 30–6) may occur in any histological variant of meningioma and may be the predominant architectural pattern encountered. Such papillary tumors are often, but not invariably, associated with other histological features suggesting aggressive behavior, and are associated with more aggressive local growth, distant metastases, and

death than meningiomas lacking papillary change. A significant number of the reported papillary meningiomas have occurred in children and young adults (Ludwin et al., 1975; Pasquier et al., 1986).

More recently, proliferation indices have been studied in meningiomas. As might be expected, there is a general increase in the expression of proliferation markers (e.g., Ki-67) with the emergence of more aggressive histological features, although there is considerable overlap within individual grades (Prayson, 1996).

FIBRILLARY ASTROCYTIC NEOPLASMS

Inflitrating fibrillary astrocytomas account for roughly 90% of astrocytic tumors. Fibrillary astrocytomas, also termed "diffuse" astrocytomas, are characterized by an infiltrative growth pattern and a prognosis that is influenced by age, location, and the histological grade of the tumor (Burger et al., 1985; Cohadon et al., 1985; Kernohan et al., 1949; Schiffer et al., 1988). Although no universally accepted grading scheme exists for these neoplasms, some form of the three-tiered system adapted by the World Health Organization (WHO) is most often employed (Kleihues et al., 1993). The salient features of this system are summarized in Table 30–2. In this scheme, the most differentiated forms of these lesions are designated simply as *astrocytoma* and the least differentiated examples as *glioblastoma multiforme*. The term *anaplastic astrocytoma* is used for intermediate-grade lesions exhibiting nuclear atypia and mitoses, but lacking the

Table 30–2. Histological Grading of Infiltrating Astrocytic Neoplasms

Tumor Type	Pleomorphism/ Nuclear Atypia	Mitotic Activity	Vascular Proliferation	Necrosis
Well differentiated astrocytoma	Usually present (often subtle)	Absent	Absent	Absent
Anaplastic astrocytoma	Present	Present (may require careful search)	Absent	Absent
Glioblastoma multiforme	Preesnt	Present	Usually present (vascular proliferation *and/or* necrosis must be present for diagnosis)	Usually present (vascular proliferation *and/or* necrosis must be present for diagnosis)

necrosis and vascular proliferation of glioblastoma multiforme.

Well-differentiated astrocytomas (WHO grade II) may occur at any age, with a peak incidence during the fourth decade. Most cases arise in the cerebral hemispheres, although any site, including the brainstem and spinal cord, may be affected. Radiographically, well-differentiated astrocytomas appear as an ill-defined area of decreased intensity in CT and T1-weighted MRI scans, which fails to enhance following the administration of contrast material. Grossly, astrocytomas are poorly demarcated, expansile lesions that tend to obliterate normal gray-white landmarks (Fig. 30–7). Their consistency may be either firmer or softer than that of the surrounding brain. Microscopically, well-differentiated astrocytomas are characterized by a mild, irregular increase in cellularity, accompanied by some degree of nuclear atypia (Fig. 30–8). In nonfrozen material, the neoplastic astrocytic nuclei tend to be somewhat angulated, in contrast to the more rounded nuclei seen in oligodendroglial tumors (discussed below). Microcystic change is uncommon and, when present, may help to distinguish low-grade neoplasms from reactive gliosis. Mitotic activity and endothelial proliferation are absent. As the neoplasm infiltrates normal gray matter, individual neoplastic cells may surround native neurons, a phenomenon known as satellitosis. Such satellitosis is generally far less conspicuous than that encountered in oligodendrogliomas, however.

Anaplastic astrocytomas (WHO grade III) are infiltrative neoplasms that exhibit a degree of malignancy between that of well-differentiated astrocytoma and glioblastoma multiforme. Overt anaplasia may be present at the time of initial diagnosis or may arise in the context of a previously well-differentiated tumor. Anaplastic change in an infiltrating astrocytoma is suggested by the presence of edema and contrast enhancement in radiographic imaging studies, although the absence of such changes does not preclude anaplasia. Microscopically, the distinction between well-differentiated and anaplastic astrocytomas is based upon the presence of mitotic activity in the latter lesions (Fig. 30–9). The presence of gemistocytic astrocytes, so named because of the abundant eosinophilic cytoplasm, may also be an indicator of anaplasia and poor prognosis, particulary when such cells represent the predominant cell type (Krouwer et al., 1991). A spectrum of differentiation is often apparent in anaplastic lesions, which, with

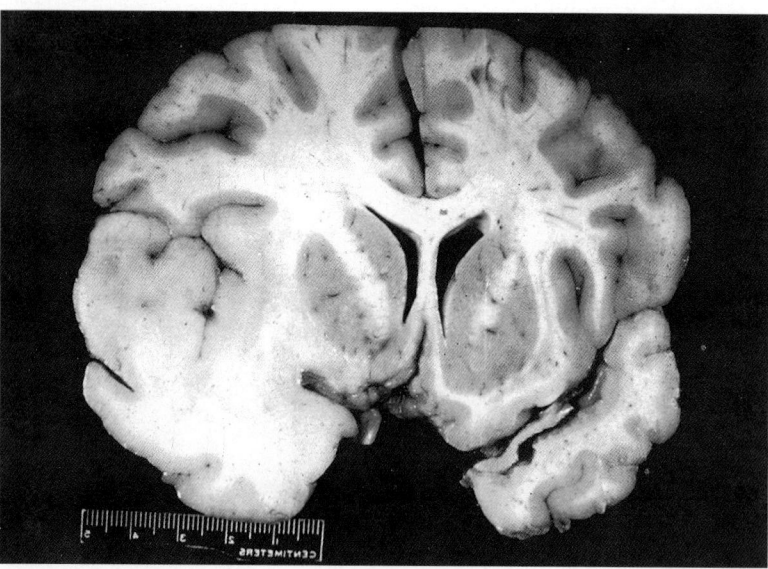

Fig. 30–7. Gross photograph of a well-differentiated fibrillary astrocytoma arising in the right temporal lobe. The neoplasm expands the involved lobe and blurs gray-white landmarks in many areas, a reflection of infiltrative growth. Hemorrhage, necrosis, and radiographic contrast enhancement are absent in such well-differentiated lesions.

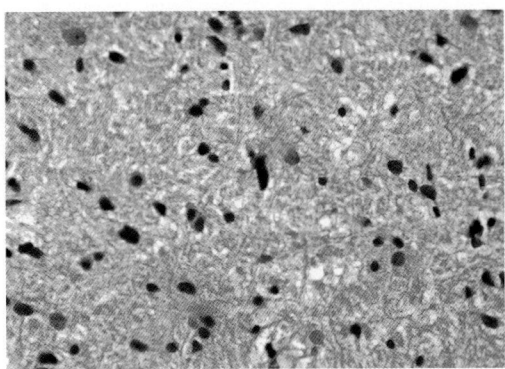

Fig. 30–8. Photomicrograph of a well-differentiated infiltrating astrocytoma. Cellularity is increased, and a mild degree of nuclear hyperchromasia and pleomorphism is present. Well-differentiated astrocytomas may be extremely difficult to distinguish from reactive gliosis in some cases. Whether reactive gliosis serves as a precursor to infiltrating astrocytic neoplasms remains uncertain, however.

increasing degrees of anaplasia, merge with glioblastoma multiforme.

Glioblastoma multiforme (WHO grade IV) is the most common infiltrating glial neoplasm in adults. Although the term "glioblastoma multiforme" has been applied in the past to a variety of gliomas exhibiting malignant

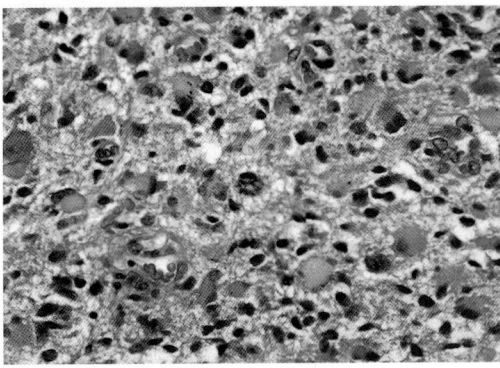

Fig. 30–9. Anaplastic astrocytoma. These lesions are distinguished from their better-differentiated counterparts by increased cellularity, nuclear pleomorphism and, most significantly, mitotic activity. Many of the cells in this lesion possess abundant, eosinophilic ("gemistocytic") cytoplasm, a feature usually associated with biologically aggressive lesions. Anaplastic change may be encountered as a focal phenomenon in otherwise well-differentiated lesions, indicating that well-differentiated astrocytomas serve as a precursor to at least some higher-grade lesions.

cytological features, necrosis, and vascular proliferation, the term is now restricted to lesions of predominantly, or exclusively, astrocytic lineage. As with the better-differentiated infiltrating astrocytic tumors, glioblastoma multiforme may arise anywhere along the central neuraxis but is most commonly encountered in the cerebral hemispheres. An exception to this are the glioblastomas arising in childhood which, for reasons that remain unclear, have a predilection for the brainstem (Albright et al., 1983; Berger et al., 1983). As noted in the introduction to this chapter, glioblastoma multiforme may arise *de novo* or may develop in a patient with a previously documented lower-grade neoplasm. Imaging studies demonstrate the presence of contrast enhancement, often in a ring-like configuration, associated with substantial edema and mass effect (Fig. 30–10). Grossly, the appearance is typically described as variegated, with irregular areas of necrosis, cystic change, and hemorrhage (Fig. 30–11). Some glioblastomas appear deceptively circumscribed, although infiltrative growth is invariably present microscopically. Histologically, a remarkable variety of cell types and architectural patterns may be encountered, including small, anaplastic cells, bizarre, multinucleated giant cells, and polygonal epithelioid cells sometimes resembling metastatic carcinoma. Substantial nuclear atypia and mitotic activity are a feature of all tumors. The glioblastoma multiforme is distinguished from anaplastic astrocytoma by the presence of vascular proliferation and necrosis, the latter often surrounded by a peripheral palisade of neoplastic nuclei (Fig. 30–12). Vascular proliferation is often striking, resulting in the formation of so-called glomeruloid bodies, which have superficial resemblance to renal glomeruli. Proliferative activity, as assessed by Ki-67 expression, is regionally heterogeneous in glioblastomas, as well as other infiltrating gliomas. Although considerable overlap exists among the various grades, Ki-67 expression is typically highest in glioblastomas, particularly in areas containing smaller, highly anaplastic cells. In the majority of cases studied, increased frequency of Ki-67 labeling has been shown to correlate in a positive fashion with tumor recurrence and decreased survival (Kirkegaard et al., 1998).

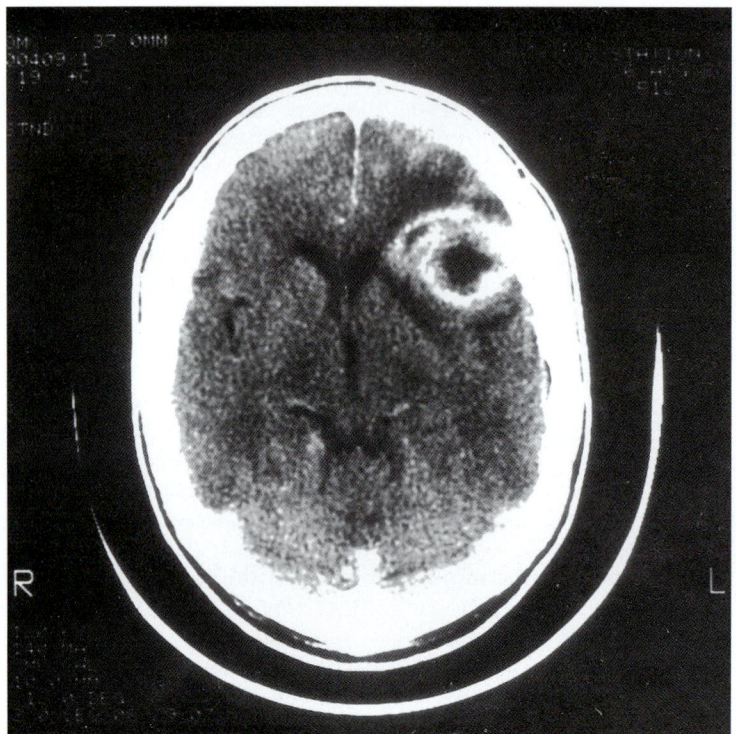

Fig. 30–10. Contrast-enhanced computed tomographic (CT) scan of a cerebral glioblastoma, demonstrating a characteristic ring-like pattern of contrast enhancement. While some glioblastomas arise in patients with a preexisting lower-grade astrocytoma, other examples apparently arise *de novo*, without a clearly defined precursor lesion.

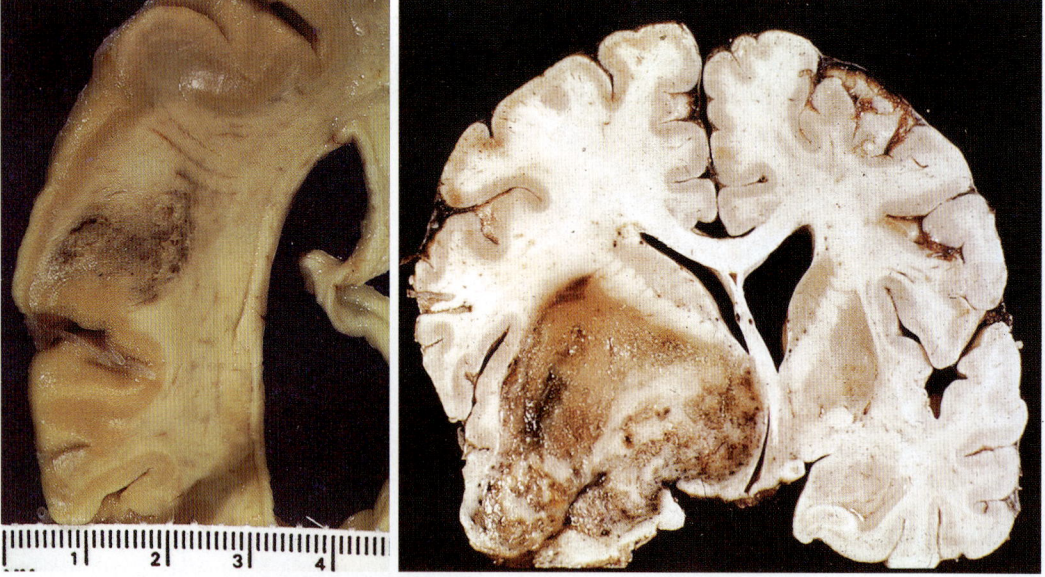

Fig. 30–11. *Right*: Gross photograph of a typical glioblastoma multiforme, demonstrating the characteristic variegated appearance of these lesions, imparted by the presence of irregular areas of hemorrhage, necrosis, and cystic change. *Left*: Gross photograph of a small, and presumably early, glioblastoma multiforme discovered as an incidental lesion in a patient with Alzheimer's disease. The histological appearance of this small lesion was indistinguishable from other glioblastomas. [Photograph courtesy of Dr. Eileen Bigio, Department of Pathology, The University of Texas Southwestern Medical Center.]

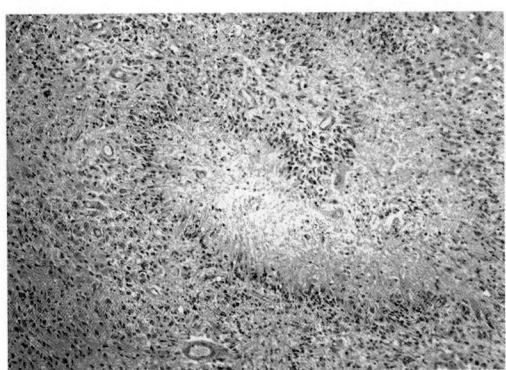

Fig. 30–12. Microscopic appearance of a glioblastoma multiforme, demonstrating substantial hypercellularity and necrosis, the latter surrounded by a palisade of neoplastic nuclei. The presence of necrosis microscopically distinguishes the glioblastoma from anaplastic astrocytoma.

On occasion, glioblastoma multiforme may be accompanied by a sarcomatous component, most frequently in the form of a fibrosarcoma. Such lesions, designated *gliosarcomas*, have a predilection for the temporal lobe, where they may present as a well-circumscribed mass mimicking either a metastatic carcinoma or meningioma (Dwyer et al., 1996). Although proliferating vascular elements have been suggested as possible precursors of the sarcomatous component of these tumors, a recent investigation documented similar genetic alterations in both the sarcomatous and glial components of gliosarcoma, suggesting that the origin of both elements is from a common progenitor cell (Boerman et al., 1996).

The pathogenesis of infiltrating astrocytic tumors has remained frustratingly elusive. The *TP*53 (*p53*) gene, located on the short arm of chromosome 17, plays a key role in cell cycle regulation and in tumorigenesis. Mutations of the *TP*53 gene are one of the more frequent genetic alterations in adult human cancers, including infiltrating astrocytic neoplasms, with reported frequencies of *p53* mutations in grades II, III, and IV astrocytic tumors of 24%, 34%, and 31%, respectively. It is postulated that mutations in the *TP*53 gene represent an early event in the development of astrocytic neoplasms. *TP*53 mutations are much less frequent in other gliomas (Del Arco et al., 1993; Maintz et al., 1998).

PILOCYTIC ASTROCYTOMA

The term *pilocytic astrocytoma* ("juvenile" pilocytic astrocytoma) encompasses a group of related astrocytic neoplasms arising most commonly in the cerebellum, third ventricular region, and optic pathways. These neoplasms differ from the infiltrating astrocytic tumors described previously by virtue of their more discrete nature and, in most cases, more indolent behavior. The prevalence of these neoplasms is increased in patients with neurofibromatosis. Mutations of the NF1 gene are extremely rare, however, and do not appear to play a role in the pathogenesis of these tumors (Platten et al., 1996). Unlike the diffusely infiltrating low-grade astrocytomas, *p53* mutations are generally absent in pilocytic astrocytomas, including the rare examples of these tumors that undergo malignant progression (Ishii et al., 1998). At present, there are no specific cytogenetic or molecular markers associated with these tumors.

Grossly and radiographically, pilocytic astrocytomas are often comparatively circumscribed. Cystic change is quite common, particularly in lesions arising within the cerebellum. An enhancing nodule is often present in imaging studies (Fig. 30–13) and, in contrast to the situation in diffuse astrocytomas, does not signify malignant change. Microscopically, the pilocytic astrocytoma derives its name from the presence of variable numbers of cells with elongated, bipolar, "hair-like" cytoplasmic processes, classically admixed with more loosely arrayed areas containing foci of microcystic change (Fig. 30–14). In practice, a significant range of histological patterns may be seen in pilocytic astrocytomas, the recognition of which is important if one is to avoid misdiagnosing these lesions as other types of glioma (Giannini and Scheithauer, 1997). Brightly eosinophilic, corkscrew-shaped Rosenthal fibers are common, particularly in the more compact areas of the neoplasm (Fig. 30–15). It is important to remember, however, that Rosenthal fibers are not restricted to pilocytic astrocytomas but may also be encountered in association with a number of other indolent lesions in the CNS. Eosinophilic, hyaline granular bodies are another common degenerative change in pilocytic astrocytomas and may be a very important clue

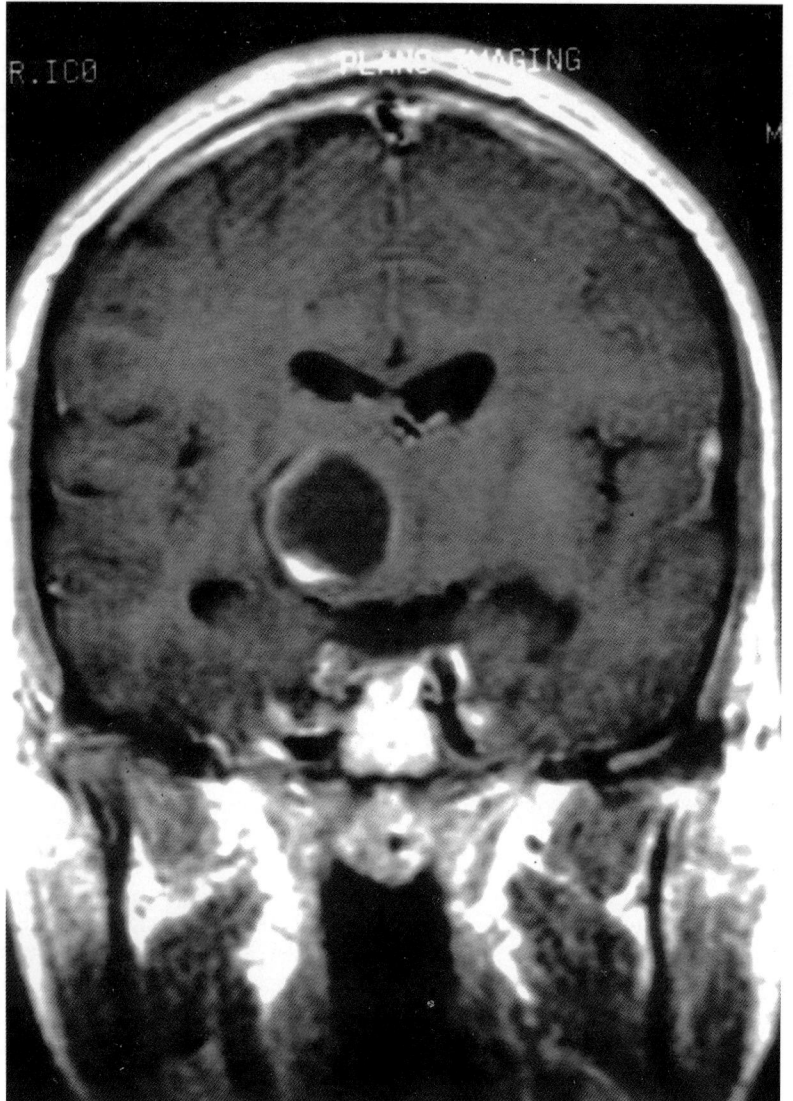

Fig. 30–13. Radiographic appearance of a pilocytic astrocytoma, demonstrating characteristic cystic change associated with an enhancing mural nodule. In contrast to the situation in infiltrating gliomas, radiographic enhancement does not signify malignancy in pilocytic lesions.

to the indolent nature of the lesion, particularly in small biopsies. A significant degree of nuclear atypia and vascular proliferation may be present but, in the absence of high mitotic activity and hypercellularity, does not signify aggressive growth potential (Giannini and Scheithauer, 1997; Giannini et al., 1999; Tomlinson et al., 1994). Extension into the subarachnoid space is quite common and, similarly, does not usually portend aggressive

behavior. In exceptional cases, however, otherwise typical pilocytic astrocytomas may disseminate inexplicably throughout the subarachnoid space (Gajjar et al., 1995). The prognosis of pilocytic astrocytoma is influenced primarily by the location of the lesion and its amenability to surgical excision. Malignant change is exceptional but documented in rare cases (Forsyth et al., 1993; Nishio et al., 1988a; Wilson et al., 1976).

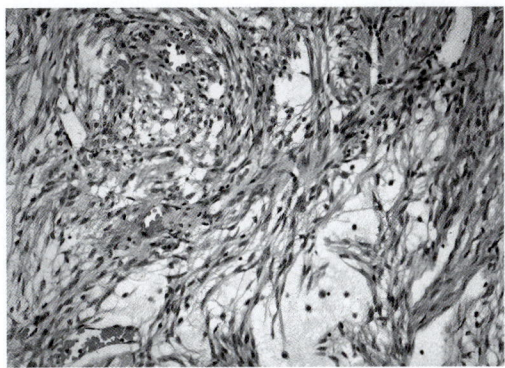

Fig. 30–14. Photomicrograph of a pilocytic astrocytoma, demonstrating interlacing fascicles of bland astrocytes with elongated, bipolar cell processes, associated with areas of microcystic change. Coalescence of microcystic areas accounts for the larger cysts evident radiographically and grossly in some lesions.

SUBEPENDYMAL GIANT CELL ASTROCYTOMA

The subependymal giant cell astrocytoma (SEGA) is characteristically associated with tuberous sclerosis, although some cases occur as apparently isolated, sporadic lesions. Although traditionally regarded as an astrocytic neoplasm, because of the dual expression of glial and neuronal markers in some

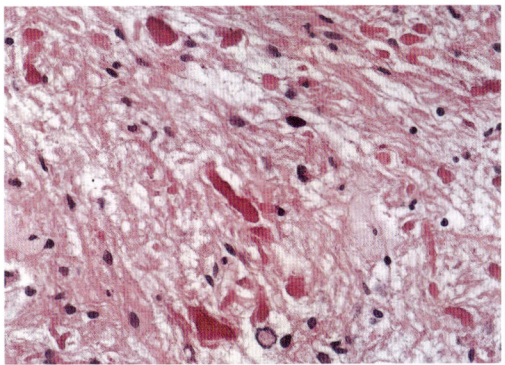

Fig. 30–15. Photomicrograph of a brightly eosinophilic Rosenthal fiber. These structures represent coalescent bundles of intermediate filaments (glial fibrillary acidic protein). While commonly encountered in pilocytic astrocytomas and other slow-growing neoplasms, they may also be seen in areas of reactive gliosis and do not, by themselves, signify a neoplastic process.

cases, it has been suggested that these lesions might be more appropriately classified as mixed glial–neuronal neoplasms (Lopez et al., 1996). The neoplasm originates in the small, but histologically identical, subependymal hamaratomas ("candle drippings") commonly encountered in the lateral ventricular walls in patients with tuberous sclerosis (Boesel et al., 1979; Fig. 30–16). The SEGAs grow slowly and typically come to attention because of increased intracranial pressure secondary to obstruction of one of the foramina of Monro. Grossly, the SEGA is a rounded, well-demarcated, frequently calcified lesion that protrudes into the ventricular lumen. Microscopically, the lesion is composed of large cells with abundant eosinophilic cytoplasm, often arrayed in ill-defined fascicles and perivascular pseudo-rosettes (Fig. 30–17). Although a disturbing degree of nuclear pleomorphism may be present in some cases, mitotic activity is characteristically absent. As might be expected from their indolent behavior, reported Ki-67 labeling indices are characteristically quite low (Gyure and Prayson, 1997). The discrete, noninfiltrating character of the lesion and its characteristic subependymal location further distinguish the SEGA from gemistocytic astrocytomas and other aggressive astrocytic neoplasms. Molecular genetic studies suggest that tumor suppressor genes on chromosomes 9q and 16p may play a role in the genesis of this neoplasm (Conner et al., 1987; Kandt et al., 1992).

OLIOGODENDROGLIOMAS

Although oligodendrogliomas were felt to represent anywhere from 5% to 15% of gliomas in older series (Russell and Rubenstein, 1989), more recent observations suggest that these neoplasms are actually much more common than previously thought (Coons et al., 1996). Oligodendrogliomas may occur at any age but are most common in younger to middle-aged adults. Most lesions arise in the cerebral hemispheres, with some predilection for the frontal lobe. Seizures are a common presenting manifestation, and may antedate the diagnosis of tumor by months to years. Radiographically, well-differentiated oligodendrogliomas tend

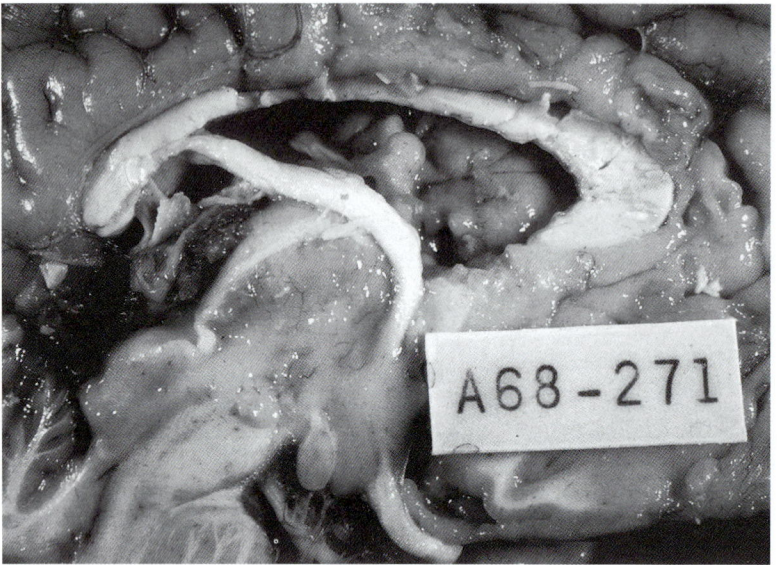

Fig. 30–16. Gross photograph of so-called candle drippings in the walls of the lateral ventricles in a patient with tuberous sclerosis. Histologically, such structures represent focal proliferations of large astrocytic cells with abundant eosinophilic cytoplasm, indistinguishable from the cells of subependymal giant cell astrocytoma.

to be low-density lesions, typically associated with calcification. Higher-grade lesions typically contain areas of enhancement following the adminstration of contrast material. Grossly, some oligodendrogliomas may appear comparatively circumscribed, despite the invariable presence of infiltrative growth microscopically. In material that has not been subjected to prior freezing, the neoplastic nuclei are comparatively rounded, in contrast to the angular configuration of neoplastic astrocytic nuclei. In material that has

been previously frozen, however, the nuclei typically assume a more irregular, angular appearance, which may be impossible to distinguish from astrocytic nuclei. Clear perinuclear "halos" are common in routine formalin-fixed tissue and are another helpful diagnostic feature (Fig. 30–18) but tend to be absent in specimens that have been promptly fixed or previously frozen. Some oligodendrogliomas contain cells with abundant eosinophilic cytoplasm reminiscent of that seen in gemistocytic astrocytes. Such

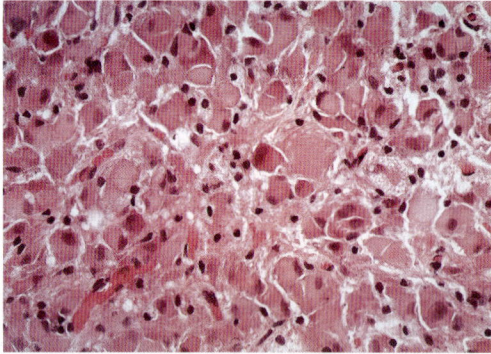

Fig. 30–17. Subependymal giant cell astrocytoma in a patient with tuberous sclerosis, demonstrating the large cells similar to those found in the hamartomatous "candle drippings" associated with this condition. Although commonly regarded as astrocytic proliferations, some evidence suggests the presence of neuronal differentiation in such cells.

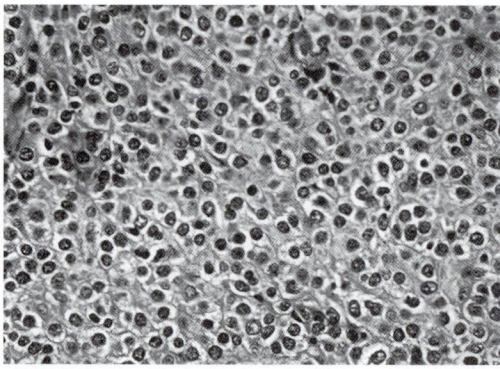

Fig. 30–18. Microscopic appearance of a well-differentiated oligodendroglioma, demonstrating characteristic rounded, uniform nuclei and conspicuous perinuclear halos. Perinuclear halos are an artifact of delayed fixation, and are absent in previously frozen material and in promptly fixed specimens.

cells, termed *microgemistocytes,* are distinguished from gemistocytic astrocytes by the more rounded appearance of their nuclei and by the absence of well-developed stellate cytoplasmic processes. Oligodendrogliomas usually contain a delicate, branching vascular network, which, in some cases, compartmentalizes the neoplastic cells into fairly distinct lobules. Although cell density is often uniform throughout the tumor, some examples contain circumscribled zones referred to as "clonal" nodules. Oligodendrogliomas have a stiking tendency to infiltrate the cerebral cortex, where they are produce prominent perineuronal satellitosis and hypercellular subpial infiltrates. The neoplasms may infiltrate overlying dura and, on rare occasions, bone. Although the criteria for grading oligodendrogliomas remain less well defined than those for infiltrating astrocytic neoplasms, nuclear pleomorphism, hypercellularity, significant mitotic activity, vascular proliferation, and necrosis have all been associated with more aggressive behavior (Burger et al., 1987; Daumas-Duport et al., 1997; Kros et al., 1988; Mork et al., 1986; Smith et al., 1983) (Fig. 30–19). Although the morphological features of anaplastic oligodendroglioma may merge with that of glioblastoma multiforme, from a prognostic and therapeutic standpoint, it is important to distinguish oligodendroglial tumors associated with microvascular proliferation, brisk mitotic activity, and necrosis from the glioblastoma multiforme, a predominantly astrocytic tumor. The latter lesions generally have a worse prognosis than malignant oligodendroglial neoplasms and, of practical importance, respond much more poorly to chemotherapy than high-grade oligodendrogliomas (Cairncross et al., 1998).

Recent studies have identified genetic alterations in oligodendrogliomas that differ from those commonly found in astrocytomas. Typical molecular alterations in oligodendrogliomas include 1p and 19q deletions, the most frequent being loss of heterozygosity (LOH) on the long arm of chromosome 19 (Reifenberger et al., 1994). In contrast to the situation in astrocytic tumors, LOH on the short arm of chromosome 17 (17p) and mutations in the *TP53* gene at 17p13.1 are uncommon in oligodendrogliomas, regardless of grade (Maintz, 1997). The identification of a characteristic molecular profile further validates the separation of oligodendroglial from astrocytic tumors, a distinction previously based on potentially subjective morphological criteria.

EPENDYMOMAS

Ependymomas are found at any age and any site within the CNS, often in a periventricular location. Rare ectopic examples arise in pre- or postsacral soft tissue, the mediastinum, lung, ovary, or broad ligament (Nobles et al., 1991). Intracranial examples occur most often during the first two decades of life, whereas intraspinal lesions predominate in adults (Lyons and Kelley, 1991; Mork and Loken, 1977). Intracranial tumors occur most commonly in the vicinity of the fourth ventricle, where cerebospinal fluid outflow obstruction and elevated intracranial pressure commonly bring the neoplasm to clinical attention. Grossly, most ependymomas present as lobulated, predominantly intraventricular proliferations, which are relatively well demarcated from the adjacent brain parenchyma (Fig. 30–20). Posterior fossa lesions may protrude into the cerebellopontine angle, mimicking either meningioma or schwannoma. Intraspinal

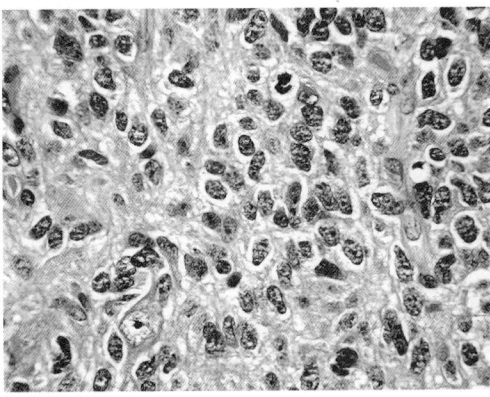

Fig. 30–19. Photomicrograph of anaplastic oligodendroglioma. Such lesions are characterized by greater cellularity, pleomorphism, and mitotic activity than well-differentiated oligodendrogliomas but often retain a generally rounder nuclear morphology than anaplastic astrocytomas. Extremely poorly differentiated lesions may be difficult to distinguish histologically from high-grade astrocytic tumors, however.

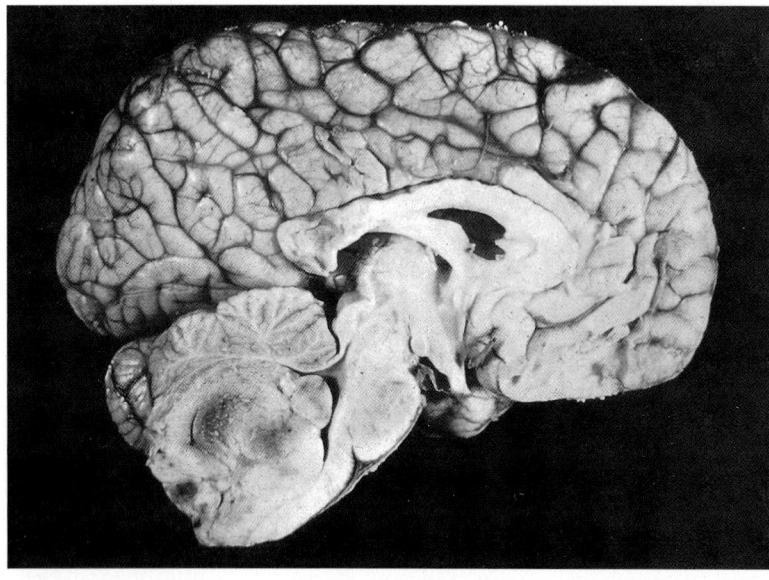

Fig. 30–20. Gross photograph of an ependymoma arising in the fourth ventricle. Such lesions typically remain well-demarcated from the adjacent brain parenchyma, in contrast to astrocytomas and oligodendrogliomas.

ependymomas present as circumscribed, elongated intramedullary tumors or, particularly in the case of myxopapillary variants, as a fusiform mass expanding the cauda equina. An associated syrinx is common.

The microscopic patterns encountered in ependymomas are quite variable, even within different regions of the same tumor. The nuclei tend to be uniform and ovoid, with a finely stippled chromatin pattern. In most cases, the processes of the neoplastic cells radiate toward vessels to form perivascular pseudorosettes. Less commonly, the neoplastic cells may surround a true lumen, recapitulating the appearance of the normal ventricular lining (Fig. 30–21). In *cellular ependymomas*, the patttern is that of a comparatively monomorphous proliferation of small, closely apposed cells forming only subtle pseudorosettes and tiny true rosettes. Clear cells mimicking oligodendroglioma are common in ependymomas; when predominant, such lesions are sometimes designated *clear cell ependymomas* (Kawano et al., 1989). Well-developed papillary structures reminiscent of choroid plexus papilloma are also common. The *myxopapillary ependymoma* is a distinctive variant of papillary ependymoma that presents as a well-defined, fusiform mass in the filum terminale or conus medullaris (Sonneland et al., 1985; Fig. 30–22). Criteria for the diagnosis of anaplasia in ependymomas remain frustratingly vague, and, not surprisingly, data re-

garding the outcome of conventional and anaplastic grade lesions vary considerably. Of the various changes associated with malignant change in other gliomas, brisk mitotic activity, usually in association with significant hypercellularity (crowded, overlapping nuclei), appears to be the most reliable predictor of aggressive behavior. Although necrosis and pleomorphism are common high-grade lesions, in the absence of significant mitotic activity, these appear to have little, if any, predictive value in ependymal neoplasms (Ross and Rubinstein, 1989). As in the case of many other CNS neoplasms,

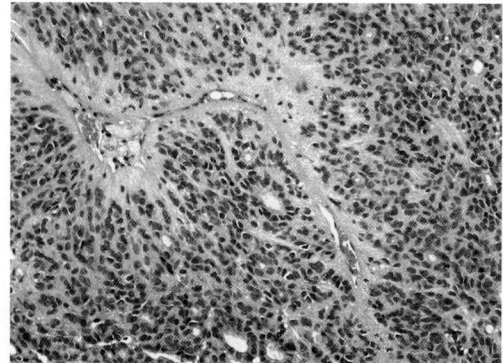

Fig. 30–21. Photomicrograph of ependymoma, demonstrating typical perivascular pseudorosettes as well as true ependymal rosettes, the latter recapitulating the morphology of native, non-neoplastic ependyma.

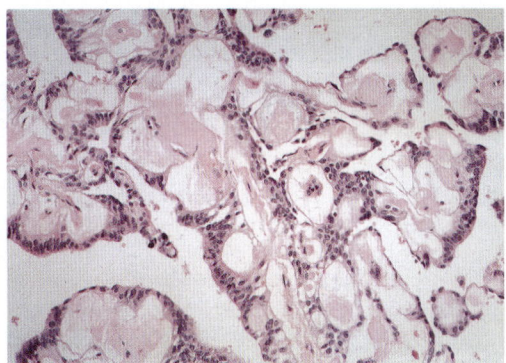

Fig. 30–22. Microscopic appearance of a myxopapillary ependymoma, containing well-developed papillae with loose, myxomatous cores. Such lesions occur most frequently as expansile masses in the region of the filum terminale.

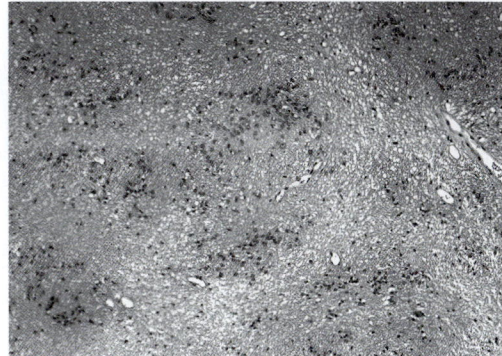

Fig. 30–24. Histological appearance of a subependymoma, with nests of bland nuclei separated by abundant fibrillar matrix, and ill-defined perivascular pseudorosettes.

assessment of Ki-67 antigen expression may prove to be of additional value in predicting the behavior of ependymal neoplasms (Karamitopoulou et al., 1994; Rushing et al., 1997, 1998). The biological significance of small foci of anaplastic change in otherwise well-differentiated ependymomas remains unclear. Approximately 30% of ependymomas show cytogenetic changes, most commonly, monosomy of chromosome 22 (Hamilton and Pollock, 1997).

The *supependymoma* is a well-circumscribed, indolent lesion usually discovered as an incidental mass in older individuals at the time of autopsy (Boykin et al., 1954; Russell and Rubenstein, 1989). On occasion, however, on account of its intraventricular location, subependymomas may come to clinical attention because of cerebrospinal fluid outflow obstruction and elevated intracranial pressure. Grossly, the typical subependymoma is a well-defined nodule attached to the ventricular wall or, less commonly, the septum pellucidum or choroid plexus (Fig. 30–23). Calcification is common. Histologically, the subependymoma is characterized by clusters of comparatively uniform, ovoid ependymal nuclei separated by an abundant fibrillar matrix (Fig. 30–24). Some attempts

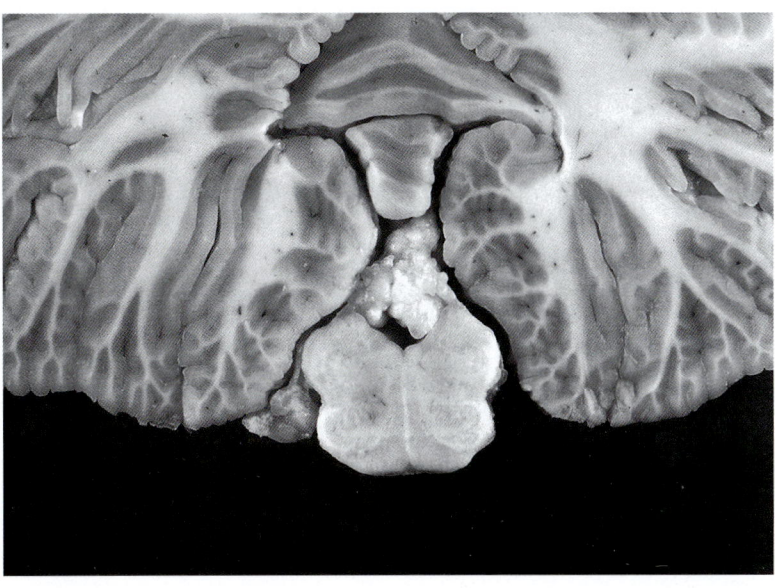

Fig. 30–23. Gross appearance of a subependymoma, discovered as an incidental finding at the time of autopsy. Such lesions are usually asymptomatic, but may, by virtue of the intraventricular location, cause cerebrospinal fluid outflow obstruction and elevated intracranial pressure.

at perivascular pseudorosette formation may be present, but true ependymal rosettes are usually absent. Increased cellularity approaching that of conventional ependymomas has been noted in some cases, particularly in younger patients, and has been associated with more aggressive behavior (Scheithauer, 1978).

PRIMITIVE NEUROEPITHELIAL TUMORS

The primitive neuroepithelial neoplasms belong to a family of embryonal small cell malignant neoplasm occurring predominantly, although not exclusively, in childhood. A considerable spectrum of neuronal, glial, and even mesenchymal differentiation may be encountered in these lesions, the nosology of which, predictably, has engendered spirited debate among pathologists. Depending upon the scheme employed, primitive neuroepithelial tumors are classified on the basis of the morphological and/or immunocytochemical characteristics of the constituent cells and the location of the neoplasm. As noted, the classification of these neoplasms remains quite controversial. On the basis of the occurrence of histologically similar tumors at different sites in the neuraxis and the assumption that such tumors arise from a common, primitive

progenitor cell, some writers have advocated designating all such central embryonal neoplasms *primitive neuroectodermal tumors* (PNETs) (Becker and Hinton, 1983; Rorke, 1983). Subclassification of the PNETs is based, in turn, on the presence or absence of differentiation along neuronal, glial, or other lines, as determined by histological, immunocytochemical, and/or ultrastructural evaluation. Critics of this classification scheme have argued forcefully that the assumption of a common cell of origin for all such neoplasms is not supported by experimental data, and that the PNET concept may represent an artificial almalgamation of biologically distinct lesions (Rubinstein, 1985).

The *medulloblastoma* is the most common primitive neuroepithelial neoplasm of the CNS (Becker and Hinton, 1983; Rubinstein, 1985). By definition, it originates, from the cerebellum. The tumor is found predominantly in childhood and adolescence, with a peak incidence during the first decade of life. Most cases are sporadic, although associations with Wilms' tumor (Rainov et al., 1995), rhabdoid tumor of the kidney (Fort et al., 1994), and Turcot syndrome (Paraf et al., 1997) have been documented. Grossly, most medulloblastomas arise in the cerebellar vermis, where they present as soft, friable masses that infiltrate and efface the normal foliar architecture. The neoplasm may protrude into the fourth ventricle (Fig. 30–25)

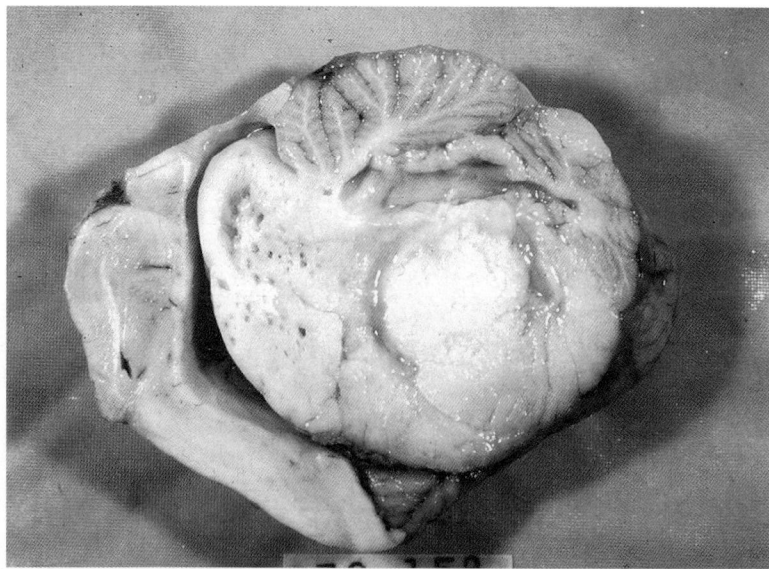

Fig. 30–25. Gross photograph of a medulloblastoma arising in and obliterating the cerebellar vermis. Such neoplasms may seed the subarachnoid space early in their course.

and frequently inflitrates the adjacent leptomeninges. Microscopically, the medulloblastoma is composed of primitive, closely
packed cells containing small, hyperchromatic, mitotically active nuclei and scant cytoplasm (Fig. 30–26). The mitotically active
external granular layer of the cerebellum,
which persists for up to 18 months after
birth, has been proposed as the likely site of
origin of the medulloblastoma (Kadin et al.,
1970; Fig. 30–27). In the case of the least-dif-
ferentiated medulloblastomas, the primitive
neoplastic cells proliferate in sheets, interrupted by scattered areas of necrosis. Occasional cells with perinuclear halos
reminiscent of oligodendroglioma are commonly encountered. In many tumors,
Homer Wright rosettes, formed by neoplastic cells arrayed around a small fibrillar core,
are present and indicate early neuronal
differentiation. In other cases, a nodular architecture is conspicuous, creating a superficial resemblance to lymphoid follicles. Like
the Homer Wright rosettes, such nodules
likely reflect the presence of neuronal differentiation (Katsetos et al., 1989). In a minority of cases, more fully developed
gangliocytic elements may be encountered.
The term *desmoplastic medulloblastoma* has
been applied to those medulloblastomas accompanied by a well-developed connective
tissue reaction (Rubinstein and Northfield,
1964). Such a reaction is seen most fre-

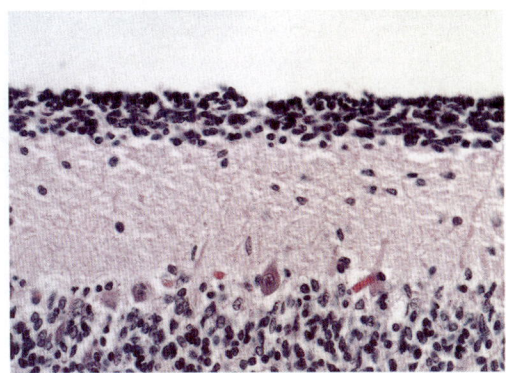

Fig. 30–27. Photomicrograph of neonatal cerebellar cortex, demonstrating the superficial external granular layer. Such primitive progenitor
cells persist in some regions into the second year
of postnatal life and are the likely cells of origin
of cerebellar medulloblatomas.

quently in medulloblastomas arising superficially in the lateral cerebral hemispheres of
older children and young adults. Desmoplastic change is common in medulloblastomas exhibiting a nodular architecture
(described above).

The atypical teratoid/rhabdoid tumor of
the CNS is a recently characterized small cell
neoplasm that should be distinguished from
medulloblastoma and other primitive neuroepithelial neoplasms (Rorke at al, 1996).
Atypical teratoid/rhabdoid tumors have a
complex immunohistochemical profile,
reflecting considerable diversity in the constituent cells. Although the immunohistochemical profile may vary considerably from
case to case, there is general agreement that
vimentin, epithelial membrane antigen, glial
fibrillary acidic protein, cytokeratins, synaptophysin, and actin are commonly expressed.
The microscopic diagnosis of atypical tera-
toid/rhabdoid tumor is suggested by the
presence of haphazardly arranged medium-
sized cells with prominent nucleoli and an
eosinophilic cytoplasmic inclusion, sometimes designated a "pink body" (Fig. 30–28).
Other features sometimes encountered in
these tumors include prominent embryonal,
PNET-like components, mesenchymal differentiation, and epithelial areas (Rorke et
al., 1996). Cytogenetic analysis reveals monosomy of chromosome 22 in a high percentage of these tumors (Biegel et al., 1992).

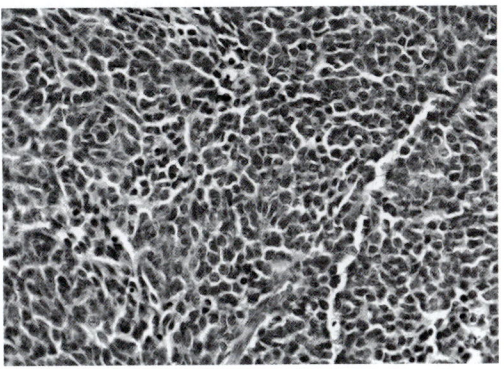

Fig. 30–26. Light microscopic appearance of an
undifferentiated medulloblastoma, characterized
by sheets of primitive cells with dense, hyperchromatic nuclei and inconspicuous cytoplasm.
Varying degrees of neuronal differentiation are a
feature of some cases.

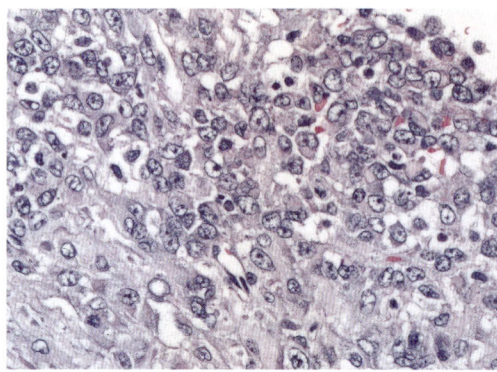

Fig. 30–28. Photomicrograph of an atypical teratoid/rhabdoid tumor, demonstrating characteristic prominent nucleoli and eccentric, eosinophilic cytoplasm. These aggressive neoplasms occur most frequently in the posterior cranial fossa and may contain areas that are difficult to distinguish from medulloblastoma and other primitive neuroectodermal tumors.

NEURONAL AND MIXED NEURONAL-GLIAL NEOPLASMS

In addition to appearing in an occasional differentiating primitive neuroepithelial tumor, mature neurons participate in the formation of a number of other interesting CNS neoplasms, including gangliogliomas, central neurocytomas, the dysembryoplastic neuroepithelial tumor, and the desmoplastic infantile ganglioglioma.

Ganglion cell tumors are generally indolent lesions, occurring predominantly in children and young adults. These neoplasms can arise anywhere in the central neuraxis but are especially common in the temporal lobe, where seizures are a common presenting manifestation. Grossly and radiographically, ganglion cell tumors are generally well circumscribed, sometimes cystic, and frequently calcified. The proportion of glial and neuronal elements varies considerably from case to case. The identification of at least some neoplastic neurons, however, is essential for the diagnosis of ganglion cell tumor. Such cells may be inconspicuous in lesions dominated by glial elements and must be clearly distinguished from both entrapped native neurons, or bizarre, neoplastic astrocytes that may bear a striking resemblance to ganglion cells. The presence of neurons in abnormal locations, e.g., the cortical molecular layer or the leptomen-

inges, and the presence of cytologically atypical, multinucleate forms help to establish the neoplastic nature of the neurons in a suspected ganglion cell tumor (Fig. 30–29). Immunohistochemical stains for neuronal markers, including synaptophysin and neurofilament protein, are a valuable supplement to routine histological sections in the identification of atypical gangliocytic elements (Miller et al., 1990; Wolf et al., 1994). More recent investigations have demonstated a splice site–associated DNA polymorphism in sporadic gangliogliomas identical to that seen in the tuberous sclerosis gene (Platten, 1997). The prognosis of ganglion cell tumors is generally favorable, with many lesions exhibiting a static course over many years. In occasional cases, aggressive behavior has been documented, sometimes in association with "dedifferentiation" of the glial component (Russell and Rubinstein, 1962).

The *central neurocytoma* characteristically presents as a well-defined, sometimes calcified, intraventricular mass in adolescents and young adults, often attached to the septum pellucidum (Hassoun et al., 1982; Nishio et al., 1988b; Townsend and Seaman, 1986) (Fig. 30–30). An origin from the

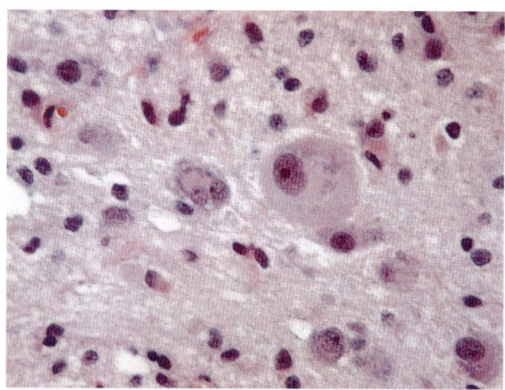

Fig. 30–29. Photomicrograph of a ganglioglioma, demonstrating atypical gangliocytic elements. The diagnosis of ganglion cell tumor rests on the demonstration of dysplastic neuronal elements, which must be distinguished from native, non-neoplastic neurons entrapped in an infiltrating glioma and from bizarre neoplastic astrocytes superficially resembling ganglion cells that may be encountered in some high-grade gliomas. The distinction between small ganglion cell neoplasms and dysplastic lesions may be difficult in some cases.

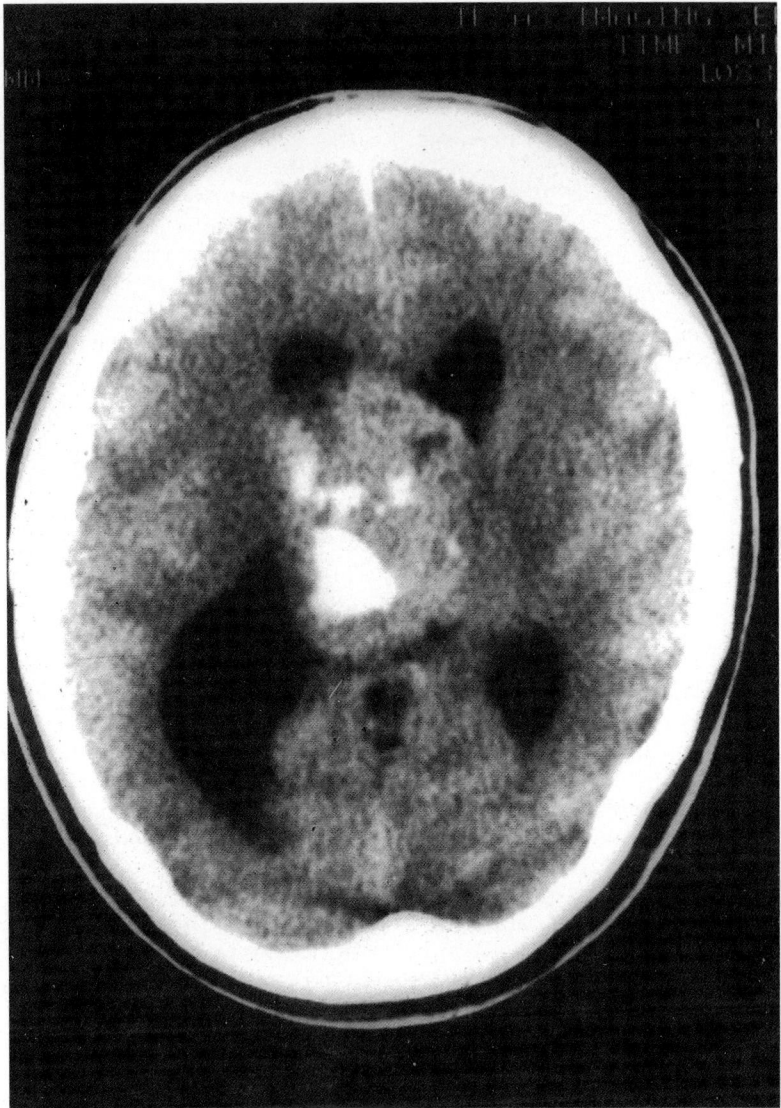

Fig. 30–30. Radiographic appearance of a central neurocytoma. These lesions classically arise in the lateral cerebral ventricles, where they may come to clinical attention by causing cerebrospinal outflow obstruction and elevated intracranial pressure. Calcification is often apparent radiographically in these neoplasms.

periventricular germinal matrix has been proposed, on account of the paraventricular location of most tumors and the concomitant expression of neuronal and glial markers in some cases (von Deimling et al., 1991). Histologically, the neurocytoma is composed of cells with strikingly uniform, round nuclei, perinuclear halos reminiscent of oligodendroglioma, occasional perivascular pseudorosettes, and variably developed fibrillar zones reminiscent of pineocytic rosettes (Fig. 30–31). Neuronal markers are

usually demonstrable in immunohistochemical preparations and help to distinguish the central neurocytoma from histologically similar lesions, such as oligodendroglioma and clear cell ependymoma. Ultrastructural studies have confirmed the neuronal character of these neoplasms.

The *dysembryoplastic neuroepithelial tumor* (DNT) is a recently described mixed neuronal–glial neoplasm that is notable for highly characteristic clinical and morphological features (Daumas-Duport, 1993; Dau-

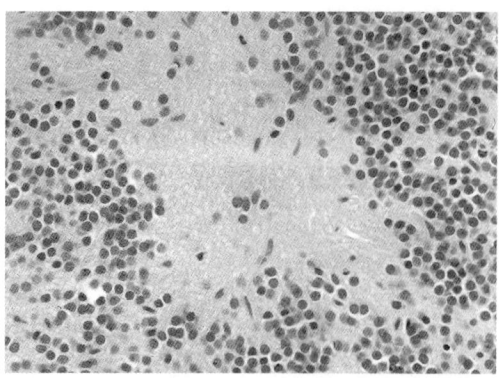

Fig. 30–31. Central neurocytoma. The histological appearance of these neoplasms may mimic that of oligodendroglioma or clear cell ependymoma. The presence of broad fibrillar areas reminiscent of pineocytic rosettes in some variants distinguishes the neurocytoma from histologically similar "clear cell" tumors.

mas-Duport et al., 1988). Most cases occur in the first two decades of life and are typically associated with a long history of medically intractable seizures, often of the complex-partial type. The most common site for these tumors is the medial temporal lobe, where it appears as a multinodular, intracortical lesion, frequently associated with cortical dysplasia in adjacent areas. Radiographic imaging studies often demonstrate characteristic "scalloping" of the adjacent calvarium, a testament to the chronic nature of these lesions (Fig. 30–32). Microscopically, the DNT is distinguished by a mixture of astrocytic, oligodendroglial, and neuronal elements, the last often appearing as "free-floating" cells in areas of microcystic change (Fig. 30–33). In contrast to the conventional ganglion cell tumors described previously, the neurons of the DNT do not appear dysplastic. The prognosis is excellent following surgical resection. The exact nature of the DNT remains incompletely understood, with some observers suggesting that it might represent more of a malformative lesion than a true neoplasm. It is important that this lesion be distinguished from infiltrating gliomas, particularly mixed oligoastrocytomas, neoplasms with a radically different prognosis. Although this may be difficult in small biopsies, careful correlation of histological findings with radiographic imaging studies and clinical information is usually of

great help in the proper diagnosis of these tumors.

Another mixed neuronal–glial neoplasm, mentioned here only for completeness, is the uncommon *desmoplastic infantile ganglioglioma* (VandenBerg, 1993). These tumors typically present as massive cerebral hemispheric lesions in infants. Histologically, neuronal cells may be inconspicuous in a background of proliferating glial cells and mesenchymal elements (Paulus et al., 1992). Nests of small primitive cells may be present but surprisingly, do not have an adverse impact on the uniformly excellent prognosis of these lesions (Parisi et al., 1992).

HEMANGIOBLASTOMA

The hemangioblastoma is predominantly a lesion of adulthood. Most examples arise in the cerebellum, with an additional minority of cases originating in the brainstem and spinal cord (Banerjee and Hunt, 1972; Cramer and Kimsey, 1952). In addition, histologically and biologically identical lesions may occur in the meninges, where they have sometimes been designated hemangioblastic variants of so-called angioblastic meningioma. Although the hemangioblastoma may develop as an isolated, apparently sporadic neoplasm, its presence should prompt the search for other stigmata of the von Hippel–Lindau syndrome. This syndrome is characterized by the presence of hemangioblastomas, often multiple, in a variety of sites, including the brain, spinal cord, optic nerve, and retina (Kerr et al., 1995). The syndrome is associated with a number of other interesting lesions, including pancreatic and hepatic cysts, cystic epididymal tumors, benign and malignant renal neoplasms, pheochromocytomas, and aggressive papillary neoplasms of the middle ear (Ouallet, 1997). Inherited in an atuosomal dominant pattern (Latif et al., 1993), the von Hippel–Lindau (VHL) gene locus resides on the short arm of chromosome 3 (Lerman et al., 1991).

Grossly, the hemangioblastoma is a well-demarcated, richly vascular mass, often presenting as a nodule in the wall of an associated cyst or syrinx. Microscopically, the tumor contains an abundant, delicate capillary network separated by intervening stro-

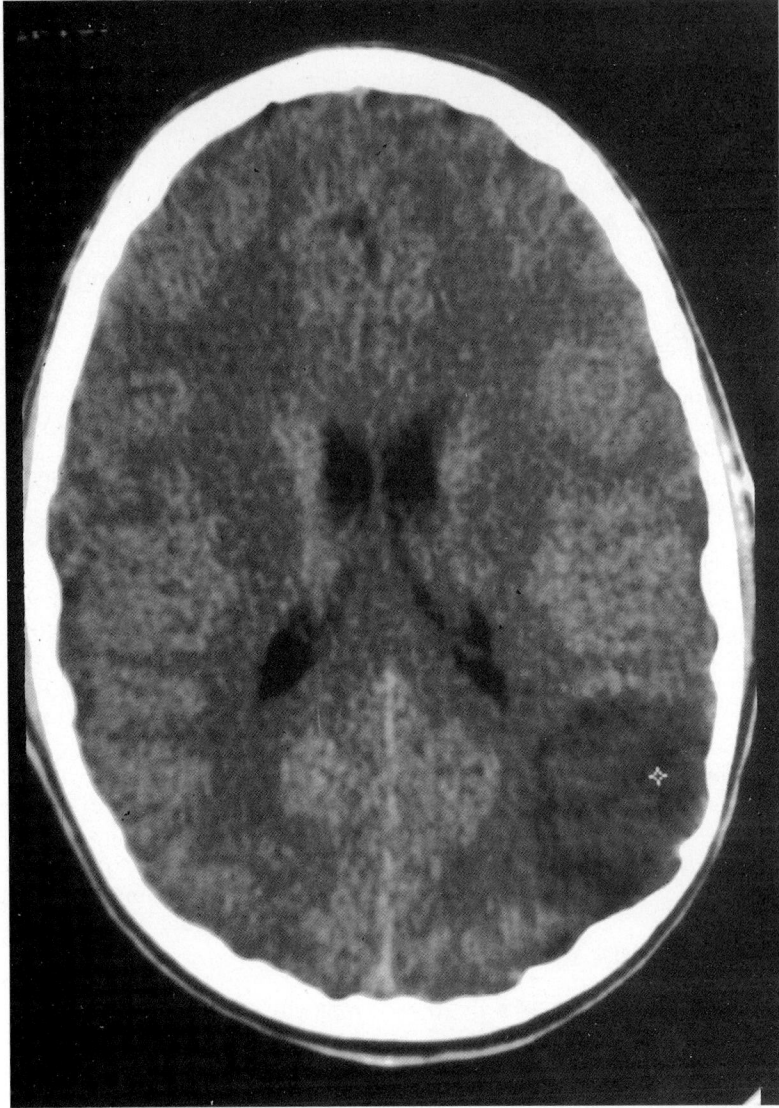

Fig. 30–32. Computed tomography scan of a dysembryoplastic neuroepithelial tumor, demonstrating characteristic "scalloping" of the inner table of the skull. A long history of complex partial seizures is often present in such cases and may provide an important clue to the diagnosis of the lesion prior to biopsy.

mal cells (Fig. 30–34). The origin of the stromal cells remains enigmatic, although the recent observation of factor XIIIa reactivity has suggested the possibility of a fibrohistiocytic origin (Nemes, 1992). Neutral fat is readily demonstrable within the cytoplasm of the stromal cells at the time of frozen section in most cases, an observation that may help one distinguish the hemangioblastoma from pilocytic astrocytoma. Significant nuclear pleomorphism may be present in the

stromal cells but does not imply aggressive behavior. Foci of extramedullary hematopoiesis are common, reflecting production of erythropoietin by the tumor. A vigorous astrocytic reaction, often accompanied by Rosenthal fiber formation, is commonly encountered at the periphery of hemangioblastomas, creating the potential for confusion with pilocytic astrocytoma. Distinguishing hemangioblastoma from metastatic renal cell carcinoma histologically may also

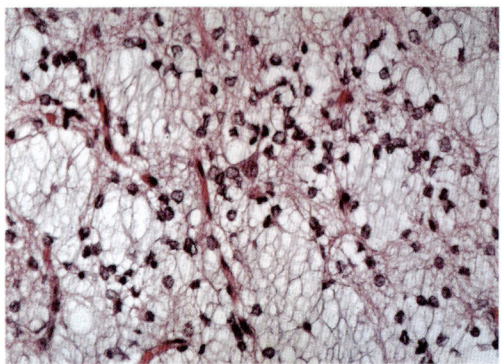

Fig. 30–33. Dysembryoplastic neuroepithelial tumor. Such lesions are characterized by a multinodular, intracortical growth pattern. Many different histological patterns may be encountered, including, as illustrated here, extensive microcystic change with "free-floating" neurons. Many examples contain prominent oligodendroglia-like areas, which should not be confused with oligodendroglioma. [Case courtesy of Dr. Linda Margraf, Children's Medical Center, Dallas, TX.]

pose a diagnostic challenge, a problem compounded by the increased frequency of renal cell carcinomas in patients with the von Hippel–Lindau syndrome. Immunohistochemical staining for epithelial membrane

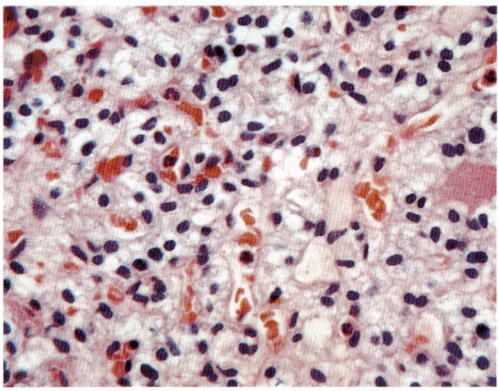

Fig. 30–34. Photomicrograph of a hemangioblastoma, demonstrating characteristic lipid-laden, foamy stromal cells separated by a delicate capillary network. The cell of origin of the stromal elements remains controversial. A significant number of these lesions are associated with the von Hippel–Lindau syndrome. Hemangioblastomas may be difficult to distinguish histologically from metastatic renal cell carcinoma, another important consideration in patients with this hereditary syndrome.

antigen (EMA) may be of value in distinguishing these latter two lesions, with most renal cell carcinomas expressing EMA, whereas the stromal cells of hemangioblastoma are typically nonreactive (Clelland and Treip, 1989; Gouldesbrough et al., 1988; Grant et al., 1988). Another recent study has suggested that Ki-67 (MIB-1) labeling indices may be of additional value in distinguishing hemangioblastomas from renal cell carcinomas (Brown et al., 1997).

SCHWANNOMAS

Schwannomas are generally benign neoplasms arising from the Schwann cells of the peripheral nerve sheath. Because Schwann cells begin to invest cranial nerve processes within a few millimeters of the pial surface of the brain and spinal cord, these neoplasms may arise within the spinal canal and cranial cavity, as well as in more peripheral locations. Although schwannomas are often sporadic, their frequency is markedly increased in patients with neurofibromatosis, particularly in those with the central form of the disease (NF2) (Riccardi, 1987). Loss of the NF2 gene and its protein product, merlin, have been implicated in the development of sporadic schwannomas (Jacoby et al., 1994).

In the intracranial compartment, the vast majority of schwannomas arise in the eighth cranial nerve near the internal auditory meatus, where hearing loss and vertigo may call attention to the lesion at an early stage (Fig. 30–35). Expansion of the meatus is often evident radiographically and, when present, helps to distinguish the schwannomas from other cerebellopontine angle tumors, including meningiomas and ependymomas. Less commonly, intracranial schwannomaas may arise in the trigeminal, or other cranial nerves. Within the spinal canal, most schwannomas arise in association with dorsal spinal nerve roots, where they present as circumscribed intradural masses, or as "dumbell"-shaped lesions protruding through adjacent intervertebral foramina. Rarely, they may present as a well-circumscribed mass within the spinal cord proper, sometimes in association with a syrinx. Minute of foci Schwann cell proliferation within the substance of the spinal cord, designated in-

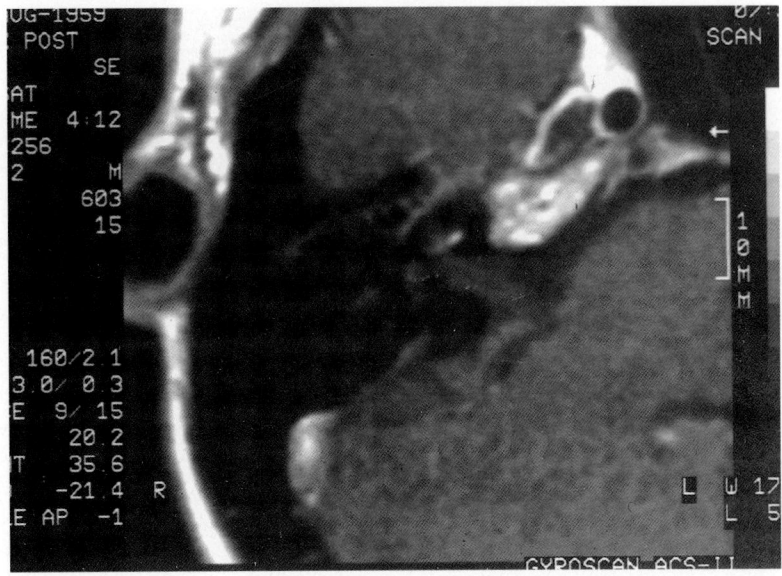

Fig. 30–35. Post-contrast-enhanced radiograph of a minute schwannoma arising within the cochlea of the inner ear. Involvement of temporal bone structures is a characteristic feature of schwannomas and helps to distinguish them from meningiomas arising in this region. [Case courtesy of Dr. Peter Rolland, Department of Otorhinolaryngology, University of Texas Southwestern Medical School.]

tramedullary "schwannosis," have been suggested as the likely precursor to such intramedullary tumors (Fig. 30–36). Most schwannomas are solitary, although multiple lesions occur in some patients, especially in association with the central form of neurofibromatosis.

Microscopically, schwannomas consist of a mixture of compact, fibrillar Antoni-A tissue and more loosely structured Antoni-B tissue. Foci of nuclear palisading, known as *Verocay bodies,* are a conspicuous feature of some tumors (Fig. 30–37). Some schwannomas, particularly those dominated by compact Antoni-A architecture, may be difficult to differentiate from meningiomas. Demonstra-

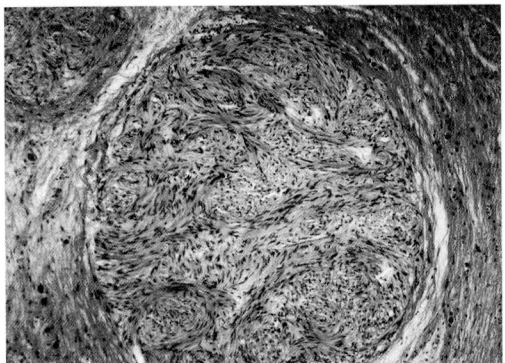

Fig. 30–36. Photomicrograph of intramedullary schwannosis, characterized by nests of proliferating Schwann cells within the substance of the spinal cord. Such microscopic lesions may occur in patients with neurofibromatosis and sporadically adjacent to other focal spinal cord lesions. These minute foci may serve as the precursor to the occasional schwannoma arising within the spinal cord.

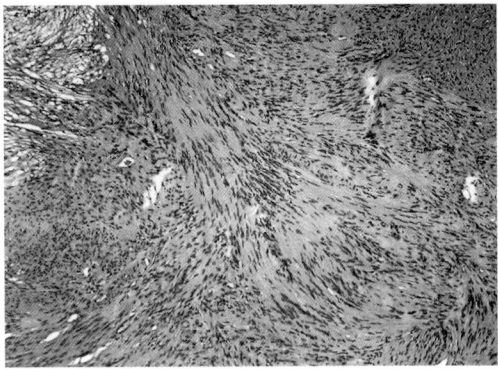

Fig. 30–37. Schwannoma. These neoplasms are composed of compact, interlacing fascicles of elongated Schwann cells (Antoni A foci), often associated with more loosely textured Antoni B tissue. Prominent palisades of closely spaced nuclei, designated Verocay bodies, are present in this example.

tion of EMA may be of great help in differentiating these two lesions, with EMA expression restricted to meningiomas. Electron microscopy may also be of value in problematic cases, with meningiomas exhibiting complex interdigitating cell processes and desmosomal attachments and lacking the well-developed pericellular basement membrane of schwannomas. An important variant to recognize is the so-called *cellular schwannoma* (Casadei et al., 1995), which may be confused with well-differentiated forms of malignant peripheral nerve sheath tumor (MPNST). As in the case of other schwannomas, cellular variants may also arise in the CNS, particularly in association with the fifth or eighth cranial nerve. Cellular schwannomas, like their more conventional counterparts, are typically encapsulated lesions. Mitotic figures may be present, although mitotic rates are generally low. The presence of Antoni B tissue and hyalinized vessels and an absence of necrosis are additional features that help to distinguish cellular schwannomas from MPNSTs. Like more conventional schwannomas, the cellular variant exhibits robust S-100 reactivity and may also express GFAP.

REFERENCES

Albright AL, Price RA, Guthkelch AN. (1983) Brain stem gliomas in children: a clinicopathologic study. *Cancer* 52:2313–2319.

Anderson JR, Treip CS. (1986) Radiation-induced intracranial neoplasms. A report of three possible cases. *Cancer* 53:426–429.

Anderson M, Hughes B, Jefferson M. et al. (1980) Gliomatous transformation and demyelinating diseases. *Brain* 103:603–622.

Arnoldus EP, Wolters LB, Voormolen JH, et al. (1992) Interphase cytogenetics: a new tool for the study of genetic changes in brain tumors. *J Neurosurg* 78: 997–1003.

Banerjee T, Hunt WE. (1972) A case of spinal cord hemangioblastoma and review of the literature. *Am J Surg* 38:460–464.

Becker LE, Hinton D. (1983) Primitive neuroectodermal tumors of the central nervous system. *Hum Pathol* 14: 538–550.

Berger MS, Edwards MSB, LaMasters D, et al. (1983) Pediatric brain stem tumors: radiographic, pathological, and clinical correlations. *Neurosurgery* 12: 298–302.

Biegel JA, Rorke LB, Packer RJ, Emanuel BS. (1992) Monosomy 22 in rhabdoid or atypical teratoid tumors of the brain. *Neurosurgery* 73:710–714.

Boerman RH, Anderl K, Herath J, et al. (1996) The glial and mesenchymal elements of gliosarcomas share similar genetic alterations. *J Neuropathol Exp Neurol* 55:973–981.

Boesel CP, Paulson GW, Kosnik EJ, Earle KM. (1979) Brain hamartomas and tumors associated with tuberous sclerosis. *Neurosurgery* 4:410–417.

Boykin FC, Cowan D, Iannucci CAJ, Wolf A. (1954) Subependymal glomerate astrocytomas. *J Neuropathol Exp Neurol* 13:30–49.

Brown DF, Gazdar AF, White CL, III, et al. (1997) Human telomerase RNA expression and MIB-1 (Ki-67) proliferation index distinguish hemangioblastomas from metastatic renal cell carcinomas. *J Neuropathol Exp Neurol* 56:1349–1355.

Burger PC, Rawlings CE, Cox EB, et al. (1987) Clinicopathologic correlations in the oligodendroglioma. *Cancer* 59:1345–1352.

Burger PC, Vogel FS, Green SB. (1985) Glioblastoma and anaplastic astrocytoma: pathologic criteria and prognostic implications. *Cancer* 56:1106–1111.

Cahill DW, Bashirelahi H, Solomon LW, et al. (1984) Estrogen and progesterone receptors in meningiomas. *J Neurosurg* 60:985–993.

Cairncross JG, MacDonald D, Ludwin S, et al. (1994) Chemotherapy for anaplastic oligodendroglioma. *J Clin Oncol* 12:2013–2021.

Cairncross JG, Ueki K, Zlatescu MC, et al. (1998) Specific genetic predictors of chemotherapeutic response and survival in patients with anaplastic oligodendrogliomas. *J Natl Cancer Inst* 7:1473–1479.

Casadei GP, Scheithauer BW, Hirose T, et al. (1995) Cellular schwannoma. A clinicopathologic, DNA flow cytometric, proliferation marker study of 70 patients. *Cancer* 75:1109–1119.

Cavanaugh JB. (1958) On certain small tumors encountered in the temporal lobe. *Brain* 81:389–405.

Choi NW, Schumann LM, Gullen WH. (1970) Epidemiology of primary central nervous system neoplasms. *Am J Epidemiol* 91:467–485.

Clelland CA, Treip CS. (1989) Histological differentiation of metastatic renal cell carcinoma of the cerebellum from cerebellar hemangioblastoma in von Hippel–Lindau's disease. *J Neurol Neurosurg Psychiatr* 52:162–166.

Cohadon F, Aouad N, Rougier A, et al. (1985) Histologic and non-histologic factors correlated with survival time in supratentorial astrocytic tumors. *J Neurooncol* 3:105–111.

Conner JM, Pirrit LA, Yates JR, et al. (1987) Linkage of the tuberous sclerosis locus to a DNA polymorphism detected by v-abl. *J Med Genet* 24:544–546.

Coons SW, Johnson PC, Scheithauer BW, et al. (1996) Improving diagnostic accuracy and interobserver concordance in the classification and grading of primary gliomas. *Cancer* 79:1381–1393.

Cramer F, Kimsey W. (1952) The cerebellar hemangioblastomas—review of 53 cases, with special reference to cerebellar cysts and the association of polycythemia. *Arch Neurol Psychiatr* 67:237–252.

Daumas-Duport C. (1993) Dysembryoplastic neuroepithelial tumors. *Brain Pathol* 3:283–295.

Daumas-Duport C, Scheithauer BW, Chodkiewicz J-P, et al. (1988) Dysembryoplastic neuroepithelial tumor: a surgically curable tumor of young patients with intractable partial seizures. *Neurosurgery* 23: 545–556.

Daumas-Duport C, Tucker ML, Kolles H, et al. (1997) Oligodendrogliomas. Part II: A new grading system based on morphological and imaging criteria. *J Neurooncol* 34:61–78.

De la Monte SM, Flickinger J, Linggood RM. (1986) Histopathologic features predicting recurrence of meningiomas following subtotal excision. *Am J Surg Pathol* 10:836–843.

Del Arco A, Garcia J, Arribas C, et al. (1993) Timing of p53 mutations during astrocytoma tumorigenesis. *Hum Mol Genet* 2:1687–1690.

Dorhmann GJ, Rubin JM. (1985) Dynamic intraoperative imaging and instrumentation of brain and spinal cord using ultrasound. *Neurol Clin* 3:425–437.

Dwyer KW, Naul LG, Hise JH. (1996) Gliosarcoma: MR features. *J Comput Assist Tomogr* 20:719–723.

Eppenberger U, Mueller H. (1994) Growth factor receptors and their ligands. *J Neurooncol* 22:249–254.

Forsyth PA, Shaw EG, Scheithauer BW, et al. (1993) Supratentorial pilocytic astrocytomas. A clinicopathologic, prognostic, and flow cytometric study of 51 patients. *Cancer* 72:1335–1342.

Fort DW, Tonk VS, Tomlinson GE, et al. (1994) Rhabdoid tumor of the kidney with primitive neuroectodermal tumor of the central nervous system: associated tumors with different histologic, cytogenetic, and molecular findings. *Genes Chromosomes Cancer* 11:146–152.

Gajjar A, Bhargava R, Jenkins JJ, et al. (1995) Low-grade astrocytoma with neuraxis dissemination at diagnosis. *J Neurooncol* 83:67–71.

Giannini C, Scheithauer BW. (1997) Classification and grading of low-grade astrocytic tumors in children. *Brain Pathol* 7:785–798.

Giannini C, Scheithauer BW, Burger PC, et al. (1999) Cellular proliferation in pilocytic and diffuse astrocytomas. *J Neuropathol Exp Neurol* 58:46–53.

Gouldesbraugh DR, Bell JE, Gordon A. (1988) Use of immunohistochemical methods in the differential diagnosis between primary cerebellar hemangioblastoma and metastatic renal cell carcinoma. *J Clin Pathol* 41:861–865.

Grant JW, Gallagher PJ, Hedinger C. (1988). Hemangioblastoma. An immunohistochemical study of ten cases. *Acta Neuropathol (Berl)* 76:82–86.

Gyure KA, Prayson RA. (1997) Subependymal giant cell astrocytoma: a clinicopathologic study with HMB-45 and MIB-1 immunohistochemical analysis. *Mod Pathol* 4:313–317.

Hamilton IF, Pollock IF. (1997) The molecular biology of ependymomas. *Brain Pathol* 7:807–822.

Harrison MJ, Wolfe DE, Lau TS, et al. (1991) Radiation-induced meningiomas: experience at the Mount Sinai Hospital and review of the literature. *J Neurosurg* 75:564–574.

Hassoun J, Gambarelli D, Grisoli F, et al. (1982) Central neurocytoma. An electron-microscopic study of two cases. *Acta Neuropathol (Berl)* 76:151–156.

Hope JK, Armstrong DA, Babyn PS, et al. (1992) Primary meningeal tumors in children: correlation of clinical and CT finding with histologic type and prognosis. *Am J Neuroradiol* 13:1353–1364.

Iglasias-Rozas JR, Collia-Fernandez F. (1980) Early proliferations of the nervous system tumors in man. *Morfolog Norm Patolog B* 4:511.

Ironside JW, Battersby RDE, Dangerfield VJM, et al. (1986) Cryostat section assay of oestrogen and progesterone receptors in meningiomas: a clinicopathological study. *J Clin Pathol* 39:44–50.

Ishii N, Sawamura Y, Tada M, et al. (1998) Absence of p53 gene mutations in a tumor panel representative of pilocytic astrocytoma diversity using a p53 functional assay. *Int J Cancer* 76:797–800.

Jaaskelainen J. (1986) Seemingly complete removal of histologically benign intracranial meningioma: late recurrence rate and factors predicting recurrence in 657 patients. A multivariate analysis. *Surg Neurol* 26:461–469.

Jacoby LB, MacCollin M, Louis DN, et al. (1994) Exon scanning for mutation of the NF2 gene in schwannomas. *Hum Mol Genet* 3:413–419.

Kadin ME, Rubinstein LJ, Nelson JS. (1970) Neonatal cerebellar medulloblastoma originating from the fetal external granular layer. *J Neuropathol Exp Neurol* 29:583–600.

Kandt RS, Haines JL, Smith M, et al. (1992) Linkage of an important gene locus for tuberous sclerosis to a chromosome 16 marker for polycystic kidney disease. *Nat Genet* 2:37–41.

Karamitopoulou E, Perentes E, Diamantis I, Maraziotis T. (1994) Ki-67 immunoreactivity in human central nervous system tumors: a study with MIG-1 monclonal antibody on archival material. *Acta Neuropathol Berl* 87:47–54.

Katsetos CD, Herman MM, Frankfurter A, et al. (1989) Cerebellar desmoplastic medulloblastomas. A further immunohistochemical characterization of the reticulin-free pale islands. *Arch Pathol Lab Med* 113:1019–1029.

Kawano N, Yada K, Yagashita S. (1989) Clear cell ependymoma. A histologic variant with diagnostic implications. *Virchows Arch A Pathol Anat* 415:467–472.

Kepes JJ. (1982) *Meningiomas. Biology, Pathology and Differential Diagnosis.* Masson, New York.

Kepes JJ, Chen WY, Connors MH, Vogel FS. (1988) "Chordoid" meningeal tumors in young individuals with peritumoral lymphoplasmacellular infiltrates causing systemic manifestations of the Castleman syndrome. A report of seven cases. *Cancer* 62:391–406.

Kernohan JW, Mabon RF, Svien HJ, et al. (1949) A simplified classification of the gliomas. *Proc Staff Meeting Mayo Clinic* 24:71–75.

Kerr DJ, Scheithauer BW, Miller GM, et al. (1995) Hemangioblastoma of optic nerve: a case report. *J Neurosurg* 36:573–581.

Kirkegaard LJ, DeRose PB, Yao B, et al. (1998) Image cytometric measurement of nuclear proliferation markers (MIB-1, PCNA) in astrocytomas. Prognostic significance. *Am J Clin Pathol* 109:69–74.

Kleihues P, Burger PC, Scheithauer BW. (1993) *Histological Typing of Tumors of the Central Nervous System. World Health Organization International Histological Classification of Tumors,* 2nd ed. Springer-Verlag, Heidelberg.

Kleinman GM, Liszezak T, Tarlov E, Richardson EP. (1980) Microcystic variant of meningioma. A light microscopic and ultrastructural study. *Am J Surg Pathol* 4:383–389.

Kros JM, Troost D, van Eden GC, et al. (1988) Oligodendroglioma: a comparison of two grading systems. *Cancer* 61:2251–2259.

Krouwer HG, Davis RL, Silver P, et al. (1991) Gemistocytic astrocytomas: a reappraisal. *J Neurosurg* 74:399–406.

Latif F, Tory K, Gnarra J, et al. (1993) Identification of the von Hippel disease tumor suppressor gene. *Science* 260:1317–1320.

Lerman MI, Latif F, Glenn GM, et al. (1991) Isolation and regional localization of a large collection (2,000) of single-copy DNA fragments on human chromosome 3 for mapping and cloning tumor suppressor genes. *Hum Genet* 86:567–577.

Linwicz BH, Berger TS, Linwicz RG, Aron BS. (1985) Radiation-associated gliomas: a report of four cases and analysis of postradiation tumors of the central nervous system. *Neurosurgery* 17:436–445.

Lopez MB, Altermatt HJ, Scheithauer BW, et al. (1996) Immunohistochemical characterization of subependymal giant cell astrocytomas. *Acta Neuropathol* 86:368–375.

Louis DN, Ramesh V, Gusella JF. (1995) Meuropathology and molecular genetics of neurofibromatosis 2 and related tumors. *Brain Pathol* 5:163–172.

Ludwin SK, Rubinstein LJ, Russell DS. (1975) Papillary meningiomas: a malignant variant of meningioima. *Cancer* 36:1363–1373.

Lyons MK, Kelly PJ. (1991) Posterior fossa ependymomas: report of 30 cases and review of the literature. *Neurosurgery* 28:659–665.

Mack E, Wilson C. (1993) Meningioma induced by high-dose cranial irradiation. *J Neurosurg* 79:28–31.

Maintz D, Fiedler K, Koopman J, et al. (1997) Molecular genetic evidence for subtypes of oligoastrocytomas. *J Neuropathol Exp Neurol* 56:1098–1104.

Miller DC, Koslow M, Budzilovich GB, Burstein DE. (1990) Synaptophysin: a sensitive and specific marker for ganglion cells in central nervous system neoplasms. *Hum Pathol* 21:271–276.

Modan B, Baidatz D, Mart H, et al. (1974) Radiation-induced head and neck tumors. *Lancet* 1:277–279.

Moore M, Black PM, Ellenbogen R, et al. (1989) Stereotactic craniotomy: Methods and results using the Brown-Roberts-Wells stereotactic frame. *Neurosurgery* 25:572–577.

Mork SJ, Halvorsen TB, Lindegaard K-F, Eide GE. (1986) Oligodendroglioma. Histologic evaluation and prognosis. *J Neuropathol Exp Neurol* 45:65–78.

Mork SJ, Loken AC. (1977) Ependymoma. A follow-up study of 101 cases. *Cancer* 40:907–915.

Nemes Z. (1992) Fibrohistiocytic differentiation to capillary hemangioblastoma. *Hum Pathol* 23:805–810.

Ng HK, Lam PY. (1998) The molecular genetics of central nervous system tumors. *Pathology* 30:196–202.

Nishio S, Takeshita I, Fukui M, et al. (1988a) Anaplastic evolution of childhood optico-hypothalamic pilocytic astrocytoma. Report of an autopsy case. *Clin Neuropathol* 7:254–258.

Nishio S, Takeshita I, Fukui M, et al. (1988b) Intraventricular neurocytoma: clinicopathological features of six cases. *J Neurosurg* 68:665–670.

Nobles E, Lee R, Kircher T. (1991) Mediastinal ependymoma. *Hum Pathol* 22:94–96.

Ouallet JC, Marsot-Dupuch K, van Effenterre R, et al. (1997) Papillary adenoma of endolymphatic sac origin: temporal bone tumor in von Hippel–Lindau disease. Case report. *J Neurosurg* 87:445–449.

Paraf F, Jothy S, Van Meir EG. (1997) Brain tumor–polyposis syndrome: two genetic diseases? *J Clin Oncol* 7:2744–2758.

Parisi JE, Scheithauer BW, Priest JR, et al. (1992) Desmoplastic infantile ganglioglioma (DIG): a form of ganglioglioma. *J Neuropathol Exp Neurol* 51:365.

Pasquier B, Gasnier F, Pasquier D, et al. (1986) Papillary meningioma: clinicopathologic study of seven cases and review of the literature. *Cancer* 58:299–305.

Paulus W, Schlote W, Perentes E, et al. (1992) Desmoplastic supratentorial tumors of infancy. *Histopathology* 21:43–49.

Perez-Diaz C, Cabello A, Lobato RD, et al. (1985) Oligodendrogliomas arising in the scar of a brain contusion. Report of two surgically verified cases. *Surg Neurol* 24:581–586.

Peters N, Wellenreuther R, Rollbrocker B, et al. (1998) Analysis of the PTEN gene in human meningiomas. *Neuropathol Appl Neurobiol* 24:3–8.

Platten M, Giordano MJ, Dirven CM, et al. (1996) Upregulation of specific NF-1 gene transcripts in sporadic pilocytic astrocytoma. *Am J Pathol* 149:621–627.

Platten M, Meyer-Puttlitz B, Blumcke I, et al. (1997) A novel splice gene associated polymorphism in the tuberous sclerosis 2 (TSC2) gene may predispose to the development of sporadic gangliogliomas. *J Neuropathol Exp Neurol* 56:806–810.

Prayson RA. (1996) Malignant meningioma: a clinicopatholgoic study of 23 patients including MIB-1 and p53 imunohistochemistry. *Am J Clin Pathol* 105:719–726.

Rachlin JR, Rosenblum ML. (1991) Etiology and biology of meningiomas. In: *Meningiomas* (Al-Mefty O, ed.). Raven Press, New York.

Rainov NG, Lubbe J, Renshaw J, et al. (1995) Association of Wilms' tumor with primary brain tumor in siblings. *J Neuropathol Exp Neurol* 54:214–223.

Reifenberger J, Reifenberger G, Liu L, et al. (1994) Molecular genetic analysis of oligodendroglial tumors shows preferential allelic deletions of 19q and 1p. *Am J Pathol* 145:1175–1190.

Riccardi VM. (1987) Neurofibromatosis. *Neurol Clin* 5:337–345.

Ron E, Modan B, Boice JD Jr, et al. (1988) Tumors of the brain and nervous system after radiotherapy in childhood. *N Engl J Med* 319:1033–1039.

Rorke LB. (1983) Presidential address: the cerebellar medulloblastoma and its relationship to primitive neuroectodermal tumors. *J Neuropathol Exp Neurol* 42:1–15.

Rorke LB, Packer RJ, Biegel JA. (1996) Central nervous system atypical teratoid/rhabdoid tumors of infancy and childhood: definition of an entity. *J Neurosurg* 85:56–65.

Ross GW, Rubinstein LJ. (1989) Lack of histopathological correlation of malignant ependymomas with postoperative survival. *J Neurosurg* 70:31–36.

Rubinstein LJ. (1985) Embryonal central neuroepthelial tumors and their differenting potential: review article. *J Neurosurg* 62:795–805.

Rubinstein LJ, Northfield DW. (1964) Medulloblastoma and the so-called "arachnoidal cerebellar sarcoma." A critical reexamination of a nosological problem. *Brain* 87:379–412.

Rushing EJ, Brown DF, Hladik CL, et al. (1998) Correlation of bcl-2, p53, and MIB-1 expression with ependymoma grade and subtype. *Mod Pathol* 11:464–470.

Rushing EJ, Yashima K, Brown DF, et al. (1997) Expression of telom,erase RNA component correlates with the MIB-1 proliferation index in ependymomas. *J Neuropathol Exp Neurol* 56:1142–1146.

Russell DS, Rubinstein LJ. (1962) Ganglioglioma: a case with long history and malignant evolution. *J Neuropathol Exp Neurol* 21:185–193.

Russell DS, Rubinstein LJ. (1989) *Pathology of Tumors of the Nervous System*, 5th ed. Williams and Wilkins, Baltimore.

Schiffer D, Chio A, Gordana T, et al. (1988) Prognostic value of histologic factors in adult cerebral astrocytoma. *Cancer* 61:1386–1393.

Scheithauer BW. (1978) Symptomatic subependymoma: report of 21 cases with review of the literature. *J Neurosurg* 49:689–696.

Sima AAF, Finkelstein SD, McLachlin DR. (1983) Multiple malignant astrocytomas in a patient with spontaneous progressive multifocal leukoencephalopathy. *Ann Neurol* 14:183–188.

Simon M, von Deimling A, Arson J, et al. (1995) Allelic losses on chromosomes 14, 10, and 22 in atypical and malignant menigiomas: a genetic model of meningioma progression. *Cancer Res* 55:4696–4701.

Sloof JL, Kernohan JW, MacCarty CS. (1964) *Primary Intramedullary Tumors of the Spinal Cord and Filum Terminale.* W. B. Saunders, Philadelphia.

Smith MT, Ludwig CL, Godfrey AD, Armbrustmacher VW. (1983) Grading of oligodendrogliomas. *Cancer* 52:2107–2114.

Sznajder L, Abrahams C, Parry DM, et al. (1996) Multiple schwannomas and meningiomas associated with irradiation in childhood. *Arch Intern Med* 156: 1873–1878.

Sonneland PR, Scheithauer BW, Onofrio BM. (1985) Myxopapillary ependymoma. A clinicopathologic and immunocytochemical study of 77 cases. *Cancer* 56:883–893.

Tilzer LL, Plapp FV, Evans JP, et al. (1982) Steroid receptor proteins in human meningiomas. *Cancer* 49: 633–636.

Tomlinson FH, Scheithauer BW, Hayostek CJ, et al. (1994) The significance of atypia and histologic malignancy in pilocytic astrocytoma of the cerebellum: a clinicopathologic and flow cytometric study. *J Child Neurol* 9:301–310.

Townsend JJ, Seaman JP. (1986) Central neurocytoma—a rare benign intraventricular tumor. *Acta Neuropathol (Berl)* 71:167–179.

VandenBerg SR. (1993) Desmoplastic infantile ganglioglioma and desmoplastic cerebral astrocytoma of infancy. *Brain Pathol* 3:275–281.

Von Deimling A, Kleihues P, Saremaslani P, et al. (1991) Histogenesis and defferentiation potential of central neurocytomas. *Lab Invest* 64:585–591.

Von Deimling A, Louis DN, Wiestler OD. (1995) Molecular pathways in the formation of gliomas. *Glia* 15:328–338.

Wellenreuther R, Kraus JA, Lenartz D, et al. (1995) Analysis of the neurofibromatosis 2 gene reveals molecular variants of meningioma. *Am J Pathol* 146:827–832.

Wellenreuther R, Waha A, Vogel Y, et al. (1997) Qantitative analysis of neruofibromatosis type 2 gene transcripts in meningiomas supports the concept of distinct molecular variants. *Lab Invest* 77:601–606.

Westermark B, Nister M. (1995) Molecular genetics of human glioma. *Curr Opin Oncol* 7:220–225.

Wilson SB, Feinsod M, Hoyt WF, Nielsen SL. (1976) Malignant evolution of childhood chiasmal pilocytic astrocytoma. *Neurology* 26:322–325.

Wolf HK, Muller MB, Spanle M, et al. (1994) Ganglioglioma: a detailed histopathological and immunohistochemical analysis of 61 cases. *Acta Neuropathol* 88:166–173.

Zorludemir S, Scheithauer BW, Hirose T, et al. (1995) Clear cell meningioma. A clinicopathologic sutdy of a potentially aggressive variant of meningioma. *Am J Surg Pathol* 19:493–505.

Zucarello M, Sawaya R, deCourten-Myers G. (1986) Glioblastoma occurring after fadiation therapy for meningioma. *Neurosurgery* 19:114–119.

31

EYE

R. Nick Hogan

Both the external ocular adnexa (eyelids and associated structures, periorbital tissues) as well as the intraocular tissues of the eye are known to exhibit several types of lesions documented to represent incipient neoplasia. Because of higher clinical visibility, preneoplastic lesions are more frequently noted in the external compartments than intraocularly. The exception is when preneoplastic processes within the globe alter visual function, thereby leading to early professional evaluation, or when lesions are found incidentally on routine ophthalmic examination. Unfortunately, once vision is affected, it is often late in the game, and neoplastic dynamics may then be well past the incipient stage. The end result is often loss of the eye, a highly dramatic and potentially disabling consequence. The obvious goal of the clinician is to be aware of the appearance of preneoplastic lesions so that treatment can be instituted early or the lesion can be watched very closely. The pathologist, therefore, is a key figure in the patient care team. Pathologists, by defining the cytologic characteristics of clinically suspicious lesions after biopsy, aid in development of cogent treatment plans. By defining lesions as preneoplastic, the pathologist furthers the education of the clinician in the early recognition of such lesions. External tissues of the eye include the eyelids, lacrimal gland, lacrimal drainage apparatus, extraocular musculature, palpebral and bulbar conjunctiva, cornea, and sclera. Preneo-

plastic lesions of the lids are similar to those of sun-exposed skin elsewhere and are covered in Chapter 2 of this volume. Lacrimal gland processes are similar to those of the major salivary glands and are discussed in Chapters 5 and 28. The focus of this section, therefore, will be on incipient lesions of tissues of the ocular globe itself, both upon its surface and within the globe.

CONJUNCTIVA

SQUAMOUS DYSPLASIA

Epithelial dysplasia is one of the most frequent clinical concerns resulting in conjunctival biopsy. It is well recognized that some dysplastic processes in the conjunctiva can progress to more aggressive neoplastic lesions including invasive squamous cell carcinoma (Grossniklaus et al., 1987; Spencer, 1996). That conjunctival epithelial tumors are second only to lid tumors in frequency validates the need for scrutiny (McLean et al., 1994a).

Dysplasia can occur anywhere in the conjunctiva but is seen more often in the sun-exposed regions of interpalpebral bulbar conjunctiva than in the fornices or palpebral conjunctiva. Significant dysplasia of the conjunctiva of the fornices or palpebral regions is more prognostically ominous. Association with other actinic lesions such as pinqueculae and pterygia is frequent. Biopsies from males are more frequently dysplastic than those from females and are performed more commonly in older individuals. Patient geographic location relative to sun exposure probably plays a role in the development of dysplastic changes; conjunctival epithelial tumors appear more frequently in patients from countries near the equator (Brazil, 48.9%) than those in northern latitudes (England, 33.8%) (McLean et al., 1994a).

Conjunctival dysplasia appears clinically as an ill-defined, elevated, gelatinous-appearing region, often attendant with prominent vasculature, blending with the surrounding conjunctiva, and without leukoplakia (Fig. 31–1). Lack of a well-demarcated lesion frequently results in only partial excision. While usually appearing sessile, lesions with severe degrees of cytologic atypia often appear papilliform, making biopsy of any such lesion appearing close to the corneal limbus mandatory. Benign conjunctival papillomas are usually not located adjacent to the limbus (Waring et al., 1984). Infectious papillomas of the conjunctiva can exhibit varying degrees of mild pleomorphism and dysplasia, but usually koilocytes are apparent. DNA from human papillomavirus types 11, 16,

and 18 have been detected in some lesions through molecular hybridization and immunohistochemical techniques (Lass et al., 1983; Lauer et al., 1990; McDonnell et al., 1986, 1992).

Like the uterine cervix, intraepithelial extent of dysplasia is the key factor relative to the incipient nature of neoplastic transformation. A scheme for gradation into mild, moderate, and severe forms is routinely employed (McLean et al., 1994a; Spencer, 1996). Dysplastic lesions display relative acanthosis and atypia with loss of the usual maturational progression from basal to superficial layers. Nuclei become larger, more hyperchromatic, and pleomorphic. When confined to the basalar regions, dysplasia is graded as mild (Fig. 31–2). Involvement of up to two-thirds of the epithelium qualifies as moderate grade (Fig. 31–3). When dysplasia occupies all but the most superficial epithelial cell layer, it is classed as severe (Fig. 31–4). Only true full-thickness lesions should be called carcinoma *in situ*, and are often attended with prominent mitoses in all cell layers (Fig. 31–5). Typically, as the grade worsens, so does the degree of cellular atypia, the overall risk of recurrence after re-

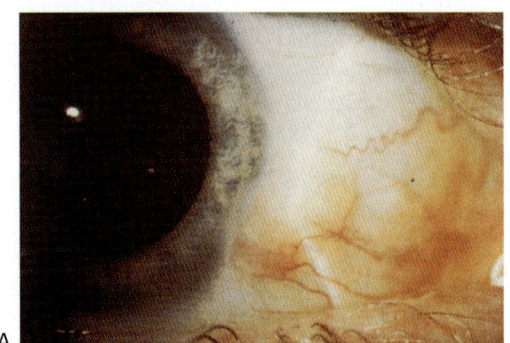
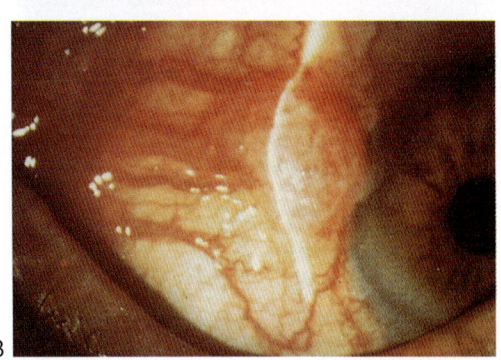
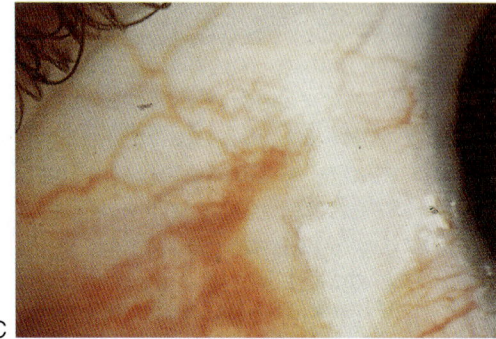

A

C

B

Figure 31–1. Clinical photomicrographs of conjunctival intraepithelial neoplasia (CIN; squamous carcinoma *in situ*). *Left*: Typical presentation of gelatinous mass at the corneoscleral limbus. *Center*: Papillomatous presentation of CIN. Similar lesions further posterior to the limbus are more likely to be benign papillomata. *Right*: CIN with leukoplakia (surface keratinization). [From Conlon MR, Alfonso EC, Starck T, Albert DM. (1994) Tumors of the cornea and conjunctiva. In: *Principles and Practice of Ophthalmology* (Albert DA, Jakobiec FA, eds.) p. 283, W.B. Saunders, Philadelphia, with permission.]

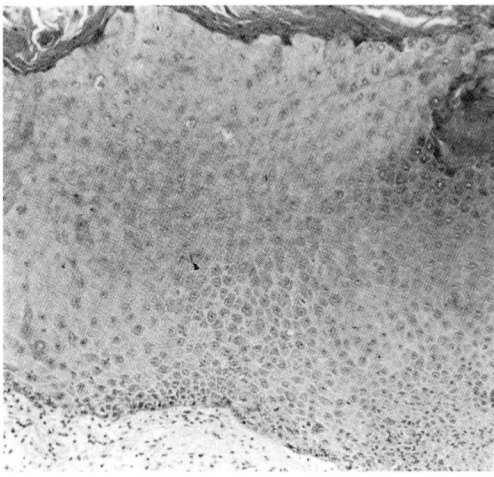

Figure 31–2. Mild conjunctival dysplasia. Epithelium is acanthotic with hyperkeratosis and parakeratosis. Dysplastic features are limited to the basal third of the epithelium. [From Grossniklaus HE, Green WR, Luckenbach M, Chan CC. (1987) Conjunctival lesions in adults. A clinical and histopathologic review. *Cornea* 6:110, with permission.]

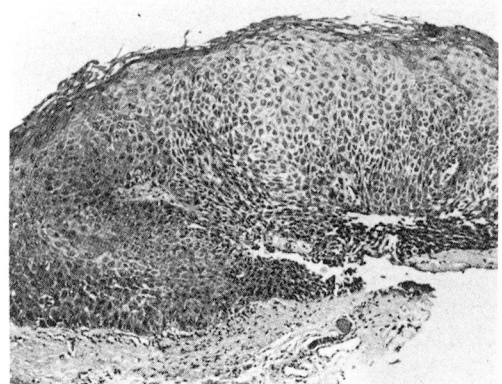

Figure 31–4. Severe conjunctival dysplasia. Pleomorphic, dysplastic cells occupy nearly all but the most superficial epithelial layers. [From Grossniklaus HE, Green WR, Luckenbach M, Chan CC. (1989) Conjunctival lesions in adults. A clinical and histopathologic review. *Cornea* 6:110, with permission.]

section, and the probability of malignant transformation. When dysplastic cells breach the basement membrane and invade the substantia propria, the line is crossed into invasive squamous cell carcinoma.

While imprint cytology has been utilized in a nonsurgical attempt to diagnose conjunctival dysplasia, sampling errors have precluded routine use. The relative grade cannot be evaluated and dysplastic epithelium can also be seen in otherwise benign conjunctival papillomas (Dykstra and Dyk-

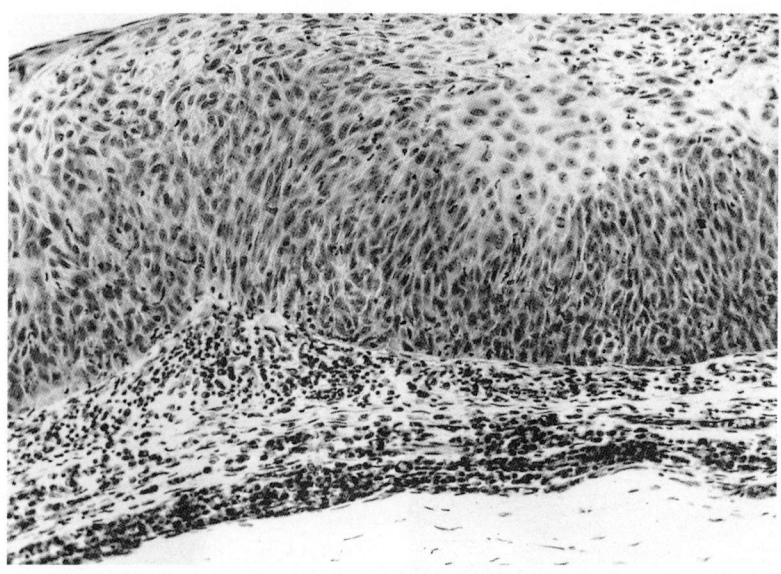

Figure 31–3. Moderate conjunctival dysplasia. Dysplastic features are limited to the basal two-thirds of the acanthotic epithelium. [From McLean IW, Burnier MN, Zimmerman LE, Jakobiec FA. (1994) Tumors of the conjunctiva. In: *Atlas of Tumor Pathology. Tumors of the Eye and Ocular Adnexa.* p. 59, Armed Forces Institute of Pathology, Washington, DC, with permission).

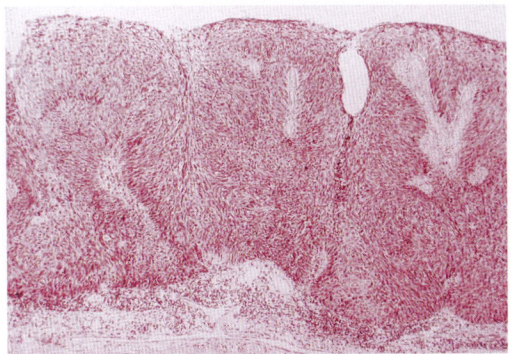

Figure 31–5. Conjunctival squamous carcinoma *in situ*, or conjunctival intraepithelial neoplasia (CIN). The entire epithelial thickness contains dysplastic cells without invasion of the underlying substantia propria. [From Zimmerman LE. (1980) *Histological Typing of Tumours of the Eye and its Adnexa.* p. 28, World Health Organization, Geneva, with permission.]

stra, 1969). Accepted diagnostic techniques for clinically suspicious lesions include excisional biopsy with cryoablation of the surgical margins and bed using a double freeze-thaw technique (Jakobiec et al., 1989). Additional regions of suspicious conjunctiva should be biopsied and regionally mapped on a drawing relayed to the pathologist. In this manner, possible contiguous spread can be regionally analyzed and monitored.

ACTINIC KERATOSIS

Actinic keratosis of the conjunctiva usually appears in the interpalpebral and perilimbal regions of the eye, and hence has been linked to prolonged exposure to ultraviolet light (Clear et al., 1979). Geographically they occur more frequently in patients living near the equator and in the elderly. Lesions appear clinically as well-demarcated, raised, well vascularized masses with a white surface due to keratinization (leukoplakia) (Fig. 31–6). Differentiation on clinical grounds from more aggressive epithelial tumors is difficult. Hence, all such lesions should be excised.

Actinic keratoses exhibit a wide range of histologic variability, but all demonstrate acanthotic epithelium with hyperkeratosis and parakeratosis (Fig. 31–7). Cellular atypia, dysplasia, and mitotic activity are variable, but the basement membrane is always intact. They frequently are attended by evidence of actinic damage to the collagen of the underlying substantia propria with attendant elastotic degeneration (Ledoux-Corbusier and Danis, 1979; McLean et al., 1994a; Spencer, 1996).

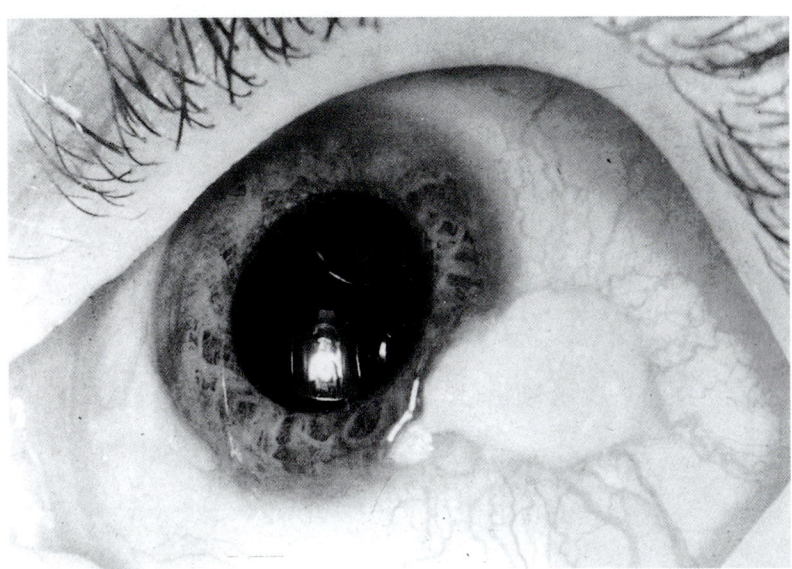

Figure 31–6. Clinical photograph of conjunctival actinic keratosis showing elevated limbal mass with leukoplakia (keratinization) in the interpalpebral zone. [From McLean IW, Burnier MN, Zimmerman LE, Jakobiec FA. (1994) Tumors of the conjunctiva. In: *Atlas of Tumor Pathology. Tumors of the Eye and Ocular Adnexa,* p. 56, Armed Forces Institute of Pathology, Washington, DC, with permission.]

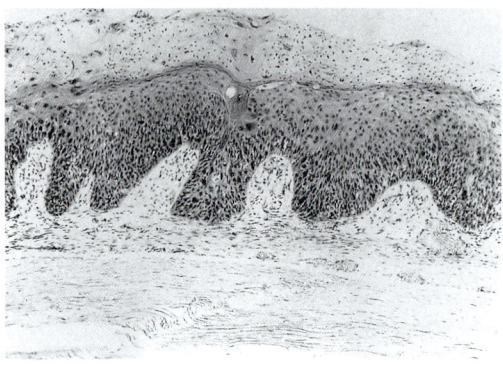

Figure 31–7. Actinic keratosis showing severe intraepithelial atypia with parakeratosis in conjunctiva and cornea. [From McLean IW, Burnier MN, Zimmerman LE, Jakobiec FA. (1994) Tumors of the conjunctiva. In: *Atlas of Tumor Pathology. Tumors of the Eye and Ocular Adnexa*, p. 57, Armed Forces Institute of Pathology, Washington, DC, with permission.]

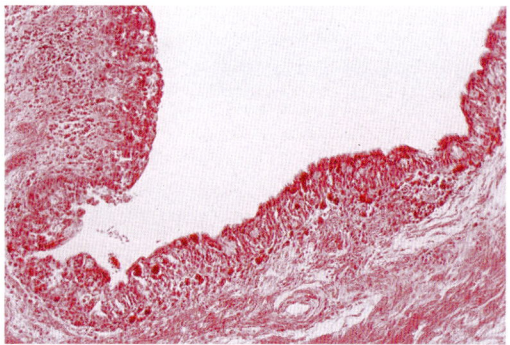

Figure 31–8. Primary acquired melanosis (PAM) of the conjunctiva. Increased number of melanocytic cells in the basalar epithelium without significant cytologic atypia. [From Zimmerman LE. (1980) *Histological Typing of Tumours of the Eye and its Adnexa.* p. 30, World Health Organization, Geneva, with permission.]

Melanocytosis

As summarized in the classification adopted by the World Health Organization (WHO) (Zimmerman and Sobin, 1980), intraepithelial melanocytic lesions of the conjunctiva are divided into two groups based on the cytologic atypia of the melanocytes. *Primary acquired melanosis (PAM) without atypia* appears histologically as increased numbers of benign-appearing melanocytes, mostly located in the basilar region of the epithelium, and without significant nesting patterns (Fig. 31–8). In this regard, there is overlap with the microscopic findings of an ephilis (Folberg, 1996). *Conjunctival ephilae,* however are usually smaller, well circumscribed, and lack history of growth. Ephilae occur in sun-exposed regions and not in the fornices or on palpebral conjunctiva, whereas PAM can occur anywhere on the conjunctiva.

Folberg et al. (1985) examined the epidemiology of PAM in long-term follow-up of specimens submitted to the Armed Forces Institute of Pathology (AFIP). None of those designated as PAM without atypia showed progression to melanoma, and only one recurred after excision; thus PAM without atypia is not representative of an incipient neoplastic process (Folberg, 1996). Primary acquired melanosis with atypia, however, progressed to melanoma in 46.4% of cases and 60.7% recurred (Folberg et al., 1985).

Unfortunately, there are no reliable clinical criteria for judging atypia on the basis of inspection of the lesions alone, hence biopsy and histologic analysis is mandatory (Folberg et al., 1984, 1985; Jakobiec et al., 1989).

Primary acquired melanosis with atypia occurs when the melanocytic cells and pattern of growth appear atypical (Fig. 31–9). Four melanocytic cell configurations are prominent, including spindle-shaped, dendritiform, small epitheliod, and large epitheliod cells (Jakobiec et al., 1989). Growth patterns of atypical cells fall into five cate-

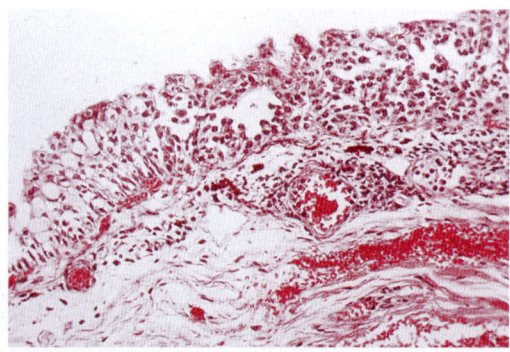

Figure 31–9. Primary acquired melanosis (PAM) of the conjunctiva, with atypia. The epithelium is nearly totally replaced by atypical melanocytic proliferation. [From Zimmerman LE. (1980) *Histological Typing of Tumours of the Eye and its Adnexa.* p. 30, World Health Organization, Geneva, with permission.]

gories: basilar hyperplasia, basilar nesting, intraepithelial nesting, full epithelial replacement, and pagetoid spread. Several cell types and patterns of growth may be present in a single specimen (Grossniklaus and Cameron, 1993). Junctional nevi are histologically similar to the basilar hyperplasia growth pattern of PAM with atypia, although junctional nevi are typically not found after young adulthood. The atypical melanocytes in PAM tend to fall away from one another and the adjacent epithelium (dyscohesiveness), whereas nevus cells tend to adhere to one another and to surrounding squamous cells. Furthermore, the epithelial cells adjacent to melanocytes may be significantly pigmented in PAM with atypia, whereas in junctional nevi, they usually are not. Pagetoid spread will only be seen in PAM with atypia (Folberg, 1996). Basilar projections of melanocytic nests into the substantia propria can simulate invasion, hence search for an intact basement membrane is important; PAM with atypia is, by definition, noninvasive (Folberg, 1996). Presence of melanin-containing macrophages in the substantia propria underlying PAM, or presence of PAM within the epithelium of pseudoglands of Henle (pouch-like epithelial infoldings into the substantia propria) should not be confused with invasive melanoma (Elsas et al., 1974; Folberg, 1996). Likewise, goblet cell ingestion of pigment may be confused with pagetoid spread. Bleaching specimens with potassium permanganate may be helpful in this regard. Pagetoid spread in PAM with atypia must be differentiated from the pagetoid cells of sebaceous carcinoma. A search should be made for HMB-45- and MART-1-negative cells, with large, "smudged" nuclei, foamy cytoplasm containing fats, surrounded by epithelial membrane antigen (EMA)-positive immunostaining. These are suggestive of sebaceous carcinoma cells.

Primary acquired melanosis with atypia results in progression to melanoma at a median rate of 2.5 years after the defining biopsy (Folberg et al., 1985). Most melanoma cases develop within 6 years, although one case developed as late as 10 years after diagnosis of PAM with atypia (Folberg, 1996). Presence of atypical melanocytes in any epithelial location other than the basilar regions promulgates the highest likelihood of progression to melanoma as does full-thickness epithelial involvement (90%) (Folberg et al., 1985). Lesions containing epitheliod-type melanocytes, often with prominent, eosinophilic nucleoli, result in progression to melanoma in 75% of cases (Folberg, 1996). Suspicious lesions, therefore, should be totally excised (Folberg and McLean, 1986; Jakobiec et al., 1989). Cryoablation of the surrounding edges and the tumor bed after lesion excision has been advocated (Brownstein et al., 1981; Jakobiec, et al., 1980, 1988). Localized irradiation of large diffuse lesions (Lommatzsch et al., 1990) and laser treatment are not widely employed (Jakobiec et al., 1989). Topical use of antimitotics such as mitomycin C in adjunctive treatment of PAM with atypia has shown promise and is currently being investigated (Folberg, 1996; Frucht-Perry and Ilsar, 1994; Frucht-Perry and Rozenman, 1994).

CORNEA

Because the cornea is avascular, neoplastic processes in the cornea are, with few exceptions, extension of disease from adjacent conjunctiva and/or eyelid (Waring et al., 1984). Occasionally, corneal tumors are metastatic from distant primary sites. Incipient neoplasia in corneal tissue is therefore generally indicative of problems elsewhere. However, when preneoplastic lesions are isolated to the cornea, they most commonly are related to varying degrees of intraepithelial dysplasia Corneal intraepithelial dysplasia appears clinically as a gray plaque on the corneal surface, with the central leading edge often arranged in finger-like projections that are sharply demarcated (Fig. 31–10). Histologic categorization is similar to that for conjunctival lesions; full-thickness dysplasia is designated carcinoma *in situ* or corneal intraepithelial neoplasia (CIN).

UVEAL TRACT

Uveal Tract Melanocytomas

Melanocytomas are essentially benign nevi that arise most commonly from uveal melanocytes adjacent to the optic nerve head, although they can be found in any re-

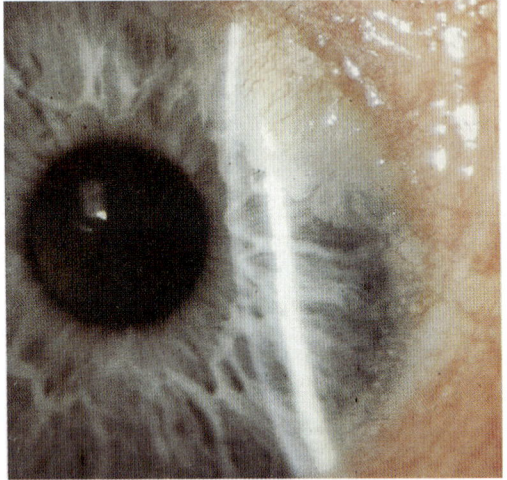

A

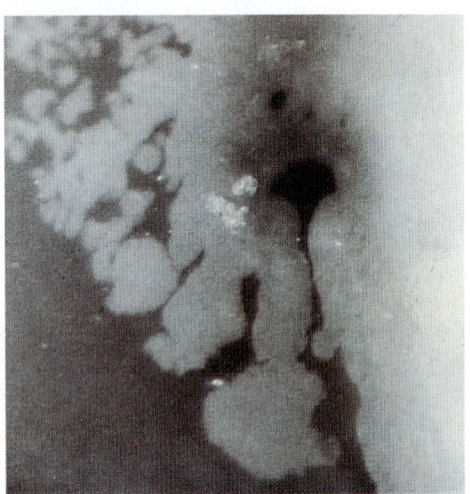

B

Figure 31–10. Clinical photograph of corneal intraepithelial neoplasia. *Left:* Translucent fingers of affected corneal epithelium are seen at 2:00 at the limbal margin. *Right:* Close-up of corneal intraepithelial neoplasia showing fimbrinated tongues of dysplastic epithelium with sharp demarcation from the nonaffected epithelium. [From Waring GO, Roth AM, Ekins MB. (1984) Clinical and pathologic description of 17 cases of corneal intraepithelial neoplasia. *Am J Ophthalmol* 97:547–559, with permission.]

gion of the uveal tract including the iris, ciliary body, and choroid (Reidy et al., 1985). They have also been reported in the conjunctiva (Folberg, et al., 1989; Verdaguer et al., 1974) and sclera (Lee et al., 1982; Reese, 1974). These lesions deserve consideration

in the present context because of rare reports of malignant transformation of uveal melanocytomas to melanoma (Apple et al., 1984; Barker-Griffith et al., 1976; Cialdini et al., 1989; Roth 1978). It should be noted, however, that controversy exists regarding the malignant potential of most of these lesions (LE Zimmerman comments following Roth, 1978). Nevertheless, the pathologist should be aware of the possible incipient neoplastic nature of melanocytomas, as concerning clinical characteristics frequently lead to biopsy or extirpation.

Uveal melanocytomas are deeply pigmented masses that usually remain quiescent or exhibit only very slow growth over years. Although melanocytomas are sometimes quite large and can be seen to locally infiltrate surrounding tissues, they never metastasize. Large amounts of intracellular pigment is seen in virtually every cell. On bleached sections, melanocytomas are composed of plump polyhedral cells containing abundant cytoplasm, small nuclei, and inconspicuous nucleoli (Fig. 31–11). They never demonstrate mitotic figures. Ultrastructurally, melanosomes are much larger than in cells from melanomas (Juarez and Tso, 1980). Pigment shedding sometimes occurs, especially from necrotic lesions, which can result in obstruction of filtration at the trabecular meshwork and secondary pigmentary glaucoma (Fineman et al., 1998; Nakazawa and Tamai, 1984; Shields et al., 1977; Teichmann and Karcioglu, 1995; Yamaguchi et al., 1987).

Iris Melanocytoma

Two cases of malignant transformation of melanocytoma of the iris have been reported by Thomas and Purnell (1969) and Cialdini et al. (1989). Two additional cases of iris plus ciliary body lesions were presented by Roth (1978). Neoplastic dedifferentiation was surmised in these masses because of the coexistence of typical melanocytoma cells admixed with spindle B melanoma cells with "a few" mitoses (Cialdini et al., 1989), or with cells possessing exceptionally large and prominent nucleoli (Thomas and Purnell, 1969) (Fig. 31–12). Reidy et al. (1985) point out that it is often difficult at the light microscopic level to define the presence of spindle-shaped cells at the periphery of a melanocytoma as being true malignant spin-

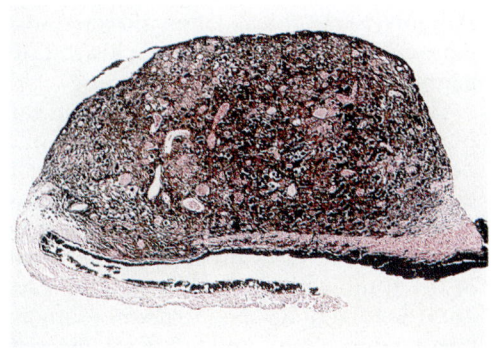
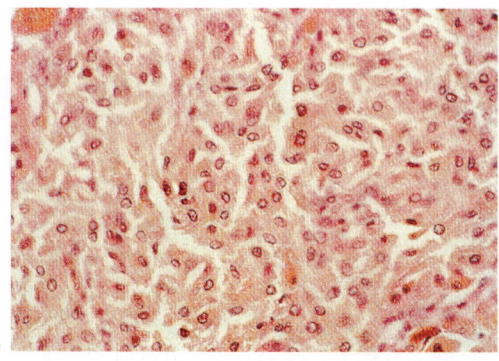

A

B

Figure 31–11. Melanocytoma of the iris. *Left*: Low-power photomicrograph of heavily pigmented iris nodule with prominent stromal vessels. *Right*: High-power micrograph of same tumor after bleaching, showing uniform polyhedral cells with abundant cytoplasm and benign-appearing nucleoli. [From Campbell RJ. (1998) *Histological Typing of Tumours of the Eye and Its Adnexa*, p. 33, 2nd ed., Springer-Verlag, Berlin, with permission.]

dle B cells as opposed to compressed melanocytoma cells, although nucleolar characteristics may help. As is often the case in pathology, clinical history describing rate of growth can be diagnostically useful.

Ciliary Body Melanocytoma

Malignant change in two ciliary body melanocytomas has been presented in the aforementioned series by Roth (1978). Histopathologic characteristics are similar to

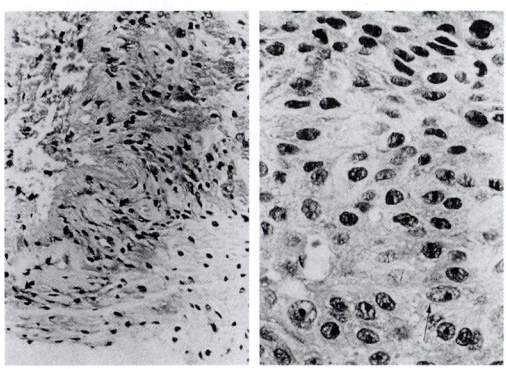

Figure 31–12. Photomicrograph of bleached sections of iris melanocytoma with malignant transformation. *Left*: Spindle-shaped nevus cells intermixed with plump polyhedral cells. *Right*: Region of tumor showing spindle B melanoma cells with prominent nucleoli and high nuclear-to-cytoplasmic ratio (arrow). [From Cialdini AP, Sahel JA, Jalkh AE, Weiter JJ, Zakka K, Albert DA. (1989) Malignant transformation of an iris melanocytoma. *Graefe's Arch Clin Exp Ophthalmol* 227:148–354, with permission.]

those described in dedifferentiated iris melanocytomas as summarized above.

Several cases of otherwise benign melanocytomas of the ciliary body have been described with associated extrascleral extension (Biswas et al., 1998; Rummelt et al., 1994; Stokes et al., 1993). However, the extrascleral lesions contained only cells consistent with melanocytoma, underscoring the locally invasive nature of some of these lesions despite the lack of rapid growth and significant mitotic activity. Ultrastructural studies have shown abundant endoplasmic reticulum and mitochondria within melanocytoma cells, indicating significant metabolic activity, which is believed to account for the local growth and invasiveness of some melanocytomas (Juarez and Tso, 1980).

Choroidal Melanocytoma

Eight cases of malignant melanoma arising in choroidal melanocytomas have been reported (Barker-Griffith et al., 1976; Heitman et al., 1988; Leidenix et al., 1994; Roth, 1978). Another case of presumed neoplastic transformation was published by Loeffler and Tecklenborg (1992). In the latter case, clinical criteria were used to initially diagnose the choroidal lesion as melanocytoma, including funduscopic appearance, lack of dye leakage on fluorescein angiography, and by ultrasound characteristics. On enucleation 7 years later, after a period of tumor growth, only spindle B melanoma cells were found; no melanocytoma cells were noted. This case therefore may not represent ma-

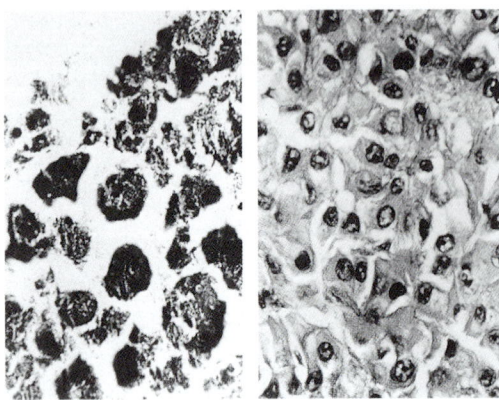

Figure 31–13. Photomicrographs of choroidal melanocytoma with malignant transformation. *Left:* Deeply pigmented polyhedral cells with small, round, centrally located nuclei. *Right:* Same tumor in region showing epitheliod-type melanoma cells. [From Leidenix M, Mamalis N, Goodart R, Harrie R, Kjeldsberg C. (1994) Malignant transformation of a necrotic melanocytoma of the choroid in an amblyopic eye. *Ann Ophthalmol* 26:42–46, with permission.]

lignant transformation but rather an unusually protracted growth of a spindle B melanoma. Likewise, Zimmerman has disagreed with the interpretation of what were called "melanocytoma cells" among the melanoma cells in the five cases presented by Roth (Zimmerman as discussion in Roth, 1978). The other two remaining cases appear to represent an admixture of melanocytoma and melanoma cells, suggesting possible transformation of a previous benign lesion (Fig. 31–13). Dedifferentiation of optic nerve melanocytomas is discussed below.

CILIARY BODY

MEDULLOEPITHELIOMA

These tumors emanate from the medullary epithelium, usually of the ciliary body but occasionally of the retina or optic nerve (McLean et al., 1994b). They represent heteroplastic dedifferentiation occurring either during or after embryonic development (congenital forms and adult forms, respectively). Both benign and malignant forms are observed. While frequently assumed, it

remains unclear how often direct transformation of the benign form yields the more aggressive and malignant form.

Historically, these lesions have been called both diktyomas and teratoneuromas, emphasizing the neuroepithelial banding patterning and neural nature of the masses (Green, 1996). Neither of these terms, however, fully embrace the heterologous nature of the tumors, which can include differentiation toward nonpigmented and pigmented ciliary epithelium, retinal pigment epithelium, retinal neurons, neuroglia, and vitreous. Tumors containing skeletal muscle, cartilage, and brain tissues are *teratoid* (McLean et al., 1994b). Malignancy is designated by anaplastic cellular appearance with high mitotic activity and presence of poorly differentiated neuronoid cells resembling retinoblastoma (McLean et al., 1994b).

In medulloepitheliomas, ciliary epithelium is seen to proliferate in sheets and cords of columnar epithelium and can vary from a single cell layer to multilaminate configurations reminiscent of immature retina (Fig. 31–14). Occasionally these structures can mimic the histologic findings of retinoblastoma including Homer Wright and Flexner-Wintersteiner rosettes, potentially causing diagnostic confusion (Green, 1996). Rudimentary external limiting membrane frequently appears along the apical borders of the cells. Both pigmented and nonpig-

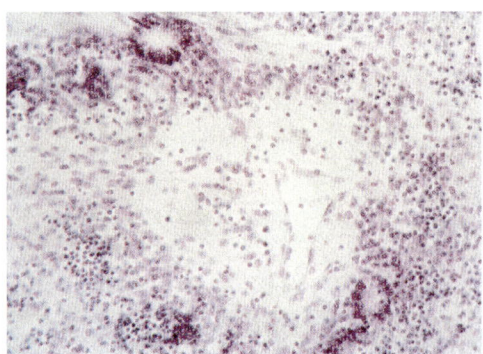

Figure 31–14. Benign medulloepitheliom of the ciliary body (nonteratoid). Ciliary muscle is replaced by small, dark, neuroepithelial cells with rosette formation. [From Campbell RJ. (1998) *Histological Typing of Tumours of the Eye and Its Adnexa,* p. 73, 2nd ed. Springer-Verlag, Berlin, with permission.]

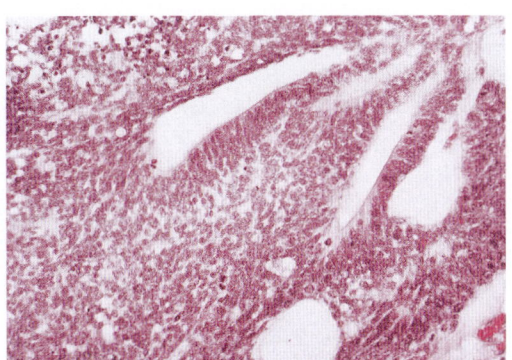

Figure 31–15. Malignant medulloepithelioma of the ciliary body. Sheets of multilayered undifferentiated neuroepithelial cells, similar to those of primative medullary epithelium, replace the ciliary muscle. [From Zimmerman LE. (1980) *Histological Typing of Tumours of the Eye and its Adnexa.* p. 74, World Health Organization, Geneva, with permission.]

mented epithelium can be seen. A basement membrane is elaborated basally separating cells from cystic spaces containing hyaluronidase-sensitive vitreous.

Malignancy is best determined by degree of invasiveness including extraocular extension (Green, 1996). Considerable pleomorphism and mitotic activity may be present and lesions can recur after excision (Fig. 31–15; Kivelä and Tarkkanen, 1988; Wakakura and Lee, 1990). Broughton and Zimmerman evaluated 56 medulloepitheliomas in the Registry of Ophthalmic Pathology for malignant features and survivability (Broughton and Zimmerman, 1978; Zimmerman and Broughton, 1978). Sixty-six percent of cases were malignant and 12.1% of these died of metastatic disease, with 4 cases lost to follow-up. Teratoid features were found in 21 cases (37.5%). Extraocular extension was present in 10 cases at the time of initial presentation. These tumors can mimic other intraocular lesions, including ciliary body melanoma, primary hyperplastic vitreous, and even ocular perforation with presumed infection (Brownstein et al., 1984; Shields et al., 1989; Virgi, 1977).

ADENOMAS OF NONPIGMENTED AND PIGMENTED CILIARY EPITHELIUM

Adenomas of ciliary neuroepithelium can also be mistaken clinically for melanoma (Green, 1996). They exhibit a spectrum from well-differentiated and low-grade lesions to pleomorphic and poorly differentiated features reminiscent of sarcoma (McLean et al., 1994). Ocular trauma or chronic inflammation is frequently antecedent in more pleomorphic tumors, suggesting a form of "scar carcinoma" and neoplastic transformation of hyperplastic reactive epithelium (McLean et al., 1994).

Histopathologically, these tumors appear as focal ciliary nodules of hyperplastic nonpigmented ciliary epithelium arranged in tubules and sheets, with intervening regions of basement membrane–like material (Fig. 31–16; Green, 1996). They may appear as papillary, tubuloacinar, or solid masses (Shields et al., 1983). Cellular characteristics include (*1*) glandular and papillary forms with low-grade pleomorphism, (*2*) moderately pleomorphic variants with hyalinized stroma, and (*3*) anaplastic forms (Fig. 31–17; Green, 1996). Tumors in the latter category are uncommon (Grossniklaus et al., 1990; Jakobiec et al., 1987; Rodriguez et al., 1988; Streeten and McGraw, 1972). Twenty-one cases of malignant forms have been registered with the Registry of Ophthalmic Pathology, with follow-up available for 16 cases (Green, 1996). Median time of follow-up was 5.7 years. Eight patients were well, although two had recurrent tumors, one of

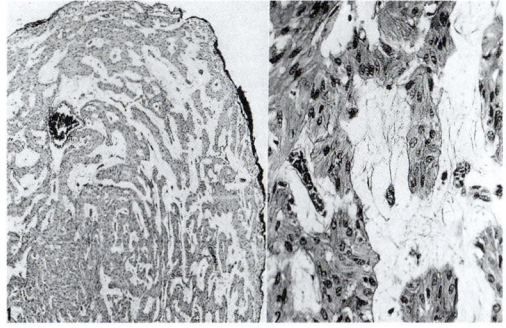

Figure 31–16. Benign adenoma of the nonpigmented ciliary epithelium. *Left*: Low-power view showing hyperplastic nonpigmented epithelium arranged in cords, with intervening basement membrane–like material. *Right*: High-power view of same tumor. [From Hogan MJ, Zimmerman LE. (1962) *Ophthalmic Pathology. An Atlas and Textbook*, 2nd ed., p. 438, W.B. Sanders, Philadelphia, with permission.]

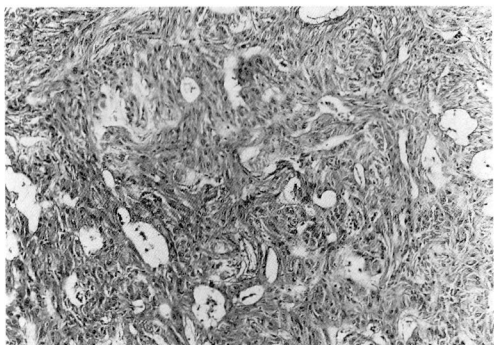

Figure 31–17. Adenocarcinoma of nonpigmented ciliary epithelium. High-power photomicrograph shows pleomorphic mixture of spindle and epithelial-shaped neoplastic cells. [From McLean IW, Burnier MN, Zimmerman LE, Jakobiec FA. (1994) Tumors of the conjunctiva. In: *Atlas of Tumor Pathology. Tumors of the Eye and Ocular Adnexa,* p. 147, Armed Forces Institute of Pathology, Washington, DC, p 147, with permission.]

which was metastatic to the parotid gland. Death due to tumor extension to the central nervous system or other sites occurred in 31.2% (5 patients). All of these had preexistent orbital lesions.

Precancerous lesions of the *pigmented* ciliary epithelium are rare. Anderson's (1962) survey of 30 adult epithelial tumors of the ciliary body found that 23% arose from pigmented epithelium. Most of these were benign but displayed some localized infiltration. Cellular patterns can appear as solid, tubular, papillary, or vacuolated. The latter is most characteristic, with large pigmented epithelial cells arranged in sheets, lobules, or nodules (Fig. 31–18; McLean et al., 1994). Cystic spaces within cellular regions contain mucopolysaccharide substances that are insensitive to digestion with hyaluronidase (Green, 1996). Electron microscopy has shown the vacuolated cysts to be lined with cilia and microvilli (Lieb et al., 1990; Streeten and McGraw, 1972). Varying degrees of anaplastic features including accelerated mitotic activity, pleomorphism, and invasiveness can be found and, if prominent, suggest classification as adenocarcinoma (Fig. 31–19; Papale et al., 1984). Metastatic activity of these lesions has not been reported (Green, 1996).

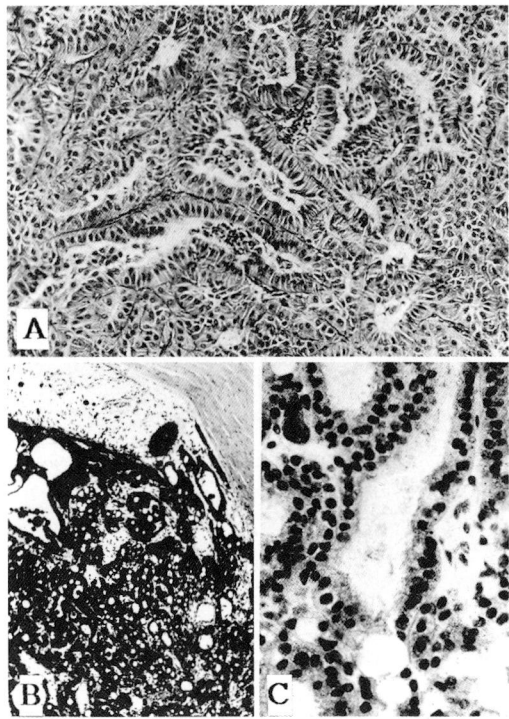

Figure 31–18. Epithelial tumors of the ciliary body. *A:* Adenoma of nonpigmented ciliary epithelium. *B:* Adenocarcinoma (well differentiated) of pigmented ciliary epithelium showing ciliary invasion. *C:* High-power bleached preparation of well-differentiated adenocarcinoma of pigmented ciliary epithelium showing high nuclear-to-cytoplasmic ratio. [From Hogan MJ, Zimmerman LE. (1962) *Ophthalmic Pathology. An Atlas and Textbook,* 2nd ed., p. 441, W.B. Sanders, Philadelphia, with permission.]

RETINA

RETINOCYTOMA

Neoplastic transformation of otherwise benign retinal tumors is controversial. Small, histologically benign retinal tumors have been identified and classified on the basis of their cytologic appearance as retinoma or retinocytomas (Balmer et al., 1991; Gaillie et al., 1982; Margo et al., 1983). Because they have been found in otherwise visually and structurally intact eyes and appear histologically similar to retinoblastomas that have regressed following irradiation, the issue of possible incipient neoplasia in these lesions

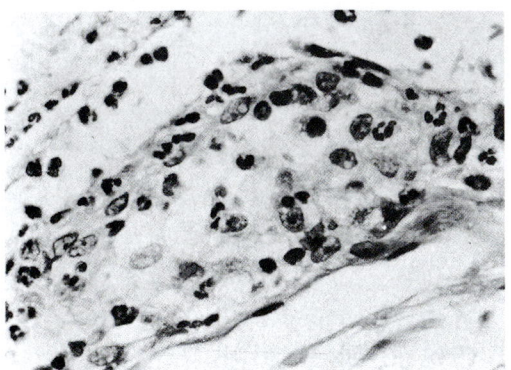

Figure 31–19. Adenocarcinoma of the pigmented ciliary epithelium in a 7-year-old boy. Large pleomorphic cells with prominent nucleoli can be seen invading an episcleral vessel. [From Papale JJ, Akiwama K, Hirose T, Tsubota K, Hanaoka K, Albert DA. (1984) Adenocarcinoma of the ciliary body pigment epithelium in a child. *Arch Ophthalmol* 102:100–103, with permission.]

has arisen (McLean et al., 1994). Malignant transformation is supported by a single case that was followed for 3 years without growth, but which then expanded rapidly. On enucleation, the cytologic appearance was that of retinocytoma in all locations except where growth was seen. In that region, poorly differentiated retinoblastoma was found (Fig. 31–20; Eagle et al., 1989). Retinocytomas appear as masses of retinal cells with low nuclear-to-cytoplasmic ratio, bland nuclear characteristics, no mitoses, and photoreceptor differentiation with fluerette formation (Margo et al., 1983). Occasional differentiation into glial cells has been reported, although reactivity of nontumorous adjacent retinal glia as the origin for these cells cannot be excluded (Margo et al., 1983; McLean et al., 1994). The epidemiologically rare cases of retinoblastoma in adults have been suggested to represent retinocytomas that have undergone neoplastic transformation (McLean et al., 1994a). The rarity of these tumors has unfortunately precluded precise elucidation of this possibility.

OPTIC NERVE

OPTIC NERVE MELANOCYTOMA

Benign melanocytomas of the optic disc are uncommon but not rare (Fig. 31–21). Reports of pigmented tumors of the optic nerve head began appearing shortly after the development of the ophthalmoscope in 1851 (Helmholtz, 1851), and by 1965 there were 42 cases of optic nerve melanocytoma on file at the Registry of Ophthalmic Pathol-

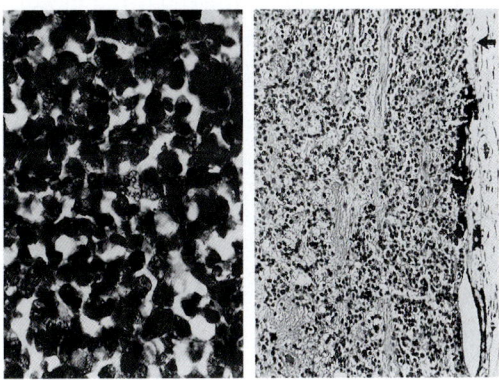

Figure 31–20. Retinocytoma with malignant transformation to retinoblastoma. *Left*: Highly cellular inner portion of tumor composed of poorly differentiated neuoblastic cells with scanty cytoplasm and hyperchromatic nuclei consistent with retinoblastoma. *Right*: Basal portion of tumor showing paucicellular accumulation of cells with abundant cytoplasm and bland nuclei consistent with retinocytoma (arrow). [From Eagle RC, Shields JA, Donoso L, Milner RS. (1989) Malignant transformation of spontaneously regressed retinoblastoma, retinoma/retinocytoma variant. *Ophthalmology* 96:1389–1395, with permission.]

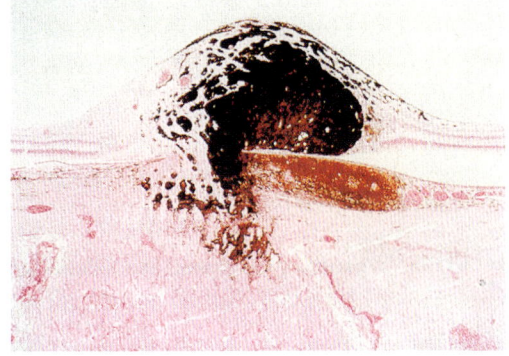

Figure 31–21. Melanocytoma of the optic disk. Heavily pigmented tumor at the optic papilla, with extension into adjacent retina and choroid. [From Campbell RJ. (1998) *Histological Typing of Tumours of the Eye and Its Adnexa*, p. 104, 2nd ed. Springer-Verlag, with permission.]

ogy at the AFIP (Zimmerman, 1965). Reports on the benign nature of most of these lesions has resulted in few enucleations since that time, and the precise incidence is therefore not currently known (I. McLean, personal communication). Melanocytomas appear with slightly greater frequency in darkly complected races than in Caucasians (Joff et al., 1979; Zimmerman, 1965). This is in contrast to the incidence of uveal melanoma in Blacks, which occurs only once for every 150 cases in Whites (Paul et al., 1962). While optic nerve melanocytomas usually do not grow, or show only very slight growth, documented cases of enlargement in histopathologically confirmed cases are available (*vide infra*). Normally these lesions are asymptomatic or only result in slight enlargement of the blind spot on visual field testing (Osher et al., 1979). However, encroachment upon optic nerve fibers or its vascular supply has resulted in profound visual loss (Takahashi et al., 1984; Usui et al., 1990).

Uveal melanocytes are normally present in the choroidal portion of the lamina cribosa in many species, including humans, and are grossly visible funduscopically in some highly pigmented human populations (Reidy, et al., 1985; Zimmerman, 1965). Zimmerman and Garron (1962) called these melanocytes "melanotic progonoma" and proposed that these cells might serve as the focus for potential nonmalignant growth resulting in a clinically recognizable optic nerve melanocytoma. Alternatively, juxtapapillary choroidal uveal melanocytes could also serve as a nidus for development of melanocytomas not intrinsically derived from the nerve but appearing to do so clinically (Reidy et al., 1985; Zimmerman, 1965).

The first case purporting to document malignant transformation of an optic nerve melanocytomas was described by Apple et al. in 1984. However, this case has been criticized as actually representing a juxtapapillary choroidal melanoma and not a tumor arising from the optic nerve proper (Monsour et al., 1989; Shields et al., 1990). As in other cases of presumed malignant transformation (*vide supra*), such lesions should possess both "melanocytoma cells" as well as either spindle B or epitheliod melanoma cells. Presumed cases of malignant transformation presented by Zografos et al. (1982)

and Erzurum et al. (1992) did not show evidence of typical melanocytoma cells within serial sections of the lesions (De Potter et al., 1996). Shields et al. (1990) reported a case with the above required histopathologic characteristics, but similarly suggested it may have arisen in the juxtapapillary choroid rather than primarily in the nerve. Another juxtapapillary melanocytoma that appeared to dedifferentiate to a melanoma over 7 years was presented by Loeffler and Tecklenborg (1992). A sixth case believed to represent malignant transformation from melanocytoma, this time strictly confined to the nerve head without choroidal involvement, was reported by De Potter et al. (1996). Again, however, extensive necrosis precluded clear elucidation of admixed melanocytoma cells within the mixed-type melanoma cells. A seventh recently published case demonstrated admixture of malignant spindle B cells with typical melanocytoma cells in an optic nerve tumor that had grown fourfold over a 2-year period. However, presence of a juxtapapillary choroidal component, could not be excluded as the site of malignant transformation (Meyer et al., 1999).

Thus, it appears that the statement made by Monsour et al. in 1989 still holds true, "there is still no documented case of malignant melanoma arising from an optic nerve melanocytoma." However, given the reasonable evidence for transformation of uveal melanocytomas in the juxtapapillary choroid, and elsewhere in the uveal tract, it is probably only a matter of time until one is discovered.

REFERENCES

Anderson SR. (1962) Medulloepithelioma of the retina. *Int Ophthalmol Clin* 2:483–506.

Apple DJ, Craythorn JM, Riedy JJ, Steinmetz RL, Brady SE, Bohart WA. (1984) Malignant transformation of an optic nerve melanocytoma. *Can J Ophthalmol* 19:320–325.

Balmer A, Munier F, Gailloud C. (1991) Retinoma. Case studies. *Ophthalm Paediatr Genet* 12:131–137.

Barker-Griffith AE, McDonald PR, Green WR. (1976) Malignant melanoma arising in a choroidal magnocellular nevus (melanocytoma). *Can J Ophthalmol* 11:140–146.

Biswas J, D'Souza C, Shanmugam MP. (1998) Diffuse melanotic lesion of the iris as a presenting feature of ciliary body melanocytoma: report of a case and review of the literature. *Surv Ophthalmol* 42:378–382.

Broughton WL, Zimmerman LE. (1988) A clinicopathologic study of 56 cases of intraocular medulloepithelioma. *Am J Ophthalmol* 85:407–418.

Brownstein S, Barsoum-Homsy M, Conway VH, et al. (1984) Nonteratoid medulloepithelioma of the ciliary body. *Ophthalmology* 91:1118–1122.

Brownstein S, Jakobiec FA, Wilkinson RD, et al. (1981) Cryotherapy for precancerous melanosis (atypical melanocytic hyperplasia) of the conjunctiva. *Arch Ophthalmol* 99:1224–1231.

Cialdini AP, Sahel JA, Jalkh AE, Weiter JJ, Zakka K, Albert DM. (1989) Malignant transformation of an iris melanocytoma. A case report. *Graefes Arch Clin Exp Ophthalmol* 227:348–354.

Clear AS, Chirambo MC, Hutt MS. (1979) Solar keratosis, pterygium, and squamous cell carcinoma of the conjunctiva in Malawi. *Br J Ophthalmol* 63:102–109.

De Potter P, Shields CL, Eagle RC, Shields JA, Lipkowitz JL. (1996) Malignant melanoma of the optic nerve. *Arch Ophthalmol* 114:608–612.

Dykstra PC, Dykstra BA. (1969) The diagnosis of carcinoma and related lesions of the ocular conjunctiva and cornea. *Trans Am Acad Ophthalmol Otolaryngol* 73:979–994.

Eagle RC, Shields JA, Donoso L, Milner RS. (1989) Malignant transformation of spontneously regressed retinoblastoma, retinoma/retinocytoma variant. *Ophthalmology* 96:1389–1395.

Elsas FJ, Green WR, Ryan SJ. (1974) Benign pigmented tumors arising in acquired conjunctival melanosis. *Am J Ophthalmol* 78:229–232.

Erzurum SA, Jampol LE, Territo C, O'Grady R. (1992) Primary malignant melanoma of the optic nerve simulating a melanocytoma. *Arch Ophthalmol* 110: 684–686.

Fineman MS, Eagle RC, Shields JA, Shields CL, DePotter P. (1998) Melanocytomalytic glaucoma in eyes with necrotic iris melanoctyoma. *Ophthalmology* 105:492–496.

Folberg R. (1996) Melanocytic lesions of the conjunctiva. In: *Ophthalmic Pathology. An Atlas and Textbook,* 2nd ed. (Spencer WH, ed.) pp. 125–155. W.B. Saunders, Philadelphia.

Folberg R, Jakobiec FA, Bernardino VB, Iwamoto T. (1989) Benign conjunctival melanocytic lesions. Clinicopathologic features. *Ophthalmology* 96:436–461.

Folberg R, McLean IW, Zimmerman LE. (1984) Conjunctival acquired melanosis and malignant melanoma. *Ophthalmology* 91:673–678.

Folberg R, McLean IW, Zimmerman LE. (1985) Malignant melanoma of the conjunctiva. *Hum Pathol* 16:136–143.

Frucht-Pery J, Ilsar M. (1994) The use of low dose mitomycin C for prevention of recurrent pterygium. *Ophthalmology* 101:759–762.

Frucht-Pery J, Rozenman Y. (1994) Mitomycin C therapy for corneal intraepithelial neoplasia. *Am J Ophthalmol* 117:164–168.

Gallie BL, Phillips RA, Ellsworth RM, et al. (1982) Significance of retinoma and phthisis bulbi for retinoblastoma. *Ophthalmology* 89:1393–1399.

Green RW. (1996) Retina. In: *Ophthalmic Pathology. An Atlas and Textbook* (Spencer WH, ed.) pp. 667–1331. W.B. Sauders, Philadelphia.

Grossniklaus HE, Cameron JD. (1993) Eye. In: *Pathology of Incipient Neoplasia,* 2nd ed. (Henson DE, Albores-Saavedra, eds.) pp. 544–556. W.B. Saunders, Philadelphia.

Grossniklaus HE, Green WR, Luckenbach M, Chan CC. (1987) Conjunctival lesions in adults. A clinical and histopathologic review. *Cornea* 6:78–116.

Grossniklaus HE, Zimmerman LE, Kachmer ML. (1990) Pleomorphic adenocarcinoma of the ciliary body. Immunohistochemical and electron microscopic features. *Ophthalmology* 97:763–768.

Heitman KF, Kindaid, MC, Steahly L. (1988) Diffuse malignant change in a chiliochoroidal melanocytoma in a patient of mixed racial background. *Retina* 8:67–72.

Helmholtz H v. (1851) *Beschreibung eines Augen-Spiefels zur Untersuchung der Netzhaut im lebenden Auge.* A. Forstner, Berlin.

Jakobiec FA, Folberg R, Iwamato T. (1989) Clinicopathologic characteristics of premalignant and malignant melanocytic lesions of the conjunctiva. *Ophthalmology* 96:147–166.

Jakobiec FA, Brownstein S, Wilkinson, et al. (1980) Combined surgery and cryotherapy for diffuse malignant melanoma of the conjunctiva. *Arch Ophthalmol* 98:1390–1396.

Jackobiec FA, Rini FJ, Fraunfelder FT, et al. (1988) Cryotherapy for conjunctival primary acquired melanosis and melanoma. Experience with 62 cases. *Ophthalmology* 95:1058–1070.

Jakobiec FA, Zimmerman LE, Spencer WH, et al. (1987) Metastatic colloid carcinoma versus primary carcinoma of the ciliary epithelium. *Ophthalmology* 94: 1469–1480.

Joffe L, Shields JA, Osher RH, Gass JDM. (1979) Clinical and follow-up studies of melanocytomas of the optic disc. *Ophthalmology* 86:1067–1078.

Juarez CP, Tso MO. (1980) An ultratructural study of melanocytomas (magnocellular nevi) of the optic disk and uvea. *Am J Ophthalmol* 90:48–62.

Kivelä T, Terkkanen A. (1978) Recurrent medulloepithelioma of the ciliary body. *Ophthalmology* 95:1565–1575.

Lass JH, Grove AS, Papale JJ, Albert DM, Jenson AB. (1983) Detection of human papillomavirus DNA sequences in conjunctival papilloma. *Am J Ophthalmol* 96:670–674.

Lauer SA, Malter JS, Meier JR. (1990) Human papillomavirus type 18 in conjunctival intraepithelial neoplasia. *Am J Ophthalmol* 110:23–27.

Ledoux-Corbusier M, Danis P. (1979) Pinguecula and actinic elastosis. An ultrastructural study. *J Cutan Pathol* 6:404–413.

Lee JS, Smith RE, Mickler DS. (1982) Scleral melanocytoma. *Ophthalmology* 89:178–182.

Leidenix M, Mamalis N, Goodart R, Harrie R, Kjeldsberg C. (1994) Malignant transformation of a necrotic melanocytoma of the choroid in an amblyopic eye. *Ann Ophthalmol* 26:42–46.

Lieb WE, Shields JA, Eagle RC, et al. (1990) Cystic adenoma of the pigmented ciliary epithelium. Clinical, pathologic, and immunohistopathologic findings. *Ophthalmology* 97:1489–1493.

Loeffler KU, Tecklenborg H. (1992) Melanocytoma-like growth of a juxtapapillary malignant melanoma. *Retina* 12:29–34.

Lommatzsch PK, Lommatzsch RE, Kirsch I, et al. (1990) Therapeutic outcome of patients suffering from malignant melanomas of the conjunctiva. *Br J Ophthalmol* 74:615–619.

Margo C, Hidayat A, Kopelman J, Zimmerman LE.

(1983) Retinocytoma: a benign variant of retinoblastoma. *Arch Ophthalmol* 101:1519–1531.

McDonnell JM, McDonnel PJ, Mounts P, et al. (1986) Demonstration of papillomavirus capsid antigen in human conjunctival neoplasia. *Arch Ophthalmol* 104:1801–1805.

McDonnell JM, McDonnel PJ, Sun YY. (1992) Human papillomavirus DNA in tissues and ocular surface swabs of patients with conjunctival epithelial neoplasia. *Invest Ophthalmol Vis Sci* 33:184–189.

McLean IW, Burnier MN, Zimmerman LE, Jakobiec FA. (1994a) *Atlas of Tumor Pathology. Tumors of the Eye and Ocular Adnexa*, Fascicle 12. Armed Forces Institute of Pathology, Washington DC.

McLean IW, Burnier MN, Zimmerman LE, Jakobiec FA. (1994b) Tumors of the uveal tract. In: *Atlas of Tumor Pathology. Tumors of the Eye and Ocular Adnexa*, Fascicle 12, pp. 155–214. Armed Forces Institute of Pathology, Washington DC.

Meyer D, Ge J, Blinder KJ, Sinard J, Xu S. (1999) Malignant transformation of an optic disk melanocytoma. *Am J Ophthalmol* 127:710–714.

Monsour AM, Zimmerman L, La Piana FG, Beauchamp GR. (1989) Clinicopthological findings in a growing optic nerve melanocytoma. *Br J Ophthalmol* 73:410–415.

Nakazawa M, Tamai M. (1984) Iris melanocytoma with secondary glaucoma. *Am J Ophthalmol* 97:797–799.

Osher RH, Shields JA, Layman PR. (1979) Pupillary and visual field evaluation in patients with melanocytoma of the optic disc. *Arch Ophthalmol* 97:1096–1099.

Paple JJ, Akiwama K, Hirose T, et al. (1984) Adenocarcinoma of the ciliary body pigment epithelium in a child. *Arch Ophthalmol* 102:100–103.

Paul EV, Parnell BL, Fraker M. (1962) Prognosis of malignant melanoma of the choroid and ciliary body. *Int Ophthalmol Clin* 2:387–402.

Reese AB. (1974) Congenital melanomas. *Am J Ophthalmol* 77:798–808.

Reidy JJ, Apple DJ, Steinmetz RL, Caythorn JM, Loftfield K, Gieser SC, Brady SE. (1985) Melanocytoma: nomenclature, pathogenesis, natureal history and treatment. *Surv Ophthalmol* 29:319–327.

Rodriquez M, Hidayat A, Karesh J. (1988) Peopmorphic adenocarcinoma of ciliary epithelium simulating an epibulbar tumor. *Am J Ophthalmol* 106:595–600.

Roth AM. (1978) Malignant change in melanocytomas of the uveal tract. *Surv Ophthalmol* 22:404–412.

Rumelt V, Maumann GO, Folberg R, Weingeist TA. (1994) Surgical management of melanocytoma of the ciliary body with extrascleral extension. *Am J Ophthalmol* 117:169–176.

Shields JA, Annesley WH, Spaeth GL. (1977) Necrotic melanocytoma of iris with secondary glaucoma. *Am J Ophthalmol* 84:826–829.

Shields JA, Augsberger JJ, Waller PH, et al. (1983) Adenoma of the nonpigmented epithelium of the ciliary body. *Ophthalmology* 90:1528–1530.

Shields JA, Shields CL, Eagle RC, Leib WE, Stern S.

(1990) Malignant melanoma associated with melanocytoma of the optic disc. *Ophthalmology* 97:225–230.

Shields JA, Shields CL, Schwartz RL. (1989) Malignant teratoid melulloepithelioma of the ciliary body simulating persistent hyperplastic primary vitreous. *Am J Ophthalmol* 107:297–298.

Spencer WH. (1996) Conjunctiva. In: *Ophthalmic Pathology. An Atlas and Textbook* (Spencer WH, ed.) pp 38–155. W.B. Saunders, Philadelphia.

Stokes DW, O'Day DM, Glick AD. (1993) Melanocytoma of the ciliary body with scleral extension. *Ophthalm Surg* 24:200–202.

Streeten BF, McGraw JL. (1972) Tumor of the ciliary pigment epithelium. *Am J Ophthalmol* 74:420–429.

Takahashi T, Isayama Y, Okuzawa I. (1984) Unusual case of melanocytoma in optic disk. *Jpn J Ophthalmol* 28:171–175.

Teichmann KD, Karcioglu ZA. (1995) Malanocytoma of the iris with rapidly developing secondary glaucoma. *Surv Ophthalmol* 40:136–144.

Thomas CI, Purnell EW. (1969) Ocular melanocytoma. *Am J Ophthalmol* 67:79–86.

Usui T, Shirakashi M, Kurosawa A, Abe H, Iwata K. (1990) Visual disturbance in patients with melanocytoma of the optic disk. *Ophthalmologica* 201:92–98.

Verdaguer J, Valenzuela H, Strozzi L. (1974) Melanocytoma of the conjunctiva. *Arch Ophthalmol* 91:363–366.

Virgi MA. (1977) Medulloepithelioma (diktyoma) presenting as a perforated infected eye. *Br J Ophthalmol* 61:229–232.

Wakakura M, Lee WR. (1990) Ultrasturctural pleomorphism in medulloepithelioma of the ciliary body: a comparative study of tumor cells and fetal ciliary epithelium. *Jpn J Ophthalmol* 34:364–380.

Waring GO, Roth AM, Ekins MB. (1984) Clinical and pathologic description of 17 cases of corneal intraepithelial neoplasia. *Am J Ophthalmol* 97:547–559.

Yamaguchi K, Shiono T, Mizuno K. (1987) Pigment deposition in the anterior segment caused by melanocytoma of the optic disc. *Ophthalmologica* 194:191–193.

Zimmerman LE. (1965) Melanocytes, melanotic nevi, and melanocytomas. The Jonas S. Friedenwald Memorial Lecture. *Invest Ophthalmol Vis Sci* 4:11–41.

Zimmerman LE, Broughton WL. (1978) A clinicopathologic and follow-up study of fifty-six intraocular medulloepitheliomas. In: *Ocular and Adnexal Tumors* (FA Jakobiec, ed.) pp. 181–195. Aesculapius, Birmingham, AL.

Zimmerman LE, Garron LK. (1962) Melanocytoma of the optic disc. *Int Ophthalmol Clin* 2:431–440.

Zimmerman LE, Sobin LH. (1980) *Histologic Typing of Tumors of the Eye and its Adnexa: International Histological Classification of Tumors No. 24*, pp. 23–34. World Health Organization, Geneva.

Zografos L, Uffer S, Gailloud C, Kohli M. (1982) Le mélanome de la papille, nouvelle observation. *Klin Monatsbl Augenheilkd* 180:503–509.

INDEX

Page numbers followed by f and t indicate figures and tables, respectively.